MW01152762

Vascular Decision Making

- Medical
- Endovascular
- Surgical

Vascular Decision Making

Medical

Endovascular

Surgical

EDITORS: **Jack L. Cronenwett, MD**

Emeritus Professor, Surgery
Geisel School of Medicine at Dartmouth
Lebanon, New Hampshire

Alik Farber, MD, MBA

Chief, Division of Vascular and Endovascular Surgery
Associate Chair for Clinical Operations, Department of Surgery
Boston Medical Center
Professor of Surgery and Radiology
Boston University School of Medicine
Boston, Massachusetts

Erica L. Mitchell, MD, MEd

Emeritus Professor, Surgery
Oregon Health and Science University
Portland, Oregon

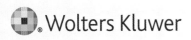 Wolters Kluwer

Philadelphia • Baltimore • New York • London
Buenos Aires • Hong Kong • Sydney • Tokyo

Acquisitions Editor: Keith Donnellan
Development Editor: Sean McGuire
Editorial Coordinator: Ashley Pfeiffer
Marketing Manager: Phyllis Hitner
Production Project Manager: Bridgett Dougherty
Design Coordinator: Stephen Druding
Illustrator: Jennifer Clements
Manufacturing Coordinator: Beth Welsh
Prepress Vendor: S4Carlisle Publishing Services

Copyright © 2021 Wolters Kluwer.

All rights reserved. This book is protected by copyright. No part of this book may be reproduced or transmitted in any form or by any means, including as photocopies or scanned-in or other electronic copies, or utilized by any information storage and retrieval system without written permission from the copyright owner, except for brief quotations embodied in critical articles and reviews. Materials appearing in this book prepared by individuals as part of their official duties as U.S. government employees are not covered by the above-mentioned copyright. To request permission, please contact Wolters Kluwer at Two Commerce Square, 2001 Market Street, Philadelphia, PA 19103, via email at permissions@lww.com, or via our website at shop.lww.com (products and services).

9 8 7 6 5 4 3 2 1

Printed in China

Library of Congress Cataloging-in-Publication Data

Names: Cronenwett, Jack L., editor. | Mitchell, Erica, editor. | Farber,
   Alik, editor.
Title: Vascular decision making: medical, endovascular, surgical /
   editors, Jack L. Cronenwett, Erica L. Mitchell, Alik Farber.
Description: Philadelphia: Wolters Kluwer Health, [2020] | Includes index.
Identifiers: LCCN 2019055170 | ISBN 9781975115814 (casebound)
Subjects: LCSH: Blood-vessels—Diseases—Diagnosis—Handbooks, manuals,
   etc. | Blood-vessels—Diseases—Treatment—Handbooks, manuals, etc. |
   Clinical medicine—Decision making—Handbooks, manuals, etc. |
   Blood-vessels—Surgery—Decision making—Handbooks, manuals, etc. |
   Blood-vessels—Endoscopic surgery—Decision making—Handbooks, manuals,
   etc.
Classification: LCC RC691.5 .V364 2020 | DDC 616.1/3—dc23
LC record available at https://lccn.loc.gov/2019055170

This work is provided "as is," and the publisher disclaims any and all warranties, express or implied, including any warranties as to accuracy, comprehensiveness, or currency of the content of this work.

This work is no substitute for individual patient assessment based upon healthcare professionals' examination of each patient and consideration of, among other things, age, weight, gender, current or prior medical conditions, medication history, laboratory data and other factors unique to the patient. The publisher does not provide medical advice or guidance and this work is merely a reference tool. Healthcare professionals, and not the publisher, are solely responsible for the use of this work including all medical judgments and for any resulting diagnosis and treatments.

Given continuous, rapid advances in medical science and health information, independent professional verification of medical diagnoses, indications, appropriate pharmaceutical selections and dosages, and treatment options should be made and healthcare professionals should consult a variety of sources. When prescribing medication, healthcare professionals are advised to consult the product information sheet (the manufacturer's package insert) accompanying each drug to verify, among other things, conditions of use, warnings and side effects and identify any changes in dosage schedule or contraindications, particularly if the medication to be administered is new, infrequently used or has a narrow therapeutic range. To the maximum extent permitted under applicable law, no responsibility is assumed by the publisher for any injury and/or damage to persons or property, as a matter of products liability, negligence law or otherwise, or from any reference to or use by any person of this work.

shop.lww.com

This book is dedicated to the students, residents, and fellows whose questions have enriched our careers and enhanced our learning. It was stimulated by their requests for a clear delineation of vascular decision making.

I also dedicate this book to all the people who have supported my personal and professional decision making throughout my life: teachers, friends, and family. I am grateful for their guidance and for the opportunity to have practiced vascular surgery during a time of complex but rewarding clinical decision making.

Jack L. Cronenwett

I dedicate this book to my mother Bella and my brother Senia, who helped me to get to where I am today; and to my wife Carolyn and my children Elina and Jake, for providing me with daily support, love, and inspiration.

Alik Farber

I am grateful to the strong women in my life, my mother Lynn, my sisters Dana and Pilar, and my lifelong best friend Caro. I also thank my husband Jon, for opening my eyes to new horizons. This book is dedicated to them.

Erica L. Mitchell

SECTION EDITORS

James H. Black, III, MD

The David Goldfarb MD Professor of Surgery
Department of Surgery
Johns Hopkins University School of Medicine
Chief
Vascular Surgery and Endovascular Therapy
Johns Hopkins Hospital
Baltimore, Maryland

Section XVI, Complications

Adam W. Beck, MD, FACS

Associate Professor
Department of Surgery
University of Alabama at Birmingham
Division Director, Vascular Surgery and
Endovascular Therapy
Department of Surgery
UAB Hospital
Birmingham, Alabama

Section IV, Thoracic Aortic Disease

Ruth L. Bush, MD, JD, MPH

Associate Dean
Office of Medical Education
University of Houston College of Medicine
Houston, Texas
Vascular Surgeon
Department of Vascular Surgery
Olin E. Teague Veterans' Medical Center
Temple, Texas

Section III, Non-Atherosclerotic Cerebrovascular Disease

Mark F. Conrad, MD, MMSc

Associate Professor
Department of Surgery
Harvard University
Program Director
Division of Vascular and Endovascular Surgery
Massachusetts General Hospital
Boston, Massachusetts

Section II, Atherosclerotic Cerebrovascular Disease

Matthew A. Corriere, MD, MS

Frankel Professor of Cardiovascular Surgery,
    Associate Professor
Department of Surgery, Section of Vascular Surgery
University of Michigan
Ann Arbor, Michigan

Section VIII, Renovascular Diseases

Robert T. Eberhardt, MD

Associate Professor
Department of Medicine and Surgery
Boston University
Director of Vascular Medicine
Department of Medicine
Boston Medical Center
Boston, Massachusetts

Section I, Preoperative Evaluation and Medical Treatment

Mohammad H. Eslami, MD, MPH

Professor of Surgery
Division of Vascular Surgery
Department of Surgery
University of Pittsburgh Medical School
Chief of Vascular Surgery
Division of Vascular Surgery
Department of Surgery
UPMC Mercy
Pittsburgh, Pennsylvania

Section VI, Other Aneurysms

Thomas L. Forbes, MD, FRCSC, FACS

Professor and Chair
Department of Vascular Surgery
University of Toronto
R. Fraser Elliott Chair and Division Head
Department of Vascular Surgery
University Health Network
Toronto, ON, Canada

Section XVI, Complications

Philip Goodney, MD, MS

Professor of Surgery
Section of Vascular Surgery
Geisel School of Medicine at Dartmouth
Hanover, New Hampshire

Section IX, Atherosclerotic Lower Extremity Disease

Thomas S. Huber, MD, PhD

Edward R. Woodward Professor and Chief
Division of Vascular Surgery
University of Florida College of Medicine
Gainesville, Florida

Section XIII, Hemodialysis Access

William A. Marston, MD

George Johnson Jr. Distinguished Professor
Department of Surgery
University of North Carolina School of Medicine
Chapel Hill, North Carolina

Section XIV, Venous Insufficiency, Lymphatic Diseases and Malformations

Marc A. Passman, MD

Professor
Division of Vascular Surgery and Endovascular
Therapy
Department of Surgery
University of Alabama at Birmingham
Birmingham, Alabama

Section XV, Venous Thrombosis

David Rigberg, MD

Professor
Department of Surgery (Vascular)
UCLA David Geffen School of Medicine
Vascular Surgeon
Department of Surgery (Vascular)
UCLA Ronald Reagan Medical Center
Los Angeles, California

Section XI, Upper Extremity Disease

Vincent L. Rowe, MD

Professor
Department of Surgery
Keck School of Medicine at University of Southern California
Los Angeles, California

Section XII, Vascular Trauma

Andres Schanzer, MD

Professor of Surgery
Division of Vascular Surgery
University of Massachusetts Medical School
Chief
Division of Vascular Surgery
UMass Memorial Medical Center
Worcester, Massachusetts

Section V, Aortoiliac Aneurysms

Marc L. Schermerhorn, MD

George H.A. Clowes Jr Professor of Surgery
Harvard Medical School
Chief, Division of Vascular and Endovascular
   Surgery
Beth Israel Deaconess Medical Center
Boston, Massachusetts

Section VII, Visceral Artery Disease

Niten Singh, MD

Professor of Surgery
Department of Surgery
University of Washington
Seattle, Washington

Section X, Non-Atherosclerotic Lower Extremity Disease

AUTHORS

Ahmed M. Abou-Zamzam, Jr, MD

Professor of Surgery
Department of Surgery
Loma Linda University Health
Chief
Division of Vascular Surgery
Loma Linda University Medical Center
Loma Linda, California

Chapter 48, Lower Extremity Amputation

Cherrie Abraham, MD

Associate Professor
Department of Surgery
Oregon Health and Sciences University
Director, Aortic Center
OHSU Department of Surgery
Oregon Health and Sciences University
Portland, Oregon

Chapter 19, Aortic Arch Aneurysm

Christopher J. Abularrage, MD, DFSVS, FACS

Associate Professor of Surgery
Vascular Surgery and Endovascular Therapy
The Johns Hopkins Hospital
Johns Hopkins Medical Institutions
Baltimore, Maryland

Chapter 18, Large Artery Vasculitis

Ali F. AbuRahma, MD

Professor of Surgery
Department of Surgery
West Virginia University-Charleston Division
Chief, Vascular and Endovascular Surgery
Department of Vascular Surgery
Charleston Area Medical Center
Charleston, Virginia

Chapter 14, Carotid Fibromuscular Disease

Stefan Acosta, MD, PhD

Professor of Vascular Surgery
Department of Clinical Sciences, Malmö
Lund University
Senior Consultant
Vascular Centre, Department of Thoracic and Vascular Surgery
Skåne University Hospital
Malmö, Sweden

Chapter 38, Mesenteric Vein Thrombosis

Cassra N. Arbabi, MD

General Surgery Resident
Department of Surgery
Loma Linda University Health
Loma Linda, California

Chapter 48, Lower Extremity Amputation

David G. Armstrong, DPM, MD, PhD

Professor of Surgery and Director
Southwestern Academic Limb Salvage
    Alliance (SALSA)
Keck School of Medicine at University of
    Southern California
Los Angeles, California

Chapter 52, Assessment of the Diabetic Foot: Wound, Ischemia, and Foot Infection

Ehrin J. Armstrong, MD, MSc, MAS, FACC, FSCAI, FSVM

Director, Interventional Cardiology
Director, Vascular Laboratory
Rocky Mountain Regional VA Medical Center
Professor of Medicine
Division of Cardiology
University of Colorado School of Medicine
Aurora, Colorado

Chapter 3, Smoking Cessation Management

Edward J. Arous, MD, MPH

Assistant Professor
Division of Vascular Surgery
University of Massachusetts Medical School
UMass Memorial Medical Center
Worcester, Massachusetts

Chapter 29, Endoleak after Endovascular Aortic Aneurysm Repair

Afsha Aurshina, MD

Research Fellow
Department of Surgery
Vascular Institute of New York
Brooklyn, New York
General Surgery Resident
Department of Surgery
Yale New Haven Hospital
New Haven, Connecticut

Chapter 81, Catheter-Associated Upper Extremity Deep Venous Thrombosis

Micheal T. Ayad, MD

Associate Chief
Division of Vascular Surgery
Co-Director of the Vascular Lab
Mount Sinai Medical Center
Miami Beach, Florida

Chapter 60, Neck Vascular Trauma

Ali Azizzadeh, MD, FACS

Professor and Director, Division of Vascular Surgery
Vice Chair, Department of Surgery for Programmatic
    Development
Associate Director, Heart Institute for Vascular
    Therapeutics
Los Angeles, California

Chapter 61, Thoracic Vascular Trauma

Robert J. Beaulieu, MD, MSE
Vascular Fellow
Section of Vascular Surgery
University of Michigan
Ann Arbor, Michigan
Chapter 6, Identifying Cerebrovascular Disease

Adam W. Beck, MD, FACS
Associate Professor
Department of Surgery
University of Alabama at Birmingham
Division Director, Vascular Surgery and Endovascular
    Therapy
Department of Surgery
UAB Hospital
Birmingham, Alabama
Chapter 20, Descending/Thoracoabdominal Aneurysm

Scott A. Berceli, MD, PhD
Professor of Surgery
Department of Surgery
University of Florida
Chief, Vascular Surgery
Department of Surgery Service
North Florida/South Georgia Veterans
    Health Service
Gainesville, Florida
Chapter 66, Failing or Thrombosed Access

James H. Black, III, MD
The David Goldfarb MD Professor of Surgery
Department of Surgery
Johns Hopkins University School of Medicine
Chief
Vascular Surgery and Endovascular Therapy
Johns Hopkins Hospital
Baltimore, Maryland
Chapter 90, Arterial Graft Infection

Joseph-Vincent V. Blas, MD
Associate Fellowship Director, Vascular Surgery
    Fellowship
Assistant Professor of Surgery
Faculty, Vascular Surgeon
Department of Surgery
University of South Carolina School of Medicine-
    Greenville
Greenville, South Carolina
Chapter 68, Hemodialysis Access Infection

Raphael Blochle, MD, FACS
Clinical Assistant Professor
Department of Surgery
Suny Buffalo
Attending
Department of Surgery
Erie County Medical Center
Buffalo, New York
Chapter 67, Aneurysms and Pseudoaneurysms of AV Access

Laura T. Boitano, MD, MPH
Vascular Surgery Integrated Resident
Vascular and Endovascular Surgery
Harvard University
Massachusetts Hall
Cambridge, Massachusetts
Vascular Surgery Integrated Resident
Vascular and Endovascular Surgery
Massachusetts General Hospital
Boston, Massachusetts
Chapter 7, Management of Asymptomatic Carotid Stenosis

Michael C. Bounds, MD
Assistant Professor of Surgery
Department of Surgery
University of Kentucky College of Medicine
Faculty, Section of Vascular Surgery
Department of Surgery
University of Kentucky Chandler Medical Center
Lexington, Kentucky
Chapter 85, Abdominal Compartment Syndrome After Aortic Operation

Thomas C. Bower, MD
Professor of Surgery
Consultant, Mayo Clinic College of Medicine and Science
Division of Vascular and Endovascular Surgery
Mayo Clinic
Rochester, Minnesota
Chapter 28, Aortoenteric Fistula

James D. Brooks, MD
Assistant Professor of Surgery
USF Heath Division of Vascular Surgery
Staff Surgeon James Haley VA Hospital
Tampa, Florida
Chapter 53, Acute Limb Ischemia

Kellie R. Brown, MD
Professor, Division of Vascular and Endovascular Surgery
Vascular Division Chief, Zablocki VA Medical Center
The Medical College of Wisconsin
Milwaukee, Wisconsin
Chapter 11, Combined Carotid and Coronary Disease

Anne Burdess, MD, PhD, FRCS
Consultant Vascular and Endovascular Surgeon
Department of Vascular Surgery
The Northern Vascular Unit, The Freeman Hospital
Newcastle Upon Tyne, United Kingdom
Chapter 23, Penetrating Aortic Ulcer, Intramural Hematoma, and Isolated Abdominal Aortic Dissection

Ruth L. Bush, MD, JD, MPH
Associate Dean
Office of Medical Education
University of Houston College of Medicine
Houston, Texas
Vascular Surgeon
Department of Vascular Surgery
Olin E. Teague Veterans' Medical Center
Temple, Texas
Chapter 17, Carotid Artery Aneurysm

Rabih A. Chaer, MD
Professor of Surgery
Division of Vascular Surgery, Department of Surgery
University of Pittsburgh Medical Center
Pittsburgh, Pennsylvania
Chapter 82, Pulmonary Embolism

W. Darrin Clouse, MD
Professor, Department of Surgery
Chief, Vascular and Endovascular Surgery
University of Virginia Health System
Charlottesville, Virginia
Chapter 13, Innominate, Common Carotid, and Subclavian Disease

Dawn M. Coleman, MD
Handleman Research Professor of Surgery
Associate Professor of Surgery and Pediatrics and
    Communicable Diseases
Program Director, Vascular Surgery
University of Michigan/Michigan Medicine
Ann Arbor, Michigan
Chapter 41, Nonatherosclerotic Renal Artery Occlusive Disease

Jill J. Colglazier, MD
Assistant Professor, Vascular Surgeon
Division of Vascular and Endovascular Surgery
Mayo Clinic
Rochester, Minnesota
Chapter 28, Aortoenteric Fistula

Mark F. Conrad, MD, MMSc

Associate Professor
Department of Surgery
Harvard University
Program Director
Division of Vascular and Endovascular Surgery
Massachusetts General Hospital
Boston, Massachusetts

Chapter 7, Management of Asymptomatic Carotid Stenosis

Matthew A. Corriere, MD, MS

Frankel Professor of Cardiovascular Surgery, Associate Professor
Department of Surgery, Section of Vascular Surgery
University of Michigan
Ann Arbor, Michigan

Chapter 42, Acute Renovascular Ischemia

David L. Cull, MD, MBA

Professor, Department of Surgery
University of South Carolina School of Medicine-Greenville
Vice President of Academic and Clinical Integration
Prisma Health
Greenville, South Carolina

Chapter 68, Hemodialysis Access Infection

David L. Dawson, MD

Clinical Professor
Department of Surgery
Texas A&M University College of Medicine
Vascular Surgeon
Department of Surgery
Baylor Scott and White Health
Temple, Texas

Chapter 63, Extremity Vascular Trauma

Thomas G. DeLoughery, MD, MACP, FAWM

Professor of Medicine, Pathology, and Pediatrics
Department of Hematology
Oregon Health and Science University
Portland, Oregon

Chapter 5, Hypercoagulability Assessment and Management

Hasan H. Dosluoglu, MD, FACS

Professor, Chief of Vascular Surgery
Department of Surgery
Jacobs School of Medicine and Biomedical Sciences
State University of New York at Buffalo
Chief
Surgery and Vascular Surgery
VA Western New York Healthcare System
Buffalo, New York

Chapter 47, Infra-Inguinal Arterial Occlusive Disease

Anahita Dua, MD, MS, MBA

Assistant Professor
Division of Vascular Surgery
Department of Surgery
Massachusetts General Hospital
Boston, Massachusetts

Chapter 58, Arterial Thoracic Outlet Syndrome

Audra A. Duncan, MD, FACS, FRCSC

Professor
Department of Surgery
University of Western Ontario
Chair/Chief
Division of Vascular and Endovascular Surgery
London Health Sciences
London, Ontario, Canada

Chapter 75, Lymphedema

Matthew J. Eagleton, MD

Robert R. Linton—Professor of Surgery
Harvard Medical School
Chief, Division of Vascular and Endovascular Surgery
Department of Surgery
Massachusetts General Hospital
Boston, Massachusetts

Chapter 86, Spinal Cord Ischemia After Aortic Operation

Robert T. Eberhardt, MD

Associate Professor
Department of Medicine and Surgery
Boston University
Director of Vascular Medicine
Department of Medicine
Boston Medical Center
Boston, Massachusetts

Chapter 1, Perioperative Cardiac Assessment and Management

Matthew S. Edwards, MD

Richard H. Dean Professor and Chair
Department of Vascular and Endovascular Surgery
Wake Forest University School of Medicine
Medical Center Boulevard
Richard H. Dean Professor and Chair, Attending Surgeon
Department of Vascular and Endovascular Surgery
Wake Forest University Baptist Medical Center
Winston Salem, North Carolina

Chapter 40, Atherosclerotic Renal Artery Disease

Steven Elias, MD, FACS, FAVLS, DABVLM

Director, Center for Vein Disease
Englewood Health Network
Englewood, New Jersey
Medical Editor, VEIN Magazine
Editor, Vein Specialist American Venous Forum

Chapter 72, Varicose Veins

Eric D. Endean, MD

Professor of Surgery
Department of Surgery
University of Kentucky College of Medicine
Chief, Section of Vascular Surgery
Department of Surgery
University of Kentucky Chandler Medical Center
Lexington, Kentucky

Chapter 85, Abdominal Compartment Syndrome After Aortic Operation

Mohammad H. Eslami, MD, MPH

Professor of Surgery
Division of Vascular Surgery
Department of Surgery
University of Pittsburgh Medical School
Chief of Vascular Surgery
Division of Vascular Surgery
Department of Surgery
UPMC Mercy
Pittsburgh, Pennsylvania

Chapter 31, Popliteal Artery Aneurysm

Marissa Famularo, DO

Vascular Surgeon
Department of Vascular Surgery
Bassett Medical Center
Cooperstown, New York

Chapter 21, Acute Aortic Dissection

Alik Farber, MD, MBA

Chief, Division of Vascular and Endovascular Surgery
Associate Chair for Clinical Operations, Department of Surgery
Boston Medical Center
Professor of Surgery and Radiology
Boston University School of Medicine
Boston, Massachusetts

Chapter 45, Chronic Atherosclerotic Leg Ischemia

Thomas L. Forbes, MD, FRCSC, FACS

Professor and Chair
Department of Vascular Surgery
University of Toronto
R. Fraser Elliott Chair and Division Head
Department of Vascular Surgery
University Health Network
Toronto, ON, Canada

Chapter 87, Post Revascularization Leg Ischemia

Jorge Fuentes, MD

Clinical Instructor
Department of Medicine
NYU Grossman School of Medicine
NYU Langone Health
New York, New York

Chapter 1, Perioperative Cardiac Assessment and Management

Daniel F. Geersen, MPAP, PA-C

Associate Director PA Surgical Residency Program
Division of Vascular and Endovascular Surgery
Duke University Medical Center
Durham, North Carolina

Chapter 76, Vascular Malformations

Hugh A. Gelabert, MD

Professor of Surgery
Division of Vascular Surgery
David Geffen School of Medicine at UCLA
Attending Surgeon
Division of Vascular Surgery
Ronald Reagan UCLA Medical Center
Los Angeles, California

Chapter 56, Management of Neurogenic Thoracic Outlet Syndrome

David L. Gillespie, MD, RVT, DMCC, FACS

Chief
Department of Vascular and Endovascular Surgery
Southcoast Health System
Dartmouth, Massachusetts
Affiliated Professor of Surgery
Department of Surgery
Uniformed Services University
Bethesda, Maryland

Chapter 60, Neck Vascular Trauma

Katherine Giuliano, MD

Department of Surgery
Johns Hopkins University School of Medicine
Baltimore, Maryland

Chapter 90, Arterial Graft Infection

Philip Goodney, MD, MS

Professor of Surgery
Section of Vascular Surgery
Geisel School of Medicine at Dartmouth
Hanover, New Hampshire

Chapter 44, Diagnosing Lower Extremity Vascular Disease

Sarah E. Gray, MD

Surgery Resident
Department of Surgery
University of Florida
Gainesville, Florida

Chapter 66, Failing or Thrombosed Access

Derek de Grijs, MD

Staff Surgeon
Baptist Heart
Jackson, Mississippi

Chapter 46, Aortoiliac Disease

Sung Ham, MD, MS

Assistant Professor of Surgery
Department of Surgery
Keck School of Medicine at the University of Southern
    California
Los Angeles, California

Chapter 33, Renal Artery Aneurysm

Mark R. Harrigan, MD

Professor
Department of Neurosurgery
The University of Alabama at Birmingham
Medical Director
Department of Neurosurgery
The University of Alabama Hospital at
    Birmingham
Birmingham, Alabama

Chapter 9, Acute Ischemic Stroke

Linda M. Harris, MD

Professor
Department of Surgery
Jacobs School of Medicine and Biomedical Sciences
University at Buffalo, SUNY
Program Director Vascular Residency and Fellowship
Department of Surgery
Kaleida Health
Buffalo, New York

Chapter 67, Aneurysms and Pseudoaneurysms of AV Access

Jake F. Hemingway , MD

Integrated Vascular Surgery Resident
Department of Surgery
University of Washington
Seattle, Washington

Chapter 49, Popliteal Entrapment and Adventitial Cyst Disease

Peter Henke, MD

Professor of Surgery
Department of Surgery
Section of Vascular Surgery
Ann Arbor, Michigan

Chapter 78, Lower Extremity Deep Venous Thrombosis

Dirk M. Hentschel, MD

Assistant Professor
Department of Medicine
Harvard Medical School
Director, Interventional Nephrology
Renal Division, Department of Medicine
Brigham and Women's Hospital
Boston, Massachusetts

Chapter 65, Nonmaturing Arteriovenous Fistula

Christine R. Herman, MD, MSc, FRCSC

Cardiac, Vascular, and Endovascular Surgeon
Divisions of Cardiac and Vascular Surgery
Queen Elizabeth II Health Science Center
Halifax, Nova Scotia, Canada

Chapter 19, Aortic Arch Aneurysm

Caitlin W. Hicks, MD, MS

Assistant Professor
Division of Vascular Surgery and Endovascular Therapy
Johns Hopkins University School of Medicine
Attending Physician
Division of Vascular Surgery and Endovascular
    Therapy
Johns Hopkins Hospital
Baltimore, Maryland

Chapter 18, Large Artery Vasculitis

Anil Hingorani, MD

Clinical Assistant Professor
Division of Vascular Surgery
New York University Langone-Brooklyn
Brooklyn, New York

*Chapter 81, Catheter-Associated Upper Extremity Deep Venous
Thrombosis*

Thomas S. Huber, MD, PhD
Edward R. Woodward Professor and Chief
Division of Vascular Surgery
University of Florida College of Medicine
Gainesville, Florida

Chapter 24, Abdominal Aortic Aneurysm
Chapter 69, Access-Related Hand Ischemia

Misty D. Humphries, MD, MAS, RPVI, FACS
Associate Professor of Surgery
Director of Vascular Training
Department of Surgery
University of California, Davis
Sacramento, California

Chapter 30, Femoral Artery Aneurysm

Karl A. Illig, MD
Dialysis Access Institute
Regional Medical Center
Orangeburg, South Carolina

Chapter 70, Failing Hemodialysis Access Due to Central Vein or Venous Outflow Lesions

Douglas Jones, MD
Assistant Professor of Surgery
Division of Vascular Surgery
University of Massachusetts Medical School
Worcester, Massachusetts

Chapter 88, Arterial Access Complications

Jeffrey Kalish, MD
Associate Professor of Surgery and Radiology
Department of Surgery
Boston University School of Medicine
Director of Endovascular Surgery
Department of Surgery
Boston Medical Center
One Boston Medical Center Place
Boston, Massachusetts

Chapter 88, Arterial Access Complications

Manju Kalra, MBBS
Professor of Surgery
Division of Vascular and Endovascular Surgery
Mayo Clinic and Foundation
Consultant Vascular Surgeon
Division of Vascular and Endovascular Surgery
Rochester, Minnesota

Chapter 80, Vena Caval Thrombosis/Obstruction

Jeanwan Kang, MD
Assistant Professor of Surgery
Section of Vascular Surgery
Geisel School of Medicine at Dartmouth
Hanover, New Hampshire
Staff Vascular Surgeon
Section of Vascular Surgery
Dartmouth-Hitchcock
Lebanon, New Hampshire

Chapter 8, Symptomatic Carotid Disease

Vikram S. Kashyap, MD, FACS
Professor
Chief, Vascular Surgery
Department of Surgery
University Hospitals
Case Western Reserve University
Cleveland, Ohio

Chapter 34, Splenic Artery Aneurysm

Sikandar Z. Khan, MBBS, RPVI
Clinical Assistant Professor of Surgery, Department of Surgery
Jacobs School of Medicine and Biomed. Sciences, SUNY at Buffalo
Attending Vascular Surgeon, Department of Surgery
Erie County Medical Center
Buffalo, New York

Chapter 47, Infra-Inguinal Arterial Occlusive Disease

Martyn Knowles, MD, MBA
Adjunct Assistant Professor
University of North Carolina
Raleigh, North Carolina

Chapter 32, Upper Extremity Artery Aneurysm

Jonathan Kwong, MD
Staff Surgeon
Department of Vascular Surgery
Louis Stokes Cleveland VA Medical Center
Cleveland, Ohio

Chapter 34, Splenic Artery Aneurysm

Brajesh K. Lal, MD
Professor
Department of Vascular Surgery
University of Maryland School of Medicine
Baltimore, Maryland

Chapter 83, Stroke after Carotid Intervention

Glenn LaMuraglia, MD
Professor of Surgery
Department of Vascular and Endovascular Surgery
Massachusetts General Hospital
Boston, Massachusetts

Chapter 16, Carotid Body Tumor

Gregory J. Landry, MD
Professor
Chief of Vascular Surgery
Department of Surgery
Oregon Health and Science University
Portland, Oregon

Chapter 50, Thromboangiitis Obliterans (Buerger's Disease)

Jeffrey H. Lawson, MD, PhD
Adjunct Professor of Surgery
Department of Surgery
Duke University
President and Chief Executive
Humacyte, Inc.
Durham, North Carolina

Chapter 92, Intraoperative Bleeding

Peter J. Lawson, BS
Student
Department of Bioengineering
University of Colorado – Anschutz Medical Campus
Aurora, Colorado

Chapter 92, Intraoperative Bleeding

Ashton Lee, MD
Integrated Vascular Surgery Resident
Department of Surgery
University of Arizona
Vascular Surgery Resident
Department of Surgery
Banner University Medical Center
Tucson, Arizona

Chapter 27, Acquired Abdominal Arteriovenous Fistula

Jason T. Lee, MD
Professor of Vascular Surgery
Department of Surgery
Stanford University School of Medicine
Director of Endovascular Surgery
Division of Vascular Surgery
Stanford Hospital and Clinics
Stanford, California

Chapter 58, Arterial Thoracic Outlet Syndrome

Patric Liang, MD

Vascular Surgery Resident
Department of Vascular and Endovascular Surgery
Harvard Medical School
Vascular Surgery Resident
Department of Vascular and Endovascular Surgery
Beth Israel Deaconess Medical Center
Boston, Massachusetts

Chapter 36, Acute Mesenteric Ischemia

Timothy K. Liem, MD, MBA, FACS

Professor
Division of Vascular Surgery
School of Medicine
Oregon Health & Science University
Portland, Oregon

Chapter 91, Heparin-Induced Thrombocytopenia

Evan Lipsitz, MD

Professor and Chief
Division of Vascular and Endovascular Surgery
Department of Cardiothoracic and Vascular Surgery
Montefiore Medical Center and the Albert Einstein
    College of Medicine
Bronx, New York

Chapter 84, Colonic Ischemia after Aortoiliac Operation

Joseph V. Lombardi, MD

Professor, Department of Surgery
Cooper Medical School of Rowan University
Chief, Department of Surgery
Cooper University Healthcare
Camden, New Jersey

Chapter 21, Acute Aortic Dissection

Christine Lotto, MD

Vascular Surgery Fellow
Department of Vascular and Endovascular Surgery
Brigham and Women's Hospital
Boston, Massachusetts

Chapter 43, Renal Vein Compression Syndrome

Justin K. Lui, MD

Fellow, Pulmonary and Critical Care Medicine
Department of Medicine
Section of Pulmonary, Allergy, Sleep and Critical Care
    Medicine
Boston University School of Medicine
Boston, Massachusetts

Chapter 2, Perioperative Pulmonary Risk Assessment and Management

Michael C. Madigan, MD

Assistant Professor of Surgery
Division of Vascular Surgery, Department of
    Surgery
University of Pittsburgh
Pittsburgh, Pennsylvania

Chapter 31, Popliteal Artery Aneurysm

Gregory A. Magee, MD, MSc, FACS

Assistant Professor of Surgery
Division of Vascular Surgery and Endovascular
    Therapy
Keck Medical Center of USC
Los Angeles, California

Chapter 62, Abdominal Vascular Trauma

Mahmoud B. Malas, MD, MHS, RPVI, FACS

Professor-in-Residence
Department of Surgery
University of California San Diego
Chief
Division of Vascular and Endovascular
    Surgery
University of California San Diego Health System
La Jolla, California

Chapter 6, Identifying Cerebrovascular Disease

Fatemeh Malekpour, MD, MSc

Assistant Professor
Department of Surgery
University of Texas Southwestern Medical Center
Assistant Professor
Division of Vascular Surgery, Department
    of Surgery
Parkland Memorial Hospital
Dallas, Texas

Chapter 51, Compartment Syndrome

Kimberly T. Malka, MD, PhD

Assistant Professor
Department of Surgery
Tufts University School of Medicine
Boston, Massachusetts
Attending Physician
Department of Vascular and Endovascular
    Surgery
Maine Medical Partners Surgical Care
Portland, Maine

Chapter 89, Late Arterial Graft/Stent Thrombosis

Kevin Mani, MD, PhD

Professor of Vascular Surgery
Department of Surgical Sciences
Uppsala University
Uppsala, Sweden

Chapter 23, Penetrating Aortic Ulcer, Intramural Hematoma, and Isolated Abdominal Aortic Dissection

William A. Marston, MD

George Johnson Jr. Distinguished Professor
Department of Surgery
University of North Carolina School of Medicine
Chapel Hill, North Carolina

Chapter 73, Chronic Venous Insufficiency

Robert B. McLafferty, MD, MBA

Chief of Surgery
Veterans Affairs Health Care System
Professor of Surgery
Division of Vascular Surgery
Oregon Health & Sciences University
Portland, Oregon

Chapter 74, Pelvic Congestion Syndrome

Katharine L. McGinigle, MD, MPH

Assistant Professor
Department of Surgery
University of North Carolina
Chapel Hill, North Carolina

Chapter 73, Chronic Venous Insufficiency

Robert C. McMurray, MD

Teaching Fellow
Department of Surgery
F. Edward Herbert School of Medicine, Uniformed Services
    University of the Health Sciences
Fellow
Department of Vascular Surgery
Walter Reed National Military Medical Center
Bethesda, Maryland

Chapter 15, Carotid and Vertebral Artery Dissection

Matthew T. Menard, MD

Associate Professor
Department of Surgery
Harvard Medical School
Co-Director, Endovascular Surgery
Division of Vascular and Endovascular Surgery
Brigham and Women's Hospital
Boston, Massachusetts

Chapter 43, Renal Vein Compression Syndrome

Aleem K. Mirza, MD
Instructor of Surgery
Division of Vascular and Endovascular
    Surgery
Mayo Clinic
Rochester, Minnesota

Chapter 80, Vena Caval Thrombosis/Obstruction

Erica L. Mitchell, MD, MEd
Emeritus Professor, Surgery
Oregon Health and Science University
Portland, Oregon

Chapter 55, Hand Ischemia

J. Gregory Modrall, MD
Professor
Division of Vascular and Endovascular
    Surgery
University of Texas Southwestern Medical Center
Chief
Department of Surgical Services
Dallas Veterans Affairs Medical Center
Dallas, Texas

Chapter 51, Compartment Syndrome

Jahan Mohebali, MD, MPH
Assistant Professor of Surgery
Department of Surgery
Harvard Medical School
Division of Vascular and Endovascular Surgery
Massachusetts General Hospital
Boston, Massachusetts

Chapter 86, Spinal Cord Ischemia After Aortic Operation

Mark D. Morasch, MD, FACS
Chief,
Department of Vascular Surgery
St. Marks Hospital
Salt Lake City, Utah

Chapter 12, Vertebral Artery Disease

Rameen S. Moridzadeh, MD
Chief Resident, Vascular Surgery
Division of Vascular and Endovascular Surgery
David Geffen School of Medicine, UCLA
Ronald Reagan UCLA Medical Center
Los Angeles, California

Chapter 57, Venous Thoracic Outlet Syndrome

Matthew Nayor, MD, MPH
Instructor
Department of Medicine
Harvard Medical School
Assistant Physician
Department of Cardiology
Massachusetts General Hospital
Boston, Massachusetts

Chapter 4, Hyperlipidemia Assessment and Management

Michael Neilson, MD
Attending Vascular Surgeon
Department of Vascular and Endovascular Surgery
Maine General Medical Center
Augusta, Maine

Chapter 26, Iliac Artery Aneurysm

Erica E. Nelson, MD
Associate Professor
Department of OBGYN
Southern Illinois University School of Medicine
Springfield, Illinois

Chapter 74, Pelvic Congestion Syndrome

Brian W. Nolan, MD, MS
Chief
Department of Vascular and Endovascular
    Surgery
Maine Medical Center
Portland, Maine

Chapter 26, Iliac Artery Aneurysm

Gustavo S. Oderich, MD
Professor of Surgery
Chair
Division of Vascular and Endovascular Surgery
Mayo Clinic Hospital, Saint Mary's Campus
Rochester, Minnesota

Chapter 22, Chronic Thoracic Aortic Dissection

C. Keith Ozaki, MD
Professor of Surgery
Department of Surgery
Harvard Medical School
John A. Mannick Professor of Surgery
Department of Surgery
Brigham and Women's Hospital
Boston, Massachusetts

Chapter 65, Nonmaturing Arteriovenous Fistula

Marc A. Passman, MD
Professor
Division of Vascular Surgery and Endovascular Therapy
Department of Surgery
University of Alabama at Birmingham
Birmingham, Alabama

Chapter 79, Acute Iliofemoral Deep Venous Thrombosis

Amani D. Politano, MD, MS
Assistant Professor
Vascular Surgeon
Vascular and Endovascular Surgery
Oregon Health and Science University
Portland, Oregon

Chapter 55, Hand Ischemia

Richard J. Powell, MD
Chief, Section of Vascular Surgery
Dartmouth Hitchcock Medical Center
Lebanon, New Hampshire
Professor of Surgery and Radiology
Dartmouth Geisel School of Medicine
Hanover, New Hampshire

Chapter 39, Celiac Artery Compression Syndrome

William J. Quinones-Baldrich, MD
Professor of Surgery
Department of Vascular Surgery
David Geffen School of Medicine at UCLA
Director UCLA Aortic Center
Ronald Reagan UCLA Medical Center
Los Angeles, California

Chapter 10, Recurrent Carotid Stenosis

Vasan S. Ramachandran, MD, DM, FACC, FAHA
Professor of Medicine and Epidemiology
Department of Medicine and Epidemiology
Boston University Schools of Medicine and Public Health
Boston, Massachusetts

Chapter 4, Hyperlipidemia Assessment and Management

Todd E. Rasmussen, MD
Professor of Surgery, Associate Dean for Research
F. Edward Hebert School of Medicine
Uniformed Services University of the Health Sciences
Attending Vascular Surgeon
Department of Surgery
Walter Reed National Military Medical Center
Bethesda, Maryland

Chapter 59, Initial Management of Life-Threatening Trauma

David Rigberg, MD

Professor
Department of Surgery (Vascular)
UCLA David Geffen School of Medicine
Vascular Surgeon
Department of Surgery (Vascular)
UCLA Ronald Reagan Medical Center
Los Angeles, California

Chapter 57, Venous Thoracic Outlet Syndrome

William P. Robinson III, MD

Professor and Chief, Division of Vascular Surgery
Program Director, Vascular Surgery Fellowship
East Carolina University Brody School of Medicine
Greenville, North Carolina

Chapter 46, Aortoiliac Disease

Sean P. Roddy, MD

Professor of Surgery
Department of Surgery
Albany Medical College
Albany, New York

Chapter 54, Upper Extremity Occlusive Disease

Thom Rooke, MD

Professor
Consultant
Division of Vascular Medicine
Mayo Clinic School of Medicine
Mayo Clinic Hospital
Rochester, Minnesota

Chapter 71, Diagnosing Lower Extremity Venous and Lymphatic Disease

Vincent L. Rowe, MD

Professor
Department of Surgery
Keck School of Medicine at University of Southern
    California
Los Angeles, California

Chapter 62, Abdominal Vascular Trauma

Zein M. Saadeddin, MD

Vascular Resident
Department of Surgery
University of Cincinnati Medical Center
College of Medicine
Academic—Medical Sciences Building
Cincinnati, Ohio

Chapter 82, Pulmonary Embolism

Timur P. Sarac, MD

Professor and Chief of Vascular Surgery, Director
    of the Aortic Center
Department of Vascular Surgery
The Ohio State University School of Medicine
Columbus, Ohio

Chapter 35, Celiac, Hepatic, and Mesenteric Artery Aneurysms

Salvatore T. Scali, MD, FACS

Associate Professor of Surgery
Division of Vascular Surgery and Endovascular Therapy
University of Florida College of Health Science
UF Health Shands Hospital at the University of Florida
Gainesville, Florida

Chapter 24, Abdominal Aortic Aneurysm
Chapter 69, Access-Related Hand Ischemia

Andres Schanzer, MD

Professor of Surgery
Division of Vascular Surgery
University of Massachusetts Medical School
Chief
Division of Vascular Surgery
UMass Memorial Medical Center
Worcester, Massachusetts

Chapter 29, Endoleak after Endovascular Aortic Aneurysm Repair

Frank Schembri, MD

Adjunct Assistant Professor
Department of Medicine
Section of Pulmonary, Allergy, Sleep and Critical Care
    Medicine
Boston University School of Medicine
Boston, Massachusetts

Chapter 2, Perioperative Pulmonary Risk Assessment and Management

Marc L. Schermerhorn, MD

George H.A. Clowes Jr Professor of Surgery
Harvard Medical School
Chief, Division of Vascular and Endovascular Surgery
Beth Israel Deaconess Medical Center
Boston, Massachusetts

Chapter 37, Chronic Mesenteric Ischemia

Philip G. Schmalz, MD

Neurosurgery Resident
Department of Neurosurgery
The University of Alabama at Birmingham
Birmingham, Alabama

Chapter 9, Acute Ischemic Stroke

Peter A. Schneider, MD

Professor of Surgery
Division of Vascular and Endovascular Surgery
University of California, San Francisco
San Francisco, California

Chapter 15, Carotid and Vertebral Artery Dissection

Samuel I. Schwartz, MD

Assistant Professor
Department of Vascular and Endovascular Surgery
Massachusetts General Hospital
Boston, Massachusetts

Chapter 16, Carotid Body Tumor

Murray L. Shames, MD

Professor and Chief Division of Vascular Surgery
Vice Chair of Research, Department of Surgery
Program Director Vascular Surgery Residency
USF Health Morsani School of Medicine
Director, Tampa General Hospital Aorta Center
Tampa, Florida

Chapter 53, Acute Limb Ischemia

Palma M. Shaw, MD, FACS, RPVI

Professor of Surgery
Director of Venous Program
Department of Surgery
Upstate Medical University
Syracuse, New York

Chapter 10, Recurrent Carotid Stenosis

Laura Shin, DPM, PhD

Assistant Professor
Department of Vascular Surgery
Keck School of Medicine at University of Southern California
Los Angeles, California

Chapter 52, Assessment of the Diabetic Foot: Wound, Ischemia, and Foot Infection

Cynthia Shortell, MD

Professor and Chief of Vascular and Endovascular Surgery
Chief of Staff, Department of Surgery
Duke University Medical Center
Durham, North Carolina

Chapter 76, Vascular Malformations

Jessica P. Simons, MD, MPH

Associate Professor
Division of Vascular and Endovascular Surgery, Department
    of Surgery
University of Massachusetts Medical School
Worcester, Massachusetts

Chapter 89, Late Arterial Graft/Stent Thrombosis

Niten Singh, MD

Professor of Surgery
Department of Surgery
University of Washington
Seattle, Washington

Chapter 49, Popliteal Entrapment and Adventitial Cyst Disease

Jeffrey Siracuse, MD, MBA

Program Director
Vascular Surgery Fellowship
Boston Medical Center
Associate Professor of Surgery and Radiology
Boston University School of Medicine
Boston, Massachusetts

Chapter 45, Chronic Atherosclerotic Leg Ischemia

Margaret E. Smith, MD, MS

General Surgery Resident
Department of General Surgery
University of Michigan
Ann Arbor, Michigan

Chapter 77, Superficial Thrombophlebitis

Benjamin W. Starnes, MD, DFSVS

Professor
Department of Surgery
University of Washington
Chief
Division of Vascular Surgery
Harborview Medical Center
Seattle, Washington

Chapter 25, Ruptured Abdominal Aortic Aneurysm

David Stone, MD

Professor of Surgery
Section of Vascular Surgery
Geisel School of Medicine at Dartmouth
Hanover, New Hampshire
Program Director, Vascular Surgery
Dartmouth-Hitchcock Medical Center
Lebanon, New Hampshire

Chapter 8, Symptomatic Carotid Disease

Nicholas J. Swerdlow, MD

Clinical Fellow in Surgery
Department of Surgery
Harvard Medical School
General Surgery Resident
Department of Surgery
Beth Israel Deaconess Medical Center
Boston, Massachusetts

Chapter 37, Chronic Mesenteric Ischemia

Emanuel R. Tenorio, MD, PhD

Aortic Research Fellow
Division of Vascular and Endovascular Surgery
Mayo Clinic Hospital, Saint Mary's Campus
Rochester, Minnesota

Chapter 22, Chronic Thoracic Aortic Dissection

Jonathan R. Thompson, MD, RPVI

Assistant Professor of Surgery
Division of Vascular Surgery, Department of Surgery
University of Nebraska Medical Center
Omaha, Nebraska

Chapter 42, Acute Renovascular Ischemia

Carlos Timaran, MD

Professor of Surgery
Chief, Endovascular Surgery
Department of Surgery
UT Southwestern Medical Center
Dallas, Texas

Chapter 32, Upper Extremity Artery Aneurysm

Bruce Tjaden, MD

Assistant Professor
Department of Vascular Surgery
Cooper University Hospital
Camden, New Jersey

Chapter 61, Thoracic Vascular Trauma

Thomas W. Wakefield, MD

Professor of Surgery
Surgeon
Section of Vascular Surgery
Department of Surgery
University of Michigan
Ann Arbor, Michigan

Chapter 77, Superficial Thrombophlebitis

Fred A. Weaver, MD, MMM

Professor
Division of Vascular Surgery and Endovascular Therapy,
    Department of Surgery
Keck School of Medicine at University of Southern California
Chief, Division of Vascular Surgery and Endovascular Therapy
Director of Vascular Surgery
Department of Surgery
Keck Hospital, University of Southern California
Los Angeles, California

Chapter 33, Renal Artery Aneurysm

Paul W. White, MD

Associate Professor
Department of Surgery
Uniformed Services University of the Health Sciences
Consultant to the Surgeon General for Vascular Surgery
United States Army
Walter Reed National Military Medical Center
Bethesda, Maryland

Chapter 59, Initial Management of Life-Threatening Trauma

Karen Woo, MD, MS

Associate Professor
Department of Surgery
University of California
Vascular Surgeon
Department of Surgery
University of California
Los Angles, California

Chapter 64, New Hemodialysis Access

Mark C. Wyers, MD, FACS

Assistant Professor of Surgery
Harvard Medical School
Vascular Surgery Program Director
Department of Vascular and Endovascular Surgery
Beth Israel Deaconess Medical Center
Boston, Massachusetts

Chapter 36, Acute Mesenteric Ischemia

Michael Yacoub , MD, FACS, RPVI

Assistant Professor of Surgery
Department of Vascular and Endovascular Surgery
West Virginia University
Charleston, West Virginia

Chapter 14, Carotid Fibromuscular Disease

Wei Zhou, MD

Professor of Surgery
Department of Surgery
University of Arizona
Chief
Department of Vascular Surgery
Banner-University Medical Center
Tucson, Arizona

Chapter 27, Acquired Abdominal Arteriovenous Fistula

PREFACE

Optimal medical decision making requires that knowledge from multiple sources be integrated and applied to individual patients. It is one of the most challenging but rewarding aspects of clinical care and has become increasingly more complex as more treatment options are developed with varying degrees of evidence. This is particularly true for vascular disease, where many new medical, endovascular, and surgical treatments have been introduced over the past 20 years. These varying treatment options not only provide an important opportunity for individualized patient care based on the details and disease burden of each patient, but also make decision making more difficult.

Decision algorithms are intended to provide a clear structure or map that includes the key clinical elements to be considered when selecting treatment, so that each can be applied to individual patients without overlooking important factors involved in a complex decision. Ideally, they are based on high levels of evidence, but in many cases experience and collective understanding are all that is available. Each algorithm in this textbook represents the opinions of the authors, who were selected based on their acknowledged clinical experience and academic expertise. Their work has been reviewed by the section editors and editors in an attempt to create broadly accepted recommendations. In cases where uniform opinion based on clear evidence was not available, the accompanying text was designed to point out the basis for different decisions or different applications to specific patients.

Decision algorithms are difficult to create. They require us to express our approach to specific diseases in a logical, linear format, where in reality we may often use a nonlinear, gestalt method of decision making. For this reason, we are especially grateful to authors and section editors who have had to endure multiple revisions of their work as we attempted to create a homogeneous textbook. While decision algorithms are sometimes criticized as promoting "cookbook" medicine that stifles individual judgment, we believe that such algorithms simply highlight the logical steps that need to be considered and informed by each clinician's experience and knowledge, so that they can be successfully applied to individual patients.

This book is not an exhaustive review of every vascular disease process, but we have selected 92 key topics which in our experience represent the most common scenarios that confront vascular practitioners. It is impossible to consider the nuance of every clinical scenario in each decision tree, so there will be specific patients where the algorithms in this book may not completely apply. Further, there are evidence gaps that are described in this book, which hopefully will stimulate future research. Nonetheless, we hope and believe that *Vascular Decision Making* will be useful to trainees and practicing physicians. We are excited to include an electronic, smart phone version of these decision trees, which we hope will promote their use in direct clinical care settings.

Finally, we acknowledge the tremendous support of Wolters Kluwer in creating the print and e-book formats, and Zingtree for providing the platform to support the smart phone version.

Jack L. Cronenwett, MD
Alik Farber, MD, MBA
Erica L. Mitchell, MD, MEd

CONTENTS

Jorge Fuentes • Robert T. Eberhardt

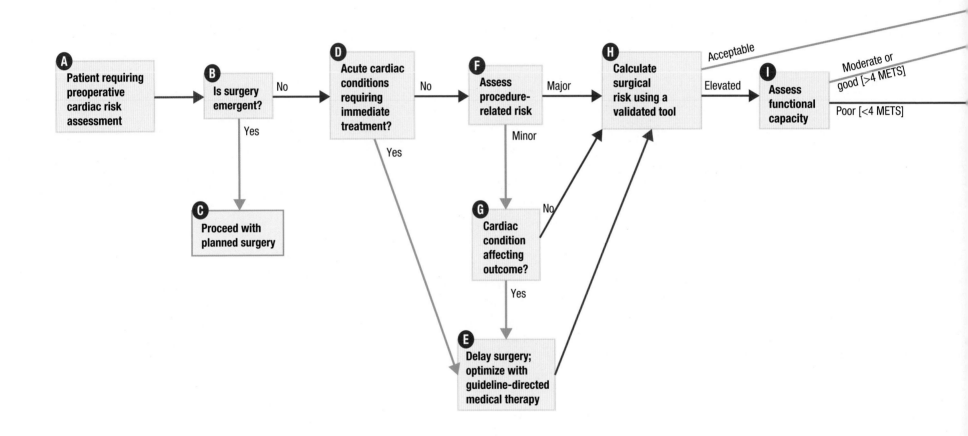

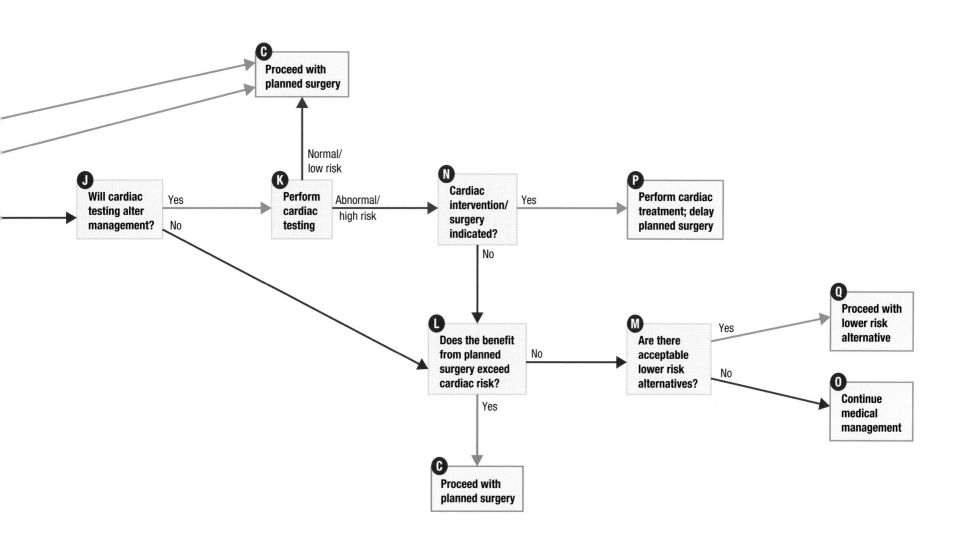

Ⓐ Patient requiring preoperative cardiac risk assessment

It is estimated that >200 million adults undergo major noncardiac surgery each year, with approximately 10 million suffering a major cardiac complication in the first 30 days.[1] These complications include MI, CHF, ventricular fibrillation, primary cardiac arrest, complete heart block, and even cardiac death. An accurate estimation of the risk of these cardiac complications is important to provide clinicians and patients with a better understanding and to allow for consideration of measures to reduce the risk, including alternative procedures with lower inherent risk. Cardiac risk should be assessed in every patient undergoing a noncardiac operation, but particular attention should be paid to those with a history of heart disease (including CAD, CHF, valvular heart disease, and arrhythmias) and those with symptoms or signs to suggest their presence.

Ⓑ Is surgery emergent?

The first step in assessing the perioperative cardiac risk is to decide whether there is an immediate need for surgery. Surgery that is required within 6 hours of an acute event for a life- or limb-threatening condition is defined as emergent.[2] Typically, there is very limited time for cardiac evaluation and few risk factors can be improved emergently. Regardless of the patient's baseline risk, emergency surgery increases the risk of perioperative cardiovascular events by 2- to 5-fold. An urgent procedure is defined as one required between 6 and 24 hours after presentation, which can provide time for a limited cardiac evaluation.[2] An elective procedure may be delayed to allow for sufficient time for evaluation without a negative impact on outcomes. The surgeon must estimate the urgency of the operation and decide whether to proceed with or delay surgery for further cardiac evaluation.

Ⓒ Proceed with planned surgery

When planned surgery is undertaken, it is important to employ intraoperative and postoperative measures to minimize cardiac complications, including appropriate monitoring and medical strategies based on anticipated complications.[2]

Ⓓ Acute cardiac conditions requiring immediate treatment?

There are acute cardiac conditions that are associated with extraordinarily poor perioperative cardiac outcomes. These include recent MI (within 30 days), unstable angina, decompensated heart failure, high-grade arrhythmias, and hemodynamically significant valvular heart disease (particularly aortic stenosis).[2,3] The presence of any of these acute cardiac conditions requires active efforts to optimize these conditions before undergoing noncardiac surgery.

Ⓔ Delay surgery; optimize with guideline-directed medical therapy

Acute cardiac conditions should be evaluated and optimized according to guideline-directed medical therapy (GDMT) before surgery.[2,4] Treatment for these acute cardiac conditions should be performed in conjunction with a cardiology consultant. Primary percutaneous coronary intervention is the preferred reperfusion approach for ST-elevation MI.[5] An invasive strategy using diagnostic angiography with intention to revascularize in the setting of suitable coronary anatomy is considered with acute coronary syndromes, including non-ST-elevation MI in association with an elevated risk for clinical events.[6] Treatment of decompensated heart failure involves management of volume overload and determining left ventricular systolic function to help guide further medical therapies (such as use of angiotensin-converting enzyme inhibitor, β-blockers, and others).[7] Treatment of high-grade arrhythmias such as sustained ventricular tachycardia may involve use of antiarrhythmic agents, cardiac ablation, or even implantable cardioverter defibrillator (ICD) based on the underlying etiology and presentation.[8] Valve intervention (such as surgical aortic valve replacement or transcatheter aortic valve replacement based on risk) may be considered if the patient meets the standard indication for valve intervention based on the symptoms and severity (such as severe symptomatic aortic stenosis).[9]

The role of optimization for nonacute cardiac conditions should be considered particularly if these are known to affect outcomes. In general, therapies for nonacute cardiac conditions should be based on guidelines used in the absence of planned surgery.[6-9] There is limited role for prophylactic therapies specifically to reduce the operative risk, but some interventions may influence long-term outcomes. The role of prophylactic β-blocker therapy was met with initial enthusiasm until the results of the early trials were invalidated. Furthermore, the POISE trial (which randomized 8351 patients undergoing noncardiac surgery to prophylactic perioperative β-blocker therapy) found that mortality and stroke were significantly increased with prophylactic metoprolol use compared with placebo (3.1% vs. 2.3% and 1% vs. 0.5%, respectively).[10] These findings were attributed to an increased risk of hypotension with β-blocker use (15% vs. 9.7% in placebo). This association of increased mortality with prophylactic preoperative β-blocker use has been confirmed by systematic reviews.[11]

Ⓕ Assess procedure-related risk

Each surgical procedure has an associated cardiac risk that varies in magnitude depending on factors inherent to the procedure. Factors that contribute to this surgical risk include anesthetic-related effects, fluid shifts, blood loss, increased catecholamines, and ventilation effects. It is helpful to categorize procedural-related risk as minor versus major.

Minor risk procedures are those associated with a low rate (typically <1%) of major adverse cardiac event (MACE) including death or MI.[2,12] These procedures generally include those performed under local anesthesia or utilizing a minimally invasive approach. Common vascular-related procedures within this category include AVF placement, venous ligation/phlebectomy, and even endarterectomies performed under local anesthesia.

Major risk procedures are associated with a higher rate of perioperative cardiac complications (typically >5%).[2] These procedures include AAA repair, arterial bypass, and arterial reconstructions. There are intermediate risk procedures (with a 1%-5% rate of MACE) including CEA (performed under general anesthesia), EVAR, and local peripheral arterial revisions (PSA repair, femoral patch angioplasty, etc). However, the preoperative cardiac assessment workup for these is typically managed in a manner similar to that for major operations.

Ⓖ Cardiac condition affecting outcome?

A clinical assessment should be performed to determine whether an underlying nonacute cardiac condition (such as CAD, CHF, valvular heart disease, or arrhythmias) requires intervention or medical optimization to reduce the likelihood of a cardiovascular complication in the perioperative period, or in the ensuing year.

Ⓗ Calculate surgical risk using a validated tool

Two of the most frequently used preoperative cardiac risk stratification tools are the revised cardiac risk index (RCRI) (https://www.mdcalc.com/revised-cardiac-risk-index-pre-operative-risk) and the Gupta model derived from the National Surgical Quality Improvement Program (NSQIP) (https://riskcalculator.facs.org/RiskCalculator/PatientInfo.jsp).[13,14] These models take into account the specific procedure performed and patient-related factors, including functional status, ASA class, BMI, and surgical factors such as urgency of procedure. It is important to understand the limitations of each risk tool to accurately assess an individual patient's preoperative risk. The RCRI includes factors of ischemic heart disease, heart failure, cerebrovascular disease, insulin-requiring diabetes mellitus, CKD, and high-risk surgery.[13] The adverse cardiac event rate has been shown to increase as the number of factors increases. A newer NSQIP risk calculator is more comprehensive and specific for a particular type of operation.[14] However, both the RCRI and the NSQIP model may underestimate risk and appear to be less predictive with vascular surgery.

Owing to these limitations, the Vascular Study Group of New England (VSGNE) developed a risk index derived specifically for patients undergoing vascular surgery to predict the risk of adverse cardiac events (including MI, arrhythmia, and heart failure, but not mortality).[15] These factors included increasing age (odds ratio [OR] 1.7-2.8), smoking (OR 1.3), insulin-dependent diabetes mellitus (OR 1.4), CAD (OR 1.4),

CHF (OR 1.9), abnormal cardiac stress test (OR 1.2), long-term β-blocker therapy (OR 1.4), COPD (OR 1.6), and creatinine ≥1.8 mg/dL (OR 1.7). Prior cardiac revascularization was protective (OR 0.8). The VSGNE calculators for various vascular surgical procedures are available online (https://qxmd.com/vascular-study-group-new-england-decision-support-tools).

A refinement of the risk of postoperative MI associated with various vascular procedures was developed from the Vascular Quality Initiative (VQI).[16] The most important predictor of postoperative MI was operation type, with MI rates of 0.9% after CEA, 1.1% after EVAR, 2.75 after supra- or infrainguinal bypass, and 4.8% after open AAA repair. Other independent factors associated with postoperative MI for all these operation types were older age, creatinine > 1.8 mg/dL, abnormal stress test, insulin-dependent diabetes, and CHF. There are unique factors associated with risk for specific procedure types, so risk prediction is most accurate when using an online calculator available at https://www.vqi.org/vqi-resource-library/vqi-risk-calculators-2.

Patients with a calculated risk of a cardiac complication <1% are typically deemed to be acceptable risk.[2] These patients may proceed with planned surgery without further diagnostic testing.

Patients with a calculated risk of a cardiac complication of >1%, or above the standard risk for planned surgery, are deemed to be at elevated risk.[2] These patients should undergo an assessment of their functional capacity to further assess their cardiovascular risk.

● Assess functional capacity

Functional status has been shown to be a useful predictor of both short- and long-term perioperative outcomes.[2,17] This may be assessed using an objective scale or measure, such as the Duke Activity Status Index, to determine functional capacity.[18] It is determined on the basis of the highest activity a patient can perform without symptoms. The energy expenditure during such activity is expressed as metabolic equivalents (METs). As a frame of reference, one MET is defined as the amount of oxygen utilized in the resting state (or 3.5 mL/kg/min). A common activity used to estimate a threshold level of functional capacity in perioperative assessment is the ability to climb one flight of stairs at a normal pace or walk on level ground at a speed of 3 to 4 mph.[2] The ability to perform this level of physical activity corresponds to four METs.

A patient is considered to have moderate functional capacity if he/she is able to achieve four METs of physical activity without symptoms. Those with a moderate or greater functional capacity typically do well with surgery and are not required to undergo further cardiac testing (class IIb).[2] Furthermore, those with a high functional capacity of above 10 METs have even better outcomes and thus provide greater confidence to proceed without further cardiac testing (class IIa).[2]

Functional Status (METs)[2]	
Exercise Level	Equivalent Activity
1-4 METs	Standard light home activities Walk around the house Take care of yourself—eating, bathing, and using the toilet
5-9 METs	Climb flight of stairs, walk up hill Walk one or two blocks on ground level at speed 4 mph Run short distance Moderate activity (golf, dancing, and mountain walk) Sexual relations
>10 METs	Strenuous sports (swimming, tennis, and cycling) Heavy professional/domestic work (scrubbing floors and lifting heavy furniture)

A poor functional capacity is considered the inability to perform four METs of physical activity without the development of limiting symptoms (of any nature). Such patients are at increased risk for an adverse cardiac event with surgery and thus require consideration for further cardiac testing.[2,4]

● Will cardiac testing alter management?

Medical and surgical clinicians involved in a patient's care should discuss whether diagnostic testing (including stress testing, ECHO, or others) will impact the decision to proceed with surgery or influence perioperative care.[2] It is important to also determine a patient's willingness to proceed with potential cardiac intervention (either percutaneous or surgical revascularization) that may be indicated on the basis of results of cardiac testing. If results of this information may influence care, then it is appropriate to proceed with testing. If such results are unlikely to alter the plan to proceed with surgery, then testing is not warranted.

● Perform cardiac testing

Cardiac testing may be performed for further perioperative cardiovascular risk assessment. The most common studies are noninvasive cardiovascular tests to assess for ischemia, but others may include ECHO to assess ventricular and valve function, and even coronary angiography in selected situations.[2] Noninvasive ischemic testing may include exercise treadmill test, stress ECHO, or nuclear, or pharmacologic, imaging studies. The specific stress testing modality should be made on an individual basis considering the patient's baseline functional status and associated comorbidities. However, the most common tests for patients undergoing

vascular procedures are pharmacologic imaging studies, either vasodilator nuclear studies (such as adenosine SPECT or PET) or DSE.[19-21] The selection of modality should consider local expertise and clinical variables (such as avoiding dobutamine with uncontrolled arrhythmias or ventricular ectopy, and avoiding adenosine with advanced conduction system disease or active bronchospasm).

The lack of findings of ischemia on stress testing, including reversible myocardial perfusion defects on vasodilator nuclear stress testing or inducible wall motional abnormalities on DSE, has an excellent negative predictive value of about 99%.[2] Patients with "normal" test results have a very low frequency (<1%) of perioperative cardiac events (MI or cardiac death).[2,19] These patients may proceed with planned surgery according to GDMT.

Patients with inducible ischemia on stress testing, including reversible perfusion defects on vasodilator nuclear stress testing and inducible wall motion abnormalities on DSE, are at increased risk for adverse cardiac events. An abnormal preoperative stress test result has been shown to have a positive predictive value of about 10% to 15% for developing a subsequent cardiac event.[2,19] According to a prospective study evaluating the prognostic value of dipyridamole rubidium PET stress test, severity of resting perfusion abnormality directly correlated with composite endpoint of cardiac death and MI.[20] A large area of ischemia (defined by a sum stress score of >8) was associated with annual risk of death or MI of approximately 7%.[20] Thus, such findings are predictive not only of perioperative cardiac events but also of long-term outcomes. Independent predictors of cardiac events on myocardial perfusion imaging include number and severity of reversible perfusion defects, heart rate achieved during stress, and extent of regional wall motion abnormalities.[19-21] In a large study (involving 1432 patients), the prognostic value of myocardial perfusion imaging using PET demonstrated that the severity of myocardial ischemia and depressed left ventricular EF at peak stress were associated with increased cardiac events and all cause death over 1 year.[21] In patients with certain so-called high-risk abnormal stress test results, coronary angiography and revascularization should be considered before surgery to further gauge and possibly optimize risk.

● Does the benefit from planned surgery exceed cardiac risk?

For a patient with poor or unknown functional status in whom testing will not impact decision making, the clinical team needs to determine whether the benefit of planned surgery exceeds the estimated cardiac risk. If the benefits of proceeding with surgery outweigh the cardiac risk, then proceeding with the planned surgical procedure with optimized GDMT is recommended.[2] If the benefit of surgery does not outweigh the risk, then considering alternative lower risk treatment options is appropriate.

Ⓜ Are there acceptable lower risk alternatives?

It is essential for the clinical care team, ideally one that is multidisciplinary, to consider alternative interventions or procedures with lower risk that may provide acceptable outcomes for the vascular condition being treated.

Ⓝ Cardiac intervention/surgery indicated?

If the cardiac testing result is considered to be high-risk abnormal, then coronary angiography is recommended with a view toward coronary revascularization if there is suitable anatomy. Revascularization should be considered in patients with stable ischemic heart disease and left main CAD, three-vessel CAD (particularly with EF <50%), and two-vessel CAD with proximal left anterior descending coronary artery involvement (particularly with EF <50%) (class I).[22] Percutaneous coronary intervention is considered if the procedural risk is low and likelihood of good long-term outcome is high (class IIa).[22,23] However, it should be emphasized that there is limited role for prophylactic revascularization to reduce operative risk, because the CARP trial showed no reduction in the risk of major cardiac events with routine cardiac revascularization before major vascular surgery in a group of high-risk patients.[24] In addition to considering coronary revascularization, medical optimization using GDMT should be pursued.

Optimal medical management at the time of surgery may include β-blockers, diuretics, statins, and antiplatelet therapy. β-Blockers should be continued at the time of noncardiac surgery if patient is chronically on β-blockers (class I).[2] The withdrawal of β-blockers before noncardiac surgery is not favored and may be associated with an increase in mortality.[25,26] It may be reasonable to start β-blocker therapy perioperatively in patients with intermediate- or high-risk features of myocardial ischemia noted during perioperative stratification tests or in patients with three or more RCRI risk factors (diabetes, heart failure, CAD, renal insufficiency, or cerebrovascular accident) (class IIb).[2,25] However, it is important not to start β-blockers on the same day of surgery because of increased cardiovascular risk (class III).[2,27] This seems to be mitigated by starting the β-blocker 2 to 7 days before surgery; however, some data support the need to start β-blockers >30 days beforehand. This is further supported by the finding that prophylactic use of β-blockers within 30 days did not decrease rates of MACEs or mortality after major vascular surgery and increased the rates of some adverse events in several subgroups.[28] Clinical assessment of volume status to ensure that the patient is euvolemic before surgery is recommended. Pulmonary artery catheterization may be considered when underlying medical conditions that significantly affect hemodynamics (decompensated heart failure or severe valvular disease) cannot be corrected before

surgery, but generally serves a limited role. If patients are on chronic diuretic therapy, diuretic therapy is generally continued with close monitoring of hemodynamics and fluid status in the postoperative period.[2,4] Statins should be continued at the time of surgery if chronically on statin therapy (class I).[22] Initiation of statin is reasonable in patients undergoing vascular or high-risk procedures (class IIa-IIb).[22,29] The use of antiplatelet therapy in the perioperative period should be made by the clinical team, preferably one that is multidisciplinary, weighing the risks of bleeding and coronary thrombosis. The data regarding the continued use of aspirin are conflicting with evidence discouraging its routine use, but less certainty in those with prior established atherosclerosis or ischemic cardiovascular events, and a clear benefit in those with prior coronary intervention.[30,31]

Ⓞ Continue medical management

It is recommended to continue medical treatments for the vascular condition for which surgery was being considered until there is a change in the clinical status that may alter the risk-benefit analysis. This includes close outpatient follow-up for continued medical treatment and risk factor modification.

Ⓟ Perform cardiac treatment; delay planned surgery

Cardiac treatment may involve either surgical or percutaneous strategies depending on the coronary anatomy and other clinical features. Following CABG, noncardiac surgery is typically delayed for several weeks to allow for healing and recovery, but the procedure can been done sooner depending on the need for surgery. Following percutaneous coronary intervention, noncardiac surgery should be delayed because of an increased risk of coronary thrombosis, particularly after stent implantation. It is recommended that surgery should be delayed for 14 days after balloon angioplasty, 30 days after bare metal stent implantation, and 3 to 6 months after drug-eluting stent (DES) implantation.[30] These recommendations impact the type of revascularization chosen in comparison with the urgency of the planned noncardiac operation. Dual antiplatelet therapy following placement of a DES may typically be discontinued after 6 months with a prior acute coronary syndrome or MI, and 3 to 6 months with stable ischemic heart disease.[30] If the risk of surgical delay is greater than the risk of coronary thrombosis within this time frame, then proceeding with continued use of dual antiplatelet therapy should be considered, but balanced against the risk of bleeding. If discontinuation of $P2Y_{12}$ inhibitors is required for the surgery, aspirin should be continued and $P2Y_{12}$ inhibitor should be restarted as soon as possible after surgery (class I).[30]

Ⓠ Proceed with lower risk alternative

If lower risk alternative vascular procedures are possible in patients with high cardiac risk, these should be pursued.

REFERENCES

1. Devereaux PJ, Sessler DI. Cardiac complications in patients undergoing major noncardiac surgery. *N Engl J Med.* 2015;3373:2258-2269.
2. Fleisher LA, Fleischmann KE, Auerbach AD, et al. 2014 ACC/AHA guideline on perioperative cardiovascular evaluation and management of patients undergoing noncardiac surgery: a report of the American College of Cardiology/American Heart Association Task Force on Practice Guidelines. *Circulation.* 2014;130:e278-e333.
3. Tashiro T, Pislaru SV, Blustin JM, et al. Perioperative risk of major non-cardiac surgery in patients with severe aortic stenosis: a reappraisal in contemporary practice. *Eur Heart J.* 2014;35:2372-2381.
4. Kristensen SD, Knuuti J, Saraste A, et al. 2014 ESC/ESA Guidelines on non-cardiac surgery: cardiovascular assessment and management: The Joint Task Force on non-cardiac surgery: cardiovascular assessment and management of the European Society of Cardiology (ESC) and the European Society of Anaesthesiology (ESA). *Eur Heart J.* 2014;35:2383-2431.
5. O'Gara PT, Kushner FG, Ascheim DD, et al. 2013 ACCF/AHA guideline for the management of ST-elevation myocardial infarction: a report of the American College of Cardiology Foundation/American Heart Association Task Force on Practice Guidelines. *Circulation.* 2013;127:529-555.
6. Amsterdam EA, Wenger NK, Brindis RG, et al. 2014 AHA/ACC guideline for the management of patients with non–ST-elevation acute coronary syndromes: a report of the American College of Cardiology/American Heart Association Task Force on Clinical Practice Guidelines. *J Am Coll Cardiol.* 2014;64:e139-e228.
7. Yancy CW, Jessup M, Bozkurt B, et al. 2017 ACC/AHA/HFSA focused update of the 2013 ACCF/AHA guideline for the management of heart failure: a report of the American College of Cardiology/American Heart Association Task Force on Clinical Practice Guidelines and the Heart Failure Society of America. *Circulation.* 2017;70:776-803.
8. Al-Khatib SM, Stevenson WG, Ackerman MJ, et al. 2017 AHA/ACC/HRS guideline for management of patients with ventricular arrhythmias and the prevention of sudden cardiac death: a report of the American College of Cardiology Foundation/American Heart Association Task Force on Clinical Practice Guidelines and the Heart Rhythm Society. *Circulation.* 2018;138:e272-e391. doi:10.1161/CIR.0000000000000549.
9. Nishimura RA, Otto CM, Bonow RO, et al. 2017 AHA/ACC focused update of the 2014 AHA/ACC guideline for the management of patients with valvular heart disease: a report of the American College of Cardiology/American Heart

Association Task Force on Clinical Practice Guidelines. *J Am Coll Cardiol*. 2017;70:252-289.

10. POISE Study Group, Devereaux PJ, Yang H, Guyatt G, et al. Effects of extended-release metoprolol succinate in patients undergoing non-cardiac surgery (POISE trial): a randomized controlled trial. *Lancet*. 2008;371:1839-1847.

11. Blessberger H, Kammler J, Domanovits H, et al. Perioperative beta-blockers for preventing surgery-related mortality and morbidity. *Cochrane Database Syst Rev*. 2018;(3):CD004476.

12. Smilowitz NR, Gupta N, Ramakrishna H, Guo Y, Berger JS, Bangalore S. Perioperative major adverse cardiovascular and cerebrovascular events associated with noncardiac surgery. *JAMA Cardiol*. 2017;2:181-187.

13. Thomas L, Marcantonio E, Mangione C, et al. Derivation and prospective validation of a simple index for prediction of cardiac risk of major noncardiac surgery. *Circulation*. 1999;100:1043-1049.

14. Gupta PK, Gupta K, Sundaram A, et al. Development and validation of a risk calculator for prediction of cardiac risk after surgery. *Circulation*. 2011;124:381-387.

15. Bertges DJ, Goodney PP, Zhao Y, et al. The Vascular Study Group of New England Cardiac Risk Index (VSG-CRI) predicts cardiac complications more accurately than the Revised Cardiac Risk Index in vascular surgery patients. *J Vasc Surg*. 2010;52:674-683.

16. Bertges DJ, Neal D, Schanzer A, et.al. The Vascular Quality Initiative cardiac risk index for prediction of myocardial infarction after vascular surgery. *J Vasc Surg*. 2016;64:1411-1421.

17. Wilson RJT, Davies S, Yates D, Redman J, Stone M. Impaired functional capacity is associated with all-cause mortality after major elective intra-abdominal surgery. *Br J Anaesth*. 2010;105:297-303.

18. Hlatky MA, Boineau RE, Higginbotham MB, et al. A brief self-administered questionnaire to determine functional capacity (The Duke Activity Status Index). *Am J Cardiol*. 1989;64:651-654.

19. Yoshinaga K, Chow BJ, Williams K, et al. What is the prognostic value of myocardial perfusion imaging using rubidium-82 positron emission tomography? *J Am Coll Cardiol*. 2006;48:1029-1039.

20. Cohen MC, Siewers AE, Dickens JD, Hill T, Muller JE. Perioperative and long-term prognostic value of dipyridamole Tc-99m sestamibi myocardial tomography in patients evaluated for elective vascular surgery. *J Nucl Cardiol*. 2003;10:464-472.

21. Dorbala S, Hachamovitch R, Curillova Z, et al. Incremental prognostic value of gated Rb-82 positron emission tomography myocardial perfusion imaging over clinical variables and rest LVEF. *JACC Cardiovasc Imaging*. 2009;2:846-854.

22. Fihn SD, Gardin JM, Abrams J, et al. 2012 ACCF/AHA/ACP/AATS/PCNA/SCAI/STS guideline for the diagnosis and management of patients with stable ischemic heart disease: a report of the American College of Cardiology Foundation/American Heart Association Task Force on, American Association for Thoracic Surgery, Preventive Cardiovascular Nurses Association, Society for Cardiovascular Angiography and Interventions, and Society of Thoracic Surgeons. *J Am Coll Cardiol*. 2012;60:e44-e164.

23. Levine GN, Bates ER, Blankenship JC, et al. 2011 ACCF/AHA/SCAI guideline for percutaneous coronary intervention: a report of the American College of Cardiology Foundation/American Heart Association Task Force on Practice Guidelines and the Society for Cardiovascular Angiography and Interventions. *J Am Coll Cardiol*. 2011;58:e44-e122.

24. McFalls EO, Ward HB, Moritz TE, et al. Coronary-artery revascularization before elective major vascular surgery. *N Engl J Med*. 2004;351:2795-2804.

25. Kertai MD, Cooter M, Pollard RJ, et al. Is compliance with Surgical Care Improvement Project Cardiac (SCIP-Card-2) measures for perioperative β-blockers associated with reduced incidence of mortality and cardiovascular-related critical quality indicators after noncardiac surgery? *Anesth Analg*. 2018;126:1829-1838.

26. Friedell ML, Van Way CW 3rd, Freyberg RW, Almenoff PL. β-Blockade and operative mortality in noncardiac surgery: harmful or helpful? *JAMA Surg*. 2015;150:658-663.

27. Wijeysundera DN, Duncan D, Nkonde-Price C, et al; ACC/AHA Task Force Members. Perioperative beta blockade in noncardiac surgery: a systematic review for the 2014 ACC/AHA guideline on perioperative cardiovascular evaluation and management of patients undergoing noncardiac surgery: a report of the American College of Cardiology/American Heart Association Task Force on Practice Guidelines. *Circulation*. 2014;130:2246-2264.

28. Scali S, Patel V, Neal D, et al. Preoperative β-blockers do not improve cardiac outcomes after major elective vascular surgery and may be harmful. *J Vasc Surg*. 2015;62:166-176.

29. Antoniou GA, Hajibandeh S, Hajibandeh S, Vallabhaneni SR, Brennan JA, Torella F. Meta-analysis of the effects of statins on perioperative outcomes in vascular and endovascular surgery. *J Vasc Surg*. 2015;61:519-532.

30. Levine GN, Bates ER, Bittl JA, et al. 2016 ACC/AHA guideline focused update on duration of dual antiplatelet therapy in patients with coronary artery disease: a report of the American College of Cardiology/American Heart Association Task Force on Clinical Practice Guidelines. *Circulation*. 2016;134:e123-e155.

31. Devereaux PJ, Mrkobrada M, Sessler DI, et al; POISE-2 Investigators. Aspirin in patients undergoing noncardiac surgery. *N Engl J Med*. 2014;370:1494-1503.

Justin K. Lui • Frank Schembri

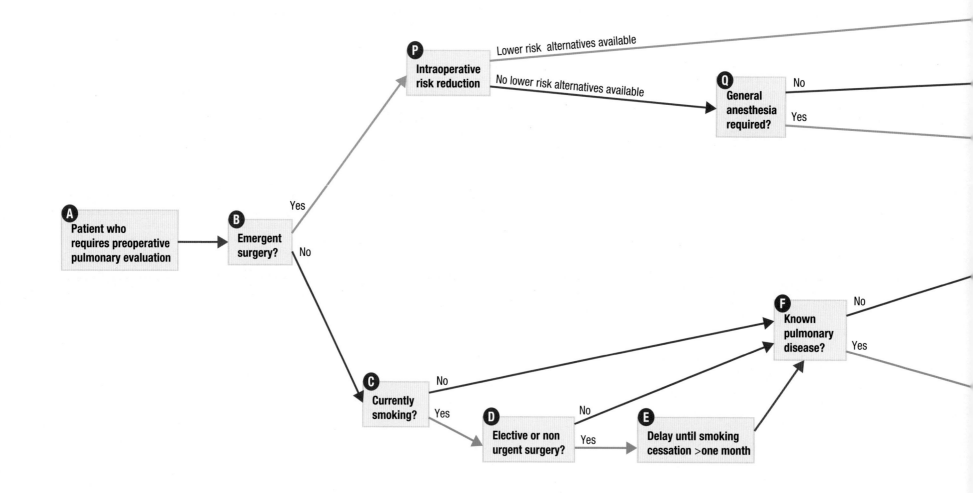

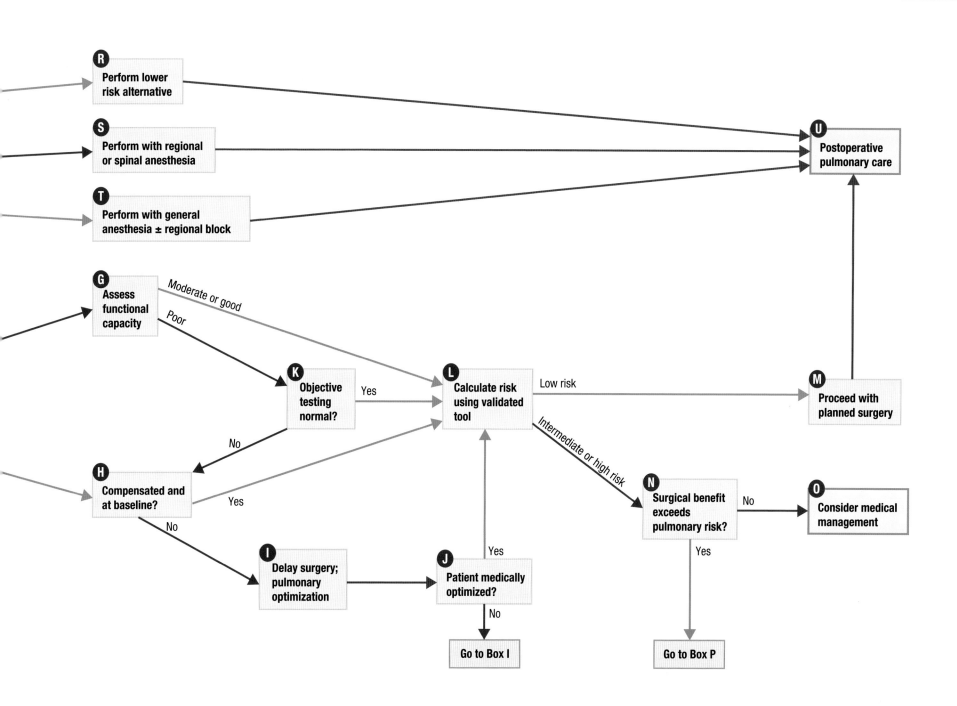

Ⓐ Patient who requires preoperative pulmonary evaluation

Postoperative pulmonary complications (PPCs) embody a key consideration in the decision to proceed with surgical intervention. There are many physiologic changes during surgery that lead to increased risks of PPCs, including reduced lung volumes/atelectasis, diaphragm dysfunction, prolonged bed rest, and impaired mucociliary clearance. The reported incidence of PPCs after major surgery ranges widely, from <1% to 23%,[1] partly because of the historical lack of definitions that makes systematic study difficult. For this reason, a European Perioperative Clinical Outcome (EPCO) definition of PPCs was recently established, which includes respiratory infection (bronchitis, tracheitis, pneumonia), respiratory failure, pleural effusion, atelectasis, pneumothorax, bronchospasm, and aspiration pneumonitis.[2] Notably, it does not include acute respiratory distress syndrome (ARDS), PE, upper airway obstruction, pulmonary edema, abdominal compartment syndrome, or exacerbation of preexisting lung disease.

Similar to other operative risk algorithms, pulmonary risk assessment includes patient- and procedure-related factors. Clinical guidelines from the American College of Physicians (ACP)[3] have recommended that *all* patients undergoing vascular surgery (or other noncardiothoracic operations) should be evaluated for significant patient-related risk factors for PPCs. These include advanced age, active smoking, poor general health status (which includes exercise capacity), a higher ASA classification, obesity, and the presence of preexisting lung disease. Furthermore, ACP guidelines also recommend that patients undergoing procedures with higher risks, expected duration >3 hours, emergent surgery, those under general anesthesia, or involving certain areas of the body (ie, vascular, thoracic, or abdominal) should undergo a more detailed pulmonary assessment.

Ⓑ Emergent surgery?

Emergent surgery is considered to be an intervention that is needed to save life or a major organ/extremity and is expected to be performed within 6 hours. Emergent surgery is associated with a 2- to 6-fold higher risk of developing PCCs as compared to elective surgery.[4] In cases of emergent surgery, it is appropriate to proceed directly with the surgical procedure while focusing on intra- and postoperative risk reduction measures.

Ⓒ Currently smoking?

Smoking is associated with an increased incidence of PPCs, and current smokers are more likely to develop these than do former smokers, who are themselves at higher risk than never smokers.[5] Furthermore, smoking cessation before surgery reduces PPCs.[6] Smoking cessation approaches are discussed in Chapter 3.

Ⓓ Elective or nonurgent surgery?

In clinical situations where life or limb is not at imminent risk, surgery should be timed to allow for sufficient optimization of underlying pulmonary conditions and smoking abstinence. However, if such delay (ie, like a suggested 4- to 8-week period of cigarette abstinence) exposes patients to additional harm, it must be reconciled with the risk of proceeding without medical optimization.

Ⓔ Delay until smoking cessation >1 month

Smoking cessation before elective or nonurgent operations drastically decreases PPCs. For instance, quitting smoking >4 weeks before surgery decreases the incidence of PPCs by 23% and abstinence of >8 weeks decreases complication rates by 47%.[6] The need for surgery therefore can be considered as an opportunity for a physician to engage a patient to commit to a smoking cessation program ideally involving counseling, pharmacotherapy, and other adjunctive aids. Smoking cessation is discussed in detail in Chapter 3.

Ⓕ Known pulmonary disease?

The relationship between preexisting pulmonary disease and the development of PPCs is disease specific. There is strong evidence that COPD increases the risk of PPCs. Data from the American College of Surgeons National Surgical Quality Improvement Program (NSQIP)[7] found that patients with COPD undergoing a variety of different elective and emergency operations had an independently increased risk of postoperative pneumonia and respiratory failure. Despite this, there is no degree of severity of COPD measured via PFTs that would yield an absolute contraindication to surgery and, as such, the decision to proceed is based on an individualized risk-benefit analysis.

The diagnosis of asthma does not itself increase the rate of PPCs. Among a pooled analysis of nearly 900 patients with asthma,[4] the rate of PPCs was 3.0%, compared to 3.4% overall, although patients with asthma tended to be of younger age and in better health. However, it is prudent to ensure that a patient with asthma is not actively having an acute exacerbation before undergoing anesthesia, because complications in asthmatic patients were almost exclusively bronchospasm or laryngospasm.[8] Factors associated with bronchospasm after surgery were older age, higher ASA score, recent use of asthma drugs, recent report of asthma symptoms, and recent treatment in a medical facility for asthma.

Chronic restrictive lung disease or neuromuscular weakness leads to lower lung volumes as measured by PFTs, but data linking these to increased risk of PPCs is lacking. Restrictive lung diseases that are advanced enough to impair functional status and lead to higher ASA classification or hypoxemia do increase the risk

associated with surgery because such components are included in many pulmonary risk-prediction algorithms.[9]

Pulmonary hypertension (PHTN), even of mild-to-moderate severity, represents a significant risk for PPCs regardless of the underlying etiology.[10] Complications include prolonged hypoxemia/respiratory failure, acute right heart failure, cardiogenic shock, and arrhythmias. Patients with PHTN at high risk include those with elevated right atrial pressure, impaired functional status, use of vasopressors, and prolonged (>3 hours) anesthesia time or emergency surgery. Similar to right heart dysfunction, there is good-quality evidence that chronic (or acute on chronic) left heart dysfunction leads to higher incidences of PPCs. In fact, in a comprehensive systemic review,[4] three studies reported a pooled odds ratio (OR) of 2.93 for PPCs in the setting of CHF, which was higher than the estimated OR for COPD (OR = 2.36).

Obstructive sleep apnea (OSA) also significantly increases the pulmonary risks of surgery. Numerous trials and systematic reviews[11] have shown that those with OSA are at increased risk for ARDS, aspiration pneumonia, and prolonged or recurrent respiratory failure. Obesity alone in the absence of OSA has not been shown consistently to be a risk factor for PPCs despite being associated with decreased lung volumes, hypoxemia, and hypercarbia.[4] In contrast, underweight patients are at higher risk for postoperative complications.[12]

Ⓖ Assess functional capacity

General health and functional capacity are critical factors in preoperative pulmonary risk assessment and should be assessed on every patient regardless of known underlying cardiopulmonary disease. Assessment includes the patients' ability to perform activities of daily living (ADLs), estimation of patients' metabolic equivalent (MET) capacity, assessment during a 6-minute walk test (6MWT), or assignment of ASA classification (assessing overall health). In two large studies,[13,14] patients who required assistance with ADLs were at significantly higher risk (OR 1.65-2.51) for developing PPCs. On 6MWT, shorter walking distance was directly correlated to overall PPCs and inversely correlated to length of stay.[15] Although the capacity to undertake activities with greater than four METs (ie, leisure cycling) has been used as an important threshold in cardiac risk-prediction models, such a lower limit threshold is not known for pulmonary risk-prediction. It is safe, however, to assume that the ability to perform any of the moderate intensity activities (three to six METs) would imply that enough capacity to perform ADLs therefore would be the lowest risk. ASA classification, which assesses overall health, is intimately tied to both overall mortality and rate of PPCs. Those undergoing surgery with ASA class II or greater have an OR of 4.87 for development of PPCs. On the basis of these considerations, functional capacity can be stratified as good, moderate, or poor: Poor functional capacity is an indication for objective pulmonary testing.

Ⓗ Compensated and at baseline?

Although known pulmonary diseases are considered nonmodifiable risk factors, it is important to medically optimize patients before surgery. Patients who are not compensated or at baseline for their pulmonary disease should have surgery delayed so that pulmonary status can be optimized. If baseline status is unclear, objective pulmonary function testing is indicated.

Ⓘ Delay surgery; pulmonary optimization

Despite limited studies comparing patients undergoing surgery with optimized and nonoptimized underlying lung disease, it is prudent when possible to treat exacerbations of pulmonary conditions before proceeding to the operating room. Depending on the urgency of the intervention and underlying conditions, this optimization may take variable amounts of time, even weeks to months. The goal is to maximally improve (but not necessarily normalize) clinical and other objective parameters.

Patients with recent or active asthma or COPD exacerbations (within 1-6 months) have increased PPCs,[16] and so should not be operated upon if they are having an acute exacerbation (ie, wheezing, dyspnea). Treatment for both revolves around bronchodilators and short courses of systemic corticosteroids, which perioperatively have not been shown to increase the risk of infection or other complications.[17] In patients with stable symptoms of asthma or COPD, bronchodilators such as inhaled β_2-adrenergic agonists (ie, albuterol, salbuterol) and antimuscarinic agents (ie, ipratropium, tiotropium), should be continued in both the immediate preoperative and postoperative periods.[18] Patients with active respiratory tract infections should also have their conditions optimized, which may require preoperative antibiotic treatment. Patients with PHTN and CHF should have hemodynamics and volume status optimized before surgery (see Chapter 1 for cardiac optimization). This may include the use of diuretics, rate control or afterload reduction agents, inotropes, or even pulmonary vasodilators. In patients with OSA, preoperative medical optimization involves institution of noninvasive positive-pressure ventilation (NiPPV), use of oral appliances or mandibular advancement devices, recognition of susceptibility to medications (ie, sedatives, opiates, and inhaled anesthetics), and preoperative weight loss, when feasible.

Ⓙ Patient medically optimized?

It may be difficult to tell whether an individual patient is medically optimized from a pulmonary perspective. Although protocols may be in use at different institutions, some facts are clear about pre-procedure medical optimization. The patient subjectively should feel at their "baseline" respiratory status, be smoke-free ideally for >4 to 8 weeks, not be in the midst of or have a recent (1-month) exacerbation of COPD or upper/lower tract infection, and be on optimal medications for underlying lung disease. Furthermore, in higher risk patients, numerous studies have shown that a preoperative education and exercise program reduces PPCs.[19]

Ⓚ Objective testing normal?

A thorough H&P, including specific screening questions regarding underlying pulmonary disease, symptoms, and exercise tolerance, remains the most comprehensive method of assessing postoperative pulmonary risks. Objective PFTs are not recommended routinely for predicting risk of PPCs because they rarely add to risk prediction over clinical impression alone and are economically wasteful.[3,4] There are certain situations when preoperative PFTs may be helpful, which include (1) when it is unclear whether symptoms or examination findings are related to lung disease or other causes; (2) when it is unknown whether a patient with lung disease is at their baseline; and (3) in patients undergoing lung resection surgery. In the first two situations, by identifying a previously undiagnosed disease or determining that a patient is not currently at their baseline, PFTs can influence the clinical treatment course before surgery. It should be stressed that there exists no consensus opinion as to which measurements obtained on PFTs should absolutely preclude surgery.

Similar to routine PFTs, routine use of preoperative chest x-rays (CXRs) should be avoided and add little incremental benefit over clinical impression alone.[4] A reasonable approach would be to limit preoperative CXR to patients who are >50 years undergoing abdominal or thoracic surgery, those who have underlying cardiopulmonary disease, or those with concerning pulmonary symptoms on preoperative history taking.

Laboratory tests are also a routine part of preoperative risk assessment, although most are irrelevant to predicting PPCs. The notable exception to this rule is preoperative albumin, which has been definitively correlated with PPCs and is recommended by the ACP guidelines[4] in all patients suspected of having low albumin or with one or more other pulmonary risk factors. A low serum albumin (<3.6 g/L) is associated with pulmonary complication rates of 27% versus 7% in those with higher levels. Although preoperative hypoxemia and hypercarbia clearly increase PPC rates,[20] ordering routine blood gases is not supported by published data. Most information can be garnered from oxygen saturations and identifying clinical risk factors for elevated blood carbon dioxide levels as in COPD or neuromuscular disease. Quantifying hypoxemia and hypercarbia may be useful in establishing a baseline for a specific patient, along with determining whether a patient is at such a baseline preoperatively or preparing the surgical team for the appropriate postoperative management.

Ⓛ Calculate risk using validated tool

A number of tools have been developed for preoperative risk stratification for the development of PPCs. Each model includes specific clinical, laboratory, or procedure-related factors, which are associated with a relative weight. The definitions of PPCs vary across models, but all provide a calculated risk that can be used in preoperative decision making to set patient or family expectations for the postoperative course or to guide the aggressiveness of postoperative pulmonary care. The widely used ARISCAT model relies on readily accessible clinical information, and is easily calculated on the basis of age, preoperative oxygen saturation, surgical site, duration, urgency, preoperative anemia, and recent respiratory infection (see table). It has a wide definition of PPCs including respiratory failure, but also some of lesser severity such as pleural effusion and atelectasis. Low-risk patients are defined as having accrued <26 points (calculated by summing the points for each risk factor in the table), which is associated with a 1.6% chance of PCCs of any severity. Intermediate-risk category (with 26-44 points) has a 13.3% risk of developing PPCs, and high-risk category (>44 points) of 42.1%. The two other most popular models[9,14] utilize postoperative respiratory failure as a primary outcome.

Variable	Points Toward Risk Score
Age	
≤50	0
51-80	3
>80	16
Preoperative SpO$_2$%	
≥96	0
91-95	8
≤90	24
Pulmonary infection in past 1 month	17
Preoperative Hb%	
>10	0
≤10	11
Surgical incision	
Peripheral	0
Upper abdomen	15
Thoracic	24
Surgical duration (h)	
≤2	0
>2-3	16
>3	23
Emergency procedure	8

Ⓜ Proceed with planned surgery

A low-risk determination for PPCs via rigorously defined and validated risk calculators should encourage the patient and surgeon to proceed with the planned operation, with subsequent focus on peri- and postoperative management.

Ⓝ Surgical benefit exceeds pulmonary risk?

Individualized and shared decision making must account for both the risk of delaying and proceeding with surgery depending on validated tools. For patients at intermediate or high risk of PPCs, discussions must include the expected benefits of the surgery that outweigh the risks and stressing the importance of pre- and postoperative measures to minimize risk. It is important to note that predictive risk indices do not have a threshold value above which surgery is unacceptable if the benefits of surgery are substantial or lifesaving.

Ⓞ Consider medical management

If the pulmonary risks of any procedure are prohibitively high compared to the expected benefits, then medical management is appropriate. Medical therapies vary depending on the underlying disease process. In the management of vascular disease, medical therapies and lifestyle modification such as exercise, smoking cessation, antiplatelet medications, lipid-lowering drugs, and blood pressure control are all important and may provide benefit.[21]

Ⓟ Intraoperative risk reduction

Once the decision has been reached to proceed with surgery, the care team should focus on intraoperative risk reduction, with the first consideration being whether lower risk alternatives are available. This may involve alternative anesthetic or paralytic choices, operative approaches, abbreviated procedures (<3 hours) or less invasive therapies such as endovascular versus open aortic aneurysm repair. In patients undergoing abdominal surgery, lung protective ventilation—including tidal volumes 6 to 8 mL/kg ideal body weight, PEEP 6 to 8 cm H_2O, along with recruitment maneuvers—has been shown to reduce a composite measure of PPCs within 7 days of surgery along with decreased hospital length of stay.[22] It is not clear whether this benefit persists for vascular procedures, although it appears safe for patients to tolerate.

Ⓠ General anesthesia required?

In patients at high risk for PPCs, general anesthesia should be avoided if possible. General anesthesia is associated with a 2.35-fold increased incidence of PPCs compared to neuraxial or regional anesthesia.[4] In a study of >2600 patients with severe COPD undergoing surgery,[23] regional or neuraxial anesthesia was correlated with lower rates of postoperative pneumonia, unplanned intubation, and prolonged mechanical ventilation. Furthermore, general anesthesia is often paired with neuromuscular

blockade to facilitate intubation or eliminate patient movement. Evidence suggests that long-acting paralytics such as pancuronium are associated with a higher incidence of residual blockade after surgery[24] and that these patients had a 3-fold increased incidence of PPCs. For that reason, shorter acting paralytics are preferred, with prompt and complete reversal after the procedure.

Ⓡ Perform lower risk alternative

Accounting for all of the benefits and risks of proceeding with surgery through preoperative tools, lower risk alternatives should always be considered when at all possible. The key considerations are that operations >3 hours long and those at certain sites (upper abdominal, aortic repair, thoracotomy, head and neck) are associated with a higher risk of PPCs. Lower risk alternatives, therefore, may include operations with different operative approaches or fields, those that are minimally invasive, or abbreviated procedures to minimize operative time.

Ⓢ Perform with regional or spinal anesthesia

In patients awaiting vascular surgery who are deemed high risk for general anesthesia, local or regional anesthesia should be considered. An increasing number of invasive procedures can safely be performed under regional or local anesthesia, including EVAR. A recent study[25] that compared general anesthesia to local anesthesia for EVAR repair showed similar short-term and 30-day surgical outcomes for both groups. Spinal or epidural anesthesia should be considered in revascularization of the lower extremities when there are no contraindications (ie, local infection at the level of the lumbar spine, indeterminate neurologic disease and/or anatomic disorders of the spine, increased intracranial pressure or evidence of space-occupying lesions in the brain, bleeding disorders or coagulopathies, hypovolemia, aortic stenosis). Regional nerve blocks are useful in revascularization of an isolated upper or lower limb in which the selection of the local anesthetic should be tailored toward the procedure on a case-by-case basis.

Ⓣ Perform with general anesthesia ± regional block

When the risks of general anesthesia are low, nerve blocks can be used together with general anesthesia to minimize both intraoperative pain (which can lead to patient movement during the procedure) and postoperative pain (which can impact deep breathing exercises). Several studies including a Cochrane Database Review of open AAA repair have shown a beneficial effect of epidural anesthesia when added to general anesthesia by improving pain relief and decreasing duration of intubation.[26]

Ⓤ Postoperative pulmonary care

Postoperative pulmonary care begins in the recovery room and includes methods to counteract negative physiologic effects from atelectasis, prolonged bed rest, impaired mucociliary clearance, and diaphragmatic dysfunction. The core tenets of postoperative

care are (1) various methods of encouraging deep breathing (ie, incentive spirometry, early ambulation, adequate pain control, deep breathing exercises, and continuous positive-pressure ventilation) and (2) secretion management via chest physiotherapy (ie, cough, postural drainage, percussion/vibration, frequent suctioning, and therapeutic bronchoscopy). Historically, incentive spirometry has been commonly used because it has been shown to be effective and the least invasive modality in reducing PPCs.[27] Additional studies have showed some reduction in PPCs with continuous positive-pressure ventilation,[28] early mobilization,[29] and adequate pain control.[30] Furthermore, secretion management modalities such as coughing and vibration of the chest wall have been shown to decrease the incidence of PPCs.[31] Although routine endotracheal or nasotracheal suction is usually adequate, a postoperative bronchoscopy can be considered for patients in whom this is inadequate and have significant areas of atelectasis. However, postoperative bronchoscopy has not been shown to be superior to noninvasive modalities. At Boston Medical Center, the abovementioned methods have been combined into a multifaceted approach referred to by the acronym ICOUGH (*i*ncentive spirometry, *c*oughing and deep breathing, *o*ral care, *u*nderstanding, *g*etting out of bed at least three times daily, and *h*ead-of-bed elevation).[32] This combined approach has been shown to decrease rates of postoperative pneumonia and unplanned intubation. Lastly, adequate pain control, which permits deep breathing and early ambulation, is an important part of reducing postoperative PPCs. Postoperative pain control has traditionally involved opiates, although epidural and regional (intercostal) nerve blocks have been shown to consistently improve pain along with decreasing PPCs especially in higher risk operations such as abdominal aortic surgery.[30]

REFERENCES

1. Miskovic A, Lumb AB. Postoperative pulmonary complications. *Br J Anaesth.* 2017;118:317-334. doi:10.1093/bja/aex002.
2. Jammer I, Wickboldt N, Sander M, et al. Standards for definitions and use of outcome measures for clinical effectiveness research in perioperative medicine: European Perioperative Clinical Outcome (EPCO) definitions: a statement from the ESA-ESICM joint taskforce on perioperative outcome measure. *Eur J Anaesthesiol.* 2015;32:88-105. doi:10.1097/EJA.0000000000000118.
3. Qaseem A, Snow V, Fitterman N, et al. Risk assessment for and strategies to reduce perioperative pulmonary complications for patients undergoing noncardiothoracic surgery: a guideline from the American College of Physicians. *Ann Intern Med.* 2006;144(8):575-580. doi:10.7326/0003-4819-144-8-200604180-00008.
4. Smetana GW, Lawrence VA, Cornell JE. Preoperative pulmonary risk stratification for noncardiothoracic

surgery: systematic review for the American College of Physicians. *Ann Intern Med.* 2006;144:581-595. doi:10.7326/0003-4819-144-8-200604180-00009.

5. Schmid M, Sood A, Campbell L, et al. Impact of smoking on perioperative outcomes after major surgery. *Am J Surg.* 2015;210:221-229.e6. doi:10.1016/j.amjsurg.2014.12.045.

6. Mills E, Eyawo O, Lockhart I, Kelly S, Wu P, Ebbert JO. Smoking cessation reduces postoperative complications: a systematic review and meta-analysis. *Am J Med.* 2011;124:144-154. doi:10.1016/j.amjmed.2010.09.013.

7. Gupta H, Ramanan B, Gupta PK, et al. Impact of COPD on postoperative outcomes: results from a national database. *Chest.* 2013;143:1599-1606. doi:10.1378/chest.12-1499.

8. Warner DO, Warner MA, Barnes RD, et al. Perioperative respiratory complications in patients with asthma. *Anesthesiology.* 1996;85:460-467.

9. Gupta H, Gupta PK, Fang X, et al. Development and validation of a risk calculator predicting postoperative respiratory failure. *Chest.* 2011;140:1207-1215. doi:10.1378/chest.11-0466.

10. Meyer S, McLaughlin VV, Seyfarth HJ, et al. Outcomes of noncardiac, nonobstetric surgery in patients with PAH: an international prospective survey. *Eur Respir J.* 2013;41:1302-1307. doi:10.1183/09031936.00089212.

11. Memtsoudis SG, Besculides MC, Mazumdar M. A rude awakening—the perioperative sleep apnea epidemic. *N Engl J Med.* 2013;368:2352-2353. doi:10.1056/NEJMp1302941.

12. Sood A, Abdollah F, Sammon JD, et al. The effect of body mass index on perioperative outcomes after major surgery: results from the National Surgical Quality Improvement Program (ACS-NSQIP) 2005-2011. *World J Surg.* 2015;39:2376-2385. doi:10.1007/s00268-015-3112-7.

13. Arozullah AM, Daley J, Henderson WG, Khuri SF. Multifactorial risk index for predicting postoperative respiratory failure in men after major noncardiac surgery. The National Veterans Administration Surgical Quality Improvement Program. *Ann Surg.* 2000;232:242-253. doi:10.1097/00000658-200008000-00015.

14. Arozullah AM, Khuri SF, Henderson WG, Daley J. Development and validation of a multifactorial risk index

for predicting postoperative pneumonia after major noncardiac surgery. *Ann Intern Med.* 2001;135:847-857. doi:10.7326/0003-4819-135-10-200111200-00005.

15. Awdeh H, Kassak K, Sfeir P, Hatoum H, Bitar H, Husari A. The SF-36 and 6-minute walk test are significant predictors of complications after major surgery. *World J Surg.* 2015;39:1406-1412. doi:10.1007/s00268-015-2961-4.

16. Smetana GW. Preoperative pulmonary evaluation. *N Engl J Med.* 1999;340(12):937-944. doi:10.1056/NEJM199903253401420.

17. Pien LC, Grammer LC, Patterson R. Minimal complications in a surgical population with severe asthma receiving prophylactic corticosteroids. *J Allergy Clin Immunol.* 1988;82:696-700. doi:10.1016/0091-6749(88)90985-2.

18. Lui J, Spaho L, Holzwanger E, et al. Intensive care of pulmonary complications following liver transplantation. *J Intensive Care Med.* 2018;33:595-608. doi:10.1177/0885066618757410.

19. Hulzebos EHJ, Smit Y, Helders PPJM, van Meeteren NLU. Preoperative physical therapy for elective cardiac surgery patients. *Cochrane Database Syst Rev.* 2012;(11):CD010118. doi:10.1002/14651858.CD010118.pub2.

20. Tisi GM. Preoperative evaluation of pulmonary function: validity, indications and benefit. *Am Rev Respir Dis.* 1979;119(2):293-310.

21. Malgor RD, Alalahdab F, Elraiyah TA, et al. A systematic review of treatment of intermittent claudication in the lower extremities. *J Vasc Surg.* 2015;61:54S-73S. doi:10.1016/j.jvs.2014.12.007.

22. Futier E, Constantin J-M, Paugam-Burtz C, et al. A trial of intraoperative low-tidal-volume ventilation in abdominal surgery. *N Engl J Med.* 2013;369:428-437. doi:10.1056/NEJMoa1301082.

23. Hausman MS, Jewell ES, Engoren M. Regional versus general anesthesia in surgical patients with chronic obstructive pulmonary disease: does avoiding general anesthesia reduce the risk of postoperative complications? *Anesth Analg.* 2015;120:1405-1412. doi:10.1213/ANE.0000000000000574.

24. Berg H, Viby-Mogensen J, Roed J, et al. Residual neuromuscular block is a risk factor for postoperative pulmonary complications. A prospective, randomised, and

blinded study of postoperative pulmonary complications after atracurium, vecuronium and pancuronium. *Acta Anaesthesiol Scand.* 1997;41:1095-1103. doi:10.1111/j.1399-6576.1997.tb04851.x.

25. Noh M, Choi B, Kwon H, et al. General anesthesia versus local anesthesia for endovascular aortic aneurysm repair. *Medicine (Baltimore).* 2018;97(32):e11789. doi:10.1097/MD.0000000000011789.

26. Nichimori M, Low J, Ballantyne JC. Epidural pain relief versus systemic opioid-based pain relief for abdominal aortic surgery. *Cochrane Database Syst Rev.* 2006;(19):CD005059. doi:10.1002/14651858.CD005059.

27. Agostini P, Naidu B, Cieslik H, et al. Effectiveness of incentive spirometry in patients Following thoracotomy and lung resection including those at high risk for developing pulmonary complications. *Thorax.* 2013;68:580-585. doi:10.1136/thoraxjnl-2012-202785.

28. Zarbock A, Mueller E, Netzer S, Gabriel A, Feindt P, Kindgen-Milles D. Prophylactic nasal continuous positive airway pressure following cardiac surgery protects from postoperative pulmonary complications: a prospective, randomized, controlled trial in 500 patients. *Chest.* 2009;135:1252-1259. doi:10.1378/chest.08-1602.

29. van der Leeden M, Huijsmans R, Geleijn E, et al. Early enforced mobilisation following surgery for gastrointestinal cancer: feasibility and outcomes. *Physiotherapy.* 2016;102:103-110. doi:10.1016/j.physio.2015.03.3722.

30. Liu SS, Wu CL. Effect of postoperative analgesia on major postoperative complications: a systematic update of the evidence. *Anesth Analg.* 2007;104:689-702. doi:10.1213/01.ane.0000255040.71600.41.

31. Morran CG, Finlay IG, Mathieson M, McKay AJ, Wilson N, McArdle CS. Randomized controlled trial of physiotherapy for postoperative pulmonary complications. *Br J Anaesth.* 1983;55:1113-1117. doi:10.1093/bja/55.11.1113.

32. Cassidy MR, Rosenkranz P, McCabe K, Rosen JE, McAneny D. I COUGH: Reducing postoperative pulmonary complications with a multidisciplinary patient care program. *JAMA Surg.* 2013;148:740-745. doi:10.1001/jamasurg.2013.358.

Ehrin J. Armstrong

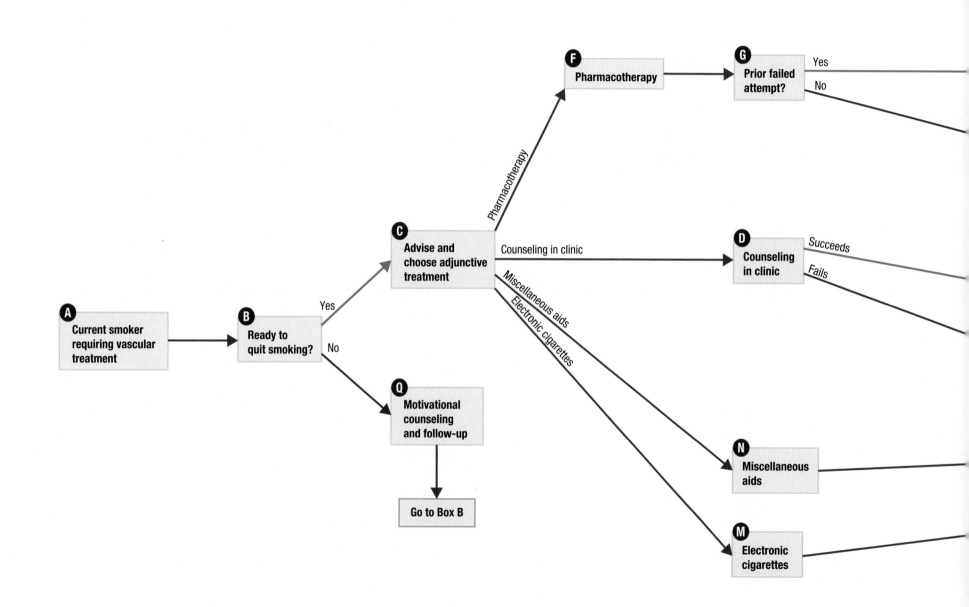

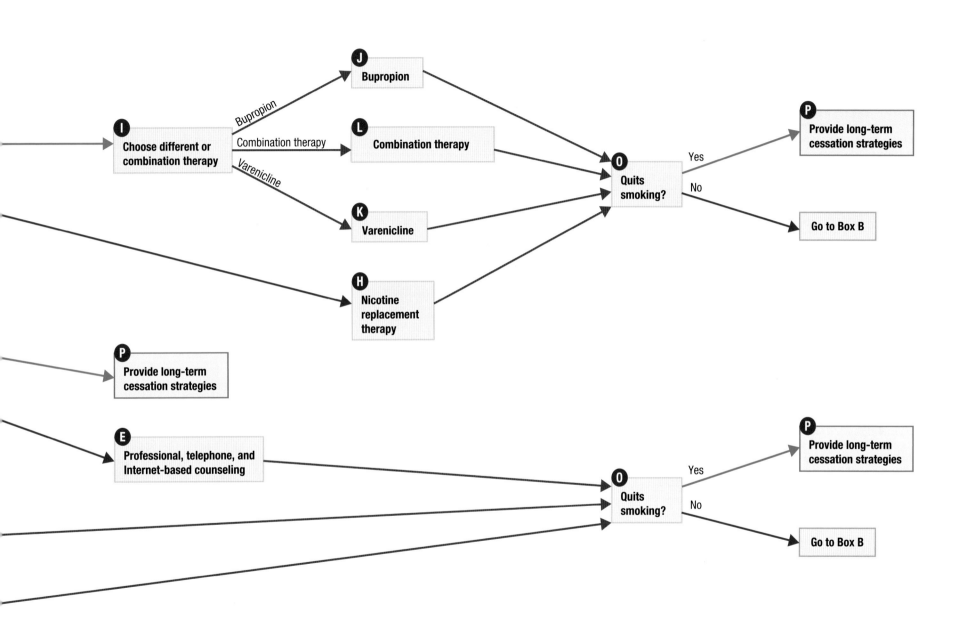

A Current smoker requiring vascular treatment

Smoking is the single most important risk factor for the development and progression of PAD. There is a 2-fold increase in the prevalence of symptomatic PAD among smokers[1] and 80% of patients with PAD report either a current or past smoking history. Smokers with PAD are more likely to be hospitalized than are nonsmokers with PAD and have worse outcomes after surgical or interventional vascular procedures.[2] Preoperative smoking cessation has been associated with a 40% relative risk reduction in postoperative complications following vascular surgery[3]; following lower extremity bypass surgery, continued smoking is associated with diminished graft patency and increased amputation rate.[4] Smokers with PAD who quit after undergoing peripheral angiography had a 17% reduction in all-cause mortality and a 21% improvement in amputation-free survival rates.[4] The risks of cardiovascular disease progression, increased hospitalization rates, worse outcomes following surgery, and high costs associated with tobacco use underscore the importance of aggressively promoting smoking cessation and abstinence from all tobacco products.[5]

B Ready to quit smoking?

Immediate smoking cessation is a class I recommendation for all patients with PAD. All physicians, including vascular specialists, should enquire about tobacco use in all patients, at every visit.[6] Although it is not uncommon for specialists to defer smoking cessation discussion to their patients' primary physicians, patients who are exposed to frequent and consistent reminders to stop smoking are more likely to actually do so. Vascular specialists, in particular, are provided with a unique opportunity to emphasize the importance of cessation, because they engage in conversations with patients who have already witnessed, firsthand, the negative impacts of smoking on their health. Patients are more likely to quit smoking after undergoing a procedure for treatment of vascular disease, and after more invasive procedures (eg, AAA repair or lower extremity bypass grafting) than after less invasive procedures (eg, CAS or CEA).[3]

C Advise and choose adjunctive treatment

Simply providing brief advice to quit smoking, as opposed to not providing any advice, was found to have a significant increase in quit rates, with a pooled risk ratio (RR) for smoking cessation of 1.66 to 1.76.[7,8] More intensive advice process (eg, longer consultations, additional visits, or self-help manuals) was found to have an even greater increase in quit rates, with a pooled RR of 1.84, although a direct comparison between brief advice versus intensive advice found no statistically significant difference between the two interventions.[7] All patients who have progressed to the point where they are willing to quit should be offered counseling.[6] Patients are more likely to quit when encouraged or assisted by each of their providers, including being 15% more likely to

quit smoking if their surgeons are the ones to offer them smoking cessation aids.[3] Brief counseling intervention for tobacco users who are willing to quit should include "5 A's": (1) **A**sk about tobacco use, (2) **A**dvise tobacco users to quit, (3) **A**ssess readiness to quit, (4) **A**ssist with quit attempt by offering medications and counseling, and (5) **A**rrange follow-up to emphasize smoking cessation and to assess progress.[9] Two of the proposed benefits of counseling are the ability to educate patients on the efficacy of various pharmacotherapeutic agents and the ability to address patient concerns regarding these agents' perceived adverse effects. Both aspects of counseling are crucial in facilitating smoking cessation, because many smokers have a poor understanding of the risks and benefits of pharmacotherapy,[10] which makes them much less likely to consider using it. As such, counseling is a reasonable first step in treating tobacco abuse, making patients 20% more likely to choose a pharmacologic agent to aid in their cessation attempt.[1] Not only can counseling increase the likelihood that smokers will go on to choose pharmacotherapy but it can also be continued alongside pharmacotherapy to potentially increase quit rates beyond those seen when either intervention is used alone.[8] Although counseling and pharmacotherapy are the pillars of smoking cessation, other interventions are available and include the highly controversial electronic cigarettes as well as the use of miscellaneous aids for those patients who refuse or fail to quit with counseling and pharmacotherapy and for those patients who wish to supplement more conventional therapies with alternative treatment strategies.

D Counseling in clinic

Counseling in clinic may consist of any of a variety of interventions, including physician- or nurse-driven counseling, provision of self-help materials, cognitive behavioral therapy to help develop a quit plan, problem-solving skills training to help select a quit date, behavioral support, motivational interviewing, and stage-based support. Counseling interventions, consisting of physician advice delivered in a single session lasting <20 minutes plus at least one follow-up session, increase the success rates for smoking cessation.[8] When counseling sessions were run by a nurse rather than by a physician, quit rates were still significantly increased. However, when adjunctive support aids such as brochures, handouts, and audio or videotape self-help materials were provided without in-person counseling, there was no significant impact on quit rates.[8] Physician- or nurse-driven counseling with or without the provision of self-help materials is easy to implement in most physicians' daily practice. The addition of follow-up visits to assess patients' progress with smoking cessation and to reaffirm the benefits of cessation also increases rates of smoking cessation. A combination of providing advice in clinic plus sending follow-up letters tailored to the patient's stage of change has been suggested to improve rates of smoking cessation; however, the benefit of adding follow-up letters to in-clinic counseling has

not been well studied, and the significance of providing follow-up letters has yet to be determined.[7]

E Professional, telephone, and Internet-based counseling

When counseling in clinic fails, patients can be referred to a specialist for more intensive counseling interventions that include cognitive behavioral therapy, problem-solving skills training, motivational interviewing, and other behavioral modification techniques. Another popular option is for patients to participate in telephone counseling. Telephone counseling can be divided into two categories: "smoker-initiated contact," where smokers reach out to telephone counseling services for assistance with smoking cessation, and "recruiter-initiated contact," where counselors reach out to smokers. Smoker-initiated telephone counseling consisting of multisession telephone counseling is more effective for smoking cessation than are interventions with minimal over-the-phone counseling (eg, one-time counseling or an automated provision of standardized self-help materials).[8] The use of recruiter-initiated telephone counseling was more effective for smoking cessation than was no intervention, but only if such interventions consisted of more than two sessions.[8] In addition, mobile phone–, computer-, and Internet-based interventions have been suggested. There are limited data on the use of mobile phone–based smoking cessation interventions. Interventions using Internet- or email-based smoking cessation programs, such as Smokefree.gov, had a modest effect on quit rates.[8]

F Pharmacotherapy

There are multiple medications available to help with smoking cessation: a variety of nicotine replacement therapies (NRTs), bupropion, and varenicline. Successful 6-month quit rates are approximately 20% when any of these agents are used, which is approximately two times greater than the quit rates observed when patients attempt to quit without assistance.[11-13] Despite the significant increase in quit rates, there is a reluctance among many smokers to try pharmacologic aids for smoking cessation, and those who do try it often fail to use it long enough or in sufficient quantity.[1,5,10] Furthermore, there are many misperceptions surrounding the various medications that may dissuade smokers from using them, such as the widespread myth that NRT is just as likely as cigarette smoking to cause MI or cancer.[5] Although some agents, such as varenicline, may be slightly more effective than others, there is no preferred initial agent, and the focus should be placed on finding the agent that is most suitable for each patient and should take into consideration factors such as cost, additional benefits, potential adverse effects, and patient preference.

G Prior failed attempt?

NRT is often the first agent chosen to help with smoking cessation because of its low cost and favorable adverse effect profile, as well as a general patient preference to start with NRT rather than with other pharmacologic aids. When patients fail to quit smoking or relapse while receiving NRT, it may be reasonable to consider an alternative agent or combination therapy, which may consist of NRT in conjunction with other pharmacologic agents.

Nicotine replacement therapy

A variety of NRT formulations are available, including patch, gum, lozenge, inhaler, and nasal spray. Because all NRT agents deliver nicotine more slowly and at lower levels, these agents are far less likely to be associated with dependence than are actual tobacco products.[14] The choice of which formulation to use should reflect patient needs, tolerability, and cost considerations. Patches are often the first-choice therapy for NRT. For patients who smoke <10 cigarettes daily, the patch can be prescribed at a dose of 14 mg daily for 6 weeks, followed by 7 mg daily for 2 weeks. For patients who smoke >10 cigarettes daily, the dose is 21 mg daily for 5 weeks, followed by 14 mg daily for 2 weeks, and 7 mg daily for an additional 2 weeks. Nicotine patches are easy to use and are the least expensive agent; however, patches cannot be used for relief of acute cravings. There is evidence that combining the nicotine patch with a more rapidly absorbing form of NRT (gum or nasal spray, also known as "patch plus" therapy) is more effective than is NRT monotherapy, because the patch can help reduce the risk and severity of withdrawal symptoms, whereas the more rapidly absorbing agents help fight acute cravings. A major benefit of the nicotine gum is that it may promote weight loss. The nasal spray may be more effective than the other agents, but it is also significantly more expensive than the cheapest alternatives: the patch and gum. Adverse effects of NRT are related to the specific type of product and include irritation to the skin (patches) and the inside of the mouth (gum and lozenges). NRT can also cause HTN, tachycardia, and anxiety in high doses; there is no evidence that NRT increases the risk of MI or cancer[11]; however, NRT is contraindicated in the setting of a recent MI, severe angina, or life-threatening arrhythmias because of its stimulatory effects on the sympathetic nervous system. The pooled RR for sustained abstinence for the various formulations of NRT versus control ranges between 1.49 and 2.02.[11,13] There is some evidence to suggest that the use of nicotine patches as precessation therapy may be more effective than is waiting until the intended quit date to start wearing the patch, although this only applies to the patch and not to other forms of NRT.[11] Benefits of NRT over bupropion and varenicline include low cost, the ability to purchase these agents without a prescription, and minimal adverse effect profile. Unfortunately, despite NRT's significant beneficial impact on smoking cessation, only 16% to 28% of smokers thought that NRT would be helpful in their quit attempts, and only 24% of smokers who intended to quit smoking intended to use NRT.[5,10]

Choose different or combination therapy

Bupropion and varenicline have both been shown to result in superior quit rates when compared with NRT and are appropriate for use both as initial therapy and when patients fail to quit smoking with NRT.[12,13] These agents can be used alone or in combination with each other or with NRT, which may yield superior results to monotherapy with any one agent.[11,15] The choice between bupropion, varenicline, and combination therapy is made on an individual patient basis after discussing the details of each treatment. If none of these options is acceptable, other adjunctive treatments can be reconsidered (C).

J Bupropion

Bupropion was the first non-nicotine medication approved for smoking cessation. It is a selective dopamine and norepinephrine uptake inhibitor. Bupropion acts as an antidepressant, facilitating smoking cessation through three mechanisms: replacement of the antidepressant effects produced by nicotine, relief from the depressive symptoms caused by nicotine withdrawal, and blockade of the neural pathways underlying nicotine addiction.[12] The adverse effects of bupropion include insomnia, dry mouth, nausea, and, rarely, seizures (~1 in 1000 cases).[12] Bupropion should be started at 150 mg daily for 3 days, then increased to 150 mg twice daily 1 to 2 weeks before the quit date and continued at this dose for 8 to 12 weeks following the quit date. Bupropion was approximately two times more effective in achieving sustained abstinence compared with placebo.[12,13] One benefit of bupropion over other pharmacologic aids is that because bupropion acts as an antidepressant, it may be ideal for patients with concurrent depression. Bupropion may also assist with weight loss, making it more desirable to patients also hoping to lose weight and for patients concerned that smoking cessation may result in overeating and weight gain.

K Varenicline

Varenicline is a partial nicotine receptor agonist that helps treat nicotine addiction through two mechanisms. First, by partially activating the nicotine receptor, craving and withdrawal symptoms may be blunted following abrupt cessation or reduction of nicotine consumption. Second, by occupying part of the receptors and blocking nicotine binding, varenicline acts as a partial antagonist, resulting in reduced satisfaction achieved through the act of smoking.[13] The most common adverse effect of varenicline is nausea, and although there is also a boxed warning regarding various psychiatric symptoms (depression, agitation, and suicidal behavior), these symptoms have not been well substantiated by the medical literature.[13] However, given this potential, patients taking varenicline should be monitored for symptoms of depression, mania, paranoia, suicidal behavior, and sleep disturbances, although a confirmed association between varenicline and these

symptoms has not been established. Varenicline should be started at 0.5 mg daily for 3 days, then increased to 0.5 mg twice daily for the remainder of the first week, and finally increased to 1 mg twice daily for an additional 11 weeks. If varenicline was helpful during the first 12 weeks, it should be continued at 1 mg twice daily for an additional 12 weeks. Smokers who used varenicline were twice as likely to quit smoking compared with smokers who attempted to quit without assistance.[13] In addition, varenicline compared favorably with both bupropion and NRT for successful smoking cessation.[13]

Combination therapy

A common question among patients is whether there is utility to combining multiple medications, particularly because it relates to combining various types of NRT. Combination therapy with NRT plus bupropion was more effective than NRT alone, although no significant benefits were seen when NRT was combined with varenicline.[11] Combination therapy with bupropion and varenicline is yet to be well studied; current evidence suggests that there may be an increase in long-term quit rates, although there is a potential risk of additive psychiatric adverse effects that needs to be explored further.[15]

M Electronic cigarettes

For patients who decline pharmacotherapy and cannot quit smoking after counseling, electronic cigarettes (e-cigarettes) can be considered. Some studies suggest that e-cigarettes can be at least as effective as other forms of NRT; however, further work is required to establish their efficacy on nicotine addiction and withdrawal.[16] Smokers who wanted to quit without professional help were significantly more likely to report abstinence using e-cigarettes than with traditional cessation aids or by quitting without any assistance.[17] E-cigarette users have reported finding the devices helpful in for reducing cigarette cravings and helping them remain tobacco-free for a period of at least several weeks to months.[18] In contrast, other users reported being less likely to be tobacco abstinent and were no more likely to have quit permanently.[16] In a large randomized controlled trial, e-cigarettes were found to be comparable to nicotine patches in helping smokers quit (7.3% quit rate for e-cigarettes vs. 5.8% for nicotine patches); among ongoing tobacco cigarette smokers, concurrent use of e-cigarettes led to a reduction in total number of tobacco cigarettes smoked per day.[19] The American Heart Association released a statement stating that there is insufficient evidence for physicians to counsel smokers to use e-cigarettes as a primary means of smoking cessation. The American Heart Association does acknowledge that e-cigarettes appear to be at least as effective as nicotine patches, and that they may be considered for patients who have failed or absolutely refused conventional smoking cessation medications. However, this statement also comes with the recommendation that patients should quit smoking conventional cigarettes as soon as possible and to set a quit date for their e-cigarettes as well and to not plan to use them indefinitely, unless as a last resort to prevent relapse to conventional cigarettes.[16]

N Miscellaneous aids

There are several other interventions available to assist with smoking cessation, including biomedical risk assessment and complementary and alternative therapies. Biomedical risk assessment interventions utilize some form of physical measurement to increase motivation to quit smoking, such as exhaled carbon monoxide, spirometry data, atherosclerotic plaque imaging, or genetic testing. Only two interventions were found to confer any benefit in smoking cessation: in one, patients were provided with results from their spirometry testing and given an explanation in the form of their "lung age" relative to their actual age, and in the other, patients were counseled on the importance of smoking cessation after undergoing carotid and femoral artery DUS to stratify their risk for future vascular disease.[8] The use of complementary and alternative therapy such as acupuncture was found to provide an increased rate of short-term smoking cessation, although this was not maintained at long-term follow-up. Other alternative therapies such as acupressure, laser therapy, and hypnotherapy did not provide any significant increase in cessation rates.[8]

O Quits smoking?

Patients who successfully quit smoking require long-term strategies to prevent relapse. Patients who continue smoking can be challenging to manage, and although it may not be possible to encourage all smokers to quit, physicians should do their best to identify patients' rationale for their ongoing tobacco abuse and to address those issues as best as they are able to, such as through providing education and dispelling myths surrounding available treatments and aiming to treat or remove triggers for ongoing tobacco abuse. Smokers who are adamant about not quitting should still have their smoking status assessed and be encouraged to quit at every clinic visit. It is important for both patients and physicians to realize that relapse is incredibly common. Most smokers will attempt to quit smoking five to eight times before achieving sustained abstinence, although this number is variably reported and may occur upward of even 10 or 20 quit attempts.[20] Regardless of the actual number, this knowledge is important because it should be dispensed to patients who relapse to assure them that relapse is common and that relapse does not equate to failure, because patients who relapse are more likely to successfully quit on subsequent attempts. This information also serves as a reminder to physicians that they should expect many of their patients to relapse and that they should avoid the unfortunate tendency many physicians have wherein they become frustrated with their patients who relapse. Physicians should not give up on patients who suffer from one or multiple relapses and should instead maintain the same approach of reassessing smoking status and willingness

to quit at each clinic visit and continue to offer interventions targeted at each individuals' stage of change.

P Provide long-term cessation strategies

Once patients have successfully quit smoking, the next step is to help them maintain abstinence and prevent relapse. This can be achieved by remaining cognizant of patients' former smoking history and reassessing their smoking status at every clinic visit, while being sure to recognize patients at risk for relapse. Sustained abstinence can be promoted by providing former smokers with positive reinforcement, either in clinic or through personalized letters or phone calls.[7] Extended use of pharmacotherapy may also help prevent relapse. Having a strong support system is also paramount in achieving and maintaining abstinence. Family or loved ones can help patients identify reasons to quit and emphasize the importance of long-term smoking cessation. Similarly, loved ones should also be encouraged to quit smoking, because patients are more likely to remain abstinent when removed from the stimulus of being exposed to other smokers. Most medications are approved for 12 weeks of continuous use, although they may be continued for longer periods (or restarted if previously discontinued) for patients who are at risk for relapse. Life stressors and psychiatric disorders are frequent triggers for relapse, and targeted interventions such as cognitive behavioral therapy and the antidepressant bupropion can be quite helpful in treating these triggers. Unlike bupropion, other antidepressants such as selective serotonin or norepinephrine reuptake inhibitors have not been shown to be effective in the primary treatment of tobacco abuse, although they may be helpful in treating the depression and anxiety that often underlie relapse.[12] Finally, although not preferred, for patients who remain at high risk for relapse despite the aforementioned therapies, e-cigarettes may be used if they are the only option that successfully staves off relapse to tobacco use.[17]

Q Motivational counseling and follow-up

Treatments for tobacco abuse are only effective when smokers are interested and motivated to quit, which makes those who are unwilling to quit the most challenging group of patients to treat. However, frequent encouragement to quit smoking, education on the association between smoking and vascular disease, and providing information on the various pharmacologic therapies available to assist with cessation are three effective interventions at the physician's disposal to help motivate patients to consider quitting. The "5 R's" method is a brief counseling intervention recommended for tobacco users who are unwilling to quit. It is designed to help clinicians better understand patients' motivations for smoking and why they value the habit: (1) **R**elevance of perceived benefits of smoking cessation to the patient, (2) **R**isks perceived by the patient of what ongoing smoking may do to their bodies, (3) **R**ewards that the patient considers they may receive if they stop smoking, (4) **R**oadblocks to quitting that the patient

struggles with, and (5) **R**epetition of this assessment at subsequent office visits. A simple way of assessing the 5 R's for clinicians with a time constraint consists of asking patients to go home and come up with a list of reasons why they like smoking and reasons why they don't like smoking that they can bring back at their next visit; this strategy may increase the transparency of potential roadblocks to smoking cessation and provide opportunities for the clinician to help patients move toward the decision to quit. Identification of a support person to help them through the quitting process may also be helpful.[1,6] Although the risks associated with tobacco use are highest for patients who use tobacco in greater quantities, the ultimate goal for physicians should be to encourage complete cessation of all tobacco products, rather than just a reduction in their use. Finally, hospitalizations provide opportunities for smokers to quit, especially for patients admitted for smoking-related illnesses. However, hospital-delivered interventions for smoking cessation are effective only when treatment continues for at least 1 month following discharge. Therefore, simply providing patients with NRT or other pharmacotherapies during admission is unlikely to be successful in facilitating long-term smoking cessation. Unfortunately, sustained use of medications for smoking cessation following discharge is often hindered by the fact that NRT is not covered by most health insurers, leading many patients to discontinue their use. Systems designed to provide patient outreach and offer smoking cessation aids following hospital discharge resulted in a 20% increase in the long-term use of smoking cessation aids and a 10% increase in successful smoking cessation.[21]

REFERENCES

1. Hennrikus D, Joseph AM, Lando HA, et al. Effectiveness of a smoking cessation program for peripheral artery disease patients. Peripheral artery disease. *J Am Coll Cardiol*. 2010;56(25):2105-2112.
2. Duval S, Long KH, Roy SS, et al. The contribution of tobacco use to high health care utilization and medical costs: a state based cohort analysis. *J Am Coll Cardiol*. 2015;66(14):1566-1574. doi:10.1016/j.jacc.2015.06.1349.
3. Hoel AW, Nolan BW, Goodney PP, et al. Variation in smoking cessation after vascular operations. *J Vasc Surg*. 2013;57:1338-1344. doi:10.1016/j.jvs.2012.10.130.
4. Armstrong EJ, Wu J, Singh, GD, et al. Smoking cessation is associated with decreased mortality and improved amputation free survival among patients with symptomatic peripheral artery disease. *J Vasc Surg*. 2014;60:1565-1571.
5. Shiffman S, Ferguson SG, Rohay J, et al. Perceived safety and efficacy of nicotine replacement therapies among US smokers and ex-smokers: relationship with use and compliance. *Addiction*. 2008;103(8):1371-1378. doi:10.1111/j.1360-0443.2008.02268.x.
6. Gerhard-Herman MD, Gornik HL, Barrett C, et al. 2016 AHA/ACC guidelines on the management of patients with

lower extremity peripheral artery disease. *J Am Coll Cardiol.* 2017;69:e71-e126. doi:10.1016/j.jacc.2016.11.007.

7. Stead LF, Buitrago D, Preciado N. Physician advice for smoking cessation 2013. *Cochrane Database Syst Rev.* 2013;(5):CD000165. doi:10.1002/14651858.CD000165. pub4.

8. Patnode CD, Henderson JT, Thompson JH, et al. *Behavioral Counseling and Pharmacotherapy Interventions for Tobacco Cessation in Adults, Including Pregnant Women: A Review of Reviews for the U.S. Preventive Services Task Force.* Rockville, MD: Agency for Healthcare Research and Quality; 2015. http://www.ncbi.nlm.nih.gov/books/NBK321744/. Accessed January 2, 2018.

9. Fiore MC, Jaén CR, Baker TB, et al. *Treating Tobacco Use and Dependence: 2008 Update. Clinical Practice Guideline.* Rockville, MD: U.S. Department of Health and Human Services. Public Health Service. 2008.

10. Etter JF, Perneger TV. Attitudes toward nicotine replacement therapy in smokers and ex-smokers in the general public. *Clin Pharmacol Ther.* 2001;69(3):175-183. doi: 10.1067/mcp.2001.113722.

11. Stead LF, Perera R, Bullen C, et al. Nicotine replacement therapy for smoking cessation. *Cochrane Database Syst Rev.* 2012;(11):CD000146. doi:10.1002/14651858.CD000146. pub4.

12. Hughes JR, Stead LF, Hartmann-Boyce J, et al. Antidepressants for smoking cessation. *Cochrane Database Syst Rev.* 2014;(1):CD000031. doi:10.1002/14651858.CD000031.pub4.

13. Cahill K, Lindson-Hawley N, Thomas KH, et al. Nicotine receptor partial agonists for smoking cessation. *Cochrane Database Syst Rev.* 2016;(5):CD006103. doi:10.1002/14651858. CD006103.pub7.

14. Schneider NG, Olmstead RE, Franzon MA, et al. The nicotine inhaler: clinical pharmacokinetics and comparison with other nicotine treatments. *Clin Pharmacokinet.* 2001;40:661-684.

15. Vogeler T, McClain C, Evor KE. Combination bupropion SR and varenicline for smoking cessation: a systematic review. *Am J Drug Alcohol Abuse.* 2016;42(2):129-139. doi:10.3109/00 952990.2015.1117480.

16. Bhatnagar A, Whitsel LP, Ribisl KM, et al. Electronic cigarettes: a policy statement from the American Heart Association. *Circulation.* 2014;130:1418-1436.

17. Brown J, Beard E, Kotz D, et al. Real-world effectiveness of e-cigarettes when used to aid smoking cessation: a cross-sectional population study. *Addiction.* 2014;109:1531-1540. doi:10.1111/add.12623.

18. Dawkins L, Turner J, Roberts A, et al. 'Vaping' profiles and preferences: an online survey of electronic cigarette users. *Addiction.* 2013;108(6):1115-1125. doi: 10.1111/add. 12150.

19. Bullen C, Howe C, Laugesen M, et al. Electronic cigarettes for smoking cessation: a randomised controlled trial. *Lancet.* 2013;382:1629-1637.

20. Chaiton M, Diemert L, Cohen JE, et al. Estimating the number of quit attempts it takes to quit smoking successfully in a longitudinal cohort of smokers. *BMJ Open.* 2018;6(6):e011045. doi:10.1136/bmjopen-2016-011045.

21. Rigotti NA, Regan S, Levy DE, et al. Sustained care intervention and postdischarge smoking cessation among hospitalized adults: a randomized clinical trial. *JAMA.* 2014;312:719-728. doi:10.1001/jama.2014.9237.

Matthew Nayor • Vasan S. Ramachandran

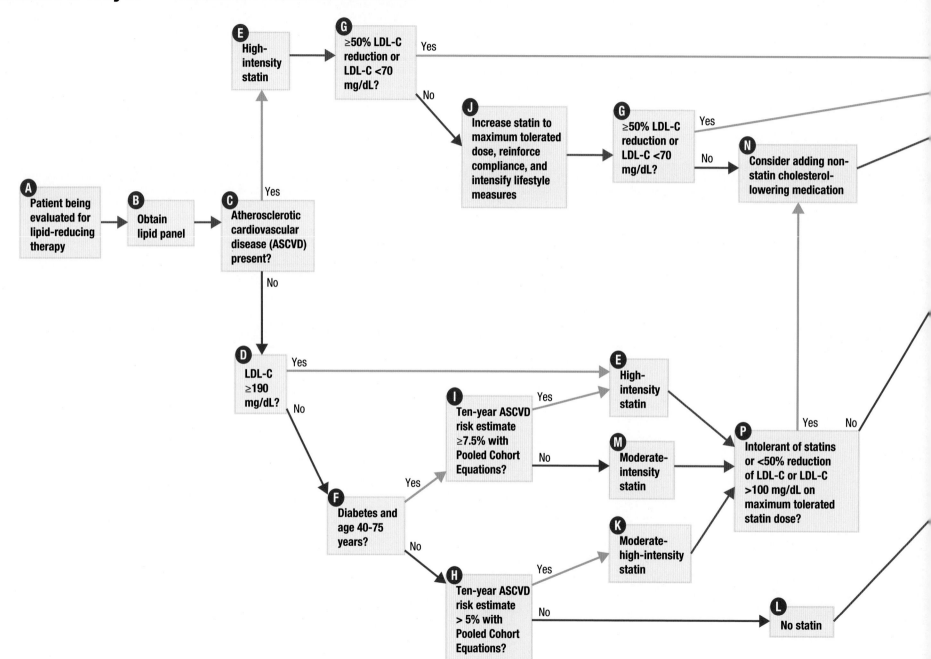

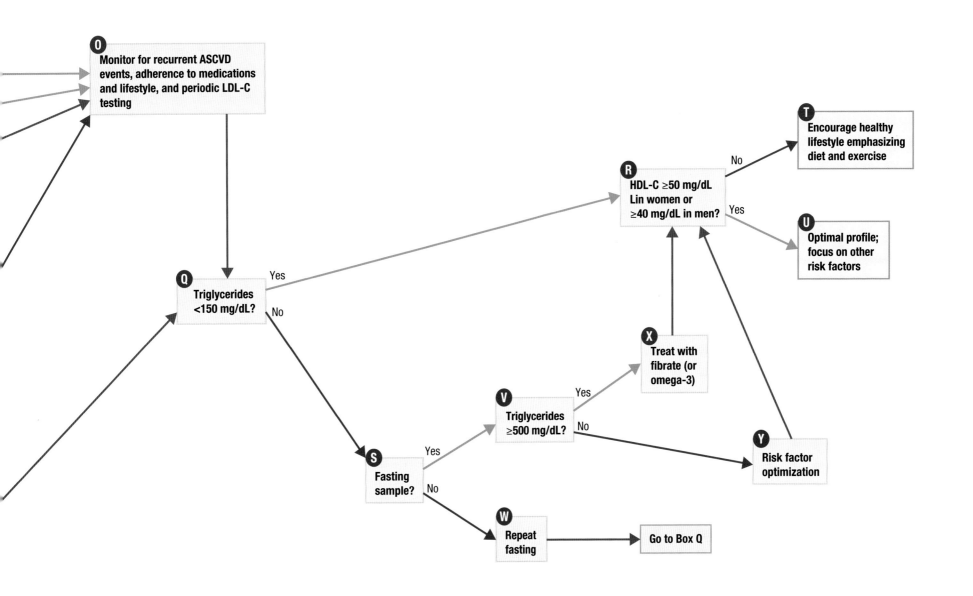

Ⓐ Patient being evaluated for lipid-reducing therapy

A blood lipid panel should be obtained for individuals of any age who are diagnosed with atherosclerotic cardiovascular disease (ASCVD).[1] For adults aged 40 to 75 years without ASCVD but with average risk, screening lipid panels are recommended every 5 years.[2] More frequent evaluation should be considered in those at increased risk because of a family history of early ASCVD or severely elevated lipid levels.[2] In adults <40 years or >75 years, the US Preventive Services Task Force recommends that clinician judgment be used to determine the appropriateness of screening lipid panel assessment.

Ⓑ Obtain lipid panel

A fasting or nonfasting blood lipid panel may be obtained as initial testing.[3,4] Nonfasting lipid panels are accurate for estimating HDL-C and LDL-C concentrations, but may overestimate triglyceride concentrations depending on the timing and composition of recent food intake.[3]

Ⓒ Atherosclerotic cardiovascular disease present?

ASCVD is defined as a history of MI, angina, coronary or other arterial revascularization, stroke, TIA, or PAD of presumed atherosclerotic origin.[1] Individuals with manifest ASCVD are at increased risk for ischemic events and have higher absolute risk reductions with statin therapy.[4] Therefore, treatment recommendations for those with clinical ASCVD (ie, secondary prevention) endorse more aggressive application of lipid-lowering therapy.[4]

Ⓓ LDL-C ≥ 190 mg/dL

Individuals with very high LDL-C levels are at increased lifetime risk for ASCVD[4] and many are heterozygous for inherited hypercholesterolemia syndromes.[5] The 2013 American College of Cardiology (ACC)/American Heart Association (AHA) Guidelines on the Treatment of Blood Cholesterol to Reduce Atherosclerotic Cardiovascular Risk in Adults (2013 ACC/AHA Guidelines) recommended initiating statin therapy for all adults with LDL-C ≥190 mg/dL to reduce their risk of developing future ASCVD.[1]

Ⓔ High-intensity statin

High-intensity statins are expected to lower LDL-C by an average of ≥50% and are recommended for patients with LDL-C >190 mg/dL.[1] They are also recommended in patients who have ASCVD, regardless of LDL-C levels. The medications included in this category are atorvastatin 40 to 80 mg/d and rosuvastatin 20 to 40 mg/d. On the basis of data from both primary and secondary prevention trials, each 38.7 mg/dL reduction in LDL-C is associated with a 20% to 30% relative risk reduction in the incidence of major cardiovascular events.[4] Monitoring for potential adverse effects from statins should include blood creatinine kinase

measurement before starting statin therapy and if muscle pain symptoms develop, and liver function tests before starting medication, at approximately 3 months after starting statin therapy, and annually thereafter.[6]

Ⓕ Diabetes and age 40 to 75 years?

Diabetes mellitus is associated with a significantly elevated lifetime risk of developing ASCVD. In fact, 40-75 years type 2 diabetes increases the risk of cardiovascular mortality by 2- to 4-fold.[7] Statin therapy reduces cardiovascular risk in individuals with diabetes but without overt ASCVD[8] and is therefore recommended for all adults 40 to 75 years of age with diabetes.

Ⓖ ≥50% LDL-C reduction or LDL-C <70 mg/dL?

The 2013 ACC/AHA Guidelines recommended specific intensities of statin therapy to be initiated depending on absolute ASCVD risk but did not identify specific LDL-C treatment targets.[1] This approach was based on the absence of clinical trial evidence supporting a treat-to-target approach[1] and represented an important departure from previous US guideline documents[6] as well as those from other leading international societies.[9] Since the publication of these guidelines, several clinical trials have demonstrated improved cardiovascular outcomes with further lipid lowering in patients already treated with statin therapy. Appropriate utilization of these therapies is challenging in the absence of treatment targets. The ACC Task Force has hence published two focused updates outlining decision pathways for considering non-statin therapies.[10,11] Notably, these updates specify a treatment target of ≥50% blood LDL-C reduction (or LDL-C < 70 mg/dL). Although specific LDL-C targets have not been rigorously tested in clinical trials, recent clinical trial data suggest that the monotonic relation between achieved LDL-C concentrations and major cardiovascular events exists all the way down to extremely low LDL-C concentrations (<10 mg/dL) without observed adverse effects.[12,13] These data, therefore, support the practice of aggressive LDL-C lowering in individuals who are at particularly high risk of ASCVD events; it remains to be seen how these data will be further incorporated into future US cholesterol treatment guidelines.

Ⓗ Ten-year ASCVD risk estimate > 5% with Pooled Cohort Equations?

The Pooled Cohort Equations leverage data from four National Heart, Lung, and Blood Institute–sponsored cohort studies to estimate ASCVD risk on the basis of the values of eight risk factors: age, sex, total cholesterol, HDL-C, SBP, blood pressure treatment status, diabetes mellitus, and current smoking status.[14] Different equations are available for white and black individuals and both lifetime and 10-year risk can be calculated. The dynamic calculator that allows entry of the above variable values can be found at: http://tools.acc.org/ASCVD-Risk-Estimator-Plus/.

Ⓘ 10-year ASCVD risk estimate ≥7.5% with Pooled Cohort Equations?

A ten-year risk of ASCVD of ≥7.5% among those with (and without) diabetes is considered "high risk" and warrants a discussion regarding aggressive lipid-lowering therapy. This "high-risk" threshold is lower than those proposed by some other leading international guidelines,[9] but it may be appropriate given the overall safety profile of statin therapies.[15] The dynamic calculator that allows entry of the abovementioned variable values can be found at: http://tools.acc.org/ASCVD-Risk-Estimator-Plus/.

Ⓙ Increase statin to maximum tolerated dose, reinforce compliance, and intensify lifestyle measures

In individuals with ASCVD who do not demonstrate the expected ≥50% reduction in blood LDL-C with high-intensity statin therapy, several measures are recommended to optimize the treatment effect. Increasing to the maximum tolerated statin dose should be undertaken. Barriers to medication adherence should be assessed and full medication compliance reinforced. Patients should also be counseled on lifestyle measures that can reduce blood LDL-C concentrations. Reduced dietary intake of saturated fats, weight loss, and physical exercise may have a positive impact on blood LDL-C concentrations, although the effects of weight loss and exercise on LDL-C itself are often modest.[3]

Ⓚ Moderate-high-intensity statin

Moderate-high-intensity statins are recommended for primary prevention of ASCVD for individuals aged 40 to 75 years without diabetes and with an estimated 10-year risk of ≥7.5%.[1] For individuals with an estimated 10-year ASCVD risk of 5% to <7.5%, moderate-high-intensity statin therapy can be considered after a clinician-patient discussion regarding the potential benefits and risks of treatment. Owing to the limited data on the benefit of statin therapy for primary prevention in individuals >75 years, guideline recommendations advocate shared decision making and clinical judgment in deciding on statin therapy for elderly individuals.[1] Moderate-intensity statins are expected to reduce blood LDL-C concentrations by 30% to 50% and include the following: atorvastatin 10 mg/d, fluvastatin 80 mg/d, lovastatin 40 mg/d, pravastatin 40 mg/d, rosuvastatin 10 mg/d, and simvastatin 40 mg/d.[1]

Ⓛ No statin

Individuals with a low estimated 10-year risk of ASCVD (<5%) are recommended to not initiate statin therapy and to focus on optimizing other ASCVD risk factors. Repeat screening lipid panel assessment should be performed approximately every 5 years.

Ⓜ Moderate-intensity statin

Moderate-intensity statins (atorvastatin 10 mg/d, fluvastatin 80 mg/d, lovastatin 40 mg/d, pravastatin 40 mg/d, rosuvastatin 10 mg/d, and simvastatin 40 mg/d) are recommended for individuals aged 40 to 75 years with diabetes who have estimated ASCVD risk <7.5%.

Ⓝ Consider adding non-statin cholesterol-lowering medication

Two medication classes have recently been shown to reduce cardiovascular events when added to statin therapy in high-risk patients.[13,16,17] In the IMPROVE-IT trial, a moderate-intensity statin plus ezetimibe (which reduces intestinal absorption of cholesterol) was associated with a lower LDL-C concentration (54 mg/dL in the statin + ezetimibe group vs. 70 mg/dL in the statin-alone group) and a 2% absolute risk reduction in cardiovascular events in individuals enrolled after an acute coronary syndrome.[13] In the FOURIER trial, evolocumab (an inhibitor of proprotein convertase subtilisin/kexin type 9 [PCSK9]) in addition to statin therapy led to a substantial reduction in LDL-C (30 vs. 92 mg/dL in the statin-alone group) and a 15% relative risk reduction in cardiovascular endpoints in patients with established ASCVD.[16] On the basis of these findings, addition of ezetimibe or a PCSK9 inhibitor should be considered in high-risk individuals who do not have adequate LDL-C lowering with statins, cannot tolerate sufficient statin doses, or have recurrent ASCVD events despite statin therapy.[11]

Ⓞ Monitor for recurrent ASCVD events, adherence to medications and lifestyle, and periodic LDL-C testing

Individuals treated with statin therapy should be monitored periodically for recurrent events, medication adherence and tolerance, and treatment response. Clear recommendations for how often to monitor lipid panels on lipid-lowering therapy are lacking, but annual assessment is reasonable in most patients once target doses of the appropriate medications have been reached.

Ⓟ Intolerant of statins or <50% reduction of LDL-C or LDL-C >100 mg/dL on maximum tolerated statin dose?

The most common reason for statin intolerance is muscle pain without muscle damage.[3] Although meta-analyses of randomized trials found no difference in muscle symptoms between statin-treated individuals and controls,[18] muscular symptoms are reported in approximately 10% of patients in real-world observational studies.[19] Often these symptoms can be managed with substituting a different statin medication, lowering the dose, or alternate day dosing. Serious muscle damage (ie, rhabdomyolysis) and liver injury are rare, but routine monitoring for these adverse effects should be performed.[18] Data on other potential adverse effects including an increased risk of cancer, diabetes, and dementia are controversial, and the benefits of statin therapy outweigh these risks for most patients.[20] If statins are not tolerated or effective at tolerated doses, treatment with non-statin medications should be considered.

Ⓠ Triglycerides < 150 mg/dL?

Observational and genetic studies suggest that triglyceride concentrations are likely to be causally related to ASCVD risk.[21] This risk appears to be relatively linear[22] and although discrete cutpoints for ideal blood triglyceride concentrations are not empirically proved, a concentration <150 mg/dL is considered optimal.[3,6]

Ⓡ HDL-C ≥50 mg/dL in women or ≥40 mg/dL in men?

HDL-C values ≥50 mg/dL in women and ≥40 mg/dL in men are considered optimal. These are the concentrations below which cardiovascular risk has been noted to increase in observational studies.[23] Despite the robust and convincing evidence that a lower HDL-C is associated with an increased risk of ASCVD, several trials of novel HDL-C raising medications have failed to show benefit,[3] and Mendelian randomization studies have questioned the causal relationship between HDL-C and ASCVD.[24]

Ⓢ Fasting sample?

Fasting triglyceride concentrations are recommended if initial assessment is elevated. Nonfasting and fasting lipid panels demonstrate similar assessments of LDL-C and HDL-C, but triglycerides are often higher on nonfasting assessments depending on the timing and composition of recent food intake.[3] On average, triglyceride levels increase 26 mg/dL and remain elevated for 1 to 7 hours after a usual meal.[25] Hence an 8- to 12-hour fast is recommended before repeat lipid panel assessment in individuals with high triglycerides to exclude the potential confounding effects of recent food intake.

Ⓣ Encourage healthy lifestyle emphasizing diet and exercise

Pharmacologic elevation of HDL-C levels has not resulted in improved outcomes; therefore, lifestyle interventions are the primary treatment for low HDL-C. Improved diet, weight loss, smoking cessation, and aerobic exercise may all have beneficial effects on HDL-C.[3] These effects are modest but potentially additive. A 0.4 mg/dL increase in HDL-C has been observed for each kilogram weight loss,[3] and the equivalent of 25 to 30 km of brisk walking weekly is expected to result in a 3.1 to 6 mg/dL rise in HDL-C.[3]

Ⓤ Optimal profile; focus on other risk factors

An optimal HDL profile includes a blood HDL-C ≥50 mg/dL in women and ≥40 mg/dL in men. Once these concentrations are achieved, attention should be focused on modifying other ASCVD risk factors.

Ⓥ Triglycerides ≥ 500 mg/dL?

Fasting triglyceride levels > 500 mg/dL increase the risk of pancreatitis. Investigation for secondary causes (such as poor glycemic control, excessive alcohol intake, thyroid, hepatic or renal dysfunction) and treatment with triglyceride-lowering medications (as reviewed below in Box X) is recommended.

Ⓦ Repeat fasting

Nonfasting triglyceride measurements can be elevated depending on recent meal composition or timing (discussed in more detail in Box S).

Ⓧ Treat with fibrate (or omega-3)

Treatment is recommended for triglyceride concentrations ≥500 mg/dL to prevent pancreatitis. Statin medications can have significant triglyceride-lowering effects and are usually an appropriate consideration as first-line therapy because many patients with severely elevated triglycerides will have an elevated estimated ASCVD risk. If triglyceride concentrations remain elevated despite statin therapy, or for patients with only elevated triglycerides with low LDL-C, fibrates (proliferator-activated receptor-α agonists) should be considered. Although the data that fibrates reduce cardiovascular outcomes in patients already treated with statins are lacking,[26] these medications can have robust triglyceride-lowering effects. Indeed, fibrates and statins can be used in combination for patients with severely elevated triglyceride levels. However, extra caution and laboratory monitoring is recommended because of an increased risk of hepatic and muscle toxicity. Omega-3 fatty acids used at pharmacologic doses (2-4 g/d) reduce triglyceride levels by up to 45% and may also be considered in this setting.[27]

Ⓨ Risk factor optimization

For individuals with fasting high triglyceride concentrations 150 to 500 mg/dL, the optimal treatment is institution of lifestyle-based measures. Insulin resistance is strongly related to triglyceride metabolism, so serum glucose lowering should be undertaken (through medications or by diet). Alcohol intake can have a major impact on triglyceride levels and should be minimized. Weight reduction and physical exercise can also have positive effects on triglyceride levels.[3]

REFERENCES

1. Stone NJ, Robinson JG, Lichtenstein AH, et al. 2013 ACC/AHA guideline on the treatment of blood cholesterol to reduce atherosclerotic cardiovascular risk in adults: a report of the American College of Cardiology/American Heart Association Task Force on Practice Guidelines. *Circulation*. 2014;129:S1-S45. doi:10.1161/01.cir.0000437738.63853.7a.
2. Bibbins-Domingo K, Grossman DC, Curry SJ, et al. Statin use for the primary prevention of cardiovascular disease in

adults: US Preventive Services Task Force Recommendation statement. *JAMA*. 2016;316(19):1997-2007. doi:10.1001/jama.2016.15450.

3. Catapano AL, Graham I, De Backer G, et al. 2016 ESC/EAS guidelines for the management of dyslipidaemias. *Eur Heart J*. 2016;37(39):2999-3058. doi:10.1093/eurheartj/ehw272.

4. Silverman MG, Ference BA, Im K, et al. Association between lowering LDL-C and cardiovascular risk reduction among different therapeutic interventions. *JAMA*. 2016;316(12):1289-1297. doi:10.1001/jama.2016.13985.

5. Ryan A, Byrne CD. Importance of early recognition of heterozygous familial hypercholesterolaemia. *Curr Opin Lipidol*. 2015;26(4):298-303. doi:10.1097/MOL.0000000000000196.

6. Expert Panel on Detection, Evaluation, and Treatment of High Blood Cholesterol in Adults. Executive summary of the Third Report of the National Cholesterol Education Program (NCEP) Expert Panel on detection, evaluation, and treatment of high blood cholesterol in adults (Adult Treatment Panel III). *JAMA*. 2001;285:2486-2497.

7. Stamler J, Vaccaro O, Neaton JD, Wentworth D. Diabetes, other risk factors, and 12-yr cardiovascular mortality for men screened in the Multiple Risk Factor Intervention Trial. *Diabetes Care*. 1993;16(2):434-444.

8. Colhoun HM, Betteridge DJ, Durrington PN, et al. Primary prevention of cardiovascular disease with atorvastatin in type 2 diabetes in the Collaborative Atorvastatin Diabetes Study (CARDS): multicentre randomised placebo-controlled trial. *Lancet*. 2004;364(9435):685-696. doi:10.1016/S0140-6736(04)16895-5.

9. Nayor M, Vasan RS. Recent update to the US cholesterol treatment guidelines: a comparison with international guidelines. *Circulation*. 2016;133(18):1795-1806. doi:10.1161/CIRCULATIONAHA.116.021407.

10. Writing Committee; Lloyd-Jones DM, Morris PB, Ballantyne CM, et al. 2016 ACC Expert Consensus decision pathway on the role of non-statin therapies for LDL-cholesterol lowering in the management of atherosclerotic cardiovascular disease risk. *J Am Coll Cardiol*. 2016;68(1):92-125. doi:10.1016/j.jacc.2016.03.519.

11. Lloyd-Jones DM, Morris PB, Ballantyne CM, et al. 2017 Focused update of the 2016 ACC Expert Consensus decision pathway on the role of non-statin therapies for LDL-cholesterol lowering in the management of atherosclerotic cardiovascular disease risk: a report of the American College of Cardiology Task Force on Expert Consensus Decision Pathways. *J Am Coll Cardiol*. 2017;70(14):1785-1822. doi:10.1016/j.jacc.2017.07.745.

12. Giugliano RP, Pedersen TR, Park J-G, et al. Clinical efficacy and safety of achieving very low LDL-cholesterol concentrations with the PCSK9 inhibitor evolocumab: a prespecified secondary analysis of the FOURIER trial. *Lancet*. 2017;390(10106):1962-1971. doi:10.1016/S0140-6736(17)32290-0.

13. Cannon CP, Blazing MA, Giugliano RP, et al. Ezetimibe added to statin therapy after acute coronary syndromes. *N Engl J Med*. 2015;372(25):2387-2397. doi:10.1056/NEJMoa1410489.

14. Goff DC, Lloyd-Jones DM, Bennett G, et al. 2013 ACC/AHA guideline on the assessment of cardiovascular risk: a report of the American College of Cardiology/American Heart Association Task Force on Practice Guidelines. *J Am Coll Cardiol*. 2014;63:2935-2959. doi:10.1016/j.jacc.2013.11.005.

15. Cholesterol Treatment Trialists' (CTT) Collaboration; Baigent C, Blackwell L, Emberson J, et al. Efficacy and safety of more intensive lowering of LDL cholesterol: a meta-analysis of data from 170 000 participants in 26 randomised trials. *Lancet*. 2010;376(9753):1670-1681. doi:10.1016/S0140-6736(10)61350-5.

16. Sabatine MS, Giugliano RP, Keech AC, et al. Evolocumab and clinical outcomes in patients with cardiovascular disease. *N Engl J Med*. 2017;376(18):1713-1722. doi:10.1056/NEJMoa1615664.

17. Ridker PM, Revkin J, Amarenco P, et al. Cardiovascular efficacy and safety of bococizumab in high-risk patients. *N Engl J Med*. 2017;376(16):1527-1539. doi:10.1056/NEJMoa1701488.

18. Naci H, Brugts J, Ades T. Comparative tolerability and harms of individual statins: a study-level network meta-analysis of 246 955 participants from 135 randomized, controlled trials. *Circ Cardiovasc Qual Outcomes*. 2013;6(4):390-399. doi:10.1161/CIRCOUTCOMES.111.000071.

19. Bruckert E, Hayem G, Dejager S, Yau C, Begaud B. Mild to moderate muscular symptoms with high-dosage statin therapy in hyperlipidemic patients—the PRIMO study. *Cardiovasc Drugs Ther*. 2005;19(6):403-414. doi:10.1007/s10557-005-5686-z.

20. Landmesser U, Chapman MJ, Stock JK, et al. 2017 Update of ESC/EAS Task Force on practical clinical guidance for proprotein convertase subtilisin/kexin type 9 inhibition in patients with atherosclerotic cardiovascular disease or in familial hypercholesterolaemia. *Eur Heart J*. 2017;376:1713. doi:10.1093/eurheartj/ehx549.

21. Do R, Willer CJ, Schmidt EM, et al. Common variants associated with plasma triglycerides and risk for coronary artery disease. *Nat Genet*. 2013;45(11):1345-1352. doi:10.1038/ng.2795.

22. Assmann G, Schulte H, Funke H, von Eckardstein A. The emergence of triglycerides as a significant independent risk factor in coronary artery disease. *Eur Heart J*. 1998;19(suppl M):M8-M14.

23. Chapman MJ, Ginsberg HN, Amarenco P, et al. Triglyceride-rich lipoproteins and high-density lipoprotein cholesterol in patients at high risk of cardiovascular disease: evidence and guidance for management. *Eur Heart J*. 2011;32(11):1345-1361. doi:10.1093/eurheartj/ehr112.

24. Voight BF, Peloso GM, Orho-Melander M, et al. Plasma HDL cholesterol and risk of myocardial infarction: a Mendelian randomisation study. *Lancet*. 2012;380(9841):572-580. doi:10.1016/S0140-6736(12)60312-2.

25. Nordestgaard BG. A test in context: lipid profile, fasting versus nonfasting. *J Am Coll Cardiol*. 2017;70(13):1637-1646. doi:10.1016/j.jacc.2017.08.006.

26. Keene D, Price C, Shun-Shin MJ, Francis DP. Effect on cardiovascular risk of high density lipoprotein targeted drug treatments niacin, fibrates, and CETP inhibitors: meta-analysis of randomised controlled trials including 117 411 patients. *BMJ*. 2014;349:g4379. doi:10.1136/bmj.g4379.

27. Wei MY, Jacobson TA. Effects of eicosapentaenoic acid versus docosahexaenoic acid on serum lipids: a systematic review and meta-analysis. *Curr Atheroscler Rep*. 2011;13(6):474-483. doi:10.1007/s11883-011-0210-3.

Thomas G. DeLoughery

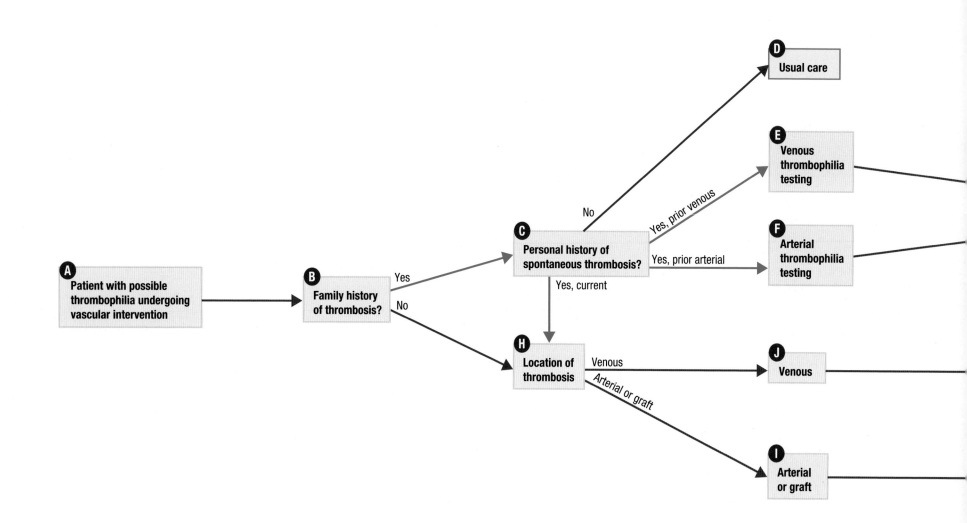

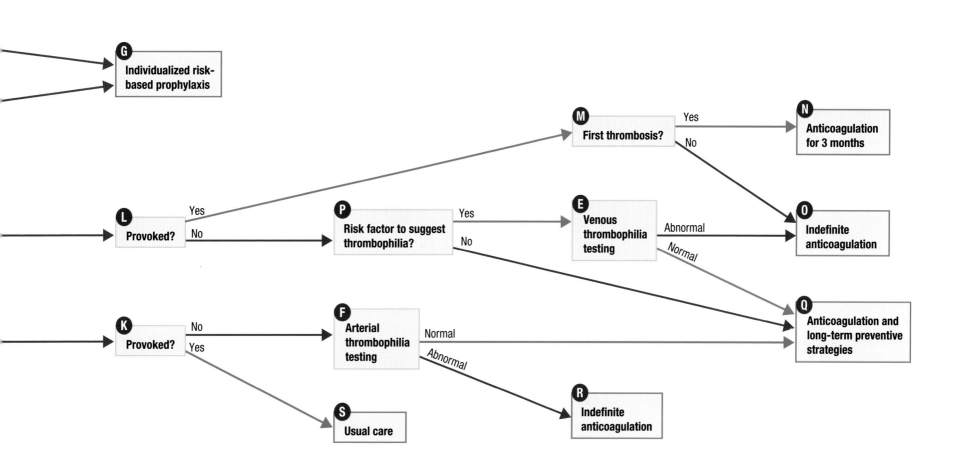

A Patient with possible thrombophilia undergoing vascular intervention

A hypercoagulable state (thrombophilia) is a condition associated with an increased propensity to develop thrombosis due to an inherited or acquired disorder.[1,2] For venous thrombosis, this state is manifested clinically by (1) thrombosis at a young age (usually considered <40 years) especially if not provoked; (2) recurrent thromboses; (3) unusual location, such as visceral vein thrombosis; or (4) a family history of thrombosis. For arterial disease, this is manifested by premature ischemic vascular disorders, such as stroke, MI, or sudden arterial occlusion or unexplained graft thrombosis. Although testing can help identify[3] a specific hypercoagulable disorder, the result is often negative, in which case a nonspecific hypercoagulable state becomes a diagnosis based on the history. It is important to assess patients with possible thrombophilia who are undergoing vascular interventions to optimize care, including preventive strategies.

B Family history of thrombosis?

A positive family history is defined as thrombosis in two or more first-degree relatives or if one relative had a venous thrombosis before age 50.[4] Inherited thrombophilias often have an incomplete penetrance and, as such, taking a detailed family history is important. Family history of thrombosis alone is a significant risk factor for thrombosis with relative risk estimated to be approximately 3.[5]

C Personal history of spontaneous thrombosis?

Personal history should include the exact location of any prior thrombosis and its extent. For venous thrombosis, the circumstance of thrombosis, with a focus on provoked or unprovoked, is also important to ascertain. Circumstances considered to be provoking factors for venous thrombosis include trauma (especially lower limb), surgery, hospital stay >72 hours, pregnancy, airplane travel over 4 hours, and estrogen use.[6]

D Usual care

Patients with a family history but without a personal history of spontaneous thrombosis should receive age- and situation-appropriate venous thrombosis prophylaxis for surgery.[7] Venous thrombosis risk can be determined by scoring systems such as the Caprini Score (see G).

E Venous thrombophilia testing

Testing for venous thrombophilia consists of blood tests to evaluate factors involved in inherited disorders. These include the following: antithrombin III, factor V Leiden, free protein S level, protein C activity, and prothrombin gene mutation. In addition, screening for antiphospholipid antibody syndrome should be conducted.[8] This should consist of the following: lupus inhibitor

testing, anticardiolipin antibodies, and anti-β_2-glycoprotein antibodies. Importantly, a positive test needs to be repeated after 12 weeks to ensure persistent presence of these antibodies. Often—especially with acute illness—these tests can be transiently positive.

There is limited utility in measuring homocysteine levels. For select patients, more thorough testing can be performed. Patients with visceral vein thrombosis should undergo testing for myeloproliferative syndrome with JAK2 mutation testing, and screening for paroxysmal nocturnal hemoglobinuria. A common issue raised is the need to search for an occult cancer. The incidence of cancer is higher in patients with idiopathic thrombosis, but trials have not shown convincing benefit of detailed cancer screening with CT or PET scans. Rather, age-appropriate cancer screening in recommended.[9]

F Arterial thrombophilia testing

Testing for arterial thrombophilia should include screening for antiphospholipid antibody syndrome. This consists of lupus inhibitor testing and measurement of anticardiolipin antibodies plus anti-β_2-glycoprotein antibodies. Patients with premature atherosclerosis should also have a lipid panel performed as well as measure of lipoprotein(a). Patients with embolic disease should have an ECHO to look for cardiac sources of embolism and extended

cardiac monitoring to rule out paroxysmal atrial fibrillation.[10] In addition, testing for heparin-induced thrombocytopenia should be considered in those who received any recent heparin products. This involves measuring antiplatelet factor 4 (PF4) antibodies first and, if the result is positive, confirming with a serotonin release assay.[11] Testing for other inherited hypercoagulable disorders is low yield because these are typically conditions affecting the venous system.

G Individualized risk-based prophylaxis

An individualized VTE risk assessment should be performed using a validated tool, such as the Caprini Score (see Table 5-1).[5] This score is then used to determine the approach for prophylaxis (see Table 5-2). Patients at increased risk of venous thrombosis (score of 3 or more) should receive chemical prophylaxis, if feasible. If there is a high bleeding risk or high risk of venous thrombosis (score of 5 or more), then pneumatic compression should be applied before surgery and continued for the duration of the hospital stay. Pharmacologic prophylaxis should also be strongly considered including standard unfractionated heparin (UFH), or LWMH, as well as factor Xa inhibitors or warfarin. In general, UFH is used in standard-risk patients, LMWH in higher risk surgery such as in patients with a history of thrombosis or those with cancer. The use of factor Xa inhibitors or warfarin is typically

Table 5-1. Caprini Score—Risk Factors Relevant for Vascular Procedures

1 Point/Risk Factor Present	2 Points/Factor	3 Points/Factor	5 Points/Factor
• Age 41-60 • Minor surgery planned • History of recent major surgery (<1 mo) • Varicose veins • History of inflammatory bowel disease • Swollen legs • Obesity (body mass index > 25) • Acute MI • CHF • Sepsis (<1 mo) • Serious lung disease (including pneumonia, <1 mo) • Abnormal pulmonary function (COPD) • Medical patient currently on bed rest • Oral contraceptive or HRT • Pregnancy or postpartum (<1 mo) • History of unexplained stillbirth or recurrent spontaneous abortion (>3), premature birth	• Age 60-74 • Malignancy (present or previous) • Major surgery (>45 min) • Laparoscopic surgery (>45 min) • Patient confined to bed (>72 h) • Immobilizing plaster cast (<1 mo) • Central venous access	• Age > 75 • History of DVT/PE • Family history of thrombosis • Factor V Leiden • Positive prothrombin 20210A • Elevated homocysteine • Positive lupus anticoagulant • Elevated anticardiolipin antibodies • Heparin-induced thrombocytopenia	• Hip, pelvis, or leg fracture (<1 mo) • Stroke (<1 mo) • Multiple trauma (<1 mo) • Acute spinal cord injury (<1 mo)

HRT, hormone replacement therapy.

Table 5-2. Prophylaxis Approach Based on Caprini Score

Score	Prophylaxis Approach
2	IPC perioperatively and during hospitalization
3-4	UFH, LMWH, or DOAC during hospitalization—start 12-24 h postop, IPC if high risk of bleeding
5-8	UFH, LMWH, or DOAC plus IPC during hospitalization—start 12-24 h postop for 7-10 d, IPC if high risk of bleeding
>8	UFH, LMWH, or DOAC plus IPC during hospitalization—start 12-24 h postop for 14-30 d, ICP if high risk of bleeding

DOAC, direct oral anticoagulant; IPC, intermittent pneumatic compression stockings; UFH, unfractionated heparin.

restricted to patients undergoing orthopedic surgery. The duration of the chemical prophylactic regimen may be guided by the risk; such that those at intermediate risk (score 3-4) receive the agent during their hospitalization, those at higher risk (score 5-7) receive the agent for 7 to 10 days, and those at extremely high risk (score of 8 or more) receive the agent for up to 30 days post procedure.

H Location of thrombosis

The location of thrombosis, either arterial or venous, is a crucial decision point for guiding the workup of thrombophilia. Inherited thrombophilias, such as factor V Leiden, are strong risk factors for venous thrombosis but are not significant risk factors for arterial thrombosis. Traditional arterial risk factors such as abnormal lipids, smoking, and elevated blood pressure are major contributors to atherosclerotic disease and associated thrombosis.[12]

I Arterial or graft

Evaluation of premature (before age 40) or unusual arterial thrombosis, in the absence of preexistent arterial pathology, is not as well defined as for venous thrombosis. The first step is determining whether the thrombosis is due to cardiac or noncardiac embolic disease, arterial issues (such as atherosclerosis, vasculitis, or trauma), or is spontaneous. For graft thrombosis, it is essential to assess mechanical factors such as inflow, graft conduit, or outflow disease that would explain the thrombosis. These tend to be much more frequently seen than is associated thrombophilia. History should include past vascular events, both arterial and venous, plus family history—especially of premature atherosclerosis.

J Venous

An important consideration in venous thrombosis is location. Lower extremity DVT (or a PE) would be considered "usual" locations. However, visceral, renal, or cerebral veins would be

unusual locations and, unless due to local factors (such as infection or surgery), would warrant a thrombophilia workup. Upper extremity venous thrombosis is almost always due to mechanical factors (such as catheters or compression within the thoracic outlet). These risk factors should be actively sought out, reserving thrombophilia evaluation for truly idiopathic thrombosis.[13]

K Provoked?

Risk factors for provoked arterial thrombosis are less well defined than for venous thrombosis but include atherosclerosis, local trauma, perivascular infections, and vasculitis.[3] For sudden arterial or graft thrombosis in a hospitalized patient on heparin, heparin-induced thrombocytopenia must be considered.

L Provoked?

It is important to consider whether a venous thrombosis was precipitated or provoked by a reversible or transient risk factor, which includes the following[6]: surgery within the past 6 weeks, hospital stay within the past 6 weeks, lower limb trauma, leg immobilization, estrogen contraception (rings, patches, or pills), pregnancy or air travel longer than 4 to 6 hours.

M First thrombosis?

The duration of anticoagulation recommended for a provoked venous thrombosis depends on whether there is a history of prior events. Randomized trials have shown that 3 months of anticoagulation suffices for first provoked venous thrombosis or PE.[14] The risk of recurrence falls back to baseline after 3 months, such that its risk is outweighed by the risk of continued anticoagulation.[15] In contrast, a randomized trial showed that patients with two or more episodes of provoked venous thrombosis (proximal DVT or PE) benefited from indefinite anticoagulation with an absolute 18% risk reduction in recurrent thrombosis.[16] Although most were idiopathic, 25% of patients in this trial had provoked thrombosis.

N Anticoagulation for 3 months

In the past, the only option was to start warfarin and LMWH together, stopping LMWH when the INR was above 2.0 for 24 hours. However, recently, data have emerged to support the use of direct oral anticoagulants (DOACs) in treatment. Advantages of DOACs include no need for monitoring, no food interactions, few drug interactions, and less bleeding. For edoxaban and dabigatran, a 5-day course of LMWH needs to be given before the DOAC is started because this was the protocol in the clinical trials. Both apixaban and rivaroxaban can be immediately started without LMWH overlap but need an initiation at a higher dose. Apixaban is started at 10 mg twice daily for 7 days and then continued at 5 mg twice daily. Rivaroxaban is started at 15 mg twice daily for 21 days and then continued at 20 mg once daily.

O Indefinite anticoagulation

Indefinite anticoagulation is recommended for patients with either multiple provoked episodes of venous thrombosis or for patients with prior unprovoked VTE. In patients at unusual risk of bleeding (eg, dialysis patients, recurrent GI bleeding), a shorter course of anticoagulation can be considered. There are also now trial data to support using lower doses of the DOACs (including apixaban 2.5 mg twice daily and rivaroxaban 10 mg once daily) for long-term secondary prevention, further strengthening the recommendation for indefinite therapy.[17]

P Risk factor to suggest thrombophilia?

Factors suggestive of venous thrombophilia are (1) thrombosis at a young age (usually considered <40 years), (2) multiple thromboses, (3) unusual location such as visceral vein thrombosis, or (4) family history of two or more first-degree relatives with VTE.

Q Anticoagulation and long-term preventive strategies

For patients with unprovoked venous thrombosis and negative thrombophilia test results, anticoagulation is required for at least 3 months. However, long-term prevention with anticoagulation is typically advocated in patients with low bleeding risk, because up to 30% of people with thrombophilia will have negative test results. After completion of initial therapy, some may utilize one of several tools to predict the risk of recurrence. This includes the Herdoo-2, Vienna, and DASH scores—which include features of age, gender and posttreatment D-dimer levels off therapy. If the risk of recurrence is deemed to be low, then anticoagulation may be discontinued. However, one drawback of these scoring systems is that even in low-risk patients, the risk of thrombosis is often higher than is the risk of long-term anticoagulation, estimated as high as 5% per year. In addition, other long-term risk reduction strategies should be employed including maintenance of ideal body weight and regular exercise.

For arterial occlusive disease, long-term therapy depends on the underlying etiology. Those with atherosclerotic disease should receive antiplatelet agents and atherosclerotic risk factors modification. Embolic disease or acute arterial thrombosis without preexisting arterial pathology even with normal thrombophilia testing is treated with long-term anticoagulation.

R Indefinite anticoagulation

Unexplained arterial (or graft) occlusion with persistently positive test results for antiphospholipid antibodies (defined as positive repeat test results 12 weeks apart) should be treated with long-term anticoagulation. The use of warfarin is advocated because data for the DOACs are concerning for increased risk of recurrent thrombosis.[18] If the cause is explained by atherosclerosis, then therapy should include long-term antiplatelet agents (such as aspirin, clopidogrel, and other newer agents) along with statins and other risk factor modification. Events due to embolic disease should receive lifelong anticoagulation with warfarin or DOACs. Heparin-induced thrombocytopenia is treated with either parenteral direct thrombin inhibitors, or increasingly with DOACs.[19]

Ⓢ Usual care

Patients with atherosclerosis should receive long-term antiplatelet agents along with statins and other risk factor modification. Patients with embolic disease should receive lifelong anticoagulation.

REFERENCES

1. Connors JM. Thrombophilia testing and venous thrombosis. *N Engl J Med.* 2017;377:1177-1187.
2. Polycythemia vera: the natural history of 1213 patients followed for 20 years. Gruppo Italiano Studio Policitemia [see comments]. *Ann Intern Med.* 1995;123:656-664.
3. Previtali E, Bucciarelli P, Passamonti SM, Martinelli I. Risk factors for venous and arterial thrombosis. *Blood Transfus.* 2011;9:120-138.
4. Bezemer ID, van der Meer FJ, Eikenboom JC, Rosendaal FR, Doggen CJ. The value of family history as a risk indicator for venous thrombosis. *Arch Intern Med.* 2009;169:610-615.
5. Sorensen HT, Riis AH, Diaz LJ, Andersen EW, Baron JA, Andersen PK. Familial risk of venous thromboembolism: a nationwide cohort study. *J Thromb Haemost.* 2011;9:320-324.
6. Kearon C, Ageno W, Cannegieter SC, et al. Categorization of patients as having provoked or unprovoked venous thromboembolism: guidance from the SSC of ISTH. *J Thromb Haemost.* 2016;14:1480-1483.
7. Gould MK, Garcia DA, Wren SM, et al. Prevention of VTE in nonorthopedic surgical patients: Antithrombotic Therapy and Prevention of Thrombosis, 9th ed: American College of Chest Physicians Evidence-Based Clinical Practice Guidelines. *Chest.* 2012;141:e227S-e77S.
8. Garcia D, Erkan D. Diagnosis and management of the antiphospholipid syndrome. *N Engl J Med.* 2018;378:2010-2021.
9. Delluc A, Antic D, Lecumberri R, Ay C, Meyer G, Carrier M. Occult cancer screening in patients with venous thromboembolism: guidance from the SSC of the ISTH. *J Thromb Haemost.* 2017;15:2076-2079.
10. Kamel H. Heart-rhythm monitoring for evaluation of cryptogenic stroke. *N Engl J Med.* 2014;370:2532-2533.
11. Arepally GM. Heparin-induced thrombocytopenia. *Blood.* 2017;129:2864-2872.
12. Boekholdt SM, Kramer MH. Arterial thrombosis and the role of thrombophilia. *Semin Thromb Hemost.* 2007;33:588-596.
13. Blom JW, Doggen CJ, Osanto S, Rosendaal FR. Old and new risk factors for upper extremity deep venous thrombosis. *J Thromb Haemost.* 2005;3:2471-2478.
14. Kearon C, Akl EA, Ornelas J, et al. Antithrombotic therapy for VTE disease: CHEST Guideline and Expert Panel Report. *Chest.* 2016;149:315-352.
15. Kearon C. A conceptual framework for two phases of anticoagulant treatment of venous thromboembolism. *J Thromb Haemost.* 2012;10:507-511.
16. Schulman S. Optimal duration of oral anticoagulant therapy in venous thromboembolism. *Thromb Haemost.* 1997;78:693-698.
17. Vasanthamohan L, Boonyawat K, Chai-Adisaksopha C, Crowther M. Reduced-dose direct oral anticoagulants in the extended treatment of venous thromboembolism: a systematic review and meta-analysis. *J Thromb Haemost.* 2018;16:1288-1295.
18. Pengo V, Denas G, Zoppellaro G, et al. Rivaroxaban vs warfarin in high-risk patients with antiphospholipid syndrome. *Blood.* 2018;132:1365-1371.
19. Shatzel JJ, Crapster-Pregont M, Deloughery TG. Non-vitamin K antagonist oral anticoagulants for heparin-induced thrombocytopenia. A systematic review of 54 reported cases. *Thromb Haemost.* 2016;116:397-400.

Robert J. Beaulieu • Mahmoud B. Malas

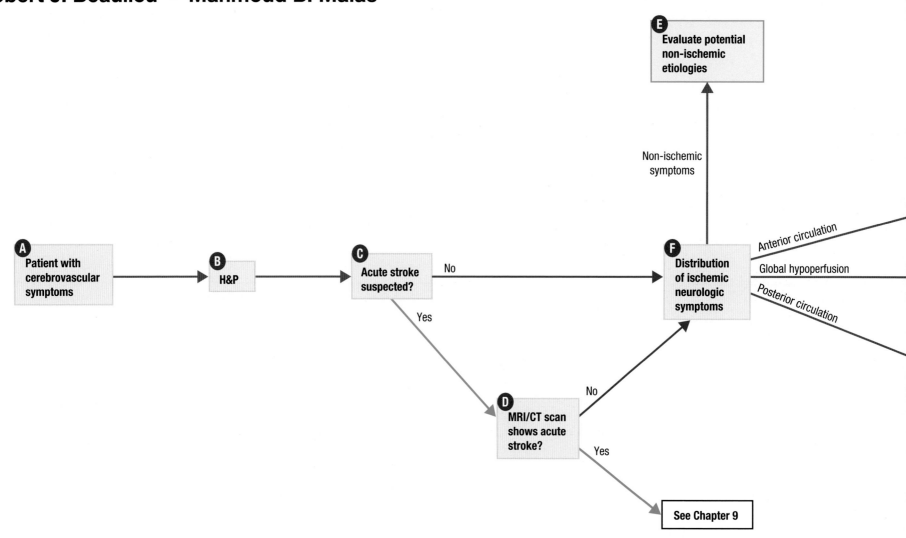

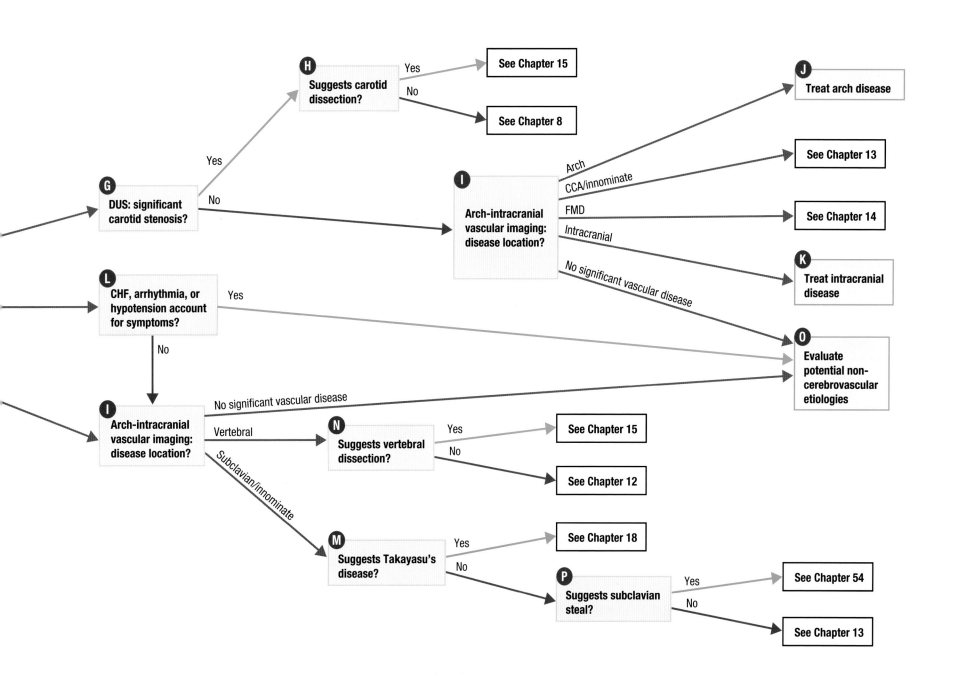

(A) Patient with cerebrovascular symptoms

In 2016, cerebrovascular disease and subsequent stroke accounted for over 140,000 patient deaths per year in the United States, making it the overall fifth leading cause of death.[1] As such, the burden and prevalence of patients with cerebrovascular disease remains daunting and requires a high index of suspicion when approaching patients with a multitude of symptoms.

(B) H&P

A focused history should be elicited from patients complaining of new-onset neurologic symptoms, particularly those that can be attributed to a defined neurovascular distribution. Important elements of the history should include time of onset, previous symptoms, known cerebrovascular disease (such as carotid disease or previous stroke/TIA), and progression of symptoms. Anterior circulation neurologic symptoms include acute-onset motor or sensory loss in upper or lower extremities, dysarthria, word-finding difficulties, amaurosis, and facial droop. Posterior circulation symptoms are more varied and can include dizziness, drop attacks, diplopia, gait disturbance, dysphagia, and bilateral hemianopia. Less frequent symptoms include confusion, global amnesia, syncope, occipital headaches, nausea, vomiting, nystagmus, bilateral facial numbness, cortical blindness, and altered mental status. The physical examination should begin with observation of the face for any facial asymmetry. This can be followed by auscultation of the chest and neck to determine irregular heart beat and cardiac or vascular murmurs. A comprehensive neurologic examination should be performed. This examination should document the patient's mental status to include orientation to person, place, time, and situation. In addition, test of the cranial nerves should be performed to help localize any neurologic deficit.

Once this is completed, the motor strength in each extremity should be assessed for weakness (paralysis, movement against gravity, or movement against resistance). The sensory strength (to both light and deep palpation) in each upper and lower extremity should also be noted. Finally, an examination for cerebellar defects should be completed and includes gait examination, finger-nose-finger testing, and the heel to shin test. After a thorough H&P is completed, imaging modalities that will assist in the specific diagnosis and treatment need to be ordered.

(C) Acute stroke suspected?

Any patient with neurologic symptoms and deficits that have persisted since onset or are progressing should raise concern for acute stroke. Although the distinction between stroke and TIA relies on symptoms lasting longer than 24 hours, this determination cannot often be made at initial evaluation except in select patients who present after this time frame. Patients with presentations concerning for acute stroke, regardless of the 24-hour mark, should immediately undergo brain imaging to allow expedited

progression to thrombolytics, anticoagulants, and stroke-directed therapy.

(D) MRI/CT scan shows acute stroke?

Patients with suspected acute stroke should undergo brain imaging with diffusion-weighted MRI (dwMRI) or noncontrast computed tomography (NCCT). DwMRI is a more sensitive modality to detect acute stroke but is less cost-effective than NCCT, primarily because NCCT allows for rapid diagnosis (compared with dwMRI or delayed NCCT) and avoidance of thrombolytic therapy in patients with hemorrhagic stroke.[2] Brain imaging should be performed within 20 minutes of arrival to the emergency department, because the subsequent treatment with alteplase or thrombectomy is time-sensitive.[2] If acute ischemic or hemorrhagic stroke is detected, management is discussed in Chapter 9. If acute stroke is not detected on initial imaging, further evaluation of the recent neurologic symptoms is performed.

(E) Evaluate potential non-ischemic etiologies

For patients without positive findings for ischemic or hemorrhagic stroke on NCCT or dwMRI, alternative etiologies should be entertained. As many as 5% of the patients admitted because of concern for acute stroke have an alternate diagnosis, with the most common symptoms among this population being aphasia, dizziness, headache, confusion, and dysarthria.[3] In these patients, the most common causes are epileptic seizures and intracranial tumors such as adenomas or metastatic disease, which are at particularly high risk for bleeding and may rapidly develop symptoms mimicking hemorrhagic stroke. Patients presenting with disturbed levels of consciousness can have an infectious etiology, such as meningoencephalitis, causing meningeal irritation. On the basis of the patient characteristics, additional causes can include thyroid storm (particularly in the elderly) or migraines.

(F) Distribution of ischemic neurologic symptoms

In patients with suspected ischemic neurologic symptoms, a thorough evaluation can help localize the neurologic territory affected to focus diagnostic imaging. If after careful evaluation, non-ischemic etiologies are suspected, these should be separately evaluated. For purposes of subsequent evaluation, ischemic symptoms are best categorized as related to the anterior, posterior, or global cerebral circulation.

Anterior circulation symptoms involve higher cerebral dysfunction such as dysphasia, homonymous visual field defect, and motor or sensory defect of the face, arm, or leg. These symptoms arise from infarcts of middle cerebral artery distribution. An additional finding of anterior circulation involvement is amaurosis fugax, or transient monocular blindness, typically described as "curtain coming down" over the affected eye. By far, the most common cause of this symptom is ipsilateral carotid artery atherosclerotic emboli; however, it should be noted that this finding

can be due to a wide variety of vascular diseases, including embolic disease from the heart/heart valves (second most common cause) lacunar infarcts in the deep perforating artery territory[4] hypercoagulable states, Takayasu's arteritis, exercise-induced vasospasm, ophthalmic artery atherosclerosis, and closed-angle glaucoma.[5]

The *posterior circulation* has more variable anatomy than does the anterior circulation but overall corresponds to the area of the brainstem, cerebellum, and occipital lobes. Posterior circulation symptoms include ipsilateral cranial nerve palsies with a contralateral motor or sensory deficit, bilateral motor or sensory deficits, disconjugate eye movement, and ataxia.[4] However, these conclusions should be interpreted in the setting of more recent data as well, which suggests that symptoms, especially those related to the posterior circulation, alone have a low accuracy for localizing neurologic distribution.[6] Homolateral hemiplegia, central face or lingual palsy, and hemisensory deficits represent symptoms associated with both the posterior and anterior circulation. Symptoms and signs that may be more suggestive of a posterior distribution origin include Horner syndrome, crossed motor and sensory deficits (such as ipsilateral motor with contralateral hemiplegia), and oculomotor nerve palsy, all of which only occur in a subset of patients with posterior circulation disease but rarely, if ever, in patients with anterior circulation disease.[6]

Finally, the diagnosis of *global hypoperfusion* should be entertained in patients with poorly localized deficits and symptoms and signs of systemic cardiovascular disease. Symptoms can include worsening dementia, amnesia, alterations in sensorium, and even hemispheric symptoms mimicking a stroke. As such, it is critical to rule out other causes of the neurologic deficit before assigning the diagnosis of global hypoperfusion.

(G) DUS: significant carotid stenosis?

DUS remains the first-line imaging method for identifying clinically significant carotid artery disease (ICA stenosis of 50%-99%) because of its low cost, high accessibility, and comparable sensitivity compared to the "gold standard" of selective DSA.[7] Additional imaging with CTA or MRA is beneficial for identifying patients with 50% to 69% ICA stenosis because the sensitivity of ultrasound in this range falls precipitously, but patients with symptomatic lesions in this range benefit most from early intervention.[7] Consensus guidelines define the anticipated level of stenosis based on DUS characteristics (see Table 6-1).[8] In addition to velocity criteria, recent evidence suggests that plaque morphology has a role in predicting subsequent stroke. The Imaging in Carotid Angioplasty and Risk of Stroke (ICAROS) study examined the impact of preoperative DUS findings on the ability to predict periprocedural stroke in patients undergoing carotid intervention. It used gray-scale median as a measure of plaque echolucency on B-mode images to define an "unstable carotid plaque" as one with a gray-scale median of 25 or less, which was found

Table 6-1. Consensus Guidelines for Grading Severity of Carotid Stenosis Based on DUS Findings

Degree of Stenosis (%)	Primary Parameters		Additional Parameters	
	ICA PSV (cm/s)	Plaque Estimate (%)[a]	ICA/CCA PSV Ratio	ICA EDV (cm/s)
Normal	<125	None	<2.0	<40
<50	<125	<50	<2.0	<40
50-69	125-230	≥50	2.0-4.0	40-100
≥70 but less than near occlusion	>230	≥50	>4.0	>100
Near occlusion	High, low, or undetectable	Visible	Variable	Variable
Total occlusion	Undetectable	Visible, no detectable lumen	Not applicable	Not applicable

[a]Plaque estimate (diameter reduction) with gray-scale and color Doppler ultrasound.
CCA, common carotid artery; DUS, Doppler ultrasound; ICA, internal carotid artery; PSV, peak systolic velocity.
Reprinted with permissions from Grant EG, Benson CB, Moneta GL, et al. Carotid artery stenosis: gray-scale and Doppler US diagnosis—Society of Radiologists in Ultrasound Consensus Conference. *Radiology*. 2003;229:340-346.

to be independently predictive of stroke.[9] Although the ICAROS study examined periprocedural patients, it confirmed the findings of earlier literature showing a high preponderance of echolucent plaques among symptomatic patients with <70% ICA stenosis, suggesting the benefit of incorporating plaque morphology into both screening and procedural planning DUS reports.[10] A recent consensus statement from the American Society of Neuroradiology highlights the ability of DUS to identify several additional factors associated with a vulnerable plaque, including luminal morphology, ulcerations, neovascularization, and inflammation.[11] However, the statement further emphasizes the low sensitivity of DUS to detect some features of vulnerable plaque, such as intraplaque hemorrhage and the status of the fibrous cap.[11] If these latter features become better established as valuable for plaque scoring systems, additional imaging studies such as CTA or MRI may be required to obtain this information.

Although DUS provides information about the presence and direction of flow in the vertebral arteries, it is neither sensitive nor specific enough to accurately diagnose or exclude significant vertebral artery lesions. In the setting of patients with suspected vertebrobasilar disease, DUS helps establish the presence of concomitant carotid disease or reversed vertebral flow.

H Suggests carotid dissection?

The use of DUS for the detection of carotid artery dissection is limited because dissections usually involve the distal ICA, which may not be visualized with DUS. Indirect DUS findings such as a minimally diseased carotid bulb despite absent or reduced ICA flow or high-resistance waveforms in the proximal ICA may suggest the presence of an ICA dissection.[12] For practitioners adept at DUS and transcranial Doppler, detection rates for carotid

dissection with complete occlusion can approach 100%.[12] However, DSA remains the "gold standard" for detection of carotid artery dissection, with MRA and CTA becoming increasingly popular methods of noninvasive imaging that allow for better determination of flap characteristics and delineation of extravascular anatomy.

I Arch-intracranial vascular imaging: disease location?

DUS may provide insight into disease anatomy even when the carotid artery is not involved. Indeed, it is well suited to *rule out* the presence of clinically significant carotid artery disease if there is question about the disease localization based on symptoms. In the presence of anterior cerebrovascular symptoms without carotid artery disease, or in the presence of posterior cerebrovascular symptoms, additional imaging such as CTA or MRA of the arch, arch vessels, neck, and intracranial arteries should be obtained. In addition to arch and intracranial disease, arch vessel disease, carotid FMD (Chapter 14), Takayasu's disease (Chapter 18), and vertebral artery disease (Chapters 12 and 15) may be identified, and their management is discussed in other chapters as referenced. If no significant vascular disease is detected on additional imaging, potential nonvascular etiologies should be evaluated.

CTA is often employed for imaging the aortic arch, especially because noncontrast CT may underestimate the quantity of noncalcified atherosclerosis.[13] If calcifications are incidentally imaged as part of a coronary CT scan, dedicated imaging of the thoracic aorta should be performed because nearly 60% of calcifications may be within the arch and proximal descending aorta, segments not well visualized on coronary CT.[13] MRA has also demonstrated high sensitivity and high interobserver agreement for aortic arch disease.[14] When conducting MRA of the arch, sensitivity is

significantly increased by breath holding, which also allows for lower doses of contrast administration.[15] Transesophageal ECHO (TEE) can be used to evaluate for thoracic aortic source of neurovascular symptoms, particularly through the identification of thoracic aortic calcifications or atheromas. There are strong correlations between protruding arch atheromas (>4 mm) and risk of stroke from a noncarotid cause.[16]

Multiple forms of intracranial vascular abnormalities can lead to neurologic deficits, and a wide array of imaging modalities can be employed to characterize these lesions. DSA remains the gold standard for evaluation of intracranial disease. However, it is associated with several limitations including need for contrast, risk of periprocedural stroke, and access site complications. Most physicians use less invasive CTA or MRA first to evaluate intracranial arterial disease. Transcranial Doppler (TCD) can also detect intracerebral vascular disease, including occlusions or stenoses in middle cerebral artery distributions as well as increases in the pulsatility index and presence of microembolizations; however, insonation through the transtemporal window may not be possible in up to 15% of patients.[17] Brain CTA is especially useful for the identification of intracranial vascular anatomic variants and abnormalities, including AVM, cavernous malformations, aneurysms, and venous malformations.[18] Comparison of CTA with DSA has demonstrated superior sensitivity of CTA for intracranial aneurysm, with CTA affording the additional benefits of identifying mural thrombus and calcifications.[19] MRA is also employed for the identification of intracranial lesions. Compared with MRA and DSA, CTA has increased sensitivity and positive-predictive value for the detection of intracranial stenosis and occlusion.[20] It should be noted that with improved MRI protocols, particularly the MR intracranial vessel wall (IVW) imaging protocols, characteristics of intracranial vascular walls can be evaluated, making this a useful modality to evaluate for intracranial vasculopathy and vasculitis.[21]

J Treat arch disease

Management of the neurovascular sequelae of thoracic aortic disease is based on the location and nature of underlying disease. In particular, acute aortic syndromes, such as intramural hematoma, penetrating aortic ulcer, dissection, and rupture, have a complex management strategy that incorporates aggressive blood pressure control with emergent surgical management, especially in the setting of ascending aortic disease. Acute aortic syndrome resulting in neurologic dysfunction may demonstrate progression of the disease into the proximal carotid or innominate arteries, or may be the result of systemic hypotension resulting from hemorrhagic shock. Aortic atheromas >4 mm have demonstrated an increased risk of subsequent stroke.[16] Various treatment strategies have been suggested once an atheroma is identified, yet the overall treatment algorithm remains controversial. The Aortic Arch-Related

Cerebral Hazard trial attempted to evaluate the effectiveness of anticoagulation with warfarin versus dual antiplatelet therapy with aspirin and clopidogrel in the management of patients with cerebrovascular symptoms, an aortic atheroma >4 mm thick, and no other identifiable source of the disease.[22] Although there were "trends" toward improved outcome with dual antiplatelet therapy for the primary combined end point of cerebral infarction, MI, peripheral embolism, vascular death, or intracranial hemorrhage (7.6% vs. 11.3%, $P = 0.2$), the trial was underpowered to detect a difference and therefore was not able to guide management.[22] Retrospective trials appear to support the use of statins for their plaque stabilization properties in these patients.[23] Atherosclerotic disease of the supra-aortic trunks may warrant intervention to prevent embolization, in particular when disease involves the innominate, left CCA, or vertebral arteries. Historically, extra-anatomic bypass replaced direct open repair for patients with atherosclerotic lesions in this area because of the high operative morbidity and mortality associated with direct repair. More recently, endovascular management with stenting has become widely accepted because of its efficacy, safety, and long-term results.[24] Owing to the potential risk of distal embolization associated with the procedure, some advocate for the use of embolic protection devices, although further studies are necessary to evaluate the utility of this strategy.

K Treat intracranial disease

There are multiple pathologies that account for intracranial disease as a source of neurovascular symptoms. As previously mentioned, there are intracranial arterial and venous abnormalities that can result in cerebrovascular symptoms, including AVMs, aneurysms, and venous fistulae.[18] The anterior circulation is the most common site for intracerebral aneurysmal degeneration, which is the most common acquired cause of subarachnoid hemorrhage (SAH).[19] When diagnosed, clinicians must assess the risk of rupture, which seems most highly correlated with aneurysm location and size at the time of diagnosis. For patients presenting with unruptured aneurysm, surgical clipping is associated with the lowest risk of recurrence compared with endovascular coiling, but carries a higher morbidity and mortality.[19] The role of flow diversion devices (stents) remains controversial, although they may be employed in selected patients.

Intracranial atherosclerotic disease is another important cause of cerebrovascular symptoms. Diabetes, HTN, and hyperlipidemia all contribute to an increased risk of disease. The risk of intracranial atherosclerotic disease appears to be highest among African American, Asian, and Hispanic populations compared with that in Caucasian populations.[25] The rate of stroke in the subsequent 2 years after diagnosis in patients with >50% luminal stenosis can approximate 20%, with worse collateral circulation being the largest predictor of developing cerebral ischemia.[25] Patients should be counseled on smoking cessation, blood sugar

control, and management of HTN. On the basis of randomized control data, anticoagulation with aspirin has similar stroke rates compared to warfarin, although warfarin is associated with a higher risk of major hemorrhage and MI.[25] Both surgical bypass and endovascular management strategies are available, although trials have not proved a benefit compared to maximal medical management. Although there is an increased risk of stroke with luminal narrowing above 50%, it is unclear whether newer technologies will be beneficial in the asymptomatic population. In symptomatic patients (ie, those with TIA or stroke within 30 days), results from the Stenting versus Aggressive Medical Management for Preventing Recurrent Stroke in Intracranial Stenosis (SAMMPRIS) trial failed to demonstrate a benefit of endovascular therapy compared with aggressive medical management (dual antiplatelet therapy with clopidogrel and aspirin, lifestyle interventions, statin therapy, and goal-directed antihypertensive management) alone, and was actually stopped early because of the much higher rates of ischemic stroke or death in 30 days after stenting compared with patients managed medically (14.7% vs. 5.8%).[26]

A potential, but uncommon, cause of neurovascular symptoms can be intracranial arterial dissection.[27] Intracranial dissections appear to be more common among patients of Asian descent, where as many as 70% of all cervicocephalic arterial dissections occur in the intracranial arteries. In adults, intracranial dissections appear to more commonly affect the posterior circulation (intradural [V4] portion of the vertebral artery) as opposed to the anterior circulation, although the opposite may be true for children.[27] Treatment of intracranial dissections is based on retrospective reports and anecdotal evidence, but follow the general pattern of managing SAH with surgical (open or endovascular) methods to reduce the risk of rebleeding and employing antithrombotic therapy for the management of dissections associated with cerebral ischemia.[27]

L CHF, arrhythmia, or hypotension account for symptoms?

Global hypoperfusion, or "misery" perfusion, results from a state of decreased cerebral blood flow during which compensatory mechanisms fail to keep up with the cerebral oxygen demand. In the setting of decreased cerebral blood flow, the cerebral vasculature vasodilates to compensate. In addition, oxygen extraction increases to compensate for the overall lower flow rate. However, as a persistent hypoperfusion state continues, cognitive decline and neurologic deficits can develop.[28] Chronic hypoxia and impaired neurovascular signaling can result in impaired response to stimulation in the affected cortex.[28] This can result in symptoms of neurologic deficit on its own, but also portends an increased risk of subsequent stroke.[29] Multiple cardiovascular comorbidities may be associated with hypoperfusion including CHF, cardiac arrhythmias, and valvular disease (severe aortic valve stenosis and mitral valve annular stenosis). Patients

presenting in cardiogenic, hypovolemic, or septic shock may, in addition, present with neurovascular symptoms due to global hypoperfusion. The patient's clinical picture and associated history, including premorbid conditions that increase cardiovascular risk such as diabetes, HTN, hyperlipidemia, and tobacco use, will help identify the potential risk for hypoperfusion. In the setting of cerebrovascular symptoms, however, dedicated arch and intracranial imaging should be performed to rule out a primary lesion in these distributions.

M Suggests Takayasu's disease?

The diagnosis of Takayasu's arteritis involves demonstrating criteria from three clinical categories: history, physical examination, and laboratory/radiologic analysis.[30] Among the radiographic evidence of the disease includes arteriographic narrowing or occlusion of the entire aorta, its primary branches, or large arteries in the proximal upper and lower extremities not due to atherosclerosis or FMD.[30] These findings may result from a combination of carotid DUS, CTA, or MRA, with the recent use of PET scan being used to evaluate for inflammation, as well (see Chapter 18).

N Suggests vertebral dissection?

Because of the multiple intraosseous segments of the vertebral artery, DUS has limitations with the ability to diagnose vertebral artery stenosis or dissection. In this case, MRA or CTA is better suited for identifying vertebral disease and has the added benefit of being able to delineate extra-arterial anatomy, such as osteophytic lesions from the cervical spine, that may be contributing to dissection or stenosis. Patients undergoing MRI/MRA may have the added benefit of helping to determine chronicity of any associated intracranial infarcts (see Chapters 12 and 15 for discussion of vertebral artery occlusive disease and dissection, respectively).

O Evaluate potential non-cerebrovascular etiologies

If cerebrovascular disease potentially responsible for symptoms is not identified on imaging, other etiologies should be investigated. Cardiac evaluation (ECG, ECHO) should be performed to identify a potential cardiac embolic source for cerebrovascular symptoms, including the potential for paradoxic embolization of venous thrombus through a patent foramen ovale. Other potential etiologies include a hypercoagulable state resulting in arterial occlusion, intracranial tumor or aneurysm, AVM, and cerebral venous sinus thrombosis. Migraine aura or postictal symptoms following a seizure may also mimic hemispheric symptoms. Neurologic consultation should be obtained, and other etiologies treated, if found.

P Suggests subclavian steal?

Posterior neurologic symptoms can result from SCA stenosis proximal to the vertebral artery origin, which can result in "steal" of blood from the opposite vertebral artery to increase arm blood flow, while reducing basilar artery flow. In such cases, there will be a resting pressure gradient in the affected side, which is more often the left side, because of its greater propensity for subclavian atherosclerosis. This syndrome is called subclavian steal and is always associated with reversed flow in the ipsilateral vertebral artery. However, reversed or to-and-fro vertebral flow is often not associated with symptoms. When posterior cerebrovascular symptoms accompany reversed vertebral flow and subclavian stenosis, treatment is indicated. See Chapter 54 for more details. If a patient has posterior cerebrovascular symptoms accompanied by innominate or subclavian atherosclerotic disease without reversed vertebral artery flow, these lesions can be a source of atheroembolism that requires treatment. See Chapter 13 for more details.

REFERENCES

1. Murphy SL, Xu J, Kochanek KD, Curtin SC, Arias E. National vital statistics reports November 27, 2017. *Natl Vital Stat Reports*. 2015;66(6):1-75.
2. Powers WJ, Rabinstein AA, Ackerson T, et al. 2018 Guidelines for the early management of patients with acute ischemic stroke: a guideline for healthcare professionals from the American Heart Association/American Stroke Association. *Stroke*. 2018;49:e46-e110.
3. Hatzitolios A, Savopoulos C, Ntaios G, et al. Stroke and conditions that mimic it: a protocol secures a safe early recognition. *Hippokratia*. 2008;12:98-102.
4. Bamford J, Sandercock P, Dennis M, Burn J, Warlow C. Classification and natural history of clinically identifiable subtypes of cerebral infarction. *Lancet*. 1991;337:1521-1526.
5. Hayreh SS. Acute retinal arterial occlusive disorders. *Prog Retin Eye Res*. 2011;30:359-394.
6. Tao WD, Liu M, Fisher M, et al. Posterior versus anterior circulation infarction how different are the neurological deficits? *Stroke*. 2012;43:2060-2065. doi:10.1161/STROKEAHA.112.652420
7. Wardlaw JM, Chappell FM, Stevenson M, et al. Accurate, practical and cost-effective assessment of carotid stenosis in the UK. *Health Technol Assess*. 2006;10:iii-iv, ix-x, 1-182.
8. Grant EG, Benson CB, Moneta GL, et al. Carotid artery stenosis: gray-scale and Doppler US diagnosis—Society of Radiologists in Ultrasound Consensus Conference. *Radiology*. 2003;229:340-346.
9. Biasi GM, Froio A, Diethrich EB, et al. Carotid plaque echolucency increases the risk of stroke in carotid stenting: the Imaging in Carotid Angioplasty and Risk of Stroke (ICAROS) Study. *Circulation*. 2004;110:756-762.
10. Geroulakos G, Ramaswami G, Nicolaides A, et al. Characterization of symptomatic and asymptomatic carotid plaques using high-resolution real-time ultrasonography. *Br J Surg*. 1993;80:1274-1277.
11. Saba L, Yuan C, Hatsukami TS, et al. Carotid artery wall imaging: perspective and guidelines from the ASNR Vessel Wall Imaging Study Group and Expert Consensus Recommendations of the American Society of Neuroradiology. *AJNR Am J Neuroradiol*. 2018;39:E9-E31.
12. Sturzenegger M, Mattle HP, Rivoir A, Baumgartner RW. Ultrasound findings in carotid artery dissection: analysis of 43 patients. *Neurology*. 1995;45:691-698.
13. Desai MY, Cremer PC, Schoenhagen P. Thoracic aortic calcification. *JACC Cardiovasc Imaging*. 2018;11:1012-1026.
14. Carpenter JP, Holland GA, Golden MA, et al. Magnetic resonance angiography of the aortic arch. *J Vasc Surg*. 1997;25:145-151.
15. Krinsky GA, Reuss PM, Lee VS, Carbognin G, Rofsky NM. Thoracic aorta: comparison of single-dose breath-hold and double-dose non-breath-hold gadolinium-enhanced three-dimensional MR angiography. *Am J Roentgenol*. 1999;173:145-150.
16. Amarenco P, Cohen A, Tzourio C, et al. Atherosclerotic disease of the aortic arch and the risk of ischemic stroke. *N Engl J Med*. 1994;331:1474-1479.
17. Alexandrov AV, Demchuk AM, Wein TH, Grotta JC. Yield of transcranial Doppler in acute cerebral ischemia. *Stroke*. 1999;30:1604-1609.
18. Pérez-Carrillo GJ, Hogg JP. Intracranial vascular lesions and anatomical variants all residents should know. *Curr Probl Diagn Radiol*. 2010;39:91-109.
19. Thompson BG, Brown RD Jr, Amin-Hanjani S, et al. Guidelines for the management of patients with unruptured intracranial aneurysms: a guideline for healthcare professionals from the American Heart Association/American Stroke Association. *Stroke*. 2015;46:2368-2400.
20. Bash S, Villablanca JP, Jahan R, et al. Intracranial vascular stenosis and occlusive disease: evaluation with CT angiography, MR angiography, and digital subtraction angiography. *AJNR Am J Neuroradiol*. 2005;26:1012-1021.
21. Alexander MD, Yuan C, Rutman A, et al. High-resolution intracranial vessel wall imaging: imaging beyond the lumen. *J Neurol Neurosurg Psychiatry*. 2016;87:589-597.
22. Amarenco P, Davis S, Jones EF, et al. Clopidogrel plus aspirin versus warfarin in patients with stroke and aortic arch plaques. *Stroke*. 2014;45:1248-1257.
23. Vizzardi E, Gelsomino S, D'Aloia A, Lorusso R. Aortic atheromas and stroke: review of literature. *J Investig Med*. 2013;61:956-966.
24. Peterson BG, Resnick SA, Morasch MD, Hassoun HT, Eskandari MK. Aortic arch vessel stenting. *Arch Surg*. 2006;141:560.
25. Lenart CJ, Binning MJ, Veznedaroglu E. Endovascular treatment of intracranial atherosclerotic disease. *Neuroimaging Clin N Am*. 2013;23:653-659.
26. Derdeyn CP, Chimowitz MI, Lynn MJ, et al. Aggressive medical treatment with or without stenting in high-risk patients with intracranial artery stenosis (SAMMPRIS): the final results of a randomised trial. *Lancet*. 2014;383:333-341.
27. Debette S, Compter A, Labeyrie MA, et al. Epidemiology, pathophysiology, diagnosis, and management of intracranial artery dissection. *Lancet Neurol*. 2015;14:640-654.
28. Nishino A, Tajima Y, Takuwa H, et al. Long-term effects of cerebral hypoperfusion on neural density and function using misery perfusion animal model. *Sci Rep*. 2016;6:25072.
29. Yamauchi H, Higashi T, Kagawa S, et al. Is misery perfusion still a predictor of stroke in symptomatic major cerebral artery disease? *Brain*. 2012;135:2515-2526.
30. Arend WP, Michel BA, Bloch DA, et al. The American College of Rheumatology 1990 criteria for the classification of takayasu arteritis. *Arthritis Rheum*. 2010;33:1129-1134.

Laura T. Boitano • Mark F. Conrad

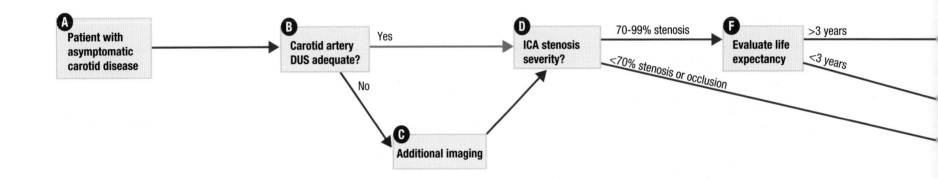

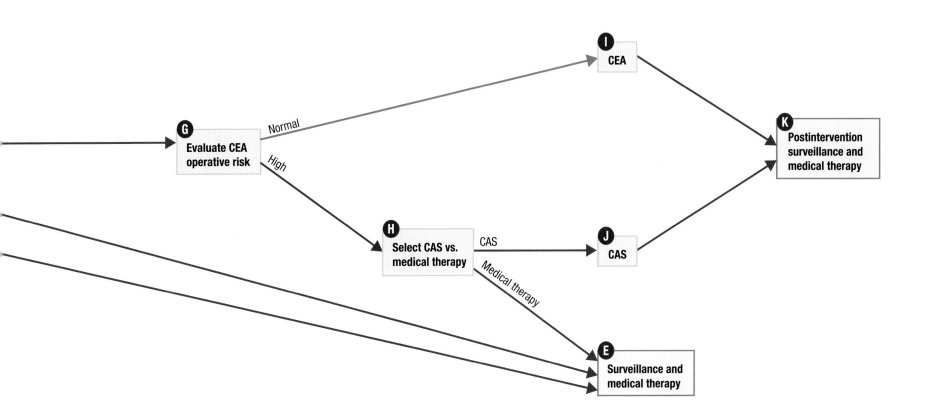

A Patient with asymptomatic carotid disease

Neurologically asymptomatic patients who are at increased risk for carotid artery stenosis sometimes undergo screening with DUS.[1,2] Factors that increase the risk of asymptomatic carotid stenosis include symptomatic PAD and age ≥65 years with a history of CAD, cigarette smoking, or hypercholesterolemia.[1,2] Although the prevalence of carotid artery stenosis in the general population is low (0.5%-1%), reports suggest that it is much higher in those with risk factors.[3,4] A study evaluating the prevalence of carotid artery stenosis reported 12.5% of patients with HTN and 18.2% with heart disease had >50% ICA stenosis.[3] Prevalence also increases with age; an analysis of patients undergoing DUS screening for vascular disease reported 11% of men over age 80 years had >50% carotid artery stenosis versus 0.9% in men 40 to 50 years of age. Prevalence was slightly lower in women but still increased with age: 7.8% in women >80 years versus 0.8% in those 40 to 50 years old.[4] Patients with multiple risk factors may be candidates for DUS screening, but most guidelines agree that routine screening is not recommended for the general population because it is not cost-effective in reducing the risk of stroke.[1,2] Detection of a carotid bruit has been suggested as an indication for DUS, but the Society for Vascular Surgery (SVS) guidelines recommend against this.[1] This chapter focuses on ICA and carotid bulb atherosclerosis (see Chapter 13 for CCA disease).

B Carotid artery DUS adequate?

DUS is the noninvasive modality of choice for initial imaging of the carotid artery.[1,5,6] This type of imaging should be conducted in an accredited vascular laboratory because there is variability in technique.[1] The sensitivity and specificity for detecting 70% to 99% ICA stenosis using DUS are 89% and 84%, respectively.[5] DUS alone can be utilized for preoperative imaging, and when only one imaging modality is utilized, DUS is the one most commonly selected.[7] Limitations of DUS include dependence on the sonographer's technique, limited visualization of the proximal and intracranial carotid artery, difficulty distinguishing between 99% stenosis and complete occlusion, and inability to insonate a severely calcified artery.[1,2] Should there be any concern about the adequacy of imaging or inflow/outflow issues identified on the DUS, additional imaging is recommended.

C Additional imaging

Three main options exist for additional carotid artery imaging to clarify DUS findings, each of which has its own advantages and disadvantages. DSA is still described as the gold standard for the evaluation of carotid artery stenosis, but owing to the cost, invasive nature, and associated risks (especially risk of stroke), its use is usually reserved for cases with conflicting imaging before CEA or as part of a CAS procedure.[1,2,6] MRA can visualize proximal

and intracranial lesions that are not visualized in DUS; however, it has a limited ability to identify calcium within plaque and tends to overestimate the degree of stenosis in highly calcified lesions.[1] CTA can visualize both intrathoracic and intracranial lesions, and compared with MRA is better at assessing the degree of stenosis, is less expensive, and can visualize calcification. However, CTA is inferior to both MRA and DUS in categorizing plaque morphology.[1,6] Axial imaging may identify lesions in the proximal CCA or innominate artery (see Chapter 13 for management of such lesions).

D ICA stenosis severity?

It is difficult for DUS to differentiate the degree of stenosis when a carotid lesion has <50% diameter reduction because there is no hemodynamic significance, so most vascular laboratories report these patients as simply <50%. More severe stenoses are differentiated using a combination of B-mode and color flow Doppler velocity measurements and are stratified into moderate stenosis (50%-69%), severe stenosis (70%-99%), and arterial occlusion (see Chapter 6 for details of DUS criteria for different degrees of carotid stenosis). CTA and MRA can also be used to estimate the degree of stenosis. ICA stenosis is expressed as the narrowest diameter of the stenosis divided by the distal normal ICA lumen diameter (referred to as the NASCET method).

<50% ICA stenosis

Asymptomatic patients with <50% diameter reduction of their ICA are at low risk for developing TIA or stroke. A natural history study of patients with mild carotid artery stenosis (<50%) found the risk of stroke was <0.5% per year in those who did not progress.[8] These patients should be treated medically with risk factor modification.

50% to 69% ICA stenosis

Although the Asymptomatic Carotid Atherosclerosis Study (ACAS) and the Asymptomatic Carotid Surgery Trial (ACST-1) demonstrated an advantage of CEA over best medical therapy in the prevention of stroke for patients with a 60% or greater stenosis, most surgeons reserve intervention for asymptomatic plaques with 70% to 99% stenosis. Recently, in patients with <70% stenosis, best medical therapy has shown good outcomes, comparable to CEA.[1,9-12] Patients with an asymptomatic moderate stenosis should undergo continued surveillance with DUS because these patients are at risk for progression and development of neurologic symptoms. This was further exemplified by a contemporary analysis of 900 patients with asymptomatic, moderate stenosis that found that optimal medical therapy was unable to halt progression from moderate to severe stenosis or the development of neurologic symptoms in 45% of patients.[13] In addition, a study of 523 subjects with asymptomatic, moderate (50%-69%) carotid artery stenosis found that stenosis progression was a significant

predictor of vascular events (hazard ratio 22). Among those with progressive carotid stenosis, 54% experienced a vascular event and 27% experienced an ipsilateral stroke during a median period of follow-up of 42 months.[14] Mansour et al. reported the natural history of patients with moderate asymptomatic stenosis followed for a 6-year period; disease progression occurred in 16% of patients and of those who progressed to severe stenosis or occlusion, the ipsilateral stroke rate was 38%.[15]

70% to 99% ICA stenosis

Patients with a 70% to 99% ICA stenosis should be evaluated for potential prophylactic CEA or CAS.[1,2] This is supported by two large-scale randomized controlled trials, ACAS and ACST-1, which compared CEA with optimal medical therapy.[9,10] The ACAS trial demonstrated that in patients with ≥60% asymptomatic carotid artery stenosis, CEA was associated with an aggregate risk reduction over 5 years of 53% for ipsilateral stroke and any perioperative stroke or death.[10] The ACST-1 demonstrated in asymptomatic patients <75 years old with ≥60% stenosis that immediate CEA reduces the 10-year risk of stroke (10.8% vs. 16.9%, $P = 0.0004$) when compared with deferred CEA and does not significantly increase perioperative morbidity or mortality.[9] Critics of these trials suggest that the medical arms do not hold up to modern-day standards, and advances in medical therapy, namely, statins, have reduced the risk of stroke such that CEA is not indicated for asymptomatic patients.[12] However, in the later years of the ACST trial, 80% of patients were on statin therapy, and CEA was found to significantly protect from stroke in such patients.[9] Furthermore, Conrad et al. studied 126 carotid arteries with severe asymptomatic stenosis and found that 25% developed ipsilateral neurologic symptoms with a mean follow-up of 27 months; 74% of these patients developed symptoms in the first 12 months after the initial DUS.[16] Thus, current recommendations support CEA for severe asymptomatic carotid artery stenosis and the results of contemporary series are in agreement with this.[1,13,16] Currently, the carotid revascularization for primary prevention of stroke (CREST-2) trial is underway to evaluate both CEA and CAS versus optimal medical therapy in the modern era.[17] In the United States, CEA is the current standard of care in these patients, because the benefit of CAS is not as clear (see H).[1,2]

ICA occlusion

The management of asymptomatic ICA occlusion includes risk factor modification with optimal medical therapy. Current practice guidelines do not recommend operative intervention because of high stroke risk with the procedure.[2,18] A recent systematic review evaluated 13 studies of 718 patients with asymptomatic ICA occlusion and found that the annual rate of ipsilateral stroke was 1.3%.[19] Such patients should undergo DUS to evaluate the contralateral carotid artery for stenosis. Acute stroke in the setting of ICA occlusion is related to low flow, intracranial embolization from the occluded ICA, intracranial clot propagation, or embolization from the ICA stump through collateral vessels.[18] Such symptomatic occlusion increases the future risk of stroke and select patients may benefit from external carotid endarterectomy with ligation of the ICA.[18] Some recommend anticoagulation to prevent distal thrombus propagation after ICA occlusion; however, there is no clear data to support this. When ICA occlusion is found on DUS, a confirmatory CTA should be considered (see C).

E Surveillance and medical therapy

Although the current standard by which carotid intervention is recommended is largely based on the degree of stenosis (and stenosis progression), further studies will likely elucidate the role of plaque characteristics on development of neurologic symptoms.[1,2] The asymptomatic internal carotid artery stenosis and cerebrovascular risk stratification (ACSRS) followed asymptomatic patients with ICA stenosis between 50% and 99% on DUS. This study demonstrated that plaque characteristics significantly improved the ability to predict ipsilateral neurologic events when added to a model with degree of stenosis and clinical characteristics.[20] Such plaque features include low gray-scale median, plaque area, and the presence of discrete white areas without acoustic shadowing on DUS. Furthermore, clinically silent emboli seen on CT or MRI in asymptomatic patients have been associated with a higher rate of neurologic events.[21] There are additional characteristics that may be associated with an increased risk of stroke. Contralateral ICA occlusion may be associated with increased risk of stroke (both contralateral and ipsilateral events).[22]

Asymptomatic patients with ICA stenosis who do not meet the criteria for revascularization are at risk for disease progression and thus require routine surveillance with DUS. A greater degree of ICA stenosis is associated with higher risk of disease progression and neurologic events.[16] In a study evaluating patients with asymptomatic stenosis of <60%, 1.8% of patients with mild stenosis and peak systolic velocity (PSV) <175 cm/s progressed to ≥60% stenosis versus 31% of those with PSV >175 cm/s.[23] Furthermore, Bertges et al. conducted a natural history study of asymptomatic carotid arteries and found that progression of carotid artery stenosis was a significant predictor of neurologic events. The effect of progression was more important than baseline stenosis.[24]

We recommend patients with moderate stenosis to be followed with DUS every 6 to 12 months to evaluate for potential disease progression. This recommendation is predicated on the stability of the lesion and the number of years that the patient has been followed. In those with <50% ICA stenosis, annual DUS imaging is adequate, and if DUS has been stable over several years and the degree of stenosis remains <50%, the time interval between DUS can be spaced out to every 2 years. DUS should always include evaluation of the contralateral carotid artery.

Optimal medical therapy is an integral aspect of treating patients with ICA stenosis and is aimed at reducing the risk of stroke and cardiovascular events.[1,2] Management is directed toward the treatment of risk factors, including HTN, diabetes, lipid disorders, and lifestyle modifications, especially smoking cessation.[1,2,13] HTN is an independent risk factor for stroke and has been associated with the development of carotid atherosclerosis.[25] Target blood pressure is <140/90 mm Hg.[1,2] Among patients with carotid artery stenosis, elevated fasting glucose is associated with increased stroke risk. Target hemoglobin A_{1C} should be <7%; however, there is no evidence that tighter glucose control is beneficial in preventing stroke.[1,2] Patients with dyslipidemia should be treated with lipid-lowering therapy to reduce the risk of stroke and cardiovascular events. Statins are the first-line therapy because they have both lipid-lowering and anti-inflammatory properties.[1,2] Tobacco cessation is paramount to stroke prevention, and counseling has been shown to reduce smoking by 10% to 20%.[1,2,13] Although antiplatelet agents have not been associated with primary stroke prevention, antiplatelet therapy (eg, aspirin) is recommended in asymptomatic patients to prevent cardiovascular morbidity and mortality.[1,2]

F Evaluate life expectancy

An evaluation of a patient's life expectancy is an important aspect of determining the appropriateness of CEA or CAS in patients with asymptomatic carotid artery stenosis.[26] In the ACAS trial, the benefit of CEA overcame the initial perioperative risk at 3 years after surgery.[10] In accordance with this, the SVS guidelines recommend CEA only in patients with at least 3-year life expectancy.[1] Conrad et al. created a validated scoring system to predict 5-year survival after CEA and included age (by decade), CAD, statin use, diabetes, neck radiation, COPD, and creatinine >1.5.[26] Scoring was as follows: age < 50 years (0 points), 50 to 59 years (2 points), 60 to 69 years (4 points), 70 to 79 years (6 points), 80 to 89 years (8 points), >90 years (10 points), CAD (2 points), no statin (2 points), diabetes (2 points), neck radiation (3 points), COPD (3 points), and creatinine >1.5 (3 points). The authors concluded that patients with 0 to 8 points are excellent candidates for CEA (>83% 5-year survival), whereas patients with ≥12 points (46% survival) should be managed medically. A recent report from Goodney et al. evaluated the outcomes of CEA in patients with life-limiting conditions.[27] In this study, life-limiting conditions included ASA IV, DNR status, age ≥90 years, disseminated cancer, advanced liver disease, symptomatic CHF, dialysis dependence, and severe COPD. These patients accounted for 20% of the CEAs and were associated with higher perioperative morbidity and mortality. In addition, the 3-year predicted mortality in patients with these conditions ranged from 37% in severe COPD to 76% with disseminated cancer. Because the outcomes of CEA and CAS are similar in asymptomatic patients, a similar argument

is applied to CAS, namely that patients with life expectancy <3 years should be managed medically.

G Evaluate CEA operative risk

CEA is recommended in asymptomatic patients if the predicted combined stroke and death rate is <3%.[1] High-risk criteria for CEA are based on randomized controlled trial exclusion criteria and are divided into those that are physiologic and anatomic. Physiologic criteria include clinically significant cardiac disease (CHF, abnormal stress test or need for open-heart surgery) and severe pulmonary disease.[28] Anatomic high-risk criteria include contralateral carotid occlusion, contralateral laryngeal-nerve palsy, previous radical neck surgery or radiation therapy to the neck, and recurrent stenosis after CEA. Furthermore, the Centers for Medicare and Medicaid Services (CMS) have adopted these high-risk criteria as requirements for reimbursement for CAS in asymptomatic patients with ≥80% stenosis who are enrolled in clinical trials.[29] It should be noted that these high-risk criteria have never been evaluated prospectively. A review of CEAs performed for asymptomatic patients found female gender, age >75 years, CHF, and combined carotid-coronary artery surgery to be associated with increased perioperative stroke and death.[30] In asymptomatic patients, it is reasonable to consider CAS if high-risk factors for CEA are present.[1]

H Select CAS vs. medical therapy

Asymptomatic patients with severe ICA stenosis deemed too high risk for CEA should be considered for CAS or primary medical management.[1] Recent data comparing outcomes of CEA versus CAS in comparable medical risk patients found normal- and high-risk asymptomatic patients to have comparable outcomes following CEA or CAS.[31] Specifically, in-hospital stroke or death rates were 0.7% with CEA and 1.1% with CAS among the normal-risk cohort and 1.2% (CEA) versus 1.6% (CAS) in the high-risk cohort. Currently, for asymptomatic patients with ICA stenosis, CAS is recommended if the patient is part of a clinical trial; it is otherwise not recommended or reimbursed by CMS.[1,29] Transcarotid artery revascularization (TCAR) is an alternative to transfemoral CAS. TCAR incorporates direct access of the CCA and utilizes a reversal of flow technique to prevent emboli to the brain during the procedure. TCAR is indicated in asymptomatic patients at high risk for CEA and with ≥80% stenosis. Kashyap et al. compared TCAR with CEA and found similar 30-day stroke rates (2.4% CEA vs. 1.8% TCAR).[32] As of September 2016, reimbursement for TCAR for high-risk symptomatic and asymptomatic patients is provided by CMS when performed at hospitals participating in the SVS Vascular Quality Initiative TCAR Surveillance Project. Patients are eligible for TCAR if ICA diameter is 4 to 9 mm, and clavicle to CCA bifurcation distance is at least 5 cm. In addition, there must be an area in the CCA that is safe to access.

❶ CEA

The recommendation of CEA for severe asymptomatic carotid artery stenosis is predicated on low perioperative morbidity, mortality, and stroke rates of <3%.[1,2] CEA with patch angioplasty or eversion endarterectomy is recommended over primary carotid arterial closure as these are associated with lower rate of neurologic events and restenosis.[1,2,33] Eversion technique is useful in treating tortuous or redundant ICA. Studies have shown no significant difference in long-term rates of restenosis between eversion and conventional CEA.[34] The anesthetic technique utilized can include general, regional, or local anesthesia. The GALA trial, a prospective multinational randomized controlled trial of general versus local anesthesia, found no difference in morbidity or mortality between these anesthetic techniques.[35] However, general anesthesia should be utilized in difficult anatomy or anxious patients. CEA can be performed with the use of routine shunting, routine nonshunting, or selective shunting and there is debate regarding best strategy. Selective shunting can be utilized with any anesthetic technique; with general anesthesia, patients are monitored with stump pressure, EEG monitoring, somatosensory evoked potentials, transcranial Doppler, or monitoring cerebral oximetry. With local or regional anesthesia, intraoperative neurologic changes determine shunt need.[1]

❿ CAS

Diagnosis of high-grade carotid artery stenosis must be confirmed on either preoperative or intraoperative angiography.[29] A type III aortic arch is associated with more difficult access resulting in increased manipulation; an arch with significant calcification or thrombus presents an increased stroke risk with manipulation.[1] Thus, in these two instances, TCAR may be a better approach over transfemoral CAS. Vessel tortuosity can also be a challenge for CAS; previous study has found that ICA–CCA angulation ≥60° increased the relative risk of stroke or death following CAS.[1,36] Other morphologic features that make CAS difficult and high risk include unstable plaque, circumferential calcification or plaque burden (because of issues with compliance), very stenotic lesions (risk of partial stent expansion), and longer lesions (risk of stroke is greater than it is with CEA).[1,37] If CAS is selected for the patient, it is recommended that the procedure is performed with the patient awake to allow for neurologic evaluation. For transfemoral CAS, embolic protection is recommended; during TCAR, reversal of flow is the mechanism by which the brain is protected by emboli.[1] Patients should be managed with dual antiplatelet therapy, including aspirin (325 mg) and clopidogrel (75 mg) or ticlopidine (250 mg), for at least 4 days before and a minimum 30 days postoperatively.

ⓀPostintervention surveillance and medical therapy

A DUS within 30 days of CEA is recommended to evaluate for residual or recurrent stenosis (intimal hyperplasia).[1] The rate of recurrent stenosis varies in the literature; however, a systematic review found that the risk in the first year after CEA was 10%, in the second year 3%, and 1% after 2 years.[38] In addition, the risk of associated stroke is lower than that for a primary lesion.[39] Following CAS, restenosis is rare; however, a recent single-institutional study found that the rate was higher after CAS than after CEA.[40] Stent fracture is another concern in follow-up. However, the rate is low and has not been associated with major adverse clinical events or in-stent restenosis.[41] If the DUS study is normal at 1 month, further imaging can be considered if the patient has risk factors for progression of atherosclerosis.[1] Continued carotid DUS is performed more for surveillance of the contralateral untreated carotid artery disease than for detection of ipsilateral recurrent stenosis.[42] The interval at which DUS should be performed is based on the findings for both the treated ICA and contralateral carotid artery. If the treated ICA is widely patent, and the contralateral artery has mild stenosis, DUS can be performed at 2-year intervals.[42]

Perioperative medical management after CEA should target blood pressure control (<140/80 mm Hg), beta blockade (HR 60-80), and statin therapy (LDL < 100 mg/dL). There is evidence to suggest statin therapy, regardless of LDL, is beneficial in patients.[2] Aspirin should be continued during the perioperative period and indefinitely.[1] Regarding clopidogrel and other P2Y inhibitors, there is no consensus regarding perioperative continuation or cessation and should be individualized for the patient. However, dual antiplatelet therapy is associated with a 0.4% to 1.0% higher risk of major bleeding compared with aspirin alone.[1]

REFERENCES

1. Ricotta JJ, Aburahma A, Ascher E, et al. Updated Society for Vascular Surgery guidelines for management of extracranial carotid disease. *J Vasc Surg*. 2011;54(3):e1-e31.
2. Brott TG, Halperin JL, Abbara S, et al. 2011 ASA/ACCF/AHA/AANN/AANS/ACR/ASNR/CNS/SAIP/SCAI/SIR/SNIS/SVM/SVS guideline on the management of patients with extracranial carotid and vertebral artery disease. A report of the American College of Cardiology Foundation/American Heart Association Task Force on Practice Guidelines, and the American Stroke Association, American Association of Neuroscience Nurses, American Association of Neurological Surgeons, American College of Radiology, American Society of Neuroradiology, Congress of Neurological Surgeons, Society of Atherosclerosis Imaging and Prevention, Society for Cardiovascular Angiography and Interventions, Society of Interventional Radiology, Society of NeuroInterventional Surgery, Society for Vascular Medicine, and Society for Vascular Surgery. *Circulation*. 2011;124(4):e54-e130.
3. Rockman CB, Jacobowitz GR, Gagne PJ, et al. Focused screening for occult carotid artery disease: patients with known heart disease are at high risk. *J Vasc Surg*. 2004;39(1):44-51.
4. Rockman CB, Hoang H, Guo Y, et al. The prevalence of carotid artery stenosis varies significantly by race. *J Vasc Surg*. 2013;57(2):327-337.
5. Wardlaw JM, Chappell FM, Stevenson M, et al. Accurate, practical and cost-effective assessment of carotid stenosis in the UK. *Health Technol Assess*. 2006;10(30):iii-iv, ix-x, 1-182.
6. Gronholdt ML. B-mode ultrasound and spiral CT for the assessment of carotid atherosclerosis. *Neuroimaging Clin N Am*. 2002;12(3):421-435.
7. Arous EJ, Simons JP, Flahive JM, et al. National variation in preoperative imaging, carotid duplex ultrasound criteria, and threshold for surgery for asymptomatic carotid artery stenosis. *J Vasc Surg*. 2015;62(4):937-944.
8. Johnson BF, Verlato F, Bergelin RO, Primozich JF, Strandness E Jr. Clinical outcome in patients with mild and moderate carotid artery stenosis. *J Vasc Surg*. 1995;21(1):120-126.
9. Halliday A, Harrison M, Hayter E, et al. 10-year stroke prevention after successful carotid endarterectomy for asymptomatic stenosis (ACST-1): a multicentre randomised trial. *Lancet*. 2010;376(9746):1074-1084.
10. Endarterectomy for asymptomatic carotid artery stenosis. Executive Committee for the Asymptomatic Carotid Atherosclerosis Study. *JAMA*. 1995;273(18):1421-1428.
11. Abbott AL, Paraskevas KI, Kakkos SK, et al. Systematic review of guidelines for the management of asymptomatic and symptomatic carotid stenosis. *Stroke*. 2015;46(11):3288-3301.
12. Abbott AL. Medical (nonsurgical) intervention alone is now best for prevention of stroke associated with asymptomatic severe carotid stenosis: results of a systematic review and analysis. *Stroke*. 2009;40(10):e573-e583.
13. Conrad MF, Boulom V, Mukhopadhyay S, Garg A, Patel VI, Cambria RP. Progression of asymptomatic carotid stenosis despite optimal medical therapy. *J Vasc Surg*. 2013;58(1):128-135.e1.
14. Balestrini S, Lupidi F, Balucani C, et al. One-year progression of moderate asymptomatic carotid stenosis predicts the risk of vascular events. *Stroke*. 2013;44(3):792-794.
15. Mansour MA, Mattos MA, Faught WE, et al. The natural history of moderate (50% to 79%) internal carotid artery stenosis in symptomatic, nonhemispheric, and asymptomatic patients. *J Vasc Surg*. 1995;21(2):346-356; discussion 56-57.
16. Conrad MF, Michalczyk MJ, Opalacz A, Patel VI, LaMuraglia GM, Cambria RP. The natural history of asymptomatic severe carotid artery stenosis. *J Vasc Surg*. 2014;60(5):1218-1226.
17. Howard VJ, Meschia JF, Lal BK, et al. Carotid revascularization and medical management for asymptomatic carotid stenosis: protocol of the CREST-2 clinical trials. *Int J Stroke*. 2017;12(7):770-778.
18. Thanvi B, Robinson T. Complete occlusion of extracranial internal carotid artery: clinical features, pathophysiology, diagnosis and management. *Postgrad Med J*. 2007;83(976):95-99.

19. Hackam DG. Prognosis of asymptomatic carotid artery occlusion: systematic review and meta-analysis. *Stroke.* 2016;47(5):1253-1257.

20. Nicolaides AN, Kakkos SK, Kyriacou E, et al. Asymptomatic internal carotid artery stenosis and cerebrovascular risk stratification. *J Vasc Surg.* 2010;52(6):1486-1496.e1-e5.

21. Kakkos SK, Sabetai M, Tegos T, et al. Silent embolic infarcts on computed tomography brain scans and risk of ipsilateral hemispheric events in patients with asymptomatic internal carotid artery stenosis. *J Vasc Surg.* 2009;49(4): 902-909.

22. AbuRahma AF, Metz MJ, Robinson PA. Natural history of ≥60% asymptomatic carotid stenosis in patients with contralateral carotid occlusion. *Ann Surg.* 2003; 238(4): 551-561; discussion 61-62.

23. Nehler MR, Moneta GL, Lee RW, Edwards JM, Taylor LM Jr., Porter JM. Improving selection of patients with less than 60% asymptomatic internal carotid artery stenosis for follow-up carotid artery duplex scanning. *J Vasc Surg.* 1996;24(4):580-585; discussion 5-7.

24. Bertges DJ, Muluk V, Whittle J, Kelley M, MacPherson DS, Muluk SC. Relevance of carotid stenosis progression as a predictor of ischemic neurological outcomes. *Arch Intern Med.* 2003;163(19):2285-2289.

25. Wilson PW, Hoeg JM, D'Agostino RB, et al. Cumulative effects of high cholesterol levels, high blood pressure, and cigarette smoking on carotid stenosis. *N Engl J Med.* 1997;337(8):516-522.

26. Conrad MF, Kang J, Mukhopadhyay S, Patel VI, LaMuraglia GM, Cambria RP. A risk prediction model for determining appropriateness of CEA in patients with asymptomatic carotid artery stenosis. *Ann Surg.* 2013;258(4):534-538; discussion 8-40.

27. Wallaert JB, De Martino RR, Finlayson SR, et al. Carotid endarterectomy in asymptomatic patients with limited life expectancy. *Stroke.* 2012;43(7):1781-1787.

28. Yadav JS, Wholey MH, Kuntz RE, et al. Protected carotid-artery stenting versus endarterectomy in high-risk patients. *N Engl J Med.* 2004;351(15):1493-1501.

29. CMS.gov. Decision memo for carotid artery stenting (CAG-00085R). 2005. https://www.cms.gov/medicare-coverage-database/details/nca-decision-memo.aspx?NCAId =157&ver=29&NcaName=Carotid+Artery+Stenting+(1st +Recon). Accessed November 1, 2019.

30. Goldstein LB, Samsa GP, Matchar DB, Oddone EZ. Multicenter review of preoperative risk factors for endarterectomy for asymptomatic carotid artery stenosis. *Stroke.* 1998;29(4):750-753.

31. Spangler EL, Goodney PP, Schanzer A, et al. Outcomes of carotid endarterectomy versus stenting in comparable medical risk patients. *J Vasc Surg.* 2014;60(5):1227-1231.e1.

32. Kashyap VS, King AH, Foteh MI, Jim J, Kumins NH. A multi-institutional analysis of contemporary outcomes after transcarotid artery revascularization versus carotid endarterectomy. *J Vasc Surg.* 2018;67(6):e191-e192.

33. Bond R, Rerkasem K, Naylor AR, Aburahma AF, Rothwell PM. Systematic review of randomized controlled trials of patch angioplasty versus primary closure and different types of patch materials during carotid endarterectomy. *J Vasc Surg.* 2004;40(6):1126-1135.

34. Crawford RS, Chung TK, Hodgman T, Pedraza JD, Corey M, Cambria RP. Restenosis after eversion vs patch closure carotid endarterectomy. *J Vasc Surg.* 2007;46(1):41-48.

35. Group GTC, Lewis SC, Warlow CP, et al. General anaesthesia versus local anaesthesia for carotid surgery (GALA): a multicentre, randomised controlled trial. *Lancet.* 2008;372(9656):2132-2142.

36. Naggara O, Touze E, Beyssen B, et al. Anatomical and technical factors associated with stroke or death during carotid angioplasty and stenting: results from the endarterectomy versus angioplasty in patients with symptomatic severe carotid stenosis (EVA-3S) trial and systematic review. *Stroke.* 2011;42(2):380-388.

37. Moore WS, Popma JJ, Roubin GS, et al. Carotid angiographic characteristics in the CREST trial were major contributors to periprocedural stroke and death differences between carotid artery stenting and carotid endarterectomy. *J Vasc Surg.* 2016;63(4):851-857, 858.e1.

38. Frericks H, Kievit J, van Baalen JM, van Bockel JH. Carotid recurrent stenosis and risk of ipsilateral stroke: a systematic review of the literature. *Stroke.* 1998;29(1):244-250.

39. Mackey WC, Belkin M, Sindhi R, Welch H, O'Donnell TF Jr. Routine postendarterectomy duplex surveillance: does it prevent late stroke? *J Vasc Surg.* 1992;16(6):934-939; discussion 9-40.

40. Heo SH, Yoon KW, Woo SY, et al. Editor's choice—Comparison of early outcomes and restenosis rate between carotid endarterectomy and carotid artery stenting using propensity score matching analysis. *Eur J Vasc Endovasc Surg.* 2017;54(5):573-578.

41. Weinberg I, Beckman JA, Matsumura JS, et al. Carotid stent fractures are not associated with adverse events: results from the ACT-1 multicenter randomized trial (carotid angioplasty and stenting versus endarterectomy in asymptomatic subjects who are at standard risk for carotid endarterectomy with significant extracranial carotid stenotic disease). *Circulation.* 2018;137(1):49-56.

42. Ricotta JJ, DeWeese JA. Is routine carotid ultrasound surveillance after carotid endarterectomy worthwhile? *Am J Surg.* 1996;172(2):140-142; discussion 3.

Jeanwan Kang • David Stone

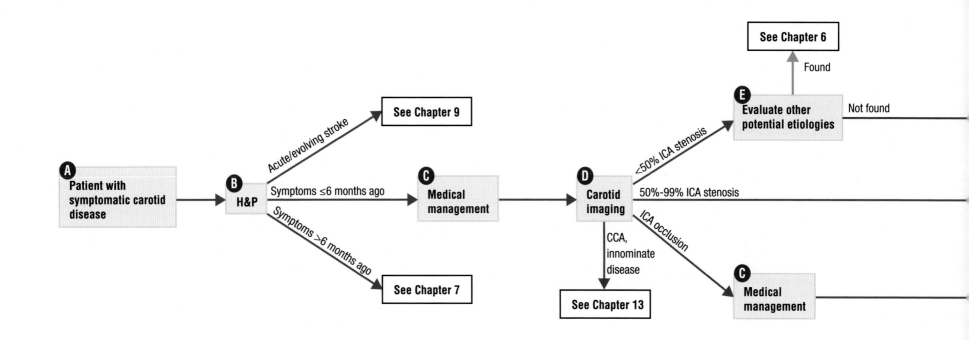

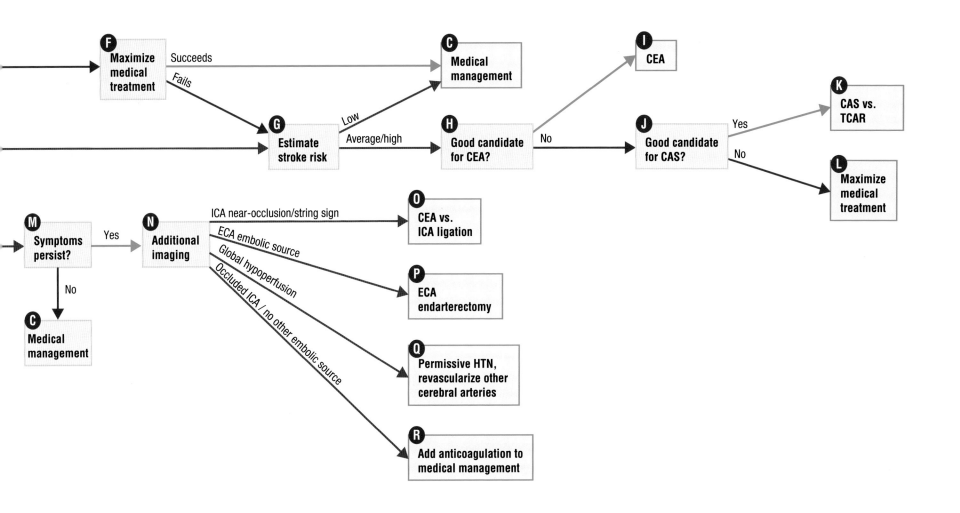

A Patient with symptomatic carotid disease

Approximately 68% of strokes worldwide are ischemic, of which about 25% are attributable to atherosclerosis involving the carotid artery, most often occurring at the carotid bifurcation.[1] Progressive narrowing of the arterial lumen can result in embolization, thrombosis, or hemodynamic compromise resulting in ischemic stroke or TIA. Risk factors associated with symptomatic carotid disease include increasing age, male sex, HTN, hyperlipidemia, diabetes, smoking, and physical inactivity.[1]

B H&P

Patients presenting with neurologic deficits referable to the carotid artery should undergo a careful H&P, including detailed neurologic evaluation, routine laboratory testing, and ECG. Neurology consultation may be appropriate for patients presenting with atypical symptoms (see Chapter 6).

Patients with acute stroke require emergent management (see Chapter 9). Those presenting with a history of only remote carotid symptoms (>6 months ago) should be considered asymptomatic and managed as such (see Chapter 7) because benefit for carotid revascularization following an ischemic stroke or TIA declines over time.[2-5] Pooled data from RCTs comparing CEA versus best medical therapy (BMT) showed that in patients with 70% to 99% ICA stenosis, the absolute risk reduction when CEA was performed within 2 weeks of randomization was 23%, whereas the absolute risk reduction was only 7.4% when CEA was delayed beyond 12 weeks following randomization.[5,6] This decrease in benefit over time was especially true for female patients with moderate symptomatic carotid stenosis where the data failed to show any benefit of CEA over BMT when CEA was delayed beyond 12 weeks.[6]

Patients with more recent carotid symptoms require medical management and additional evaluation to determine whether CEA or CAS is indicated.

C Medical management

Medical management for secondary ischemic stroke prevention (after initial stroke or TIA) includes treatment with antiplatelet therapy and statins, HTN management, and diabetes control as well as lifestyle modifications such as smoking cessation, weight loss, and regular exercise.[7,8]

Recommended antiplatelet therapy in secondary stroke prevention include aspirin monotherapy, clopidogrel monotherapy, or the combination of aspirin–extended-release dipyridamole.[7-11] A short duration (21 days) of dual antiplatelet therapy (DAPT) with aspirin and clopidogrel may reduce the risk of a recurrent ischemic event if initiated early (<24 hours) following a minor stroke or TIA.[7] Long-term use of DAPT, however, is associated with an increased risk of bleeding complications without definitive added benefit and is currently not recommended.[7,12] Early initiation of antiplatelet therapy is of critical importance in preventing recurrent stroke. Pooled analysis of data from nearly 16,000 patients in 12 trials evaluating aspirin for secondary stroke prevention demonstrated that the early benefit of aspirin was even higher than previously noted, with nearly 60% reduction in risk of recurrent ischemic stroke during the initial 6 weeks following the index event. The reduction in risk of disabling or fatal stroke was even higher at 71%.[9]

Along with antiplatelet therapy, statins are a mainstay of medical management in secondary prevention of stroke.[7,8,13-15] In the Stroke Prevention by Aggressive Reduction in Cholesterol Levels (SPARCL) trial, patients randomized to high-dose atorvastatin had 16% reduction in stroke recurrence compared with those randomized to placebo.[13] Although the degree of reduction in LDL cholesterol level correlates with the degree of protection from recurrent stroke or TIA,[14,15] statins also lower the risk of recurrent ischemic stroke through alternative mechanisms such as plaque stabilization, anti-inflammatory effect, and improved endothelial function. As such, the current recommendation regarding statin therapy following an ischemic stroke is to initiate high-dose statin therapy (eg, atorvastatin 80 mg daily), regardless of the baseline cholesterol level and aim to achieve an LDL level of <70 mg/dL (see Chapter 4).

D Carotid imaging

Carotid DUS is often the first imaging modality used to assess the severity of carotid disease. It is noninvasive, safe, and comparatively inexpensive, although it remains somewhat dependent on the experience and expertise of the ultrasonographer. Established DUS criteria (see Chapter 6) allow the severity of ICA stenosis to be characterized as <50%, 50% to 69%, 70% to 99%, or occlusion. Furthermore, plaque characteristics can be evaluated by calculating the gray-scale median score, which helps define stroke risk (see Chapter 6). CTA and MRA are often obtained to confirm DUS findings. In addition, they allow evaluation of both proximal arch vessel and intracranial anatomy/pathology that are not evaluable by DUS (see Chapter 6 for details).

For patients with nonoccluded ICA disease, the next steps depend primarily on the severity of ICA stenosis. If ICA occlusion is identified, medical management is recommended. Imaging may also reveal direct or indirect evidence of CCA origin or innominate artery tandem lesions, which are discussed in Chapter 13.

E Evaluate other potential etiologies

When carotid territory symptoms occur with <50% ICA stenosis, other potential causes should be carefully evaluated, as most minimal carotid stenoses do not produce atheroemboli to cause carotid symptoms. Cardiac evaluation (eg, ECG) should be done to identify a potential cardiac embolic source for carotid territory symptoms (eg, atrial fibrillation, dilated cardiomyopathy, endocarditis). If occult cardiac embolism is suspected, transthoracic or transesophageal ECHO, ambulatory cardiac monitoring, or transcranial Doppler (TCD) may be helpful. Paradoxical embolism of venous thrombus through a patent foramen ovale (PFO) should be evaluated and treated if found. For patients younger than or equal to 60 years old who are found to have a PFO without documented DVT, percutaneous PFO closure in addition to antiplatelet therapy may be indicated.[16]

If no cardiac source is found, additional imaging with CTA or MRA is indicated to detect other potential embolic sources in the aortic arch, CCA, or innominate artery, as well as intracranial arterial disease. If these other causes are detected, they are managed as described in Chapter 6. Other potential etiologies include a hypercoagulable state resulting in extra- or intracranial arterial occlusion, dissection, FMD, intracranial tumor, aneurysm, AVM, or cerebral venous sinus thrombosis. Migraine aura or postictal symptoms following a seizure may also mimic hemispheric symptoms.

F Maximize medical treatment

If no source for carotid territory symptoms, except a carotid bifurcation plaque causing <50% stenosis, is found, medical treatment should be augmented, as such lesions have not been shown to benefit from CEA. Pooled data from RCTs, including the North American Symptomatic Carotid Endarterectomy Trial (NASCET), European Carotid Surgery Trial (ECST), and Veterans Affairs Trial 309 (VA 309), demonstrated that CEA increased the 5-year risk of ipsilateral ischemic stroke in those with <30% stenosis and had no effect in those with 30% to 49% stenosis, compared with BMT.[17,18] Although both NASCET and ECST[5,6] demonstrated that the presence of plaque irregularity or ulceration increased the incidence of ipsilateral stroke among patients on medical therapy with severe carotid stenosis, there is no evidence to suggest benefit of CEA or CAS over BMT in those with ulcerated lesions in the setting of a <50% ICA stenosis. This argues for a trial on maximal medical treatment. If a given patient is not on appropriate antiplatelet therapy or statin at the time of carotid symptoms, these should be added. If the patient is already taking these medications, the intensity of treatment should be maximized, including dual antiplatelet and high-dose statin therapy. If such treatment prevents further carotid symptoms, medical treatment is continued. If symptoms recur on maximal medical therapy, and no other source of symptoms can be identified, further stroke risk stratification is done to determine if CEA or CAS is indicated.[6]

G Estimate stroke risk

The degree of carotid stenosis has been shown to affect the risk of a recurrent stroke and hence the benefit from carotid intervention. Pooled data from RCTs, including the NASCET, ECST, and VA 309, demonstrated that CEA compared favorably to BMT in reducing the 5-year risk of ipsilateral ischemic stroke in patients with symptomatic 50% to 99% ICA stenosis. The degree of benefit from CEA was much higher among those patients with 70% to 99% ICA stenosis (absolute risk reduction of 16%) compared to those with moderate 50% to 69% ICA stenosis (absolute risk reduction of 4.6%). In contrast, CEA had no effect in those with 30% to 49% stenosis and increased the 5-year risk of ipsilateral ischemic stroke in those with <30% stenosis compared with BMT.[17,18]

In addition to the severity of carotid stenosis, subgroup analysis of pooled data from the same RCTs demonstrated that certain clinical and anatomic features were associated with a higher risk of late stroke on BMT in patients with 50% to 99% stenosis. These included increasing age (5-year absolute risk reduction in ipsilateral stroke CEA vs. BMT: <65 years = 5.6%; 65-74 years = 8.6%; >75 years = 19.2%), recent symptoms (<2 weeks = 18.5%; 2-4 weeks = 9.8%; 4-12 weeks = 5.5%; >12 weeks 0.8%), male sex (male = 11%; female = 2.8%), hemispheric symptoms (ocular = 5%; TIA = 15%; stroke = 18%), increasing medical comorbidity (0-5 comorbidities = 17%; 6 = 23%; 7+ = 39%), plaque surface irregularity (smooth plaques = 8%; irregular plaques = 17%), and contralateral occlusion (contralateral occlusion = 24%; no occlusion = 13%).[6]

Some patients with symptomatic carotid stenosis appear to be at a particularly high risk of early recurrent stroke, with 11% to 25% having recurrent stroke within 14 days of the index event.[6] The ABCD[2] score is a validated prognostic scoring system developed for predicting 2- and 7-day risk of stroke in patients presenting with a TIA. The scoring system is based on patient age, blood pressure, clinical presentation, duration of symptoms, and the presence of diabetes mellitus, with a score of 6 to 7 being associated with 8% risk of stroke at 2 days and 12% at 7 days.[19]

	Parameter	Score
Age	>60 y	1
Blood pressure	>140/90 mm Hg	1
Clinical presentation	Unilateral leg weakness	2
	Speech impairment	1
Duration of symptoms	>60 min	2
	10-59 min	1
Diabetes mellitus	Yes	1

There are also a number of imaging findings that may predict the presence of an unstable plaque and increased risk of early recurrent stroke. These include low gray-scale median value of the carotid plaque noted on carotid DUS (reflecting hypoechoic lesions), intraplaque hemorrhage noted on MRI, evidence of embolization on TCD, and high fluorodeoxyglucose uptake in the carotid plaque on PET (indicative of increased macrophage activity or inflammation).[6]

Good candidate for CEA?

Perioperative morbidity and mortality rates >6% eliminate the stroke-reducing benefit of CEA in patients with symptomatic carotid stenosis.[7] Currently, there is no reliable, validated prediction model for identifying patients who may be too "high risk" for CEA, but contemporary CEA outcomes would suggest only a select group of very high-risk patients would be categorized as such.[20-22]

Early enthusiasm for CAS was due at least in part to the potential for diminished morbidity and mortality in patients deemed "high risk" for CEA. Thus far, studies have failed to demonstrate superiority of CAS over CEA among such patients. The Stenting and Angioplasty with Protection in Patients at High Risk for Endarterectomy (SAPPHIRE) trial was an RCT designed to test the noninferiority of CAS over CEA in both symptomatic and asymptomatic, high-risk surgical patients.[23] Although the study reported no difference in outcomes between the two treatment groups, it has been criticized for its documented high 30-day stroke/death rate in the CEA group despite the fact that more than 70% of patients were those with asymptomatic disease.

The remainder of RCTs comparing CAS versus CEA have been limited to non–high-risk patients. Meta-analysis of 11 RCTs comparing CAS versus CEA demonstrated that among symptomatic patients with standard surgical risk, CAS was associated with significantly higher rate of periprocedural stroke or death at 30 days (8.2% vs. 5.0%, OR 1.72) as well as combined 30-day stroke, MI, or death (OR 1.44).[24] The Carotid Revascularization Endarterectomy versus Stenting Trial (CREST) comparing CAS versus CEA in both symptomatic and asymptomatic patients reported no difference in their composite endpoint of 30-day combined stroke, MI, or death between the two groups.[25,26] However, it should be noted that the 30-day stroke or death rate was significantly higher in the CAS group compared with the CEA group (4.4% vs. 2.3%, HR 1.9), whereas the 30-day MI rate was significantly lower in the CAS group (1.1% vs. 2.3%, HR 0.5).[25] Subgroup analysis of symptomatic patients demonstrated a significantly higher risk of 30-day stroke or death in the CAS group compared with the CEA group (6.0% vs. 3.2%, HR 1.89) and no difference in 30-day rate of MI between the two groups (1.0% vs. 2.3%, HR 0.45).[27]

Accordingly, based on currently available data, most patients with symptomatic carotid stenosis would be safe to undergo CEA, whereas patients with high-risk anatomic features (eg, recurrent carotid stenosis, prior neck radiation, prior radical neck dissection, or surgically inaccessible lesions) or significant cardiac or pulmonary comorbidities may be better candidates for CAS or BMT.[7]

CEA

CEA may be performed under general anesthesia, regional anesthesia with cervical block, or in some instances with local anesthesia. There are no data to suggest superior outcome with one mode of anesthesia over the others and the choice is largely dependent on the preferences of the patient, the anesthesiologist, and the surgeon.

The two basic techniques for CEA are conventional and eversion with no consistent evidence showing superiority of one technique over the other. In conventional CEA, a longitudinal arteriotomy is made beginning in the CCA and extended to the ICA beyond the lesion. Following endarterectomy, a patch closure is carried out with vein, bovine pericardium, or prosthetic patch. Patch closure has been shown to be associated with decreased risk of perioperative stroke as well as recurrent stenosis during long-term follow-up compared with primary closure.[28,29] A recent analysis of more than 70,000 patients undergoing primary CEA in the Vascular Quality Initiative registry showed that 94% were patched, usually with bovine pericardium (77%) followed by Dacron (19%), ePTFE (2%), and vein (2%). By multivariable analysis, bovine pericardium was significantly associated with less reoperation for bleeding (OR 0.7, $P < 0.01$), fewer postoperative neurologic events (OR 0.6, $P < 0.01$), and less restenosis at 1 year (OR 0.6, $P < 0.01$) compared with no patch.[30]

In eversion endarterectomy, the ICA is transected transversely at its origin and everted to remove the plaque that is transected or feathered at its distal endpoint. The ICA is then anastomosed to its origin in an end-to-end manner. This technique may be attractive for patients with short focal lesions at the bifurcation and is particularly useful in patients with a redundant ICA as it avoids potential kinking. In these cases, the ICA can be pulled down, straightened, and the redundant portion excised before the reanastomosis.

An intravascular shunt is used by many surgeons during CEA to decrease the risk of perioperative stroke related to the period of potential cerebral ischemia during carotid artery clamping. However, because the use of shunts may increase the risk of an embolic stroke, some prefer selective rather than routine use of shunts. Measurement of carotid stump pressure, intraoperative neurologic monitoring with electroencephalogram or somatosensory evoked potentials, measurement of middle cerebral artery flow by TCD, and monitoring with cerebral oximetry have been used to identify patients at risk for ischemic stroke during carotid clamping to determine when to selectively shunt. There has been no convincing evidence to suggest significant difference in outcomes between routine versus selective use of shunt during CEA.[31,32]

Good candidate for CAS?

CAS has been associated with increased risk of 30-day stroke or death compared with CEA in those with symptomatic carotid stenosis. Certain clinical features seem to increase this risk even more. A meta-analysis of pooled patient data from four RCTs comparing CAS and CEA demonstrated that while there was no difference in 30-day stroke/death rate between CAS and CEA in those <70 years of age, CAS was associated with higher risk of 30-day stroke/death for patients aged 70 to 74 years (HR 2.1) and even higher for those above the age of 80 years (HR 2.4) compared with CEA.[33]

Another clinical feature associated with higher risk of stroke/death following CAS compared with CEA may be early intervention following symptom onset. A meta-analysis of three RCTs comparing CAS and CEA in patients with symptomatic carotid stenosis demonstrated that those undergoing CAS within 0 to 7 days after the index event had more than a 3-fold increase in 30-day stroke/death rate compared with those undergoing CEA (9.4% vs. 2.8%; $P = 0.03$). Patients undergoing CAS within 8 to 14 days after symptom onset were also significantly more likely to suffer a perioperative stroke compared with CEA (8.1% vs. 3.4%; $P = 0.04$).[34] This finding may be of particular importance because the early recurrent stroke risk appears to be higher than initially thought for those with symptomatic carotid stenosis, and there is a move for earlier intervention following onset of symptoms in these patients.

Various anatomic features have also been identified as increasing the associated periprocedural stroke risk for CAS, many of which have been identified on secondary analyses of major CAS trials.[35,36] These include aortic arch calcification, type II or III aortic arch, carotid lesions with circumferential calcification or ulceration, long lesion length, tandem lesions, or tortuous ICA anatomy. Increased risk of perioperative stroke among older patients undergoing CAS compared with CEA may, in part, be because of the increased prevalence of some of these high-risk anatomic features.[25,26]

K   CAS vs. TCAR

CAS is usually performed via percutaneous retrograde access to the CFA. Following an aortic arch angiogram, the CCA is selected and a sheath is advanced into the distal CCA. The diseased ICA is then crossed and a filter is deployed distal to the lesion for embolic protection. The carotid lesion is then usually predilated before placement of a self-expandable stent.

Issues related to access, including severe aortoiliac and femoral occlusive disease, or hostile arch anatomy, may preclude patients from being able to undergo CAS via a transfemoral approach. In response to this issue, transcarotid artery revascularization (TCAR) has emerged as an alternative CAS paradigm that obviates many of the associated morbidity related to femoral arterial access as well as embolic potential from hostile arch anatomy. In addition, TCAR offers embolic protection via the initiation of flow reversal from the CCA to the femoral vein, thereby avoiding the need to cross or manipulate the symptomatic lesion. TCAR may accordingly be associated with potentially decreased perioperative stroke risk compared with transfemoral CAS and, as such, assume a larger role in treating patients with high-risk anatomic features for CEA.[37] A retrospective cohort study comparing the outcomes of the initial 646 patients enrolled in the Society for Vascular Surgery VQI TCAR Surveillance Project and those who underwent transfemoral CAS showed that TCAR was associated with lower risk of any in-hospital neurologic event (stroke/TIA) or death compared with transfemoral CAS (2.2% vs. 3.8%; $P = 0.03$).

This difference in risk-adjusted, in-hospital outcomes was mainly because of the increased risk of TIA (rather than stroke) in the transfemoral CAS group.[38] A more recent study using the same registry reported similar in-hospital outcomes between those who underwent TCAR and those who underwent CEA despite the fact that the TCAR cohort was older and had higher medical risk factors.[39] Further studies are needed to confirm these early results.

L   Maximize medical treatment

In the rare instances where the periprocedural morbidity and mortality risk is prohibitively high for both CEA and CAS, the patient may be better managed by maximizing medical treatment. Antiplatelet and high-dose statin therapy should be maintained (as described in C). There continues to be debate over the optimal BP goals for secondary stroke prevention, but, in general, SBP <140 mm Hg and diastolic blood pressure <90 mm Hg are recommended. In addition, all patients should be screened for diabetes if no previous diagnosis exists and treated as needed. Additional counseling or a support group may be helpful in achieving successful lifestyle modifications such as weight loss, improved nutrition, and increased physical activity.[7]

M   Symptoms persist?

If ipsilateral carotid symptoms persist despite BMT in a patient with ICA occlusion, several causes are possible, which should be evaluated with additional imaging. If symptoms cease, BMT is continued.

N   Additional imaging

Potential causes for continued carotid symptoms in a patient with ICA occlusion include a nearly but not occluded ICA that was undetected by DUS or other imaging, embolization from carotid bifurcation plaque via the ECA, global hypoperfusion in the setting of severe contralateral disease, or embolization from the occluded ICA thrombus. To evaluate these potential etiologies, additional imaging may be required, including catheter-directed DSA. Treatment then depends on the potential etiology detected.

O   CEA vs. ICA ligation

Very low flow through the ICA can be caused by a near-occlusive lesion of the carotid bifurcation, which can over time lead to diffuse narrowing or fibrosis of the ICA (also called "string sign" on DSA). In the first instance, DSA or CTA with delayed venous phase can reveal a narrow but smooth-walled ICA distal to the area of the focal severe stenosis. In such cases, CEA can usually be performed with the expectation that the narrowed but thin-walled ICA will gradually dilate. In contrast, if the distal ICA is thickened, fibrotic, and irregularly narrowed throughout, it will not likely dilate after CEA, but rather lead to occlusion. In such cases, ICA ligation with ECA endarterectomy, as needed, is recommended. Sometimes this decision cannot be made before intraoperative ICA inspection.

P   ECA endarterectomy

In the setting of confirmed ICA occlusion, a patent ECA can provide a collateral route for atheroembolization from the carotid bulb through the ophthalmic artery and be responsible for recurrent ipsilateral ischemic events. TCD can be used to demonstrate reversal of flow in the ipsilateral ophthalmic artery as well as microembolic signals or high-intensity transient signals in the more distal arteries.[40] Patients suspected of having recurrent ischemic symptoms from such a mechanism despite BMT are candidates for ECA endarterectomy with flush oversewing of the ICA stump to eliminate a nidus for thrombus accumulation.

Q   Permissive HTN, revascularize other cerebral arteries

Although most patients develop adequate distal cerebral collateral circulation following ICA occlusion, a select cohort will continue to experience ischemic symptoms because of cerebral hypoperfusion (see also Chapter 6). This scenario is more likely to be observed in patients with multivessel disease (eg, contralateral carotid stenosis, vertebral artery stenosis) or significant intracranial vascular disease. Symptoms are typically transient, occurring in periods of relative hypotension or stress (eg, amaurosis fugax in response to bright light that stresses retinal metabolism). CT or MR perfusion studies can assess baseline cerebral blood flow. TCD measurement of flow velocities in the middle cerebral artery or single-photon emission CT (SPECT) before and after a vasodilatory stimulus (eg, CO_2 or acetazolamide) may be helpful in assessing cerebrovascular reserve.[40,41]

Patients with recurrent ischemic symptoms because of hypoperfusion can be treated with permissive HTN, contralateral CEA, or arch vessel or vertebral artery revascularization, if indicated. ECA endarterectomy has been shown to improve cerebral blood flow in some studies,[42] although whether this leads to demonstrable stroke prevention is uncertain. ECA–ICA bypass has been performed for select patients with recurrent or progressive ischemic symptoms associated with ICA occlusion and no other artery revascularization options, but its value has not been proven.[7]

R   Add anticoagulation to medical management

Patients with an occluded ICA may have recurrent ischemic symptoms because of propagation of clot intracranially. TCD may be useful in detecting the presence of microembolic signals or high-intensity transient signals in the distal circulation.[40] In cases of ongoing symptoms from emboli despite aggressive antiplatelet therapy without any other source, the addition of an oral anticoagulant for a period of 3 to 6 months while the thrombus matures is sometimes recommended, but without sound evidence.

REFERENCES

1. Benjamin EJ, Blaha JM, Chiuve SE, et al. Heart disease and stroke statistics-2017 update: a report from the American Heart Association. *Circulation.* 2017;135:e146-e603.

2. North American Symptomatic Carotid Endarterectomy Trial Collaborators, Barnett HJM, Taylor DW, et al. Beneficial effect of carotid endarterectomy in symptomatic patients with high-grade carotid stenosis. *N Engl J Med.* 1991;325:445-453.

3. Barnett HJM, Taylor DW, Eliasziw M, et al. Benefit of carotid endarterectomy in patients with symptomatic moderate or severe stenosis. North American Symptomatic Carotid Endarterectomy Trial Collaborators. *N Engl J Med.* 1998;339:1415-1425.

4. The European Carotid Surgery Trialists' Collaborative Group. Randomised trial of endarterectomy for recently symptomatic carotid stenosis: final results of the MRC European Carotid Surgery Trial. *Lancet.* 1998;351:1379-1387.

5. Naylor AR, Rothwell PM, Bell PRF. Overview of the principal results and secondary analyses from the European and North American randomized trials of endarterectomy for symptomatic carotid stenosis. *Eur J Vasc Endovasc Surg.* 2003;26:115-129.

6. Naylor AR, Sillesen H, Schroeder TV. Clinical and imaging features associated with an increased risk of early and late stroke in patients with symptomatic carotid disease. *Eur J Vasc Endovasc Surg.* 2015;49:513-523.

7. Kernan WN, Ovbiagele B, Black HR, et al. Guidelines for the prevention of stroke in patients with stroke and transient ischemic attack: a guideline for healthcare professionals from the American Heart Association/American Stroke Association. *Stroke.* 2014;45:2160-2236.

8. Rothwell PM, Algra A, Amarenco P. Medical treatment in acute and long-term secondary prevention after transient ischemic attack and ischemic stroke. *Lancet.* 2011;377:1681-1692.

9. Rothwell PM, Algra A, Chen Z, et al. Effects of aspirin on risk and severity of early recurrent stroke after transient ischemic attack and ischemic stroke: time-course analysis of randomized trials. *Lancet.* 2016;388:365-375.

10. CAPRIE Steering Committee. A randomized, blinded, trial of clopidogrel versus aspirin in patients at risk of ischemic events (CAPRIE). CAPRIE Steering Committee. *Lancet.* 1996;348:1329-1339.

11. Verro P, Gorelick PB, Nguyen D. Aspirin plus dipyridamole versus aspirin for prevention of vascular events after stroke or TIA: a meta-analysis. *Stroke.* 2008;39:1358-1363.

12. Diener HC, Bogoussalavsky J, Brass LM, et al, on behalf of the MATCH investigators. Aspirin and clopidogrel compared with clopidogrel alone after recent ischemic stroke or transient ischemic attack in high-risk patients (MATCH): randomized, double-blind, placebo-controlled trial. *Lancet.* 2004;364:331-337.

13. Amarenco P, Bogousslavsky J, Callahan A 3rd, et al. High-dose atorvastatin after stroke or transient ischemic attack. Stroke Prevention by Aggressive Reduction in Cholesterol Levels (SPARCL). *N Engl J Med.* 2006;355:549-559.

14. Amarenco P, Labreuche J. Lipid management in the prevention of stroke: review and updated meta-analysis of statins for stroke prevention. *Lancet Neurol.* 2009;8:453-463.

15. Cholesterol Treatment Trialists' (CTT) Collaboration, Baigent C, Blackwell L, Emberson J, et al. Efficacy and safety of more intensive lowering of LDL cholesterol: a meta-analysis of data from 170,000 participants in 26 randomized trials. *Lancet.* 2010;376:1670-1681.

16. Saver JL. Clinical practice: cryptogenic stroke. *N Engl J Med.* 2016;374:2065-2074.

17. Rothwell PM, Eliasziw M, Gutnikov SA, et al. Analysis of pooled data from the randomized controlled trials of endarterectomy for symptomatic carotid stenosis. *Lancet.* 2003;361:107-116.

18. Orrapin S, Rerkasem K. Carotid endarterectomy for symptomatic carotid stenosis. *Cochrane Database Syst Rev.* 2017;(6):CD001081.

19. Johnston SC, Rothwell PM, Nguyen-Huynh MN, et al. Validation and refinement of scores to predict very early stroke risk after transient ischaemic attack. *Lancet.* 2007;369:283-292.

20. Kang J, Chung TK, Lancaster RT, Lamuraglia GM, Conrad MF, Cambria RP. Outcomes after carotid endarterectomy: is there a high-risk population? A National Surgical Quality Improvement Program Report. *J Vasc Surg.* 2009;49:331-339.

21. Schermerhorn ML, Fokkema M, Goodney P, et al. The impact of Centers for Medicare and Medicaid Services high-risk criteria on outcome after carotid endarterectomy and carotid artery stenting in the SVS Vascular Registry. *J Vasc Surg.* 2013;57:1318-1324.

22. Paraskevas KI, Kalmykov EL, Naylor AR. Stroke/death rates following carotid artery stenting and carotid endarterectomy in contemporary administrative dataset registries: a systematic review. *Eur J Vasc Endovasc Surg.* 2016;51:3-12.

23. Yadav JS, Wholey MH, Kuntz RE, et al. Protected carotid-artery stenting versus endarterectomy in high-risk patients. *N Engl J Med.* 2004;351:1493-1501.

24. Bonati LH, Lyrer P, Ederle J, et al. Percutaneous transluminal balloon angioplasty and stenting for carotid artery stenosis. *Cochrane Database Syst Rev.* 2012;(12):CD000515.

25. Brott TG, Hobson RW II, Howard G, et al. Stenting versus endarterectomy for treatment of carotid-artery stenosis. *N Engl J Med.* 2010;363:11-23.

26. Brott TG, Howard G, Roubin GS, et al. Long-term results of stenting versus endarterectomy for carotid-artery stenosis. *N Engl J Med.* 2016;374:1021-1031.

27. Silver FL, Mackey A, Clark WM, et al. Safety of stenting and endarterectomy by symptomatic status in the Carotid Revascularization Endarterectomy Versus Stenting Trial (CREST). *Stroke.* 2011;42:675-680.

28. Rerkasem K, Rothwell PM. Patch angioplasty versus primary closure for carotid endarterectomy. *Cochrane Database Syst Rev.* 2009;(4):CD000160.

29. Goodney PP, Nolan BW, Eldrup-Jorgensen J, Likosky DS, Cronenwett JL; Vascular Study Group of Northern New England. Restenosis after carotid endarterectomy in a multicenter regional registry. *J Vasc Surg.* 2010;52:897-905.

30. Edenfield L, Blazick E, Aranson N, et al. Outcomes of carotid endarterectomy in the VQI based on patch type. Presented at: the New England Society for Vascular Surgery Annual Meeting; October 12, 2018; Cape Neddick, Maine.

31. Aburahma AF, Mousa AY, Stone PA. Shunting during carotid endarterectomy. *J Vasc Surg.* 2011;54:1502-1510.

32. Goodney PP, Wallaert JB, Scali ST, et al. Impact of practice patterns in shunt use during carotid endarterectomy with contralateral carotid occlusion. *J Vasc Surg.* 2012;55:61-71.

33. Howard G, Roubin GS, Jansen O, et al. Association between age and risk of stroke or death from carotid endarterectomy and carotid stenting: a meta-analysis of pooled patient data from four randomized trials. *Lancet.* 2016;387:1305-1311.

34. Rantner B, Goebel G, Bonati LH, et al. The risk of carotid artery stenting compared with carotid endarterectomy is greatest in patients treated within 7 days of symptoms. *J Vasc Surg.* 2013;57:619-626.

35. Muller MD, Ahlhelm FJ, von Hessling A, et al. Vascular anatomy predicts the risk of cerebral ischemia in patients randomized to carotid stenting versus endarterectomy. *Stroke.* 2017;48:1285-1292.

36. Moore WS, Popma JJ, Roubin GS, et al. Carotid angiographic characteristics in the CREST trial were major contributors to periprocedural stroke and death differences between carotid artery stenting and carotid endarterectomy. *J Vasc Surg.* 2016;63:851-858.

37. Kwolek CJ, Jaff MR, Leal JI, et al. Results of the ROADSTER multicenter trial of transcarotid stenting with dynamic flow reversal. *J Vasc Surg.* 2015;62:1227-1234.

38. Malas MB, Dakour-Aridi H, Wang GJ, et al. Transcarotid artery revascularization versus transfemoral carotid artery stenting in the Society for Vascular Surgery Vascular Quality Initiative. *J Vasc Surg.* 2019;69:92-103.

39. Schermerhorn ML, Liang P, Dakour-Aridi H, et al. In-hospital outcomes of transcarotid artery revascularization and carotid endarterectomy in the Society for Vascular Surgery Vascular Quality Initiative. *J Vasc Surg.* 2019;71:87-95.

40. Malhotra K, Goyal N, Tsivgoulis G. Internal carotid artery occlusion: pathophysiology, diagnosis, and management. *Curr Atheroscler Rep.* 2017;19:41.

41. Klijn CJM, Kappelle LJ. Haemodynamic stroke: clinical features, prognosis, and management. *Lancet Neurol.* 2010;9:1008-1017.

42. Gertler JP, Cambria RP. The role of external carotid endarterectomy in the treatment of ipsilateral internal carotid occlusion: collective review. *J Vasc Surg.* 1987;6:158-167.

Philip G. Schmalz • Mark R. Harrigan

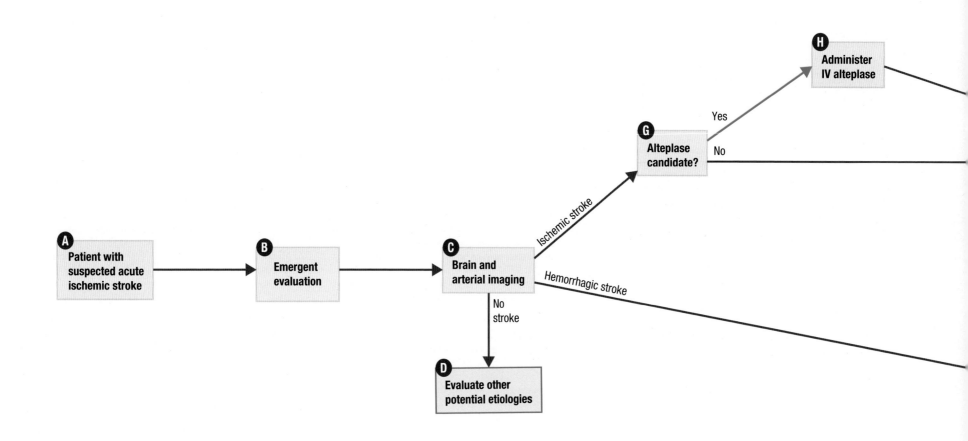

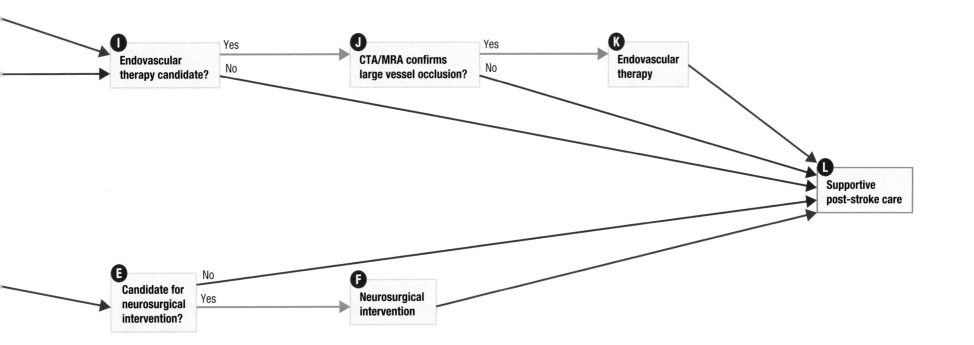

Ⓐ Patient with suspected acute ischemic stroke

Patients presenting with the abrupt onset of focal neurologic deficit, including hemi- or monoparesis, plegia, aphasia/dysphasia, or forced gaze deviation, should be emergently evaluated for acute ischemic stroke (AIS). Hemibody weakness or paralysis can suggest either an anterior or posterior circulation stroke, whereas ocular anomalies such as diplopia, visual field loss, or depression in the level of consciousness with ocular bobbing suggest posterior circulation stroke. Patients with a history of stroke or TIA raise the likelihood that the above presenting symptoms represent AIS. Patients presenting with headaches, nausea/vomiting, progressive neurologic deficit, or increasing depression in the level of consciousness may have a hemorrhagic, rather than an ischemic stroke.

Ⓑ Emergent evaluation

When a patient presents with a suspected AIS, an organized protocol for emergency evaluation ("Code Stroke") should be adopted by hospitals and emergency medical services (EMS) systems. A designated acute stroke team including physician specialists, nurses, and laboratory and radiology personnel should be established. Airway, breathing, and circulatory (ABC) assessment should begin upon arrival and airway and ventilatory support should be provided to patients with diminished level of consciousness or respiratory compromise. Supplemental oxygen in the absence of hypoxemia has not been shown to improve outcomes; it is not recommended in patients without hypoxia, and should be used only to the extent necessary to maintain oxygen saturation >94%.[1] Hypotension and hypovolemia, if present, should be corrected to levels that will maintain systemic organ perfusion. Although optimal blood pressure (BP) for patients with AIS is not established,[2] hypertensive patients who are candidates for alteplase (tissue plasminogen activator) treatment should have their BP carefully lowered to values <185/110 mm Hg before the administration of alteplase (see later).

Immediate stroke severity scoring (National Institutes of Health Stroke Score [NIHSS] preferred)[2] should be performed upon patient contact after initial ABC assessment. Although other diagnostic tests may be beneficial in the evaluation of AIS, a blood glucose value, to rule out hypoglycemic stroke mimics, is the only laboratory test required before the administration of alteplase. Baseline ECG and troponin assessment are recommended; however, these studies should not delay alteplase administration or progression to endovascular therapy (EVT).

Ⓒ Brain and arterial imaging

A noncontrast head CT scan should be obtained within 20 minutes of patient arrival and is required before the administration of alteplase. The purpose of NCCT is to exclude the presence of hemorrhage and to provide additional information about the extent and severity of the ischemic stroke. For patients who are likely to meet the criteria for EVT, additional intra- and extracranial vascular imaging, such as CTA and CT perfusion cerebral blood flow imaging, can provide complementary information and identify the etiology of stroke. Similarly, cardiac sources of embolic stroke, such as atrial fibrillation, should be investigated and treated as appropriate. However, these additional studies should *not* delay the administration of alteplase in the patient with AIS.[2]

In most cases, the diagnosis of AIS can be made on the basis of H&P and brain imaging. Although diffusion-weighted MRI (DW-MRI) is more sensitive than CT in detecting acute stroke, routine use of MRI in this setting is both cost-ineffective and time-consuming.[3,4] Clinical symptoms combined with a negative NCCT or NCCT with early ischemic changes (which can be detected with careful observation in a majority of acute stroke patients) are generally sufficient to make a diagnosis. Although DW-MRI may be of benefit in patients with puzzling presentations or those considered for early revascularization, there are inadequate criteria at this time to determine which patients will benefit from this imaging modality during the initial evaluation.[5] Based on the finding of AIS, hemorrhagic stroke, or no stroke, different treatment is pursued.

Ⓓ Evaluate other potential etiologies

The differential diagnosis for patients presenting with possible AIS includes intracerebral and subarachnoid hemorrhage, toxic or drug ingestion, and "stroke mimics" such as hemiplegic migraine or anamnestic syndromes (also termed recrudescence syndrome). Stroke teams with neurologic expertise can often distinguish these presentations from AIS by history and NCCT alone.

Ⓔ Candidate for neurosurgical intervention?

The diagnosis of hemorrhagic stroke caused by spontaneous intracerebral hemorrhage (ICH), rather than AIS, can be readily made based on clinical and radiologic information. Patients who present with a depressed level of consciousness and severe headache or who demonstrate progressive decline in neurologic function and level of consciousness are more likely to have hemorrhagic rather than ischemic stroke. The diagnosis is confirmed with an NCCT. As in ischemic stroke, baseline severity scoring is recommended in these patients. The ICH score is currently the most widely used externally validated scoring system.[6,7] After establishing the diagnosis, vascular imaging such as CTA can be beneficial for identifying patients who are likely to suffer early deterioration because of ongoing bleeding, and can be useful for identifying structural lesions in patients in whom surgical evacuation is considered.

Patient selection for surgical evacuation of clot in patients with supratentorial ICH remains controversial. Those with rapidly deteriorating neurologic status should be considered for surgical clot evacuation, or alternatively for decompressive craniectomy without clot evacuation, particularly in the case of coma from mass effect or midline shift because of a large-volume clot. In contrast, the benefit of craniotomy for evacuation of lobar hemorrhage in patients presenting without coma or rapid neurologic decline was addressed by STICH I and II trials.[8,9] Overall, no significant difference in mortality or functional outcome was seen for patients with lobar hemorrhages presenting with relatively stable neurologic status. At present, the effectiveness of surgical evacuation of supratentorial hemorrhages for most patients has not been well established in the literature and should be considered only in select cases.[10] In patients with hemorrhage into the posterior fossa, particularly those with salvageable neurologic status and hemorrhage >3 cm, emergent surgical evacuation is indicated. Attempts to control intracranial pressure or reduce brainstem compression through CSF diversion alone is not recommended and may actually cause harm.[10,11] Detailed guidelines for the management of spontaneous ICH are regularly updated by the American Heart Association (AHA)/American Stroke Association. Readers are encouraged to review these publications for changes in this rapidly developing area of stroke care.[2]

Ⓕ Neurosurgical intervention

Evacuation of lobar hematomas is accomplished via standard supratentorial craniotomy techniques. Exposure can be tailored to the lesion and need not be excessive for simple evacuation of hemorrhage without an underlying vascular lesion. Large trauma-style craniotomy flaps are not required unless the operator is planning on performing decompression as well. Corticectomy should be kept to the minimum sufficient to aspirate the clot using standard surgical suction. For deep-seated lesions or those of abnormal configuration, neuronavigation can be a helpful adjunct. In general, surgical techniques that minimize damage to surrounding brain are optimal, especially given the limited evidence for the benefits of evacuation. Posterior fossa hematoma evacuation is performed in similar fashion with a midline incision, which may be extended laterally in a "hockey stick" fashion for eccentric clots, followed by craniectomy and evacuation. External ventricular drain placement is recommended for patients with posterior fossa hemorrhages and may be placed either supine before cranial fixation using standard landmarks (preferred) or from a separate incision over the occipital region through Keen point. Currently, minimally invasive techniques are under investigation and may prove more beneficial than traditional craniotomy for supratentorial hemorrhages.

Ⓖ Alteplase candidate?

In patients who have suffered AIS, the benefit of IV tissue plasminogen activator (alteplase) administration to potentially lyse thrombus causing the stroke must be rapidly evaluated. The safety and efficacy of alteplase administration to patients with

AIS presenting within the first 3 hours from symptom onset has been well established in multiple RCTs with the greatest benefit coming from early administration (<90 minutes), which underscores the importance of rapid assessment and treatment.[12,13] IV alteplase administration is recommended for adults with disabling stroke symptoms, regardless of age or stroke severity if administered within 3 hours of symptom onset.[2] Candidates for alteplase must be able to receive therapy within 3 to 4.5 hours, have a blood glucose of at least 50 mg/dL, have not received oral anticoagulants or LMWH before 24 hours, have not had recent surgery, or experienced recent major bleeding or intracranial hemorrhage. Additionally, hypertensive patients must have a BP <185/110 mm Hg. This BP target can be achieved with IV antihypertensive medications such as labetalol or nicardipine. A detailed list of extensive inclusion/exclusion criteria can be found in Table 6 of the 2018 Guidelines for the Early Management of Patients With Acute Ischemic Stroke.[2] One study, ECASS III, demonstrated a greater likelihood of favorable neurologic outcome (odds ratio 1.34) with alteplase administration up to 4.5 hours from symptom onset without an increase in death or adverse events.[14] Stringent criteria were used for patient selection during this trial and those with severe stroke (NIHSS > 25), any prior warfarin use (even with normal INR), and patients with a prior stroke who also had diabetes were excluded from the study. Similar criteria should be used for patients presenting between 3 and 4.5 hours from symptom onset. Other IV thrombolytics have been assessed for treatment of AIS. Tenecteplase has been reported to be as safe as alteplase, but has not been shown to be superior in clinical trials. Administration of tenecteplase is an option for patients with minor deficit and without evidence of large vessel occlusion (LVO).[2]

H Administer IV alteplase

IV alteplase is indicated for patients with AIS who meet the aforementioned exclusion/inclusion criteria at doses of 0.9 mg/kg up to 90 mg, with 10% of the dose given as a bolus and the remainder administered over 60 minutes. Ancillary testing beyond blood glucose level, in the absence of a history of anticoagulant use, should not delay alteplase administration. BP should be monitored during and after alteplase administration and a target value of <180/105 mm Hg is maintained for 24 hours after alteplase administration.[2] IV alteplase is approved for use up to 3 hours after symptom onset in the United States and up to 4.5 hours after symptom onset in Europe.

I Endovascular therapy candidate?

Patients with a suspected LVO (occlusion of the ICA, M1 or A1 segments of the middle and anterior cerebral arteries) should be considered for EVT (mechanical thrombectomy). Clinical findings suggestive of LVO include NIHSS > 10, examination findings suggestive of a cortical ischemia such as aphasia, neglect, or forced gaze deviation. A hyperattenuating (hyperdense) large

vessel on initial NCCT imaging is also suggestive of LVO. Patients with a prestroke modified Rankin score of 0 to 1, with ASPECTS score of ≥6, NIHSS ≥ 6, and evidence of LVO should be considered for EVT.

Five large randomized trials have demonstrated benefit of EVT for AIS within 6 hours of symptom onset (MR CLEAN, SWIFT-PRIME, REVASCAT, ESCAPE, and EXTEND-IA[15-19]). Two more recent randomized trials using patient selection based on perfusion imaging found that selected patients may benefit from EVT up to 24 hours from symptom onset (DAWN, DEFUSE 3[20,21]). Although these two landmark trials differed slightly in selection criteria, both demonstrated that in patients with smaller core infarct volumes (<51 mL in DAWN and <70 mL in DEFUSE 3) and relatively larger regions of ischemic penumbra (DEFUSE required a ratio of at least 1.8) EVT outperformed standard treatment even up to 24 hours from symptom onset (16 hours in DEFUSE 3). Thus, patients meeting the criteria outlined in these two studies should be considered for EVT. It is important to note that selection criteria in both trials were stringent; caution is necessary when applying findings from these trials to a broader population.

Approximately 20% of patients with AIS have a posterior circulation LVO. The major trials that found benefit with thrombectomy were limited to anterior circulation lesions. Benefits of EVT for basilar and other posterior circulation LVO have not been demonstrated in RCTs; however, the 2018 AHA recommendations indicate that carefully selected patients with posterior circulation stroke who can undergo EVT within 6 hours of symptom onset should be considered for EVT (level of evidence IIb). With the advent of smaller devices and more trackable aspiration catheters, the 2018 AHA guidelines make a similar recommendation for more distal M2 or M3 segments (portion of middle cerebral artery from the MCA bifurcation to the cortical surface) (IIb).[2]

J CTA/MRA confirms large vessel occlusion?

For patients who are candidates for EVT (ie, suspected LVO, meeting functional and time window criteria or perfusion-mismatch criteria), noninvasive vascular imaging (CTA preferred) is used to confirm the presence of LVO. Ideally, vascular imaging should include the aortic arch through the intracranial circulation. This provides valuable information for planning the EVT procedure and can identify extracranial carotid atherosclerotic disease or occlusion as the cause of stroke. This finding can alert the operator that extracranial angioplasty and possible carotid stenting may be necessary before intracranial thrombectomy. This additional imaging should not delay the administration of alteplase nor should administration of alteplase be dependent on the presence of a vessel occlusion demonstrated on noninvasive imaging. Ideally, after NCCT is obtained and the decision is made to administer alteplase, the

medication can be prepared and even administered during noninvasive vascular imaging. Importantly, CTA is recommended before assessment of creatinine in patients without a history of renal disease.[2] In patients who present between 6 and 24 hours from symptom onset, perfusion imaging (CT or MR) should be performed to aid in decision making for EVT. CT perfusion software that can distinguish between core infarct and ischemic penumbra can be extremely helpful for patient selection for EVT. Emergent CEA (done within ~60-90 minutes of presentation) does not have a role in patients with LVO and is not recommended by the current AHA guidelines.[2]

K Endovascular therapy

Mechanical thrombectomy should be performed as rapidly as possible after the patient is identified and selected for this intervention. Existing guidelines recommend the use of a stent retriever as the technique of choice for EVT. A stent retriever is a microwire-mounted, nondetachable and self-expanding stent designed to be placed within an occluded vessel to engage thrombus for removal. Several devices are available, including the Trevo (Stryker Neurovascular, Fremont, CA) and Solitaire (Medtronic, Minneapolis, MN) devices. All are designed for delivery via microcatheter, self-expansion and integration into the offending thrombus, and subsequent retrieval into the guide catheter to perform thrombectomy. An alternative technique is contact aspiration alone using a large-bore distal access catheter that is placed adjacent to the thrombus while suction is applied to the hub, termed the ADAPT technique (a direct aspiration first pass technique).[22] One RCT compared contact aspiration with mechanical thrombectomy with a stent retriever[23]; although no significant difference was shown, the trial's power to detect subtle differences in efficacy has been criticized as being insufficient to establish equivalence. Regardless of the technique, the goal of EVT is successful recanalization of the affected vessel to a thrombolysis in cerebral infarction (TICI) score of at least 2B or 3 (>50% recanalization in distal vessels or complete recanalization).

Several additional technical adjuncts are currently available in addition to mechanical thrombectomy using a stent retriever. These include the use of a balloon guide catheter with proximal aspiration to reverse flow and prevent distal embolism and/or a large-bore distal access catheter beyond the cervical ICA for direct aspiration against the thrombus. Additionally, intra-arterial injection of alteplase can be used for thrombus in arteries that are too small or too difficult to reach with mechanic thrombectomy devices; this technique should not be used as a primary EVT technique.[2]

In patients who have extracranial carotid occlusion, extracranial thrombectomy and angioplasty, along with possible stent placement, may be required before intracranial EVT. There is no role for CEA in that setting.[2]

Ⓛ Supportive post-stroke care

Patients with AIS should be admitted to a specialized stroke unit or ICU with expertise in the management of neurologic disorders (neuro-ICU). Patients who receive alteplase or EVT with successful reperfusion should have BP maintained <180/105 mm Hg for the first 24 hours after treatment. Hemodilution and BP augmentation in those with normal BP is not recommended.

Antiplatelet medications should be held for 24 hours as well. Aspirin should be administered to patients with AIS, regardless of alteplase treatment or EVT, within 24 to 48 hours of admission. The benefit of other anticoagulant or antiplatelet agents is not well established at this time. Glycoprotein IIb/IIIa antagonists (particularly abciximab) have been shown to be harmful for the treatment of AIS and increase the risk of hemorrhagic transformation.[24,25]

Patients should be assessed early for rehabilitation potential and nutrition, including dysphagia screening. Depression screening should also be performed. Nutrition should be started within 7 days of admission, ideally earlier. Interestingly, the benefit of LMWH or unfractionated heparin for the prevention of VTE is not presently established in acute stroke patients.[2]

REFERENCES

1. Roffe C, Nevatte T, Sim J, et al. Effect of routine low-dose oxygen supplementation on death and disability in adults with acute stroke: the Stroke Oxygen Study Randomized Clinical Trial. *JAMA*. 2017;318(12):1125-1135.
2. Powers WJ, Rabinstein AA, Ackerson T, et al. 2018 Guidelines for the early management of patients with acute ischemic stroke: a guideline for healthcare professionals from the American Heart Association/American Stroke Association. *Stroke*. 2019;50:e344-e418.
3. Chalela JA, Kidwell CS, Nentwich LM, et al. Magnetic resonance imaging and computed tomography in emergency assessment of patients with suspected acute stroke: a prospective comparison. *Lancet*. 2007;369(9558):293-298.
4. Brazzelli M, Sandercock PA, Chappell FM, et al. Magnetic resonance imaging versus computed tomography for detection of acute vascular lesions in patients presenting with stroke symptoms. *Cochrane Database Syst Rev*. 2009;(4):CD007424.
5. Barber PA, Hill MD, Eliasziw M, et al. Imaging of the brain in acute ischaemic stroke: comparison of computed tomography and magnetic resonance diffusion-weighted imaging. *J Neurol Neurosurg Psychiatry*. 2005;76(11):1528-1533.
6. Hemphill JC III, Bonovich DC, Besmertis L, Manley GT, Johnston SC. The ICH score: a simple, reliable grading scale for intracerebral hemorrhage. *Stroke*. 2001;32(4):891-897.
7. Hemphill JC III, Farrant M, Neill TAJ. Prospective validation of the ICH score for 12-month functional outcome. *Neurology*. 2009;73(14):1088-1094.
8. Mendelow AD, Gregson BA, Fernandes HM, et al. Early surgery versus initial conservative treatment in patients with spontaneous supratentorial intracerebral haematomas in the International Surgical Trial in Intracerebral Haemorrhage (STICH): a randomised trial. *Lancet*. 2005; 365(9457):387-397.
9. Mendelow AD, Gregson BA, Rowan EN, et al. Early surgery versus initial conservative treatment in patients with spontaneous supratentorial lobar intracerebral haematomas (STICH II): a randomised trial. *Lancet*. 2013;382(9890):397-408.
10. Hemphill JC, Greenberg SM, Anderson CS, et al. Guidelines for the management of spontaneous intracerebral hemorrhage: a guideline for healthcare professionals from the American Heart Association/American Stroke Association. *Stroke*. 2015;46(7):2032-2060.
11. van Loon J, Van Calenbergh F, Goffin J, Plets C. Controversies in the management of spontaneous cerebellar haemorrhage. A consecutive series of 49 cases and review of the literature. *Acta Neurochir (Wien)*. 1993;122(3-4):187-193.
12. Wardlaw JM, Murray V, Berge E, del Zoppo GJ. Thrombolysis for acute ischaemic stroke. *Cochrane Database Syst Rev*. 2014;(7):CD000213.
13. Hacke W, Donnan G, Fieschi C, et al. Association of outcome with early stroke treatment: pooled analysis of ATLANTIS, ECASS, and NINDS rt-PA stroke trials. *Lancet*. 2004;363(9411):768-774.
14. Hacke W, Kaste M, Bluhmki E, et al. Thrombolysis with alteplase 3 to 4.5 hours after acute ischemic stroke. *N Engl J Med*. 2008;359(13):1317-1329.
15. Berkhemer OA, Fransen PSS, Beumer D, et al. A randomized trial of intraarterial treatment for acute ischemic stroke. *N Engl J Med*. 2015;372(1):11-20.
16. Saver JL, Goyal M, Bonafe A, et al. Stent-retriever thrombectomy after intravenous t-PA vs. t-PA alone in stroke. *N Engl J Med*. 2015;372(24):2285-2295.
17. Jovin TG, Chamorro A, Cobo E, et al. Thrombectomy within 8 hours after symptom onset in ischemic stroke. *N Engl J Med*. 2015;372(24):2296-2306.
18. Goyal M, Demchuk AM, Menon BK, et al. Randomized assessment of rapid endovascular treatment of ischemic stroke. *N Engl J Med*. 2015;372(11):1019-1030.
19. Campbell BCV, Mitchell PJ, Kleinig TJ, et al. Endovascular therapy for ischemic stroke with perfusion-imaging selection. *N Engl J Med*. 2015;372(11):1009-1018.
20. Nogueira RG, Jadhav AP, Haussen DC, et al. Thrombectomy 6 to 24 hours after stroke with a mismatch between deficit and infarct. *N Engl J Med*. 2018;378(1):11-21.
21. Albers GW, Marks MP, Kemp S, et al. Thrombectomy for stroke at 6 to 16 hours with selection by perfusion imaging. *N Engl J Med*. 2018;378(8):708-718.
22. Turk AS, Spiotta A, Frei D, et al. Initial clinical experience with the ADAPT technique: a direct aspiration first pass technique for stroke thrombectomy. *J Neurointerv Surg*. 2014;6(3):231-237.
23. Lapergue B, Blanc R, Gory B, et al. Effect of endovascular contact aspiration vs stent retriever on revascularization in patients with acute ischemic stroke and large vessel occlusion: the ASTER randomized clinical trial. *JAMA*. 2017;318(5):443-452.
24. Ciccone A, Motto C, Abraha I, Cozzolino F, Santilli I. Glycoprotein IIb–IIIa inhibitors for acute ischemic stroke. *Stroke*. 2014;45(8):e155.
25. Adams HP, Effron MB, Torner J, et al. Emergency administration of abciximab for treatment of patients with acute ischemic stroke: results of an international phase III trial. *Stroke*. 2008;39(1):87.

Palma M. Shaw • William J. Quinones-Baldrich

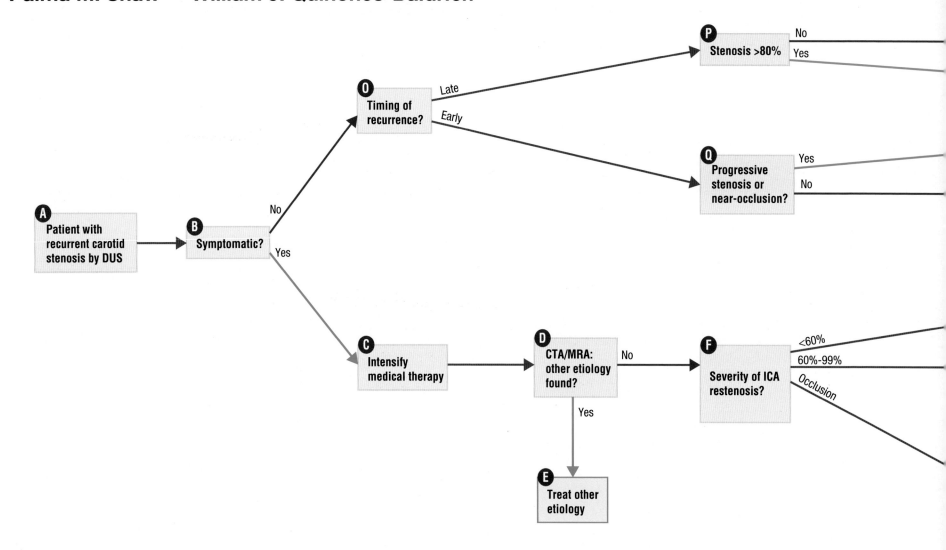

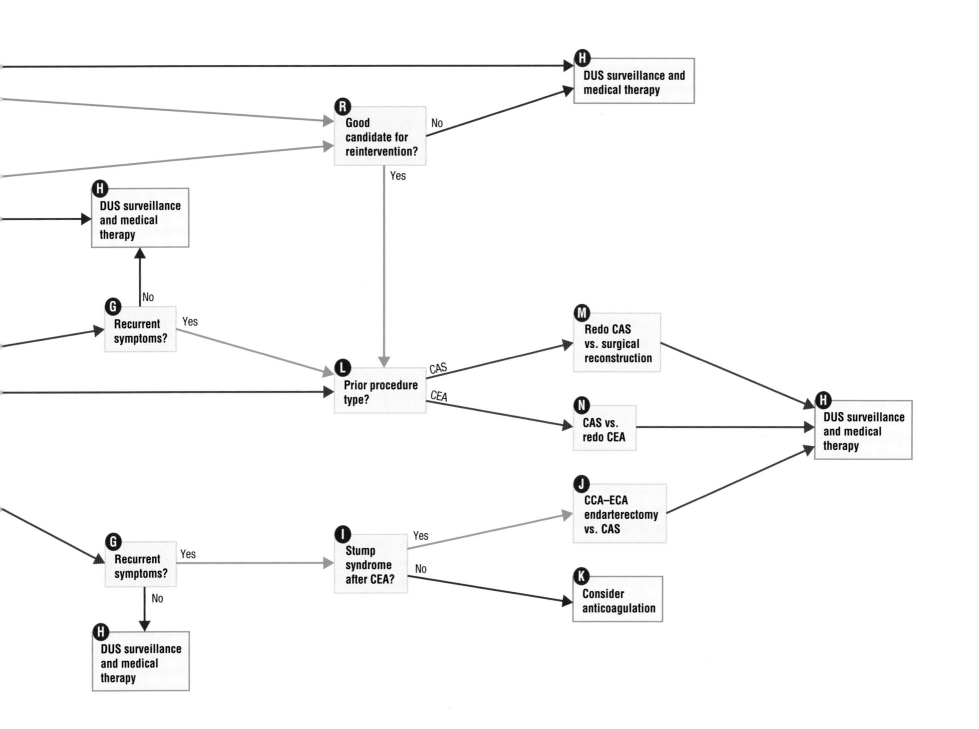

A Patient with recurrent carotid stenosis by DUS

Although the historical incidence of carotid restenosis after CEA or CAS ranged between 1% and 28% of cases,[1,2] recent studies report a lower rate, <6% of significant (>70%) restenosis.[3,4] The recurrence rate is higher with primary closure after CEA compared with patch closure,[5] and similar after CAS compared with CEA. It is our practice to obtain a baseline DUS within 6 weeks after CEA or CAS, then at 6 months, and annually thereafter, if stable.[6] Management of recurrent carotid stenosis depends primarily on whether there are associated neurologic symptoms.[7]

B Symptomatic?

Patients who develop TIA or stroke ipsilateral to a recurrent carotid stenosis should be considered symptomatic from the recurrent stenosis until proven otherwise. Symptoms are most often caused by emboli but can be related to flow restriction.

C Intensify medical therapy

For symptomatic patients with recurrent carotid stenosis on a single antiplatelet medication, dual antiplatelet therapy (usually aspirin + clopidogrel) should be initiated to reduce stroke risk. Initiation or intensification of statin therapy is also recommended.[7,8] Smoking cessation and treatment of HTN and diabetes should be optimized, as needed. Anticoagulation may be considered in symptomatic patients whose symptoms are thought to be low-flow related, but who are prohibitive candidates for intervention.[7,8]

D CTA/MRA: other etiology found?

Symptomatic patients with a recurrent carotid stenosis should be evaluated with additional imaging to confirm the severity of the recurrence and to detect other potential causes for neurologic symptoms. In heavily calcified lesions, MRA may be preferred over CTA, but CTA offers the advantage of further characterizing the plaque as there may be a significant soft component. The composition of plaque both on DUS and CTA can help in deciding whether repeat intervention is indicated. It is important to rule out other potential etiologies of ipsilateral neurologic symptoms in patients with recurrent carotid stenosis. Embolic sources other than the carotid bulb include the heart, atherosclerotic plaque in the ascending aorta, aortic arch, innominate artery, or proximal CCA. Paradoxical embolism from a venous source can occur through a patent foramen ovale. Hypertensive patients with stereotypical neurologic symptoms should be evaluated for potential lacunar events. Intracranial pathology should also be considered, particularly in patients who have other associated symptoms such as headache. Migraine equivalent syndromes can mimic TIAs. Vasculitis should be considered when the sedimentation rate is elevated.[6] If careful H&P and imaging rule out other causes for neurologic symptoms, carotid reintervention is considered.

E Treat other etiology

Patients with a cardiac source of embolization should be treated with systemic anticoagulation. Patients with a more proximal arterial source of emboli are usually managed with intensive antiplatelet medication, although stenting or open surgery is indicated for a dominant proximal lesion (see Chapter 13). The management of other etiologies responsible for the symptomatic condition of a patient with recurrent carotid stenosis depends on the specific disease responsible.[8]

F Severity of ICA restenosis?

In the absence of another explanation for a patient's symptoms, with appropriate distribution of the neurologic events, the degree of recurrent carotid stenosis and the plaque composition determine further management. Soft (echolucent) plaque has a significantly increased potential for embolization compared with calcific plaque. Complex plaques, those with both a calcific and a soft component, present an intermediate risk. In most instances, the degree of recurrent stenosis is the most determinant factor influencing the need for reintervention.[9-11]

G Recurrent symptoms?

Patients with recurrent neurologic symptoms despite maximum medical therapy should be considered for reintervention for recurrent carotid stenosis, if other potential causes have been eliminated.[7] This usually applies to patients with more than 60% recurrent ICA stenosis, but less frequently also to less severe stenosis or even occlusion. In some cases of ICA occlusion, neurologic symptoms may be secondary to hypoperfusion of the affected hemisphere because of poor collateral flow from the contralateral carotid or basilar circulation. In such cases, if stenoses can be treated in arteries responsible for collateral circulation, this should be performed. Extracranial to intracranial bypass is possible in this situation, but has not been supported by controlled trials.[12]

H DUS surveillance and medical therapy

Asymptomatic patients with <80% recurrent carotid stenosis should continue medical therapy and have DUS surveillance, initially in 6 months, and every year thereafter in absence of progression or symptoms. Symptomatic patients with <60% stenosis who become asymptomatic in response to aggressive medical therapy should also have DUS surveillance, as should patients who undergo reintervention. Continued medical treatment with antiplatelet and statin therapy, smoking cessation, and treatment of HTN and cardiac disease is essential.

I Stump syndrome after CEA?

In patients with ICA occlusion after CEA, embolization to intracranial branches of the ICA can occur through collaterals from the ECA. In the presence of an ICA occlusion, a stump or cavity can result at its origin and may lead to platelet and or thrombus aggregation that can potentially embolize through the ECA to the brain. Most important of these collaterals are the infraorbital, supraorbital, and mastoid branches of the ECA.[13,14] If symptoms persist after ICA occlusion, then consideration should be given to the presence of a stump syndrome.[8,15] This is confirmed by CTA, MRA, or DUS, and presumed to be the etiology if no other sources for symptoms have been defined. Even without an ICA stump cavity, atheroemboli from the carotid bulb or proximal ECA can cause neurologic symptoms. The exact etiology may not be clear until surgical exploration.

J CCA–ECA endarterectomy vs. CAS

Carotid stump syndrome due to ICA occlusion after CEA has been traditionally managed with surgical intervention consisting of flush ligation or resection of the ICA origin and endarterectomy of the CCA onto the ECA, with patch angioplasty. Most recently, placement of a covered stent from the CCA to the proximal ECA has been reported for treatment of an ICA stump syndrome, which needs to be evaluated based on more experience.[16-19]

K Consider anticoagulation

In patients with recurrent ipsilateral neurologic symptoms despite maximal medical therapy of ICA occlusion after CEA or CAS, anticoagulation is sometimes used. This is based on the concept that thromboemboli might arise from the distal ICA thrombus. There is no firm evidence to support this practice, but anticoagulation for 3 to 6 months while the ICA thrombus stabilizes may be the only option available.

L Prior procedure type?

Symptomatic patients unresponsive to medical therapy with appropriate symptoms ipsilateral to a recurrent carotid stenosis should be considered for reintervention. Options for reintervention depend on whether the initial procedure was CEA or CAS.

M Redo CAS vs. surgical reconstruction

Recurrent stenosis after CAS is most often treated with redo CAS. Surgical intervention for recurrent stenosis after CAS is also possible and involves removal of the stent, resection of the injured ICA, and reconstruction with prosthetic or autologous conduit.[20] In rare cases, the artery may be sufficiently intact to perform CEA with patching. Repeat endovascular therapy for carotid stenosis after CAS has been used commonly. In one review (42 articles including 239 interventions), the following techniques were used: PTA alone in 57%, repeat CAS in 21%, CEA in 16%, carotid artery bypass in 4%, and brachytherapy in 1%.[21] Variations of these techniques using cutting balloons, brachytherapy, and drug-coated balloons have been used, with repeat CAS placement reserved for when those fail.[22] No well-defined treatment algorithm is yet available. Data from a large registry showed equivalent outcomes for treating recurrent carotid stenosis after CEA versus CAS: 30-day ipsilateral stroke rate of 2.2% versus 1.3% ($P = 0.09$) for asymptomatic patients and 1.2% versus 1.6% ($P = 0.604$) for symptomatic patients. Thirty-day mortality was 1.3% versus 0.6% ($P = 0.04$) and MI in 1.4% versus 11% ($P = 0.443$), respectively. Cranial nerve injury occurred in 4.1% of redo CEA cases and access site complications occurred in 5.3% of CAS procedures. There was no significant difference in perioperative and 1-year outcomes between those treated with repeat CEA versus CAS.[23] In the group who had recurrent stenosis after prior CEA, significant predictors of perioperative stroke and death were older age, diabetes, active smoking, and preoperative ASA class IV status. When comparing patients treated for recurrent stenosis with CEA versus CAS, there was also no difference in outcome: 30-day postoperative stroke was 0% versus 0.3% ($P = 0.61$) for asymptomatic patients and 4.4% versus 3.5% ($P = 0.79$) for symptomatic patients for an overall stroke rate of 1.5% versus 1.4%. The rate of MI was 2.3% versus 1.2% ($P = 0.35$), but there was a significantly higher 30-day mortality rate of 3.7% for redo CEA versus 0.9% ($P = 0.02$) for redo CAS. However, freedom from stroke and death at 1 year was 91% for CEA and 92% for redo CAS ($P = 0.76$).[23] Because the outcomes are so similar, the choice of redo CAS versus open surgical revision should consider the patient's risk factors, location of the recurrence, operator experience, and patient's preference. High-risk patients are better candidates for repeat CAS, whereas acceptable risk patients can be considered for either. The accessibility of the stenosis to surgical treatment, surgical risk, and arch anatomy for CAS should be included in the decision between surgical or endovascular intervention. The recent introduction of transcarotid angioplasty and stenting may reduce the risk, particularly when the arch anatomy is unfavorable.[20,22-29]

ⓝ CAS vs. redo CEA

Reintervention for restenosis after CEA can be in the form of a redo CEA (or interposition graft) or CAS. Redo carotid surgery is associated with an increased risk of cranial nerve injury. Real-world data have demonstrated that CAS is used more commonly (63%) than CEA (37%) for recurrent stenosis after prior CEA. In asymptomatic patients, the difference in 30-day ipsilateral stroke rate was significant for CEA (2.2%) versus CAS (1.3%), and in symptomatic patients approached significance 1.2% versus 1.6% ($P = 0.60$). The incidence of redo-CEA cranial nerve injury is 4.1%. CEA was noted to have a higher mortality at 30 days and 1 year, 2.8% and 2.2%, respectively.[22] Early reports of CAS and stenting for treatment of recurrent carotid stenosis have

suggested acceptable results with perhaps a slightly increased risk of recurrence >50% recurrent stenosis rate of CAS versus CEA (6% vs. 0%, $P < 0.001$).[30]

ⓞ Timing of recurrence?

Asymptomatic patients with recurrent carotid stenosis can be categorized into those who experience an early recurrence (usually <2 years) and those who experience a late recurrence (>2 years). Although this division point is not precise, it is based on the fact that early recurrences are usually because of intimal hyperplasia that has a significantly lower potential for embolization. In contrast, later recurrence is more likely because of recurrent atherosclerosis, with comparable risk as de novo atherosclerotic lesions. The appearance of the stenosis on DUS can be helpful in making this differentiation, because intimal hyperplasia appears homogeneous, whereas atherosclerotic plaque is heterogeneous and often calcified.[2,11,31]

ⓟ Stenosis >80%?

Asymptomatic patients with late recurrent carotid stenosis, particularly those showing characteristics of atherosclerotic plaque on DUS, should have the stenosis severity confirmed with CTA. If ICA stenosis is more than 80%, consideration should be given for reintervention, analogous to patents with asymptomatic de novo ICA stenosis (see Chapter 7), but with higher risk of reintervention.

ⓠ Progressive stenosis or near-occlusion?

Early recurrent stenosis after CEA or CAS is usually because of intimal hyperplasia. Some have suggested that this has a more benign course than restenosis caused by atherosclerosis. These patients are usually managed with medical therapy and DUS surveillance.[6] Earlier studies suggest a 5.4% incidence of recurrent stenosis within 24 months. In the same study, two patients with early restenosis did progress to occlusion.[31] A different study reported 5-year follow-up on in-stent recurrent stenosis after CAS and found a significant restenosis rate (>80%) of 6.4% (5/122). In this small series, in-stent restenosis was not associated with neurologic symptoms.[32] Restenosis at 2 years was assessed as a secondary goal of the CREST trial. In this instance, restenosis was defined as more than 70% with PSV of 300 cm/s. Incidence of 6% noted in the CAS group and 6.3% in the CEA group was not significantly different. Of those participants who had restenosis or occlusion at 2 years, after adjustment for age, sex, and asymptomatic status, there was an increased risk for ipsilateral stroke during the follow-up period.[33] Close surveillance in hemodynamically significant lesions is still appropriate. If a lesion is clearly progressing or approaches near occlusion, most would recommend reintervention.[8,22]

ⓡ Good candidate for reintervention?

Patients with recurrent carotid stenosis who are asymptomatic must be carefully evaluated to ensure that the risk/benefit of reintervention outweighs best medical treatment alone. A randomized study comparing best medical therapy alone with redo CAS or CEA has not been conducted. Because the risk of redo treatment is generally higher than primary treatment, best medical therapy is more often used in patients with recurrent asymptomatic stenosis than with primary stenosis, particularly if the periprocedural risk of stroke is >3%.[34]

REFERENCES

1. DeGroote RD, Lynch TG, Jamil Z, Hobson RW II. Carotid restenosis: long-term noninvasive follow-up after carotid endarterectomy. *Stroke.* 1987;18(6):1031-1036.
2. Stoney RJ, String ST. Recurrent carotid stenosis. *Surgery.* 1976;80(6):705-710.
3. Carballo RE, Towne JB, Seabrook GR, Frieschlag JA, Cambria RA. An outcome analysis of carotid endarterectomy: the incidence and natural history of recurrent stenosis. *J Vasc Surg.* 1996;23:749-754.
4. Groschel K, Riecker A, Schulz JB, Ernemann U, Kastrup A. Systematic review of early recurrent stenosis after carotid angioplasty and stenting. *Stroke.* 2005;36(2):367-373.
5. AbuRahma AF, Robinson PA, Saiedy S, Richmond BK, Khan J. Prospective randomized trial of bilateral carotid endarterectomies: primary closure versus patching. *Stroke.* 1999;30(6):1185-1189.
6. Brott TG, Halperin JL, Abbara S, et al. 2011 ASA/ACCF/AHA/AANN/AANS/ACR/ASNR/CNS/SAIP/SCAI/SIR/SNIS/SVM/SVS guideline on the management of patients with extracranial carotid and vertebral artery disease: executive summary. *Catheter Cardiovasc Interv.* 2013; 81:E75-E123.
7. Ricotta JJ, AbuRahma A, Ascher E, Eskandari M, Faries P, Lal BK. Updated society for vascular surgery guidelines for management of extracranial carotid disease. *J Vasc Surg.* 2011;54:e1-e31.
8. Sacco RL, Adams R, Albers G, et al. Guidelines for prevention of stroke in patients with ischemic stroke or transient ischemic attack: a statement for healthcare professionals from the American Heart Association/American Stroke Association Council on Stroke Co-Sponsored by the Council on Cardiovascular Radiology and Intervention. *Circulation.* 2006;113:e409-e449.
9. Howard DPJ, van Lammeren GW, Rothwell PM, et al. Symptomatic carotid atherosclerotic disease correlations between plaque composition and ipsilateral stroke risk. *Stroke.* 2015;46:182-189. doi:10.1161/STROKEAHA.114.007221.

10. O'Donnell TF Jr, Rodriguez AA, Fortunato JE, Welch HJ, Mackey WC. Management of recurrent carotid stenosis: should asymptomatic lesions be treated surgically? *J Vasc Surg.* 1996;24:207-212.

11. O'Donnell TF Jr, Callow AD, Scott G, Shepard AD, Heggerick P, Mackey WC. Ultrasound characteristics of recurrent carotid disease. Hypothesis explaining the low incidence of symptomatic recurrence. *J Vasc Surg.* 1985;2:26-41.

12. Powers WJ, Clarke WR, Grubb RL Jr, Videen TO, Adams HP, Derdeyn CP; COSS Investigators. Extracranial-intracranial bypass for stroke prevention in hemodynamic cerebral ischemia: the carotid occlusion surgery study: a randomized trial. *JAMA.* 2011;306(18):1983-1992. doi:10.1001/jama.2011.1610.

13. Liberman AL, Zandieh A, Loomis C, et al. Symptomatic carotid occlusion is frequently associated with microembolization. *Stroke.* 2017;48:394-399. doi:10.1161/STROKEAHA.116.015375.

14. Thanvi B, Robinson T. Complete occlusion of extracranial internal carotid artery: clinical features, pathophysiology, diagnosis and management. *Postgrad Med J.* 2007;83:95-99. doi:10.1136/pgmj.2006.048041.

15. Omoto S, Hasegawa Y, Sakai K, et al. Common carotid artery stump syndrome due to mobile thrombus detected by carotid duplex ultrasonography. *J Stroke Cerebrovasc Dis.* 2016;25(10):e205-e207.

16. Harris M, Pillai L, Ricotta JJ. External carotid endarterectomy with internal carotid artery transposition flap angioplasty for symptomatic internal carotid artery occlusion. *Cardiovasc Surg.* 1995;3(6):625-629.

17. Baracchini C, Meneghetti G, Manara R, Ermani M, Ballotta E. Cerebral hemodynamics after contralateral carotid endarterectomy in patients with symptomatic and asymptomatic carotid occlusion: a 10-year follow-up. *J Cereb Blood Flow Metab.* 2006;26:899-905. doi:10.1038/sj.jcbfm.9600260.

18. Gertler JP, Cambria RP. The role of external carotid endarterectomy in the treatment of ipsilateral internal carotid occlusion: collective review. *J Vasc Surg.* 1987;6:158-167.

19. Naylor AR, Bell PRF, Bolia A. Endovascular treatment of carotid stump syndrome. *J Vasc Surg.* 2003;38(3):593-595.

20. Gonzalez A, Drummond M, McCord S, Garrett HE Jr. Carotid endarterectomy for treatment of in-stent restenosis. *J Vasc Surg.* 2011;54:1167-1169.

21. Pourier VEC, de Borst GJ. Technical options for treatment of in-stent restenosis after carotid artery stenting. *J Vasc Surg.* 2016;64:1486-1496.

22. Arhuidese I, Obeid T, Nejim B, Locham S, Hicks CW, Malas MB. Stenting versus endarterectomy after prior ipsilateral carotid endarterectomy. *J Vasc Surg.* 2017;65:1-11.

23. Arhuidese IJ, Nejim B, Chavali S, et al. Endarterectomy versus stenting in patients with prior ipsilateral carotid artery stenting. *J Vasc Surg.* 2017;65:1418-1428.

24. Matas M, Alvarez B, Ribo M, Molina C, Maeso J, Alvarez-Sabin J. Transcervical carotid stenting with flow reversal protection: experience in high-risk patients. *J Vasc Surg.* 2007;46:49-54.

25. Illuminati G, Belmonte R, Schneider F, Pizzardi G, Calió FG, Ricco JB. Prosthetic bypass for restenosis after endarterectomy or stenting of the carotid artery. *J Vasc Surg.* 2017;65:1664-1672.

26. Fokkema M, Jan de Borst G, Nolan BW, et al; Vascular Study Group of New England. Carotid stenting versus endarterectomy in patients undergoing reintervention after prior carotid endarterectomy. *J Vasc Surg.* 2014;59:8-15.

27. Vos JA, Jan de Borst G, Overtoom TT, et al; Antonius Carotid Endarterectomy, Angioplasty, and Stenting Study Group. Carotid angioplasty and stenting: treatment of postcarotid endarterectomy restenosis is at least as safe as primary stenosis treatment. *J Vasc Surg.* 2009;50:755-761.

28. Reichmann BL, van Laanen JHH, de Vries JP, et al. Carotid endarterectomy for treatment of in-stent restenosis after carotid angioplasty and stenting. *J Vasc Surg.* 2011;54:87-92.

29. Kwolek CJ, Jaff MR, Leal JI, et al. Results of the ROADSTER multicenter trial of transcarotid stenting with dynamic flow reversal. *J Vasc Surg.* 2015;62:1227-1235.

30. AbuRahma AF, Bates MC, Stone PA, Wulu JT. Comparative study of operative treatment and percutaneous transluminal angioplasty/stenting for recurrent carotid disease. *J Vasc Surg.* 2001;34:831-838.

31. Samson RH, Showalter DP, Yunis JP, Dorsay DA, Kulman HI, Silverman SR. Hemodynamically significant early recurrent carotid stenosis: an often self-limiting and self-reversing condition. *J Vasc Surg.* 1999;30:446-452.

32. Lal BK, Hobson RW II, Goldstein J, et al. In-stent recurrent stenosis after carotid artery stenting: life table analysis and clinical relevance. *J Vasc Surg.* 2003;38:1162-1169.

33. Lal BK, Beach KW, Roubin GS, et al; CREST Investigators. Restenosis after carotid artery stenting and endarterectomy: a secondary analysis of CREST: a randomized controlled trial. *Lancet Neurol.* 2012;11:755-763.

34. Liapis CD, Bell PRF, Mikhailidis D, et al; ESVS Guidelines Collaborators. ESVS guidelines. Invasive treatment for carotid stenosis: indications, techniques. *Eur J Vasc Endovasc Surg.* 2009;37:S1-S19.

Kellie R. Brown

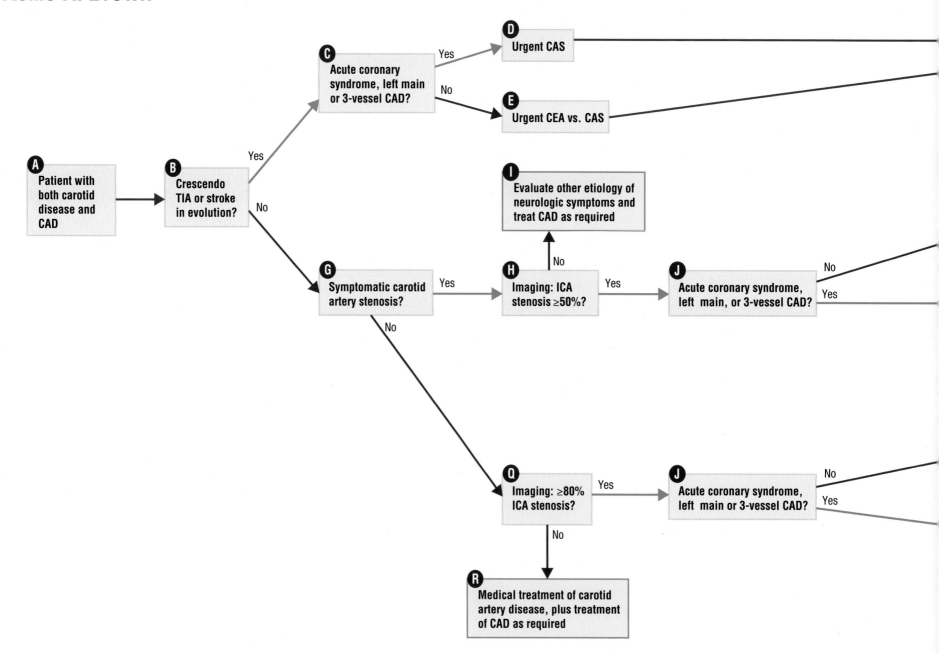

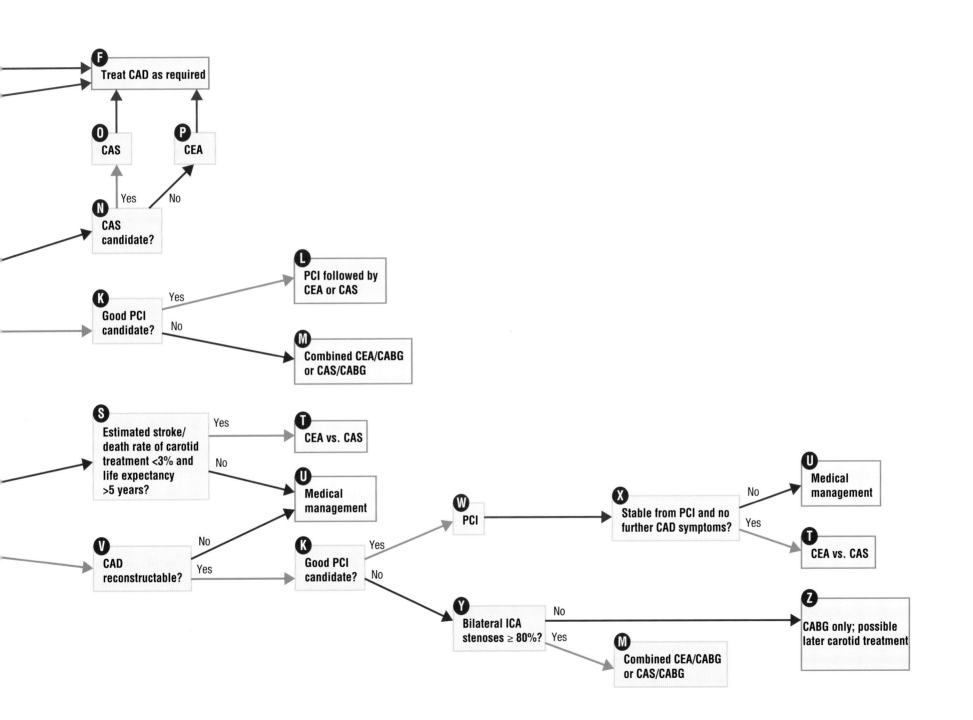

(A) Patient with both carotid disease and CAD

Combined disease in both the coronary and carotid vascular beds is common. In 1989, Hertzer et al. found 30% advanced compensated, 28% severe correctable, and 7% severe inoperable CAD in a series of 506 patients undergoing CEA and who underwent coronary arteriography.[1] Additionally, stroke is a major cause of morbidity after CABG, and patients are often screened for carotid disease before CABG. Schwartz et al. found 12% incidence of ≥80% stenosis in one or both carotid arteries in patients undergoing cardiopulmonary bypass.[2] Thus, the vascular surgeon is not infrequently confronted with a patient who has been found to have significant disease in both carotid and coronary arteries.

(B) Crescendo TIA or stroke in evolution?

Patients who present with crescendo TIAs or stroke in evolution represent a surgical emergency, generally precluding an in-depth evaluation of CAD. In addition, simultaneous correction of CAD in this situation is not feasible. Therefore, the carotid disease in these patients should be treated expeditiously understanding that they carry a higher risk of morbidity and mortality than a patient in an elective situation.

(C) Acute coronary syndrome, left main, or 3-vessel CAD?

The presence of simultaneous acute coronary syndrome, known left main CAD, or severe three-vessel CAD in a patient presenting with crescendo TIA or stroke in evolution influences the most appropriate emergent treatment of the carotid disease. These patients represent a very high-risk cohort,[3,4] and as such, the least invasive carotid treatment, namely CAS, is recommended. If markers of severe CAD are not present, urgent CAS or urgent CEA can be performed.

(D) Urgent CAS

If there is known symptomatic or severe CAD in a patient with crescendo TIA or stroke in evolution, urgent CAS is preferred for management of the carotid disease, if feasible.[3] CAS is discussed in detail in Chapters 7 and 8.

(E) Urgent CEA vs. CAS

If acute coronary syndrome, left main CAD, or severe three-vessel CAD is not present, the choice of urgent CAS versus CEA depends on several factors. If there is mobile thrombus as the cause of crescendo TIA, then CEA is more appropriate. If there is hostile neck anatomy (eg, presence of tracheostomy or history of radiation), CAS is more appropriate. As always, vessel anatomy (eg, tortuosity or calcification) and surgeon experience can determine whether CEA or CAS is more appropriate. CEA and CAS are discussed in detail in Chapters 7 and 8.

(F) Treat CAD as required

Once the carotid disease is treated appropriately in a patient with crescendo TIAs or stroke in evolution, CAD should be treated as required.

(G) Symptomatic carotid artery stenosis?

Symptoms referable to carotid stenosis generally include unilateral TIA, stroke, or amaurosis fugax (see Chapter 6). Carotid territory symptoms, especially ones that are recent, increase the benefit of carotid treatment.[5] If 6 months have passed since carotid symptoms, most would consider the patient to be asymptomatic. Carotid imaging with DUS to quantitate the severity of carotid stenosis is the next step in evaluation.

(H) Imaging: ICA stenosis ≥50%?

Initial imaging is done with DUS, and is sometimes supplemented by CTA or MRA, if needed, to more precisely define or confirm the anatomy and stenosis severity (see Chapter 8). The NASCET trial established that patients with amaurosis fugax, TIA, or stroke and who are found to have <50% stenosis do not benefit from carotid intervention.[6] However, in symptomatic patients with ≥50% ICA stenosis, the carotid disease warrants intervention in all but very high-risk patients.[6]

(I) Evaluate other potential etiologies for neurologic symptoms and treat CAD as required

If a patient with amaurosis fugax, TIA, or stroke is found to have <50% stenosis, a search for other possible causes of emboli is warranted. This would include CTA to evaluate intracranial, arch, and arch vessel disease, in addition to ECHO to exclude cardiac sources. In addition, risk factor management in the form of antiplatelet therapy, lipid lowering and blood pressure control, diabetes control, and smoking cessation is indicated.[3,4,7]

(J) Acute coronary syndrome, left main, or 3-vessel CAD?

Prophylactic coronary revascularization in patients with stable CAD is not warranted before noncardiac surgery. However, in patients with acute coronary syndromes or significant left main or three-vessel CAD, who would otherwise benefit from revascularization from the standpoint of survival or symptom improvement, coronary revascularization is warranted.[8]

(K) Good PCI candidate?

In a patient with acute coronary syndrome, left main CAD, or three-vessel CAD, coronary arteriography should be performed to determine if the patient is a good candidate for percutaneous coronary intervention (PCI), which would be performed at the time of diagnostic arteriography if appropriate.

(L) PCI followed by CEA or CAS

If the patient is a PCI candidate, then PCI should be done first, with initiation of dual antiplatelet therapy after coronary stent placement. This can be followed by CAS or CEA when the patient has recovered from PCI, unless carotid symptoms recur, or the carotid stenosis is very severe, in which case more rapid carotid treatment may be needed. This must be balanced against the risk of coronary stent thrombosis and death in patients who undergo noncardiac surgery within the first 4 weeks of coronary stenting.[8] This is an argument to pursue CAS in such patients, and allow treatment of symptomatic carotid disease within the 2-week time window recommended for maximum benefit. If CEA is needed, the timing needs to carefully balance the risk of progressive cerebrovascular symptoms versus coronary stent thrombosis. In addition, dual antiplatelet therapy should be continued during CEA or CAS if coronary stents have been placed.[8]

(M) Combined CEA/CABG or CAS/CABG

If the patient has both symptomatic coronary and carotid disease and PCI is not feasible, a combined treatment approach is favored.[3,4] Traditionally, a combined CEA/CABG is undertaken during the same anesthetic. More recently, some groups have been treating the carotid disease with CAS followed by CABG after 30 days when the clopidogrel can be stopped 5 to 7 days before CABG. In patients who cannot wait 30 days for CABG, CAS can be performed with aspirin and heparin, followed immediately by CABG. The clopidogrel is then started in the ICU after CABG.[9,10] However, recent meta-analysis found that CAS/CABG in patients with symptomatic carotid disease had a higher stroke risk than CEA/CABG.[11] Therefore, the decision to pursue CAS rather than CEA in this situation cannot be routinely recommended at this point and should depend primarily on local expertise and results.

(N) CAS candidate?

In a patient with symptomatic carotid artery stenosis and significant CAD (but without acute coronary syndrome, left main CAD, or three-vessel CAD), CAS is indicated and should be pursued in favor of CEA if anatomic assessment supports CAS. Relative contraindications to CAS include unfavorable arch anatomy, severe circumferentially calcified carotid bifurcation disease, aortoiliac occlusion, renal insufficiency, and severe allergy to contrast or antiplatelet agents.[3,4] CAS is discussed further in Chapters 7 and 8.

(O) CAS

CAS is discussed in detail in Chapters 7 and 8.

P CEA

Patients who are not CAS candidates should be considered for CEA. NASCET established that patients with symptomatic carotid disease >50% had a statistically significant benefit from CEA. However, this procedure needs to be performed by an experienced surgeon with a low stroke/death rate within 2 weeks of symptom onset to preserve the benefit.[5,6] The NASCET had a 2.1% major stroke/death rate in the perioperative period. It is necessary to perform this procedure with similar outcomes to maintain the benefit reported in that study.[6,12] CEA is discussed in detail in Chapters 7 and 8.

Q Imaging: ≥80% ICA stenosis?

The Asymptomatic Carotid Atheroslerosis Study (ACAS) and the Asymptomatic Carotid Surgery Trial (ACST) demonstrated a benefit for CEA in asymptomatic patients with a ≥60% stenosis.[13,14] However, the absolute risk reduction in ACAS at 5 years was relatively small (11% for medically treated vs. 5% for surgically treated patients). Furthermore, recent evaluation of aggressive medical management suggests a lower stroke rate, further reducing the potential benefit of prophylactic carotid treatment.[15] Therefore, CEA or CAS in asymptomatic patients has to be performed with very low morbidity and mortality if the benefit is to be maintained. It is generally accepted that the higher the risk of stroke, the greater the degree of stenosis.[13,14] Therefore, in asymptomatic patients, CEA and CAS are generally reserved for those with high-grade stenosis. What constitutes high-grade stenosis has evolved. Traditionally, ultrasound criteria included an 80% to 99% stenosis category that constituted high-grade stenosis. With the publication of the Society of Radiologists in Ultrasound consensus document, however, a 70% to 99% stenosis category has become widely adopted.[16] It seems reasonable to use whatever one's accredited vascular lab adopts as a standard for high-grade stenosis.

R Medical treatment of carotid artery disease, plus treatment of CAD as required

Medical management of risk factors in a patient with mild or moderate asymptomatic carotid disease is indicated, and is preferred over CEA or CAS.[13] Medical management should include antiplatelet therapy, lipid lowering and blood pressure control, aggressive diabetes management, and smoking cessation.[3,4,7] Although there is no confirmatory evidence that dual antiplatelet therapy is more effective than aspirin alone for prevention of stroke in asymptomatic carotid disease, dual antiplatelet therapy is beneficial in patients with acute coronary syndromes or after PCI for preventing death, reinfarction, or stroke.[7,17] Therefore, the decision for dual antiplatelet therapy should be based on its proven benefit in CAD.

S Estimated stroke/death rate of carotid treatment <3% and life expectancy >5 years?

In patients with stable CAD and asymptomatic carotid disease, the decision to move forward with CEA or CAS should be made carefully. To maintain the advantage of CEA in an asymptomatic population, the procedure has to be done with very low morbidity. In ACAS, the 6% absolute stroke rate reduction in patients undergoing CEA was dependent on a low perioperative stoke/death rate of only 2.6%.[13] If the estimated stroke and death rate from CEA or CAS is <3% and life expectancy is >5 years, then CEA or CAS can be recommended, understanding that thorough discussion of the risks and benefits with the patient is critical for decision making.[13]

T CEA vs. CAS

The choice between CEA and CAS in asymptomatic carotid disease is discussed in Chapter 7. Generally, in asymptomatic patients, CEA is preferred as long as the patient has a low risk of coronary complications with surgery.[13,14] In patient with combined coronary and carotid disease, there may be elevated coronary risk; therefore, in certain cases CAS may be preferred, as CAS has been shown to have lower risk of MI after intervention than CEA.[18] However, strong consideration should be given to medical management in patients who have asymptomatic disease if they are not suitable candidates for CEA, as the risk of stroke with CAS is higher than with CEA.[18]

U Medical management

If a patient with asymptomatic carotid stenosis has nonreconstructable symptomatic CAD or is at high risk of stroke or death from CEA or CAS, medical management of both coronary and carotid disease is the most appropriate therapy, and includes antiplatelet therapy, cholesterol and blood pressure control, aggressive diabetic management, and smoking cessation.[3,4,7,13] This is also true for patients with asymptomatic carotid stenosis who continue to have CAD symptoms despite prior PCI.

V CAD reconstructable?

In patients with asymptomatic severe carotid stenosis who also have acute coronary syndrome, left main disease, or three-vessel CAD, evaluation should be undertaken to determine if CAD is reconstructable.

W PCI

Patients with asymptomatic carotid stenosis and CAD amenable to PCI are treated with PCI, after which carotid treatment can be considered in patients with adequate CAD treatment.

X Stable from PCI and no further CAD symptoms?

After PCI, carotid intervention in asymptomatic patients should be delayed for at least 4 weeks to ensure that the CAD has been effectively treated.[8] Once the patient recovers from PCI, with no further symptoms of CAD, reevaluation and risk stratification for potential prophylactic carotid treatment should be performed.

Y Bilateral ICA stenoses ≥ 80%?

The decision to treat asymptomatic carotid disease before CABG to prevent stroke is controversial because definitive data are lacking. It is clear that the presence of carotid disease increases the risk of stroke with CABG, although stroke is highest in those patients with carotid occlusion, which cannot be remedied by CEA or CAS.[19] Additionally, many studies fail to identify whether post-CABG strokes are ipsilateral to the noted carotid disease—all of which may overestimate the benefit that carotid intervention may have on stroke prevention before CABG. In fact, the majority of strokes after CABG are not attributable to carotid disease.[20] Therefore, it seems reasonable to limit prophylactic carotid intervention in patients undergoing CABG to those who are at particularly high risk for stroke.

In that regard, there is some support in the literature for treating patients who have bilateral asymptomatic 80% to 99% ICA stenosis, or an 80% to 99% ICA stenosis with contralateral occlusion, with a combined approach, although definitive proof of benefit is lacking.[3] Patients with a history of stroke or TIA in the previous 6 months or with severe bilateral carotid disease represent those at highest risk for stroke with CABG. Carotid intervention in these patients is recommended, and synchronous CEA/CABG or CAS followed by CABG could be considered. The decision to perform CEA/CABG or CAS/CABG should be based on urgency of surgery, antiplatelet strategy, local expertise, and results.[3]

Z CABG only; possible later carotid treatment

In patients who require CABG with unilateral, asymptomatic carotid stenosis, the stroke risk after surgery is ≤2%.[20] Thus, it is not currently recommended that these patients undergo prophylactic CEA or CAS before, or in conjunction with, CABG.[3,4] In such patients, future potential treatment of carotid stenosis would be evaluated independently, taking into consideration the effectiveness of CAD treatment and the potential progression of carotid stenosis or symptom development.

REFERENCES

1. Hertzer NR, Loop FD, Beven EG, et al. Surgical staging for simultaneous coronary and carotid disease: a study including prospective randomization. *J Vasc Surg.* 1989;9:455-463.

2. Schwartz LB, Bridgman AH, Kieffer RW, et al. Asymptomatic carotid artery stenosis and stroke in patients undergoing cardiopulmonary bypass. *J Vasc Surg*. 1995;21(1):146-153.

3. Naylor AR, Ricco JB, deBorst GJ, et al. Management of atherosclerotic carotid and vertebral artery disease: 2017 clinical practice guidelines of the European Society for Vascular Surgery. *Eur J Vasc Endovasc Surg*. 2018;55:3-81.

4. Brott TG, Halperin JL, Abbara S, et al. 2011 ASA/ACCF/AHA/AANN/AANS/ACR/ASNR/CNS/SAIP/SCAI/SIR/SNIS/SVM/SVS guideline on the management of patients with extracranial carotid and vertebral artery disease. *J Am Coll Cardiol*. 2011;57:e16-e94.

5. Rothwell PM, Eliasziw M, Gutnikov SA, Warlow CP, Barnett HJ; Carotid Endarterectomy Trialists Collaboration. Endarterectomy for symptomatic carotid stenosis in relation to clinical subgroups and diming of surgery. *Lancet*. 2004;363(9413):915-924.

6. Barnett HJM, Taylor DW, Eliasziw M, et al. North American Symptomatic Carotid Endarterectomy Trial Collaborators. Benefit of carotid endarterectomy in patients with symptomatic moderate or severe stenosis. *N Engl J Med*. 1998;339:1415-1425.

7. Cheng SF, Brown MM. Contemporary medical therapies of atherosclerotic carotid artery disease. *Semin Vasc Surg*. 2017;30(1):8-16.

8. Levine GN, Bates ER, Blankenship JC, et al. 2011 ACCF/AHA/SCAI Guidelines for percutaneous coronary intervention. *J Am Coll Cardiol*. 2011;58(24):e44-e122.

9. Velissaris J, Kiskinis D, Anastasiadis K. Synchronous carotid artery stenting and open heart surgery. *J Vasc Surg*. 2011;53:1237-1241.

10. Versaci F, Reimers B, Del Giudice C, et al. Simultaneous hybrid revascularization by carotid stenting and coronary artery bypass grafting: the SHARP study. *JACC Cardiovasc Interv*. 2009;2:393-401.

11. Paraskevas KL, Nduwago S, Saratzis AN, et al. Carotid stenting prior to coronary bypass surgery: an updated systemic review and meta-analysis. *Eur J Endovasc Surg*. 2017;53:309-319.

12. North American Symptomatic Carotid Endarterectomy Trial Collaborators; Barnett HJM, Taylor DW, Haynes RB, et al. Beneficial effect of carotid endarterectomy in symptomatic patients with high-grade carotid stenosis. *N Engl J Med*. 1991;325:445-453.

13. Executive Committee for the Asymptomatic Carotid Atherosclerosis Study. Endarterectomy for asymptomatic carotid artery stenosis. *JAMA*. 1995;273(18):1421-1428.

14. Halliday A, Harrison M, Hayter E, et al. 10-year stroke prevention after successful CEA for asymptomatic stenosis (ACST-1): a multicenter randomized trial. *Lancet*. 2010;376(9746):1074-1084.

15. Abbott AL. Medical (non-surgical) intervention alone is now best for prevention of stoke associated with asymptomatic severe carotid stenosis: results of a systematic review and analysis. *Stroke*. 2009;40:e573-e583.

16. Grant EG, Benson CB, Moneta GL, et al. Carotid artery stenosis: Gray-scale and Doppler US diagnosis—Society of Radiologists in Ultrasound consensus conference. *Radiology*. 2003;229(2):340-346.

17. Bowry AD, Brookhart A, Chaudhry NK. Meta-analysis of the efficacy and safety of Clopidogrel plus aspirin as compared to antiplatelet monotherapy for the prevention of vascular events. *Am J Cardiol*. 2008;101(7):960-966.

18. Brott TG, Hobson RW, Howard G, et al; CREST Investigators. Stenting versus endarterectomy for the treatment of carotid-artery stenosis. *N Engl J Med*. 2010;363:11-23.

19. Naylor AR. Managing patients with symptomatic coronary and carotid disease. *Perspect Vasc Surg Endovasc Ther*. 2010;22(2):70-76.

20. Naylor AR, Mehta Z, Rothwell PM, Bell PRF. Carotid artery disease and stroke during coronary artery bypass: a critical review of the literature. *Eur J Vasc Endovasc Surg*. 2002;23:283-294.

Mark D. Morasch

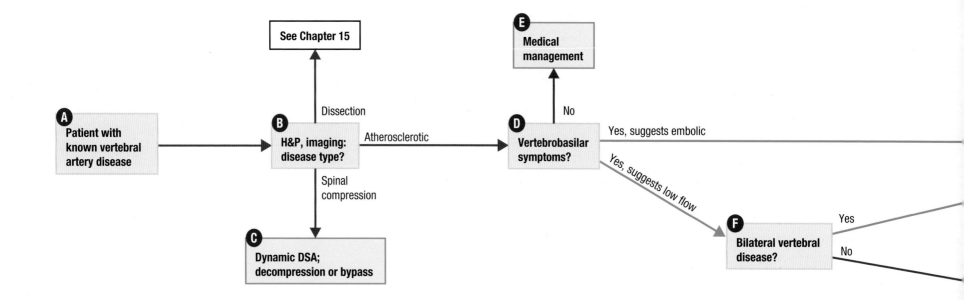

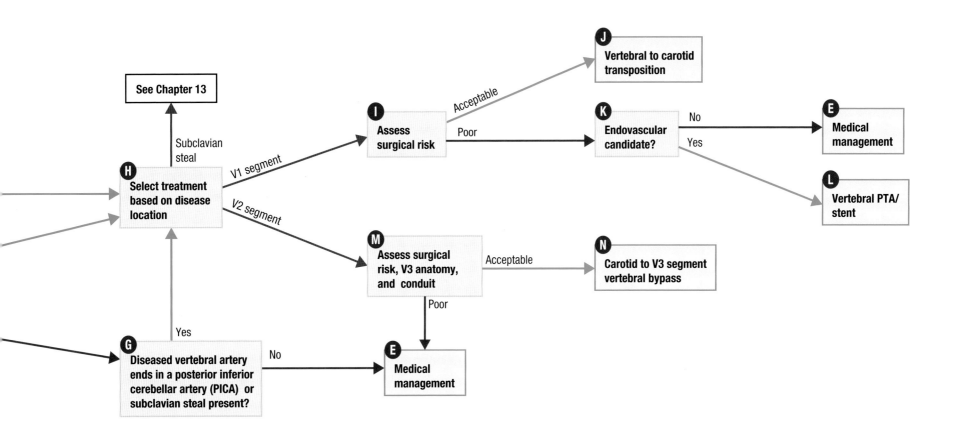

A Patient with known vertebral artery disease

Although it is not uncommon, on imaging, to identify vertebral pathologic lesions (atherosclerotic, dissection, osteophytic compression, dysplasia, arteritis, or aneurysm), it is uncommon for these lesions to require surgical or endoluminal treatment. Despite this, up to 20% of ischemic strokes involve the posterior circulation of the brain and half of these are attributable to large artery occlusive or embolic disease.[1] Symptoms of ischemia of the posterior circulation are often vague and nonspecific but warrant additional workup as symptomatic vertebral artery stenosis is associated with a 5-year stroke risk of 30%.[2]

B H&P, imaging: disease type?

Vertebral artery stenosis is a common arteriographic finding, and dizziness is a common complaint. However, the presence of both cannot be assumed to have a cause–effect relationship. Ischemia affecting the temporo-occipital areas of the cerebral hemispheres or segments of the brain stem and cerebellum characteristically produces bilateral symptoms. The classic symptoms of vertebrobasilar ischemia are dizziness, vertigo, drop attacks, diplopia, perioral numbness, alternating paresthesia, tinnitus, dysphasia, dysarthria, and ataxia. When patients present with two or more of these symptoms, vertebrobasilar ischemia is likely the cause.[3] Symptoms or signs consistent with posterior circulation ischemia warrant adequate imaging by CTA, MRA, or DSA. DUS may be helpful to identify physiologic steal (reversed flow in one vertebral artery). MRI may be necessary to appropriately image the posterior brain for infarcts as well as to rule out other pathology that could explain symptoms. The surgical anatomy of the paired vertebral arteries has traditionally been divided into four segments: V-1, the origin of the vertebral artery arising from the subclavian artery to the point at which it enters the C6 transverse process; V-2, the segment of the artery buried deep within intertransversarii muscles and the cervical transverse processes of C6–C2; V-3, the extracranial segment between the transverse process of the C2 and the base of the skull before it enters the foramen magnum; and V-4, the intracranial portion beginning at the atlantooccipital membrane and terminating as the two vertebral arteries converge to form the basilar artery. Management of vertebral artery pathology, identified by imaging, depends on the etiology. Atherosclerosis is the most common cause of vertebral artery disease and is discussed in detail in this chapter. Vertebral artery dissection is discussed in detail in Chapter 15. Vertebral artery compression syndromes caused by cervical spine degeneration or osteophytes may also require neuro- or vascular surgical intervention.

C Dynamic DSA; decompression or bypass

In circumstances when symptoms suggest episodic, positional ischemia but static images of the vertebral artery appear normal, dynamic DSA with provocative positioning may become necessary. If osteophytic compression is identified, neurosurgical decompression or V3 segment bypass may be indicated.[4]

D Vertebrobasilar symptoms?

Most patients with atherosclerotic vertebral artery lesions are asymptomatic because of well-compensated collateral circulation from the contralateral vertebral, cervical collaterals or carotid arteries via an intact circle of Willis. A single, normal vertebral artery is sufficient to adequately perfuse the basilar artery, regardless of the patency status of the contralateral vertebral artery. Asymptomatic patients are managed medically. Patients with identified vertebral artery disease who have vertebrobasilar circulation symptoms require further evaluation. These symptoms can be caused by embolization or low flow. Patients who experience emboli have varied symptoms that are unpredictable regarding their timing and can cause a stroke. In contrast, symptoms from low flow tend to be short-lived and repetitive, and are predictably caused by maneuvers that reduce cardiac output (such as rising quickly from a recumbent position). Fortunately, these hemodynamic mechanisms rarely result in a stroke, but the symptoms can be disabling in some cases and require treatment. Patients with embolic symptoms who fail antiplatelet therapy should be considered for intervention. Similarly, patients with incapacitating hemodynamic symptoms should also be considered for intervention.

E Medical management

Surgical or endovascular treatment is not indicated in an asymptomatic patient with stenotic or occlusive atherosclerotic vertebral artery lesions. These patients are managed medically, with antiplatelet agents and statins, smoking cessation, and treatment of any associated HTN, diabetes, and heart disease (see Chapters 1 and 2).

F Bilateral vertebral disease?

Because a single normal vertebral artery is sufficient to normally perfuse the basilar artery, symptoms because of low flow require bilateral significant vertebral stenosis or occlusion, unless subclavian steal or anomalous anatomy is present (see G). When hemodynamic symptoms are sufficiently severe and both of the paired vertebral arteries have significant disease, intervention is appropriate.

G Diseased vertebral artery ends in a posterior inferior cerebellar artery (PICA) or subclavian steal present?

Hemodynamic vertebrobasilar symptoms can arise without bilateral vertebral artery disease in patients with subclavian occlusive disease, leading to vertebral steal phenomena, or in patients where one vertebral artery does not join the basilar, but rather ends in a posterior inferior cerebellar artery (PICA). In these circumstances, despite a normal, patent single or bilateral (steal) vertebral artery, intervention is appropriate if warranted by symptom severity.

H Select treatment based on disease location

Patients with posterior circulation symptoms of either hemodynamic or embolic origin and appropriate identifiable occlusive lesions should be placed on appropriate antiplatelet and statin therapy and considered for surgical or endovascular intervention. The optimal type of treatment depends on whether the V1 versus the V2 segment, or a subclavian stenosis causing the steal requires treatment. In patients with subclavian artery stenosis, DUS demonstrating reversed or to-and-fro flow in the ipsilateral vertebral artery[5] and appropriate posterior circulation symptoms should be considered for subclavian artery revascularization if considered a reasonable risk for surgery or stenting (see Chapter 13).

I Assess surgical risk

Appropriate surgical risk assessment should be undertaken to help determine whether open surgical or endovascular treatment is more appropriate. Patients with reasonable exercise tolerance who would be considered appropriate for CEA should be considered appropriate for open vertebral artery revascularization procedures if performed in a center of excellence by experienced vertebral surgeons.

J Vertebral to carotid transposition

Proximal vertebral artery stenosis, confined to the vertebral artery origin from the subclavian artery (in the V1 segment), is best treated surgically with a vertebral to CCA transposition. The approach to the proximal vertebral artery is the same as the approach for a subclavian to carotid transposition, between the two heads of the sternocleidomastoid, with the CCA reflected medially with the vagus nerve and the jugular vein retracted laterally. Once identified, the vertebral artery, found deep to the vertebral vein and cervical sympathetic plexus, is dissected superiorly up to the level of the tendon of the longus colli and inferiorly to its origin from the subclavian artery, exposing 2 to 3 cm of its length. When fully exposed, an appropriate site for reimplantation in the CCA is selected. The distal portion of the V1 segment of the vertebral artery is clamped below the edge of the longus colli. The proximal vertebral artery is ligated immediately above the stenosis using a small monofilament suture as a transfixion stitch. The artery is divided at this proximal level. The CCA artery is then cross-clamped. An elliptical 5-to-7-mm arteriotomy is created in the posterolateral wall of the CCA with an aortic punch. The anastomosis is performed in a parachute fashion with continuous 7-0 polypropylene suture, avoiding any tension on the vertebral artery, which may tear easily. Before completion of the anastomosis, standard flushing maneuvers are performed, the suture is tied, and flow is reestablished.[6]

Combined death and stroke rates reported for vertebral to carotid transposition are 1% in centers of excellence.[7,8] Risk is generally increased when patients undergo a combination of both vertebral and carotid revascularization. Surgical morbidity includes risk for stroke (<1%), immediate thrombosis (1.4%), vagus and recurrent laryngeal nerve palsy (2%), Horner syndrome (8%-28%), lymphocele (4%), and chylothorax (5%).[8] Long-term outcomes of open revascularization for vertebral artery disease are generally excellent with high stroke-free survival rates and patency as high as 90% at 10 years.[9] Although the number of studies are limited and these reports consist of only medium-sized case series, the results seen with open vertebral reconstruction should be considered benchmarks upon which endovascular therapy should be compared.

Ⓚ Endovascular candidate?

Patients with proximal vertebral artery stenosis, confined to the vertebral artery origin from the subclavian artery (in the V1 segment), who are not surgical candidates can be considered for proximal vertebral angioplasty and stenting. Endovascular intervention should be considered a second choice because of durability inferior to surgical transposition and a relatively high stent fracture rate. However, because relatively few surgeons are expert in open surgical treatment of vertebral artery disease, much V1 segment vertebral disease is now treated with an endovascular approach. More distal vertebral lesions should be approached with caution as arterial thrombosis rates after intervention are high.

Ⓛ Vertebral PTA/stent

In the past decade, endovascular treatment of vertebral artery disease, usually with stent placement, has gained favor as an alternative to surgery. Endovascular access to the vertebral artery is relatively straightforward. The procedure can be performed under local anesthesia, enabling continuous neurologic monitoring of the patient. Most cases are performed from a femoral approach, although transbrachial and transradial access has also been used. The stenotic lesions are crossed using 0.014 or 0.018 in. guidewires and treated with small coronary-diameter balloons and stents. Procedures can be performed with or without the assistance of embolic protection devices. Periprocedural risks include embolization, rupture, thrombosis, arterial dissection, and stent malposition or fracture.

In their series of 105 patients who underwent endovascular stenting for symptomatic vertebral artery disease, Jenkins et al. achieved 100% radiographic improvement (residual stenosis ≤ 30%). The authors reported immediate (30-day) periprocedural risk of death of 1% and periprocedural complication rate of 4.8%. At 1 year of follow-up, six patients had died and five had experienced a vertebrobasilar stroke. At 2.5 years of follow-up, 70% of patients remained symptom-free, but 13% of patients had restenosis requiring re-treatment.[10] Eighteen patients with extracranial vertebral artery disease in the Stenting of Symptomatic Atherosclerotic Lesions in the Vertebral or Intracranial Arteries (SSYLVIA) Trial underwent PTA and stenting. Technical success was achieved in 17 (94%) of the 18 patients. There were no periprocedural neurologic complications. The investigators, however, reported 6-month restenosis rates of 50%. These recurrences were symptomatic in 39% of cases.[11] Ogilvy et al. reported a series of patients with 21-month follow-up in whom drug-eluting stents were used in vertebral artery origin stenoses. They found decreased incidence of in-stent restenosis (>50% diameter) from 38% in patients who received non-drug-eluting stents to 17% in those who received drug-eluting stents.[12] Other reports also suggest decreased restenosis rates with drug-eluting stents; however, majority of the studies have mean patient follow-up times <1 year.[13,14] In addition, a 2014 meta-analysis of 480 lesions compared bare metal stents (BMS) (309) with the use of drug-eluting stents (175) and found a significant improvement in angiographic restenosis (8.2% DES vs. 23.7% for BMS, $P < 0.001$).[15] Finally, a recent meta-analysis of vertebral artery stenting included 980 patients and reported a favorable 30-day stroke rate of 1.1% and low symptomatic recurrence of 6.5% at 21 months.[16]

Endovascular treatment of vertebral artery disease is associated with high technical success rates and, newer technologies such as drug-eluding stents have led to an improvement in restenosis rates when compared with the initial reports that used PTA alone. Although adjuvant stent placement improves clinical durability, it does add an inherent morbidity such as malposition and late stent fracture; however, these have been rare in contemporary studies. Treatment with drug-eluting stents requires long-term dual antiplatelet therapy and it remains unclear to date whether differing stent makeup will have a significant impact in outcomes. There are currently no level I data to support the routine application of PTA and stenting of the vertebral artery over best medical therapy.

Ⓜ Assess surgical risk, V3 anatomy, and conduit

Reasonable surgical candidates with symptomatic lesions extending beyond the vertebral artery origin, including patients with complete V1 and V2 segment occlusion, can be considered for CCA to distal vertebral artery bypass provided the V3 segment is reconstituted and is a reasonable target for reconstruction. Adequate GSV or radial artery conduit must be available for the bypass.

Ⓝ Carotid to V3 segment bypass

This reconstruction is performed as a bypass, usually from the CCA to the V3 segment at the C1-C2 spinal level. The skin incision is placed in the upper neck anterior to the sternocleidomastoid muscle, similar to the incision used for CEA. The dissection proceeds between the jugular vein and the anterior edge of the sternocleidomastoid, exposing and protecting the retrojugular portion of the spinal accessory nerve. The levator scapula muscle is identified by removal of the fibrofatty tissue overlying it. Once the anterior edge of the levator muscle is exposed, the anterior ramus of C2 will be visible. With the ramus as a guide, a right-angle clamp is slid under the levator scapula and over the ramus, and the muscle is transected from its insertion on the C1 transverse process. The vertebral artery between C1 and C2 can easily be identified after dividing the C2 ramus. Once the vertebral artery is exposed circumferentially at this level, the CCA is dissected and prepared as inflow for a bypass graft. The vertebral artery is elevated gently and controlled using a small J-clamp. This isolates a short segment for an end-to-side anastomosis. The vertebral artery is opened longitudinally over a short length adequate to accommodate the spatulated end of the bypass conduit. The end-to-side anastomosis is completed with a continuous 8-0 monofilament suture. The proximal end of the graft is passed behind the jugular vein, the carotid controlled, and the proximal anastomosis completed. Before the anastomosis is completed, standard flushing maneuvers are performed. Although GSV is optimal, other conduits such as radial artery have been successfully used.[7,17]

Combined death and stroke rates reported for carotid to V3 bypass is 4% in centers of excellence.[7,8] Risk is generally increased when patients undergo a combination of both vertebral and carotid revascularization. Surgical morbidity includes risk for stroke (<1%), immediate thrombosis (1.4%), and vagus and recurrent laryngeal nerve palsy (2%).[8] Long-term outcomes of open revascularization for vertebral artery disease are generally excellent with high stroke-free survival rates and patency as high as 90% at 10 years.[9] Although the number of studies are limited and these reports consist of only medium-sized case series, the results seen with open vertebral reconstruction should be considered benchmarks to which endovascular therapy should be compared.

REFERENCES

1. Jenkins JS, Stewart M. Endovascular treatment of vertebral artery stenosis. *Prog Cardiovasc Dis.* 2017;59:619-625.
2. Crowley F, Brown MM. Percutaneous transluminal angioplasty and stenting for vertebral artery stenosis. *Cochrane Database Syst Rev.* 2000;(2):CD000516.
3. Morasch MD. Vertebral artery revascularization. UpToDate; 2017. https://www.uptodate.com/contents/vertebral-artery-revascularization.
4. Bauer R. Mechanical compression of the vertebral arteries. In: Berguer R, Bauer R, eds. *Vertebrobasilar Arterial Occlusive Disease: Medical and Surgical Management.* New York, NY: Raven; 1984:45-71.
5. Berguer R, Higgins R, Nelson R. Noninvasive diagnosis of reversal of vertebral-artery blood flow. *N Engl J Med.* 1980;302(24):1349-1351.
6. Roon AJ, Ehrenfeld WK, Cooke PB, Wylie EJ. Vertebral artery reconstruction. *Am J Surg.* 1979;138(1):29-36.

7. Berguer R. Complex carotid and vertebral revascularizations. In: Pearce WH, Matsumura JS, Yao JST, eds. *Vascular Surgery in the Endovascular Era*. Evanston, IL: Greenwood Academic; 2008:344-352.

8. Berguer R, Morasch MD, Kline RA. A review of 100 consecutive reconstructions of the distal vertebral artery for embolic and hemodynamic disease. *J Vasc Surg*. 1998;27(5):852-859.

9. Berguer R, Flynn LM, Kline RA, Caplan L. Surgical reconstruction of the extracranial vertebral artery: management and outcome. *J Vasc Surg*. 2000;31(1 pt 1):9-18.

10. Jenkins JS, Patel SN, White CJ, et al. Endovascular stenting for vertebral artery stenosis. *J Am Coll Cardiol*. 2010;55(6):538-542.

11. SSYLVIA Study Investigators. Stenting of symptomatic atherosclerotic lesions in the vertebral or intracranial arteries (SSYLVIA): study results. *Stroke*. 2004;35(6):1388-1392.

12. Ogilvy CS, Yang X, Natarajan SK, et al. Restenosis rates following vertebral artery origin stenting: does stent type make a difference? *J Invasive Cardiol*. 2010;22(3):119-124.

13. Steinfort B, Ng PP, Faulder K, et al. Midterm outcomes of paclitaxel-eluting stents for the treatment of intracranial posterior circulation stenoses. *J Neurosurg*. 2007;106(2):222-225.

14. Vajda Z, Miloslavski E, Guthe T, et al. Treatment of stenoses of vertebral artery origin using short drug-eluting coronary stents: improved follow-up results. *Am J Neuroradiol*. 2009;30(9):1653-1656.

15. Langwieser N, Buyer D, Schuster T, et al. Bare metal vs. drug-eluting stents for extracranial vertebral artery disease: a meta-analysis of nonrandomized comparative studies. *J Endovasc Ther*. 2014;21(5):683-692.

16. Stayman AN, Nogueira RG, Gupta R. A systematic review of stenting and angioplasty of symptomatic extracranial vertebral artery stenosis. *Stroke*. 2011;42(8):2212-2216.

17. Berguer R. Distal vertebral artery bypass: technique, the "occipital connection," and potential uses. *J Vasc Surg*. 1985;2(4):621-626.

Jahan Mohebali • W. Darrin Clouse

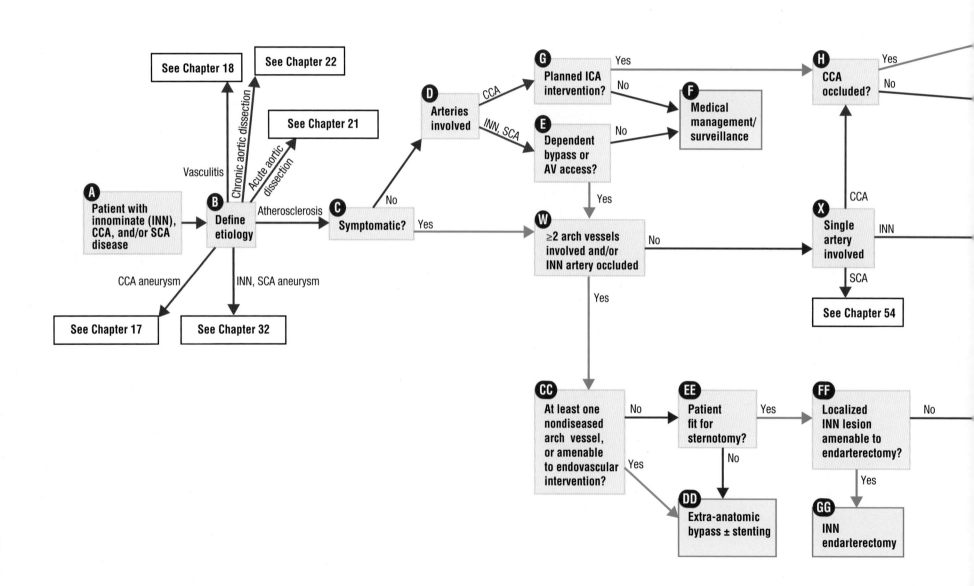

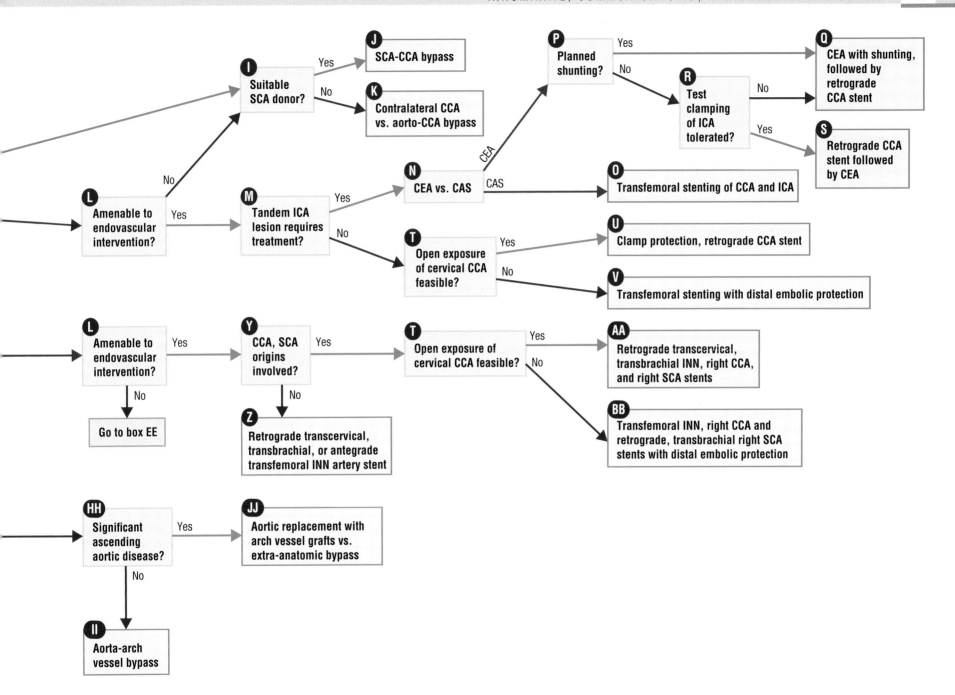

(A) Patient with innominate (INN), common carotid (CCA), and/or SCA disease

Occlusive disease of the INN, CCA, or SCA is uncommon, accounting for <9% of cerebrovascular lesions. Further, these arch vessels are involved in <5% of cerebrovascular operations. Most patients with arch vessel disease are in their early 60s and younger than those with isolated carotid bifurcation disease. They are typically Caucasian and have an extensive smoking history with multiple risk factors for atherosclerosis.[1,2]

(B) Define etiology

Most arch vessel disease is caused by atherosclerosis. However, arch vessels can also be affected by aneurysmal disease (see Chapters 17 and 32), vasculitis, and associated aortic dissection. Vasculitis should be considered in patients with arch vessel disease where there is multivessel involvement (see Chapter 18 for details of large vessel vasculitis). Thoracic aortic dissection can result in stenosis or occlusion of arch vessel ostia and/or extension into these vessels (see Chapters 22 and 23 for details of acute and chronic aortic dissection).

(C) Symptomatic?

The primary decision point for management of patients with arch vessel atherosclerotic occlusive disease is to determine whether they are symptomatic. This is of paramount importance given the frequent finding of incidentally discovered disease in today's era of routine axial imaging (see Chapter 6 for details of identifying cerebrovascular symptoms).

(D) Arteries involved

Management recommended for asymptomatic but significant (>50% flow reducing diameter reduction) stenosis depends on whether the INN, CCA, or SCA is involved.

(E) Dependent bypass or AV access?

If an asymptomatic >50% stenosis involves the INN or SCA that provides inflow to an internal mammary artery graft for CAD, an axillofemoral bypass, an upper extremity bypass graft, or dialysis access AVF/AVG, prophylactic revascularization is usually recommended.[3-5] Another indication for considering intervention in asymptomatic patients is the need for accurate blood pressure monitoring in those with bilateral upper extremity disease.[6,7] If these conditions are not present, or if the patient is too high risk to consider intervention, medical management and surveillance is indicated.

(F) Medical management/surveillance

Asymptomatic patients with INN, CCA, or SCA stenosis who do not meet the criteria for intervention are medically managed with cardiovascular risk-reduction, including antiplatelet and statin therapy, to stabilize these lesions.[8,9] Although no clear guideline recommendations on surveillance of these lesions have been published, annual clinical assessment with arm blood pressure assessment supplemented by DUS or CTA is performed, as needed.

(G) Planned ICA intervention?

If an asymptomatic, but significant (>50%), CCA stenosis is present in a patient with an ICA stenosis for which treatment (CEA or CAS) is planned, the CCA lesion must be evaluated for potential treatment to avoid compromising the outcome of the ICA intervention. This CCA treatment can take the form of open anatomic or extra-anatomic revascularization (see J, K, II), hybrid revascularization, or endovascular intervention (see L). Performing hybrid concomitant, proximal CCA endovascular intervention in tandem with a bifurcation CEA in asymptomatic patients is controversial. Some studies have shown outcomes similar to isolated CEA, whereas others have found that addition of proximal CCA intervention to a bifurcation CEA is associated with an increased risk of stroke (3%-10%) when compared with results of isolated CEA.[10-13] However, recent data from the Vascular Quality Initiative (VQI) describe an acceptably low risk of stroke and death (2%), in asymptomatic patients treated with this hybrid procedure.[10] Therefore, we recommend proximal, asymptomatic CCA intervention selectively when the CCA stenosis is of obvious hemodynamic significance,[13] as confirmed by physical examination (poor pulse and upstroke) and DUS findings, including tardus and parvus waveforms in the distal CCA and ICA.[13-17] Such findings provide sufficient concern that poor inflow may adversely affect outcome and durability of bifurcation reconstruction. However, the need for treatment of ICA and CCA tandem lesions occurs in <1% of CEAs.[13] Benefits of simultaneous reconstruction when indicated include distal ICA surgical clamp cerebral embolic protection and aggressive flushing of any debris from the arterial lumen following CCA stenting. In addition, because our preferred method for CCA and INN treatment is via cervical, retrograde approach (see W and GG), concomitant intervention avoids staged, reoperative cervical exposure following CEA.

If ICA intervention is not needed, medical management and surveillance is indicated for an asymptomatic CCA lesion. No good evidence to support treatment of proximal asymptomatic CCA stenosis is available, although some will consider intervention for nearly occlusive stenoses.[10,18,19]

(H) CCA occluded?

CCA occlusion is rare and its incidence in asymptomatic patients is unknown. Less than 4% of stroke patients will have CCA occlusion.[20] In the case of occluded CCA lesions requiring treatment, open revascularization should be undertaken.

(I) Suitable SCA donor?

The ipsilateral SCA is the inflow choice for revascularizing an occluded CCA, but it is often itself affected by atherosclerotic stenosis. It must therefore be evaluated for suitability as a donor vessel. This requires CTA or MRA and bilateral arm pressure measurements supporting normal perfusion. Systolic arm pressure difference compared with a normal contralateral arm should be <15 mm Hg. If concern remains, arteriography with pressure measurements can be performed. Endovascular intervention of the SCA at same time can provide for donor suitability.

(J) SCA-CCA bypass

A nondiseased ipsilateral SCA should be used to restore CCA inflow via bypass. This can be performed at the time of planned CEA if this is required. The bypass may be to the CCA or to the CEA site. Endovascular intervention can also be utilized to treat concerning mild-to-moderate SCA disease to allow it to be used as a donor vessel. Prosthetic conduit for subclavian-carotid bypass is superior to saphenous vein.[21-23] Operative stroke rates are generally ≤5% with 5-year patency using prosthetic graft approximating 90%.[23] A transverse incision above the clavicle over the sternocleidomastoid clavicular head is used. This is slightly more lateral than that used for arm revascularization using transposition. The CCA is exposed behind this muscle and the internal jugular vein. The phrenic nerve is identified on the anterior scalene muscle and protected while the muscle is divided. The brachial plexus lies lateral to the dissection and is protected. The SCA is mobilized and the bypass is usually brought underneath the jugular vein.[24] Similar to CEA with proximal endovascular intervention, CEA with added subclavian bypass (SCB) has higher stroke and death rates (3%-6%) compared with isolated CEA.[25,26] However, adding CEA to a required SCB does not significantly alter the stroke risk of 4%.[27]

(K) Contralateral CCA vs. aorto-CCA bypass

If the ipsilateral SCA is not a suitable donor for CCA bypass, the contralateral CCA can be used as a donor vessel if it does not have a significant proximal stenosis. CCA-CCA bypass is usually performed using a prosthetic graft, through a retropharyngeal route over the prevertebral fascia, placed obliquely from the base of the neck on the donor side to an anastomosis on the CCA or the bifurcation with CEA.[28,29] Alternatively, sternotomy and direct anatomic aorto-CCA reconstruction with aorto-carotid bypass can be considered in appropriate patients (see II).

(L) Amenable to endovascular intervention?

The first-line treatment for focal, nonoccluded arch vessel disease should be the less invasive endovascular intervention. Factors reducing endovascular suitability include total occlusion, eccentric or long lesions, and complex lesion spillover into the arch that may result in embolization and dissection. Calcification in these lesions can be long, bulky, eccentric or circumferential, and, as such, also contraindicate endovascular therapy. Lesions not amenable to endovascular therapy can be treated with open surgical reconstruction.[18,30,31]

M Tandem ICA lesion requires treatment?

Preoperatively, the ipsilateral ICA should be evaluated to determine if simultaneous treatment of the CCA and an ICA lesion is indicated. Generally, indication to manage the ICA lesion should be considered on its own merit. Anyone with ipsilateral symptoms and ≥50% ICA stenosis should be considered for tandem treatment because understanding which lesion is responsible is difficult. Asymptomatic patients with significant ICA stenosis and a proximal CCA or INN lesion severe enough to be treated should undergo tandem treatment.

N CEA vs. CAS

If intervention for the ICA lesion is indicated, this can be addressed with either CEA or CAS. CEA allows for open cervical access to address the CCA/INN stenosis and is preferred in those with tortuous and calcified ICA lesions, and difficult arch anatomy. The authors consider CAS for high lesions, hostile necks after irradiation, stoma, or before surgery. For details of CEA versus CAS selection, see Chapters 6, 7, 8, and 10.

O Transfemoral stenting of CCA and ICA

The authors believe that concomitant ICA and CCA stenting is best accomplished via a transfemoral approach with cerebral embolic protection in a sequence previously described by Moore and Schneider.[32] This technique consists of crossing and predilating the CCA lesion, if necessary, to accept a delivery sheath, deploying an embolic protection device (EPD) in the ICA, stenting the ICA lesion and then stenting the CCA lesion to complete the procedure.[32] As most arch vessel lesions are continuous with aortic arch disease, all stents in arch vessels should be placed several millimeters into the aorta proximal to all disease and flared into the arch. We prefer to use stent grafts. In 2% to 6% of individuals, the left vertebral artery may originate from the aortic arch at or near the CCA origin, and in such patients open revascularization may be the best option.

P Planned shunting?

If shunting is planned during CEA for anatomic/perfusion reasons, the authors recommend performing the CEA first to allow for expeditious shunt placement and to minimize cerebral ischemia, after which a retrograde CCA stent is placed. If shunting is not planned during CEA, we recommend retrograde CCA intervention before CEA.

Q CEA with shunting, followed by retrograde CCA stent

To use this approach, the CCA lesion to be treated must be located below the proximal extent of the planned shunt, to avoid embolization during shunt placement. Because most CCA lesions are orificial, this is not usually an issue; but if the CCA lesion is longer or more central, shunting should be avoided, if possible.

Alternatively, a looped shunt may be used, which requires less CCA purchase. The procedure starts with CEA and shunting is performed with the surgeon's standard technique. After completing the CEA and removing the shunt, the proximal CCA lesion can be stented with retrograde access via the patch, the patch suture line, or the CCA proximal to the patch, while the ICA remains clamped. We prefer to place the retrograde access through the cinched lateral patch suture line secured tightly on each side of the sheath to separate, tied sutures, because it allows us to establish antegrade ECA flow during intervention and easily flush any debris from the CCA. After the sheath is withdrawn, standard flushing is done and the last few bites are taken completing the repair. Care must be taken not to create a dissection with initial retrograde CCA wire passage. Other methods require enlarging the puncture site in the patch or CCA to ensure adequate flushing, and then closing this defect.

R Test clamping of ICA tolerated?

If shunting during CEA is not planned, test clamping the distal ICA should be performed prior to committing to CCA stenting before CEA. During this interval, systemic blood pressure is raised to optimize cerebral blood flow via collateral circulation. The ICA is clamped for 1 to 2 minutes, while neurologic status (if awake) or electroencephalogram (EEG) change or stump pressure (if under general anesthesia) is monitored. Any EEG lateralized slowing or a systolic stump pressure <50 mm Hg is considered intolerance to the clamp. If test clamping is tolerated, we proceed with CCA stenting followed by CEA. If not tolerated, CEA with shunting is performed before CCA stenting (see Q).

S Retrograde CCA stent followed by CEA

With this approach, retrograde CCA stenting is performed first, with temporary ICA clamping to prevent cerebral embolization. To prevent cerebral embolization, care should be taken to clamp the normal ICA distal to the plaque. The CCA puncture is done so that it will be incorporated into the planned arteriotomy for CEA. In this manner, debris can be flushed from the extended arteriotomy following stent deployment. Some recommend use of a shunt during CEA with this sequence to allow CCA flow and avoid potential debris accumulation at the stent site while the CEA is being performed.[33] Alternatively, we use proximal copious flushing with heparin solution as the CCA clamp is placed, and brisk, antegrade CCA flushing after CEA but before completing the patch closure and restoring ICA blood flow. This method also avoids manipulation of the CEA site after completion.

T Open exposure of cervical CCA feasible?

The neck should be evaluated for the feasibility of open cervical carotid exposure and retrograde access. Before neck irradiation or surgery, significant cervical CCA disease and low carotid bifurcations may make cervical access less attractive. The authors

believe that open cervical exposure with retrograde great vessel stenting provides superior cerebral embolic protection because of the ability to directly clamp the carotid artery, which is our preferred approach. Furthermore, cervical access allows for shorter, more direct working length for crossing the lesion and stent introduction, while avoiding crossing the arch and other supra-aortic trunk ostia. However, concurrent transfemoral access for adequate imaging to define the exact great vessel origin and lesion anatomy may be required, which eliminates some of the advantage of avoiding arch manipulation and increasing stroke risk.

U Clamp protection, retrograde CCA stent

For full cerebral protection, the mid- or distal CCA and disease-free ICA origin and ECA are exposed. The ICA is clamped and retrograde CCA sheath placement and intervention accomplished. At completion, the intervention is flushed with heparinized saline, and the CCA proximal to the access and the ECA are clamped. The sheath is removed, the puncture site enlarged, vigorous flushing performed, and the arteriotomy primarily repaired. Similar to CEA unclamping, antegrade flow in the ECA is allowed before reestablishing ICA flow. Alternatively, some simply clamp the CCA distal to access, perform the intervention, remove the sheath, and clamp the CCA below. This allows for retrograde and antegrade CCA flushing through an enlarged CCA site; however, the ICA is not independently protected.

V Transfemoral stenting with distal embolic protection

Similar to endovascular treatment of tandem lesions (see P), we recommend crossing the CCA lesion and predilating if necessary to accept a delivery sheath. An EPD is placed in the ICA, then the CCA lesion is stented to complete the procedure. Some report selective use, or no use of embolic protection.[10,30-32]

W ≥2 arch vessels involved and/or INN artery occluded

Between 25% and 85% of symptomatic patients with great vessel disease have severe multivessel disease.[34] Unlike asymptomatic arch vessel disease, which is often incidentally discovered on imaging, symptomatic disease attributed to these lesions should be treated in appropriate candidates. The complexity of treatment and optimal reconstruction depends on the patient, the number of vessels involved, and distribution of disease.

X Single artery involved

Given the challenging location of these vessels and the resultant morbidity from open exposure, most single arch vessel disease should be managed with an "endovascular-first" approach as described for each artery (INN, CCA, and SCA).

Y CCA, SCA origins involved?

Planning for endovascular INN intervention should focus on the extent of disease and whether the INN trunk is diseased in isolation. Plaque/atheroma may extend into the aortic arch, CCA, and SCA origins that could necessitate treatment. Considerations for tandem ICA/INN stenoses requiring treatment should undergo the same considerations as those with proximal CCA lesions (see G–V). Anomalous anatomy of the supra-aortic trunks may affect planning and options. Bovine arch anatomy may require open operation; however, novel endovascular approaches for accessing the INN and CCA from the right arm, left neck, and/or groin are possible. Another common arch anomaly is direct left vertebral origin from the aortic arch. Such anomalies can frequently complicate INN, CCA, or SCA intervention and may require open reconstruction.

Ⓩ Retrograde transcervical, transbrachial, or antegrade transfemoral INN artery stent

If the CCA or SCA origins are not involved in the INN lesion, transcervical, transbrachial access, antegrade transfemoral access, or a combination of these are all options and can be employed. Open, retrograde transcervical access is accomplished similar to that for CCA lesions (see U). This can be accompanied by brachial or femoral access for imaging. This is our preferred approach for isolated INN lesions. Along with brachial access it provides two direct routes to cross and treat the INN lesion, as well as surgical cerebral protection and ease dealing with any bifurcation dissection or embolic arm complication.[12] When cervical access is not used, transfemoral access provides the ability to deploy an EPD in the ICA before ballooning and stent placement (see O, V). Some instances may require both femoral and brachial access for complete diagnostic and interventional capability. As with the transcervical approach, we prefer to use brachial access along with the transfemoral approach for imaging and an alternative treatment pathway. Others do not routinely use multiple access or EPDs for INN lesions.[30,31] The INN lesion usually is continuous with disease spilling into the aortic arch. Predilation is generally required with little role for angioplasty alone. Balloon-expandable stenting is used almost universally because of bulky disease in the INN. The stent should be placed several millimeters into the aorta proximal to all disease and flared in the arch. We recommend using stent grafts.

ⒶⒶ Retrograde transcervical, transbrachial INN, right CCA, and right SCA stents

INN lesions may be continuous with CCA and SCA disease. In this instance, the authors prefer cervical and transbrachial access for retrograde INN stenting as well as distal embolic cerebral protection with surgical carotid clamping. Open CCA access along with brachial access provides for INN stent placement followed by retrograde CCA/SCA origin angioplasty and stenting in a kissing fashion into the INN stent. The INN stent should be placed beyond all disease several millimeters into the aortic arch and flared. Occasionally, transfemoral access for full arch imaging may

be necessary to fully define the INN lesion and arch wall. We recommend stent grafts in these locations.

ⒷⒷ Transfemoral INN, right CCA and retrograde, transbrachial right SCA stents with distal embolic protection

When cervical CCA exposure is not possible, INN stenting and kissing stents of the right CCA and right SCA can be deployed via the right brachial and the femoral artery, again employing an ICA EPD. The INN stent is deployed first from the femoral access with the CCA stent then from the femoral access and the SCA stent from the right brachial access.

ⒸⒸ At least one nondiseased arch vessel, or amenable to endovascular intervention?

Symptomatic, multi-arch vessel disease can be treated with extra-anatomic bypass if one nondiseased donor arch vessel is available as a donor site for bypass origin. If all arch vessels are diseased, but one can be treated with stenting, this can then serve as the "undiseased" donor artery. Although some have reported superior patency and similar morbidity/mortality in treatment of multivessel disease employing a transthoracic, direct aortic origin bypass when compared with extrathoracic/extra-anatomic reconstruction, these data usually come from experienced centers before the incorporation of hybrid (ie, stent plus extra-anatomic bypass) techniques.[34] Furthermore, others have reported a higher risk of transthoracic reconstruction, including pulmonary complications, sternal wound infections, and recurrent laryngeal nerve injury,[35] as well as higher resource utilization.[2] Therefore, each patient's presentation, fitness, anatomy, and extent of disease should be considered carefully with the goal of minimizing operative morbidity and mortality, but also accounting for long-term durability and patency. This is particularly true for patients in whom multiple cervical extra-anatomic bypasses would be inflow-dependent on a single diseased arch vessel that has been first treated with an endovascular approach who may be better served with anatomic reconstruction. In summary, it must be recognized that endovascular approaches, while accompanied by less operative morbidity and mortality, are generally less durable.[36,37] In direct comparison, total extrathoracic/cervical reconstruction morbidity and mortality has been demonstrated to be modestly lower than open, direct reconstruction.[2,34,35,38-40] The transthoracic approach provides better durability and patency in over 95% at 5 years compared with 80% to 94% for isolated extra-anatomic bypass.[23,34-44] This difference, however, is not prohibitive, and extra-anatomic revascularization is a viable alternative.[23,28] Yet, in properly selected patients, with little comorbidity, open, direct reconstruction is appropriate and enduring.

ⒹⒹ Extra-anatomic bypass ± stenting

In patients with one normal, or endovascular treatment–amenable arch vessel, extra-anatomic reconstruction taking the form of

SCA, CCA-CCA bypass, alone or together, with or without donor inflow intervention is appropriate. No specific outcome data discussing extra-anatomic reconstruction with inflow endovascular intervention in occlusive disease are available. Durability likely depends on the endovascular component and should be considered heavily in choosing this treatment modality. The 5-year primary patency for great vessel stents is 60% to 75%.[18,31,45] Contemporary series of SCA and CCA-CCA bypass indicate operative mortality of <2%. Perioperative stroke is slightly more common in CCA-CCA bypass at 4% to 6% compared with <3% in recent SCA bypass series.[23,28,39,43] In rare cases where none of the arch vessels can serve as a donor artery, and the patient cannot tolerate direct aortic reconstruction via sternotomy, a femoral to axillary extra-anatomic bypass can be performed, with supplemental bypass from the SCA on the revascularized side to the carotid artery as necessary.

ⒺⒺ Patient fit for sternotomy?

If all arch vessels are heavily diseased and one is not readily amenable to endovascular treatment to allow hybrid reconstruction, the patient's fitness for sternotomy and open, direct aortic anatomic reconstruction should be assessed. Many patients with arch vessel occlusive disease will have significant cardiac pathology, and cardiopulmonary risk stratification must be accomplished before any anatomic reconstructive approach (see Chapter 1).[34] Furthermore, many of these patients might have already undergone sternotomy for coronary revascularization and the increased morbidity risk of redo sternotomy and mediastinal dissection must be considered and can be prohibitive. If a patient cannot undergo sternotomy and direct repair, and hybrid repair constructs are not possible, extra-anatomic femoral to axillary bypass can be considered.

ⒻⒻ Localized INN lesion amenable to endarterectomy?

Localized INN disease can be amenable to INN endarterectomy rather than bypass. However, most such lesions can be treated with an endovascular approach, so this technique is seldom used today.

ⒼⒼ INN endarterectomy

The features of the INN stenosis that are important in consideration for endarterectomy are the degree of disease in the aortic arch and the proximity of the left CCA. If the lesion is focal and the arch is without debris and calcification, and is suitable for side-biting clamp placement encompassing the origin of the INN without LCCA compromise for proximal control, endarterectomy can then be performed without the need for cardiopulmonary bypass. However, the INN lesion frequently is part of aortic arch atherosclerosis, making adequate clamping, clamp injury, embolization, aortic dissection, or adventitial thinning problematic. When a bovine arch configuration is present, endarterectomy should be avoided because it would unnecessarily render both brain hemispheres ischemic. Similarly, it is common for the left CCA to be very close to the INN origin such that adequate placement of a J clamp on the arch compromises of LCCA flow. The ascending aorta is most often soft and amenable as inflow for a technically more straightforward bypass. When feasible, endarterectomy is performed via median sternotomy with thymic and pericardial fat division. The left brachiocephalic vein is mobilized and usually able to be preserved; however, division may be required. Depending on anatomy, the pericardial sac may be opened to facilitate exposure and clamping. The INN must be fully mobilized. Depending on the INN length, bifurcation control may be needed, taking care not to injure the right vagus and recurrent laryngeal nerves. Endarterectomy is performed from distal to proximal toward the aorta. Care must be taken not to create too thin an endarterectomy plane. Freedom from restenosis and recurrent symptoms are over 90%.[46-48]

HH Significant ascending aortic disease?

The ascending aorta must be evaluated with preoperative imaging, usually CTA, to determine suitability for clamping and construction of an ascending aorta to arch vessel bypass. The ascending aorta is usually spared of atherosclerotic disease. Atherosclerotic plaque or calcification along the anterior and right lateral walls precludes clamp placement for inflow anastomosis.

II Aorta-arch vessel bypass

Similar to exposure for INN endarterectomy, median sternotomy is used, thymus and pericardial fat divided, pericardium opened, and left brachiocephalic vein mobilized. If needed, it can be divided but grafts can generally be placed underneath without difficulty. The ascending aorta is inspected, and clamp site confirmed. Dissection of the arch vessels is done to the level of appropriate clamp sites. Depending on the level, further cervical incision extensions or separate cervical incisions can be performed. Aorto-arch vessel bypass is accomplished using prosthetic conduit with no differences between Dacron and ePTFE.[49] Blood pressure is reduced to 80 to 90 mm Hg systolic for ascending clamping with a reinforced side-biting clamp. The proximal ascending aortic anastomosis is placed on the antero-right lateral wall to allow for a better, deep course to the vessels to avoid kinking or compression. Multivessel reconstruction can be done with bifurcated grafts, but the larger main bodies can be compressed in the closed mediastinum and the authors prefer smaller 8 mm and 10 mm diameter grafts with sewn branches. Removal of thymic and fatty tissue can help create mediastinal space. The left SCA can be difficult to expose from sternotomy, but anastomosis is usually feasible to the main trunk. Revascularization into more distal portions of the left SCA may require separate incision or staged extra-anatomic reconstruction. At centers accustomed to transthoracic revascularization,

outcomes in appropriately selected patients can approach that of extra-anatomic reconstruction with mortality and stroke rates of 2% or less.[2,34,35,39,40]

JJ Aortic replacement with arch vessel grafts vs. extra-anatomic bypass

If both the ascending aorta and arch are too diseased to clamp for aortic origin bypass or INN endarterectomy, the patient should be referred for cardiac surgical evaluation and consideration for arch and/or ascending aortic replacement with concomitant direct great vessel reconstruction because this will require full cardiopulmonary bypass, possibly with hypothermic circulatory arrest and cerebral perfusion. If this is not possible, femoral-axillary bypass with additional required extrathoracic arch branch bypass can be considered in select patients (see CC).

REFERENCES

1. Blaisdell FW, Hall AD, Thomas AN, Ross SJ. Cerebrovascular occlusive disease. *Cal Med*. 1965;103:321-329.
2. Daniel VT, Madenci AL, Nguyen LL, et al. Contemporary comparison of supra-aortic trunk surgical reconstructions for occlusive disease. *J Vasc Surg*. 2014;59(6):1577-1582, 1582.e1-e2.
3. Cua B, Mamadani N, Halpin D, Jhamnani S, Jayasuriya S, Mena-Hurtado CM. Review of coronary subclavian steal syndrome. *J Cardiol*. 2017;70:432-437.
4. Che W, Dong H, Jiang X, et al. Stenting for left subclavian artery stenosis in patients scheduled for left internal mammary artery-coronary artery bypass grafting. *Catheter Cardiovasc Interv*. 2016;87:579-588.
5. Potter BJ, Pinto DS. Subclavian steal syndrome. *Circulation*. 2014;129(22):2320-2323.
6. Afari ME, Wylie JV Jr, Carrozza JP Jr. Refractory hypotension as an initial presentation of bilateral subclavian artery stenosis. *Case Rep Cardiol*. 2016;2016:1-3.
7. Huibers A, Hendrikse J, Brown MM, et al. Upper extremity blood pressure difference in patients undergoing carotid revascularization. *Eur J Vasc Endovasc Surg*. 2017;53(2):153-157.
8. Artom N, Montecucco F, Dallegri F, Pende A. Carotid atherosclerotic plaque stenosis: the stabilizing role of statins. *Eur J Clin Invest*. 2014;44(11):1122-1134.
9. Kaneko K, Saito H, Sasaki T, et al. Rosuvastatin prevents aortic arch plaque progression and improves prognosis in ischemic stroke patients. *Neurol Res*. 2017;39(2):133-141.
10. Paukovits TM, Haász J, Molnár A, et al. Transfemoral endovascular treatment of proximal common carotid artery lesions: a single-center experience on 153 lesions. *J Vasc Surg*. 2008;48(1):80-87.
11. Naylor AR, Ricco JB, de Borst GJ, et al. Editor's choice—Management of atherosclerotic carotid and vertebral artery disease: 2017 clinical practice guidelines of the European Society for Vascular Surgery (ESVS). *Eur J Vasc Endovasc Surg*. 2018;55(1):3-81.
12. Wang LJ, Ergul E, Conrad MF, et al. Addition of proximal intervention to carotid endarterectomy increases risk of stroke and death. *J Vasc Surg*. 2019;69:1102-1110.
13. Sfyroeras GS, Karathanos C, Antoniou GA, Saleptsis V, Giannoukas AD. A meta-analysis of combined endarterectomy and proximal balloon angioplasty for tandem disease of the arch vessels and carotid bifurcation. *J Vasc Surg*. 2011;54(2):534-540.
14. Clouse WD, Ergul EA, Wanken ZJ, et al. Risk and outcome profile of carotid endarterectomy with proximal intervention is concerning in multi-institutional assessment. *J Vasc Surg*. 2018;68(3):760-769.
15. Clouse WD, Ergul EA, Cambria RP, et al. Retrograde stenting of proximal lesions with carotid endarterectomy increases risk. *J Vasc Surg*. 2016;63(6):1517-1523.
16. Matos JM, Barshes NR, Mccoy S, et al. Validating common carotid stenosis by duplex ultrasound with carotid angiogram or computed tomography scan. *J Vasc Surg*. 2014;59(2):435-439.
17. Pisimisis GT, Katsavelis D, Mandviwala T, Barshes NR, Kougias P. Common carotid artery peak systolic velocity ratio predicts high-grade common carotid stenosis. *J Vasc Surg*. 2015;62(4):951-957.
18. Slovut DP, Romero JM, Hannon KM, Dick J, Jaff MR. Detection of common carotid artery stenosis using duplex ultrasonography: a validation study with computed tomographic angiography. *J Vasc Surg*. 2010;51(1):65-70.
19. Grant EG, El-Saden SM, Madrazo BL, Baker JD, Kliewer MA. Innominate artery occlusive disease: sonographic findings. *AJR Am J Roentgenol*. 2006;186(2):394-400.
20. Klonaris C, Kouvelos GN, Kafeza M, Koutsoumpelis A, Katsargyris A, Tsigris C. Common carotid artery occlusion treatment: revealing a gap in the current guidelines. *Eur J Vasc Endovasc Surg*. 2013;46:291-298.
21. Perler BA, Williams GM. Carotid-subclavian bypass—a decade of experience. *J Vasc Surg*. 1990;12(6):716-722; discussion 722-723.
22. Ziomek S, Quiñones-Baldrich WJ, Busuttil RW, Baker JD, Machleder HI, Moore WS. The superiority of synthetic arterial grafts over autologous veins in carotid-subclavian bypass. *J Vasc Surg*. 1986;3(1):140-145.
23. Cinà CS, Safar HA, Laganà A, Arena G, Clase CM. Subclavian carotid transposition and bypass grafting: consecutive cohort study and systematic review. *J Vasc Surg*. 2002;35(3):422-429.
24. Morasch MD. Technique for subclavian to carotid transposition, tips and tricks. *J Vasc Surg*. 2009;49:251-254.
25. Risty GM, Cogbill TH, Davis CA, Lambert PJ. Carotid-subclavian arterial reconstruction: concomitant

ipsilateral carotid endarterectomy increases risk of perioperative stroke. *Surgery.* 2007;142(3):393-397.

26. Goudreau BJ, Wang LJ, Tanious A, et al. The impact of adding supra-aortic trunk surgical reconstruction to carotid endarterectomy. In: *48th Annual Symposium, Society for Clinical Vascular Surgery.* Huntington Beach, CA; March 14-18, 2020.

27. Wang LJ, Crofts SC, Nixon TP, et al. Addition of carotid endarterectomy to supra-aortic trunk surgical reconstruction does not increase risk. In: *Accepted to the 47th Annual Symposium of the Society for Clinical Vascular Surgery.* Boca Raton, FL; March 16-20, 2019.

28. Ozsvath KJ, Roddy SP, Darling RC III, et al. Carotid-carotid crossover bypass: is it a durable procedure? *J Vasc Surg.* 2003;37(3):582-585.

29. Berguer RM, Gonzalez JA. Revascularization by the retropharyngeal route for extensive disease of the extracranial arteries. *J Vasc Surg.* 1994;19:217-225.

30. van de Weijer MA, Vonken EJ, de Vries JP, Moll FL, Vos JA, de Borst GJ. Technical and clinical success and long-term durability of endovascular treatment for atherosclerotic aortic arch branch origin obstruction: evaluation of 144 procedures. *Eur J Vasc Endovasc Surg.* 2015;50(1):13-20.

31. Paukovits TM, Lukács L, Bérczi V, Hirschberg K, Nemes B, Hüttl K. Percutaneous endovascular treatment of innominate artery lesions: a single-centre experience on 77 lesions. *Eur J Vasc Endovasc Surg.* 2010;40(1):35-43.

32. Moore JD, Schneider PA. Management of simultaneous common and internal carotid artery occlusive disease in the endovascular era. *Semin Vasc Surg.* 2011;24(1):2-9.

33. Payne DA, Hayes PD, Bolia A, Fishwick G, Bell PR, Naylor AR. Cerebral protection during open retrograde angioplasty/stenting of common carotid and innominate artery stenoses. *Br J Surg.* 2006;93(2):187-190.

34. Takach TJ, Reul GJ, Cooley DA, et al. Brachiocephalic reconstruction I: operative and long-term results for complex disease. *J Vasc Surg.* 2005;42(1):47-54.

35. Berguer R, Morasch MD, Kline RA. Transthoracic repair of innominate and common carotid artery disease: immediate and long-term outcome for 100 consecutive surgical reconstructions. *J Vasc Surg.* 1998;27(1):34-41; discussion 42.

36. AbuRahma AF, Bates MC, Stone PA, et al. Angioplasty and stenting versus carotid-subclavian bypass for the treatment of isolated subclavian artery disease. *J Endovasc Ther.* 2007;14(5):698-704.

37. Takach TJ, Duncan JM, Livesay JJ, et al. Brachiocephalic reconstruction II: operative and endovascular management of single-vessel disease. *J Vasc Surg.* 2005;42(1):55-61.

38. Berguer R, Morasch MD, Kline RA, Kazmers A, Friedland MS. Cervical reconstruction of the supra-aortic trunks: a 16-year experience. *J Vasc Surg.* 1999;29(2):239-246; discussion 246-248.

39. Aziz F, Gravett MH, Comerota AJ. Endovascular and surgical treatment of brachiocephalic arteries. *Ann Vasc Surg.* 2011;25:569-581.

40. Farina C, Sterpetti AV, Schultz RD, Feldhaus RJ, Davenport KD. Extrathoracic and transthoracic management of vascular disease of the aortic arch branches: a 16-year experience. *Ann Thorac Surg.* 1989;47:580-585.

41. Abou-Zamzam AM, Moneta GL, Edwards JM, et al. Extrathoracic arterial grafts performed for carotid artery occlusive disease not amenable to endarterectomy. *Arch Surg.* 1999;134:952-957.

42. Fry WR, Martin JD, Clagett PG, Fry WJ. Extrathoracic carotid reconstruction: the subclavian-carotid artery bypass. *J Vasc Surg.* 1992;15:83-89.

43. Takach TJ, Duncan JM, Livesay JJ, Ott DA, Cervera RD, Cooley DA. Contemporary relevancy of carotid-subclavian bypass defined by an experience spanning five decades. *Ann Vasc Surg.* 2011;25:895-901.

44. Song L, Zhang J, Li J, et al. Endovascular stenting vs. extrathoracic surgical bypass for symptomatic subclavian steal syndrome. *J Endovasc Ther.* 2012;19:44-51.

45. Palchik E, Bakken AM, Wolford HY, Saad WE, Davies MG. Subclavian artery revascularization: an outcome analysis based on mode of therapy and presenting symptoms. *Ann Vasc Surg.* 2008;22:70-78.

46. Cherry KJ, McCullough JL, Hallett JW Jr, Pairolero PC, Gloviczki P. Technical principles of direct innominate artery revascularization: a comparison of endarterectomy and bypass grafts. *J Vasc Surg.* 1989;9:718-724.

47. Brewster DC, Moncure AC, Darling RC, Ambrosino JJ, Abbott WM. Innominate artery lesions: problems encountered and lessons learned. *J Vasc Surg.* 1985;2:99-112.

48. Carlson RE, Ehrenfeld WK, Stoney RJ, Wylie EJ. Innominate artery endarterectomy. *Arch Surg.* 1977;112:1389-1393.

49. Cormier F, Ward A, Cormier JM, Laurian C. Long-term results of aortoinnominate and aortocarotid polytetrafluoroethylene bypass grafting for atherosclerotic lesions. *J Vasc Surg.* 1989;10:135-142.

Michael Yacoub • Ali F. AbuRahma

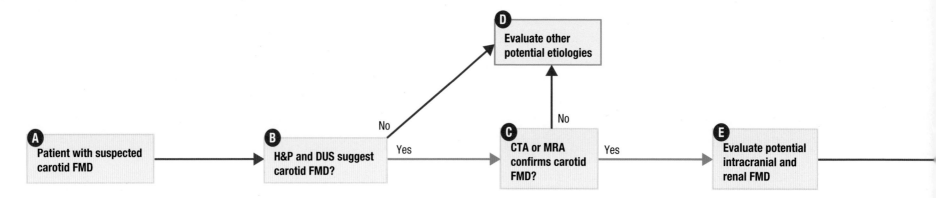

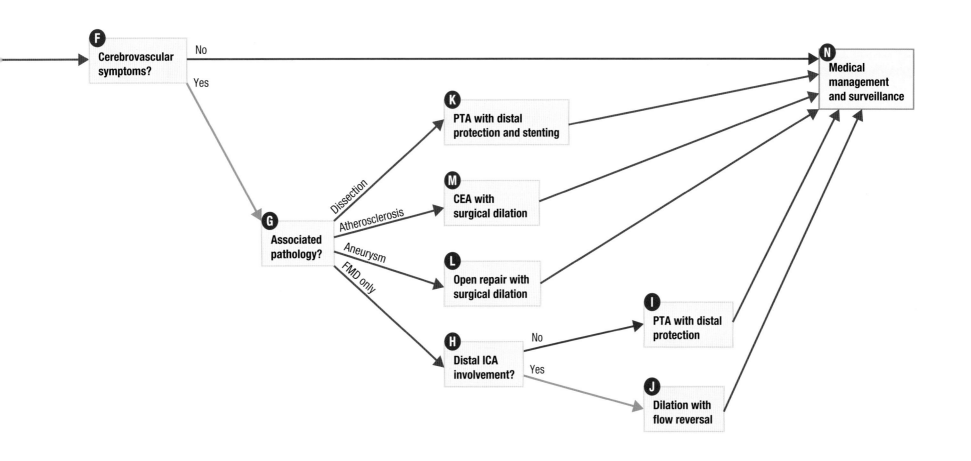

A Patient with suspected carotid FMD

Carotid artery FMD is an uncommon pathology found in 0.25% to 0.68% of consecutive cerebral angiograms.[1,2] This disease entity occurs bilaterally in 39% to 86% of reported cases.[2-5] In most series, it is predominately seen in women (60%-90%) between 40 and 60 years of age.[3,4,6,7] Medial fibroplasia is the most common type of carotid FMD, accounting for 80% to 95% of disease.[1,6,7,8] Carotid FMD can present as an asymptomatic incidental finding on an imaging study, or with cerebrovascular symptoms. The natural history of the disease is not well understood. Multiple studies have followed up small groups of asymptomatic patients, and <10% ever developed neurologic symptoms. However, these studies failed to include a significant number of patients with high-grade asymptomatic stenosis that is considered at high risk for developing a cerebral ischemic event.[4,9,10]

B H&P and DUS suggest carotid FMD?

Carotid FMD can be an incidental imaging finding in asymptomatic patients, or it may be associated with cerebrovascular symptoms. In series of patients treated for carotid FMD, hemispheric stroke was the initial finding in 12% to 27%, TIA in 31% to 42%, and amaurosis fugax in 22% to 28%.[11-13] In some cases, nonspecific symptoms such as dizziness, altered mentation, neck pain, and headache have led to imaging that revealed the diagnosis.

Physical examination findings reported in the U.S. FMD registry included Horner syndrome in 12%, cranial nerve abnormality in 9%, focal neurologic deficits in 14%, carotid bruits in 31%, epigastric bruit in 18%, and flank bruit in 6% of patients.[14]

DUS is the initial imaging modality of choice for patients suspected of potential FMD, although it cannot always image pathology in the more distal ICA. The disease process results in weblike stenotic segments, creating a "string of beads" appearance. The beads are best visualized using color or power Doppler showing the irregular interface between the vessel wall and the lumen.

C CTA or MRA confirms carotid FMD?

If H&P and DUS suggest carotid FMD, cross-sectional imaging with CTA or MRA is indicated to more precisely define the anatomy and pathology, and to plan potential treatment. If carotid FMD is not confirmed by this imaging, other potential etiologies for the presenting symptoms should be evaluated.

D Evaluate other potential etiologies

If carotid FMD is not confirmed by imaging, other etiologies for cerebrovascular symptoms should be pursued (see Chapter 6).

E Evaluate potential intracranial and renal FMD

Intracranial aneurysms and renal artery FMD can be present in up to 51%[4,15] and 40% of patients with carotid FMD, respectively.[6,15,16] Therefore, patients with carotid FMD should be

evaluated with a cerebral CTA or MRA to rule out cerebral aneurysms, and renal DUS should be considered in patients with significant HTN. Intracranial aneurysms tend to be located on the same side as does the extracranial carotid FMD, and some pose a risk of rupture with subsequent intracranial hemorrhage related to location, size, and presence of HTN.

Intracranial aneurysms should be treated separately, based on their own clinical presentation and indications. The presence of a small asymptomatic intracranial aneurysm does not preclude patients with symptomatic carotid FMD from receiving appropriate treatment. The presence of renovascular HTN can complicate the clinical course of patients with carotid FMD, especially if they also have intracranial aneurysms. Therefore, renal artery FMD should be treated before carotid FMD unless cerebrovascular symptoms warrant urgent treatment of carotid FMD. Renal FMD is discussed in detail in Chapter 41.

F Cerebrovascular symptoms?

If cerebrovascular symptoms referable to carotid FMD are present (see Chapter 6), interventional or surgical treatment is indicated.[3,6] If the patient is asymptomatic, treatment of carotid FMD is not recommended because its natural history is relatively benign.

G Associated pathology?

The presence of concomitant pathology may complicate the treatment of carotid FMD. This includes atherosclerotic occlusive disease of the carotid bifurcation, extracranial carotid artery aneurysms, carotid artery dissection, and vertebral artery FMD. The presence of these associated findings dictates specific treatment approaches. Additional information about these associated pathologies can be found in Chapters 8, 12, 15, and 17.

H Distal ICA involvement?

Interventional treatment for carotid FMD is currently preferred over open surgical exposure and dilation, but placement of a distal ICA embolic protection device is required. FMD or severe tortuosity in the distal ICA may prevent placement of an embolic protection device, in which case flow reversal is required during dilation, either by open carotid exposure or endovascular techniques.[17-20]

I PTA with distal protection

PTA with distal embolic protection has become the preferred approach for treating symptomatic carotid artery FMD.[21-25] However, there are no large studies that report on the efficacy and long-term outcomes of endovascular treatment of carotid artery FMD. Most centers rationalize the use of this approach, relying on the data from balloon PTA of the renal artery in patients with renal artery FMD, which has fewer complications than does an open surgical approach. A diagnostic carotid arteriogram is performed, and, depending on the patient's anatomy, a sheath is

placed in the CCA using an anchoring or telescoping technique. Distal embolic protection is obtained using a filter and PTA of the ICA is performed using the appropriate balloon size.[17,23-25] Unlike carotid atherosclerotic disease, stenting is not performed unless a flow-limiting dissection results after PTA.

J Dilation with flow reversal

If a distal embolic protection device cannot be placed, flow reversal is implemented to prevent distal embolization during dilation. This can be done with open surgery or endovascular techniques. Open surgical graduated rigid dilatation has been utilized for treating symptomatic carotid FMD for several decades. The carotid artery is dissected out in the same manner as for a CEA. Proximal and distal control is obtained, the ICA is straightened using a silastic loop, an arteriotomy is created at the base of the ICA, and surgical dilatation of the FMD in the ICA is performed using 1.5-mm probe, progressing to a 3.5-mm probe. After each dilation, back-bleeding of the ICA is performed to prevent distal embolization. Multiple studies have reported excellent outcomes for open surgical graduated rigid dilatation,[6,16,26] with an incidence of perioperative stroke ranging from 1.4% to 2.6%, and TIAs ranging from 1.4% to 7.7%. The long-term follow-up was excellent, and the late stroke rate ranged from 1.2% to 3.8%. The primary patency and stroke-free survival rates were both 94% at 5 years.

Flow reversal can also be accomplished with a transfemoral approach using devices that employ balloon occlusion of the proximal CCA and ECA, while allowing retrograde ICA flow during balloon angioplasty of the FMD lesions.[27] In addition, a transcarotid approach developed for carotid stenting could be adapted to FMD treatment, allowing ICA flow reversal during balloon PTA (without stenting).[28]

K PTA with distal protection and stenting

Patients diagnosed with carotid artery FMD may develop spontaneous dissection of the carotid artery. Open surgical and endovascular approaches have been described in the literature. See Chapter 15 for further details. See Box I for details of balloon angioplasty for carotid FMD. In the setting of a dissection complicating typical FMD, placement of a carotid stent is recommended.

L Open repair with surgical dilation

In a published series of patients with extracranial carotid artery aneurysms, 2.3% were associated with carotid artery FMD.[13] These patients are best treated with open surgical repair of the aneurysm and rigid graduated dilatation of any associated carotid FMD. See Chapter 17 for details of aneurysm treatment. See Box J for details of rigid graduated dilation.

M CEA with surgical dilation

Patients with carotid artery FMD may also show evidence of carotid artery atherosclerosis. In good surgical candidates, the preferred approach is CEA with open surgical graduated rigid dilatation. In case of redundancy with severe kinking, a shortening procedure for the ICA may be required. In poor surgical candidates, a combination of carotid bifurcation stenting and balloon angioplasty of ICA FMD not encompassed within the stent could be considered.

Ⓝ Medical management and surveillance

Patients with asymptomatic carotid FMD, or previously treated FMD, are treated with medical therapy and surveillance. An antiplatelet regimen should be started once carotid FMD is diagnosed; however, there is no evidence to suggest a role for cholesterol-lowering agents. Patients with more than 50% carotid artery stenosis should be monitored at 6- to 12-month intervals with DUS, with less frequent surveillance if the stenosis stabilizes, and more frequent if it progresses.

REFERENCES

1. Houser OW, Baker HL. Fibrovascular dysplasia and other uncommon diseases of the cervical carotid artery: angiographic aspects. *AJR Am J Roentgenol.* 1968;104:201-212.
2. Osborn AG, Anderson RE. Angiographic spectrum of cervical and intracranial fibromuscular dysplasia. *Stroke.* 1977;8:617-626.
3. Slovut DP, Olin JW. Fibromuscular dysplasia. *N Engl J Med.* 2004;350:1862-1871.
4. Mettinger KL, Ericson K. Fibromuscular dysplasia and the brain I: observations on angiographic, clinical, and genetic characteristics. *Stroke.* 1982;13:46-52.
5. Schievink WI, Björnsson J. Fibromuscular dysplasia of the internal carotid artery: a clinicopathological study. *Clin Neuropathol.* 1996;15:2-6.
6. Moreau P, Albat B, Thevenet A. Fibromuscular dysplasia of the internal carotid artery: long-term results. *J Cardiovasc Surg.* 1993;34:465-472.
7. Furie DM, Tien RD. Fibromuscular dysplasia of arteries of the head and neck: imaging findings. *AJR Am J Roentgenol.* 1994;162:1205-1209.
8. Fisicaro M, Tonizzo M, Pozzi Mucelli R, et al. Fibromuscular dysplasia: a case report of multivessel vascular involvement. *Int Angiol.* 1994;13:347-350.
9. Zhou W, Bush RL, Lin PL, Lumsden AB. Fibromuscular dysplasia of the carotid artery. *J Am Coll Surg.* 2005;200:807.
10. Corrin LS, Sandok BA, Houser OW. Cerebral ischemic events in patients with carotid artery fibromuscular dysplasia. *Arch Neurol.* 1981;38:616-618.
11. Stanley JC, Fry WJ, Seeger JF, Hoffman GL, Gabrielsen TO. Extracranial internal carotid and vertebral artery fibrodysplasia. *Arch Surg.* 1974;109:215-222.
12. Stahlfeld KR, Means JR, Didomenico P. Carotid artery fibromuscular dysplasia. *Am J Surg.* 2007;193:71-72.
13. Miyauchi M, Shionoya S. Aneurysm of the extracranial internal carotid artery caused by fibromuscular dysplasia. *Eur J Vasc Surg.* 1991;5:587-591.
14. Olin JW, Froehlich J, Gu X, et al. The United States Registry for fibromuscular dysplasia: results in the first 447 patients. *Circulation.* 2012;125:3182-3190.
15. So EL, Toole JF, Dalal P, Moody DM. Cephalic fibromuscular dysplasia in 32 patients: clinical findings and radiologic features. *Arch Neurol.* 1981;38:619-622.
16. Schneider PA, Cunningham CG, Ehrenfeld WK, et al. Fibromuscular dysplasia of the carotid artery. In: Veith FJ, Hobson RW, Williams FA, Wilson SE, eds. *Vascular Surgery: Principles and Practice.* New York, NY: McGraw-Hill; 1994:711-717.
17. Smith LL, Smith DC, Killeen JD, Hasso AN. Operative balloon angioplasty in the treatment of internal carotid artery fibromuscular dysplasia. *J Vasc Surg.* 1987;6:482-487.
18. de Smul G, Bostoen H. Operative balloon dilatation of fibromuscular dysplasia of the internal carotid artery: two case reports. *Acta Chir Belg.* 1995;95:139-143.
19. Ballard JL, Guinn JE, Killeen JD, Smith DC. Open operative balloon angioplasty of the internal carotid artery: a technique in evolution. *Ann Vasc Surg.* 1995;9:390-393.
20. Lord RS, Graham AR, Benn IV. Radiologic control of operative carotid dilation: aneurysm formation following balloon dilation. *J Cardiovasc Surg.* 1986;27:158-162.
21. Brown MM. Balloon angioplasty for cerebrovascular disease. *Neurol Res.* 1992;14:159-163.
22. Motarjeme A. Percutaneous transluminal angioplasty of the supra-aortic vessels. *J Endovasc Surg.* 1996;3:171-181.
23. Hasso AN, Bird CR, Zinke DE, Thompson JR. Fibromuscular dysplasia of the internal carotid artery: percutaneous transluminal angioplasty. *AJNR Am J Neuroradiol.* 1981;2:175-180.
24. Tsai FY, Matovich V, Hieshima G, et al. Percutaneous transluminal angioplasty of the carotid artery. *AJNR Am J Neuroradiol.* 1986;7:349-358.
25. Theron JG, Payelle GG, Coskun O, Huet HF, Guimaraens L. Carotid artery stenosis: treatment with protected balloon angioplasty and stent placement. *Radiology.* 1996;201:627-636.
26. Haldeman S, Kohlbeck FJ, McGregor M. Risk factors and precipitating neck movements causing vertebrobasilar artery dissection after trauma and spinal manipulation. *Spine.* 1999;15:785-794.
27. Clari DG, Hopkins LN, Mehta M; EMPIRE Clinical Study Investigators. Neuroprotection during carotid artery stenting using GORE flow reversal system: 30-day outcomes in the EMPIRE Clinical Study. *Catheter Cardiovasc Interv.* 2011;77:420-429.
28. Malas MB, Dakour-Aridi H, Wang GJ, et al. Transcarotid artery revascularization versus transfemoral carotid artery stenting in the Society for Vascular Surgery Vascular Quality Initiative. *J Vasc Surg.* 2019;69(1):92.e2-103.e2. doi:10.1016/j.jvs.2018.05.011.

Robert C. McMurray • Peter A. Schneider

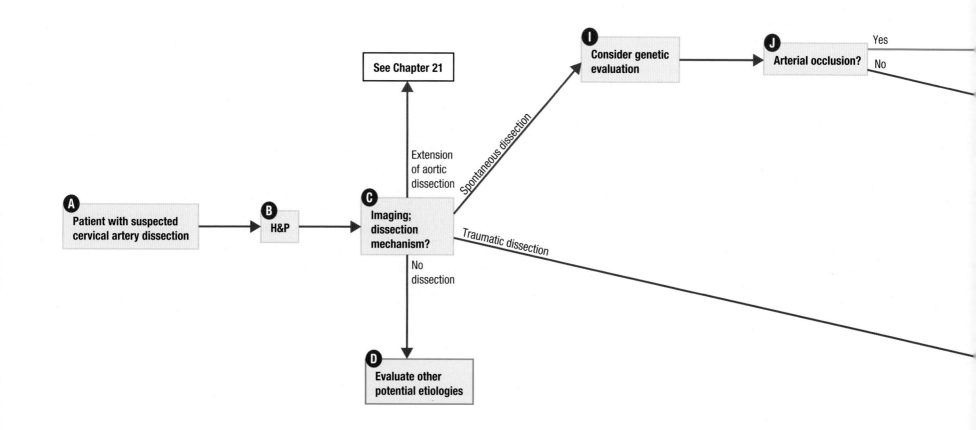

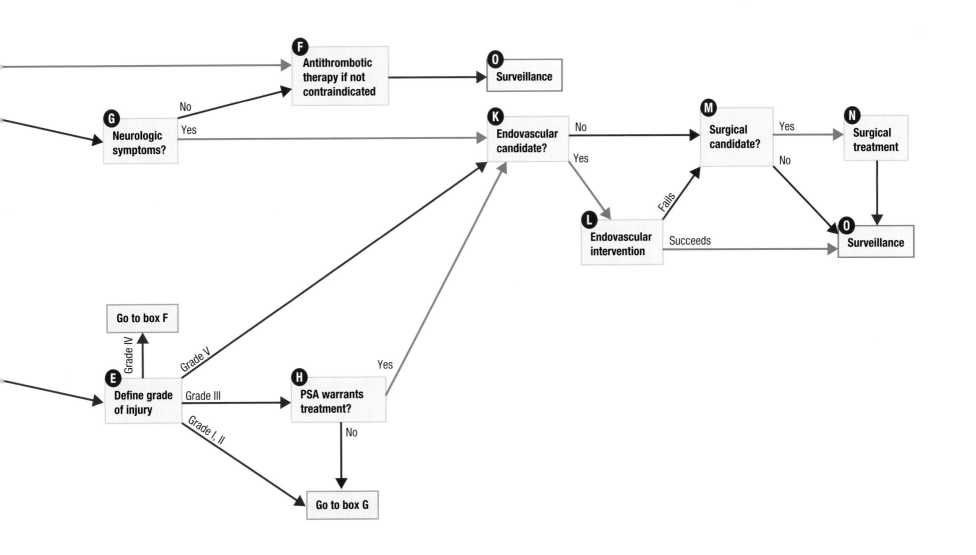

A. Patient with suspected cervical artery dissection

Carotid and vertebral artery dissection is a relatively uncommon condition that occurs spontaneously or as the result of traumatic injury. In patients experiencing spontaneous dissection, there is often no clear-cut cause identified. The overall incidence of clinically significant carotid artery dissection has been reported to be 1.72 per 100,000 and the incidence of vertebral artery dissection is noted at 0.97 per 100,000 for a combined incidence of 2.6 per 100,000 individuals.[1] The true incidence is likely higher because many dissections are without clinical symptoms and go undetected. Spontaneous carotid artery dissection occurs most frequently between the third and fifth decades of life, with a mean age of 45 years. There is no sex difference in occurrence, but women are affected, on average, about 5 years younger than are men.[2]

The percentage of blunt traumatic carotid dissection in all trauma patients is 0.08%,[3] and higher with specific injury patterns. Patients with head and neck trauma have an incidence of carotid artery dissection of 0.86% per 100,000.[4] If the patient also has an altered level of consciousness, then the incidence increases to 3.2% per 100,000.[5] Historically, untreated blunt carotid injury was associated with a mortality rate from 23% to 28%, with 48% to 58% of survivors sustaining permanent neurologic deficits.[6] More recent data suggest that with extracranial cervical artery dissection, poor outcome (a modified Rankin Scale score >2) at 3 months among patients with ischemic stroke was more likely with ICA dissection compared with vertebral artery dissection (25% vs. 8%).[7] Complete or excellent recovery occurs in 70% to 85% of patients with extracranial dissection, with major disabling deficits in 10% to 25% and mortality in 5% to 10% of cases.[8]

B. H&P

The "classic" presentation of cervical carotid artery dissection includes headache, neck pain, cerebral or retinal ischemia, and a partial Horner syndrome (oculosympathetic palsy). The patient may have miosis and ptosis caused by injury to the sympathetic fibers running along the ICA, but they will not have anhidrosis because this is mediated by sympathetic fibers running along the ECA. The most common initial symptom in patients with spontaneous carotid artery dissection is headache. Patients can also present with amaurosis fugax, anisocoria, pulsatile tinnitus, and cranial nerve palsies.[2] The classic triad of symptoms is present in less than one-third of patients with carotid artery dissection and, as such, a high index of suspicion is needed to make the diagnosis.

Vertebral artery dissection can present with head or neck pain. More severe lesions may lead to lateral medullary infarction (Wallenberg syndrome), other posterior circulation territory infarction, or spinal cord ischemia.[9]

The majority of patients with traumatic carotid dissection from blunt injury have no obvious symptoms at presentation.[10] A latent period between the time of injury and the onset of symptoms is typically seen. Among those who develop symptoms, approximately 10% to 15% have lateralizing neurologic symptoms and at least 50% develop a completed stroke.[11] Certain clinical signs are so suggestive of blunt cervical vascular injury that they warrant emergent diagnostic evaluation. These signs include active bleeding from the neck, mouth, nose, or ear; expanding cervical hematoma; a cervical bruit in a patient <50 years of age, and focal or lateralizing neurologic deficits. Symptoms such as pain may be difficult to elicit in the multiply injured trauma patient.

The following risk factors to pursue further workup for potential cervical (carotid or vertebral) artery dissection have been agreed upon by both the Eastern and Western Trauma Associations:

- Injury mechanism compatible with severe cervical hyperextension/flexion or rotation
- Severe facial trauma and subcondylar fractures
- Basilar skull fracture involving the carotid canal
- Closed head injury consistent with a diffuse axonal injury and GCS <6
- Cervical vertebral body or transverse foramen fracture, subluxation or ligamentous injury at any level, or any fracture of C1 to C3
- Near hanging resulting in cerebral anoxia
- Clothesline-type injury or seat-belt sign associated with significant cervical pain, swelling, or altered mental status[12-14]

C. Imaging; dissection mechanism?

The approach to diagnostic imaging is the same regardless of the mechanism of the dissection (spontaneous, traumatic, or as an extension of aortic dissection). Extracranial carotid dissections usually occur in the ICA, 2 to 4 cm distal to the bifurcation near the level of the skull base.[15] Vertebral dissections usually occur in the V3 segment at the C1 to C2 level.

CTA and MRA are used to evaluate potential cervical artery dissections, not only because their resolution approaches that of DSA in detecting luminal defects but also because they are superior to DSA in the evaluation of intramural hematomas and perivascular hematomas and evaluation of injury to surrounding structures.[16] CTA demonstrates a sensitivity and specificity of 97% and 100%, respectively, in diagnosing blunt carotid and vertebral artery injuries.[17] CTA has proved to be reliable, fast, safe, and cost-effective, although results may be limited secondary to timing of contrast, artifact, and the amount of contrast necessary for the study. MRA is able to show ischemic changes in the brain the earliest as well as demonstrate a hyperintense crescent-shaped intramural hematoma and eccentric flow usually seen in a dissection, although the time required to perform the study and the risk of image distortion secondary to external fixation devices limit its usage in trauma patients. A systematic review published in 2009 found that the sensitivity and specificity of CTA and MRA were roughly equivalent.[18]

Although selective cerebral DSA is the "gold standard," less invasive CTA or MRA is preferred because of less frequent complications. Angiographic findings of dissection include a string sign, tapered stenosis, flame-shaped occlusion, intimal flap, aneurysm, or intramural hematoma. DSA allows visualization and characterization of the arterial lumen, although it carries a 1% to 2% risk of hematoma or PSA at the access site, a 1% to 2% risk of contrast nephropathy, and a 1% risk of stroke.[19] DSA is recommended only if intervention is planned, or if it is required for other arterial evaluation.

Carotid DUS detects abnormalities in only 65% to 95% of cervical artery dissections and is suboptimal in identifying dissections near the skull base and vertebral artery dissection within the vertebral foramina.[20] It also is unreliable in detecting dissections in patients with isolated Horner syndrome.[21] For these reasons, it is not used to rule out cervical artery dissections, but dissections are sometimes seen on DUS when this is performed for new cerebrovascular symptoms.

D. Evaluate other potential etiologies

The differential diagnosis among patients with suspected cervical artery dissection is broad. Symptoms of head and neck pain can be caused by various types of headache, migraines, and cluster headaches. Horner syndrome, lower cranial nerve palsies, cerebral ischemia, and subarachnoid hemorrhage should also be considered because they may manifest with symptoms similar to cervical artery dissections.

E. Define grade of injury

The grading scale for blunt cerebrovascular injury was created to guide therapy (Table 15-1). For the vertebral artery, stroke rates and neurologic outcome are independent of injury grade. For the carotid

Table 15-1. Grading Scale for Blunt Cerebrovascular Injury

Grade of Injury	Imaging Findings	Percentage of Injuries
I	Intimal irregularity or dissection with <25% luminal narrowing	58
II	Intramural hematoma or dissection with >25% luminal narrowing, visible intimal flab or intraluminal clot	22
III	Pseudoaneurysm or hemodynamically insignificant AVF	14
IV	Complete occlusion	11
V	Transection with active extravasation or hemodynamically significant AVF	3

AVF, arteriovenous fistula.
From Biffl WL, Ray CE Jr, Moore EE, et al. Treatment-related outcomes from blunt cerebrovascular injuries: importance of routine follow-up arteriography. *Ann Surg.* 2002;235:699.

artery, stroke rate increases as injury severity increases.[22] Treatment, then, depends on the grade of injury. Indications for endovascular or surgical treatment of acute traumatic cervical artery dissections include deteriorating or unstable neurologic symptoms despite medical therapy, symptomatic or expanding aneurysms or PSAs, and transection (grade V).[23-25] In the case of grade IV total occlusion, anticoagulation alone is recommended. Most (82%) of grade IV injuries do not recanalize after traumatic dissection.[10] There are no data demonstrating a benefit of endovascular intervention.

F Antithrombotic therapy if not contraindicated

Anticoagulation, unless contraindicated, has been the primary treatment for carotid and vertebral artery dissection, because of the associated increased risk of stroke with worsening grade of arterial damage. Concerns regarding initiating anticoagulation in this setting include possible worsening of intramural bleeding, bleeding from concomitant traumatic injuries, and bleeding from unrelated sources. Currently, there is no level 1 evidence to support the use of either anticoagulant versus antiplatelet therapy. In 2003, a Cochrane Database Review was unable to find any randomized control trials that compared antiplatelet drugs and anticoagulation. Recently, the CADISS trial randomized patients with acute carotid or vertebral dissection to antiplatelet therapy (aspirin-dipyridamole, or clopidogrel alone or in combination) or anticoagulation (heparin followed by warfarin with an INR goal of 2-3) for at least 3 months.[19] There was no difference in efficacy between antiplatelet and anticoagulant drugs in preventing stroke and death in patients with symptomatic vertebral artery or carotid artery dissection, although stroke was rare in both groups, much lower than previously reported in observational studies.[26] In contrast, a large retrospective review of patients who sustained blunt trauma at high risk for cerebrovascular injury found that asymptomatic patients treated with antithrombotic therapy had a lower incidence of neurologic events compared to the patients who did not receive anticoagulation (0.5% vs. 21%).[27] Overall, despite the lack of level 1 evidence, most patients receive heparin followed by warfarin for 3 to 6 months. There are as yet no data to support the use of direct oral anticoagulants, although by extension from other pathologies, these might be considered.

G Neurologic symptoms?

If the patient develops new or progressing neurologic symptoms (see Chapter 9) despite anticoagulation or antiplatelet therapy after cervical artery dissection, and has compromised cerebral blood flow, contraindications to anticoagulation, or develops a symptomatic or expanding PSA, then endovascular or surgical therapy should be considered.[23]

H PSA warrants treatment?

PSAs in the setting of dissection (grade III) are less likely to heal compared with lower grade injuries.[28] Although PSAs rarely

rupture, they can be a source of distal embolization.[29] Once diagnosed, antithrombotic therapy with heparin should be initiated. In one study, over half of PSAs remained the same size or enlarged at a mean of 6 months. Intervention is generally warranted for symptomatic PSAs or those that are >1.0 to 1.5 cm in diameter (carotid) or 2× the normal arterial diameter. Treatment options include endovascular repair (stent grafts, bare-metal stent, or coil embolization) or resection and repair, if surgically accessible.[30,31]

I Consider genetic evaluation

The proportion of patients with spontaneous cervical artery dissection who are also affected by known connective tissue or vascular disorders is low.[32] However, various connective tissue and vascular disorders have been associated with dissections including FMD, Ehlers-Danlos syndrome, Marfan syndrome, osteogenesis imperfecta, cystic medial necrosis, and autosomal dominant polycystic kidney disease.[2] The most common association is FMD, which accounts for 15% to 20% of all cases of cervical artery dissection.[33] Ehlers-Danlos is found in less than 2% of cases.[32] All other remaining connective tissue disorders are rare, and it remains uncertain whether these disorders truly directly increase the risk of dissection. In addition to monogenic connective tissue disorders, it is believed that polygenic factors may play a role with a family predisposition to dissection secondary to inherited weakness in the wall of the artery, although no specific genetic markers have been found to date. These genetic alterations leading to a family history of dissections are suspected to be inherited in an autosomal dominant manner.[34] Despite the scarcity of evidence, there are valid reasons to suspect that genetic factors are related to the pathophysiology of spontaneous cervical artery dissection. For example, patients with a family history of arterial dissections involving cervicocephalic arteries, renal arteries, or the aorta appear to be at increased risk for recurrent arterial dissection.[35] Genetic evaluation may help diagnose connective tissue disorders that were inherited and further genetic testing may help identify further genetic markers that predispose patients to arterial dissection.

J Arterial occlusion?

For patients with arterial occlusion after spontaneous cervical dissection, the neurologic outcome is proportional to the degree of neurologic deficit on presentation.[36] Patients with arterial occlusion should be treated with antithrombotic therapy. In most cases, arteries with stenosis or luminal irregularities undergo recanalization and healing in the first months after spontaneous dissection. In a report of 61 patients with acute vertebral artery dissection who presented with symptoms of vertebrobasilar territory ischemia, complete recanalization of the vertebral artery was observed at 6 months in 62% of patients.[37] In another study that followed up 76 patients with spontaneous cervical artery dissection involving

105 vessels, complete recanalization was noted in 51% of vessels, nearly all occurring within the first 9 months.[38]

K Endovascular candidate?

Initially, endovascular treatment of cervical artery dissection was limited to lesions that were inaccessible via an open approach. However, endovascular therapies have been increasingly employed because they have less associated morbidity than do open surgical techniques. Favorable results have been reported in both traumatic and spontaneous dissections.[39] Symptomatic patients with dissection should be evaluated for the potential of endovascular repair. In the setting of severe neurologic deficit and evidence of major intracranial artery occlusion (eg, occluded carotid siphon or middle cerebral artery), consideration should be given to catheter-based intracranial neurologic rescue. This is performed in most institutions by or in conjunction with a neurointerventional team. Technical considerations of the procedure are the main determinants of whether a patient is an endovascular candidate. If the dissection is identified within the extracranial carotid artery and the artery remains patent, it is usually possible to improve intraluminal patency with stent placement. If the extracranial carotid artery is occluded or it is unclear whether the artery is occluded, the likelihood of technical failure of an attempt at recanalization is increased. If the distal cervical ICA in the petrous segment is patent and of normal caliber, it is worth considering an attempt at endovascular repair. This is an area where personal clinical experience is key because there is no substantial published data to inform treatment decisions. If the carotid lesion has progressed to occlusion, crossing the lesion is not a foregone conclusion. An advantage in approaching an occlusion is that the lesions are typically focal, which makes blind passage of the wire a little more likely with gentle probing. The key feature regarding clinical decision making is the desire to avoid making the patient's neurologic status worse. Patients must be candidates for anticoagulation that accompanies interventional treatment.

L Endovascular intervention

Endovascular therapies include stenting of the dissection with either bare-metal or covered stents and coiling of PSAs. Patients are treated with heparin intraoperatively, 4 days of aspirin and clopidogrel postoperatively, 6 weeks of clopidogrel after the procedure, and kept on aspirin indefinitely.[24] A recent systematic review demonstrated a technical success rate of 99% with a 1.3% procedural complication rate. At follow-up at a mean of 12.8 months' follow-up, in-stent stenosis or occlusion was seen in only 2% of patients.[40] Currently, there are no data to support endovascular intervention in asymptomatic patients. Intraarterial and intravenous thrombolytic agents can also be used for the treatment of carotid or vertebral artery dissections associated with ischemic symptoms secondary to thromboembolism. Thrombolytic therapy is usually contraindicated in the setting of trauma, although for spontaneous dissections there is still a concern that thrombolytic therapy can lead to expansion of a subintimal hematoma leading to aneurysm formation, vessel occlusion, or to a subarachnoid hemorrhage. However, there is currently no evidence to support these concerns. The CADISP multicenter study demonstrated that thrombolysis was not associated with significant bleeding or other poor outcomes.[41]

Ⓜ Surgical candidate?

Grade II-V injuries should be considered for surgical repair if surgically accessible, in agreement with major Trauma Society Guidelines.[12,13] However, most injuries are near the skull base and are not accessible. Surgical treatment may also be considered after 6 months of medical therapy if there is a continued high-grade stenosis, or a new or persistent aneurysm that is 1.0 to 1.5 cm in diameter. To be a candidate for surgical repair, the lesion must be accessible by an open approach.

Ⓝ Surgical treatment

Exposure of the ICA for dissection is more complicated than is exposure for normal indications of CEA because lesions are typically located in the more distal ICA. Exposure may require maneuvers for high ICA exposure such as nasal intubation, division of the posterior belly of the digastric muscle, fracture of the styloid bone, mandibular subluxation, or division. The latter usually involve participation of oral or ENT surgeons. Once exposure is achieved, open surgical options include carotid ligation, interposition vein graft, thrombectomy, or patch angioplasty. Ligation is considered reasonable if systolic stump pressure is >70 mm Hg.[42] Complications secondary to surgical intervention are common. Postoperative ipsilateral stroke rates in one group occurred in 8% of patients, cranial nerve palsies in 58% of patients, 20% of reconstructions did not have patency at discharge, and there was a 2% mortality.[23]

Ⓞ Surveillance

There are no strong long-term data to guide duration of antithrombotic therapy initiated for cervical artery dissection. For spontaneous dissections, antithrombotic therapy is continued for a minimum of 3 to 6 months. At that time, repeat imaging is performed (CTA, MRA, DSA, or DUS) and further treatment is tailored to imaging findings. Some studies have demonstrated that most arterial lesions stabilize or resolve within the first 3 months, and vessels that have failed to reconstitute by 6 months are unlikely to recover.[39] For traumatic dissections, some authors perform follow-up imaging at 7 to 10 days post injury, and if the lesion is completely healed, then antithrombotic therapy is discontinued.[10] If the lesion remains, the patient should be continued on antithrombotic therapy for at least 3 months. At that time, imaging should be repeated and therapy tailored to imaging findings. Therapy can be discontinued if healing is demonstrated. For those who demonstrate continued lesions, continued

antithrombotic therapy versus lifelong aspirin as well as endovascular intervention should be considered.[43] Note that follow-up imaging is not generally needed after grade IV traumatic dissection because the occlusion is very unlikely to recanalize.[44]

The rate of recurrence of vertebral or carotid artery dissection with or without symptoms is uncertain. Previous reports suggest that recurrent ischemic symptoms (stroke or TIA) after dissection ranges from 0% to 13%.[20] However, the CADISS trial found that the rate of recurrent ischemic stroke at 3 months was approximately 2%, and all occurrences occurred within 10 days of onset, suggesting that the risk after 2 weeks was probably low.[26] Another study demonstrated the incidence of recurrent ischemic stroke rates at 0.3% annually and a TIA incidence 0.6% annually.[45]

REFERENCES

1. Lee VH, Brown RD Jr, Mandrekar JN, Mokri B. Incidence and outcome of cervical artery dissection: a population-based study. *Neurology.* 2006;67:1809-1812.
2. Schievink WI. Spontaneous dissection of the carotid and vertebral arteries. *N Engl J Med.* 2001;344:898-906.
3. Davis JW, Holbrook TL, Hoyt DB, Mackersie RC, Field TO Jr, Shackford SR. Blunt carotid artery dissection: incidence, associated injuries, screening, and treatment. *J Trauma.* 1990;30:1514-1517.
4. Nedeltchev K, Baumgartner RW. Traumatic cervical artery dissection. *Front Neurol Neurosci.* 2005;20:54-63.
5. Hughes KM, Collier B, Greene KA, Kurek S. Traumatic carotid artery dissection: a significant incidental finding. *Am Surg.* 2000;66:1023-1027.
6. Biffl WL, Moore EE, Ryu RK, et al. The unrecognized epidemic of blunt carotid arterial injuries: early diagnosis improves neurologic outcome. *Ann Surg.* 1998;228:462.
7. Debette S, Grond-Ginsbach C, Bodenant M, et al. Differential features of carotid and vertebral artery dissections: the CADISP study. *Neurology.* 2011;77:1174.
8. Arnold M, Bousser MG, Fahrni G, et al. Vertebral artery dissection: presenting findings and predictors of outcome. *Stroke.* 2006;37:2499.
9. Crum B, Mokri B, Fulgham J. Spinal manifestations of vertebral artery dissection. *Neurology.* 2000;55:304.
10. Biffl WL, Ray CE Jr, Moore EE, et al. Treatment-related outcomes from blunt cerebrovascular injuries: importance of routine follow-up arteriography. *Ann Surg.* 2002;235:699.
11. Biffl WL, Moore EE, Elliott JP, Brega KE, Burch JM. Blunt cerebrovascular injuries. *Curr Probl Surg.* 1999;36:505.
12. Biffl WL, Cothren CC, Moore EE, et al. Western Trauma Association critical decisions in trauma: screening for and treatment of blunt cerebrovascular injuries. *J Trauma.* 2009;67:1150.
13. Bromberg WJ, Collier BC, Diebel LN, et al. Blunt cerebrovascular injury practice management guidelines: the

Eastern Association for the Surgery of Trauma. *J Trauma.* 2010;68:471.
14. Mundinger GS, Dorafshar AH, Gilson MM, Mithani SK, Manson PN, Rodriguez ED. Blunt-mechanism facial fracture patterns associated with internal carotid artery injuries: recommendations for additional screening criteria based on analysis of 4,398 patients. *J Oral Maxillofac Surg.* 2013;71:2092.
15. Downer J, Nadarajah M, Briggs E, Wrigley P, McAuliffe W. The location of origin of spontaneous extracranial internal carotid artery dissection is adjacent to the skull base. *J Med Imaging Radiat Oncol.* 2014;58:408.
16. Stallmeyer MJ, Morales RE, Flanders AE. Imaging of traumatic neurovascular injury. *Radiol Clin North Am.* 2006;44:13-39, vii.
17. Eastman AL, Chason DP, Perez CL, McAnulty AL, Minei JP. Computed tomographic angiography for the diagnosis of blunt cervical vascular injury: is it ready for prime time? *J Trauma.* 2006;60:925-929; discussion 929.
18. Provenzale JM, Sarikaya B. Comparison of test performance characteristics of MRI, MR angiography, and CT angiography in the diagnosis of carotid and vertebral artery dissection: a review of the medical literature. *AJR Am J Roentgenol.* 2009;193:1167.
19. Biffl WL. Diagnosis of blunt cerebrovascular injuries. *Curr Opin Crit Care.* 2003;9:530-534.
20. Debette S, Leys D. Cervical-artery dissections: predisposing factors, diagnosis, and outcome. *Lancet Neurol.* 2009;8:668.
21. Arnold M, Baumgartner RW, Stapf C, et al. Ultrasound diagnosis of spontaneous carotid dissection with isolated Horner syndrome. *Stroke.* 2008;39:82.
22. Biffl WL, Moore EE, Offner PJ, Brega KE, Franciose RJ, Burch JM. Blunt carotid arterial injuries: implications of a new grading scale. *J Trauma.* 1999;47:845.
23. Muller BT, Luther B, Hort W, Neumann-Haefelin T, Aulich A, Sandmann W. Surgical treatment of 50 carotid dissections: indications and results. *J Vasc Surg.* 2000;31:980-988.
24. Edgell RC, Abou-Chebl A, Yadav JS. Endovascular management of spontaneous carotid artery dissection. *J Vasc Surg.* 2005;42:854-860.
25. Cohen JE, Ben-Hur T, Rajz G, Umansky F, Gomori JM. Endovascular stent-assisted angioplasty in the management of traumatic internal carotid artery dissections. *Stroke.* 2005;36:e45-e47.
26. CADISS Trial Investigators; Markus HS, Hayter E, Levi C, Feldman A, Venables G, Norris J. Antiplatelet treatment compared with anticoagulation treatment for cervical artery dissection (CADISS): a randomised trial. *Lancet Neurol.* 2015;14(4):361-367.
27. Cothren CC, Moore EE, Biffl WL, et al. Anticoagulation is the gold standard therapy for blunt carotid injuries to reduce stroke rate. *Arch Surg.* 2004;139:540.

28. Edwards NM, Fabian TC, Claridge JA, Timmons SD, Fischer PE, Croce MA. Antithrombotic therapy and endovascular stents are effective treatment for blunt carotid injuries: results from longterm followup. *J Am Coll Surg*. 2007;204:1007.

29. Schievink WI, Piepgras DG, McCaffrey TV, Mokri B. Surgical treatment of extracranial internal carotid artery dissecting aneurysms. *Neurosurgery*. 1994;35:809-815; discussion 815-816.

30. Spanos K, Karathanos C, Stamoulis K, Giannoukas AD. Endovascular treatment of traumatic internal carotid artery pseudoaneurysm. *Injury*. 2016;47:307.

31. Cox MW, Whittaker DR, Martinez C, Fox CJ, Feuerstein IM, Gillespie DL. Traumatic pseudoaneurysms of the head and neck: early endovascular intervention. *J Vasc Surg*. 2007;46:1227.

32. Debette S, Markus HS. The genetics of cervical artery dissection: a systematic review. *Stroke*. 2009;40:e459.

33. Olin JW, Gornik HL, Bacharach JM, et al. Fibromuscular dysplasia: state of the science and critical unanswered questions: a scientific statement from the American Heart Association. *Circulation*. 2014;129:1048.

34. Grond-Ginsbach C, Klima B, Weber R, et al. Exclusion mapping of the genetic predisposition for cervical artery dissections by linkage analysis. *Ann Neurol*. 2002;52:359.

35. Martin JJ, Hausser I, Lyrer P, et al. Familial cervical artery dissections: clinical, morphologic, and genetic studies. *Stroke*. 2006;37:2924.

36. Cogbill TH, Moore EE, Meissner M, et al. The spectrum of blunt injury to the carotid artery: a multicenter perspective. *J Trauma*. 1994;37:473.

37. Arauz A, Márquez JM, Artigas C, Balderrama J, Orrego H. Recanalization of vertebral artery dissection. *Stroke*. 2010;41:717.

38. Baracchini C, Tonello S, Meneghetti G, Ballotta E. Neurosonographic monitoring of 105 spontaneous cervical artery dissections: a prospective study. *Neurology*. 2010;75:1864.

39. Nedeltchev K, Bickel S, Arnold M, et al. R2-recanalization of spontaneous carotid artery dissection. *Stroke*. 2009;40:499.

40. Pham MH, Rahme RJ, Arnaout O, et al. Endovascular stenting of extracranial carotid and vertebral artery dissections: a systematic review of the literature. *Neurosurgery*. 2011;68:856-866.

41. Engelter ST, Dallongeville J, Kloss M, et al. Thrombolysis in cervical artery dissection—data from the Cervical Artery Dissection and Ischaemic Stroke Patients (CADISP) database. *Eur J Neurol*. 2012;19:1199-1206.

42. Ehrnefeld WK, Stoney RJ, Wylie EJ. Relation of carotid stump pressure to safety of carotid artery ligation. *Surgery*. 1983;93:299-305.

43. Miller PR, Fabian TC, Croce MA, et al. Prospective screening for blunt cerebrovascular injuries: analysis of diagnostic modalities and outcomes. *Ann Surg*. 2002;236:386.

44. Wagenaar AE, Burlew CC, Biffl WL, et al. Early repeat imaging is not warranted for high-grade blunt cerebrovascular injuries. *J Trauma Acute Care Surg*. 2014;77:540.

45. Touzé E, Gauvrit JY, Moulin T, Meder JF, Bracard S, Mas JL; Multicenter Survey on Natural History of Cervical Artery Dissection. Risk of stroke and recurrent dissection after a cervical artery dissection: a multicenter study. *Neurology*. 2003;61:1347.

Samuel I. Schwartz • Glenn LaMuraglia

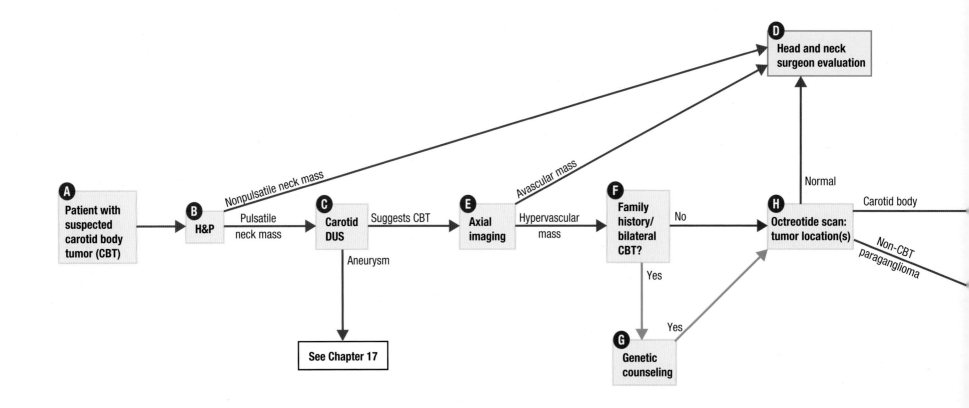

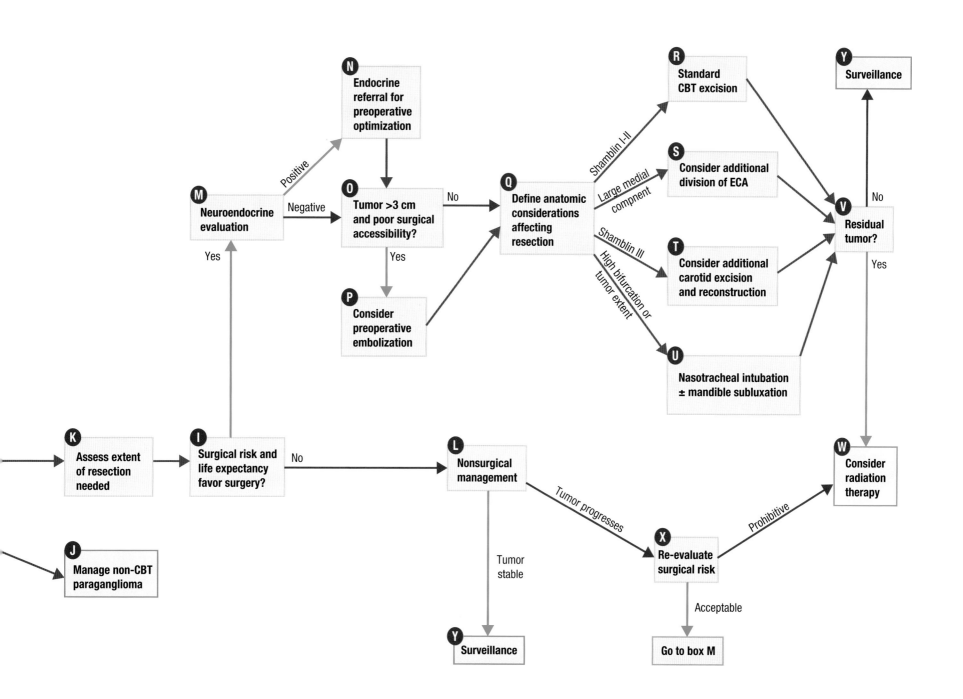

A Patient with suspected carotid body tumor (CBT)

CBTs most commonly present as a painless mass or fullness under the mandible.[1] Historically, there is a 5% incidence of bilateral tumors and a 10% familial pattern with autosomal dominant transmission.[2,3] The main environmental risk factor associated with CBTs is chronic hypoxia (COPD or living at a high altitude over 3000-4000 m).[4] There is no gender or age predilection for these tumors.

B H&P

Patients may present with hoarseness and/or dysphagia resulting from the mass effect of a large CBT. Six percent of patients experience HTN attributable to catecholamine secretion from the CBT.[5] Rarely there are nonspecific symptoms such as headaches or dizziness.

On physical examination, a CBT is an isolated mass that is pulsatile (due to adjacency to the carotid artery and transmitted pulse) but not expansive; in contrast, carotid aneurysms appear both expansive and pulsatile. Classically, the Fontaine's sign (anterior and posterior motility, but fixed in a vertical axis) is a definitive finding. Care should be taken when examining the CBT mass, because manipulation of the tumor may result in a decrease in heart rate and subsequent dizziness. Occasionally, a bruit may be heard and a CBT can be seen transorally if there is a large medial component.

C Carotid DUS

Color flow DUS imaging is the best screening study.[6] Because of a 5% incidence of bilateral CBTs, bilateral DUS should always be performed. Typical features include the presence of the solid hypervascular, hypoechoic mass directly in the carotid bifurcation, with wide splaying of the external and ICAs. Triplex color flow analysis may demonstrate a low-resistance arterial flow pattern in the mass but a high, turbulent flow pattern characteristic of a carotid aneurysm is not seen.[7] Small flow channels, if detected by DUS, favor the diagnosis of CBT given its hypervascularity. A simple DUS can prevent ill-advised biopsy—and resulting hemorrhage—during a workup of a suspected neck mass.[8] Carotid DUS can also be used for postoperative surveillance to identify recurrence.

D Head and neck surgeon evaluation

A head and neck surgeon should be involved in the workup of the patient with suspected CBT if imaging is not consistent with a CBT. The differential diagnosis is voluminous, including metastatic cancer to the cervical lymph nodes, glomus tumor, brachial cleft cyst, and low parotid tumor. The head and neck surgeon can further undertake a workup for malignancy with further imaging and biopsy as indicated.

E Axial imaging

The diagnosis of a CBT should be confirmed, and its extent and relationship to the carotid arteries be determined by axial imaging, such as CTA. Splaying of the carotid arteries and the presence of a homogeneous, highly vascularized mass between the carotid arteries is diagnostic of the lesion. MRA may also be used.

F Family history/bilateral CBT?

In patients with a positive family history or bilateral CBTs, a genetic mutation is likely present (subunits SDHB on chromosome 1p35-36 and SDHD on chromosome 11q23). SDHB mutations are more often malignant and associated with adrenal paragangliomas.[9]

G Genetic counseling

For patients with a positive family history or bilateral CBTs, referral to a genetic counselor is beneficial. These specialists will perform the genetic workup, and because there are no current guidelines recommending who should have genetic screening, they can assist in guiding familial workup of the condition.

H Octreotide scan: tumor location(s)

Regardless of the presence or absence of a positive family history or bilateral CBTs, an octreotide scan should be performed early in the evaluation of these patients to exclude synchronous lesions in other locations. An octreotide scan is performed by injecting radiotracer-labeled octreotide intravenously; cells with somatostatin receptors (seen with most neuroendocrine tumors) will bind radiolabeled octreotide, which can be visualized during serial scans. A positive octreotide scan will also validate the diagnosis of CBT in the carotid bifurcation. If synchronous lesions are found, their management depends on location.

I Surgical risk and life expectancy favor surgery?

Preoperative surgical evaluation includes an evaluation of surgical risk as well as extent of tumor burden (ie, evaluation for tumor outside of the carotid bifurcation within the head/neck region or chest and abdomen). For patients with limited life expectancy, high surgical risk, or the requirement for an extensive or morbid resection, non-surgical management is pursued.

A full head and neck evaluation should be performed in patients with CBT because cranial nerve involvement with CBTs has been estimated as high as 20%. The most common adjacent nerves involved are the vagus and hypoglossal nerves; therefore, the preoperative assessment should include laryngoscopy for documentation of vocal cord function and a careful neurologic examination of the other cranial nerves.[10]

J Manage non-CBT paraganglioma

Paragangliomas in the neck that are not in the carotid bifurcation must be particularly carefully evaluated since they often involve other cranial nerves, increasing the potential morbidity of resection. Those involving the vagus nerve (glomus vagale) or the hypoglossal nerve (glomus hypoglossi) require resection of the affected nerve, resulting in complete loss of nerve function.[11,12] For these paragangliomas not in the carotid bifurcation, surgery would usually be postponed until symptoms develop or with increasing size in a good risk patient when it threatens to make future resection more difficult. Treatment in conjunction with a head and neck surgeon is advisable as vocal cord medialization may be required to prevent aspiration after vagal nerve excision. Abdominal or thoracic paragangliomas require referral to a surgical oncologist for further management. Treatment of non-CBT paragangliomas is outside the scope of this chapter.

K Assess extent of resection needed

Large CBTs surrounding adjacent cranial nerves or neck structures may require an extensive/morbid resection that may result in neurologic or other deficits. This dissection should be weighed against the presenting symptoms and symptoms expected with continued tumor growth. This is particularly true when the tumor is very cranial in the neck. For patients with a limited life expectancy, significant medical comorbidities (see Chapters 1 and 2), or large/poorly accessible tumors with risk for poor operative outcomes, nonsurgical management with surveillance should be considered.

L Nonsurgical management

In patients excluded from surgical consideration, periodic (every 6-12 months) clinical evaluation of tumor growth and evidence of compression symptoms of adjacent structures should be undertaken. Depending on the findings and the individual patient, appropriate decisions can be made for either surgery (if disease progression now outweighs high surgical risk) or radiation therapy.

M Neuroendocrine evaluation

Neuroendocrine secretory screening is recommended for all patients with a suspected CBT, especially those with symptoms, familial/bilateral CBTs, or extracervical paragangliomas. Neuroendocrine hypersecretory activity is present in only 5% of patients who typically have paragangliomas at other locations, which can be identified with an octreotide scan.[13,14]

Testing includes a 24-hour urine collection for metanephrines and catecholamines; plasma levels can additionally be ordered per the endocrinologist's preferences.[15]

N Endocrine referral for preoperative optimization

Elevated catecholamines result in headaches, palpitations, HTN, photophobia, diaphoresis, and cardiac dysrhythmias. For patients with neuroendocrine secretory tumors, endocrinology referral may be of use for preoperative optimization and management of the active neuroendocrine symptoms. Preoperative α-blockade in the form of phenoxybenzamine followed by β-blockade is instituted; on the day of surgery, the anesthesia team needs to optimize the patient's fluid status and have nitroglycerine, labetalol, and nicardipine on standby for treatment of blood pressure elevations.

O Tumor > 3 cm and poor surgical accessibility?

Patients with CBT >3 cm, especially those difficult to access anatomically, may benefit from preoperative embolization. In some series, this has been shown to decrease the otherwise large intraoperative blood loss, facilitate the operation, and potentially diminish morbidity.[1] However, it is accompanied by a small stroke risk and, as such, is not universally used.

P Consider preoperative embolization

CBT embolization involves highly selective catheter cannulation of the arteries supplying the tumor (ascending cervical and ECA branches with occasional branches of the CCA itself). Before injecting the embolic material, the interventionalist must visualize each branch with arteriography to exclude collaterals to the vertebral or ICA circulation, which would contraindicate embolization. Ideally, preoperative embolization should be performed on the day before operative resection to minimize associated tissue inflammation and edema.[1]

Q Define anatomic considerations affecting resection

Despite the surgical challenge of CBT, surgical excision is the only curative therapy. Nearly 95% of CBT can be completely resected with rare mortality (2%).[13] Perioperative stroke affects only 2% to 3% of patients. Careful attention to the anatomy and proximity of the cranial nerves in these tumors is imperative to minimize their injury, which remains, in some series, the highest morbidity (40%) associated with this operation.[13]

Of historical significance, in 1971 Shamblin classified CBT as group I through III; group I tumors are relatively small with minimal adherence to the carotid vasculature, group II tumors are larger with moderate attachment, and group III tumors encase the carotid vasculature and potentially surrounding nerves.[5]

Surgical resection of the CBT obviously varies depending on the tumor size, location, and associated surrounding structure involvement. Dissection differs for Shamblin I-II versus Shamblin III tumors and for tumors with a large medial component versus tumors associated with a high carotid bifurcation or cephalad extension. The team approach of vascular and head and neck surgeons has been advocated, especially for large tumors, to diminish complications and to facilitate the sometimes, difficult identification and handling of nerve and artery problems. A selective lymph node dissection can also be performed to rule out malignancy.

R Standard CBT excision

Before dissecting the CBT off the artery, the surgeon should obtain proximal control of the common carotid artery. Careful periadventitial carotid dissection is important to avoid injury to the arterial wall and also avoid incision into the tumor, which can cause significant bleeding. If this occurs, arterial injury can be repaired using a stitch or patch reconstruction. In large CBTs that significantly splay and stretch the carotid bifurcation, the adventitial surface of the arteries may be attenuated , therefore, spreading during the dissection should be avoided. This principle is in contrast to the situation of a patient with atherosclerotic disease or metastatic disease in the neck when the carotid artery may be fibrotic. Therefore, the surgeon must take extra care in retracting the artery from the CBT.

S Consider additional division of ECA

Division of the ECA can be useful when the tumor is large or when there is a large medial component to a "dumbbell"-shaped tumor. Division facilitates the medial and posterior dissection of the ICA and provides valuable exposure of the posterior aspect of the carotid bifurcation, where the tumors are usually very adherent. The artery should be divided in a convenient location, and after removal of the specimen, it should be oversewn to avoid a dead space/stump arising from the carotid bifurcation that could accumulate thrombus and result in stroke.

T Consider additional carotid excision and reconstruction

With CBT encasement (*Shamblin III*) or invasion into the carotid artery wall, carotid resection and vascular reconstruction may be necessary. Because this cannot always be predicted before surgery, it is recommended that (1) a method of cerebral perfusion monitoring be available and (2) conduit issues should be planned because bypass may be needed. The GSV or ePTFE (if autogenous vein is not available) is suitable. Lastly, if the ICA is tortuous, there may be enough length for direct reimplantation after excision of the CBT *en bloc* with the carotid bifurcation.[1]

U Nasotracheal intubation ± mandible subluxation

High exposure to further improve access to the CBT can be achieved by nasotracheal intubation and anterior subluxation of the mandible, if needed. Fixed mechanical retractors always improve exposure, and with proper positioning, cranial nerve injury can be minimized. At the most cephalad and posterior point of dissection, the hypoglossal nerve, superior laryngeal nerve, vagus nerve, glossopharyngeal nerve, or mandibular branch of the facial nerve can be injured. If cranial nerves are involved in the capsule and adherent to the tumor, but not frankly invaded, it is important to identify the nerves near the tumor and to dissect them free. However, should the nerves be encased in the tumor and

be nonfunctional preoperatively, there is no evidence that freeing them from the tumor will restore their function.

V Residual tumor?

The goal of surgical resection should be to completely remove all tumor. If extenuating circumstances force residual tumor to be left at the time of surgery, radiation therapy should be considered. All patients should have medical follow-up. Tumor histology will also be confirmed; rarely, malignancy is identified by involvement of lymph nodes. This would require formal presentation at a National Comprehensive Cancer Network (NCCN) guideline governed committee meeting for consideration of additional adjuvant therapy.

W Consider radiation therapy

Radiation therapy has been used but is of only anecdotal benefit, because CBTs are thought to be radioresistant.[16] This concept has been challenged in one study in which there was complete response in 23%, partial response in 54%, and no response in the other 23% of patients treated with radiotherapy.[17] Adjuvant radiotherapy after partial resection, likewise, is of questionable benefit because most of the tumors can continue to demonstrate some enlargement.

X Re-evaluate surgical risk

If a patient judged to be at high surgical risk develops symptoms and clear tumor progression during follow-up, the potential for surgical treatment should be re-evaluated given the current tumor status.

Y Surveillance

If there is no evidence of contralateral or residual tumor on follow-up studies, the patient should be monitored clinically for evidence of a new contralateral or a recurrent CBT. Recurrence is seen in up to 6% of cases and is most commonly seen in patients with multiple paragangliomas or a positive family history.[18] If detected, surgical excision is recommended if the lesion is accessible and the patient is of appropriate risk.

In patients who have undergone a CBT resection, it is advisable to obtain baseline DUS imaging at follow up depending on the intraoperative findings. If there is no evidence of contralateral or residual tumor, the patient should be monitored clinically for evidence of a new contralateral or a recurrent CBT and imaged as indicated.

For patients who have also undergone a carotid artery reconstruction, such as a bypass or reimplantation, additional follow-up should be undertaken for this reconstruction. For a 2-year period, these patients should be evaluated with carotid DUS starting 6 weeks postoperatively and every 6 to 12 months (for 2 years), thereafter if no significant abnormalities are noted.

Acknowledgments

The authors would like to acknowledge the contributions of Dr. Daniel Deschler of Mass Eye and Ear Infirmary, Boston, and Dr. Jahan Mohebali of Massachusetts General Hospital for the conception, writing, and editing of this chapter.

REFERENCES

1. LaMuraglia GM, Fabian RL, Brewster DC, et al. The current surgical management of carotid body paragangliomas. *J Vasc Surg.* 1992;15:1038-1045.
2. Ridge BA, Brewster DC, Darling RC, Cambria RP, LaMuraglia GM, Abbott WM. Familial carotid body tumors: incidence and implications. *J Vasc Surg.* 1993;7:190-194.
3. Grufferman S, Gillman MW, Pasternak LR, Peterson CL, Young WG Jr. Familial carotid body tumors: case report and epidemiologic review. *Cancer.* 1980;46:2116-2122.
4. Farr HW. Carotid body tumors: a 40-year study. *CA Cancer J Clin.* 1980;30:260-265.
5. Shamblin WR, ReMine WH, Sheps SG, Harrison EG. Carotid body tumor (chemodectoma): clinicopathologic analysis of ninety cases. *Am J Surg.* 1971;122:732-739.
6. Steinke W, Hennerici M, Aulich A. Doppler color flow imaging of carotid body tumors. *Stroke.* 1989;20:1574-1577.
7. Muhm M, Polterauer P, Gstottner W, et al. Diagnostic and therapeutic approaches to carotid body tumors: review of 24 patients. *Arch Surg.* 1997;132:79-284.
8. Williams MD, Phillips MJ, Rainer WG. Carotid body tumor. *Arch Surg.* 1992;127:963-968.
9. Lenders JW, Duh Q, Eisenhofer G, et al. Pheochromocytoma and paraganglioma: an endocrine society clinical practice guideline. *J Clin Endocrinol Metab.* 2014;99(6):1915-1942.
10. Davidge-Pitts KJ, Pantanowitz D. Carotid body tumors. *Surg Annu.* 1984;16:203-227.
11. Fink DS, Benoit MM, LaMuraglia GM, et al. Paraganglioma of the hypoglossal nerve. *Laryngoscope.* 2011;120 Suppl 4:S147.
12. Persky M, Tran T. Acquired vascular tumors of the head and neck. *Otolaryngol Clin North Am.* 2018;51:255-274.
13. Hallett JW, Nora JD, Hollier LH, Cherry KJ Jr, Pairolero PC. Trends in neurovascular complications of surgical management for carotid body and cervical paragangliomas: a fifty-year experience with 153 tumors. *J Vasc Surg.* 1988;7:284-291.
14. Lamberts SW, Bakker WH, Reubi JC, Krenning EP. Somatostatin-receptor imaging in the localization of endocrine tumors. *N Engl J Med.* 1990;323:1246-1249.
15. Neumann HP, Eng C. The approach to the patient with paraganglioma. *J Clin Endocrinol Metab.* 2009;94(8):2677-2683.
16. Mitchell DC, Clyne CA. Chemodectomas of the neck: the response to radiotherapy. *Br J Surg.* 1985;72:903-905.
17. Evenson LJ, Mendenhall WM, Parsons JT, Cassisi NJ. Radiotherapy in the management of chemodectomas of the carotid body and glomus vagale. *Head Neck.* 1998;20:609-613.
18. Nora JD, Hallett JW, O'Brien PC, Naessens JM, Cherry KJ Jr, Pairolero PC. Surgical resection of carotid body tumors: long-term survival, recurrence, and metastasis. *Mayo Clin Proc.* 1988;63(4):348-352.

Ruth L. Bush

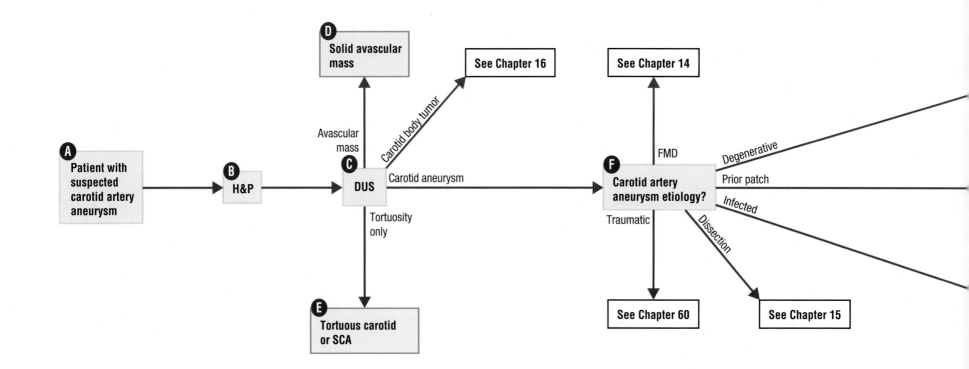

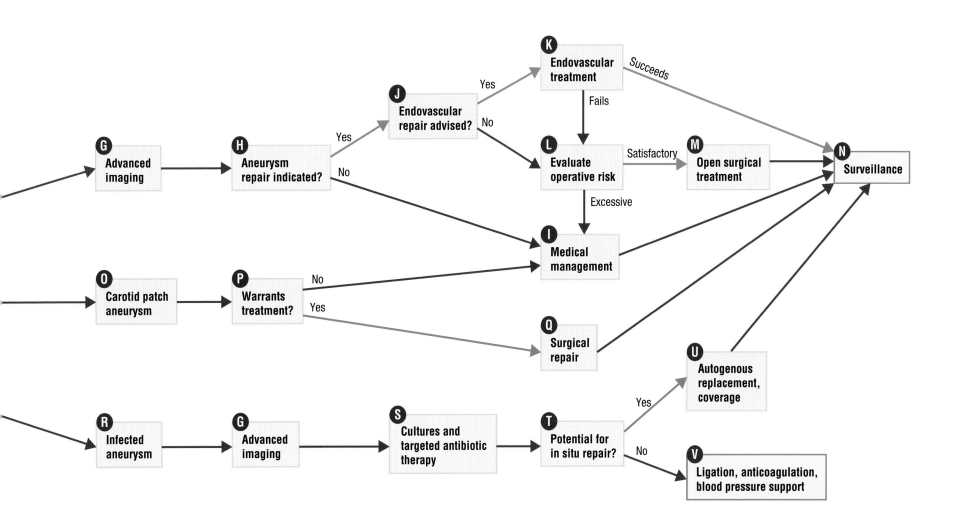

A Patient with suspected carotid artery aneurysm

Extracranial carotid artery aneurysms (ECAAs) are a rare carotid artery pathology leading to less than 2% of all extracranial carotid interventions.[1,2] ECAAs may be either true aneurysms, involving all layers of the arterial wall, or PSAs, such as occur with a disrupted patch angioplasty. Presentation may vary from an asymptomatic pulsatile neck mass, to permanent neurologic deficits from embolization of thrombus within the ECAA. Major neurologic symptoms may present in 15% to 45% of patients, including TIA or stroke.[1,3] Other symptoms, resulting from direct mass effect and compression, include dysphagia, facial or trigeminal neuralgia, hoarseness, and/or Horner syndrome. An expanding hematoma from a carotid PSA is possible but infrequent. ECAAs most commonly involve the carotid bifurcation and present as a palpable, pulsatile neck mass. Patients who have less common (higher) ICA aneurysms usually present with swelling of the posterior pharynx and/or dysphagia. ECAAs proximal to the carotid bifurcation are usually palpable.

B H&P

Initial evaluation for patients presenting with suspected ECAA should include a careful H&P including a thorough neurologic examination. The history should consider any relevant carotid artery or neck procedures, such as prior CEA with patch angioplasty, external beam radiation therapy, neck trauma, or "whiplash" that may have resulted in a carotid arterial dissection, history of a collagen-vascular disorder, or prior diagnosis of FMD. Any increase in size of the mass and time frame should be noted. On physical examination, attention should be given to size and location as well as to the mobility of the mass. Classically, ECAA can be moved from side to side in a lateral plane but not in a vertical plane. Any overlying redness or tenderness may raise concern for arterial infection.

C DUS

Initial diagnostic imaging for a suspected ECAA is usually performed using DUS. ICA aneurysms may require cross-sectional imaging (CTA or MRA) to make the diagnosis and develop a treatment plan. Accepted diagnostic criterion for an ECAA is a 200% increase in the diameter of the ICA or a 150% increase in the diameter of the CCA.[4] Other pathology that might initially be mistaken for an ECAA includes a solid avascular neck mass, a carotid body tumor, or a very tortuous but nonaneurysmal CCA or SCA. These conditions should be distinguishable depending on H&P and DUS.

D Solid avascular mass

Any solid avascular mass identified on DUS needs to be further evaluated by an appropriate specialist.

E Tortuous carotid or SCA

A tortuous carotid artery, sometimes described as "coiled," or a tortuous SCA can be palpated in the neck and mistaken for an ECAA. These entities can usually be identified with DUS, or, if unclear, by CTA. They do not require treatment in the asymptomatic patient and are rarely associated with any symptoms except a noticeable mass.

F Carotid artery aneurysm etiology?

Once the diagnosis of ECAA is made, the etiology of the aneurysm needs to be determined depending on H&P and imaging. Degenerative or "atherosclerotic" disease is the most common etiology of ECAAs.[1-3] These present as true aneurysms, usually located at sites of plaque formation such as the carotid bifurcation or proximal ICA. They can be bilateral or unilateral. Saccular-shaped aneurysms are rare and more frequently associated with HTN (especially when located in the distal ICA), or infection.

Some ECAAs represent PSAs, which may develop after trauma or iatrogenic intervention, as well as after CEA from degeneration at the site of patching. Small ECAAs may develop as a result of carotid artery dissection or FMD. Finally, an ECAA may develop as a result of localized or hematogenous infection resulting in aneurysmal degeneration. Management of ECAAs differs according to etiology.

G Advanced imaging

CTA or MRA is used to guide the treatment plan or discern details of ECAA anatomy that may influence a decision to treat. Both CTA and MRA provide more detailed representation of ECAA anatomy, presence of thrombus, or potential signs of infection such as fluid accumulation, or hyperdense wall.[5] CTA can define relationship of the ECAA to bony landmarks that determine surgical accessibility or define distorted anatomy because of mass effect, inflammation, or infection. MRA can provide information regarding cerebral circulation and possible additional lesions, or extension of the ECAA into the cranial space. DSA is no longer recommended to diagnose ECAA because of the risk, albeit small, for stroke, unless carotid ligation is a necessary definitive treatment. In this scenario, an end-hole balloon occlusion catheter may be useful for measuring carotid artery back pressure to determine adequacy of cerebral blood flow in the territory of the ICA.

H Aneurysm repair indicated?

Operative treatment is indicated for any symptomatic ECAA, ECAAs with evidence of thrombus or infection, diameter >2 cm, and/or evidence of enlargement on imaging, assuming satisfactory surgical risk.[6] Indication for repair also includes local compressive symptoms.

Surgical risk should be evaluated for in all patients with ECAAs including cardiac and pulmonary risk (Chapters 1 and 2) and balanced against the risk of not intervening.

Thromboembolic events remain of high concern for patients presenting with ECAAs. Stroke rates of 50% have recently been reported in patients receiving nonoperative treatment for ECAAs; and older studies evaluating traumatic and infected aneurysms reported mortality rates of 60% to 70% without treatment.[7,8] Although the natural history of ECAAs is difficult to elucidate from the literature, the incidence of major neurologic complications provides insight into progression of the disease and provides the indication for operative treatment, because rupture is extremely rare. The likelihood of embolization is usually associated with the extent of thrombus within the ECAA, but this is extrapolated from other aneurysm locations.

I Medical management

Conservative treatment with medical therapy and surveillance should be reserved only for patients with asymptomatic, stable ECAAs and those who are at prohibitive operative risk.[9]

Medical therapy for patients with ECAA should focus on prevention of disease progression in addition to prophylaxis for thromboembolic complications. Treatment of etiologic factors is important and should include smoking cessation, statin therapy, and control of HTN. Both single and dual antiplatelet therapy as well as anticoagulation have been reported in the literature, although the paucity of data regarding therapy specific outcomes prevents recommendation of any specific agent or course.[3] Aspirin and other antiplatelet agents have demonstrated reduced morbidity and mortality in patients with carotid stenosis and may have prophylactic value in ECAA. In patients requiring carotid ligation, anticoagulation therapy is recommended postoperatively for 6 to 12 months; however, there is no level 1 evidence to support this practice.

J Endovascular repair advised?

Anatomic considerations are critical in surgical planning as well as in determining open surgical versus endovascular therapy. Endovascular approaches prevent the need for surgical dissection and exposure, which may be challenging in cases of hostile or inaccessible anatomy with high risk of iatrogenic injury to neurovascular tissues. The surgeon needs to evaluate the access pathway, arch anatomy, tortuosity of all carotid arteries, and thrombus burden to ensure that endovascular treatment can be performed safely. ECAAs with evidence of thrombus, tortuosity, or mass effect are better managed with open surgery (see N). Further, most bifurcation and proximal ICA degenerative aneurysms are treated with open surgery except in very high-risk patients. Aneurysms of the distal ICA or with distal extension requiring complex surgical exposure, or patients with hostile neck anatomy may be better treated with endovascular techniques if experienced interventionalists are available.

Endovascular treatment

Endovascular treatment of ECAAs focuses on exclusion of the aneurysm with either a bare-metal stent (BMS) or a covered stent. Approach to the ECAA is most frequently obtained through transfemoral percutaneous access, although direct puncture of the proximal carotid artery is also an option. Distal protection devices may be deployed, if deemed necessary.

Stent and stent-graft coverage may be performed with a variety of devices, although conflicting recommendations exist regarding various indications for BMSs and covered stents. In a systematic review of 113 studies, involving a total of 224 patients, BMSs with small vessels and patent side branches were typically preferred, whereas covered stents were used in nonbranching arteries with PSAs. In one large review of ECAAs of varying etiologies, BMSs and stent grafts failed to demonstrate any significant differences in patency, stroke, or mortality. However, covered stents did demonstrate a significant decrease in reintervention and stent-graft stenosis as well as an increase in thrombosis of the aneurysm sac.[10] For saccular aneurysms in which stent coverage was inadequate for embolization, trans-stent coiling may be performed. Specific device selection should be based on manufacturer's recommendations for sizing and emphasis should be placed on using the shortest available stent with adequate seal zones to prevent future kinking and stenosis of the artery. Additional techniques including hybrid approaches, double stenting, and balloon occlusion have been described.

The major complications of endovascular repair include stent stenosis or occlusion, and neurologic complications secondary to thromboembolism. However, large reviews of endovascular treatment of ECAAs have shown favorable early- and midterm results with stroke rates ranging from 0% to 2%.[3,9,10]

Evaluate operative risk

As with all major operations involving general anesthesia, a preoperative risk assessment should be performed. If timing allows, that is, an elective operation, medical optimization of comorbidities is preferable.

Open surgical treatment

Open surgical treatment of ECAAs can be accomplished through a variety of techniques and is the treatment of choice to prevent thromboembolism-induced neurologic dysfunction and aneurysm rupture. For lesions localized to the bifurcation or proximal ICA, exposure, proximal and distal control, and routine or selective shunting can be performed in a manner similar to CEA. Distal lesions, particularly those approaching the skull base, require more complex techniques for exposure and control. Nasotracheal

intubation, mandibular subluxation, mandibulotomy, excision of the styloid process, and drilling away of the petrous portion of the temporal bone are all techniques that can be used to facilitate distal exposure. Smaller saccular aneurysms can be excised with patch angioplasty or primary closure of the artery. Fusiform aneurysms must be resected completely to prevent progression. If the ECAA is associated with tortuous or elongated carotid arteries, it may be possible to perform primary end-to-end anastomosis after resection. However, in most cases, interposition grafts are used to reconstruct the resected portion. Carotid reconstruction may be performed with either autologous vein or prosthetic grafts, which have been demonstrated to have equivalent outcomes and long-term patency rates in this location.[11,12] For smaller ICAs, the saphenous vein is usually preferred.

Carotid artery ligation should only be performed for rare cases of rupture or infection (excluding the possibility of reconstruction) because the rate of neurologic complications is high. Ensuring a back pressure >50% of MAP, as well as a satisfactory balloon occlusion test, is necessary to ensure adequacy of cerebral perfusion before ligating the distal ICA.[13]

Cranial nerve damage may occur with open reconstruction, but most reports document transient deficits rather than permanent neurologic damage.[3] Reported perioperative stroke rates for ECAA open repair range from 10% to 15%.[1,3,14]

Surveillance

Although there are no established clinical guidelines for routine follow-up surveillance imaging after conservative or invasive treatment of ECAAs, postoperative imaging should be considered. Although the number of treated ECAA aneurysms reported in current literature is small, the early and long-term outcome of operative treatment is favorable.[15] Regardless of whether definitive treatment was surgical or endovascular, DUS surveillance to evaluate graft patency, in-stent stenosis, and the presence of degenerative disease (recurrent aneurysm), should be performed on a yearly or biyearly basis. For patients undergoing conservative management, surveillance is indicated to detect aneurysm growth that may support repair.

Carotid patch aneurysm

PSA is a known, but relatively rare (<1%) complication of CEA. Despite this, CEA is the leading cause of PSA formation in the carotid artery due to disruption of the patch suture line or degeneration of either the patch or the arterial wall. Mycotic PSAs have been rarely reported.[1,3,9,14] The time interval between CEA and presentation of a PSA is highly variable and may range from a few days to many years.[9,14] Subclinical infection of the PSA wall is found to be present in up to 38% of cases, with the most common organisms reported as strains of *Staphylococcus*, *Streptococci*, *Salmonella*, and *Escherichia*.[16]

Warrants treatment?

Surgical treatment is indicated for aneurysmal degeneration of all synthetic carotid patch aneurysms when infection is suspected. Intervention is also indicated for all symptomatic patients or if imaging reveals thrombus accumulation within the aneurysmal patch. Patients with aneurysmal degeneration of vein patches should also undergo patch revision because patch rupture is a known complication of saphenous vein patches.

Surgical repair

For ECAAs due to post-CEA patch degeneration, resection of the PSA patch should be performed, followed by repeat patch angioplasty, to reduce the risk of thromboembolism or rupture. Autologous grafts are recommended in this scenario because of the high probability of an infectious etiology. For more extensive ECAAs, an interposition vein graft with end-to-end anastomosis may be necessary. Rarely, a carotid PSA infection may be so severe as to require arterial ligation (see V).

Infected aneurysm

Infected ECAAs, aside from infected post-CEA PSAs, are rare but associated with high morbidity, including rupture, bleeding, and stroke. Pathogenesis has been attributed to dental abscesses, septic emboli, penetrating trauma, immunosuppression, and iatrogenic injury from surgical or endovascular manipulation. The most common cultured organisms are *Staphylococcus*, *Salmonella*, and *Streptococcus*.[17,18] In patients with infected ECAAs, both local and systemic signs of infection are present, most frequently with pain and tenderness of the pulsatile mass.

Cultures and targeted antibiotic therapy

For infected ECAAs, long-term antibiotic therapy is warranted. Initial therapy should include broad-spectrum agents with coverage for the most commonly cultured organisms as well as for gram-negative bacteria followed by specific coverage depending on sensitivities. Recommended duration of therapy in the literature is organism specific and varies, although typical treatments consist of IV therapy lasting 4 to 6 weeks[6,16-18] with continued oral antibiotics for a period ranging from months to lifelong.

Potential for in situ repair?

The potential for in situ repair of any infected aneurysm depends on the virulence of the infecting organism and the extent of local infection that cannot be debrided. If minor local infection can be debrided, and the organism is not gram negative, in situ repair is usually recommended, because it avoids the potential risk of stroke that can occur after ICA ligation.

segmentionegment" CARTID ARTERY ANEURYSM

Autogenous replacement, coverage

For infected ECAAs, standard methods of infection control including debridement and drainage should be utilized followed by reconstruction with good-quality GSV graft. Surgical repair may be difficult because of surrounding tissue inflammation and increased risk of neurologic damage. If extensive debridement is performed, muscle flap coverage may be required to obtain adequate closure.

Ligation, anticoagulation, blood pressure support

In cases of severe infection or distal involvement, ICA ligation at a site of noninfected artery may be required. To reduce the risk of stroke in such cases, the patient's blood pressure should be pharmacologically elevated as tolerated, and gradually reduced over 1 to 2 days. Anticoagulation to reduce distal thrombus propagation is practiced by most, despite absence of literature to support this practice.

REFERENCES

1. El-Sabrout R, Cooley DA. Extracranial carotid artery aneurysms: Texas Heart Institute experience. *J Vasc Surg.* 2000;31(4):702-712.
2. Garg K, Rockman CB, Lee V, et al. Presentation and management of carotid artery aneurysms and pseudoaneurysms. *J Vasc Surg.* 2012;55(6):1618-1622.
3. Zhou W, Lin PH, Bush RL, et al. Carotid artery aneurysm: evolution of management over two decades. *J Vasc Surg.* 2006;43(3):493-496; discussion 497.
4. Li Z, Chang G, Yao C, et al. Endovascular stenting of extracranial carotid artery aneurysm: a systematic review. *Eur J Vasc Endovasc Surg.* 2011;42(4):419-426.
5. Pourier V, De Borst GJ. Which carotid artery aneurysms need to be treated (and how)? *J Cardiovasc Surg.* 2016;57(2):152-157.
6. Bush RL, Long P, Atkins MD. Carotid artery aneurysms. In: Sidawy AN, Perler BA, eds. *Rutherford's Vascular Surgery and Endovascular Therapy.* Philadelphia, PA: Elsevier Health Sciences; 2018.
7. Winslow N. Extracranial aneurysm of the internal carotid artery: history and analysis of the cases registered up to Aug. 1, 1925. *Arch Surg.* 1926;13(5):689-729.
8. Zwolak RM, Whitehouse WM, Knake JE, et al. Atherosclerotic extracranial carotid artery aneurysms. *J Vasc Surg.* 1984;1(3):415-422.
9. de Jong KP, Zondervan PE, Urk HV. Extracranial carotid artery aneurysms. *Eur J Vasc Surg.* 1989;3(6):557-562.
10. Borazjani BH, Wilson SE, Fujitani RM, Gordon I, Mueller M, Williams RA. Postoperative complications of carotid patching: pseudoaneurysm and infection. *Ann Vasc Surg.* 2003;17(2):156-161.
11. Dorafshar AH, Reil TD, Ahn SS, Quinones-Baldrich WJ, Moore WS. Interposition grafts for difficult carotid artery reconstruction: a 17-year experience. *Ann Vasc Surg.* 2008;22(1):63-69.
12. Roddy SP, Darling RC III, Ozsvath KJ, et al. Choice of material for internal carotid artery bypass grafting: vein or prosthetic? Analysis of 44 procedures. *Cardiovasc Surg.* 2002;10(6):540-544.
13. Litwinski RA, Wright K, Pons P. Pseudoaneurysm formation following carotid endarterectomy: two case reports and a literature review. *Ann Vasc Surg.* 2006;20(5):678-680.
14. Abdelhamid MF, Wall ML, Vohra RK. Carotid artery pseudoaneurysm after carotid endarterectomy: case stories and a review of the literature. *Vasc Endovascular Surg.* 2009;43(6):571-577.
15. Welleweerd JC, den Ruijter HM, Nelissen BG, et al. Management of extracranial carotid artery aneurysm. *Eur J Vasc Endovasc Surg.* 2015;50(2):141-147.
16. El-Sabrout R, Reul G, Cooley DA. Infected postcarotid endarterectomy pseudoaneurysms: retrospective review of a series. *Ann Vasc Surg.* 2000;14(3):239-247.
17. Pirvu A, Bouchet C, Garibotti FM, Haupert S, Sessa C. Mycotic aneurysm of the internal carotid artery. *Ann Vasc Surg.* 2013;27(6):826-830.
18. Jebara VA, Acar C, Dervanian P, et al. Mycotic aneurysms of carotid arteries—case report and review of the literature. *J Vasc Surg.* 1991;41(2):215-219.

Caitlin W. Hicks • Christopher J. Abularrage

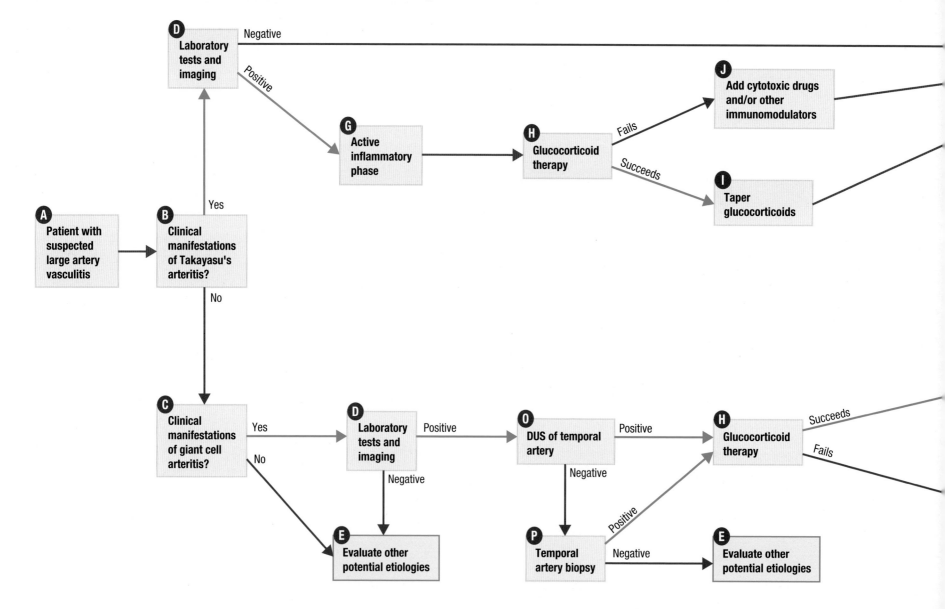

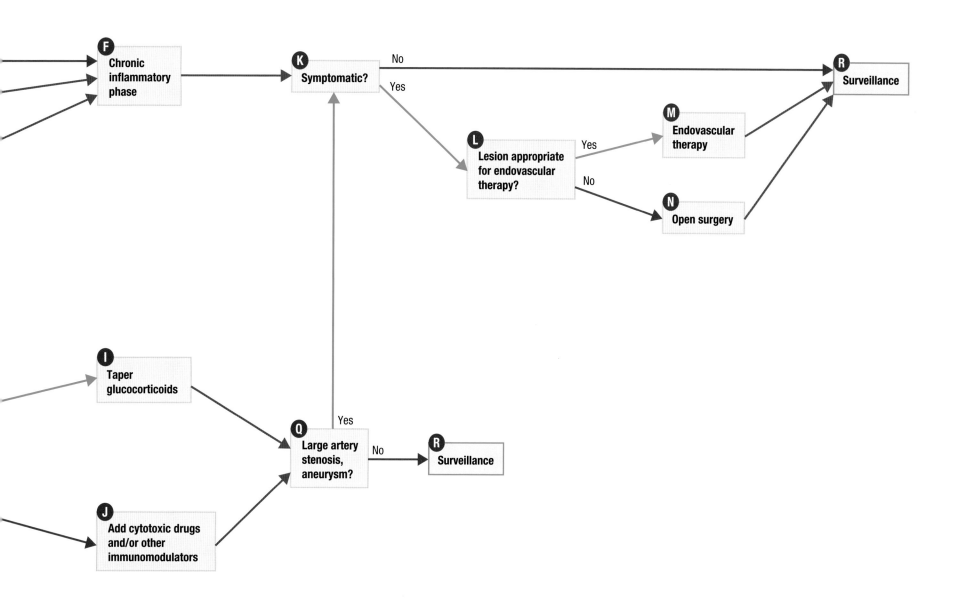

A Patient with suspected large artery vasculitis

Vasculitides are diseases defined by the presence of leukocytes in vessel walls, causing mural injury secondary to inflammation and reactive damage. Disease classification is based on the size of the affected vessels. Large artery vasculitides affect the aorta and its major branches and include Takayasu's arteritis (TA) and giant cell arteritis (GCA).

Patients with large artery vasculitis present with a variety of nonspecific, heterogeneous symptoms, making the diagnosis challenging. Most commonly, patients present with systemic or constitutional symptoms, including fatigue, fever, weight loss, and/or arthralgias. However, these symptoms are nonspecific and require a high index of clinical suspicion to make the diagnosis. A thorough medical history including birth country and travel history, physical examination, and laboratory evaluation are necessary, including WBC, complete metabolic panel (CMP), ESR, and CRP levels. Patients should also be evaluated for an infectious etiology with viral serologies, urinalysis, and blood cultures. Frequently, the diagnosis of large artery vasculitis is made on the basis of the presence of constitutional symptoms, elevated inflammatory markers, and dedicated vascular imaging. MRA, CTA, DUS, and, in some cases, PET are all useful in detecting vasculitis in the aorta and its primary branches.

B Clinical manifestations of Takayasu's arteritis?

TA affects the aorta and its primary branches. In most cases, the vasculitis is localized, but panaortitis can occur in select cases. Patients are most frequently affected at a young age (<20 years) and are female in 80% to 90% of cases.[1] TA occurs worldwide but is more common in Asian populations; approximately one to three cases per million people are affected in the United States each year.[2]

Clinical manifestations of TA include constitutional symptoms such as fever, fatigue, and/or weight loss, upper or lower extremity claudication in the absence of traditional atherosclerotic risk factors, and absent or diminished pulses in one limb compared to the contralateral limb (ie, blood pressure discrepancy between the right and left upper extremities). Patients may also experience difficult-to-control HTN and have an abdominal bruit due to renal artery involvement.[1]

In 1990, the American College of Rheumatology developed six criteria for the classification of TA[2]:

1. Onset at age ≤40 years
2. Claudication of an extremity
3. Decreased brachial artery pulse
4. >10 mm Hg difference in SBP between arms
5. Bruit over the subclavian arteries or aorta
6. Arteriographic evidence of narrowing or occlusion of the entire aorta, its primary branches, or large arteries in the proximal upper or lower extremities

The presence of three or more of these criteria has a sensitivity and specificity of 91% and 98% for TA, respectively.[2]

C Clinical manifestations of giant cell arteritis?

GCA can affect the aorta and its main branches but has a predilection for branches of the carotid artery. Classically, GCA is associated with the superficial temporal artery, which is why it is frequently called "temporal arteritis." GCA affects women more frequently than men (ratio 3:1) and rarely presents before 50 years of age; its highest incidence is in patients aged 70 to 79 years.[3] There is a strong ethnic predisposition for the disease, with persons of Scandinavian descent at highest risk.[3]

As with TA, patients with GCA frequently present with the nonspecific symptoms of fever, fatigue, and/or weight loss. Fevers are usually low grade in nature and occur in as many as 50% of affected patients. Owing to the older age of presentation, GCA should be considered in the workup of any older patient presenting with these symptoms, especially after malignancy and infectious etiology have been excluded. Polymyalgia rheumatica, characterized by morning stiffness in the shoulders and hips, frequently accompanies GCA, occurring in 40% to 50% of patients.[3]

Other symptoms that may be more specific for GCA include new-onset headaches, jaw pain with mastication, and vision changes. Headaches are estimated to occur in more than two-thirds of patients, and primarily affect the temporal regions, although they can be frontal, occipital, or generalized in nature. Jaw pain with mastication, analogous to leg claudication, is usually rapid onset and can be severe. It is thought to be the most specific symptom for GCA, because it is the symptom most highly associated with a positive temporal artery biopsy.[4] Approximately 15% of patients with GCA experience sudden, painless vision loss.[5] This can be transient or permanent, and either unilateral or bilateral. The main etiology for vision loss in these patients is anterior ischemic optic neuropathy (80%), followed by central retinal artery occlusion (10%), and posterior ischemic optic neuropathy.[6] Once established, vision loss associated with GCA is usually irreversible, making early diagnosis and treatment critical.

The diagnosis of GCA is based on a combination of clinical features with histopathology and/or imaging findings. The large vessel manifestations of GCA include aortic aneurysms and/or dissections and large artery stenoses, which are estimated to occur in 27% of patients with GCA.[7] Data from a population-based study of 168 patients with GCA showed that aortic aneurysms developed in 18%, aortic dissections occurred in 5%, and large artery stenosis occurred in 13%.[7] Aortic pathologies are most common in the thoracic aorta (11%), and large vessel stenoses usually affect the cervical arteries (9%), innominate or subclavian arteries (4%), and, less frequently, iliofemoral arteries (<1%).

D Laboratory tests and imaging

For patients with suspected large artery vasculitis, laboratory studies including a complete blood count (CBC), CMP, ESR, and CRP should be assessed. The CBC is used to assess WBC that may be elevated in inflammatory states. The CMP is useful for assessing albumin levels as well as alkaline phosphatase, which may be mildly elevated in approximately 30% of patients. ESR and CRP are inflammatory markers, and although not specific for large artery vasculitis, are helpful in making its diagnosis. An ESR as high as 100 mm/h can occur in patients with GCA, although less striking elevations may be observed.[7] Among patients with abnormal albumin levels, CRP may be more accurate for assessing inflammation, because ESR can be spuriously elevated or depressed owing to its role as an acute-phase reactant. There are some data to suggest that interleukin-6 levels may correlate closely with disease activity and treatment response in patients with GCA,[8] but this assay is not routinely available in the clinical setting.

Diagnostic imaging for large artery vasculitis is used to confirm the diagnosis, localize specific arterial lesions, and plan potential treatment. CTA and MRA provide high-quality images of the aorta and the large vessels most commonly affected, and also provide substantial information about the patient's anatomy should an endovascular or open surgical intervention be required. DUS has also been shown to be effective in identifying patients with large artery vasculitis and can provide information about both flow dynamics and the presence of a characteristic "halo sign" indicative of vasculitis.[9] DUS is less invasive than is CTA or MRA, and so can be useful for both diagnosis and surveillance of arterial lesions in patients with TA and GCA. PET-CT is used less commonly in patients with vasculitis but can be useful in distinguishing active arterial disease. Fluorodeoxyglucose (FDG) uptake in large vessels is a sensitive marker for active vasculitis and has been shown to decrease on repeat imaging after appropriate glucocorticoid therapy.[10] DSA is usually reserved for surgical planning if cross-sectional imaging is not sufficient or used during endovascular therapy.

E Evaluate other potential etiologies

When the diagnosis of large artery vasculitis is not consistent with a patient's presentation or laboratory studies, other diseases with similar presentations should be considered. Cogan syndrome, polychondritis, and spondyloarthropathy can all present with clinical and radiographic features that are similar to TA but have additional clinical features that are pathognomonic. Behçet disease can be associated with aneurysmal changes of both medium and large arteries, but classically presents with oral and/or genital ulcerations and arthritis. IgG-4-related disease is a rare cause of noninfectious aortitis but requires a diagnosis based on histologic evidence of lymphoplasmocytes and storiform fibrosis. Infectious aortitis should be excluded in all cases of large vessel vasculitis by taking blood cultures of affected patients. FMD generally affects the carotid and renal arteries, but aortic involvement is rare. The characteristic imaging lesions (ie, "beads on a string") are not seen in patients who have TA or GCA.

F Chronic inflammatory phase

Patients with TA in a chronic inflammatory phase tend to have persistent low-grade symptoms with intermittent relapses of acute disease. Inflammatory markers may be mildly elevated, but ESR and CRP levels should not be nearly as high as with active disease. There is some evidence for the use of PET-CT imaging to determine whether a low level of chronic inflammation is present, although FDG uptake may never completely normalize in affected patients.[10] Some patients require long-term treatment with low-dose glucocorticoids to prevent frequent relapses into the active inflammatory phase.

G Active inflammatory phase

There are differing definitions of active inflammation in TA, but, in general, patients in an active inflammatory phase present with systemic symptoms and elevated inflammatory markers. According to the National Institutes of Health, active disease is defined by the presence of systemic features not attributable to other causes, elevated ESR, features of vascular ischemia or inflammation, and typical angiographic changes on diagnostic imaging.[11] Patients with active inflammation should be treated with aggressive medical management in an effort to improve symptoms and halt disease progression.

H Glucocorticoid therapy

In a patient with active large vessel vasculitis, glucocorticoids are the mainstay of therapy. Glucocorticoids suppress systemic symptoms and halt the progression of disease. In patients with early inflammatory vascular lesions, the stenoses may regress if detected early. Patients with longer courses of acute and/or chronic inflammation will likely have fibrous changes to their vasculature, are more likely to have hemodynamically significant stenoses, and may not demonstrate much improvement.

The initial glucocorticoid dose is 1 mg/kg/d of prednisone (or its equivalent) for 1 to 3 months. This dose may be administered in a single morning dose or can be divided into smaller doses administered throughout the day depending on the patient's response and adverse reactions associated with treatment.

I Taper glucocorticoids

The glucocorticoid dose can be tapered gradually once a patient's symptoms and inflammatory markers show improvement. The dose should be decreased no more than 10% per week. If the patient achieves complete remission (ie, resolution of symptoms and normalization of inflammatory markers), glucocorticoid therapy

can be stopped completely, although many physicians continue low-dose prednisone (5 mg/d) long term to prevent progression of arterial lesions.

J Add cytotoxic drugs and/or other immunomodulators

As many as 50% of patients may have a form of large artery vasculitis that is refractory to glucocorticoid therapy alone.[12] In these patients, a trial of methotrexate, azathioprine, mycophenolate, tocilizumab, or leflunomide is warranted. There are open-label studies showing efficacy of methotrexate,[12] azathioprine,[13] and leflunomide,[14] in combination with glucocorticoids, for achieving disease remission in patients with TA. Methotrexate has also been shown to be effective for lowering the risk of relapse in patients with GCA.[15]

There is one randomized trial comparing tocilizumab (an anti-IL-6 agent) versus placebo in patients with refractory TA. This study did not show a significant benefit with tocilizumab, but the results were favorable in a per-protocol analysis and the trial was underpowered to demonstrate a difference.[16] However, a RCT of tocilizumab versus placebo in patients with GCA did demonstrate superior gluococorticoid-free remissions rates.[17]

There are no trial-based data on the use of mycophenolate for large vessel vasculitis, although an observational study of 21 patients demonstrated a significant improvement in disease activity.[18] There are preliminary data supporting the use of anti-tumor necrosis factor (TNF)-α agents (etanercept, infliximab) for treating large artery vasculitis, but a small series of 25 patients with refractory TA demonstrated reasonable improvement in the majority of patients following treatment with etanercept or infliximab.[19]

The use of cyclophosphamide, commonly used in many other forms of vasculitis, has not been well studied in large artery vasculitis, and is not currently recommended unless as salvage therapy after multiple other failures.

K Symptomatic?

Once a patient with large artery vasculitis achieves remission, treatment of symptomatic arterial lesions should be considered. In the United States, as many as 50% to 70% of patients with large artery vasculitis may eventually require a revascularization procedure because of symptomatic and/or progressive disease.[20] Common symptoms include lifestyle-limiting ischemic symptoms such as severe upper extremity pain with exercise or subclavian steal syndrome, cerebral ischemia (ie, TIA or stroke), refractory HTN in the setting of renal artery stenosis, and severe aortic stenosis. Asymptomatic patients with progressive aneurysmal enlargement of either the aorta or its branches, as well as those with carotid artery stenosis ≥70%, should undergo intervention in an effort to reduce risk of aneurysm rupture and cerebral ischemia, respectively. Unless symptoms are limb- or life-threatening,

interventions should be reserved for patients without active inflammation.

L Lesion appropriate for endovascular therapy?

Angioplasty, stent, and stent-graft placement have all been described as viable options for patients with large artery vasculitis. The benefit of endovascular interventions is the relatively noninvasive nature of the procedures, which can usually be performed on an outpatient basis. The major limitation, however, is that restenosis is common, likely due to recurrent inflammation of the affected arterial segment as well as circumferential fibrosis and scarring of the vessel wall.

Patients with vasculitic stenotic lesions in the subclavian and renal arteries may be good candidates for first-line endovascular revascularization depending on the potential morbidity associated with open bypass. Patients with aortic stenosis have also been shown to have reasonable short-term outcomes with an endovascular-first approach,[21] although the long-term results appear to be limited. In contrast, patients with carotid artery disease, aortic occlusive disease, and renal artery stenosis beyond the ostia may be more appropriate for open surgery because of the limited success rates with endovascular therapy and, particularly for carotid disease, the potential for serious complications.

M Endovascular therapy

Endovascular interventions for patients with large artery vasculitis were initially limited to PTA. Although short-term success rates with this approach demonstrate 74% to 100% 1-year patency, depending on the patient's disease activity and lesion being treated,[22] long-term patency is low. In one study of 42 patients with TA, restenosis following PTA occurred in 32% of patients at 2 years postoperatively, with 10-year patency rates of only 50%.[23] The use of stent grafts or drug-eluting technologies to treat TA lesions has been described and may offer a reduced risk of restenosis, but data are currently limited to small retrospective case series.

A recent meta-analysis of endovascular versus open surgical interventions in patients with TA demonstrated that approximately 48% of interventions are endovascular, and restenosis is higher among patients undergoing endovascular treatments compared to those with open revascularizations.[24] This was seen in both supra-aortic and renal artery locations, regardless of disease activity. Mortality and overall complications were similar for endovascular treatment versus open surgery, although stroke was lower in the endovascular group. Limiting interventions to patients with no evidence of active disease has been shown to reduce the degree of restenosis following endovascular interventions,[23] but the long-term patency of this approach is unknown.

N Open surgery

Open surgical revascularization is considered the "gold standard" for revascularization among patients with large artery vasculitis because lesions tend to be long, fibrotic, and therefore less amenable to endovascular treatment. Bypass grafts to the CCA are the most common open surgical procedures performed and should originate off the ascending aorta rather than the proximal CCA because the former is less likely to be diseased.[25] CEA should be avoided because the lesions are fibrotic without clear dissection planes, and endarterectomy leads to poor patency.[26] Imaging of target vessels is essential to diagnose and locate areas of arterial thickening, which is avoided; bypass should be planned to normal-appearing arteries.

Upper extremity bypass, usually with autogenous vein to the brachial artery, is also a common procedure, because stenotic lesions have a strong prevalence in the subclavian and axillary arteries.[11,20] As with carotid artery bypass, strong consideration should be given to originating the bypass off the ascending aorta to avoid areas of disease.

Renal artery bypass is usually reserved for patients who have failed endovascular therapy, as well as those with nonostial disease less amenable to stent treatment.[20] Such bypass should originate from the abdominal aorta unless the aortic tissue appears to be unhealthy, in which case an extra-anatomic (hepatorenal, splenorenal, iliorenal) bypass should be considered. Whenever possible, an autogenous conduit is preferred for bypass, especially in younger patients.

Patients with aortic stenosis induced by large artery vasculitis can be treated via an endovascular approach. However, patients with aortic occlusive disease are best managed with an open aortoaortic bypass, because the dense fibrotic aortic lesion will resist dilation with a stent graft. Inflow should be from the suprarenal or distal thoracic aorta, because it has better patency in young patients and is usually less affected by inflammatory disease than is the infrarenal aorta.

Aortic aneurysms related to large artery vasculitis should be managed via the open surgery. The indications for aneurysm repair are the same as those for other etiologies of aneurysmal disease. Because panaortitis is common, the landing zones for endovascular stent-graft repairs may be prone to degeneration and failure. Furthermore, affected patients are usually relatively young, and the longevity of most EVAR options is currently unknown.[25]

O DUS of temporal artery

DUS can be used to diagnose GCA if specific findings are identified. A circumferential hypoechogenic area surrounding the vascular lumen of the temporal artery, known as a "halo sign," is highly specific for GCA.[27] The "compression sign," which refers to persistent visibility of the halo even with compression by the ultrasound probe, is also highly specific for GCA.[28]

Compared to temporal artery biopsy, use of DUS criteria alone has a sensitivity and specificity for diagnosing GCA of 75% and 83%, respectively.[27] Although this technology is operator dependent, a positive DUS precludes the need for temporal artery biopsy if positive. However, in patients with high pretest probability of GCA, temporal artery biopsy is indicated if the DUS finding is negative.

P Temporal artery biopsy

Temporal artery biopsy is the gold standard for establishing a diagnosis of GCA.[29] The procedure should be performed as soon as possible once the diagnosis of GCA is suspected, but it should not delay initiation of glucocorticoid therapy. The histopathologic changes characteristic of GCA persist for at least 14 days after starting treatment, so glucocorticoids can be started before biopsy if it is scheduled promptly thereafter.[30]

The procedure is usually performed under local anesthesia in an outpatient setting. The superficial temporal artery is identified by palpation, and marked. Local anesthesia is administered, and a 3-cm vertical incision is made over the vessel. The artery is dissected free from surrounding tissue, and the proximal and distal ends are ligated 2 cm apart to yield sufficient (1-2 cm) specimen length. The wound is closed with subcuticular suture.

Of note, if a patient has unilateral symptoms, a unilateral temporal artery biopsy is usually sufficient. A bilateral temporal artery biopsy is favored in patients without lateralizing symptoms to increase sensitivity.

Q Large artery stenosis, aneurysm?

Because 27% of patients with GCA will have large artery aneurysms, stenoses, or dissections, some of these may be symptomatic or progress to require surgical or endovascular treatment.[8] These will be detected by symptoms, physical examination, or imaging and, if present, need to be assessed for potential need for treatment. As with TA, patients with acute GCA should be managed with aggressive medical treatment before consideration of surgery.

R Surveillance

Patients with active large artery vasculitis should be followed up regularly, with laboratory data tracked at least monthly for 6 months. Close follow-up will ensure appropriate response to medical treatment and enable the physician to assess for glucocorticoid-related adverse effects and evidence of arterial disease progression.

Once disease remission has been achieved, repeat diagnostic imaging should be obtained to establish the patient's new baseline. Imaging should be repeated at 6-month intervals and, if stable, annually thereafter. The choice of imaging modality should be based on the mutual preference of the treating physician and the patient. If long-term annual imaging is indicated, MRA or DUS imaging, avoid repeated radiation exposure.

For patients with large artery vasculitis who have undergone revascularization procedures, postoperative imaging surveillance is warranted. Given the poor patency associated with most endovascular treatment of these lesions, follow-up imaging is essential to allow for early reintervention in cases of restenosis. Even among patients undergoing revascularization via open bypass for large artery vasculitis, progression of disease may necessitate reintervention in up to 40% of patients by 6 years. The type and frequency of imaging best used for surveillance is procedure- and surgeon dependent, but patients should be seen at regular intervals to assess revascularization patency and screen for other stenotic or aneurysmal disease.

REFERENCES

1. Lupi-Herrera E, Sanchez-Torres G, Marcushamer J, Mispireta J, Horwitz S, Vela JE. Takayasu's arteritis: clinical study of 107 cases. *Am Heart J.* 1977;93(1):94-103.
2. Arend WP, Michel BA, Bloch DA, et al. The American College of Rheumatology 1990 criteria for the classification of Takayasu arteritis. *Arthritis Rheum.* 1990;33(8):1129-1134.
3. Gonzalez-Gay MA, Barros S, Lopez-Diaz MJ, Garcia-Porrua C, Sanchez-Andrade A, Llorca J. Giant cell arteritis: disease patterns of clinical presentation in a series of 240 patients. *Medicine (Baltimore).* 2005;84(5):269-276.
4. Gabriel SE, O'Fallon WM, Achkar AA, Lie JT, Hunder GG. The use of clinical characteristics to predict the results of temporal artery biopsy among patients with suspected giant cell arteritis. *J Rheumatol.* 1995;22(1):93-96.
5. Nuenninghoff DM, Hunder GG, Christianson TJ, McClelland RL, Matteson EL. Incidence and predictors of large-artery complication (aortic aneurysm, aortic dissection, and/or large-artery stenosis) in patients with giant cell arteritis: a population-based study over 50 years. *Arthritis Rheum.* 2003;48(12):3522-3531.
6. Hayreh SS, Podhajsky PA, Zimmerman B. Ocular manifestations of giant cell arteritis. *Am J Ophthalmol.* 1998;125(4):509-520.
7. Smetana GW, Shmerling RH. Does this patient have temporal arteritis? *JAMA.* 2002;287(1):92-101.
8. Roche NE, Fulbright JW, Wagner AD, Hunder GG, Goronzy JJ, Weyand CM. Correlation of interleukin-6 production and disease activity in polymyalgia rheumatica and giant cell arteritis. *Arthritis Rheum.* 1993;36(9):1286-1294.
9. Ghinoi A, Pipitone N, Nicolini A, et al. Large-vessel involvement in recent-onset giant cell arteritis: a case-control colour-Doppler sonography study. *Rheumatology (Oxford).* 2012;51(4):730-734.
10. Blockmans D, de Ceuninck L, Vanderschueren S, Knockaert D, Mortelmans L, Bobbaers H. Repetitive 18F-fluorodeoxyglucose positron emission tomography in giant cell arteritis: a prospective study of 35 patients. *Arthritis Rheum.* 2006;55(1):131-137.
11. Kerr GS, Hallahan CW, Giordano J, et al. Takayasu arteritis. *Ann Intern Med.* 1994;120(11):919-929.

12. Hoffman GS, Leavitt RY, Kerr GS, Rottem M, Sneller MC, Fauci AS. Treatment of glucocorticoid-resistant or relapsing Takayasu arteritis with methotrexate. *Arthritis Rheum.* 1994;37(4):578-582.

13. Valsakumar AK, Valappil UC, Jorapur V, Garg N, Nityanand S, Sinha N. Role of immunosuppressive therapy on clinical, immunological, and angiographic outcome in active Takayasu's arteritis. *J Rheumatol.* 2003;30(8):1793-1798.

14. de Souza AW, da Silva MD, Machado LS, Oliveira AC, Pinheiro FA, Sato EI. Short-term effect of leflunomide in patients with Takayasu arteritis: an observational study. *Scand J Rheumatol.* 2012;41(3):227-230.

15. Mahr AD, Jover JA, Spiera RF, et al. Adjunctive methotrexate for treatment of giant cell arteritis: an individual patient data meta-analysis. *Arthritis Rheum.* 2007;56(8):2789-2797.

16. Nakaoka Y, Isobe M, Takei S, et al. Efficacy and safety of tocilizumab in patients with refractory Takayasu arteritis: results from a randomized, double-blind, placebo-controlled, phase 3 trial in Japan (the TAKT study). *Ann Rheum Dis.* 2018;77(3):348-354.

17. Stone JH, Tuckwell K, Dimonaco S, et al. Trial of tocilizumab in giant-cell arteritis. *N Engl J Med.* 2017;377(4):317-328.

18. Goel R, Danda D, Mathew J, Edwin N. Mycophenolate mofetil in Takayasu's arteritis. *Clin Rheumatol.* 2010;29(3):329-332.

19. Molloy ES, Langford CA, Clark TM, Gota CE, Hoffman GS. Anti-tumour necrosis factor therapy in patients with refractory Takayasu arteritis: long-term follow-up. *Ann Rheum Dis.* 2008;67(11):1567-1569.

20. Maksimowicz-McKinnon K, Clark TM, Hoffman GS. Limitations of therapy and a guarded prognosis in an American cohort of Takayasu arteritis patients. *Arthritis Rheum.* 2007;56(3):1000-1009.

21. Perrone-Filardi P, Costanzo P, Cesarano P, et al. Long abdominal aortic stenosis: a rare presentation of Takayasu arteritis treated with percutaneous stent implantation. *J Thorac Cardiovasc Surg.* 2007;133(6):1647-1648.

22. Sharma S, Rajani M, Kaul U, Talwar KK, Dev V, Shrivastava S. Initial experience with percutaneous transluminal angioplasty in the management of Takayasu's arteritis. *Br J Radiol.* 1990;63(751):517-522.

23. Park MC, Lee SW, Park YB, Lee SK, Choi D, Shim WH. Post-interventional immunosuppressive treatment and vascular restenosis in Takayasu's arteritis. *Rheumatology (Oxford).* 2006;45(5):600-605.

24. Jung JH, Lee YH, Song GG, Jeong HS, Kim JH, Choi SJ. Endovascular versus open surgical intervention in patients with Takayasu's arteritis: a meta-analysis. *Eur J Vasc Endovasc Surg.* 2018;55(6):888-899.

25. Giordano JM. Surgical treatment of Takayasu's disease. *Cleve Clin J Med.* 2002;69(suppl 2):SII146-SII148.

26. Pajari R, Hekali P, Harjola PT. Treatment of Takayasu's arteritis: an analysis of 29 operated patients. *Thorac Cardiovasc Surg.* 1986;34(3):176-181.

27. Arida A, Kyprianou M, Kanakis M, Sfikakis PP. The diagnostic value of ultrasonography-derived edema of the temporal artery wall in giant cell arteritis: a second meta-analysis. *BMC Musculoskelet Disord.* 2010;11:44.

28. Aschwanden M, Imfeld S, Staub D, et al. The ultrasound compression sign to diagnose temporal giant cell arteritis shows an excellent interobserver agreement. *Clin Exp Rheumatol.* 2015;33(2 suppl 89):S113-S115.

29. Meisner RJ, Labropoulos N, Gasparis AP, Tassiopoulos AK. How to diagnose giant cell arteritis. *Int Angiol.* 2011;30(1):58-63.

30. Achkar AA, Lie JT, Hunder GG, O'Fallon WM, Gabriel SE. How does previous corticosteroid treatment affect the biopsy findings in giant cell (temporal) arteritis? *Ann Intern Med.* 1994;120(12):987-992.

Christine R. Herman • Cherrie Abraham

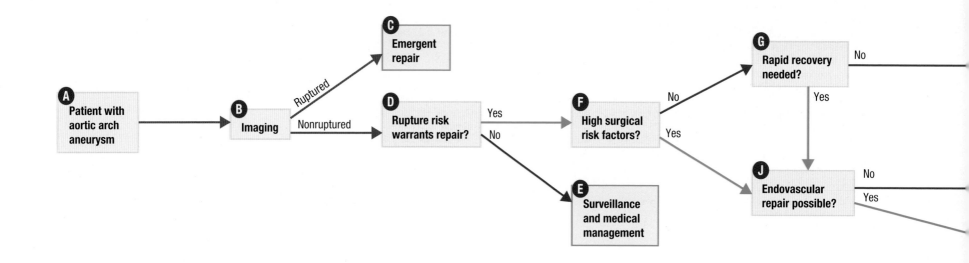

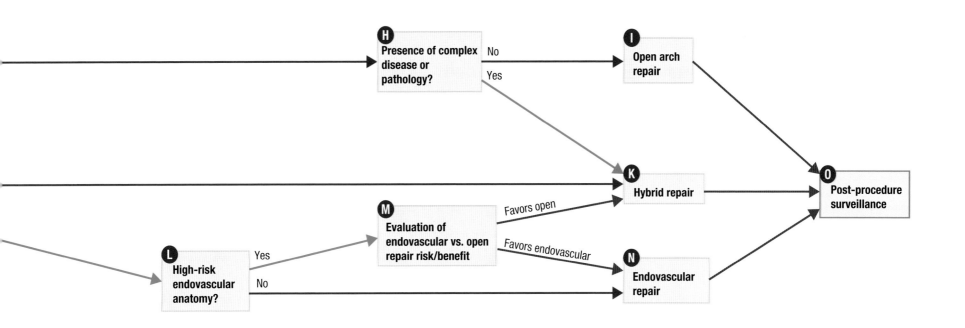

A Patient with aortic arch aneurysm

The aortic arch accounts for a short length of the aorta, but its position within the mediastinum and its complex anatomy makes surgical and endovascular access challenging. The superior attachment of the pericardial reflection just proximal to the innominate artery marks the most proximal aspect of the aortic arch. The aortic arch terminates just distal to the left SCA where it is tethered by the parietal pleura and the ligamentum arteriosum. In its most common trajectory, the left-sided arch courses posteriorly and toward the left, giving off the innominate, left carotid and left subclavian arteries.

Pathology of the arch is similar to that of most other aortic segments and includes aneurysm, acute or chronic dissection, penetrating ulcerations, and intramural hematoma. Commonly, arch aneurysms involve adjacent aortic segments and in just over 50% of cases are caused by chronic dissection.[1] Etiology of arch pathology includes connective tissue disease, medial degeneration, infection, trauma, and aortitis.[1,2]

Understanding the risk associated with complex open arch repair and challenges associated with endovascular repair is essential in treatment selection.

B Imaging

Chest CTA is the ideal imaging modality for arch aneurysm. ECG gating, either prospectively or retrospectively triggered, improves temporal resolution and reduces motion artefact, improving measurement accuracy.[3] Including imaging of proximal and mid portions of the arch branch vessels is recommended in the event that extra-anatomic revascularization is required. Although imaging of the cerebral arteries is not necessarily required preoperatively, this baseline information can be very useful postoperatively if the patient experiences neurologic sequelae and requires postoperative cerebral imaging.

Extent of arch pathology, often described in Ishimaru zones[4] (0, involving innominate origin, 1 involving CCA origin, 2 involving L SCA origin), as well as presence of normal aorta must be identified to determine suitability for treatment options. Other important considerations include arch elongation class, arch anatomic classification (bovine or right sided), and vessel aberrancy such as arch origin of the vertebral artery or aberrant SCA. Presence of dissection, rupture, atheroma, and calcification must also be identified. Ruptured aortic arch aneurysms require emergent repair unless the patient is considered unfit for attempted treatment.

C Emergent repair

In the setting of rupture of an arch aneurysm or immediately adjacent aortic segments, emergent repair is indicated. In this setting, preservation of life is the ultimate concern and the surgeon should select the safest and most efficient approach to address all ruptured segments. Assuming availability of appropriate devices, complete open, hybrid, or endovascular approaches are available options in the setting of rupture with the exception of custom arch stent grafts, which require custom manufacturing and shipment. These treatment options are discussed under nonruptured arch aneurysm treatment in this chapter (see I, K, and N). As in all cases of aortic rupture, the likelihood of survival is poor, and in poor-risk patients, palliative care can represent the best option.

D Rupture risk warrants repair?

Published guidelines for arch aneurysm intervention criteria vary widely.[2,5,6] Because isolated arch pathology is encountered less frequency than are other aortic pathologies, evidence supporting arch guidelines is lacking. Consequently, criteria are borrowed from adjacent aortic segments and applied to the arch. Generally, indications for intervention on arch aneurysms include aortic diameter ≥5.5 cm in a low-risk patient, growth rate exceeding 0.5 cm/y, symptomatic aneurysm, and ruptured aneurysm. Individual patient risk profile must be taken into consideration when determining optimal intervention and timing.

E Surveillance and medical management

Little evidence supports strict surveillance guidelines for the arch. Although yearly imaging is suggested for isolated arch dilation <4.0 cm and biyearly imaging for dilatation ≥4.0 cm,[4] these intervals may be aggressive and can likely be increased in patients with stable growth patterns and low concomitant risk. Surveillance intervals should be more frequent if there is a family history of aortic rupture.

Aggressive blood pressure management and the avoidance of isometric strain are the mainstay of medical management.[6] β-Blockers, calcium channel blockers, and angiotensin-1 antagonists[7] have all been shown to reduce aneurysm degeneration and late rupture, and improve survival in certain populations.[7-10] Management of other risk factors that may affect surgical risk profile is encouraged.

F High surgical risk factors?

Patient risk profile can greatly influence selection of treatment options. Clinical risk factors that predispose to worse outcomes after open heart surgery, in general, include age >70 years, renal dysfunction, advanced liver disease, pulmonary dysfunction, preoperative right ventricular dysfunction, and low cardiac output.[11-15] Frailty is associated with a higher rate of discharge to rehabilitation or nursing facilities and reduced perioperative and midterm survival after cardiac surgery.[16]

Scenarios that may increase surgical risk include porcelain aorta, previous mediastinitis, previous radiation, chest wall deformity, and previous surgical complications. High risk of redo sternotomy can result from the right ventricle (RV) being adhered to the sternum or patent coronary grafts in close proximity to the midline and sternum. Elevated Euroscore II calculated risk is a well-established risk predictor for patient outcomes after open heart surgery.[17]

Presence of one or more high-risk features listed earlier warrants consideration of endovascular or hybrid strategies.

G Rapid recovery needed?

On occasion, a patient may present with a clinical scenario that requires rapid recovery after arch aneurysm repair. This may include need for chemotherapy or radiation therapy, oncologic or other semiurgent intervention, and special social situations. Consideration for endovascular intervention, despite a low-risk patient profile, is appropriate in these scenarios.

H Presence of complex disease or pathology?

Certain anatomic features may increase the complexity of open repair and thus augment the risk of poor postoperative outcomes. These may include the following: absence of healthy aorta for anastomosis, as in the case of aneurysmal extension into the descending aorta; aneurysmal extension into branch vessels; ulcerated or calcified tissues; and, severely displaced and less accessible arch branch vessels or distal anastomotic sites. The presence of these risk factors should refocus the surgeon toward a hybrid repair.

Total open repair of the arch should be considered in young patients, where a long-term durable result is preferred, or in patients with a known connective tissue disorder, where use of endovascular devices is controversial given the fragility of aortic tissue at the proximal and distal seal zones.

I Open arch repair

Simple arch repairs may only require a hemiarch reconstruction under circulatory arrest. The hemiarch involves construction of an anastomosis just proximal to the innominate artery bevelled into the lesser curve of the arch, allowing for replacement of part or all of the lesser curve of the arch while preserving the branch vessels. More complex pathology may require total arch repair. Revascularization of branch vessels in total arch repair is achieved with the island technique (generally less favored), branched grafts, y-graft, or double y-grafts.[1,18] To accommodate distal arch or descending aortic pathology, the arch repair can include an elephant trunk, where a segment of the tube graft used to replace the arch is extended without fixation into the proximal descending aorta for future use in a second-stage thoracic repair, or a frozen elephant trunk, a hybrid procedure where the arch graft extension is secured with an endovascular stent placed into the descending aorta, to accommodate future additional descending thoracic aorta endovascular repair.

Cerebral perfusion strategies are strongly advised when undertaking any arch repair that requires any period of circulatory arrest.

J Endovascular repair possible?

Near-total endovascular repair of aortic arch pathology is feasible when certain criteria are met.[19] Of paramount importance is the diameter of the ascending aorta. Ideally, the diameter should be 38 mm or less, and be fairly uniform in diameter for the proximal 80% of the ascending aorta past the sinotubular junction. Suitable landing zones proximally and distally should be ≥20 mm in length, with longer seal zones always preferred. In particular, a suitable length of uniform diameter in the proximal landing zone is required for direct apposition of the aortic wall with the proximal sealing stents of the arch stent graft. Inappropriate placement of an arch stent graft into a compromised proximal landing zone will often result in a type Ia endoleak, usually due to poor apposition along the proximal inner curve of the aortic arch. In a high-risk patient, these are extremely difficult, if not impossible, to reintervene upon, highlighting the importance of sound patient selection. Other suggested anatomic criteria include innominate diameter >8 mm, left CCA diameter >6 mm, and acceptable arch tortuosity and calcification, as well as adequate iliac access.

K Hybrid repair

In hybrid repair, supra-aortic debranching is performed to provide an appropriate landing zone for the stent graft so as to preserve perfusion to the supra-aortic vessels, followed by stent-graft deployment into zone 0 to 2 of the aortic arch.[20] An advantage of hybrid procedures is that cardiopulmonary bypass and/or circulatory arrest is avoided. Such open surgical debranching may be currently combined with standard commercially approved thoracic stent grafts, and possibly in the future with single-branch (off-the-shelf) designs that reperfuse one arch branch vessel (currently in clinical trials).[20]

When ascending aortic diameters exceed 38 mm, consideration should be given to replacing the ascending aorta and debranching the supra-aortic trunk vessels off the proximal Dacron graft repair, to ensure a safe and reliable proximal seal zone for the endovascular stent graft.

L High-risk endovascular anatomy?

Significant atheromatous disease of the aortic arch, along with proximal arch branch atherosclerotic disease are relative contraindications for endovascular arch repair because of potential atheroembolization potentially caused by required manipulation of catheters and wires in such diseased arteries. Indeed, stroke has been the Achilles heel of this procedure, although encouraging reports highlighting a decreased incidence of stroke are emerging as high-volume centers gain more experience.[21]

As mentioned in Box K, a proximal seal zone diameter exceeding 38 mm is a potential pitfall leading to possible type 1a endoleak and treatment failure, and therefore should be avoided for arch branched graft technology.

The presence of a mechanical aortic valve is a relative contraindication to endovascular repair because this procedure requires the nose cone of the delivery system to cross the aortic valve, possibly resulting in inadvertent aortic valve injury. Custom modification of the delivery system may permit treatment in rare cases.[22]

M Evaluation of endovascular vs. open repair risk/benefit

If patients present with both high-risk surgical and high-risk endovascular features, a risk-benefit analysis must be performed. Expert surgeons with advanced experience in both open and endovascular techniques should select the treatment option judged to be the best for each individual patient. If an open repair is needed to eliminate the high-risk endovascular features, then a hybrid approach may be a more reasonable option over total open repair.

N Endovascular repair

Chimney/snorkel grafts may be considered as a possible endovascular option to preserve arch vessel flow when placing an aortic stent graft that must cover these important branches.[23] However, current aortic stent-graft technology has not been developed with consideration of chimney grafts for arch vessel perfusion. The authors caution against this hybrid technique in the aortic arch, because type Ia endoleak may result from incomplete proximal seal.

Reports of laser fenestration of thoracic stent grafts placed across the arch, with covered stents maintaining perfusion into the arch vessels, have been reported.[24] This technique is considered off label, and should only be performed in the context of a clinical trial that is approved by the institutional IRB and with appropriate patient consent. Laser fenestration can be successful in maintaining perfusion to an arch vessel in the sealing zone of aortic dissection treatment. Caution, however, should be exercised when using this technique in the treatment of aneurysmal pathology, especially if the laser fenestrated vessel is not in the sealing zone, because continued aneurysm sac pressurization may occur with an incomplete seal at the level of the laser fenestration. Of note, durability of the seal between the covered stent and the laser fenestration in the material of the stent graft has been questioned.[25]

Various single- and double- branched arch stent grafts are currently in clinical trials globally or available by special access. One disadvantage of the single-branch iteration, especially for zone 0 repair, is the need for extra-anatomic carotid to carotid bypass, which adds potential morbidity to the operation. Even in zone 1 and 2 repairs, the evidence supports use of left carotid to SCA bypass to maintain perfusion to the vertebral artery, as well as provide perfusion to the spinal cord in cases that require extensive thoracic aortic coverage.[26] The authors' experience in near-total aortic arch aneurysm repair has been with the custom-made double-branched aortic arch stent graft from Cook Medical, Inc (Bloomington, IN). With this device, the target

arteries and left ventricle must be in the field of view to visualize the deployment of the arch branched graft, as well as visualize the end of the delivery wire delivered deep into the left ventricle. Deployment is generally performed under rapid ventricular pacing that ideally achieves asystole to prevent a possible windsock effect during stent-graft deployment. It is vital that the proximal stent deploys distal to the coronary arteries. Meticulous planning with dedicated imaging software is essential for accurate configuration of the inner branch location on the arch stent graft. Stroke risk correlates with the time needed to catheterize the stent-graft branches from their respective supra-aortic vessel access. The authors' generally prefer direct proximal CCA access because it provides the most direct approach to the stent-graft branch openings. This technique also allows ipsilateral carotid clamping during catheterization to further decrease the risk of stroke. The authors prefer left carotid to SCA bypass in the same sitting, generally reserving proximal left subclavian occlusion or ligation as the final step in the procedure.

Initial reports of near-total endovascular repair of aortic arch aneurysm have been encouraging,[27] but additional experience is necessary to refine the technique and devices, as well as improve criteria for patient selection. Interestingly, these branched devices have recently been used successfully for patients with challenging anatomy, including aortic dissection in the arch.[28] Further study in this challenging population of patients is warranted.

O Post-procedure surveillance

In patients who undergo open repair with no residual aortopathy, CTA at 1 year should be performed to assess for PSA; subsequent surveillance imaging should be performed every 3 to 5 years.[5] If a hybrid or total endovascular approach is undertaken, imaging should be performed either before discharge or within the first month post the procedure.[2,6] The authors strongly recommend predischarge imaging if the intervention was performed for rupture or dissection. Subsequent surveillance with CTA should be scheduled at 3 months, 6 months, and then at yearly intervals.[2,6]

REFERENCES

1. Zanotti G, Reece TB, Aftab M. Aortic arch pathology surgical options for the aortic arch replacement. *Cardiol Clin.* 2017;35:367-385.
2. Hiratzka LF, Bakris GL, Beckman JA, et al; American College of Cardiology Foundation/American Heart Association Task Force on Practice Guidelines. 2010 ACCF/AHA/AATS/ACR/ASA/SCA/SCAI/SIR/STS/SVM guidelines for the diagnosis and management of patients with Thoracic Aortic Disease: a report of the American College of Cardiology Foundation/American Heart Association Task Force on Practice Guidelines, American Association for Thoracic Surgery, American College of Radiology, American Stroke Association, Society of Cardiovascular Anesthesiologists,

Society for Cardiovascular Angiography and Interventions, Society of Interventional Radiology, Society of Thoracic Surgeons, and Society for Vascular Medicine. *Circulation.* 2010;121(13):e266-e369.

3. Desjardins B, Kazerooni EA. ECG gated cardiac CT. *AJR Am J Roentgenol.* 2004;182(4):993-1010.

4. Mitchell RS, Ishimaru S, Ehrlich MP, et al. First International Summit on Thoracic Aortic Endografting: roundtable on thoracic aortic dissection as an indication for endografting. *J Endovasc Ther.* 2002;9(suppl 2):II98-II105.

5. Boodhwani M, Andelfinger G, Leipsic J, et al. Canadian Cardiovascular Society Position Statement on the management of thoracic aortic disease. *Can J Cardiol.* 2014;30:577-589.

6. Erbel R, Aboyans V, Boileau C, et al. 2014 ESC Guidelines on the diagnosis and treatment of aortic diseases: document covering acute and chronic aortic diseases of the thoracic and abdominal aorta of the adult. The Task Force for the Diagnosis and Treatment of Aortic Diseases of the European Society of Cardiology (ESC). *Eur Heart J.* 2014;35(41):2873-2926.

7. Groenink M, den Hartog AW, Franken R, et al. Losartan reduces aortic dilatation rate in adults with Marfan syndrome: a randomized controlled trial. *Eur Heart J.* 2013;34:3491-3500.

8. Genoni M, Paul M, Jenni R, Graves K, Seifert B, Turina M. Chronic beta–blocker therapy improves outcome and reduces treatment costs in chronic type B aortic dissection. *Eur J Cardiothorac Surg.* 2001;19:606-610.

9. Suzuki T, Isselbacher EM, Nienaber CA, et al. Type-selective benefits of medications in treatment of acute aortic dissection (from the International Registry of Acute Aortic Dissection [IRAD]). *Am J Cardiol.* 2012;109:122-127.

10. Brooke BS, Habashi JP, Judge DP, Patel N, Loeys B, Dietz HC III. Angiotensin II blockade and aortic–root dilation in Marfan's syndrome. *N Engl J Med.* 2008;358:2787-2795.

11. Estrera AL, Miller CC III, Huynh TT, Porat EE, Safi HJ. Replacement of the ascending and transverse aortic arch: determinants of long-term survival. *Ann Thorac Surg.* 2002;74(4):1058-1064.

12. Okita Y, Ando M, Minatoya K, et al. Early and long-term results of surgery for aneurysms of the thoracic aorta in septuagenarians and octogenarians. *Eur J Cardiothorac Surg.* 1999;16(3):317-323.

13. Yağdi T, Atay Y, Cikirikçioğlu M, et al. Determinants of early mortality and neurological morbidity in aortic operations performed under circulatory arrest. *J Cardiol Surg.* 2000;15(3):186-193.

14. Modi A, Vohra HA, Barlow CW. Do patients with liver cirrhosis undergoing cardiac surgery have acceptable outcomes? *Interact Cardiovasc Thorac Surg.* 2010;11(5):630-634.

15. Peyrou J, Chauvel C, Pathak A, Simon M, Dehant P, Abergel E. Preoperative right ventricular dysfunction is a strong predictor of 3 years survival after cardiac surgery. *Clin Res Cardiol.* 2017;106(9):734-742.

16. Lee DH, Buth KJ, Martin BJ, Yip AM, Hirsch GM. Frail patients are at increased risk for mortality and prolonged institutional care after cardiac surgery. *Circulation.* 2010;121(8):973-978.

17. Paparella D, Guida P, Di Eusanio G, et al. Risk stratification for in-hospital mortality after cardiac surgery: external validation of EuroSCOREII in a prospective regional registry. *Eur J Cardiothorac Surg.* 2014;46(5):840-848. doi:10.1093/ejcts/ezt657.

18. Spielvogel D, Strauch JT, Minanov OP, Lansman SL, Griepp RB. Aortic arch replacement using a trifurcated graft and selective cerebral antegrade perfusion. *Ann Thorac Surg.* 2002;74:S1810-S1814; discussion S1825-S1832.

19. Lioupis C, Corriveau MM, Mackenzie KS, Obrand DI, Steinmetz OK, Abraham CZ. Treatment of aortic arch aneurysms with a modular transfemoral multibranched stent graft: initial experience. *Eur J Vasc Endovasc Surg.* 2012;43:525-532.

20. Bavaria J, Vallabhajosyula P, Moeller P, Szeto W, Desai N, Pochettino A. Hybrid approaches in the treatment of aortic arch aneurysms: postoperative and midterm outcomes. *J Thorac Cardiovasc Surg.* 2013;145(3):S85-S90.

21. Haulon S, Greenberg RK, Spear R, et al. Global experience with an inner branched arch endograft. *J Thorac Cardiovasc Surg.* 2014;148:1709-1716.

22. Spear R, Azzaoui R, Maurel B, Sobocinski J, Roeder B, Haulon S. Total endovascular treatment of an aortic arch aneurysm in a patient with a mechanical aortic valve. *Eur J Vasc Endovasc Surg.* 2014;48(2):144-146.

23. Donas KP, Lee JT, Lachat M, Torsello G, Veith FJ; PERICLES investigators. Collected world experience about the performance of the snorkel/chimney endovascular technique in the treatment of complex aortic pathologies: the PERICLES registry. *Ann Surg.* 2015;262(3):546-553.

24. Bradshaw RJ, Ahanchi SS, Powell O, et al. Left subclavian revascularization in zone 2 thoracic endovascular aortic repair is associated with lower stroke risk across all aortic diseases. *J Vasc Surg.* 2017;65(5):1270-1279.

25. Jayet J, Heim F, Coggia M, Chakfe N, Coscas R. An experimental study of laser in situ fenestration of current aortic endografts. *Eur J Vasc Endovasc Surg.* 2018;56(1):68-77.

26. Weigang E, Parker JA, Czerny M, et al. Should intentional endovascular stent graft coverage of the left subclavian artery be preceded by prophylactic revascularization? *Eur J Cardiothorac Surg.* 2011;40:858-868.

27. Spear R, Hertault A, Van Calster K, et al. Complex endovascular repair of post dissection arch and thoracoabdominal aneurysms. *J Vasc Surg.* 2018;67(3):685-693.

Adam W. Beck

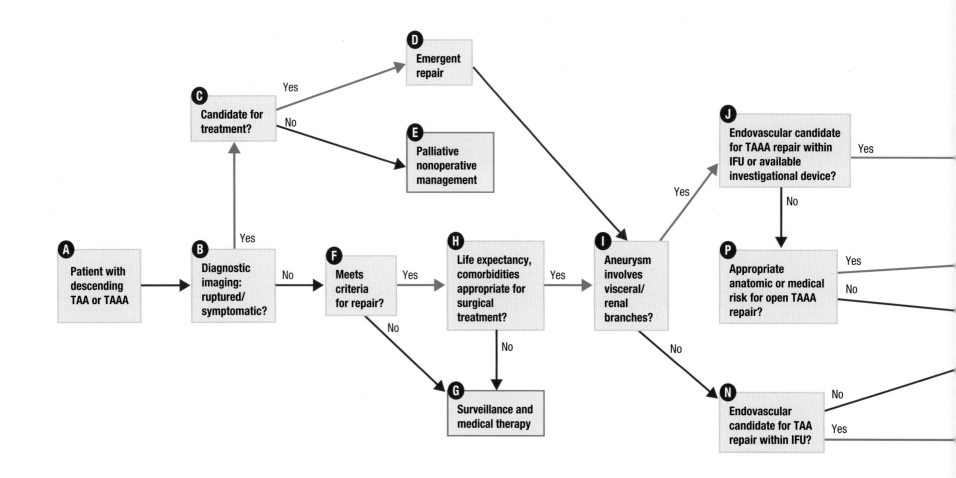

A Patient with descending TAA or TAAA

B Diagnostic imaging: ruptured/symptomatic?

C Candidate for treatment?

D Emergent repair

E Palliative nonoperative management

F Meets criteria for repair?

G Surveillance and medical therapy

H Life expectancy, comorbidities appropriate for surgical treatment?

I Aneurysm involves visceral/renal branches?

J Endovascular candidate for TAAA repair within IFU or available investigational device?

P Appropriate anatomic or medical risk for open TAAA repair?

N Endovascular candidate for TAA repair within IFU?

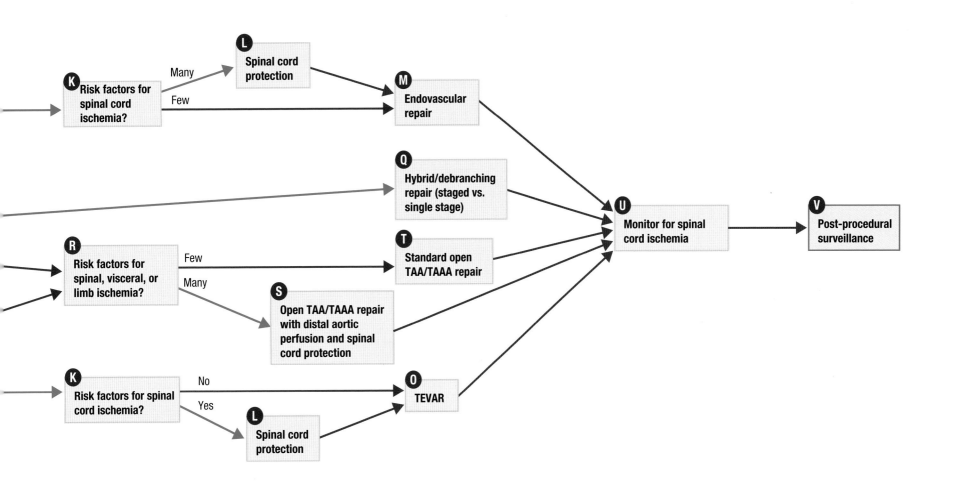

A Patient with descending TAA or TAAA

A descending TAA is a permanent, localized dilation involving the thoracic aorta distal to the left subclavian artery (LSA) and proximal to the diaphragm. A TAAA involves contiguous segments of the descending thoracic and abdominal aorta including the visceral branches of the aorta. The average thoracic aortic diameter ranges from 2.4 to 3.0 cm, whereas the abdominal aorta averages 1.7 to 2.6 cm in diameter. The normal thoracic aorta is 2 to 3 mm greater in men than in women. The majority of TAAs and TAAAs develop secondary to a degenerative etiology (~80%) or aortic dissection (~15%), with many other aortic pathologies contributing to a small portion of the overall TAA/TAAA incidence.[1] The incidence of TAA/TAAA is 16/100,000 per year for men and 9/100,000 per year for women; it is believed to be increasing secondary to an aging population and improved diagnostic techniques.[2]

B Diagnostic imaging: ruptured/symptomatic?

Any patient suspected of having a TAA/TAAA should undergo appropriate diagnostic imaging. Although multiple modalities are available, CTA is the gold standard imaging modality used to determine the extent and diameter of an aneurysm. In addition to its diagnostic capabilities, CTA provides important anatomic information needed to plan potential endovascular repair including the presence of associated occlusive disease, thrombus, associated dissection, and inflammatory changes suggestive of impending rupture. The size and patency of intercostal arteries and visceral branches can also be evaluated. Finally, CTA also allows for 3D centerline reconstruction vital for endovascular intervention planning. MRA had been historically used in patients with renal insufficiency; however, concerns for gadolinium use in patients with renal insufficiency and the development of nephrogenic systemic fibrosis combined with worse spatial resolution than with CTA has limited the use of MRA for TAA/TAAA diagnosis and operative planning. DSA, although routinely used in the past, is now limited primarily to document visceral/renal branch anatomy and potentially treat renal occlusive disease in patients with significant CKD.[1]

Patients with a ruptured TAA/TAAA present with acute-onset severe chest, back, or abdominal pain, typically associated with hemodynamic instability. Urgent evaluation with CTA can confirm rupture and allow for treatment planning. Most patients with a TAA/TAAA are asymptomatic at the time of diagnosis. Symptomatic patients without rupture may complain of vague pain in the chest, back, or abdomen, resulting from acute expansion, inflammation or compression of adjacent structures. Although the differential diagnosis for this presenting symptomatology is extensive, life-threatening conditions such as acute coronary syndrome, aortic dissection, and aortic rupture require prompt exclusion.

C Candidate for treatment?

Patients with ruptured TAA/TAAA require emergent repair because mortality exceeds 90% without surgical intervention.[3] Rapid clinical assessment of the patient, consideration of patient's and family's wishes, and management of family expectations should be performed expeditiously. The extreme elderly, those with prohibitive cardiopulmonary comorbidities, and patients with active or recurrent cardiac arrest should be advised to go in for palliative treatments, particularly if there are no straightforward endovascular repair options.

D Emergent repair

If feasible, endovascular repair should be the treatment of choice in the patient population with ruptures. A recent analysis of the National Inpatient Sample found that TEVAR was used in 13% of patients with ruptured TAA over a 20-year period. This percentage increased from 2% in 2003 to 2004 to 43% of patients in 2011 to 2012. TEVAR has resulted in an increased number of patients eligible for urgent/emergent repair, and a decreased operative mortality.[4] Treatment of ruptured TAAAs is much more complex. Open surgical intervention is associated with high mortality and morbidity for those who survive. Endovascular repair with surgeon-modified grafts, parallel grafting, or multibranched devices has limited data because these techniques have been introduced relatively recently.[5] The National Surgical Quality Improvement Project recently reported 38% mortality for open repair of ruptured TAAAs versus 26% mortality for endovascular repair of ruptured TAAAs ($P = 0.09$). Although this did not reach statistical significance, patients undergoing endovascular TAAA repair were far less likely to develop a pulmonary injury (OR 0.34, $P = 0.005$) or renal failure (OR 0.30, $P = 0.02$).[6]

E Palliative nonoperative management

Patients who decline surgical intervention or are not offered surgery because of exceedingly high perioperative risk of mortality should be offered palliative care services and appropriate pain/anxiety controlling measures. Usually nonoperative management of ruptured TAA or TAAA results in rapid death, but occasionally patients may survive several days and palliative care team support should be pursued.

F Meets criteria for repair?

For patients with asymptomatic TAA/TAAA, the decision for repair requires evaluation of the risk of rupture versus the risk of treatment. Rupture risk is primarily based on aneurysm diameter, but morphology, associated symptoms, and patient characteristics should also be considered. For descending TAA and extent I to III, V TAAA (see I), a diameter of 6 cm is generally regarded as the appropriate threshold for intervention to prevent rupture.[7] For type IV TAAA, the same 5.5 cm threshold used for infrarenal AAA repair is recommended. The decision to recommend repair should be based on individual patient factors. For instance, women have been shown to have a higher rupture risk at smaller aortic diameters as compared to men, leading some to believe that aortic size index (aortic diameter/body surface area) is a more important measure than is aortic diameter alone, particularly in women.[8] Saccular (vs. fusiform) aneurysm morphology is generally considered to have a higher rupture risk.[9] Connective tissue disorders, such as Marfan syndrome, also increase rupture risk, lowering the threshold at which repair is recommended.[10] Finally, documented growth of an aortic aneurysm ≥ 1.0 cm over the course of 1 year is an indication for earlier repair.[11]

G Surveillance and medical therapy

Patients not yet meeting criteria for surgical intervention should have optimal medical therapy and surveillance. Antihypertensive therapy with β-blockers and angiotensin-converting enzyme inhibitors should be initiated to maintain blood pressures of ≤140/90 in patients without diabetes or CKD and ≤130/80 in those with diabetes or CKD.[1] Other atherosclerotic risk reduction methods including statin therapy, aspirin, and smoking cessation are also recommended. Because there are no specific evidence-based guidelines for surveillance of TAA/TAAA, guidelines established for AAA are generally applied. Small aneurysms, <3.5 cm in diameter, are reimaged every 3 years. Larger aneurysms measuring 3.5 to 4.4 cm are reimaged annually, and those >4.5 cm should be reimaged every 6 months until definitive repair is completed. Given the limitations of DUS in the chest, CTA is the recommended modality for surveillance.

Patients considered too frail or at high risk for operative repair should be treated with best medical therapy, as described earlier. If a decision is made not to treat on the basis of these considerations, surveillance imaging is not needed.

H Life expectancy, comorbidities appropriate for surgical treatment?

Assessment of perioperative risk is vital to the successful management of TAA/TAAA patients. It involves assessment primarily of the cardiopulmonary and renal function of the patient, as well as the overall functional capacity and life expectancy. Although perioperative stress differs significantly between open and endovascular repair, basic tenets hold true for both. Cardiac disease is the leading cause of mortality following TAAA repair and therefore extensive evaluation of CAD and valvular disease should be completed (see Chapter 1).[12] Because COPD is present in up to 40% of patients with a TAAA, careful preoperative pulmonary evaluation is important (see Chapter 2). Preoperative renal dysfunction is the single strongest predictor of postoperative renal failure, which is associated with a 50% to 70% in-hospital mortality rate.[13] Preoperative hydration along with other intraoperative measures, discussed later in this chapter, can help decrease the risk of postoperative renal failure.

Overall assessment of functional status and frailty is essential. Recently, the use of a modified frailty index (mFi), consisting of 11 variables derived from the Canadian Study of Health and Aging (CSHA) frailty index, has been shown to appropriately stratify patients into high-risk categories for mortality and morbidity following vascular intervention.[14] Although no study to date has specifically evaluated the association between frailty and outcomes after open or endovascular TAA/TAAA repair, it is reasonable to extrapolate from the AAA population. In the same study by Arya et al., patients in the high mFi tertile as compared to the low mFI tertile, after multivariate regression analysis, were more likely to experience a life-threatening complication (OR 1.7 [1.4-1.9]), or die within 30 days of the operation (OR 2.0 [1.5-2.8]). This outcome was even more pronounced in the open aneurysm repair group as opposed to the EVAR group. Although advanced age can certainly contribute to overall frailty, data evaluating the risk of repair depending on age alone have been mixed, further supporting the idea that patient functional assessment is more important than is age.

ⓘ Aneurysm involves visceral/renal branches?

TAAAs are traditionally defined using the Crawford classification, which has implications as to the type/extent of operation required and to specific complications of each repair. The five types of TAAA according to the Crawford classification are as follows[15]:

Extent I: distal to the LSA extending to the visceral vessels but not involving the renal arteries; requires repair of the entire descending thoracic aorta and a varying extent of the abdominal aorta

Extent II: distal to the LSA to the aortic bifurcation; requires repair of the entire descending thoracic and abdominal aorta

Extent III: sixth intercostal space to the aortic bifurcation; requires repair of the lower half of the descending thoracic aorta and the entire abdominal aorta

Extent IV: limited to the abdominal aorta below the diaphragm; requires repair of the entire abdominal aorta beginning cephalad to the celiac axis.

Extent V: sixth intercostal space to the suprarenal aorta; requires repair of the lower half of the descending thoracic aorta and varying extent of the abdominal aorta

Ⓙ Endovascular candidate for TAAA repair within IFU or available investigational device?

Suitability for endovascular repair largely depends on aortic and branch vessel anatomy along with issues related to durability and vascular access. At the extremes of decision making, endovascular repair is best suited for elderly patients with a history of cardiopulmonary disease or other prohibitive risk factors to a more invasive open approach, as well as for patients with previous open aortic reconstructions. Conversely, younger/healthier patients, especially those with known or suspected connective tissue disorders

are best served with an open reconstruction given the question of endovascular device durability.

The most important aspect in successful endovascular repair is anatomic suitability. A healthy proximal and distal seal zone within nondiseased, parallel aorta devoid of significant thrombus or calcified plaque is the most essential factor for a durable endovascular repair. Visceral or renal arteries <4 to 4.5 mm in diameter or those with early bifurcations usually prevent endovascular branch reconstruction. Finally, appropriate access for large sheath placement is necessary and at times requires adjunct procedures, such as an iliac conduit, to achieve successful access. Adjunct procedures increase the physiologic impact of endovascular repair and, as such, are not recommended in high-risk patients. Currently, there is no endograft commercially available in the United States for treatment of a TAAA. However, surgeons with a physician-sponsored investigational device exemption (IDE) have access to investigational devices suitable for total endovascular repair or the option for surgeon-modified endograft approaches. Devices for endovascular TAAA treatment are currently in clinical trials. Their likely ultimate broad availability will significantly impact this decision tree.

Ⓚ Risk factors for spinal cord ischemia?

Spinal cord injury leading to paraplegia is one of the most severe complications of aortic surgery. The most common risk factors for SCI in TAA/TAAA repair includes aneurysm extent relating to the number of intercostal vessels compromised by the repair, aneurysm location with regard to the robustness of collateralization of the spinal cord, presence of acute aortic dissection, need for urgent/emergent repair, proximal aortic cross-clamp times >30 minutes in open repair, and perioperative hypotension.[16-18] Acher and colleagues add low cardiac index and age to the risk factors of SCI.[19] The need for left subclavian coverage or hypogastric coverage/occlusion also increases the risk of SCI given the compromise to the collateral perfusion network of the spinal cord. Other risk factors include the presence of atheromatous lesions (ie, "shaggy" atheromatous disease) within the aorta, increasing the risk of embolization to the intercostal/hypogastric arteries leading to SCI. The more risk factors present, the more spinal cord protection measures should be considered.

Ⓛ Spinal cord protection

The protocols for prevention of SCI during TAA/TAAA repair developed initially from an anatomic model of causation, primarily with focus on the artery of Adamkiewicz and reimplantation of vital intercostal branches. Recently, there has been a shift in focus of treating anatomic causes of SCI (ie, segmental artery coverage or ligation) with nonanatomic/physiologic measures, such as improving spinal perfusion pressure and increasing the tolerance of the SCI. Acher and Wynn have documented an 80% risk reduction in experimental models using primarily physiologic measures and confirmed this reduction in endovascular repair where intercostal

reimplantation is not possible.[20] With this model in mind, there are three primary areas that comprise the most successful SCI prevention protocols: improving spinal cord perfusion, increasing spinal cord oxygenation, and increasing the tolerance of the spinal cord to ischemia. All three areas, in part, focus on the importance of a robust collateral network to supplement perfusion of the spinal cord when intercostal arteries are covered during repair.

Reducing SCI time is directly related to the anatomic causes of ischemia. Specifically, limiting aortic cross-clamp time or clamping in a stepwise manner, utilizing assisted circulation, and reimplantation of intercostal arteries are effective methods of reducing SCI time and ischemic burden. Aortic cross-clamping or coverage of multiple segmental arteries with TEVAR placement acutely reduces arterial blood supply to the spinal cord leading to edema and increased CSF production, subsequently increasing CSF pressure and decreasing cerebral perfusion pressure further, leading to secondary injury. The use of somatosensory-evoked potentials (SSEPs) or motor-evoked potentials (MEPs) can provide active feedback to alert the physician to episodes of decreased spinal perfusion, allowing for directed efforts to resolve this problem in a timely manner during the operation. The most effective method for reducing this physiologic response is the use of a spinal drain for CSF drainage to lower the CSF pressure and to increase the MAP typically above 90 mm Hg to increase the cerebral perfusion pressure. The MAP should be maintained at this level for at least 48 hours postoperatively while the spinal drain remains to prevent delayed SCI. The use of vasodilators, such as nitroprusside, should be avoided during the postoperative period, and all agents used for HTN should be short-acting. The spinal drain is typically maintained for 24 to 48 hours postoperatively keeping CSF pressures <10 mm Hg (14 cm H_2O). Before removing the spinal drain, a clamping trial of at least 12 to 24 hours is completed. Methylprednisolone (30 mg/kg) can be given intraoperatively to decrease the effects of spinal cord edema after reperfusion. Sustaining adequate intravascular volume with a goal CVP of 8 to 10 mm Hg in the postoperative setting along with a goal hemoglobin of 9 to 10 g/dL is also essential to maintaining adequate spinal cord perfusion and oxygen delivery. Finally, increasing the spinal cord's tolerance of ischemia is achieved by reducing metabolic demands using mild systemic hypothermia (~34°C). In the absence of a contraindication to hypothermia (ie, coagulopathy), patients should not be actively rewarmed postoperatively. There is also evidence that naloxone reduces levels of excitatory amino acids released during the ischemic time, further decreasing the risk of SCI.[21] If used, naloxone is typically administered as a drip (1 µg/kg/h) and continued for 48 hours postoperatively. Any evidence of neurologic deficit is treated immediately by raising the MAP and urgent placement of a spinal drain, if not placed preoperatively, to improve spinal cord perfusion.

More recently, the notion that staged repair improves collateral perfusion to the spinal cord has led many to incorporate staged repair into SCI prevention protocols. O'Callaghan et al. demonstrated a significantly lower SCI rate in staged patients undergoing total endovascular repair of extent II TAAA compared to nonstaged patients (11.1% vs. 37.5%, $P = 0.03$). Furthermore, none of the staged patients experienced permanent paraplegia.[22]

Ⓜ Endovascular repair

Total endovascular repair of TAAAs is more complex than is TAA repair and is accomplished with one of three approaches to branch vessel incorporation: branched grafts (BEVAR), fenestrated grafts (FEVAR), or parallel grafting. Although BEVAR/FEVAR devices for endovascular repair of a TAAA have been used for quite some time outside of the United States, they are not currently commercially available in the United States. Owing to limited availability, data regarding the outcomes of endovascular repair of TAAAs are limited to mostly single-center, retrospective studies. Mastracci et al. found BEVAR/FEVAR treatment of type IV TAAA and juxtarenal AAA to be safe and durable. A total of 349 patients with a type IV TAAA treated with a fenestrated endograft experienced 2% aneurysm-related mortality at 8 years.[23] The same group later reported on the outcomes of BEVAR/FEVAR repair of 354 more extensive type II and III TAAAs. Technical success, defined as placement of an aortic graft with successful stenting of all target vessels was achieved in 94% of patients. Thirteen of the 21 failures involved the celiac artery with the remaining eight involving one of the renal arteries. Thirty-day mortality was 4.8%, whereas 8.8% of patients experienced at least temporary SCI, with 4% permanent SCI, more common in extent II TAAA. Hemodialysis was required postoperatively in 2.8% of patients, and branch artery patency ranged from 92% to 96% at 36 months.[24]

The results of surgeon-modified endografts for TAAA repair have been reported by surgeons with an IDE in the United States. The largest series comes from Starnes et al. of 60 consecutive patients with reported technical success of 95% and 30-day mortality of 5.1%. Freedom from migration, type I/III endoleaks, and sac enlargement at 12 months was 100%, 96%, and 98%, respectively.[25]

Ⓝ Endovascular candidate for TAA repair within IFU?

For descending TAAs, TEVAR is more straightforward because there is no need for branch artery incorporation. Current IFU criteria for commercially available thoracic endografts recommend a length of at least 2 cm for both proximal and distal landing zones to achieve an effective seal.

Available device diameters range from 21 to 46 mm, depending on the manufacturer, with recommendations of a minimal seal zone diameter of 16 mm and a maximum of 42 mm to remain within the IFU. Relative contraindications to endovascular repair of descending TAAs include excessive thrombus or calcifications of the proximal/distal landing zones, thoracic aortic tortuosity, and inadequate access vessels for device delivery. In the absence of a connective tissue disorder, anatomic contraindication, or

infectious etiology, endovascular repair of descending TAAs is the treatment of choice because of lower morbidity and mortality when compared to open repair.[26]

Ⓞ TEVAR

When planning TEVAR for a TAA, the urge to cover more aorta than is needed to successfully seal the aneurysm should be tempered by the risk of spinal cord ischemia (SCI) with longer coverage lengths. Landing the proximal portion of the endograft in a curved portion of the aorta increases the risk of poor endograft approximation or "bird beaking," which can decrease the overall durability of the repair. Endograft oversizing should generally be 10% to 20% for treatment of degenerative TAA, whereas repair of aortic dissections or blunt aortic injuries should be 0% to 10%. Patients with aortoiliac occlusive disease or small/tortuous iliac vessels pose a challenge for successful endovascular repair and often require adjunctive measures for access with either a traditional iliac conduit to the CIA or an internal "endoconduit" with covered stents and controlled rupture of the stenotic iliac vessels. Patients may require extension into the aortic arch to achieve an appropriate proximal landing zone, necessitating coverage of the brachiocephalic branch vessels. If the LSA requires coverage in the elective setting, it is generally recommended to revascularize the LSA with either a carotid to subclavian bypass or SCA transposition to decrease the risk of stroke and left arm/SCI. In the emergent setting, it is acceptable to cover the LSA, when necessary, with subsequent revascularization if complications occur. Aortic endografts with a branch for LSA have been developed and are currently under investigation, which may obviate the discussion of when/whether to revascularize the LSA. A recent meta-analysis demonstrated TEVAR to have a lower 30-day mortality when compared to open repair for intact TAA (OR, 0.6). Further, TEVAR had lower rates of SCI (OR, 0.35) and pulmonary complications (OR, 0.41).[26]

Ⓟ Appropriate anatomic or medical risk for open TAAA repair?

Patients being considered for open repair should be stratified depending on the overall risk of operative repair as well as other complicating circumstances. In general, younger patients with a life expectancy of 10 years or greater, particularly those with connective tissue disorders, should be treated with a traditional open approach. Exceptions to this rule include those with prior open repair that would make a subsequent operation more complicated and of higher risk, in which case an endovascular repair landing within existing Dacron from prior open repairs is generally considered acceptable.

Ⓠ Hybrid/debranching repair (staged vs. single stage)

Patients considered prohibitively high risk for conventional open repair of a TAAA, such as those not able to tolerate

proximal aortic clamping or single-lung ventilation, and those who are not appropriate anatomic candidates for total endovascular repair can be considered for a hybrid approach. The hybrid approach consists of open surgical visceral and renal debranching with inflow usually from the distal CIA or the proximal EIA followed by endograft aortic relining. Endograft placement can be done during the same procedure; however, performing the repair in two stages may decrease the risk of spinal cord injury and should be considered, particularly for extent I and II TAAA.[27] The proposed benefits of hybrid repair are its avoidance of thoracotomy, proximal aortic cross-clamping, and prolonged organ ischemic times. Although certain single centers with extensive experience in this technique demonstrate excellent outcomes, most reports are hampered by higher mortality and morbidity rates. A meta-analysis of 528 patients demonstrated a 14% pooled 30-day/in-hospital mortality rate. Further, permanent renal failure occurred in 7.0%, mesenteric ischemia in 4.5%, and symptomatic spinal cord injury in 7.0%, with 4.4% experiencing irreversible paraplegia. The authors concluded that although the hybrid approach offers a less invasive approach as compared to open TAAA repair, patients considered too high risk for open TAAA repair are equally likely to suffer complications from hybrid repair.[28] In our practice, debranching is limited to high-risk patients with visceral/renal occlusive disease or other anatomic contraindications to branched or fenestrated repair.

Ⓡ Risk factors for spinal, visceral, or limb ischemia?

Spinal cord ischemia (SCI) is a concern across both endovascular and open repair options, whereas visceral and limb ischemia is primarily a concern of open TAA or TAAA repair. The primary risk factors associated with SCI are discussed in further detail in section M. Clamping of the thoracic aorta can lead to significant physiologic derangements because distal tissues become ischemic throughout the length of cross-clamp time. This can lead to renal failure, bowel necrosis, coagulopathy, and liver dysfunction postoperatively, in addition to SCI. There is also significant strain placed on the left heart due to the acute rise in left ventricular afterload and increased myocardial oxygen demand. Similar to spinal cord protection, renovisceral protection follows the same tenets of decreasing ischemia time, decreasing metabolic demands, and improving ischemic tolerance of the kidneys and the viscera. The use of assisted circulation or distal aortic perfusion benefits the patient by providing retrograde perfusion to the pelvic and visceral arteries, as well as offloading the left heart during proximal aortic repair. The primary methods of assisted circulation are discussed further in section T.

Concern for visceral and limb ischemia primarily revolves around the extent of the aneurysm to be repaired and the underlying comorbid conditions of the patient. Contemporary reports show acute renal dysfunction in 9% of extents I and IV TAAA and as high as 17% in extent II TAAA. Bowel ischemia is much less frequent, occurring in approximately 1% of all TAAA repairs.[29] Further, the underlying comorbid conditions of each individual patient should be taken into account when determining which adjuncts to use. Patients with underlying cardiac disease may not be able to tolerate the stress of a proximal aortic clamp and will benefit from partial left heart bypass (LHB). Similarly, those with renal dysfunction, extents I to III aneurysms and patients with higher preoperative cardiopulmonary risk are indicated for use of distal aortic perfusion. Mohebali et al. demonstrated favorable outcomes with distal aortic perfusion as compared to the clamp-and-sew technique from the U.S. Medicare database in multiple postoperative outcomes including renal failure (14% vs. 24%, $P < 0.0001$), pulmonary complications (21% vs. 27%, $P < 0.0001$), and 30-day mortality 9.7% vs. 12.2%, $P = 0.01$).[30] The more risk factors present, the more assisted circulation, distal aortic perfusion, and spinal cord protection are favored (see S).

S Open TAA/TAAA repair with distal aortic perfusion and spinal cord protection

With the recent advancements in endovascular technologies, open repair of TAAA, and especially TAA, have become less common but still has an important role in management of these complex patients. The open surgical approach depends on the underlying aneurysm extent. More extensive repairs, including those for extent I to III TAAA, increase the risk of spinal cord (see L) and visceral/limb (see R) ischemia, often requiring the need for adjunctive measures. Although certain centers of excellence report mortality rates ranging from 5% to 15%, data using national or regional datasets show higher 30-day mortality rates of 20%.[31] This difference demonstrates the importance of treating these complex patients in high-volume centers. Specific to TAAA repair, data from the NIS demonstrated both hospital and surgeon volume to be significant predictors of mortality for elective repair. The mortality at high-volume institutions, defined as 5 to 31 cases per year, was 15% overall compared to 27% for low-volume institutions ($P < 0.001$). High-volume surgeons, defined as those with 3 to 18 cases per year, had a mortality rate of 11% compared to 26% for low-volume surgeons ($P < 0.001$).[32]

There are three primary techniques to consider when treating TAAs/TAAAs using an open approach: cross-clamp and sew plus spinal fluid drainage, assisted circulation with partial LHB/cardiopulmonary bypass and spinal fluid drainage, or hypothermic circulatory arrest. The benefits to the cross-clamp and sew plus spinal drainage are that it is the simplest and fastest of the approaches and does not require the degree of anticoagulation required for LHB or full cardiopulmonary bypass. However, this approach puts the most strain on the left heart and is not ideal for more extensive TAAAs because of the prolonged visceral/renal ischemia times. Despite these concerns, select high-volume centers have demonstrated excellent outcomes using a clamp-and-sew

technique with other adjuncts including spinal drainage, systemic hypothermia, and 4°C renal artery perfusion.[33]

LHB essentially withdraws oxygenated blood form the left side of the circulation and returns it to the distal aorta via a femoral or distal aortic cannula. The source of the oxygenated blood can be the left pulmonary vein, the left atrium via the left atrial appendage, or the apex of the left ventricle. LHB reduces strain on the left heart, but this approach adds the complexity of cannulating for bypass and requires more circulating heparin than does the clamp-and-sew technique, potentially leading to more coagulopathic bleeding at the conclusion of the procedure. Cardiopulmonary bypass with a period of hypothermic circulatory arrest allows a bloodless field for extensive aortic reconstruction and the ability to perform the proximal or distal anastomoses without a clamp. This can be very beneficial in patients with prior transverse arch replacement, connective tissue disorders leading to concern for vessel damage with clamping, or a need for an anastomosis extending into the arch necessitating cerebral circulatory arrest. This technique is preferentially used at some centers but does increase the procedure times because of prolonged cardiopulmonary bypass times with cooling and rewarming.

T Standard open TAA/TAAA repair

Standard open TAA or TAAA repair without the use of spinal protection or distal aortic perfusion adjuncts is essentially limited to treatment of type IV TAAA repair or in an isolated focal TAA patient with an underlying connective tissue disorder or pathology of infectious etiology. With type IV TAAA isolated to the abdominal aorta, the majority of the dissection is below the diaphragm and can often be completed with limited transection of the diaphragm. Renal and visceral ischemic times can be decreased by performing a beveled proximal anastomosis incorporating the right renal, SMA, and celiac arteries into the anastomosis. This lessens the need for adjunctive procedures needed to limit spinal cord, mesenteric, and renal ischemia, but may allow for late aneurysmal degeneration of this visceral patch, which should be considered in younger patients. Excellent outcomes using this inclusion technique have been reported from the Massachusetts General Hospital over a 20-year period with 30-day mortality of 2.8%, MI of 3.4%, renal failure requiring dialysis in 2.8%, and any degree of spinal cord injury of 2.2%.[34]

U Monitor for spinal cord ischemia

Postoperative SCI can be manifested as a spectrum of neurologic deficit ranging from mild unilateral leg weakness to overt paralysis with total loss of sensation. This deficit may develop acutely or can be gradual. The overall risk of SCI for TEVAR ranges from 4% to 7% for TAA, 2% to 28% for elective open TAA repair, 5% to 22% for extent II TAAA, and as high as 40% for emergent TAAA repair.[16]

Management of a patient who develops symptoms consistent with SCI postoperatively is discussed in detail in Chapter 86.

V Post-procedural surveillance

Postprocedural surveillance after TAA or TAAA endovascular repair follows guidelines similar to that of standard endovascular aortic repair with surveillance CTA at 1 month, 6 months, and then annually thereafter, assuming no evidence of endoleak, stent-graft migration, or aneurysm sac growth, and adequate renal function for CTA. For patients with branched or fenestrated grafts, use of postoperative DUS should be considered for monitoring of the abdominal component and the branch/fenestrated stents/branch vessels. Although no specific DUS criteria have been developed to demonstrate graft stenosis, significant changes in flow velocities can indicate the need for further assessment, especially if evidence of end-organ malperfusion exists (eg, elevated creatinine or chronic mesenteric ischemia symptoms).

Postprocedural surveillance following open repair is less stringent than that after endovascular repair. Routine CT follow-up is recommended at 5-year intervals following open aneurysm repair given that the risk of para-anastomotic aneurysm or metachronous aneurysm development occurs in up to 15% of patients.[35]

REFERENCES

1. Hiratzka LF, Bakris GL, Beckman JA, et al. 2010 ACCF/AHA/AATS/ACR/ASA/SCA/SCAI/SIR/STS/SVM Guidelines for the diagnosis and management of patients with Thoracic Aortic Disease: a report of the American College of Cardiology Foundation/American Heart Association Task Force on Practice Guidelines, American Association for Thoracic Surgery, American College of Radiology, American Stroke Association, Society of Cardiovascular Anesthesiologists, Society for Cardiovascular Angiography and Interventions, Society of Interventional Radiology, Society of Thoracic Surgeons, and Society for Vascular Medicine. *Circulation.* 2010;121:e266-e369.
2. Olsson C, Thelin S, Stahle E, Ekbom A, Granath F. Thoracic aortic aneurysm and dissection: increasing prevalence and improved outcomes reported in a nationwide population-based study of more than 14,000 cases from 1987 to 2002. *Circulation.* 2006;114:2611-2618.
3. Johansson G, Markstrom U, Swedenborg J. Ruptured thoracic aortic aneurysms: a study of incidence and mortality rates. *J Vasc Surg.* 1995;21:985-988.
4. Ultee KHJ, Zettervall SL, Soden PA, et al. The impact of endovascular repair on management and outcome of ruptured thoracic aortic aneurysms. *J Vasc Surg.* 2017;66:343.e1-352.e1.
5. Ricotta JJ II, Tsilimparis N. Surgeon-modified fenestrated-branched stent grafts to treat emergently ruptured and symptomatic complex aortic aneurysms in high-risk patients. *J Vasc Surg.* 2012;56:1535-1542.
6. Locham SS, Grimm JC, Arhuidese IJ, et al. Perioperative outcomes of open versus endovascular repair for ruptured

thoracoabdominal aneurysms. *Ann Vasc Surg.* 2017;44: 128-135.

7. Juvonen T, Ergin MA, Galla JD, et al. Prospective study of the natural history of thoracic aortic aneurysms. *Ann Thorac Surg.* 1997;63:1533-1545.

8. Lo RC, Lu B, Fokkema MT, et al. Relative importance of aneurysm diameter and body size for predicting abdominal aortic aneurysm rupture in men and women. *J Vasc Surg.* 2014;59(5):1209-1216.

9. Kristmundsson T, Dias N, Resch T, Sonesson B. Morphology of small abdominal aortic aneurysms should be considered before continued ultrasound surveillance. *Ann Vasc Surg.* 2016;31:18-22.

10. MacCarrick G, Black JH III, Bowdin S, et al. Loeys-Dietz syndrome: a primer for diagnosis and management. *Genet Med.* 2014;16:576-587.

11. Knyshov GV, Sitar LL, Glagola MD, Atamanyuk MY. Aortic aneurysms at the site of the repair of coarctation of the aorta: a review of 48 patients. *Ann Thorac Surg.* 1996;61:935-939.

12. Panneton JM, Hollier LH. Dissecting descending thoracic and thoracoabdominal aortic aneurysms: part II. *Ann Vasc Surg.* 1995;9:596-605.

13. Kashyap VS, Cambria RP, Davison JK, L'Italien GJ. Renal failure after thoracoabdominal aortic surgery. *J Vasc Surg.* 1997;26:949-955; discussion 955-7.

14. Arya S, Kim SI, Duwayri Y, et al. Frailty increases the risk of 30-day mortality, morbidity, and failure to rescue after elective abdominal aortic aneurysm repair independent of age and comorbidities. *J Vasc Surg.* 2015;61:324-331.

15. Crawford ES, Snyder DM, Cho GC, Roehm JO. Progress in treatment of thoracoabdominal and abdominal aortic aneurysms involving celiac, superior mesenteric, and renal arteries. *Ann Surg.* 1978;188(3):400-421.

16. Etz CD, Weigang E, Hartert M, et al. Contemporary spinal cord protection during thoracic and thoracoabdominal aortic surgery and endovascular aortic repair: a position paper of the vascular domain of the European Association for Cardio-Thoracic Surgery. *Eur J Cardiothorac Surg.* 2015;47:943-957.

17. Livesay JL, Cooley DA, Ventemiglia RA. Surgical experience in descending thoracic aneurysmectomy with and without adjuncts to avoid ischaemia. *Ann Thorac Surg.* 1985;39:37-46.

18. Katz NM, Blackstone EH, Kirklin JW, Karp RB. Incremental risk factors for spinal cord injury following operation for aortic transection. *J Thorac Cardiovasc Surg.* 1981;81:669-674.

19. Acher C, Wynn M. Outcomes in open repair of the thoracic and thoracoabdominal aorta. *J Vasc Surg.* 2010;52:3S-9S.

20. Acher CW, Wynn M. A modern theory of paraplegia in the treatment of aneurysms of the thoracoabdominal aorta: an analysis of technique specific observed/expected ratios for paralysis. *J Vasc Surg.* 2009;49:1117-1124; discussion 1124.

21. Kunihara T, Matsuzaki K, Shiiya N, Saijo Y, Yasuda K. Naloxone lowers cerebrospinal fluid levels of excitatory amino acids after thoracoabdominal aortic surgery. *J Vasc Surg.* 2004;40:681-690.

22. O'Callaghan A, Mastracci TM, Eagleton MJ. Staged endovascular repair of thoracoabdominal aortic aneurysms limits incidence and severity of spinal cord ischemia. *J Vasc Surg.* 2015;61:347.e1-354.e1.

23. Mastracci TM, Eagleton MJ, Kuramochi Y, Bathurst S, Wolski K. Twelve-year results of fenestrated endografts for juxtarenal and group IV thoracoabdominal aneurysms. *J Vasc Surg.* 2015;61:355-364.

24. Eagleton MJ, Follansbee M, Wolski K, Mastracci T, Kuramochi Y. Fenestrated and branched endovascular aneurysm repair outcomes for type II and III thoracoabdominal aortic aneurysms. *J Vasc Surg.* 2016;63:930-942.

25. Starnes BW, Heneghan RE, Tatum B. Midterm results from a physician-sponsored investigational device exemption clinical trial evaluating physician-modified endovascular grafts for the treatment of juxtarenal aortic aneurysms. *J Vasc Surg.* 2017;65:294-302.

26. Alsawas M, Zaiem F, Larrea-Mantilla L, et al. Effectiveness of surgical interventions for thoracic aortic aneurysms: a systematic review and meta-analysis. *J Vasc Surg.* 2017;66:1258.e8-1268.e8.

27. Canaud L, Karthikesalingam A, Jackson D, et al. Clinical outcomes of single versus staged hybrid repair for thoracoabdominal aortic aneurysm. *J Vasc Surg.* 2013;58:1192-1200.

28. Moulakakis KG, Mylonas SN, Antonopoulos CN, Liapis CD. Combined open and endovascular treatment of thoracoabdominal aortic pathologies: a systematic review and meta-analysis. *Ann Cardiothorac Surg.* 2012;1:267-276.

29. Aftab M, Coselli JS. Renal and visceral protection in thoracoabdominal aortic surgery. *J Thorac Cardiovasc Surg.* 2014;148:2963-2966.

30. Mohebali J, Carvalho S, Lancaster RT, et al. Use of extracorporeal bypass is associated with improved outcomes in open thoracic and thoracoabdominal aortic aneurysm repair. *J Vasc Surg.* 2018;68:941-947.

31. Rigberg DA, Zingmond DS, McGory ML, et al. Age stratified, perioperative, and one-year mortality after abdominal aortic aneurysm repair: a statewide experience. *J Vasc Surg.* 2006;43:224-229.

32. Cowan JA Jr, Dimick JB, Henke PK, Huber TS, Stanley JC, Upchurch GR Jr. Surgical treatment of intact thoracoabdominal aortic aneurysms in the United States: hospital and surgeon volume-related outcomes. *J Vasc Surg.* 2003;37:1169-1174.

33. Wynn MM, Acher C, Marks E, Engelbert T, Acher CW. Postoperative renal failure in thoracoabdominal aortic aneurysm repair with simple cross-clamp technique and 4 degrees C renal perfusion. *J Vasc Surg.* 2015;61:611-622.

34. Patel VI, Ergul E, Conrad MF, et al. Continued favorable results with open surgical repair of type IV thoracoabdominal aortic aneurysms. *J Vasc Surg.* 2011;53:1492-1498.

35. Kalman PG, Rappaport DC, Merchant N, Clarke K, Johnston KW. The value of late computed tomographic scanning in identification of vascular abnormalities after abdominal aortic aneurysm repair. *J Vasc Surg.* 1999;29:442-450.

Marissa Famularo • Joseph V. Lombardi

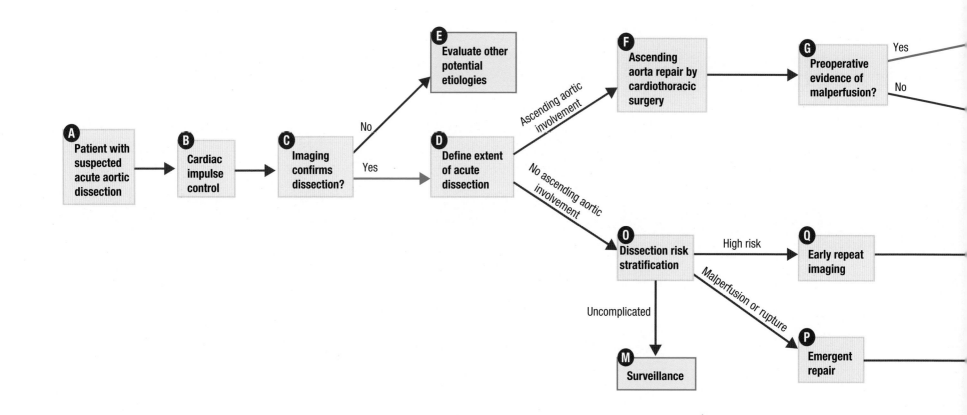

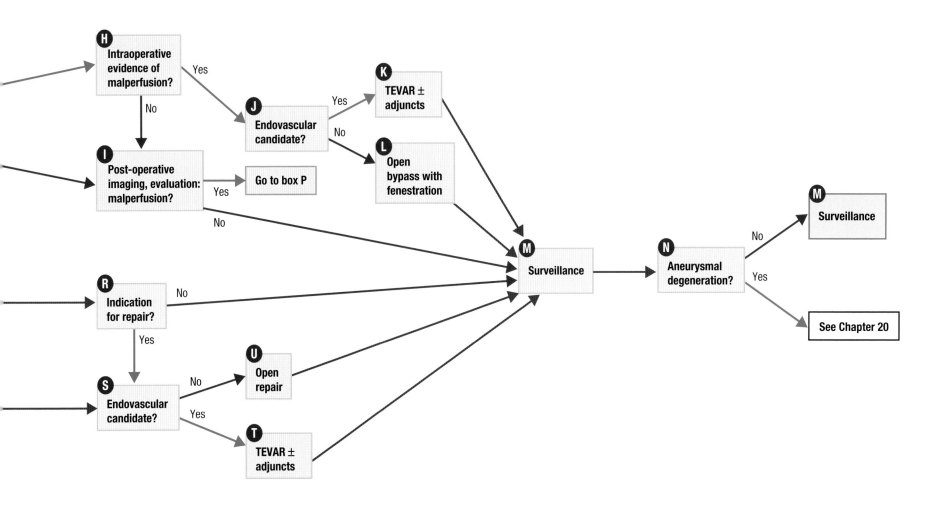

A Patient with suspected acute aortic dissection

Acute aortic dissection (AAD) is a life-threatening emergency. Symptoms mimicking other more common pathologies make AAD particularly difficult to identify. Because AAD is seen in a wide range of patients, clinical suspicion should be high for all patients presenting with pain that may be consistent with AAD. It should be noted that over 60% of patients are male and over 80% of patients are white,[1] and the mean age of presentation is in the seventh decade. Importantly, the age range is wide, and, as such, consideration of AAD in younger patients is also warranted.[1] Younger patients may have undiagnosed genetic abnormalities, HTN, or recent drug use, which increase their risk.[2] Although severe chest pain is the most common presenting symptom of AAD, this nonspecific complaint does little to pinpoint the underlying pathology. Other, more specific symptoms, such as tearing or ripping pain quality, HTN, and pulse deficits are noted in less than half of all patients.[2] A thorough H&P is necessary to identify risk factors and rule out alternative pathologies.

B Cardiac impulse control

The first step in management of any patient with AAD involves strict cardiac impulse control to reduce stress on the aortic wall in an attempt to halt progression of the dissection. This includes management of associated HTN as well as prevention of tachycardia. β-Blockers are used as a first-line drug in patients who can physiologically tolerate them. In bradycardic patients or those in whom a second agent is required, IV calcium channel blockers are frequently used. Although sodium nitroprusside has traditionally been used in this setting, it can cause reflex tachycardia and therefore is prescribed only after optimal β-blockade has been achieved. Importantly, both β-blockers and calcium channel blockers have been proved to improve outcomes in patients with type B aortic dissection.[3] Given the impact of the sympathetic response to pain and anxiety on tachycardia/HTN, control of both is an important component of early treatment. Although no blood pressure or heart rate goals have been standardized across studies, we aim for an MAP <80 mm Hg in all patients with AAD. In patients with continued chest pain, the MAP should be lowered further to <70 mm Hg, if tolerated depending on mental status and end-organ perfusion.

C Imaging confirms dissection?

CTA of the chest, abdomen, and pelvis should be obtained if AAD is suspected because it is fast, noninvasive, and provides important anatomic information regarding the dissection. In addition to confirmation of the diagnosis, CTA allows for classification of the dissection extent, which guides management. For patients who later undergo surgical or endovascular repair, CTA provides important information regarding the number and location of intimal tears and end-organ perfusion. For these reasons, CTA is the current diagnostic test of choice. When possible, a dissection protocol that includes thin cuts (<3 mm) to assess small dissection tears, cardiac gating to evaluate the proximal aorta where motion artifact is particularly problematic, and delayed imaging to look for the presence of false lumen perfusion should be used. High-quality imaging is very important to guide intervention should it be necessary.

In situations where CTA is contraindicated, transesophageal echocardiogram (TEE) can be performed intraoperatively. TEE is a useful modality to confirm questionable lesions (especially in the ascending aorta) noted on ungated CTA. Its limitations include the need for expertise to perform the study and the inability to evaluate the distal aorta, which is often involved in AAD.

D Define extent of acute dissection

Once a diagnosis of AAD is confirmed, classification of the dissection is necessary to guide management. The Stanford and DeBakey classification systems are most commonly used. The Stanford system separates patients into two categories: those with involvement of the ascending aorta (type A) and those without involvement of the ascending aorta (type B). The DeBakey classification system includes type I, involving the ascending and descending aorta, type II involving only the ascending aorta, and type III, involving only the descending aorta. Type III is further subdivided into dissection involving only the thoracic aorta (IIIa) and dissection extending through the visceral segment (IIIb). To determine an initial management strategy, it is important to quickly determine whether the ascending aorta is involved, regardless of what overall classification system is used.

E Evaluate other potential etiologies

If AAD is not confirmed on imaging, alternate etiologies must be evaluated and treated when identified. Differential diagnosis includes, but is not limited to, the following conditions: MI, aortic aneurysm, pericarditis, pneumonia, cholecystitis, pancreatitis, PE, musculoskeletal pain, and peptic ulcer disease.

F Ascending aorta repair by cardiothoracic surgery

Patients with involvement of the ascending aorta, either with a primary intimal tear in the ascending aorta or by retrograde propagation of intramural hematoma or dissection from a tear in the aortic arch or descending aorta, present a surgical emergency in most cases. Without surgery, these patients have a 1% to 2% mortality per hour for the first 24 hours,[4] and emergent cardiothoracic surgical consultation and repair is warranted unless the patient is at prohibitive surgical risk.

G Preoperative evidence of malperfusion?

A significant portion of patients with type A dissections have concomitant involvement of the descending thoracic aorta (DeBakey type I), which may lead to persistent distal end-organ malperfusion after the ascending aorta has been repaired. Identification of distal malperfusion is an essential step in the preoperative evaluation and best accomplished with preoperative CTA. Early vascular surgical consultation is essential in these patients to avoid delay should they need additional intervention after central aortic repair.

H Intraoperative evidence of malperfusion

Often, distal malperfusion is alleviated by ascending aortic repair. All patients with involvement of the more distal aorta should have a repeat examination of their distal pulses postoperatively while still in the operating room. This will allow for prompt intervention should persistent malperfusion be identified. If malperfusion of visceral/renal arteries was identified preoperatively, intraoperative arteriography can be performed after ascending aortic repair, to determine whether malperfusion still exists, and, if so, to potentially treat this with endovascular techniques (see J).

Patients with evidence of distal malperfusion after ascending aortic repair should be considered for early intervention to treat malperfusion. Although type A repair often depressurizes the false lumen, allowing expansion and pressurization of the true lumen and branch vessels, the presence of multiple intimal tears or a primary tear distal to the repaired ascending aorta can allow continued false lumen pressurization. This can cause continued malperfusion of the visceral/renal vessels and/or iliac arteries and can be a lethal complication if not identified early. Distal pulse deficits, a concerning abdominal examination for mesenteric ischemia, or unexplained persistent/worsening metabolic acidosis and oliguria should raise suspicion for malperfusion and prompt postoperative imaging.

I Post-operative imaging, evaluation: malperfusion?

Patients with no evidence of distal malperfusion on intraoperative examination after ascending aorta repair should be transferred to the ICU for resuscitation and postoperative care. After clinical stabilization, repeat CTA should be performed within 72 hours to evaluate the postoperative anatomy and evaluate for residual dissection. Unfortunately, this imaging study is often delayed secondary to postoperative acute kidney injury, which is common after type A repair. Rising creatinine unresponsive to fluid resuscitation in the postoperative patient should raise concern for renal artery malperfusion from dissection. In cases where renal malperfusion is in question, DUS imaging can be helpful in making the diagnosis of this complication. Noncontrasted MRA protocols are also available at some institutions. MRA can fully evaluate the septal motion throughout the cardiac cycle and identify end-organ malperfusion without contrast. Transfemoral IVUS can also be helpful if CTA cannot be performed. If malperfusion is detected, it must be performed.

J Endovascular candidate?

Patients with continued end-organ malperfusion after type A repair may be candidates for endovascular revascularization. If distal entry flow and pressurization of the false lumen persists, additional coverage with TEVAR may be indicated. Classic contraindications to endovascular techniques include small, calcified, or occluded access vessels. Prior open femoral operations with significant scarring or extension of dissection into the femoral vessels may present challenges to access. Although the true lumen may be entered using ultrasound guidance, femoral cutdown with direct visualization may be preferable. IVUS is helpful to determine true lumen status and to ensure that any wire placed from the femoral vessel stays within the true lumen throughout its course.

🄚 TEVAR ± adjuncts

Intimal tears in the aorta distal to a type A repair warrant immediate treatment if they lead to true lumen collapse or branch vessel malperfusion. Depending on patient anatomy, large tears may be covered with a thoracic endograft to prevent false lumen inflow/pressurization. Adjunctive stenting of branch vessels may also be required to alleviate obstruction, in combination with proximal tear coverage by TEVAR. Alternatively, endovascular fenestration may be used to equalize the pressure between the true and false lumens, effectively correcting branch vessel malperfusion.[5,6] This method is particularly helpful if the false lumen inflow source is in the arch and not amenable to coverage with an aortic endograft.

🄛 Open bypass with fenestration

If there are no viable endovascular options for reperfusion of branch vessels, or if endovascular attempts have failed, open surgical treatment of malperfusion is warranted. With visceral malperfusion, single-branch vessel obstructions can be treated with surgical bypass; however, it is essential for an uninvolved inflow site to be available (ie, iliac artery). If multiple visceral branches are involved, open aortic septal fenestration with removal of the intimal flap may be a more expeditious technique to reperfuse all involved branches. For unilateral lower extremity ischemia, a femoral-femoral bypass is a safe, relatively quick way to reestablish flow to the ischemic limb. Rare bilateral iliac occlusion that cannot be treated with endovascular techniques requires axillo-bi-femoral bypass unless aortofemoral bypass is felt to be warranted and safe. See also Box U for additional details regarding open surgical repair.

🄜 Surveillance

Uncomplicated patients, stable patients with high-risk features, and all patients treated with TEVAR for AAD should be placed on an intensive surveillance program. Patients with aortic dissection, even after successful treatment and apparent false lumen thrombosis, should be treated as patients with a chronic disease. Over 70% of patients treated medically and 60% of patients treated with TEVAR develop aneurysmal degeneration over 5 years, with 20% and 30% of each group, respectively, requiring

late intervention or reintervention in that same time period.[7] All patients should be educated on the importance of long-term surveillance and the potential need for future interventions. Repeat imaging in patients with AAD should be performed before discharge and at 6 weeks after the dissection event.[8] As with initial imaging, CTA is the preferred study of choice. However, in patients with renal insufficiency, CT scans without contrast can be used to estimate aortic diameter and monitor for aneurysmal degeneration over time. In the abdominal aorta, DUS can be used to identify false lumen flow and branch vessel patency. Noncontrasted MRA is available in some institutions, but evaluation of the treated aorta after TEVAR will be limited by the metallic components of the endograft.

🄝 Aneurysmal degeneration?

Patients with evidence of aneurysmal degeneration during surveillance may require treatment to prevent rupture. Chronic dissections are a distinct pathology and treatment guidelines specific to this challenging population are outlined in Chapter 20.

🄞 Dissection risk stratification

To guide management, all patients with type B aortic dissection (and patients with persistent descending aortic dissection after type A dissection repair) should be further classified into one of three categories: malperfusion or rupture, high risk, or uncomplicated.

Patients with evidence of malperfusion or rupture are at high risk for early mortality and should be repaired emergently, usually with TEVAR.

High-risk patients are those who exhibit characteristics that place them at high risk for early complications. The list of high-risk features reported in the literature continues to grow, but currently includes patients with the following[9-11]:

- Refractory HTN or pain
- A large (>10 mm) primary entry tear
- Total aortic diameter in the area of dissection > 40 mm
- Proximal false lumen diameter > 20 mm
- Elliptical true lumen
- Fully patent or partially thrombosed false lumen

Patients with high-risk features do not need emergent repair but should be monitored closely with frequent imaging to evaluate for potential complications. Special attention should be given to patients with refractory HTN and pain, who present an especially high risk of early rupture. These patients should be monitored closely in the ICU for early resolution of pain and HTN, which, if uncontrolled for more than 12 hours after initiation of appropriate medical therapy, should prompt consideration for early repair.

Patients without malperfusion/rupture or high-risk features are classified as uncomplicated. There are no current data to

support early intervention for truly uncomplicated AAD of the descending aorta.[12] In fact, there is more evidence contradicting the premise that TEVAR in uncomplicated patients prevents future aneurysmal degeneration.

🄟 Emergent repair

Patients with evidence of malperfusion or rupture of type B dissection are at high risk for early mortality and should proceed emergently to repair, most commonly using TEVAR. Even patients who would be considered questionable endovascular candidates in nonemergent situations (ie, patients with very small aortas, concern for infection, short proximal landing zones, etc.) should be considered for endovascular treatment in the case of rupture. This is because TEVAR is usually the most expeditious way to control hemorrhage in the case of rupture, and may be used even in imperfect candidates as a means of temporizing an often fatal clinical scenario.

As in all cases of TEVAR for dissection, a 10% maximum graft oversizing is used for choosing an endograft in emergency procedures. Whenever possible, percutaneous access is obtained via the common femoral arteries with ultrasound guidance. Percutaneous access is the quickest way to enter the endovascular space. If there is not time to place closure devices before upsizing, conversion to open cutdown can be performed later, after hemorrhage has been controlled. Unlike elective cases where extent of aortic coverage can be debated, coverage of the aorta from the left SCA to the celiac is recommended in all cases of rupture, with the goal being cessation of flow in the false lumen to prevent continued hemorrhage. Should coverage of the left subclavian be necessary to achieve a proximal seal, this should be performed without preoperative revascularization. Revascularization of the left SCA can be addressed postoperatively, if necessary.

🄠 Early repeat imaging

Early repeat imaging should be obtained on any patient deemed at high risk for complications of AAD, including those with anatomic features such as large aortic or false lumen diameter (see O). In addition, patients with refractory HTN or pain despite maximal impulse control have an increased risk of early mortality, and early repeat imaging should be obtained to evaluate for potential complications or progression of their dissection.[9] AAD can be a dynamic process during the early phase of treatment, and any clinical changes, such has a return of pain, new hypotension, or new pulse deficits, should also prompt repeat imaging to evaluate for new malperfusion, rupture/impending rupture, or other changes requiring intervention.

🄡 Indication for repair?

Patients who require repair after failing early observation include those with persistent pain or HTN, or signs of either visceral or extremity ischemia. Repeat CTA may also show rapid aneurysmal degeneration or progression of the dissection with new evidence of malperfusion. Any of these findings require prompt repair.

🅢 Endovascular candidate?

TEVAR has become the standard of care in the treatment of acute, complicated type B aortic dissection.[7,8] Complicated patients experience a high early mortality without treatment, which significantly improves to 5% to 15% after endovascular repair.[13-15] Immediate TEVAR is therefore recommended for all patients with acute type B aortic dissection and evidence of rupture or malperfusion.[7] Early TEVAR may carry an increased risk of complications, especially retrograde aortic dissection and stroke. Therefore, for high-risk patients, this increased risk must be considered when weighing the benefit of repair. Some have suggested that waiting for 14 days in high-risk patients (those without rupture/malperfusion) may be preferable to avoid early TEVAR-related complications.

With the advent of TEVAR, open procedures have become rare and are generally avoided because of their high perioperative morbidity and mortality. Patients with inadequate proximal landing zones due to aortic diameter or proximity to brachiocephalic vessels, or those with poor endovascular access options may require open repair. A lack of proximal landing zone may sometimes be managed with a proximal debranching procedure followed by TEVAR, and poor access may be mitigated by open iliac/aortic conduits. Hybrid arch procedures avoid complete replacement of the arch and may be performed with or without concomitant ascending aortic replacement, or with extra-anatomic (ie, cervical) debranching, depending on disease extent. When the distal landing zone is inadequate, visceral debranching procedures before TEVAR are also an option, but are exceedingly uncommon in the setting of acute dissection.

🅣 TEVAR ± adjuncts

The primary objectives of TEVAR for malperfusion and rupture are somewhat different. With malperfusion, the ultimate goal is to cover the primary entry tear, depressurize the false lumen, and reestablish flow to the end organs. For ruptured dissection, the goal is to stop all flow to the false lumen and prevent further hemorrhage, which may require a longer length of coverage than is necessary with malperfusion. In both cases, the primary entry tear must be covered and the endograft must land proximal to the fenestration, preferably in healthy, nondissected aorta. Endografts are selected, whenever possible, depending on preoperative imaging of the proximal landing zone, with a 0% to 10% oversizing used for diameter selection. Tapered endografts should be used whenever the proximal to distal diameter change is significant.

Importantly, landing an endograft in diseased proximal aorta (aorta with intramural hematoma present or false lumen flow) increases the risk of adverse events, including

perioperative stroke and retrograde propagation of dissection, and should be avoided if possible. Also, balloon molding of an endograft proximally in acute dissection is unnecessary and strongly discouraged.

There are proponents of maximum aortic coverage during initial TEVAR irrespective of the clinical presentation to maximize false lumen thrombosis and decrease the risk of late distal aortic aneurysmal degeneration. However, this may increase the risk of complications, specifically postoperative paralysis. For this reason, when possible, a salient strategy to minimize risk of paraplegia may involve limited coverage of the descending thoracic aorta with a plan to intervene later with additional coverage if it becomes necessary because of unfavorable remodeling on follow-up imaging.

Newer technologies that allow the use of a bare-metal stent extending into the visceral aorta to improve the true lumen diameter and potentially avoid spinal ischemia are becoming available.[16] Clinical trial data have suggested that this technique assists with total positive aortic remodeling, and allows for future interventions such as branched/fenestrated endografts on the visceral aorta should this become necessary.[13]

IVUS should be used in all cases of dissection to ensure proper wire and stent placement in the true lumen. IVUS can also be used to identify branch vessels and can demonstrate the septal dynamics throughout the cardiac cycle before and after TEVAR device placement, demonstrating successful depressurization of the false lumen. Continued compression of the true lumen after TEVAR can suggest a failure in proximal entry tear coverage or the need to extend coverage distally. Intraoperative TEE can also assist in confirming true lumen status and placement of stent grafts.

Adjunctive stenting of branch vessels may also be required to alleviate malperfusion, in combination with proximal tear coverage by TEVAR. Alternatively, endovascular fenestration may be used to equalize the pressure between the true and false lumens, effectively correcting branch vessel malperfusion.[5,6] Achieving a healthy proximal landing zone may require coverage of the left SCA. In the urgent setting, coverage can be done with a low likelihood of immediate complications. However, in the less acute setting, coverage without revascularization should generally not be performed given the higher risk of stroke, spinal cord ischemia, and arm ischemia with coverage. Importantly, those patients with a patent left internal mammary to coronary bypass should have their SCA revascularized before coverage to avoid MI. Those with a functioning dialysis access in the left arm should also have revascularization, as should patients with a dominant left vertebral artery. Postoperative monitoring for extremity ischemia, spinal cord ischemia, and subclavian steal syndrome is important to identify patients who will require postoperative subclavian revascularization. Branched aortic devices allowing for endovascular

left subclavian revascularization at the time of TEVAR are in development and will likely alter the algorithm for subclavian revascularization in the future.

Postoperatively, patients should be allowed permissive HTN to MAPs >80 to encourage spinal cord perfusion, and hypotension should be strictly avoided. Close monitoring with hourly neurologic examinations must be performed to evaluate for spinal cord ischemia. Although this dreaded complication is more common in patients with longer areas of aortic coverage, prior aortic repair, and left SCA coverage, false lumen thrombosis can lead to ischemia in patients deemed to be low risk. Evidence of weakness or paralysis should be immediately treated with spinal drain placement and induced HTN. In less urgent cases, spinal drain placement before TEVAR in patients with a planned long segment aortic coverage is advisable, especially in institutions where emergent placement is not easily obtained leading to delays (for details, see Chapter 86).

After 24 hours of neurologic stability with permissive HTN, patient blood pressure goals may be decreased. Close neurologic monitoring for at least 24 hours in the setting of normotension should be performed, and the transition to oral antihypertensive medications can begin. Finding an effective oral antihypertensive regimen is often challenging and should be a priority before discharge. Indeed, effective blood pressure management is central to long-term management and avoidance of late complications. Importantly, patients should have repeat imaging after TEVAR before discharge whenever possible.

🅤 Open repair

As with TEVAR, the goal of open repair is to reestablish primary true lumen flow. It should be noted that repair of all affected aorta is not necessary and increases the risk of spinal cord ischemia without noted benefit to the patient. In fact, persistent false lumen flow has been documented in nearly half of patients after open repair.[17] Aortic repair should be limited to proximal descending thoracic aorta except in cases of distal rupture or extensive early aneurysmal degeneration.

Repair of the dissected aorta is technically challenging because of the friable and easily injured aortic wall. Finding a healthy proximal clamp site is especially important to prevent retrograde dissection, proximal propagation of intramural hematoma, or clamp injuries to the weakened vessel wall. If a safe proximal clamp site is not identified, consideration should be given to more proximal aortic repair, possibly requiring cardiothoracic surgical involvement with or without circulatory arrest allowing for a clamp-free proximal anastomosis.

Given the high risk of spinal cord ischemia, partial left heart bypass should be strongly considered in all cases of open repair. Because of the difficulties associated with the dissected aorta, clamp times are often prolonged when compared with aneurysmal repairs, increasing the risk for distal malperfusion. In addition, bypasses to branch vessels may be required for full return of normal circulation to the viscera, which will further increase the aortic clamp time.

Reconstruction of the aorta often involves anastomosis to unhealthy tissue, so several methods have been proposed to improve the integrity of these sites. Using felt strips on both the luminal and outer surface of the anastomosis can help prevent tearing and improve hemostasis.[18] Glue aortoplasty can also be used to fuse the dissected layers of distal aorta before surgical anastomosis, strengthening the distal aorta and potentially blocking the flow of blood into the distal false lumen.[19]

REFERENCES

1. Evangelista A, Isselbacher EM, Bossone E, et al; IRAD Investigators. Insights from the international registry of acute aortic dissection: a 20-year experience of collaborative clinical research. *Circulation*. 2018;137(17):1846-1860.
2. Pape LA, Awais M, Woznicki EM, et al. Presentation, diagnosis, and outcomes of acute aortic dissection: 17-year trends from the International Registry of Acute Aortic Dissection. *J Am Coll Cardiol*. 2015;66:350-358.
3. Suzuki T, Isselbacher EM, Nienaber CA, et al. Type-selective benefits of medications in treatment of acute aortic dissection from the International Registry of Acute Aortic Dissection [IRAD]. *Am J Cardiol*. 2012;109:122-127.
4. Hagan PG, Nienaber CA, Isselbacher EM, et al. The International Registry of Acute Aortic Dissection (IRAD): new insights into an old disease. *JAMA*. 2000;283:897-903.
5. Panneton JM, Teh SH, Cherry KJ Jr, et al. Aortic fenestration for acute or chronic aortic dissection: an uncommon but effective procedure. *J Vasc Surg*. 2000;32:711-721.
6. Trimarchi S, Segreti S, Grassi V, et al. Open fenestration for complicated acute aortic B dissection. *Ann Cardiothorac Surg*. 2014;3:418-422.
7. Fattori R, Cao P, De Rango P, et al. Interdisciplinary expert consensus document on management of type B. aortic dissection. *J Am Coll Cardiol*. 2013;61:1661-1678.
8. Fattori R, Montgomery D, Lovato L, et al. Survival after endovascular therapy in patients with type B aortic dissection: a report from the International Registry of Acute Aortic Dissection (IRAD). *JACC Cardiovasc Interv*. 2013;6(8):876-882.
9. Trimarchi S, Eagle KA, Nienaber CA, et al. Importance of refractory pain and hypertension in acute type B aortic dissection insights from the International Registry of Acute Aortic Dissection (IRAD). *Circulation*. 2010; 122(13):1283-1289.
10. Durham C, Aranson NJ, Ergul EA, et al. Aneurysmal degeneration of the thoracoabdominal aorta after medical management of type B aortic dissections. *J Vasc Surg*. 2015;62:900-906.
11. Schwartz SI, Durham C, Clouse WD, et al. Predictors of late aortic intervention in patients with medically treated type B aortic dissection. *J Vasc Surg*. 2018;67(1):78-84.
12. Famularo M, Meyermann K, Lombardi JV. Aneurysmal degeneration of type B aortic dissections after thoracic endovascular aortic repair: a systematic review. *J Vasc Surg*. 2017;66(3):924-930.
13. Lombardi JV, Cambria RP, Nienaber CA. Aortic remodeling after endovascular treatment of complicated type B aortic dissection with the use of a composite device design. *J Vasc Surg*. 2014;59(6):1544-1554.
14. Cambria RP, Crawford RS, Cho J, et al. A multicenter clinical trial of endovascular stent graft repair of acute catastrophes of the descending thoracic aorta. *J Vasc Surg*. 2009;50: 1255-1264.
15. Sobocinski J, Dias NV, Berger L, et al. Endograft repair of complicated acute type B aortic dissections. *Eur J Vasc Endovasc Surg*. 2013;45(5):468-474.
16. Sobocinski J, Lombardi JV, Dias NV. Volume analysis of true and false lumens in acute complicated type B aortic dissections after thoracic endovascular aortic repair with stent grafts alone or with a composite device design. *J Vasc Surg*. 2016;63(5):1216-1224.
17. Safi HJ, Miller CC III, Reardon MJ, et al. Operation for acute and chronic aortic dissection: recent outcome with regard to neurologic deficit and early death. *Ann Thorac Surg*. 1998;66:402-411.
18. Ahmed AA, Mahadevan VS, Webb SW, MacGowan SW. Glue aortoplasty repair of aortic dissection after coronary angioplasty. *Ann Thorac Surg*. 2001;72:922-924.
19. Conrad MF, Cambria RP. Aortic dissection. In: Cronenwett J, Johnston KW, eds. *Rutherford's Vascular Surgery*. Philadelphia, PA: Elsevier Saunders; 2014:chap 138, 2169-2188.

Emanuel R. Tenorio • Gustavo S. Oderich

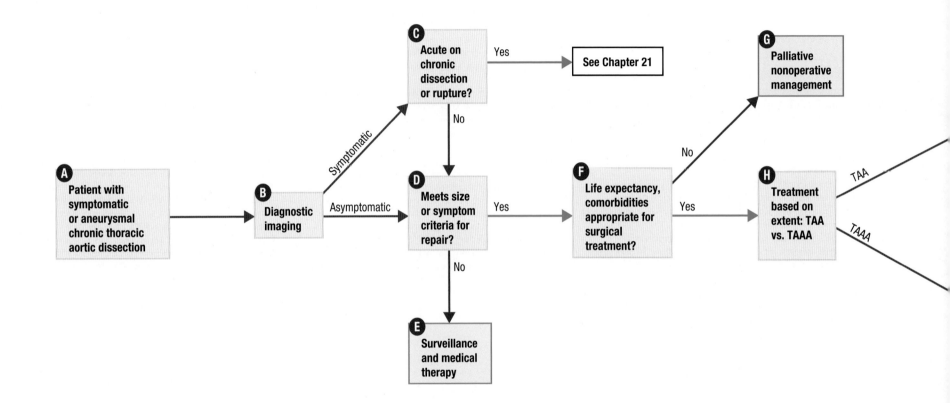

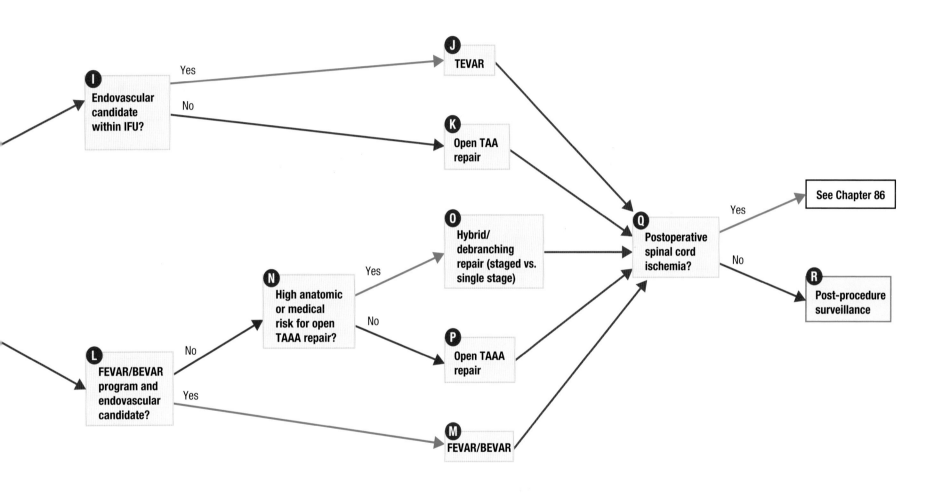

A Patient with symptomatic or aneurysmal chronic thoracic aortic dissection

Medical therapy is the standard initial treatment for all patients with type B aortic dissections and for those who undergo repair of acute type A or complicated dissections. Among survivors of acute dissections, most patients enter the subacute (15-90 days) or chronic phase (>90 days). Although medical treatment is highly effective, chronic dissection can be complicated by progressive aneurysm degeneration, chronic visceral or limb malperfusion, and recurrent pain. The average age of presentation in patients with chronic aortic dissection is 60 years, occurring approximately 10 years after the initial event. The disease affects males predominantly (70%). The risk of late rupture is largely dependent on development of postdissection TAA or TAAA. In the first year after the acute event, 20% to 45% of patients develop aortic enlargement, and 20% require an intervention. At 5 years, 75% of patients develop aortic enlargement and 40% require intervention.[1,2]

Patients with chronic aortic dissection generally follow one of two clinical patterns: those who have an acute dissection and enter the chronic phase or those who are incidentally diagnosed with chronic dissection but have no recollection of an acute event. In the latter group, dissection is usually incidentally diagnosed as mediastinal widening or prominent aortic knob on chest x-ray or by noninvasive cross-sectional imaging of the chest. The exact timing of an incidentally discovered dissection is often difficult to determine; however, careful review of the patient's history for previous acute pain events may help identify the time of the initial presentation. Symptoms are uncommon, but patients may develop local compression due to aortic enlargement (hoarseness and chest or back pain), chronic malperfusion syndrome (intestinal angina, claudication, or renal function deterioration), or acute chest pain indicating progression of dissection (acute on chronic) or rupture.

The extent of aortic dissection is defined using one of two accepted classification schemes.[3,4] The DeBakey system is based on the location of the primary intimal tear and the distal extension of dissection flap into the thoracic or thoracoabdominal aorta:

- DeBakey I: the dissection originates in the ascending aorta and propagates distally to include at least the aortic arch and descending aorta, more often extending into the abdominal aorta.
- DeBakey II: dissection is isolated to the ascending aorta.
- DeBakey IIIA: dissection originates in the descending thoracic aorta and propagates distally to the level of the diaphragm.
- DeBakey IIIB: dissection originates in the descending thoracic aorta and propagates distally into the abdominal aorta and iliac arteries.

The Stanford system divides dissections into only two categories, including those that involve the ascending aorta (*Stanford A*) and those that do not involve the ascending aorta and are primarily located distal to the left SCA (*Stanford B*), or involve the aortic arch without the ascending aorta. This chapter focuses on the management of chronic dissections that involve the thoracic or thoracoabdominal aorta (*DeBakey I or III*).

Post-dissection TAAs or TAAAs are further classified using the same classification as for thoracic aortic degenerative aneurysms.[5,6] TAAs are classified depending on extent above or below the level of the sixth thoracic vertebra into type A (proximal to T6), type B (distal to T6), and type C (entire thoracic aorta). For TAAAs, the classification proposed by E. Stanley Crawford[5] is utilized:

- Extent I TAAA: starting at the proximal thoracic aorta (above T6) and extending distally to the level of the renal arteries, but not into the infrarenal aorta
- Extent II TAAA: starting at the proximal thoracic aorta (above T6) and extending distally to the infrarenal aorta or iliac arteries
- Extent III TAAA: starting at the distal thoracic aorta (below T6) and extending distally to the renal arteries (Safi[6] extent V) or to the infrarenal aorta and iliac arteries (Safi extent III)
- Extent IV TAAA: starting at the diaphragmatic hiatus or CA and extending distally into the abdominal aorta or iliac arteries

B Diagnostic imaging

The entire aorta should be imaged with precontrast, contrast, and delayed images to define the extent of dissection, presence of calcification, and delayed flow patterns in a false lumen (FL). The angulated geometry of the aorta requires that measurements are made in planes perpendicular to the centerline of flow to determine the shape and diameter of the aorta in each segment. Meticulous side-by-side measurements and comparison with serial examinations are most useful to determine growth and exclude random error of an individual measurement. Multidetector CTA is our preferred imaging modality if the patient does not have CKD preventing use of contrast. In patients with acute symptoms, CTA is used to detect potential rupture, which requires emergent management.[7]

MRI/MRA is preferred in some centers to avoid radiation exposure or use of iodinated contrast. Gadolinium-enhanced sequences can be performed to differentiate slow flow from thrombus in the FL. Dynamic studies and four-dimensional (4D) MRA offer advantages of assessment of flow pattern between true lumen (TL) and FL and accurate visualization of re-entrance sites and dynamic obstruction by dissection flap motion.[8,9]

The most important strategic decision on planning any open surgical or endovascular aortic repair is selection of the proximal and distal anastomotic sites or landing zones, respectively. For open repair, the aortic clamp should be placed in normal or minimally ectatic segments relatively free of calcification or thrombus. Endovascular sealing should be obtained in normal segments to avoid endoleak or progression of aortic disease with continued neck enlargement that universally occurs after placement of self-expandable stent grafts.[10] Areas of the aorta that have severe tortuosity or appear noncylindrical and segments that contain atheromatous debris, thrombus, or calcification are not considered safe regions to clamp, sew a graft, or to fix and seal endovascular devices.

Extension of the dissection into the abdominal aorta is very common, affecting the origin of the renal-mesenteric arteries. Compression of the TL needs to be assessed as well as potential dynamic obstruction of vessels by the intimal flap. It is important to characterize the vessel origin with respect to the TL or FL.[11,12] The presence of occlusive or aneurysmal disease in the branch vessel should be noted, along with any extension of the dissection flap into the branch itself.

Planning fenestrated and branched stent grafts to incorporate aortic side branches requires precise measurement of the distance between the center of each aortic branch ostium using centerline of flow.[7,10] The radial position of the branch ostium is also assessed and described in relation to a clock position, angle (0°-360°), or using an arc length from the 12 o'clock position.[7,10]

C Acute on chronic dissection or rupture?

Most patients with chronic aortic dissections are asymptomatic. Symptoms, when present, indicate local compression, rapid enlargement, acute on chronic dissection, or a ruptured aneurysm. Chest and upper thoracic back pain are the most common symptoms. Rarely, dysphagia or dyspnea can occur from mass effect into the esophagus or bronchi, respectively. A ruptured aneurysm presents with acute chest or back pain, with or without associated hypotension due to hemorrhage into the pleural space or pericardium. An aortoesophageal fistula may manifest as GI hemorrhage. An unusual manifestation is hemoptysis from erosion into the left main stem bronchus.[13] Patients with chronic aortic dissection can also develop acute extension or expansion causing symptoms of acute dissection (see Chapter 21). Given that these patients have failed medical treatment and present with a recurrent event, repair is indicated after an expedited initial evaluation. Patients with acute on chronic dissection or rupture are managed as an acute primary dissection, which is discussed in detail in Chapter 21.

D Meets size or symptom criteria for repair?

Three society guidelines have outlined the evolution of treatment of acute and chronic dissections, with the 2017 Guidelines of the European Society for Vascular Surgery being most contemporary.[13-15] The goal of chronic aortic dissection treatment is to prevent or treat rupture. Repair is indicated in patients with symptoms, impending rupture, ruptured aneurysms, and in those with large or rapidly expanding aneurysms.

The risk of aortic rupture among patients with chronic aortic dissection is determined by the diameter of the postdissection aneurysm, rate of enlargement, morphology, and presence of genetically triggered aortic disorders (GENTADs). Estimation of risk is based on retrospective natural history and population-based studies that do not differentiate degenerative and postdissection aortic aneurysms. The average rate of expansion of TAAs is estimated to be 1 to 4 mm/y. Aortic-related complications occur in 20% to 50% of patients with chronic dissections.[13] Overall, approximately 20% to 40% of patients have enlargement of the FL and total aortic diameter necessitating repair, and 25% of all TAAs/TAAAs are of chronic postdissection etiology.[16] Factors associated with late aneurysm degeneration include HTN, aortic diameter > 40 mm in the acute phase, proximal entry tear >10 mm, FL diameter > 22 mm, COPD, patency, or only partial thrombosis of the FL. Conversely, complete FL thrombosis has been associated with slower aortic enlargement or aortic remodeling.[17]

Elective repair is considered if the risk of aneurysm rupture is significantly higher than the risk of operative death or major complications (stroke, paralysis, and dialysis). The last guidelines of the ACCF/AHA recommended elective repair for patients with chronic dissections with thoracic aortic diameter exceeding 55 mm, particularly if associated with GENTADs.[14] For TAAAs, the recommended diameter was 60 mm, or less in patients with Marfan or Loeys-Dietz syndromes. The European guidelines recommended repair of chronic dissections in patients with ≥60 mm of total aortic diameter or a rate of enlargement >10 mm/y, and in those with chronic symptoms of malperfusion syndrome or recurrent pain.[13,15]

E Surveillance and medical therapy

Aggressive medical therapy and close surveillance of the aorta remains of paramount importance in patients with chronic dissection who do not meet criteria for elective repair. One study showed that 80% of patients treated with β-blockers were free from aortic events at a mean of 4 years, compared to 47% of patients treated using other antihypertensive medications.[18] Blood pressure goals include a systolic below 130 mm Hg and diastolic below 85 mm Hg. Because 40% to 70% of late deaths among patients with chronic dissections are due to cardiovascular events (mainly heart disease and stroke), emphasis should be on modification of cardiovascular risk factors. As such, antiplatelet and statin therapy are recommended for primary prevention of cardiovascular events.

A conservative approach with surveillance is recommended in patients with smaller aneurysms who do not meet the minimum criteria for repair and in those patients who have limited life expectancy or are deemed high risk for any type of repair. Sequential imaging with serial CT or MRI is indicated in patients who are potential candidates for future repair.

F Life expectancy, comorbidities appropriate for surgical treatment?

A comprehensive evaluation of cardiac (see Chapter 1), pulmonary (see Chapter 2), and renal function is crucial to optimize patient selection for potential surgical treatment. Patients with chronic dissection are often elderly and high risk, so it is important to determine not only the operative risk but also the anticipated long-term survival depending on other medical comorbidities. Medical optimization is needed before entertaining surgical repair.

Approximately one-third of patients with chronic aortic dissection have renovascular involvement by either occlusive disease or the dissection flap. Open surgical repair carries excessive high risk in patients with advanced stages of CKD, and should generally not be considered in any patient with stage IV or V (dialysis dependent). Endovascular repair can be considered even in patients with advanced stages of CKD, whereas the higher risk of mortality and potential risk of progression to dialysis should be thoroughly discussed with the patient.

Genetic evaluation is recommended in younger patients or in those with familial history or phenotypic features, because GENTADS are best managed with open surgical repair. These disorders are autosomal dominant and are strongest in the younger patient population affected by aortic dissection or aneurysm. Clinically relevant disorders include Marfan, Turner, vascular Ehlers-Danlos, and Loeys-Dietz syndromes. The most common mutations are noted in the fibrillin (*FBN1*) or TGF-receptor 2 genes (*TGFBR2*) in Marfan and Loyes-Dietz syndromes, respectively. The most common nonsyndromic mutation associated with TAAs and dissections is in the SMC actin gene (*ACTA2*).[19]

G Palliative nonoperative management

Nonoperative treatment is indicated in patients with chronic aortic dissection who have limited life expectancy because of comorbidities, or when the risks of the operative procedure outweigh benefits because of anatomic or clinical factors. The most common problems are associated malignancy, advanced CHF, ischemic cardiomyopathy with nonreconstructed CAD, severe COPD, CKD requiring chronic dialysis, or CKD. In these patients, 1- and 2-year survival is limited.

H Treatment based on extent: TAA vs. TAAA

Treatment selection continues to evolve and should take into consideration the patient's clinical risk, the extent of the dissection, and the presence of suitable landing zones for stent-graft placement. In general, open surgical repair continues to be the first line of treatment for younger patients with GENTADs, except for those who present with ruptured aneurysms where endovascular therapy can sometimes be used as a bridge for open surgical repair. Although open surgical repair is considered the primary method of treatment in lower risk patients in some centers, endovascular repair has been increasingly used in patients who are intermediate or higher risk for open repair and may be considered in any patient who has a suitable proximal landing zone, regardless of surgical risk. The main advantage of endovascular repair is lower rates of mortality, stroke, paraplegia, and dialysis compared to open surgical repair. The European guidelines acknowledged that TEVAR and open surgical repair are suitable options, and that the optimal treatment remains unclear. More recently, the ESVS guidelines issued a class IIa (level of evidence C) recommendation for TEVAR in patients who are considered intermediate or high risk for open repair.[13-15]

There are no prospective randomized comparisons between TEVAR and open surgical repair for chronic dissections, and therefore treatment recommendations are based on large single-center experiences. Contemporary series of open surgical repair in large aortic centers show an operative mortality of 6% to 11%, with spinal cord ischemia (SCI) in 4% to 12% of patients. In the past decade, endovascular repair has been increasingly utilized and is currently an accepted alternative to open repair. TEVAR for chronic dissection has an operative mortality of 3%, stroke rate of 0.8%, and SCI rate of 0.4%.[13]

Treatment strategies for endovascular repair differ depending on extent of dissection and aneurysm involvement. The primary goals of therapy are to divert blood flow into the TL with coverage of the entry tear, leading to thrombosis of the FL. This strategy is different for TAAs and TAAAs.

I Endovascular candidate within IFU?

The proximal thoracic aorta or distal arch is most commonly affected by enlargement in the chronic phase of dissection resulting in TAA. Although some patients have dissections isolated to the thoracic aorta, the majority has distal extension of the dissection flap into the abdominal aorta, which may be relatively normal in diameter. An accepted strategy in these patients is to limit the surgical resection or endovascular repair to the aortic segment at risk of rupture or late complication, which is often the proximal thoracic aorta, leaving dissection in the abdomen untreated. In the case of open repair or isolated thoracic dissection, complete aneurysm exclusion can be achieved, whereas this is often not the case in patients treated using TEVAR.

The primary requirement for TEVAR is the presence of a suitable proximal landing zone. Approximately 60% of the patients have involvement of the left SCA, requiring extension of sealing into zones 1 or 2.[14] In these patients, left SCA revascularization is recommended using carotid-subclavian bypass or subclavian transposition. Worldwide, five thoracic stent grafts currently have indications for aortic dissection: Bolton Relay Plus, Conformable GORE TAG, Cook Zenith Dissection Endovascular Stent, Medtronic Valiant, and E-vita Thoracic 3G stent grafts. Current IFU of these devices cover aortic diameter ranges from 16 to 42 mm, with a minimum proximal sealing zone of 20 mm. Distal sealing zone is not a requirement for treatment of chronic dissections, given that the repair is extended into the TL.

J TEVAR

The principles of TEVAR for chronic aortic dissections include exclusion of the proximal entry tear with redirection of flow predominantly into the TL. Contrary to acute or subacute dissections where complete remodeling of the aorta is often achieved, this is not an expected outcome with chronic dissections due to fibrosis and hardening of the aortic wall. For chronic dissections, the expected goal of TEVAR is to achieve thrombosis of the FL in the thoracic aorta alongside the stented segment and stabilization of the aneurysmal aortic segment to prevent rupture.[20] Therefore, it is expected that there will usually be persistent FL flow in the distal aortic segment if it is not covered by the thoracic stent graft because of the presence of reentrance tears.

Planning needs to be completed preoperatively with selection of all anticipated modular devices. Each of the commercially available endografts has identified minimum length and diameter requirements for the proximal and distal landing zones, which are available in the IFU. There are important differences in TEVAR planning between acute and chronic dissections. Although the stent graft should be minimally oversized for acute dissection (5%-10%), in patients with chronic dissection, the device diameter is selected on the basis of the aortic diameter in the proximal landing zone with oversizing of 10% to 20%, similar to degenerative aneurysms. The length of the stent graft for acute dissection usually covers the proximal to mid portion of the thoracic aorta, averaging 15 to 20 cm in length. For chronic dissections, it is recommended that the entire descending thoracic aorta be treated by the stent graft, from the left SCA to just above the celiac axis, usually requiring a minimum of two stent grafts. Cervical debranching (eg, carotid-subclavian bypass) or total arch repair (eg, frozen elephant trunk technique) may be needed in patients with arch involvement to provide a suitable proximal landing zone for the thoracic stent graft.

The risk of SCI is generally low in patients treated using TEVAR for DeBakey I or IIIb dissections because of persistent flow into the FL distal to the repair. Therefore, we have not used CSF drainage in these patients and only recommend routine placement of CSF drainage in patients with DeBakey IIIa chronic dissections that have complete aneurysm exclusion by stent graft or in those requiring TAAA repair with fenestrated-branched stent grafts.

Endovascular aortic repair is performed in a hybrid operating room with bilateral percutaneous femoral access, using the side not involved by dissection or with access to the TL for placement of the aortic device. The use of onlay fusion CTA assists with identification of anatomic landmarks and may decrease use of contrast or radiation.[21] It is important to confirm that the initial guidewire is located within the TL throughout the entire aortic length, which is best done using IVUS. SBP is decreased to 90 to 100 mm Hg while the stent graft is deployed in the proximal landing zone. The repair usually needs to be extended distally to the level of the celiac axis, which requires placement of a second stent graft. Because the second stent graft rarely achieves distal seal at the celiac level, the distal diameter is not relevant and should ideally be around 30 mm to facilitate future visceral aortic repair with a fenestrated or branched stent graft if needed.[10] The proximal landing zone and any attachment sites are gently dilated, but we do not recommend dilatation of the distal third of the stented segment to avoid tearing the dissection septum at the termination of the stent causing a large reentrance into the FL. This approach rarely affects flow into the renal-mesenteric vessels, even when one or more vessels originate from the FL because of the presence of reentrance tears.

K Open TAA repair

Open repair should be considered in patients with TAA from chronic dissection who are good or intermediate surgical risk and do not meet anatomic requirements for TEVAR. It is also the recommended treatment option in most patients with GENTADs or those younger than 55 years of age. In most patients, the chronic dissection results in enlargement of the proximal thoracic aorta with relatively normal diameter in the abdominal aorta. In these patients, a left posterolateral thoracotomy via the fourth to fifth intercostal space is usually sufficient to expose the thoracic aorta, and division of the diaphragmatic muscle or extension into the abdomen is not necessary. Distal protection can be secured using left heart bypass or the repair can be performed using deep hypothermia and circulatory arrest with cardiopulmonary bypass.

L FEVAR/BEVAR program and endovascular candidate?

Patients with TAAAs require more extensive repair with revascularization of the renal-mesenteric vessels using open, hybrid, or total endovascular approaches. Although fenestrated and branched (FEVAR/BEVAR) stent grafts have gained acceptance, access to these devices is currently limited to a few sites with dedicated aortic programs and ongoing physician-sponsored investigational device exemption studies. In centers with access to the FEVAR/BEVAR program, this option should be considered in all patients who are anatomic candidates and have no evidence of GENTADs. For placement of bridging stents during fenestrated and branched stent grafts, minimum branch vessel requirements are diameters from 4 to 11 mm and absence of early vessel bifurcation (<13 mm).

M FEVAR/BEVAR

The technique FEVAR/BEVAR for treating chronic dissection varies with the specific stent-graft device design. General aspects of the procedure are similar to that of TEVAR for TAA (see J.) The graft delivery system of patient-specific, low-profile, fenestrated-branched stent grafts has four preloaded guidewires for the celiac axis, SMA, and renal arteries. These can be tailored for access via the brachial or femoral approach. The authors' preference is to use brachial access to leverage the limited space in the compressed TL using a staggered deployment technique. The repair is then extended distally with a universal bifurcated device and iliac limb extensions, and flow is restored to the lower extremities if the patient has any changes in neuromonitoring or near-infrared spectroscopy (NIRS). Sequential stenting is performed first for the renal arteries, followed by the SMA and celiac axis. Selection of bridging stent is usually balloon-expandable covered stents for fenestrations and self-expandable or balloon-expandable covered stents for directional branches.

The risk of SCI is high with total endovascular repair of extents I and II TAAAs (10%-20%), intermediate with extent III TAAAs (5%-10%), and low with extent IV TAAAs (1%-3%). Therefore, we apply a standardized protocol to reduce risk of SCI in all patients undergoing endovascular extent I or II TAAA repair, including staged repair, blood pressure management, CSF drainage, neuromonitoring, and limb perfusion, as appropriate.[22,23]

Staging of the repair is recommended to promote development of collateral networks to the spinal cord by avoiding simultaneous coverage of all intercostal arteries. The first-stage procedure is TEVAR to just above the celiac axis. As part of the first-stage repair, any cervical debranching or permanent iliofemoral conduit is done if needed. The second-stage procedure is performed 1 week to 2 months after the first stage, depending on availability of the patient-specific stent.

It is important to maintain adequate blood pressure during the procedure to reduce the risk of SCI. Calcium channel blockers and angiotensin inhibitors are discontinued a week before the TAAA repair if possible and slowly restarted postoperatively to avoid hypotension. The MAP is targeted at ≥80 mm Hg intraoperatively and for the first 72 hours after the operation. If there are changes in neuromonitoring detected during the operation or neurologic changes observed postoperatively, MAP goals are increased to 100 mm Hg. In addition, transfusion of blood products is indicated in the first 48 hours after the procedure to keep a target hemoglobin ≥10 mg/dL and a normal coagulation profile until the spinal drain is removed, if present.

A CSF drain is placed preoperatively in all patients with extents I and II TAAAs. Intraoperative neuromonitoring with continuous motor-evoked potential (MEP) and somatosensory-evoked potential (SSEP) is used routinely by the authors. A ≥75% reduction from baseline-evoked potential amplitude is considered significant. Immediate recognition of ischemia using neuromonitoring allows use of maneuvers to rescue the spinal cord perfusion. These maneuvers include increments in target MAP, increase in CSF drainage, and restoration of blood flow to the pelvis and lower extremities.[24] If despite the maneuvers MEP changes persist, the repair can be left incomplete with temporary aneurysm sac perfusion via the celiac branch or contralateral limb of the bifurcated stent graft.

In those who do not have any postoperative signs of SCI, have the CSF drain clamped. In those with symptoms, CSF drainage is indicated and the drain is left open with a baseline CSF pressure of 10 mm Hg for 15 minutes every hour. A maximum drainage of 20 mL/h is allowed, after which the drain is reclamped for the remaining of the hour. A maximum of 150 mL of CSF drainage is accepted for a 24-hour period. If there are changes in neuromonitoring or neurologic examination, the CSF pressure may be titrated down to 5 mm Hg or even 0 mm Hg, with careful attention to avoid excessive drainage or any blood in the CSF. CSF drainage is continued for 48 hours and the drain is removed in patients who have stable hemodynamics, NIRS, and neurologic examination after a 6-hour clamping trial. It is critical that coagulation profile be normal upon removal. If there are neurologic symptoms after removal, epidural hematoma should be rapidly ruled out by spinal cord imaging and a new drain should be placed within 1 hour.

N High anatomic or medical risk for open TAAA repair?

If patients are not candidates for FEVAR/BEVAR, they are evaluated for potential open TAAA repair versus hybrid TEVAR with visceral renal artery debranching. Surgical risk is primarily determined by evaluating their cardiac (see Chapter 1), pulmonary (see Chapter 2), and renal function, as with any major open vascular operation. Functional status, frailty, and other chronic disease must also be assessed to determine whether open TAAA can be safely performed. In some cases, anatomic factors may influence the decision between potential hybrid/debranching and full open TAAA repair. Severe pulmonary disease may favor hybrid repair that avoids thoracotomy, whereas lack of an appropriate infrarenal aortic or iliac donor site for debranching would preclude such an approach. Other anatomic factors such as prior abdominal or retroperitoneal surgery, abdominal wall hernia, obesity, and prior left chest surgery may influence this decision.

Open repair of TAAAs continues to carry significant risk of morbidity and mortality in most centers. Even in centers of excellence, mortality rate averages 5% to 10% in most series. Hybrid/debranching repair was introduced as a means to reduce the magnitude of the operation by avoiding thoracotomy, division of the diaphragmatic muscle, and, in most cases, aortic cross-clamping. Nonetheless, mortality of hybrid approach averages 15% in systematic reviews, with worse outcomes in higher risk patients.[25] Therefore, endovascular repair has been used whenever possible in patients who are anatomic candidates and do not have GENTADs.

O Hybrid/debranching repair (staged vs. single stage)

In centers without access to FEVAR/BEVAR, high-risk patients are considered for hybrid endovascular or complete surgical repair. In hybrid cases, a staged approach is preferred whenever possible. Four-vessel debranching of the celiac, SMA, and renal arteries is usually performed using midline laparotomy or retroperitoneal approach. Extra-anatomic bypass can be based on the iliac arteries, distal aorta, or one of the visceral arteries (eg, splenic, hepatic). The authors' preference is to use a polyester graft originating in the distal common or external iliac artery. The graft is covered with omentum to avoid erosion into the intestine. A second-stage procedure is then planned using thoracic and/or abdominal stent grafts with off-label indication. Several centers have used techniques of parallel stent grafts (referred to as chimneys, periscope, or sandwich) because of limited access to fenestrated and branched endografts. Problems with this technique include a higher risk of endoleaks from gutters along the chimney graft and potential risk of stroke due to multiple transbrachial sheaths. Independent of which technique is used (eg, FEVAR-BEVAR, hybrid, or parallel grafts), we consider patients with extents I to III TAAAs at higher risk of SCI. Therefore, the same measures outlined earlier for FEVAR/BEVAR are followed for hybrid or parallel stent-graft techniques (see M).

P Open TAAA repair

Open repair of chronic dissections follows the same principles already described (see Chapter 20), with emphasis on organ protection using adjunctive techniques. Most centers use intraoperative CSF drainage and left heart bypass with moderate hypothermia. Because these patients are often young and have extensive aortic branch vessel involvement and GENTADs, our approach has evolved in the past decade to allow replacement of the entire aorta with separate branch reconstruction while avoiding island or patch reconstructions. Patients are routinely treated by a dedicated team comprised of cardiac and vascular surgeons. Our approach evolved to routine use of deep hypothermia with cardiopulmonary arrest, allowing longer time for reconstruction with better organ protection and lower rates of SCI and dialysis.[26] Although we recognize that some centers avoid deep hypothermia because of coagulopathy and higher reported mortality rates, our mortality using this approach has been 11%.[27] The aorta is reconstructed using separate branches for the celiac, SMA, and left renal arteries. The right renal artery is usually reimplanted into the aortic graft or reconstructed with a separate branch. Large pairs of intercostal arteries are reimplanted as a patch, away from the renal-mesenteric bypasses to allow future coverage by stent graft if there is degeneration.

Q Postoperative spinal cord ischemia?

SCI is the most devastating complication of thoracic aortic repair. Overall, 30-day and 36-month survival in those developing SCI were 92% and 45%, respectively. In those patients who do not have resolution of their symptoms, 3-month survival is reduced from 92% to 36%.[28] If a patient develops symptoms of SCI following open or endovascular repair, immediate measures are recommended to rescue or prevent progression of injury (see Chapter 86).

R Postprocedure surveillance

Surveillance after repair of chronic aortic dissection is dependent on the type of repair. Patients treated by FEVAR/BEVAR follow a strict surveillance protocol which includes CTA of the chest, abdomen, and pelvis and DUS of the renal and mesenteric stents at 2 months, 6 months, and annually thereafter. For patients treated by TEVAR or hybrid procedures, surveillance consists of CTA at 1 to 2 months, 6 months, and annually. Among patients treated using open surgical repair, follow-up includes CTA at 1 to 2 months, 1 year, 3 years, 5 years, and at 10 years. Surveillance imaging is obtained more frequently in patients who have recurrent aneurysms or symptoms.

REFERENCES
1. Nienaber CA, Kische S, Rousseau H, et al. Endovascular repair of type B aortic dissection: long-term results of the randomized investigation of stent grafts in aortic dissection trial. *Circ Cardiovasc Interv.* 2013;6(4):407-416.
2. Hughes GC. Management of acute type B aortic dissection; ADSORB trial. *J Thorac Cardiovasc Surg.* 2015;149(2):S158-S162.
3. Debakey ME, Henly WS, Cooley DA, Morris GC Jr, Crawford ES, Beall AC Jr. Surgical management of dissecting aneurysms of the aorta. *J Thorac Cardiovasc Surg.* 1965;49:130-149.
4. Daily PO, Trueblood HW, Stinson EB, Wuerflein RD, Shumway NE. Management of acute aortic dissections. *Ann Thorac Surg.* 1970;10:237-247.
5. Crawford ES, Coselli JS. Thoracoabdominal aneurysm surgery. *Semin Thorac Cardiovasc Surg.* 1991;3(4):300-322.
6. Safi HJ, Miller CC III. Spinal cord protection in descending thoracic and thoracoabdominal aortic repair. *Ann Thorac Surg.* 1999;67(6):1937-1939.
7. Vrtiska TJ, Macedo TA, Oderich GS. *Computed Tomography/Computed Tomography Angiography for Evaluation, Planning, and Surveillance of Complex Endovascular Repair.* New York, NY: Springer; 2017:149-188.
8. François CJ, Markl M, Schiebler ML, et al. Four-dimensional, flow-sensitive magnetic resonance imaging of blood flow patterns in thoracic aortic dissections. *J Thorac Cardiovasc Surg.* 2013;145(5):1359-1366.
9. Wang Y, Alkasab TK, Narin O, et al. Incidence of nephrogenic systemic fibrosis after adoption of restrictive gadolinium-based contrast agent guidelines. *Radiology.* 2011;260(1):105-111.
10. Ribeiro M, Macedo T, Vrtiska T, Oderich G. Planning endovascular aortic repair with standard and fenestrated-branched endografts. *J Cardiovasc Surg.* 2017;58(2):204-217.
11. Verhoeven EL, Paraskevas KI, Oikonomou K, et al. Fenestrated and branched stent-grafts to treat post-dissection chronic aortic aneurysms after initial treatment in the acute setting. *J Endovasc Ther.* 2012;19(3):343-349.

12. Spear R, Sobocinski J, Settembre N, et al. Early experience of endovascular repair of post-dissection aneurysms involving the thoraco-abdominal aorta and the arch. *Eur J Vasc Endovasc Surg*. 2016;51(4):488-497.

13. Riambau V, Böckler D, Brunkwall J, et al. Editor's choice—management of descending thoracic aorta diseases: clinical practice guidelines of the European Society for Vascular Surgery (ESVS). *Eur J Vasc Endovasc Surg*. 2017;53(1):4-52.

14. Hiratzka LF, Bakris GL, Beckman JA, et al. 2010 ACCF/AHA/AATS/ACR/ASA/SCA/SCAI/SIR/STS/SVM Guidelines for the diagnosis and management of patients with thoracic aortic disease. *J Am Coll Cardiol*. 2010;55(14):e27-e129.

15. Erbel R, Aboyans V, Boileau C, et al. 2014 ESC Guidelines on the diagnosis and treatment of aortic diseases: document covering acute and chronic aortic diseases of the thoracic and abdominal aorta of the adult The Task Force for the Diagnosis and Treatment of Aortic Diseases of the European Society of Cardiology (ESC). *Eur Heart J*. 2014;35(41):2873-2926.

16. Marui A, Mochizuki T, Mitsui N, Koyama T, Kimura F, Horibe M. Toward the best treatment for uncomplicated patients with type B acute aortic dissection. *Circulation*. 1999;100(suppl 2):II275-II280.

17. Immer FF, Krähenbühl E, Hagen U, et al. Large area of the false lumen favors secondary dilatation of the aorta after acute type A aortic dissection. *Circulation*. 2005;112(9 suppl):I249-I252.

18. Genoni M, Paul M, Jenni R, Graves K, Seifert B, Turina M. Chronic β-blocker therapy improves outcome and reduces treatment costs in chronic type B aortic dissection. *Eur J Cardiothorac Surg*. 2001;19(5):606-610.

19. Albornoz G, Coady MA, Roberts M, et al. Familial thoracic aortic aneurysms and dissections—incidence, modes of inheritance, and phenotypic patterns. *Ann Thorac Surg*. 2006;82(4):1400-1405.

20. Conrad MF, Chung TK, Cambria MR, Paruchuri V, Brady TJ, Cambria RP. Effect of chronic dissection on early and late outcomes after descending thoracic and thoracoabdominal aneurysm repair. *J Vasc Surg*. 2011;53(3):600-607.

21. Tenorio ER, Oderich GS, Sandri GA, et al. Impact of onlay fusion and cone beam computed tomography on radiation exposure and technical assessment of fenestrated-branched endovascular aortic repair. *J Vasc Surg*. 2019;69:1045.e3-1058.e3.

22. Banga PV, Oderich GS, Reis de Souza L, et al. Neuromonitoring, cerebrospinal fluid drainage, and selective use of iliofemoral conduits to minimize risk of spinal cord injury during complex endovascular aortic repair. *J Endovasc Ther*. 2016;23(1):139-149.

23. Tenorio ER, Eagleton MJ, Karkkainen JM, Oderich GS. Prevention of spinal cord injury during endovascular thoracoabdominal repair. *J Cardiovasc Surg (Torino)*. 2019;60:54-65.

24. Maurel B, Delclaux N, Sobocinski J, et al. The impact of early pelvic and lower limb reperfusion and attentive peri-operative management on the incidence of spinal cord ischemia during thoracoabdominal aortic aneurysm endovascular repair. *Eur J Vasc Endovasc Surg*. 2015;49(3):248-254.

25. Bakoyiannis C, Kalles V, Economopoulos K, Georgopoulos S, Tsigris C, Papalambros E. Hybrid procedures in the treatment of thoracoabdominal aortic aneurysms: a systematic review. *J Endovasc Ther*. 2009;16(4):443-450.

26. Huang Y, Gloviczki P, Oderich GS, et al. Outcome after open and endovascular repairs of abdominal aortic aneurysms in matched cohorts using propensity score modeling. *J Vasc Surg*. 2015;62(2):304.e2-311.e2.

27. Gifford E, Kalra M, Pochettino A, et al. PC004 Early and late results of reconstruction with renal and visceral bypasses during open thoracoabdominal aortic aneurysm repair. *J Vasc Surg*. 2017;65(6):142S.

28. Estrera AL, Sandhu HK, Charlton-Ouw KM, et al. A quarter century of organ protection in open thoracoabdominal repair. *Ann Surg*. 2015;262(4):660-668.

Anne Burdess • Kevin Mani

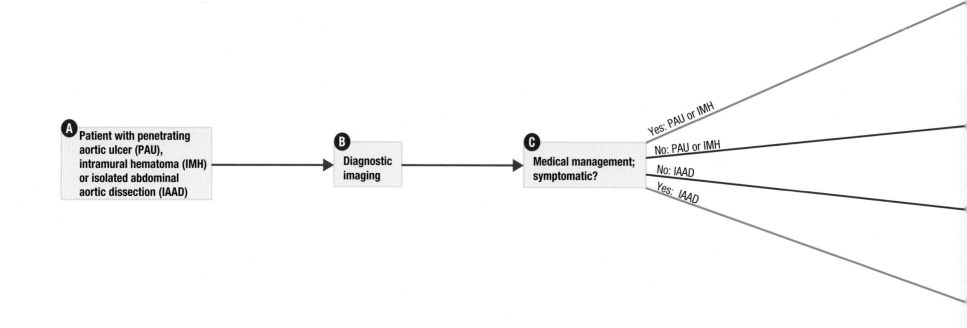

A Patient with penetrating aortic ulcer (PAU), intramural hematoma (IMH) or isolated abdominal aortic dissection (IAAD)

B Diagnostic imaging

C Medical management; symptomatic?

Yes: PAU or IMH

No: PAU or IMH

No: IAAD

Yes: IAAD

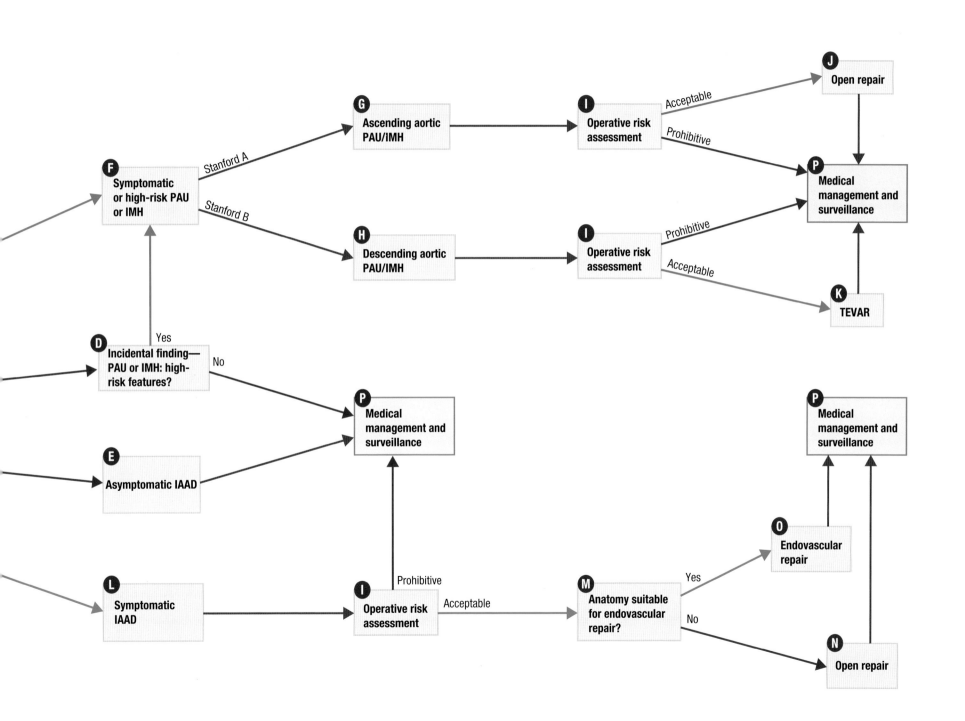

A **Patient with penetrating aortic ulcer, intramural hematoma, or isolated abdominal aortic dissection**

Advances in high-resolution imaging have identified important variants of classic aortic dissection. Acute aortic syndrome (AAS) refers to a group of conditions with similar anatomic and clinical characteristics. They include classic acute aortic dissection (AAD), intramural hematoma (IMH), and penetrating aortic ulcer (PAU). Traumatic aortic injury and isolated abdominal aortic dissection (IAAD) are also often included in this heterogeneous group. All entities involve disruption of the media of the aorta and likely represent different stages of the same pathologic process. Ultimately, all presentations can lead to aneurysm formation and/or aortic rupture and death. The true incidence of AAS is difficult to define because the diagnosis is frequently missed on initial presentation. However, the prevalence of this aortic pathology appears to be increasing.[1] AAD is by far the most common pathology causing AAS (see Chapter 21).

PAU is defined as an ulceration of an atherosclerotic plaque that penetrates through the aortic intima resulting in hematoma within the aortic wall. PAU represents 2% to 7% of AAS cases.[2]

IMH is defined as the presence of blood within the aortic wall without an identifiable entry point on imaging. The exact etiology is unknown, but it has been proposed to arise from hemorrhage of the vasa vasorum located within the medial layer or from microscopic tears in the aortic intima.[3,4] Approximately 10% to 20% of patients with a clinical picture of dissection exhibit IMH on imaging.

IAAD comprises a subgroup of aortic dissections accounting for <1.5% of all AADs.[5] The entry tear generally originates below or at the level of the renal arteries (82%). The etiology can be spontaneous, iatrogenic, or traumatic.

B **Diagnostic imaging**

CTA is the technique of choice for diagnosis of PAU. The characteristic finding is localized ulceration, penetrating through the aortic intima into the aortic wall in the mid- to distal third of the descending thoracic aorta. Focal thickening or high attenuation of the adjacent aortic wall suggests associated IMH.

An unenhanced CT acquisition is crucial for the diagnosis of IMH. A high-attenuation crescentic thickening of the aorta, extending in a longitudinal, nonspiral manner, is the hallmark of IMH. In contrast to AAD, the aortic lumen is preserved, and no intimal flap or enhancement of the aortic wall is seen after administration of contrast. IMH is also generally more localized than is classic dissection. Using CT, the combination of unenhanced followed by contrast-enhanced acquisition yields a sensitivity as high as 96% for detection of IMH.[3] Infrequently, however, the differentiation of IMH from aortic plaque, thrombus, or a thrombosed dissection may be difficult using CT. In those circumstances, MRI may provide additional differentiation of the aortic wall tissues and the age of a hematoma.

In IAAD, CTA remains the gold standard, but DUS of the abdomen can reveal the intimal flap with a sensitivity and specificity of up to 80% and 100%, respectively.[6]

C **Medical management; symptomatic?**

The aim of treatment is to prevent progression to complicated dissection, aneurysm formation, aortic rupture, and death. All patients require the same aggressive anti-impulse therapy to optimize blood pressure and heart rate as in aortic dissection (see Chapter 21), and this treatment should be lifelong. In the acute phase, SBP between 100 and 120 mm Hg is a widely accepted goal.[7] Additional evidence has demonstrated an improved outcome with a heart rate of <60 bpm.[8] IV b-adrenergic receptor blockers usually constitute the first-line treatment with IV calcium channel blockers, a second-line option. Once blood pressure and heart rate are controlled, transition to oral antihypertensives together with a statin (in the presence of CAD) constitutes optimum medical therapy in the long term.

As with aortic dissection, forms of AAS can be classified as complicated or uncomplicated, depending on their associated symptoms and clinical course. Intractable pain, uncontrollable blood pressure, development of visceral malperfusion or symptoms of impending rupture define a complicated, symptomatic presentation that provokes intervention in all but the highest risk patients. In asymptomatic patients, medical management and surveillance are recommended, unless high-risk anatomic features are present (see D).

With increasing use of cross-sectional imaging, a number of incidental presentations of AAS are diagnosed. For clinically asymptomatic patients, the decision to treat will be based on the presence or evolution of high-risk anatomic features or the development of new symptoms.

D **Incidental finding—PAU or IMH: high-risk features?**

Although the specific growth rate is unknown, 20% to 30% of asymptomatic PAUs show evidence of progression over time.[9] There is currently no evidence to support treatment of asymptomatic PAU other than with blood pressure control and surveillance. These lesions are treated as saccular aneurysms and monitored for size progression.

IMH is more often associated with dynamic evolution, with 28% to 47% leading to classical dissection and/or rupture (20%-45%). Regression is seen in 10% of patients.[10]

The presence or development of high-risk anatomic features (Table 23-1) indicates disease progression with a higher likelihood of AAD, aneurysm formation, or rupture. The decision to pursue conservative management versus surgical/endovascular intervention is based on the number of these clinical and radiologic features present in comparison with associated patient comorbidities, risk of treatment, and life expectancy.

Table 23-1. Predictors of IMH/PAU Progression to Dissection, Aneurysm, or Rupture

Ascending aortic involvement[15,18,19]

Maximum aortic diameter ≥ 50 mm[24]

Progressive aortic wall thickness (>11 mm)[25]

Enlarging aortic diameter[25]

Recurrent pleural effusion[26]

Coexistent IMH and PAU[18,26]

Focal intimal disruption in IMH[27]

IMH, intramural hematoma; PAU, penetrating aortic ulcer.

E **Asymptomatic IAAD**

Owing to its low incidence, little is known of the natural history of IAAD. Kang et al., reported on the outcomes of 210 patients identified with spontaneous IAAD and followed up with serial CT.[11] During the study period, aortic rupture occurred in two patients (0.9%), aortic intervention was required in five (2.4%), and aorta-related deaths were identified in three (1.4%). In this study, female gender, symptoms, and suprarenal IAAD were associated with an increased frequency of aorta-related mortality.[11] Concomitant AAA and IAAD may be associated with increased risk of rupture and such patients may merit intervention. Notwithstanding this, medical management is recommended for most patients with asymptomatic IAAD. Several studies have reported superior outcomes in treating chronic, asymptomatic IAAD compared with patients with acute or symptomatic IAAD.[12,13] However, at present, it is not advised to intervene in asymptomatic patients with IAAD.

F **Symptomatic or high-risk PAU or IMH**

Symptomatic PAU typically manifests in elderly patients (usually >65 years of age, with HTN and diffuse atherosclerosis) with chest or back pain without signs of aortic regurgitation or malperfusion. Symptomatic PAUs have an ominous natural history of progression and rupture, particularly if associated with IMH.[14] Less commonly, patients can present with signs of distal embolization.

Symptomatic IMH has a clinical manifestation similar to that of aortic dissection. Chest or back pain is characteristic, whereas malperfusion and pulse deficits are much less common.[15]

IMH and PAU are classified according to Stanford criteria. Type A involves the ascending aorta and type B is localized to the arch and descending aorta. The clinical course of these pathologies varies according to location, and subsequently influences their management. Conservative medical treatment (blood pressure control and intensive care monitoring, as described in C) is used for asymptomatic IMH and PAU without high-risk features for progression (see D).[16]

Ⓖ Ascending aortic PAU/IMH

Around 20% of IMH are located within the ascending aorta, whereas PAU is a rare occurrence at this site. Regression of acute IMH occurs in one-third, progression in 20%, and up to 40% evolve into aortic dissection.[17] Conversion of an IMH to a more classic picture of dissection occurs in 3% to 14% of type B IMH, but in up to 88% of cases involving the ascending aorta (IRAD series[5]). Consequently, type A IMH has a high, early risk of complication and death.[15] The greatest risk is within the first 8 days of onset of symptoms. Emergency open surgery is indicated in complicated cases with pericardial effusion, periaortic hematoma, or large aneurysms, and urgent surgery (24 hours after diagnosis) is required in most of type A IMHs. If a PAU involves the ascending aorta, urgent surgery is indicated as for other types of AAS because of an increased risk of rupture or cardiac tamponade.[18,19] Operative risk is assessed before proceeding with open surgical repair.

Ⓗ Descending aortic PAU/IMH

The majority (50%-80%) of IMH and PAU occur within the descending thoracic aorta.[15,18] In symptomatic patients, or those with high-risk factors for progression, treatment is recommended depending on assessment of operative risk.

Ⓘ Operative risk assessment

In a complicated presentation of AAS, operative intervention is indicated in all but very high-risk patients. In the high-surgical-risk patient (significant combination of comorbidity, frailty, and poor life expectancy), whose risk of surgical or endovascular treatment is prohibitive, optimal medical therapy with a "wait-and-watch strategy" (medical therapy with blood pressure and pain control and repetitive imaging as defined in the surveillance protocol for conservatively managed cases [see P] or at the clinician's discretion) may be the most appropriate option. Specific medical conditions such as connective tissue disorders must be considered in young patients and in those with relevant family history and previous medical history. The presence of such pathology carries a higher risk of disease progression to full dissection and aortic expansion and/or rupture. Optimal treatment of aortic pathology in those with connective tissue disease is open repair. However, in the emergency setting, endovascular intervention can be lifesaving and is often used as a bridge to future intervention at a more stable time. If the operative risk is deemed acceptable, endovascular or open approaches are selected depending on the specific pathology and anatomy in patients with complicated disease.

Ⓙ Open repair

Emergency open surgery is the treatment of choice in patients with a complicated type A PAU or IMH. The aim of open surgery on the ascending aorta is to avoid the risk of rupture and cardiac tamponade. In treatment, the cardiothoracic surgeons perform resection of the affected ascending aortic segment and replacement with a polyester graft through a sternotomy and under cardiopulmonary bypass. If repair requires resection and reconstruction of the aortic arch, the operation is performed under hypothermia and circulatory arrest with selective cerebral perfusion.

Ⓚ TEVAR

Although the evidence is incomplete, just as with complicated classic aortic dissection, endovascular repair is generally recommended for patients with complicated descending aortic PAU or IMH.

TEVAR is associated with a lower perioperative morbidity and mortality than is open repair for these patients.[2,20,21] IMH in a normal-caliber aorta without an apparent intimal tear presents a treatment challenge as to where to place the endograft. Although the literature provides no compelling evidence, international guidelines advise that treatment of IMH should mirror the treatment of AAD in the corresponding segment of the aorta.[10] Therefore, as with dissection, stent-graft diameter should be oversized <5% to 10% (to prevent stent-graft-induced intimal injury) and be long enough to cover 2 cm beyond the length of the involved aorta, if possible.

If a PAU is associated with clinical symptoms or radiologic evidence of associated IMH or an increase in total aortic diameter, further intervention is required. These patients are often poor candidates for conventional surgery because of age and comorbidity. Therefore, TEVAR is the preferred treatment of choice, although there are no direct randomized trials comparing TEVAR with open repair. The PAU is treated as a saccular aneurysm with 2-cm proximal and distal coverage and 10% to 20% oversizing for adequate seal.

Ⓛ Symptomatic IAAD

The presentation of symptomatic IAAD can be ambiguous, with sudden-onset sharp abdominal or lumbar pain in 80% of cases. In a review of the IRAD data,[5] abdominal pain, mesenteric ischemia or infarction, limb ischemia, and hypotension were significantly more frequent in patients with IAAD, whereas chest pain was more typical in patients with type B dissections. No neurologic symptoms, such as ischemic spinal cord damage or ischemic peripheral neuropathy, occurred in the IAAD cohort.[5]

Because IAAD usually commences below the level of the renal arteries, renal function remains unaffected. Lower extremity ischemia is reported in up to 33% of cases, and is also highly associated with the synchronous presence of AAA.

The management of IAADs is controversial because of the small number of cases and paucity of literature. In the presence of symptoms, or radiologic progression of dissection and aneurysm development, intervention is warranted. Depending on patient fitness, both endovascular and open strategies may be possible, depending on the anatomy.

Ⓜ Anatomy suitable for endovascular repair?

As in the management of infrarenal AAA, the patient's cardiopulmonary fitness and aortic anatomy are assessed to decide on the optimal treatment strategy. The anatomic constraints of standard EVAR apply to endovascular management of IAAD. An adequate length of at least 10 mm, parallel, disease-free, infrarenal neck, without excessive angulation; adequate access size of femoral and iliac vessels for graft delivery; and at least 2 cm of distal sealing vessel would be required for the use of standard endografts. If the proximal entry tear originates <10 mm below the renal arteries, then more complicated endovascular solutions could be considered, although longer manufacturing times of fenestrated devices and durability of chimneys may be drawbacks for endovascular repair in such patients.

Ⓝ Open repair

Because the majority of IAAD are infrarenal in location, traditional open surgical repair has better outcomes in comparison to thoracic dissections, and should be considered in young, fit patients, in the presence of IAAD and concomitant aneurysmal dilatation of the aorta, and in patients where the tear originates close to the renal arteries. The technique for open IAAD repair is similar to that used for open AAAs (see Chapter 24).

Ⓞ Endovascular repair

Several small series and case reports have reported the feasibility and good outcomes possible with an endovascular approach. The aim of endovascular intervention is to seal entry tears, reverse possible malperfusion, promote false lumen remodeling, and exclude any coexistent aneurysm.[12,13,22] The anatomy of IAAD may prove challenging because of small true lumen size, involvement of visceral vessels, and extension into external iliac arteries, which may require additional stenting. A meta-analysis of 92 patients demonstrated lower mortality and complication rate with endovascular in comparison to open surgical intervention (0% and 5%, vs. 2% and 13%, respectively).[23] The technique for endovascular repair of IAAD is similar to that used for EVAR (see Chapter 24).

Ⓟ Medical management and surveillance

To prevent complications and ascertain therapeutic efficacy, all patients diagnosed with or treated for aortic disease should undergo a program of systematic surveillance with lifelong medical therapy for blood pressure control and risk factor modification. The natural history of both PAU and IMH is unclear and given that morphologic changes can develop in these patients over time, close surveillance, similar to that used with AAD, is crucial. Current guidelines recommend a surveillance protocol detailed subsequently for those patients treated with initial medical therapy only (Table 23-2).[16] Patients receiving endovascular repair should undergo early postoperative imaging with CTA (within 30 days) to assess the success of the repair, including sealing zones

Table 23-2. Surveillance Protocols for Conservative Management of Penetrating Aortic Ulcer, Intramural Hematoma and Isolated Abdominal Aortic Dissection[16]

	Imaging	Surveillance Interval	Indications for Closer Follow-Up or Potential Intervention
IMH	CT or MRI	3 mo, 6 mo, yearly *If unchanged after 3 y, extend review interval to, eg, 3 y*	Extension of IMH *Presence of concomitant PAU* *Aortic growth > 5 mm/y* *Aortic diameter > 50 mm*
PAU	CT or MRI	3 mo, 6 mo, yearly *If unchanged after 3 y of follow-up, extend review interval to, eg, 3 y*	*Aortic growth > 5 mm/y* *Aortic diameter > 50 mm*
IAAD	DUS, CT or MRI	3 mo, 6 mo, yearly *If unchanged after 3 y of follow-up, extend review interval to, eg, 3 y*	*Aortic growth > 5 mm/y* *Aortic diameter > 50 mm*

IAAD, isolated abdominal aortic dissection; IMH, intramural hematoma; PAU, penetrating aortic ulcer.
From Clinical Practice Guidelines of the European Society for Vascular Surgery (ESVS). Management of descending thoracic aorta disease. *Eur J Vasc Endovasc Surg.* 2017;53:4-54.

and presence of endoleaks. Lifelong surveillance involves annual imaging with CTA after TEVAR, and CTA or DUS after endovascular repair of IAAD. Those undergoing open surgery should continue to receive medical therapy and there is no evidence or recommendation for imaging surveillance in this group.

REFERENCES

1. Olsson C, Thelin S, Ståhle E, Ekbom A, Granath F. Thoracic aortic aneurysm and dissection: increasing prevalence and improved outcomes reported in a nationwide population-based study of more than 14,000 cases from 1987 to 2002. *Circulation.* 2006;114:2611-2618.
2. Eggebrecht H, Plicht B, Kahlert P, Erbel R. Intramural hematoma and penetrating ulcers: indications to endovascular treatment. *Eur J Vasc Endovasc Surg.* 2009;38:659-665.
3. O'Gara PT, DeSanctis RW. Acute aortic dissection and its variants. Toward a common diagnostic and therapeutic approach. *Circulation.* 1995;92:1376-1378.
4. Nienaber CA, Sievers HH. Intramural hematoma in acute aortic syndrome: more than one variant of dissection? *Circulation.* 2002;106:284-285.
5. Trimarchi S, Tsai T, Eagle KA, et al. International Registry of Acute Aortic Dissection (IRAD) investigators. Acute abdominal aortic dissection: insight from the International Registry of Acute Aortic Dissection (IRAD). *J Vasc Surg.* 2007;46:913.e1-919.e1.
6. Fojtik JP, Costantino TG, Dean AJ. The diagnosis of aortic dissection by emergency medicine ultrasound. *J Emerg Med.* 2007;32:191-196.
7. Alfson D, Ham S. Type B aortic dissections. Current guidelines for treatment. *Cardiol Clin.* 2017;35:387-410.
8. Kudama K, Nishigami K, Sakamoto T, et al. Tight heart rate control reduces secondary adverse events in patients with Type B acute aortic dissection. *Circulation.* 2008;118:S169-S170.
9. Evangelista A, Czerny M, Nienaber C, et al. Interdisciplinary expert consensus on management of type B intramural haematoma and penetrating aortic ulcer. *Eur J Cardiothorac Surg.* 2015;47:1037-1043.
10. Erbel R, Aboyans V, Boileau C, et al. 2014 ESC Guidelines on the diagnosis and treatment of aortic diseases. *Eur Heart J.* 2014;35:2873-2926.
11. Kang JH, Kim YW, Heo SH, et al. Treatment strategy based on the natural course of the disease for patients with spontaneous isolated abdominal aortic dissection. *J Vasc Surg.* 2017;66(6):1668.e3-1678.e3.
12. Faries CM, Tadros RQ, Lajos PS, Vouyouka AG, Faries PL, Marin ML. Contemporary management of isolated chronic infrarenal abdominal aortic dissections. *J Vasc Surg.* 2016;64:1245-1250.
13. Jawadi N, Bisadas T, Torsello G, Stavroulakis K, Donas KP. Endovascular treatment of isolated abdominal aortic dissections: long term results. *J Endovasc Ther.* 2014;21:324-328.
14. Vilacosta I, Aragoncillo P, Cañadas V, San Román JA, Ferreirós J, Rodríguez E. Acute aortic syndrome: a new look at an old conundrum. *Heart.* 2009;95:1130-1139.
15. Evangelista A, Mukherjee D, Mehta RH, et al. Acute intramural hematoma of the aorta: a mystery in evolution. *Circulation.* 2005;111:1063-1070.
16. Clinical Practice Guidelines of the European Society for Vascular Surgery (ESVS). Management of descending thoracic aorta disease. *Eur J Vasc Endovasc Surg.* 2017;53:4-54.
17. Mussa FF, Horton JD, Moridzadeh R, Nicholson J, Trimarchi S, Eagle KA. Acute aortic dissection and intramural hematoma: a systematic review. *JAMA.* 2016;316(7):754-763.
18. Quint LE, Williams DM, Francis IR, et al. Ulcer like lesions of the aorta: imaging features and natural history. *Radiology.* 2001;218:719-723.
19. Nathan DP, Boonn W, Lai E, et al. Presentation, complications, and natural history of penetrating atherosclerotic ulcer disease. *J Vasc Surg.* 2012;55:10-15.
20. Von Kodolitsch Y, Csösz SK, Koschyk DH, et al. Intramural hematoma of the aorta: predictors of progression to dissection and rupture. *Circulation.* 2003;107:1158-1163.
21. Geisbüsch P, Kotelis D, Weber TF, Hyhlik-Dürr A, Kauczor HU, Böckler D. Early and midterm results after endovascular stent graft repair of penetrating aortic ulcers. *J Vasc Surg.* 2008;48:1361-1368.
22. Zhu QQ, Li DL, Lai MC, et al. Endovascular treatment of isolated abdominal aortic dissection and postoperative aortic remodeling. *J Vasc Surg.* 2015;61:1424-1431.
23. Jonker FH, Schlosser FJ, Moll FL, Muhs BE. Dissection of the abdominal aorta. Current evidence and implications for treatment strategies: a review and meta-analysis of 92 patients. *J Endovasc Ther.* 2009;16:71-80.
24. Evangelista A, Dominguez R, Sebastia C, et al. Prognostic value of clinical and morphologic findings in short-term evolution of aortic intramural haematoma. Therapeutic implications. *Eur Heart J.* 2004;25:81-87.
25. Song JM, Kim HS, Song JK, et al. Usefulness of the initial noninvasive imaging study to predict the adverse outcomes in the medical treatment of acute typeA aortic intramural hematoma. *Circulation.* 2003;108(suppl 1):II324-II328.
26. Ganaha F, Miller DC, Sugimoto K, et al. Prognosis of aortic intramural hematoma with and without penetrating atherosclerotic ulcer: a clinical and radiological analysis. *Circulation.* 2002;106:342-348.
27. Moral S, Cuellar H, Avegliano G, et al. Clinical implications of focal intimal disruption in patients with type B intramural hematoma. *J Am Coll Cardiol.* 2017;69(1):28-39.

Salvatore T. Scali • Thomas S. Huber

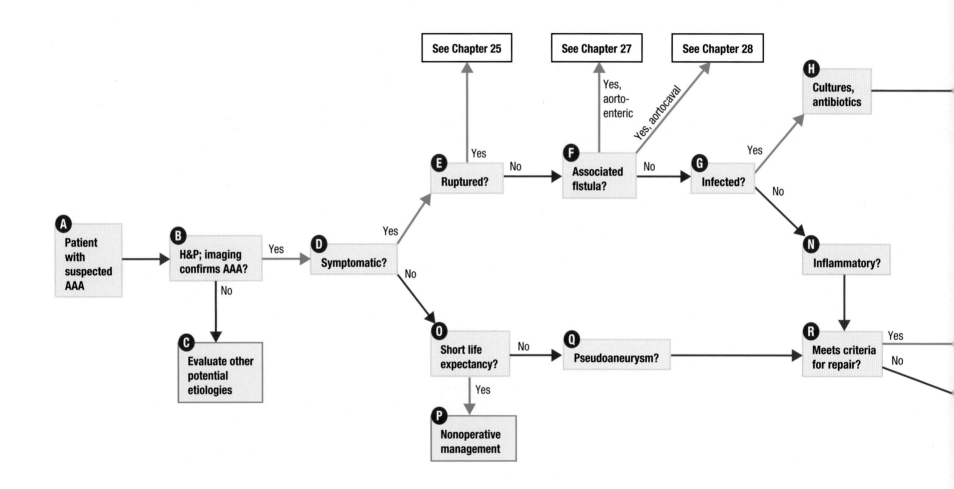

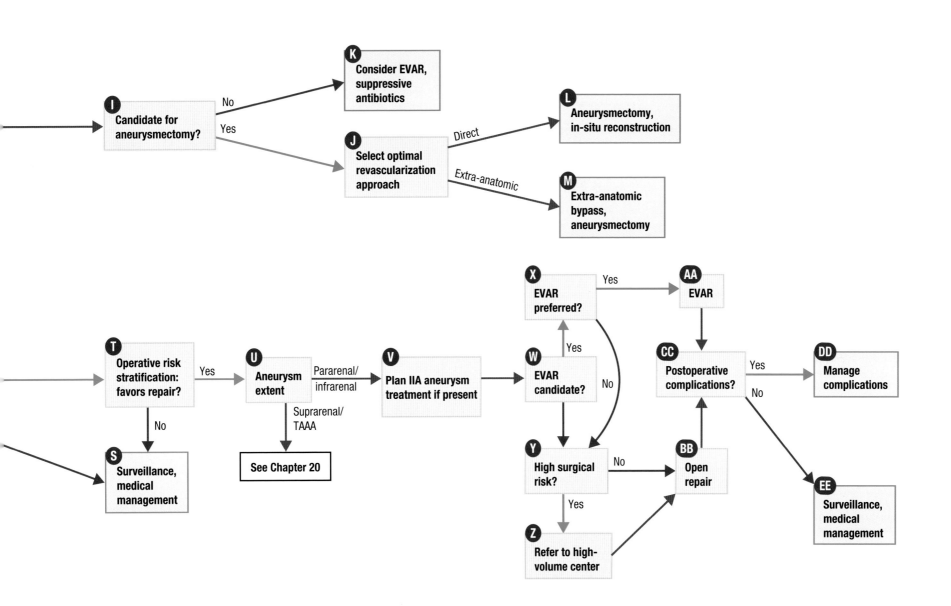

A Patient with suspected AAA

An AAA is typically defined by the presence of a focal dilatation that is at least 50% greater than the normal adjacent arterial diameter. In general, an AAA must be larger than 3 cm because the average diameter of the infrarenal aorta is approximately 2 cm (whereas the suprarenal aorta is usually ~0.5 cm larger than the infrarenal aorta). The prevalence of AAA is estimated to be approximately 4% to 10% for patients older than 60 years and several factors increase the likelihood of AAA.[1] Specifically, these include prior family history (especially ruptured AAA), male sex, and tobacco exposure. Other patient-level factors that should be documented, because they influence decisions regarding management of suspected or known AAA, include functional status, as well as the presence of concomitant cardiovascular and/or renal comorbidity.[2-4]

B H&P; imaging confirms AAA?

A patient who presents with a suspected or known AAA should undergo a thorough H&P. On examination, the existence of a pulsatile abdominal mass and whether there is associated tenderness palpated directly over the aneurysm should be determined. Although the sensitivity of the physical examination for detecting AAA is marginal, it increases with greater diameter sizes (eg, 29% for 3-3.9 cm, 50% for 4-4.9 cm, and 76% for >5 cm).[5] For this reason, abdominal DUS should be obtained in any patient with a suspected AAA. Attention should also be paid to the detection of femoral or popliteal aneurysms, which can be present in 5% to 15% of patients with AAA.[5] Documentation of the pulse examination, as well as an inventory of associated cardiopulmonary findings such as murmur and/or aberrant lung sounds, is important because these results further inform the clinician about whether additional testing is warranted to appropriately risk stratify the patient.

Imaging in asymptomatic subjects with suspected AAA can start with an abdominal DUS. Screening with DUS has been demonstrated to be cost-effective in specific patient populations (male patients, age ≥ 65, smoked >100 cigarettes during their life-time, and/or male and female patients with a positive family history).[6,7] For more precise imaging and preoperative planning, arterial contrast-enhanced, thin-cut (<1 mm) CTA is predominantly used because of its greater sensitivity and specificity compared to DUS and would be mandatory in a symptomatic patient, because DUS cannot reliably exclude rupture. Initial imaging should include the chest in addition to the abdomen and pelvis because 10% to 15% of patients can have synchronous and/or metachronous aneurysmal disease of the thoracic aorta.[1,2,5,8,9] Alternative imaging choices such as MRA or plain radiography are either too costly, time consuming or lack the sensitivity and specificity to be used for routine clinical management of AAA.

C Evaluate other potential etiologies

If the initial evaluation and imaging does not reveal presence of AAA, then other potential etiologies should be considered in the differential diagnosis. A false-positive AAA diagnosis based on physical examination can occur in a patient with a thin body habitus where the aortic pulse appears prominent, which is especially true in young adults and pediatric patients. Other abdominal arterial aneurysms (eg, renal, mesenteric) can be mistaken for AAA on physical examination. Additional diagnoses such as right heart failure with hepatomegaly (especially left lobe hypertrophy), GI tumors, pancreatic pseudocyst, and splenomegaly should be considered if AAA is not present on cross-sectional imaging after initial detection of a pulsatile abdominal mass on physical examination.

D Symptomatic?

A critical distinction in the management of AAA is whether the patient has symptoms related to the aneurysm. Typically, this would be new-onset back or abdominal pain. It can be difficult to determine whether new-onset back pain is being caused by an AAA, but if there is associated tenderness of the aneurysm on examination, the AAA is considered symptomatic. It is generally assumed that such symptoms are associated with acute expansion, such that symptomatic aneurysms are usually treated urgently. Much less commonly, AAAs can cause symptoms of acute ischemia because of distal embolization or acute aortic occlusion from in situ thrombosis. Rarer symptoms include local compression (ie, ureter), aorto-caval or -enteric fistulas associated with AAA (see Chapters 27 and 28). Symptomatic but nonruptured presentations characterize approximately 5% to 23% of all AAA cases. Historically, outcomes after symptomatic (nonruptured) AAA have been reported to be comparable or worse than elective AAA repair, with 30-day or in-hospital mortality rates ranging from 4% to 22%.

E Ruptured?

For a patient with a symptomatic AAA, CTA should be obtained urgently to determine whether the aneurysm has ruptured (see Chapter 25). Sudden onset of abdominal, back, flank, and/or inguinal pain in a patient older than age 50 that is associated with hypotension, syncope, or any signs of shock should be considered a ruptured AAA until proved otherwise. The differential diagnosis for abdominal catastrophe (eg, ruptured AAA, GI bleeding, perforated viscus, splenic rupture, etc) mandates an efficient, coordinated, and rapid evaluation if an optimal outcome is to be achieved. Significant delays in the workup for ruptured AAA can occur if this diagnosis is not considered initially, and this adversely impact outcomes.[10]

F Associated fistula?

If the symptomatic patient does not have a ruptured AAA, then any associated fistula needs to be ruled out. Primary aortoenteric fistula (AEF) from AAA erosion into the duodenum is rare but often lethal. Patients typically present with upper GI bleeding with an associated AAA, but more commonly such bleeding is due to primary GI pathology coincidentally present in a patient with AAA. The diagnosis is established with CTA or upper GI endoscopy and mandates emergent treatment (see Chapter 27). An even more rare entity is an aortocaval fistula, which occurs in <1% of all aneurysms and <3% of ruptured AAA cases. These patients can manifest with high-output cardiac failure, renal insufficiency, hematuria, lower extremity edema, and a continuous abdominal bruit. Such fistula can be suspected in the presence of a holosystolic, machinery-like abdominal bruit, and the diagnosis is usually made by CTA preoperatively, but may be an unexpected finding during symptomatic AAA repair (see Chapter 27).

G Infected?

Once a symptomatic patient is found to have a nonruptured AAA with no associated fistula, the presence of an infected aneurysm needs to be considered, especially if the presentation is associated with fever, malaise, night sweats, weight loss, abdominal/back pain, and/or failure to thrive. Infected AAA is a rare (~0.5%-1%) but very challenging clinical problem to manage because it is frequently associated with other complicating features such as rupture, sepsis, and paravisceral involvement (~50%-60% of cases).[11] Preexisting degenerative aneurysms can become secondarily infected as a result of remote hematogenous seeding from septic embolization. Aneurysms can also develop in a normal aorta as a result of local or hematogenous spread of infection. In fact, the term "mycotic aneurysm" was originally coined by Osler to describe the entity of an infected aneurysm (really a "mushroom"-shaped PSA) resulting from septic embolization originating from bacterial endocarditis.[12] Other potential risk factors that can increase a patient's risk for an infected AAA presentation include impaired immunity, prior aortic surgery, malnutrition, and arterial injury.

H Cultures, antibiotics

After initial stabilization and resuscitation of a patient with a suspected infected AAA, blood cultures followed by treatment with empiric broad-spectrum antibiotic coverage should occur. Although the bacteriology of implicated organisms in mycotic AAA cases has evolved in the past 60 years, initial antibiotic choices should still cover both gram-positive and gram-negative organisms. The value of blood cultures is underscored by positive results in 50% to 85% of cases.[13] The most common organisms that are implicated in infected AAA cases are coagulase-negative and coagulase-positive *Staphylococcus* (28%-71% of cases), as well as *Salmonella* species. However, if there is any concern of alimentary tract communication, the possibility of concurrent *Enterobacteriaceae* and even anaerobic species contamination should be considered.

Candidate for aneurysmectomy?

A complex decision-making process must be navigated to determine whether a patient is a candidate for aneurysmectomy. The surgical tenets governing the management of infected AAA are aggressive surgical debridement of all infected tissue and vascular reconstruction, as needed. Owing to the significant morbidity and mortality associated with management of infected aneurysms, thorough patient risk stratification must be completed to determine whether definitive open surgical treatment is possible, or if temporizing treatment such as endovascular graft and antibiotics is the only option. An individualized patient approach must be undertaken and is best done by an experienced surgical team. Even in the "best-case" scenario where the cases are managed in high-volume centers with a concentration on complex aortic disease, mortality rates are still 20% to 50% with morbidity approaching 75% to 100%.[14,15]

J Select optimal revascularization approach

The optimal revascularization approach in the management of an infected AAA is debated in the contemporary literature. The classic teaching for management of infected AAA is to perform extra-anatomic revascularization followed by aneurysmectomy with aortic ligation. However, for patients with paravisceral and/or thoracoabdominal involvement, this approach may not be feasible and may mandate antegrade visceral debranching or inline, anatomic revascularization. Although in situ reconstruction may be associated with increased risk of graft-related complications, it can be performed safely with reasonable durability in selected patients with infected AAA.[11,16] Several descriptions of staged reconstruction strategies have also been reported, so the timing, type, and configuration of the revascularization procedure are all details one must consider when managing this difficult clinical problem.

The authors have usually selected a direct, in situ reconstruction with rifampin-soaked Dacron graft conduit in good physiologic risk patients presenting with suspected Staphylococcal and/or biofilm infection (*S. epidermidis*; especially with associated PSA) as long as no associated vertebral osteomyelitis and/or perigraft abscess is present. Neo-aortoiliac system (NAIS) has been applied selectively in younger (eg, age < 65), good-risk (ASA ≤ III) patients with adequate preoperative femoral vein conduit (mean diameter ≥ 7 mm) and no presence of retroperitoneal abscess on CT, as well as absence of enteric communication (no AEF) and/or gram-negative infection (verified with preoperative and/or intraoperative culture). Poor physiologic-risk patients, independent of bacteriology, typically undergo axillobifemoral bypass followed by staged graft explantation and aortic ligation.

Consider EVAR, suppressive antibiotics

For patients with infected AAAs who are deemed unfit for open surgical repair, there are limited data on efficacy, but some reports have suggested the feasibility of using EVAR with lifelong suppressive antibiotics in anatomically suitable patients. Systematic reviews have identified that preoperative history of rupture and fever are independent predictors of persistent and/or recurrent infection.[17] Up to 20% of patients will die from aneurysm-related causes in reports of EVAR in the management of infected AAA. However, this may be the only option for high-risk patients. Notably, some series have found that aortic-related deaths increased after cessation of antibiotics, which argues for lifelong antibiotic suppression and CT imaging surveillance.[18]

L Aneurysmectomy, in-situ reconstruction

For good-risk patients, aneurysmectomy with in situ reconstruction can be considered. Primary mycotic aortic infections often involve *S. aureus* (especially MRSA) or gram-negative organisms, so in situ reconstruction using antibiotic impregnated prosthetic graft (eg, gelatin sealed knitted polyester Dacron graft, 60 mg/mL concentration of Rifampin, soaked × 30 minutes) or autogenous biologic conduits (eg, femoral-popliteal vein [NAIS] vs. cadaveric homograft) has been widely reported and debated. The reinfection rates with prosthetic conduit placed into the anatomic bed of a recently debrided infected AAA can range from 25% to 60% depending on the presence of gram-negative organisms.[14,19] As an alternative, graft excision and NAIS reconstruction with large-caliber, femoral-popliteal vein grafts have been shown to have favorable results compared to other revascularization strategies such as aortic ligation with extra-anatomic bypass. However, predictors of poor outcome with the NAIS procedure include presence of *Candida/Klebsiella/Bacteroides* infection and overt preoperative sepsis, so use of this strategy in the management of AEF is not typically recommended.[19]

Extra-anatomic bypass, aneurysmectomy

The procedure that is most frequently reported in the management of infected AAA is use of extra-anatomic revascularization (eg, bilateral axillofemoral or axillobifemoral bypass) followed by aortic ligation and debridement. For high-risk subjects, a strategy of performing revascularization followed by a second-stage operation for graft removal and aortic ligation can be used to reduce morbidity. Important considerations in this strategy are the quality of the patient's runoff vessels to maintain graft patency and the amount of residual noninfected aortic tissue below the renal arteries. At least 2 to 3 cm of noninfected infrarenal aorta is optimal for closure and oversewing the aorta in two layers followed by placement of an omental pedicle after wide local debridement of the retroperitoneum is classically described ("triple

ligation" = running horizontal mattress + simple running suture + omental flap). Although this strategy can take less operative time compared to some forms of in situ reconstruction (eg, NAIS), the 15% to 20% risk of aortic stump blowout remains a concern postoperatively and is almost universally fatal if it does occur.[20]

N Inflammatory?

If an infected aneurysm is not present, a symptomatic presentation can be associated with the presence of an inflammatory AAA, which accounts for 5% to 10% of symptomatic presentations.[21] The natural history of inflammatory AAA is poorly understood; however, current guidelines recommend repair at diameters similar to degenerative aneurysms.[8,21] The hallmarks of inflammatory AAA include marked aneurysm wall thickening with contrast enhancement on CTA, retroperitoneal fibrosis, and surrounding visceral adhesion to the AAA sac.

The operative approach to an inflammatory aneurysm is technically demanding as evidenced by higher blood product utilization and longer operative times compared to noninflammatory AAA cases. Optimally, an endovascular repair is selected; however, if open aortic repair is required, a retroperitoneal approach is recommended to minimize risk of injury to the duodenum and proximal jejunum that are frequently adherent to the anterior aneurysm wall. Limitations of this approach include poor access to the right iliac, right renal artery, and right ureter. In addition, this approach limits ability to manage inadvertent duodenal injury. Although aortic wall integrity may seem adequate given the dense fibrotic reaction, anastomotic dehiscence remains a concern, so a Teflon or polytetrafluoroethylene pledget-reinforced anastomosis is usually completed. Because ureteral obstruction can complicate up to 25% of cases preoperatively, ureteral stents can be placed preemptively to ensure adequate urinary drainage; they may act as a guide for localization during dissection.

O Short life expectancy?

In the patient with an asymptomatic AAA, before establishing a surveillance protocol or determining whether the aneurysm is at a size threshold that warrants elective repair, an estimation of life expectancy should be made. Because patients with AAA are generally older and frequently have associated cardiovascular comorbidities, the 5-year survival is usually predicted to be 60% to 70%.[22] However, in certain patient cohorts with advanced cardiac and/or renal disease, the 5-year survival can be <50%, which equates to a >10% annual mortality risk even without the presence of an aneurysm.[4,23,24] Repair will dramatically increase the AAA-rupture-free survival but does not reduce the risk of all-cause mortality from major adverse cardiac and oncologic events.[25] The prophylactic nature of elective AAA repair mandates that the surgeon consider four crucial variables in the decision-making algorithm: (1) patient life expectancy;

(2) annualized rupture risk, predominantly predicted by aneurysm diameter; (3) perioperative mortality risk of repair; and (4) patient preference. Patients with a reasonable life expectancy (eg, >2-5 years) will derive the greatest benefit from prophylactic AAA repair, but this determination is influenced by the diameter of the aneurysm at presentation.

❗ Nonoperative management

Although the annualized rupture risk has historically been reported to be between 3% and 15% for a 5- to 6-cm AAA, more recent analyses suggest that this overestimates the true natural history of the disease.[22,26] This is especially true for smaller diameter aneurysms (3.0-5.5 cm) where a systematic review identified an annual rupture risk of 0% to 1.6%.[26] Given these features, patients with asymptomatic AAA with short life expectancy (eg, <2 years), due to other comorbidities such as cancer or advanced cardiopulmonary/renal disease, should be counseled accordingly and offered nonoperative management. This decision can be complex and nuanced; as such, multiple visits with the patient and their health care surrogates with extensive documentation are prudent features of this management strategy. An explanation about the scenario for a ruptured AAA and a discussion about comfort measures should occur. Establishing or updating a living will with the assistance of the primary care provider and a social worker are important steps in nonoperative AAA management.

❓ Pseudoaneurysm?

On the basis of history and imaging, differentiation of a true from a false aneurysm or PSA should be made. The underlying causes of aortic PSA may be degenerative (penetrating ulcer) or nondegenerative (trauma, infection), but most frequently these are associated with a prior aortic graft anastomosis. The natural history and subsequent rupture risk of an aortic PSA is not well established, but it is generally considered *worse* than for a true AAA. Therefore, the decision to treat an AAA depends on the nature of the presentation (eg, symptomatic, infected, growth rate, diameter, anticipated complexity of the repair, patient preference/age/comorbidities, and life expectancy).

❗ Meet criteria for repair?

Current repair thresholds for asymptomatic AAA include diameter ≥5.5 cm for men and ≥5.0 cm for women.[8] These diameter thresholds are not absolute and larger thresholds may be more appropriate in high medical risk patients given their greater risk of postoperative mortality and reduced overall life expectancy. Notably, the diameter repair threshold for women is less than that for men, predominantly based on the fact that they are three to four times more likely to experience AAA rupture during surveillance.[27] Unfortunately, women also have higher postoperative

mortality, so a uniform policy of repairing all 5-cm aneurysms in women is likely not the best strategy.[28] Besides diameter criteria, AAAs that are found to have growth rates >10 mm/y are also recommended for repair.[8] Most degenerative aneurysms present with fusiform morphology; however, some patients (1%-2%) have a saccular configuration. The rupture risk of saccular aneurysms is generally thought to be greater than for comparable fusiform aneurysms because of elevated wall sheer stress, but the evidence for this is inconclusive.[8]

❗ Surveillance, medical management

For patients with AAA diameters below a size threshold for elective repair, imaging surveillance is recommended. Small AAAs are characterized by diameters from 3.0 to 5.0 cm. In asymptomatic patients with small AAAs (men, diameter <5.5 cm; women, <5.0 cm), the risk of rupture is less than is the risk of prophylactic surgery, so surveillance is indicated. Although the majority of small AAAs grow slowly, there is substantial variation between patients. For men with a 3-cm AAA, the estimated mean annual growth rate is 1.28 mm/y (95% CI 1.03-1.53; I^2 compared to 3.61 mm/y; 95% CI 3.34-3.88; I^2 = 89%) in a man with a 5-cm AAA.[29] Thus, the optimal intervals for AAA surveillance are mostly dependent on the size of the aneurysm. The recommendations for surveillance intervals vary with shorter imaging intervals as AAA diameters increase in size. The Society for Vascular Surgery currently recommends 12-month intervals for surveillance of AAAs between 4.0 and 4.9 cm and 6-month intervals for AAA >5.0 cm.[8]

Dramatic advances in medical therapy over the past two decades have led to significant improvements in longer term survival of patients through substantial reduction in major adverse cardiovascular events. These advances benefit multiple at-risk populations with patients having AAA representing an important target subgroup because of the high rates of associated cardiovascular comorbidities. Although many pharmacologic therapies aimed at reducing AAA diameter expansion and subsequent rupture risk have been examined (eg, propranolol, doxycycline, macrolides, statins), none have proved successful in achieving these goals to be recommended for this specific purpose.[8,23] Smoking is the most important modifiable risk factor to reduce AAA expansion and associated CAD, so patients should be counseled about the necessity of smoking cessation[8] (see Chapter 3). Judicious control of chronic systolic HTN and avoidance of diastolic HTN (>90 mm Hg) is important for reducing long-term cardiovascular events and may reduce AAA growth rates. Specific treatment with β-adrenergic receptor blockers, angiotensin-converting enzyme inhibitors, and angiotensin receptor blockers has been recommended, but no specific antihypertensive medication class has been proved to be optimal for all patients with AAA. Importantly, unless there is a contraindication, all patients with AAA (preoperatively and postoperatively) should be on aspirin and statin therapy (independent of their

cholesterol profile) because of long-term survival benefits.[8,24] The cardiovascular benefits of moderate exercise are well described and may portend a protective effect on AAA growth.[23]

❗ Operative risk stratification: favors repair?

The final step in preoperative decision making involves the assessment of operative risk versus the underlying risk of the AAA. Multiple publications have documented the influence of different demographic, comorbidity, and intraoperative variables affecting AAA postoperative outcomes. Similarly, the extent of the anatomic repair is an important feature to consider because open infrarenal and juxtarenal AAA repair can be expected to have similar outcomes, whereas suprarenal/thoracoabdominal aortic disease is associated with worse outcomes. Thus, larger AAA diameter thresholds (eg, ≥6.0 cm) are appropriate before elective open repair in subjects needing concurrent renal/mesenteric reconstruction.

Owing to unique patterns of these factors in different patients, an individualized approach is needed when assigning risk. The operative stratification should account for both early and late mortality risk because patients dying within the first postoperative year will not have lived long enough to derive any benefit from the decision to offer a prophylactic repair. A number of decision-aid tools are available to estimate the in-hospital, 30-day, and 1-year mortality risk after elective AAA repair.[30] In addition, postoperative risk of major adverse cardiac events can be independently estimated using multiple validated models that are available.[31] Once it is determined that a patient with reasonable life expectancy has an estimated postoperative risk of death less than the annualized rupture risk of the AAA under surveillance, recommendation for repair is justified.

❗ Aneurysm extent

Preoperative determination of the aneurysm extent and identification of normal proximal aorta is crucial to procedural planning. The distinction of infrarenal, para/juxtarenal, and suprarenal disease is important because of the implications of the different types of repair on operative complexity and outcomes. Approximately 5% to 15% of AAAs undergoing repair involve the suprarenal aorta (see Chapter 20). Suprarenal AAA disease is delineated by the requirement of reimplantation and/or bypass of at least one renal artery with open repair. In contradistinction, pararenal/juxtarenal AAA disease is classified by the need to place an aortic cross-clamp above at least one renal artery for control, but the aortic anastomosis is performed below both renal arteries.

❗ Plan IIA aneurysm treatment if present

Another important morphologic feature to consider in the preoperative planning is involvement of the iliac arteries. Between 30% and 40% of all AAAs will have CIA aneurysm disease, usually involving the CIAs, and treated simultaneously with the AAA. Presence of an IIA that requires treatment increases the operative complexity for either open or endovascular AAA repair because contingencies need to be made for iliac bifurcation management, to preserve adequate IIA circulation. This topic is discussed in more detail in Chapter 26.

W EVAR candidate?

Approximately 70% and 80% of all elective AAA cases in the United States are now performed using EVAR. Multiple large randomized trials have consistently demonstrated that EVAR is associated with lower risk of postoperative complications and mortality compared to open repair for elective AAA, even though no long-term survival advantage is evident. This early EVAR benefit is balanced against the greater long-term risk of surveillance and aorta-related reintervention. Multiple commercially available devices can safely be used, but, notably, they have important differences in their IFU (see Table 24-1). Use of high-quality thin-cut CTA with centerline reconstruction is recommended to adequately plan an EVAR. If patients are not candidates for EVAR and have anatomic features that would require using a device outside the IFU, strong consideration of open repair should occur.

X EVAR preferred?

EVAR is generally preferred in good anatomic patients with high medical risk. Patients being offered EVAR need to be counseled about the risks of the procedure with specific attention paid to contrast and radiation exposure, access vessel complications, as well as the lifelong need for imaging surveillance and potential for aorta-related reintervention. Some patients may express significant anxiety with the notion that their aneurysm is treated and not "cured" by EVAR. The mandatory requirement of lifelong postoperative imaging surveillance and/or risk of aortic-related reintervention may also influence patients to prefer open repair even when they have suitable anatomy for a stent graft. In that scenario, the patient's physiologic risk for open surgery will influence the ultimate decision.

Y High surgical risk?

Ultimately, the patients' physiologic and anatomic risk stratification strongly influences decisions surrounding choice of endovascular or open AAA repair. In contrast, to reach a decision in patients with both low/intermediate surgical risk and anatomy suitable for EVAR, the patients' preferences should be ascertained after they have been counseled objectively about the risks and benefits of both endovascular and open AAA repair using a shared decision-making model. Multiple physiologic and anatomic features can coalesce to make a surgeon designate a patient as being high risk. Although there is no standard definition for what is a high-risk patient, those with advanced age (eg, >80), poor functional status (bed bound, nonambulatory), and significant cardiac (eg, CHF, aortic valve disease, revised cardiac risk index score >5), pulmonary ($FEV_1 < 1.5$, steroid/oxygen dependence), and renal (eg, $Cr > 1.8$ mg/dL or dialysis dependence) disease invariably fall into this category. Important anatomic features such as aortic wall calcification, thrombus, associated iliac aneurysm and/or occlusive disease, as well as body habitus and prior surgical history all can contribute to elevated surgical risk, so that the unique constellation of these factors in each patient is considered to determine, in a surgeon's judgment, whether they are high risk. High-risk patients who either prefer open repair despite being candidates for EVAR or are not anatomic candidates for on-label EVAR should be offered referral to a high-volume aortic center.

Z Refer to high-volume center

Regionalization of care to high-volume centers is appropriate because they typically have expertise in "cutting-edge" aortic therapies that can accommodate complex patients with improved outcomes compared to lower volume centers. Frequently, these institutions have providers experienced with both advanced complex open and endovascular aortic surgery, investigational device exemptions for fenestrated/branched endografts, as well as strong integrated, multidisciplinary service relationships with thoracic/cardiovascular surgery, anesthesia, and critical care. Regionalization of AAA care to high-volume centers is especially important for patients undergoing open surgery. Although standard (eg, no chimney/fenestrated component), elective infrarenal EVAR does not appear to be as significantly influenced by center volume, the hospital and surgeon volume effects on open AAA outcomes are well established. High-volume centers specializing in AAA care have robust systems of care that can rescue patients who experience intraoperative or postoperative complications that are linked to poor outcomes. Current guidelines recommend that centers offering elective open AAA repair should routinely perform ≥20 cases per year.[8]

AA EVAR

Since the initial FDA approval of commercially available devices for the treatment of AAA in 1997, a variety of device choices have become available (Table 24-1). The various device companies have all modified their products over time to accommodate most of the anatomic challenges that historically prevented patients from being EVAR eligible. Treating aortic neck lengths of 7 to 15 mm (4 mm for Cook Zfen), high-angle necks (up to 90° for the AorFix device; 60° for other devices), as well as iliac vessel diameters as small as 5 mm is now commonplace. The technique for EVAR implantation can be completed using regional or general anesthesia in most cases. Fluoroscopic guidance and supplemental angiography (and/or IVUS especially in patients with renal disease) allows delineation of anatomic landmarks to facilitate graft implantation. The sequence of stent-graft implantation is unique for each device and it is incumbent upon the surgeon to select the correct anatomy that fits within the prespecified device's IFU to ensure durability of repair. When planning and subsequently performing EVAR, several important features of the repair strategy need to be considered including contrast utilization, wire manipulation of atheromatous debris causing embolization, branch vessel catheterization, aortoiliac calcification, proximal/distal landing zone morphology, tortuosity, and access vessel anatomy. Each of these factors can significantly influence the potential for postoperative complications and reintervention.

Table 24-1. Differences in Key Anatomic Features in Instruction for Use of Commercially Available Endovascular Abdominal Aortic Aneurysm Repair Devices

Device	Suprarenal Fixation	Proximal LZ (mm)	Neck Angle (Infrarenal)	Main Sheath OD (Fr)	Max Iliac (mm)	Iliac LZ (mm)
Excluder C3	No	15	60	18	25	10
Gore IBD	No	15	60	18	n/a	10
Zenith Flex	Yes	15	60	20/22/24	20	10
Z-Fen	Yes	4	45	22/24	20	10
Powerlink/AFX	Yes	15	60	19	23	15
Ovation	Yes	13	60	14	20	10
Endurant IIs	Yes	10	60	18	25	15
Aorfix	±	10	90	23	19	15
Treo	Yes	10	60	18/19	20	10
Treo	Yes	15	75	18/19	20	10

LZ, landing zone; OD, outer diameter.
Excluder C3, Gore IBD Iliac Branch Device, W.L. Gore & Associates; Zenith Flex and Cook Zfen, Cook Medical; AFX and Ovation, Endologix, Inc; Endurant IIs, Medtronic, Inc; AorFix, Lombard Medical; Treo, Bolton Medical.

BB Open repair

If the patient does not have anatomy that conforms to the IFU of a standard, commercially available endograft device but is low/intermediate surgical risk, open aortic repair should be offered. Consideration of surgical exposure using transperitoneal or left retroperitoneal aortic access should be made in each open case. The utility of the left retroperitoneal approach deserves mention given its greater flexibility to manage suprarenal disease, ability to avoid hostile tissue planes from prior abdominal surgery, association with lower pulmonary complications and reduced ileus, as well as capacity to manage aberrant anatomy such as a horse-shoe kidney. In contrast, the retroperitoneal exposure may be suboptimal compared to transperitoneal, inframesocolic aortic access in patients with left-sided vena cava, retroaortic left renal vein, right iliac aneurysm, or significant aortoiliac occlusive disease.

A variety of important technical factors need to be considered when performing open AAA repair including cross-clamp positioning precipitating renal-mesenteric ischemia, use of invasive hemodynamic monitoring, ratio of colloid:crystalloid resuscitation, utilization of blood-scavenging techniques, as well as management of IIA and IMA. Revascularization of the IMA is generally not necessary if sufficient collateral flow is present from the IIA and SMA. If patients are known to have significant occlusive disease of the SMA and/or IIAs, or have undergone prior colonic surgery that may have disrupted SMA-IMA collateralization, it is strongly recommended to factor this into the repair strategy.

CC Postoperative complications?

The incidence of complications after open and endovascular AAA repair can be significant (open repair-elective, 15%-40%; -ruptured, 50%-75%; EVAR-elective, 5%-15%; -ruptured 25%-50%). The most common complications are due to renal, cardiac, pulmonary and bleeding-related dysfunction. The initial "management" of complications should start in the preoperative period with rigorous risk stratification and operative planning.

DD Manage complications

Most postoperative complications after AAA repair are common to many procedures (cardiac, pulmonary, renal) and managed with standard therapy. Two unique complications require specific management. Colon ischemia is a rare (0.5%-3%), but devastating, complication, resulting from IMA or iliac artery occlusion during AAA repair, and is associated with a 3- to 5-fold increase in postoperative mortality. Diagnosis and treatment are discussed in Chapter 84. Abdominal compartment syndrome after EVAR or open AAA repair, especially of ruptured AAA, can also be a life-threatening complication if not recognized and treated (see Chapter 85).

EE Surveillance, medical management

Patients should be counseled preoperatively about the importance of long-term follow-up. After open AAA repair, patients are at risk for developing metachronous disease in the proximal aorta or anastomotic degeneration. In fact, 10% to 15% of patients after open AAA repair develop aneurysm formation at remote sites that warrant surgical intervention. Therefore, a follow-up CTA of the chest, abdomen, and pelvis is recommended between 3 and 5 years postoperatively.[8] Long-term follow-up after EVAR is mandatory because 15% to 20% of patients will undergo aortic-related reintervention during their lifetime, usually related to endoleak management (see Chapter 29). After EVAR, a patient without postoperative imaging is considered to be unrepaired until proved otherwise, given the late risk of aortic-related reintervention (15%-18%) and rupture (0.5%-1%). Initial recommended surveillance intervals from the FDA-sponsored pivotal device trials were CT-imaging at 1 month, 6 months, 12 months, and annually thereafter. However, multiple studies have demonstrated that if there is no endoleak on the first postoperative CTA, then the 6-month scan can safely be eliminated.[8] DUS has also been shown to be safe and cost-effective for post-EVAR surveillance and many centers have replaced their CT surveillance with this modality after the first postoperative year if no endoleak is evident and no sac enlargement has occurred. National rates of EVAR surveillance are poor, with 22% to 25% of living patients missing imaging at 1 year postoperatively and >50% have no imaging after 3 years.[8] This lack of longer term imaging surveillance has been shown to be associated with worse 5-year survival compared to subjects receiving routine imaging surveillance, especially when it is accompanied by face-to-face follow-up visits. All patients should be maintained on optimal medical therapy to increase probability of long-term survival after AAA repair. Similar to the patients with small aneurysms who are under imaging surveillance, patients with AAA should postoperatively be counseled to remain abstinent from tobacco and maintained indefinitely on an aspirin and statin agent.[8,24] Specific attention to other cardiovascular risk factor modification, as well as oncologic screening protocols is needed to optimize long-term survival.

Acknowledgment

The author acknowledges and appreciates the assistance of Thomas S. Huber, MD, PhD, who provided significant editorial oversight and mentorship in the development of this chapter.

REFERENCES

1. Gianfagna F, Veronesi G, Tozzi M, et al. Prevalence of abdominal aortic aneurysms in the general population and in subgroups at high cardiovascular risk in Italy. Results of the RoCAV population based study. *Eur J Vasc Endovasc Surg.* 2018;55:633-639.
2. Hernesniemi JA, Vänni V, Hakala T. The prevalence of abdominal aortic aneurysm is consistently high among patients with coronary artery disease. *J Vasc Surg.* 2015;62:232.e3-240.e3.
3. Takagi H, Umemoto T; ALICE (All-Literature Investigation of Cardiovascular Evidence) Group. Association of chronic obstructive pulmonary, coronary artery, or peripheral artery disease with abdominal aortic aneurysm rupture. *Int Angiol.* 2017;36:322-331.
4. Takagi H, Umemoto T; ALICE (All-Literature Investigation of Cardiovascular Evidence) Group. Coronary artery disease and abdominal aortic aneurysm growth. *Vasc Med.* 2016;21:199-208.
5. Lederle FA, Simel DL. The rational clinical examination. Does this patient have abdominal aortic aneurysm? *JAMA.* 1999;281:77-82.
6. Wanhainen A, Lundkvist J, Bergqvist D, Björck M. Cost-effectiveness of different screening strategies for abdominal aortic aneurysm. *J Vasc Surg.* 2005;41:741-751; discussion 751.
7. Medical Advisory Secretariat. Ultrasound screening for abdominal aortic aneurysm: an evidence-based analysis. *Ont Health Technol Assess Ser.* 2006;6:1-67.
8. Chaikof EL, Dalman RL, Eskandari MK, et al. The society for vascular surgery practice guidelines on the care of patients with an abdominal aortic aneurysm. *J Vasc Surg.* 2018;67:2-77.e2.
9. Moll FL, Powell JT, Fraedrich G, et al. Management of abdominal aortic aneurysms clinical practice guidelines of the European Society for Vascular Surgery. *Eur J Vasc Endovasc Surg.* 2011;41(suppl 1):S1-S58.
10. Boyle JR, Gibbs PJ, Kruger A, Shearman CP, Raptis S, Phillips MJ. Existing delays following the presentation of ruptured abdominal aortic aneurysm allow sufficient time to assess patients for endovascular repair. *Eur J Vasc Endovasc Surg.* 2005;29:505-509.
11. Oderich GS, Panneton JM, Bower TC, et al. Infected aortic aneurysms: aggressive presentation, complicated early outcome, but durable results. *J Vasc Surg.* 2001;34:900-908.
12. Osler W. The Gulstonian Lectures, on malignant endocarditis. *Br Med J.* 1885;1:467.
13. Maeda H, Umezawa H, Goshima M, et al. Primary infected abdominal aortic aneurysm: surgical procedures, early mortality rates, and a survey of the prevalence of infectious organisms over a 30-year period. *Surg Today.* 2011;41:346-351.
14. Woon CY, Sebastian MG, Tay KH, Tan SG. Extra-anatomic revascularization and aortic exclusion for mycotic aneurysms of the infrarenal aorta and iliac arteries in an Asian population. *Am J Surg.* 2008;195:66-72.
15. Hagendoorn J, de Vries JP, Moll FL. Primary infected, ruptured abdominal aortic aneurysms: what we learned in 10 years. *Vasc Endovascular Surg.* 2010;44:294-297.
16. Lee CH, Hsieh HC, Ko PJ, Li HJ, Kao TC, Yu SY. In situ versus extra-anatomic reconstruction for primary infected infrarenal abdominal aortic aneurysms. *J Vasc Surg.* 2011;54:64-70.

17. Kan CD, Lee HL, Yang YJ. Outcome after endovascular stent graft treatment for mycotic aortic aneurysm: a systematic review. *J Vasc Surg.* 2007;46:906-912.

18. Sorelius K, Mani K, Björck M, et al. Endovascular treatment of mycotic aortic aneurysms: a European multicenter study. *Circulation.* 2014;130:2136-2142.

19. Ali AT, Modrall JG, Hocking J, et al. Long-term results of the treatment of aortic graft infection by in situ replacement with femoral popliteal vein grafts. *J Vasc Surg.* 2009; 50:30-39.

20. Glimaker H, Björck CG, Hallstensson S, Ohlsén L, Westman B. Avoiding blow-out of the aortic stump by reinforcement with fibrin glue. A report of two cases. *Eur J Vasc Surg.* 1993;7:346-348.

21. Hellmann DB, Grand DJ, Freischlag JA. Inflammatory abdominal aortic aneurysm. *JAMA.* 2007;297:395-400.

22. Parkinson F, Ferguson S, Lewis P, Williams IM, Twine CP; South East Wales Vascular Network. Rupture rates of untreated large abdominal aortic aneurysms in patients unfit for elective repair. *J Vasc Surg.* 2015;61:1606-1612.

23. Dalman RL, Tedesco MM, Myers J, Taylor CA. AAA disease: mechanism, stratification, and treatment. *Ann N Y Acad Sci.* 2006;1085:92-109.

24. De Martino RR, Eldrup-Jorgensen J, Nolan BW, et al. Perioperative management with antiplatelet and statin medication is associated with reduced mortality following vascular surgery. *J Vasc Surg.* 2014;59:1615.e1-1621.e1.

25. Sonesson B, Dias N, Resch T. Is there an age limit for abdominal aortic aneurysm repair? *J Cardiovasc Surg (Torino).* 2018;59:190-194.

26. Powell JT, Gotensparre SM, Sweeting MJ, Brown LC, Fowkes FG, Thompson SG. Rupture rates of small abdominal aortic aneurysms: a systematic review of the literature. *Eur J Vasc Endovasc Surg.* 2011;41:2-10.

27. Mortality results for randomised controlled trial of early elective surgery or ultrasonographic surveillance for small abdominal aortic aneurysms. The UK small aneurysm trial participants. *Lancet.* 1998;352:1649-1655.

28. Katz DJ, Stanley JC, Zelenock GB. Gender differences in abdominal aortic aneurysm prevalence, treatment, and outcome. *J Vasc Surg.* 1997;25:561-568.

29. RESCAN Collaborators; Bown MJ, Sweeting MJ, Brown LC, Powell JT, Thompson SG. Surveillance intervals for small abdominal aortic aneurysms: a meta-analysis. *JAMA.* 2013;309:806-813.

30. Beck AW, Goodney PP, Nolan BW, Likosky DS, Eldrup-Jorgensen J, Cronenwett JL. Predicting 1-year mortality after elective abdominal aortic aneurysm repair. *J Vasc Surg.* 2009;49:838-843.

31. Bertges DJ, Neal D, Schanzer A, et al. The Vascular Quality Initiative Cardiac Risk Index for prediction of myocardial infarction after vascular surgery. *J Vasc Surg.* 2016;64:1411-1421.

Benjamin W. Starnes

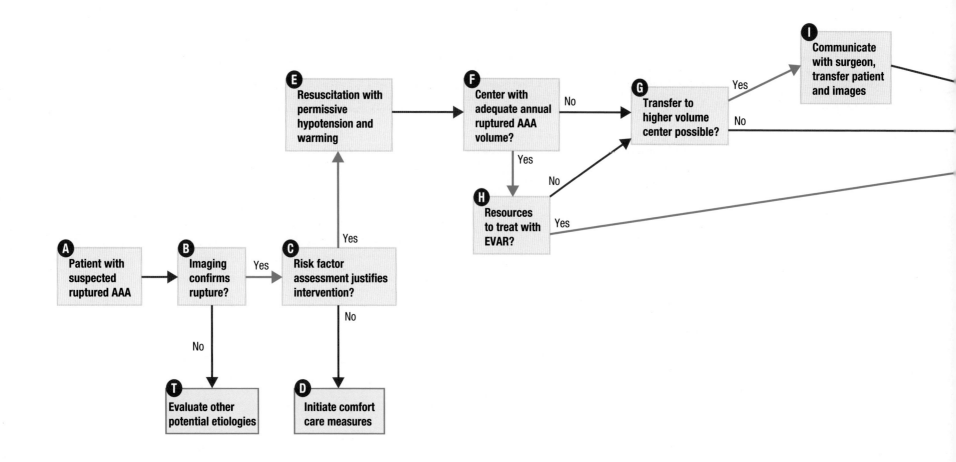

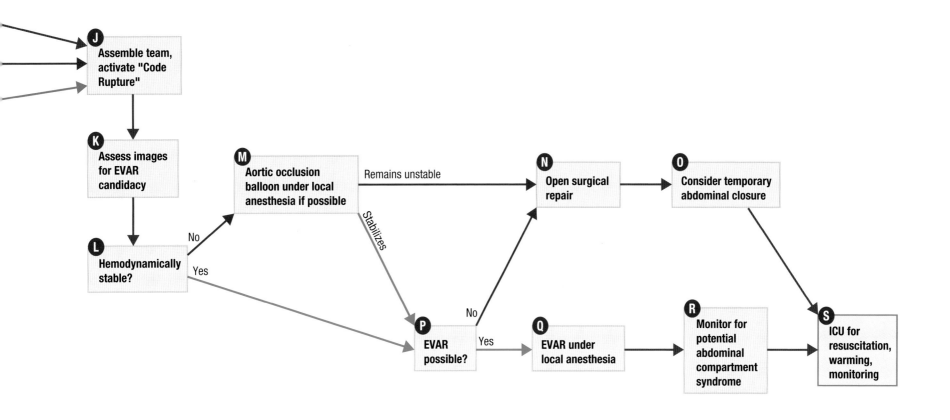

Ⓐ Patient with suspected ruptured AAA

Individuals presenting with ruptured AAA (rAAA) may have varying complaints or clinical conditions. The most typical presentation is abdominal and/or back pain with an episode of transient hypotension or syncope. However, the classic triad of back pain ± abdominal pain, hypotension, and a pulsatile abdominal mass is only present in 25% to 50% of all patients with rAAA.[1] Patients with rAAA may also present in frank hemorrhagic shock with cyanosis, tachycardia, unconsciousness, and severe hypotension.

Ⓑ Imaging confirms rupture?

The initial evaluation of a patient presenting with a suspected rAAA includes imaging to confirm rupture. CTA is the preferred imaging modality for AAA. Axial imaging provides critical information regarding aneurysm size, aortic neck angulation, and seal zone characteristics and is invaluable for operative planning, whether it be for open or endovascular repair.[2,3] Most institutions have CT scanners that are readily and rapidly available. Alternative imaging modalities that are rapidly available include bedside DUS. DUS, however, cannot reliably diagnose aortic rupture, has limited utility in patients who are morbidly obese, and offers insufficient anatomic detail for operative planning.

Ⓒ Risk factor assessment justifies intervention?

There are several risk scores that have been developed to predict mortality from a rAAA. These include the Glasgow Aneurysm Score, the Hardman Index, the Vancouver Score, the Edinburg Ruptured Aneurysm Score, the Vascular Study Group of New England (VSGNE) rAAA Risk Score, and the University of Washington rAAA Risk Score.[4-9] Many of these risk scores use a combination of preoperative and intraoperative variables to predict postoperative mortality. We favor the University of Washington rAAA Risk Score (Table 25-1).

Using this score, when all four preoperative variables are present, there is a 100% risk of mortality. Identification of factors associated with little or no chance of survival can be used to characterize patients who would not benefit from potentially futile repair of a rAAA.

Table 25-1. University of Washington rAAA Risk Score

Age > 76	1 point
SBP < 70 mm Hg at any time	1 point
Serum creatinine >2.0 mg/dL	1 point
Serum pH < 7.2	1 point

Ⓓ Initiate comfort care measures

When a decision is made not to intervene, comfort care measures may be considered. Comfort care refers to a care plan for the patient that is focused on symptom control, pain relief, and quality of life. Often support is provided to family members to help them understand the care plan and to address needs and concerns they might have. There are different forms of comfort care. Two of the best known are hospice and palliative care. Under hospice care, a person receives medical care as well as emotional, psychosocial, and spiritual care delivered by an interdisciplinary team of professionals that includes a physician, nurse, social worker, counselors, home health aides, spiritual and grief support, and trained volunteers. Each person's care plan can be tailored to his or her specific needs, with some patients requiring services that others might not need. Palliative care means patient- and family-centered care that optimizes quality of life by anticipating, preventing, and treating suffering. Palliative care involves addressing physical, intellectual, emotional, social, and spiritual needs and to facilitate patient autonomy, access to information, and choice.[10] It should be noted that some patients with rAAA may live for several days before expiring with comfort care measures in place.

Ⓔ Resuscitation with permissive hypotension and warming

The natural physiologic response to hemorrhagic shock is to become hypotensive, diaphoretic, hypothermic, and tachycardic.[11] One temptation for many physicians presented with direly ill patients in shock is to attempt to normalize the vital signs. This approach may include administering IV fluids and vasopressor agents to raise the blood pressure to normal levels. For a patient presenting with a rAAA, this may lead to catastrophic consequences.[12] Many experts have advocated "permissive hypotension" or "hypotensive hemostasis," which involves limiting resuscitation fluids in case of massive blood loss.[13-16] We use the hypotensive hemostasis protocol of Lachat that involves *permissive hypovolemia* and *controlled hypotension* that allows high enough blood pressure to maintain neurocognitive function. Permissive hypovolemia consists of minimizing administration of fluids, whereas controlled hypotension implies active lowering of SBP with vasodilators and/or beta blockers in normotensive or hypertensive patients to target an SBP < 90 mm Hg. Hypothermia (<35°) is associated with higher morbidity and mortality in patients presenting with hypotension in association with hemorrhagic shock.[17,18]

Ⓕ Center with adequate annual ruptured AAA volume?

The exact "adequate" number of rAAAs on an annual basis required to maintain proficiency has yet to be clearly defined. Surely, if an institution sees one patient per year with a rAAA, they will likely not have the streamlined process in place to deliver the best and most expedient care. Healthcare Quality Initiatives such

as the Leapfrog Group have proposed creating "evidence-based hospital" referral criteria for centers that perform *elective* AAA repair which would require an annual AAA volume (nonruptured) exceeding 50 cases and having ICUs run by board-certified intensivists.[19] It has clearly been shown that institutional volume is associated with improved outcomes.[20,21]

Ⓖ Transfer to higher volume center possible?

Transfer to a higher volume center should not be delayed if the resources and/or expertise are not readily available to perform expedited repair of a rAAA.[22,23] A goal of "door to intervention" time of *<90 minutes* is recommended by the Society for Vascular Surgery AAA Practice Guidelines.[16,24] In situations where a patient with a rAAA is unstable, transfer to a high-volume center with permissive hypotension should still be considered rather than an open operation in a low-volume center, because the outcome would likely be better.

Ⓗ Resources to treat with EVAR?

Resources to perform expedited EVAR include the personnel (surgeon, anesthesiologist, scrub nurse, circulator, radiology technician), an operating room equipped to perform both endovascular and open procedures (in case conversion is required), the appropriate wires, catheters, and sheaths as well as a robust inventory of commercially available stent grafts.[23] A recommended graft inventory of 28- to 32-mm-diameter main body grafts should be available at a minimum. Systems and protocols have been shown at many centers to make a dramatic improvement in successful outcomes and are thus an important resource to be developed.[23,25]

Ⓘ Communicate with surgeon, transfer patient and images

It is of paramount importance that the referring physician, often NOT a surgeon, speak directly with the accepting surgeon to communicate vital details about the patient to include vital signs, hematocrit, pH, and chemistries. It is also recommended that blood be available to transfer with the patient and be administered if needed.[16,22] Blood products should be administered at the discretion of the transferring team but SBPs > 100 mm Hg should be avoided, if possible. Acute pain management should not be overlooked and may be helpful in avoiding HTN during transfer. It is extremely helpful to transfer images if a CT scan has been performed, so that potential EVAR evaluation can be done before the patient arrives at the receiving hospital.

Ⓙ Assemble team, activate "Code Rupture"

Many institutions have implemented call structures for rAAAs where pages simultaneously go out to all team members on call for that particular hospital to assemble the team before the patient arrives, if possible. Team members include resident and attending surgeons, anesthesiologists, operating room nurses, and scrub and angiography technicians. By implementing an institutional rupture protocol, several authors have been able to lower the 30-day mortality rate dramatically to as low as 18%.[23,25,26]

K Assess images for EVAR candidacy

All patients with rAAA should be assessed for potential EVAR, if possible using preoperative CT imaging. Image assessment is done as soon as possible to allow adequate time for EVAR planning while the patient is being prepared for surgery. Often a CTA has been obtained at an outside hospital, but if not, it should be done preoperatively unless the patient is so unstable that emergent surgery is required. In our experience in analyzing more than 300 patients with rAAA, 73% of patients qualified for standard EVAR. Mean aortic neck diameter of these patients was 26.7 mm, neck length 17.2, and average aneurysm size 82.4 mm.[23] A suitable aortic neck of no more than 32 mm in diameter and at least 15 mm in length will lead to the best outcomes for EVAR in this setting.

L Hemodynamically stable?

Hemodynamic stability can be simply defined as stable blood flow. Hemodynamic instability is defined as any instability in blood pressure that can lead to inadequate arterial blood flow to vital organs. If the patient's SBP is 80 mm Hg, does not widely fluctuate, and he/she is cognitively intact, then the patient is *hypotensive* but hemodynamically stable. If a patient is hypotensive, not cognitively intact and requiring vasopressive medications to maintain heart rate and blood pressure, then he/she is considered hemodynamically unstable.[13]

M Aortic occlusion balloon under local anesthesia if possible

One of the most significant findings to come out of the IM-PROVE (Immediate Management of the Patient with Ruptured Aneurysm: Open Versus Endovascular Repair) trial was that patients undergoing EVAR with local anesthesia had a survival benefit.[27] Although this may represent selection bias, it does highlight that these procedures can be done entirely under local anesthesia with the patient either awake or lightly sedated. Aortic occlusion balloons can be rapidly placed once the patient has been prepared and draped.[23,28] We routinely place the balloon at the T-12 vertebral body and only inflate it if necessary to maintain blood pressure. Balloons should be inserted through long supportive sheaths (40-55 cm) over stiff wires. The balloon should initially be inflated under fluoroscopic guidance until it changes from a circular shape to a rectangular or squared shape. The volume required to attain this shape should be recorded in case blind inflation is required after an open conversion. Further, we recommend that balloon occlusion also be used in planned open repair if possible, because

this can more rapidly stabilize a patient than supraceliac clamping. General anesthesia for open repair can then be induced after aortic balloon placement.

N Open surgical repair

The most important goal of the operation is to place a clamp on the aorta above the area of rupture. If an aortic occlusion balloon has been placed before induction of anesthesia, the approach can be done more deliberately to avoid iatrogenic injuries to nearby structures.[28] Open surgical repair is performed either through a transperitoneal or retroperitoneal incision depending on surgeon experience and factors such as prior abdominal surgery. A suitable aortic clamp is then placed after deflation and retraction of the aortic occlusion balloon. If an aortic occlusion balloon has not been utilized, supraceliac control of the aorta can be rapidly obtained before infrarenal or suprarenal clamp placement. Our practice has been to administer 50 U/kg heparin when the patient presents with a contained rupture, is hemodynamically stable, and has a normal INR. We do not give heparin to patients who are hemodynamically unstable or with an INR > 2.0. Elegant descriptions of both transperitoneal and retroperitoneal repair of ruptured AAAs have been published.[29-33]

O Consider temporary abdominal closure

Depending on the amount of fluid resuscitation and the duration of the open surgical repair, it may prove difficult to close the abdominal wall fascia. In this scenario, it is highly recommended to apply a temporary dressing and leave the incision open until it can be subsequently closed 1 to 3 days later.[34] A vacuum-assisted device is recommended.[35] If this is not available, a homemade vacuum dressing can be constructed with sponges, standard suction tubing, and iodine-impregnated adhesive drapes. The last resort is to use a series of towel clips directly on the skin.

P EVAR possible?

If the patient is an EVAR candidate and the resources exist to repair the rAAA in an expedient manner, EVAR should be planned and performed unless the patient cannot be stabilized. There exist several technical tips for expediting EVAR for rAAA.[23,36] These include proper control and rapid positioning of the patient with the left arm tucked, a secure strap placed above the knees, rapid percutaneous femoral access, always placing the aortic occlusion balloon from the straightest iliac artery (to facilitate contralateral gate cannulation), and imaging focused on the proper gantry angles to maximize visualization of the aortic neck.

Q EVAR under local anesthesia

Standard EVAR can be carried out under local anesthesia with mild to moderate sedation (preferred) or under general anesthesia if the patient stabilizes.[27] The choice to place an aortic occlusion balloon can be based on the hemodynamic stability of the patient.

R Monitor for potential abdominal compartment syndrome

After EVAR repair of rAAA, abdominal compartment can develop because of hemorrhage before EVAR or potentially from ongoing bleeding from lumbar arteries into the ruptured AAA sac. The exact clinical conditions that define abdominal compartment syndrome (ACS) are controversial; however, organ dysfunction caused by intra-abdominal HTN is considered to be abdominal compartment syndrome.[34,37,38] Some authorities have recommended measuring bladder pressures to diagnose ACS. A bladder pressure of >20 mm Hg is diagnostic of ACS. Our group has a very low threshold for performing decompression in these patients and this is largely based on clinical judgment and assessment of peak airway pressures, bladder pressures, and abdominal rigidity. Details for assessment and treatment of ACS are provided in Chapter 85.

S ICU for resuscitation, warming, monitoring

In the postoperative period after rAAA repair, patients typically require massive fluid resuscitation and warming. This is true after both open repair and EVAR.[39] Close monitoring of vital signs and respiratory and renal function, with appropriate support is essential. Colon ischemia is more frequent after rAAA repair than elective repair, and should be urgently evaluated if suspected, because failure to treat promptly can be fatal (see Chapter 84).

T Evaluate other potential etiologies

If imaging does not confirm rAAA, other etiologies for the presenting symptoms should be evaluated. AAAs may be symptomatic, but not ruptured, and still require urgent treatment (see Chapter 24). Common conditions that present similarly to rAAA include MI, CHF, gastric or duodenal perforation, ureteral obstruction, diverticulitis, and lumbar spine disease.

REFERENCES

1. Marston WA, Ahlquist R, Johnson G Jr, Meyer AA. Misdiagnosis of ruptured abdominal aortic aneurysms. *J Vasc Surg.* 1992;16(1):17-22.
2. Siegel CL, Cohan RH, Korobkin M, Alpern MB, Courneya DL, Leder RA. Abdominal aortic aneurysm morphology: CT features in patients with ruptured and nonruptured aneurysms. *AJR Am J Roentgenol.* 1994;163(5):1123-1129.
3. Rakita D, Newatia A, Hines JJ, Siegel DN, Friedman B. Spectrum of CT findings in rupture and impending rupture of abdominal aortic aneurysms. *Radiographics.* 2007;27(2):497-507.
4. Ali MM, Flahive J, Schanzer A, et al. In patients stratified by preoperative risk, endovascular repair of ruptured abdominal aortic aneurysms has a lower in-hospital mortality and morbidity than open repair. *J Vasc Surg.* 2015;61(6):1399-1407.
5. Chen JC, Hildebrand HD, Salvian AJ, et al. Predictors of death in nonruptured and ruptured abdominal aortic aneurysms. *J Vasc Surg.* 1996;24(4):614-620; discussion 21-23.

6. Garland BT, Danaher PJ, Desikan S, et al. Preoperative risk score for the prediction of mortality after repair of ruptured abdominal aortic aneurysms. *J Vasc Surg*. 2018;68:991-997.

7. Hardman DT, Fisher CM, Patel MI, et al. Ruptured abdominal aortic aneurysms: who should be offered surgery? *J Vasc Surg*. 1996;23(1):123-129.

8. Samy AK, Murray G, MacBain G. Prospective evaluation of the Glasgow aneurysm score. *J R Coll Surg Edinb*. 1996;41(2):105-107.

9. Tambyraja A, Murie J, Chalmers R. Predictors of outcome after abdominal aortic aneurysm rupture: Edinburgh Ruptured Aneurysm Score. *World J Surg*. 2007;31(11):2243-2247.

10. Campbell WB. Non-intervention and palliative care in vascular patients. *Br J Surg*. 2000;87(12):1601-1602.

11. Bougle A, Harrois A, Duranteau J. Resuscitative strategies in traumatic hemorrhagic shock. *Ann Intensive Care*. 2013;3(1):1.

12. Morrison CA, Carrick MM, Norman MA, et al. Hypotensive resuscitation strategy reduces transfusion requirements and severe postoperative coagulopathy in trauma patients with hemorrhagic shock: preliminary results of a randomized controlled trial. *J Trauma*. 2011;70(3):652-663.

13. Lachat ML, Pfammatter T, Witzke HJ, et al. Endovascular repair with bifurcated stent-grafts under local anaesthesia to improve outcome of ruptured aortoiliac aneurysms. *Eur J Vasc Endovasc Surg*. 2002;23(6):528-536.

14. Moll FL, Powell JT, Fraedrich G, et al. Management of abdominal aortic aneurysms clinical practice guidelines of the European society for vascular surgery. *Eur J Vasc Endovasc Surg*. 2011;41(suppl 1):S1-S58.

15. van der Vliet JA, van Aalst DL, Schultze Kool LJ, Wever JJ, Blankensteijn JD. Hypotensive hemostatis (permissive hypotension) for ruptured abdominal aortic aneurysm: are we really in control? *Vascular*. 2007;15(4):197-200.

16. Chaikof EL, Dalman RL, Eskandari MK, et al. The Society for Vascular Surgery practice guidelines on the care of patients with an abdominal aortic aneurysm. *J Vasc Surg*. 2018;67(1):2.e2-77.e2.

17. Kozek-Langenecker SA, Afshari A, Albaladejo P, et al. Management of severe perioperative bleeding: guidelines from the European Society of Anaesthesiology. *Eur J Anaesthesiol*. 2013;30(6):270-382.

18. Quiroga E, Tran NT, Hatsukami T, Starnes BW. Hypothermia is associated with increased mortality in patients undergoing repair of ruptured abdominal aortic aneurysm. *J Endovasc Ther*. 2010;17(3):434-438.

19. Brooke BS, Perler BA, Dominici F, Makary MA, Pronovost PJ. Reduction of in-hospital mortality among California hospitals meeting Leapfrog evidence-based standards for abdominal aortic aneurysm repair. *J Vasc Surg*. 2008;47(6):1155-1156; discussion 63-64.

20. McPhee J, Eslami MH, Arous EJ, Messina LM, Schanzer A. Endovascular treatment of ruptured abdominal aortic aneurysms in the United States (2001-2006): a significant survival benefit over open repair is independently associated with increased institutional volume. *J Vasc Surg*. 2009;49(4):817-826.

21. Vogel TR, Nackman GB, Brevetti LS, et al. Resource utilization and outcomes: effect of transfer on patients with ruptured abdominal aortic aneurysms. *Ann Vasc Surg*. 2005;19(2):149-153.

22. Mell MW, Schneider PA, Starnes BW. Variability in transfer criteria for patients with ruptured abdominal aortic aneurysm in the western United States. *J Vasc Surg*. 2015;62(2):326-330.

23. Starnes BW, Quiroga E, Hutter C, et al. Management of ruptured abdominal aortic aneurysm in the endovascular era. *J Vasc Surg*. 2010;51(1):9-17; discussion 17-18.

24. Patel MS, Chaikof EL. Ruptured aneurysm systems of care: a national imperative to improve clinical outcomes. *J Vasc Surg*. 2017;65(3):589-590.

25. Mehta M, Taggert J, Darling RC III, et al. Establishing a protocol for endovascular treatment of ruptured abdominal aortic aneurysms: outcomes of a prospective analysis. *J Vasc Surg*. 2006;44(1):1-8; discussion 8.

26. Veith FJ, Lachat M, Mayer D, et al. Collected world and single center experience with endovascular treatment of ruptured abdominal aortic aneurysms. *Ann Surg*. 2009;250(5):818-824.

27. IMPROVE Trial Investigators; Powell JT, Hinchliffe RJ, Thompson MM, et al. Observations from the IMPROVE trial concerning the clinical care of patients with ruptured abdominal aortic aneurysm. *Br J Surg*. 2014;101(3):216-224; discussion 224.

28. Arthurs Z, Starnes B, See C, Andersen C. Clamp before you cut: proximal control of ruptured abdominal aortic aneurysms using endovascular balloon occlusion—case reports. *Vasc Endovascular Surg*. 2006;40(2):149-155.

29. Bahnson HT. Treatment of abdominal aortic aneurysm by excision and replacement by homograft. *Circulation*. 1954; 9(4):494-503.

30. Chang BB, Shah DM, Paty PS, Kaufman JL, Leather RP. Can the retroperitoneal approach be used for ruptured abdominal aortic aneurysms? *J Vasc Surg*. 1990;11(2):326-330.

31. Cooley DA, Debakey ME. Ruptured aneurysms of abdominal aorta; excision and homograft replacement. *Postgrad Med*. 1954;16(4):334-342.

32. Dubost C, Allary M, Oeconomos N. Resection of an aneurysm of the abdominal aorta: reestablishment of the continuity by a preserved human arterial graft, with result after five months. *AMA Arch Surg*. 1952;64(3):405-408.

33. Rob C. Extraperitoneal approach to the abdominal aorta. *Surgery*. 1963;53:87-89.

34. Kirkpatrick AW, Roberts DJ, De Waele J, et al. Intra-abdominal hypertension and the abdominal compartment syndrome: updated consensus definitions and clinical practice guidelines from the World Society of the Abdominal Compartment Syndrome. *Intensive Care Med*. 2013;39(7):1190-1206.

35. Sorelius K, Wanhainen A, Acosta S, Svensson M, Djavani-Gidlund K, Bjorck M. Open abdomen treatment after aortic aneurysm repair with vacuum-assisted wound closure and mesh-mediated fascial traction. *Eur J Vasc Endovasc Surg*. 2013;45(6):588-594.

36. Mehta M. Technical tips for EVAR for ruptured AAA. *Semin Vasc Surg*. 2009;22(3):181-186.

37. Djavani Gidlund K, Wanhainen A, Bjorck M. Intra-abdominal hypertension and abdominal compartment syndrome after endovascular repair of ruptured abdominal aortic aneurysm. *Eur J Vasc Endovasc Surg*. 2011;41(6):742-747.

38. Djavani K, Wanhainen A, Bjorck M. Intra-abdominal hypertension and abdominal compartment syndrome following surgery for ruptured abdominal aortic aneurysm. *Eur J Vasc Endovasc Surg*. 2006;31(6):581-584.

39. Bown MJ, Nicholson ML, Bell PR, Sayers RD. The systemic inflammatory response syndrome, organ failure, and mortality after abdominal aortic aneurysm repair. *J Vasc Surg*. 2003;37(3):600-606.

Michael Neilson • Brian W. Nolan

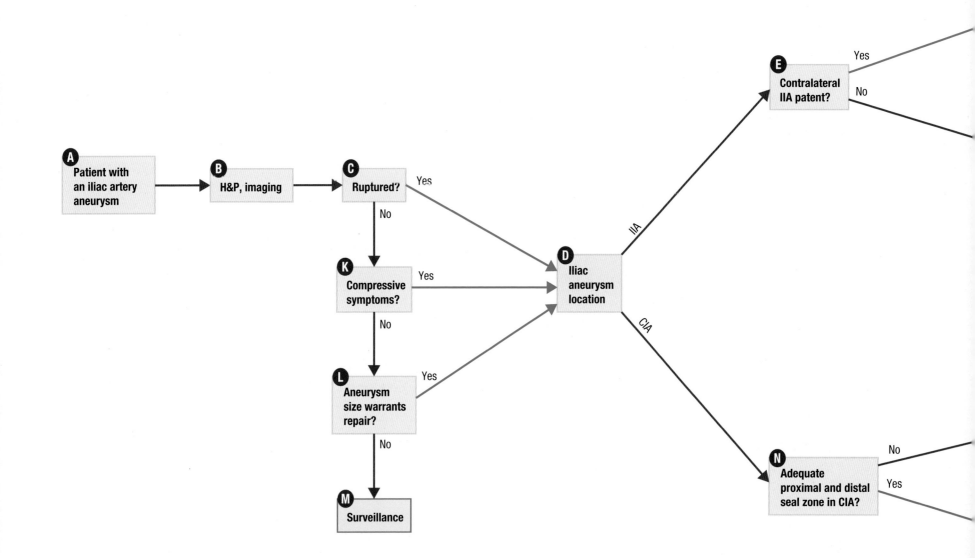

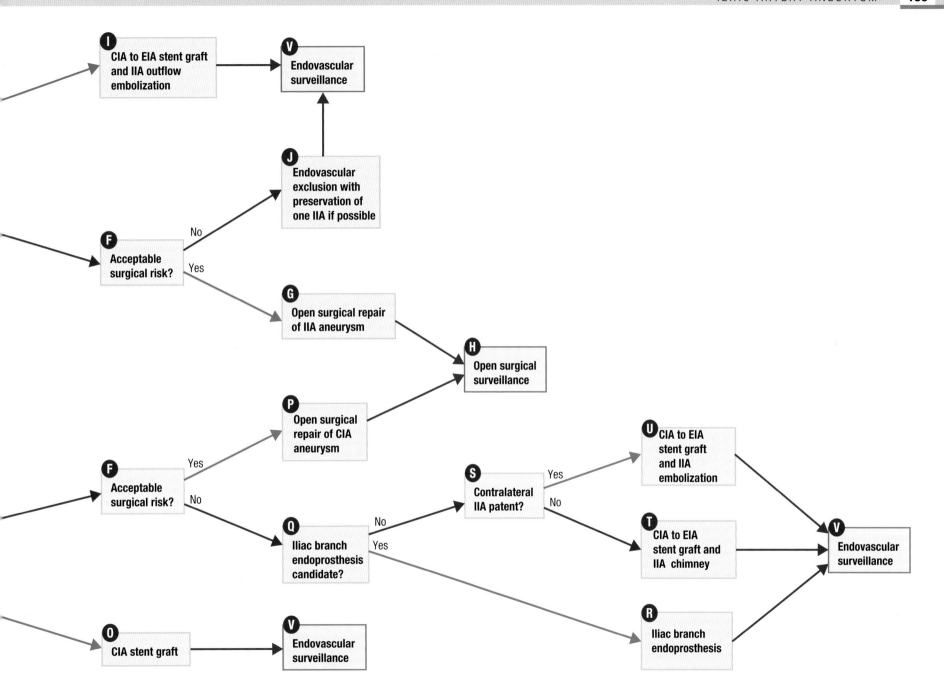

A **Patient with an iliac artery aneurysm**

Iliac artery aneurysms are usually (80%-90%) associated with AAAs.[1] Approximately 40% of AAAs undergoing repair have associated CIA aneurysms[2] and their treatment is discussed in Chapter 24. Isolated iliac artery aneurysms represent a small percentage of all aneurysms (1.3%), and their treatment is considered in detail in this chapter. Of iliac aneurysms, 70% are of the CIA. The remaining are of the IIA. Isolated EIA aneurysms are exceedingly rare. The etiology of iliac aneurysms is similar to that of other aneurysms: most are degenerative, with far fewer classified as mycotic, inflammatory, traumatic, or associated with connective tissue disease. Aneurysms of the IAA are most often unilateral, with the left being the most frequent side affected (61.8%), and fewer being bilateral (10.9%).[3]

B **H&P, imaging**

When evaluating a patient with an isolated iliac artery aneurysm, the history should focus on whether the aneurysm is symptomatic and its presumed etiology (ie, family history of aneurysmal disease, personal or family history of connective tissue disease, recent infections, trauma). Presenting symptoms can be due to the aneurysm causing compression of surrounding structures, resulting in DVT (if compressing the iliac vein), hydronephrosis (if compressing the ureter), lower extremity radiculopathy (if compressing the nerves), or abdominal/flank pain.[3,4] Pain can also be caused by rupture (see C). Symptoms can be caused by thrombosis, leading to buttock claudication or even ALI; however, this is uncommon. A complete physical examination should be undertaken, with a focus on evaluating whether the patient has other aneurysms (ie, femoral, popliteal, etc.). CTA is the preferred imaging modality to fully assess the aneurysm and pertinent anatomy (in those patients without contraindications).

C **Ruptured?**

Ruptured aneurysms of either CIA or IIA are surgical emergencies. Although little data exist regarding the mortality of a ruptured isolated CIA aneurysm, it is likely similar to that associated with a ruptured AAA.[5] Ruptured IIA aneurysms have traditionally carried a high mortality, up to 53% in one systematic review (which heavily favored open repair),[3] although more contemporary case series from large single centers[6,7] and multicenter retrospective analysis have demonstrated lower mortality rates (7%-13%).[8] Ruptured CIA aneurysms often present in a manner similar to AAA, that is, back/abdominal pain and hypotension. Ruptured IIA aneurysms can present similarly, or, due to their location deep in the pelvis, with rectal bleeding or hematuria if the rupture is associated with erosion of the aneurysm into adjacent structures.[9]

D **Iliac aneurysm location**

The location of the aneurysm is of utmost importance because the treatment differs depending on whether the isolated aneurysm is located in the CIA or IIA.

E **Contralateral IIA patent?**

Many of the treatment decisions regarding the management of isolated IIA aneurysms revolve around whether the contralateral IIA is patent. All attempts to maintain patency to at least one IIA should be undertaken to reduce the risk of pelvic ischemia, which has been reported to be as high as 75% at 24 months when both IIAs are compromised.[6]

F **Acceptable surgical risk?**

A careful assessment of the patient's fitness for open surgery should be undertaken, including cardiac, pulmonary, renal, and other major organ function.

G **Open surgical repair of IIA aneurysm**

Patients without a patent contralateral IIA who are deemed appropriate for surgery should undergo open repair of their isolated IAA aneurysm to preserve IIA, and thereby pelvic, blood flow. Exposure can be either retroperitoneal through an oblique incision in the ipsilateral lower abdomen or transperitoneal, depending on surgeon preference. These patients should undergo an interposition bypass graft of the IIA aneurysm. Distal control of the outflow branches of the IIA is obtained first, and an end-to-end anastomosis to the distal internal iliac artery is undertaken. If the distal IIA is aneurysmal, it may be possible to bypass to one or two of the largest outflow arteries, although this can be technically challenging. The proximal anastomosis is then done to the proximal IIA, EIA, or CIA depending on the quality of the vessel. If there is inadequate proximal IIA or the CIA is aneurysmal (or otherwise deemed inadequate to receive the proximal anastomosis), then we perform an end-to-end aorto to EIA bypass, which then serves as inflow for the IIA interposition bypass. Endoaneurysmorrhaphy with oversewing of all branches from within the sac is not appropriate in this setting because it would lead to bilateral internal iliac artery occlusion and increased risk of buttock claudication, pelvic necrosis, or paralysis. Large single-center experiences have shown that maintaining flow to at least one IIA is often attainable, and such bypasses have high (95%) primary patency at 1 year.[6]

H **Open surgical surveillance**

Following open repair of IIA or CIA aneurysm follow-up, we obtain imaging at 1 month and 1 year, and then as needed.

I **CIA to EIA stent graft and IIA outflow embolization**

Open surgical repair was once the standard of care for patients who presented with symptomatic or ruptured IIA aneurysms,[3,10] whereas endovascular intervention has now become standard therapy. In patients with a patent contralateral IIA, ipsilateral IIA aneurysm outflow embolization and inflow exclusion with a stent graft from the CIA to the EIA can be performed. Although there are no randomized controlled trials comparing open to endovascular

repair, there are retrospective cohort studies describing shorter hospital stay and lower morbidity with endovascular repair compared to open repair, although at the cost of potentially increased pelvic ischemia.[6] Although there have been case reports describing more creative treatment techniques such as ultrasound-guided embolization of the sac,[11] in the acute setting, distal embolization and proximal coverage is fast and effective. It should be noted that although the abovementioned technique is ideal to prevent type II endoleaks, embolization of each outflow vessel is not always possible in an emergent setting, in which case embolization of the aneurysm sac with proximal coverage may be an acceptable alternative. However, this seems to be associated with a higher risk of type II endoleak as well as secondary interventions.[12] These experiences have been mirrored in elective repair, as well. In a review of consecutive patients with a patent contralateral IIA undergoing elective endovascular repair of IIA aneurysms, the "coil and cover technique" was well tolerated and associated with decreased morbidity and length of stay as compared to open repair. In a systematic review, Antoniou et al. demonstrated a 2% 30-day mortality rate, although they reported a technical success rate of only 71%,[13] suggesting that IIA aneurysms can be difficult to treat in a purely endovascular manner. In a retrospective review of 33 patients treated with selective embolization and proximal occlusion with stent grafts, there was a 79% technical success rate as opposed to just 29% with proximal embolization.[14]

J **Endovascular exclusion with preservation of one IIA if possible**

If the patient is stable, after successfully excluding the IIA aneurysm as mentioned, endovascular treatment of the nonaneurysmal (although severely diseased or occluded) contralateral IIA can be considered to avoid pelvic ischemia. If the contralateral IIA is stenosed, although not occluded, then endovascular revascularization with either PTA or stent/stent graft can be considered. Should one place a stent graft, this may require a chimney or periscope technique into the CIA to preserve blood flow to the EIA.[15] If endovascular treatment is not possible, then an EIA to IIA bypass of the contralateral (nonaneurysmal) IIA has been shown to have excellent durability and freedom from ischemic complications, with only 4% of these patients experiencing buttock claudication, although at the cost of increased blood loss and length of stay.[16]

K **Compressive symptoms?**

As many as 53% of patients with intact isolated iliac artery aneurysms present with compressive symptoms caused by mass effect of the aneurysm. These include hydronephrosis, DVT, and radiculopathy, and are an indication for treatment.[3,17]

L **Aneurysm size warrants repair?**

For a patient presenting with an isolated asymptomatic CIA aneurysm, treatment should be considered when the diameter is >3.5 cm.

This is largely based on the retrospective analysis of 715 such aneurysms that showed no CIA aneurysm ruptured below 3.8 cm.[4] Isolated CIA aneurysms usually expand slowly (<10% per year), although this varies depending on size.[4,18] Aneurysms growing at a faster rate may be recommended for repair at a 3-cm diameter, although there is no firm evidence to support this. The decision to treat must take into consideration the risk of treatment and the life expectancy of the patient to ensure benefit of prophylactic repair. Isolated aneurysms of the IAA are less frequent than are CIA aneurysms, accounting for only 20% of isolated iliac aneurysms.[19] There have been retrospective multicenter studies showing the risk of rupture does not increase until 4 cm.[8] We consider repair once the 3.5- to 4-cm threshold has been reached, depending on the overall health and life expectancy of the patient.

Ⓜ Surveillance

Patients with small CIA and IIA aneurysms who are candidates for future treatment should be followed up with annual imaging. CIA aneurysms can be followed up with DUS, which has a high concordance with CTA measurements.[18] IIA aneurysms require CTA surveillances because DUS does not provide accurate measurement deep in the pelvis.[19] Noncontrast CT scan is adequate for surveillance of size.

Ⓝ Adequate proximal and distal seal zone in CIA?

A careful assessment of the CTA should be undertaken to determine whether there is a 1-cm length of normal CIA to provide an adequate proximal and distal seal zone for stent-graft repair of a CIA aneurysm.

Ⓞ CIA stent graft

If there is at least a 1-cm-long proximal and distal normal artery landing zone, then a simple CIA stent graft can be used for repair. Recent literature has supported improved mortality and morbidity in patients with CIA aneurysms treated using endovascular therapy versus open repair. An observational study of 33,000 CIA aneurysm repairs found that those treated endovascularly, despite being older and with more comorbidities (increased incidence of heart and renal disease) had lower mortality (1.8% vs. 0.5%), fewer complications (18% vs. 7%), and shorter length of stay.[20] Patency of CIA endovascular repair has been shown to be comparable to that seen with open repair.[21,22]

Ⓟ Open surgical repair of CIA aneurysm

If the patient does not have adequate endovascular seal zones but is a good surgical candidate, then open repair with preservation of ipsilateral IIA perfusion is warranted. Often this can be done with a tube graft from the common iliac to the iliac bifurcation. Of note, should the patient have a concomitant IIA aneurysm, then a bifurcated graft would be required unless the IIA aneurysm is simply excluded.

Ⓠ Iliac branch endoprosthesis candidate?

If the patient is not an appropriate open surgical candidate and does not have an adequate seal distal zone for isolated CIA stent grafting, then the patient's anatomy should be evaluated for an iliac branch endoprosthesis (IBE). Currently, the only device with approval in the United States is the Gore IBE, which requires a minimum CIA diameter of 17 mm, an IIA diameter of 6.5 to 13.5 mm, and EIA diameter of 6.5 to 25 mm.[23] It is only approved for aortoiliac aneurysm use, and as such, its use for an isolated CIA is technically "off label."

Ⓡ Iliac branch endoprosthesis

IBE is advocated if the patient's anatomy fits the instructions for use criteria. In a multicenter study, Schnieder et al. showed a 95% technical success rate of IBE with a 95% IIA patency rate, with 100% freedom from buttock claudication, although follow-up was limited to 6 months.[22] This experience was mirrored in a retrospective cohort of 46 patients, again with only 6 months of follow-up.[24] Verzini et al. prospectively evaluated 74 consecutive patients, treated either with IBE (Cook Medical Zenith system) or traditional endovascular means with CIA stent graft and occlusion of the ipsilateral IIA, and found similar success rates, although with a trend toward more buttock claudication in the traditional endovascular group at 1 year.[25] IBEs may become the first-line treatment choice for patients with CIA aneurysms once prospective data with longer follow-up and more devices to accommodate different iliac sizes are available.

Ⓢ Contralateral IIA patent?

If the contralateral IIA is occluded or severely diseased, revascularization should be considered, to reduce the risk pelvic ischemia which has been reported to be as high as 75% at 24 months post intervention when both IIA are occluded.[6]

Ⓣ CIA to EIA stent graft and IIA chimney

If the patient is not an acceptable candidate for open surgery, then ipsilateral IIA revascularization with a chimney (or also referred to as a "sandwich technique") has shown good midterm results with low rates of buttock claudication or pelvic ischemia.[26] This is done by placing a stent graft within the ipsilateral IIA with the proximal portion extending into the CIA. An additional stent graft is then placed from the CIA to the EIA (overlapping the IIA stent graft within the CIA), thereby maintaining flow to both the IIA and EIA.

Ⓤ CIA to EIA stent graft and IIA embolization

If the contralateral IIA is patent, then embolization of the IIA outflow branches to prevent a type II endoleak, combined with CIA to CIA iliac stent grafting should be undertaken. Embolization should be as proximal as possible in the IIA branches to preserve pelvic collateral flow. In this case, when the contralateral IIA is

patent, the risk of buttock claudication or other ischemic complications is acceptable, with 68% freedom from buttock claudication at 2 years.[6]

Ⓥ Endovascular surveillance

Much like endovascular aneurysm repair in other arterial beds, a regimented surveillance program is necessary because of the risk of endoleak and late rupture after endovascular iliac artery aneurysm repair. In a retrospective review of procedures performed with IIA branch embolization, there was a 19% endoleak rate, 9% sac enlargement, and 9% need for secondary procedures at 5 years[27] that increased to as high as 36% with patients treated for ruptured aneurysms.[7] Similarly, in one large review, there was a 10% rate of new endoleaks at an average of 15-month follow-up.[12] Although there are no published guidelines for iliac aneurysm repair, we utilize the Society for Vascular Surgery Guidelines for Endovascular Aortic Aneurysm Repair which recommend CTA and DUS at 1 month, and then yearly, with additional imaging at 6 months if type II endoleak is detected.[28]

REFERENCES

1. Lawrence PF, Gazak C, Bhirangi L, et al. The epidemiology of surgically repaired aneurysms in the United States. *J Vasc Surg*. 1999;30(4):632-640.
2. Bannazadeh M, Jenkins C, Forsyth A, et al. Outcomes for concomitant common iliac artery aneurysms after endovascular abdominal aortic aneurysm repair. *J Vasc Surg*. 2017;66(5):1390-1397.
3. Wilhelm BJ, Sakharpe A, Ibrahim G, Baccaro LM, Fisher J. The 100-year evolution of the isolated internal iliac artery aneurysm. *Ann Vasc Surg*. 2014;28(4):1070-1077.
4. Huang Y, Gloviczki P, Duncan AA, et al. Common iliac artery aneurysm: expansion rate and results of open surgical and endovascular repair. *J Vasc Surg*. 2008;47(6):1203-1210; discussion 1210-1201.
5. Shimabukuro K, Miyauchi T, Takemura H. Rupture of left common iliac artery aneurysm. *J Vasc Surg*. 2007;45(5):1083.
6. Rana MA, Kalra M, Oderich GS, et al. Outcomes of open and endovascular repair for ruptured and nonruptured internal iliac artery aneurysms. *J Vasc Surg*. 2014;59(3):634-644.
7. Hechelhammer L, Rancic Z, Pfiffner R, et al. Midterm outcome of endovascular repair of ruptured isolated iliac artery aneurysms. *J Vasc Surg*. 2010;52(5):1159-1163.
8. Laine MT, Bjorck M, Beiles CB, et al. Few internal iliac artery aneurysms rupture under 4 cm. *J Vasc Surg*. 2017;65(1):76-81.
9. Krupski WC, Bass A, Rosenberg GD, Dilley RB, Stoney RJ. The elusive isolated hypogastric artery aneurysm: novel presentations. *J Vasc Surg*. 1989;10(5):557-562.
10. Ricci MA, Najarian K, Healey CT. Successful endovascular treatment of a ruptured internal iliac aneurysm. *J Vasc Surg*. 2002;35(6):1274-1276.

11. Vaillant M, Bartoli MA, Soler R, et al. Emergency embolization of a ruptured aneurysm of the internal iliac artery by direct ultrasound-guided puncture: report of a case. *Ann Vasc Surg.* 2016;31:205.e201-204.

12. Millon A, Paquet Y, Ben Ahmed S, Pinel G, Rosset E, Lermusiaux P. Midterm outcomes of embolisation of internal iliac artery aneurysms. *Eur J Vasc Endovasc Surg.* 2013;45(1):22-27.

13. Antoniou GA, Nassef AH, Antoniou SA, Loh CY, Turner DR, Beard JD. Endovascular treatment of isolated internal iliac artery aneurysms. *Vascular.* 2011;19(6):291-300.

14. Muradi A, Yamaguchi M, Okada T, et al. Technical and outcome considerations of endovascular treatment for internal iliac artery aneurysms. *Cardiovasc Intervent Radiol.* 2014;37(2):348-354.

15. Duvnjak S. Endovascular treatment of aortoiliac aneurysms: From intentional occlusion of the internal iliac artery to branch iliac stent graft. *World J Radiol.* 2016;8(3):275-280.

16. Lee WA, Nelson PR, Berceli SA, Seeger JM, Huber TS. Outcome after hypogastric artery bypass and embolization during endovascular aneurysm repair. *J Vasc Surg.* 2006;44(6):1162-1168; discussion 1168-1169.

17. Walsh JJ, Williams LR, Driscoll JL, Lee JF. Vein compression by arterial aneurysms. *J Vasc Surg.* 1988;8(4):465-469.

18. Santilli SM, Wernsing SE, Lee ES. Expansion rates and outcomes for iliac artery aneurysms. *J Vasc Surg.* 2000;31(1, pt 1):114-121.

19. Morris ME, Huber KM, Maijub JG. Ruptured hypogastric artery aneurysms: a contemporary review. *Vasc Endovasc Surg.* 2013;47(3):239-244.

20. Buck DB, Bensley RP, Darling J, et al. The effect of endovascular treatment on isolated iliac artery aneurysm treatment and mortality. *J Vasc Surg.* 2015;62(2):331-335.

21. Fossaceca R, Guzzardi G, Di Terlizzi M, et al. Long-term efficacy of endovascular treatment of isolated iliac artery aneurysms. *Radiol Med.* 2013;118(1):62-73.

22. Schneider DB, Matsumura JS, Lee JT, Peterson BG, Chaer RA, Oderich GS. Prospective, multicenter study of endovascular repair of aortoiliac and iliac aneurysms using the Gore Iliac Branch Endoprosthesis. *J Vasc Surg.* 2017;66(3):775-785.

23. W. L. Gore & Associates. Gore Excluder iliac branch endoprosthesis instructions for use. https://www.accessdata.fda.gov/cdrh_docs/pdf2/P020004S123d.pdf. Accessed May 2020.

24. Zander T, Baldi S, Rabellino M, et al. Bifurcated endograft (Excluder) in the treatment of isolated iliac artery aneurysm: preliminary report. *Cardiovasc Intervent Radiol.* 2009;32(5):928-936.

25. Verzini F, Parlani G, Romano L, De Rango P, Panuccio G, Cao P. Endovascular treatment of iliac aneurysm: Concurrent comparison of side branch endograft versus hypogastric exclusion. *J Vasc Surg.* 2009;49(5):1154-1161.

26. Lobato AC, Camacho-Lobato L. The sandwich technique to treat complex aortoiliac or isolated iliac aneurysms: results of midterm follow-up. *J Vasc Surg.* 2013;57(2 Suppl):26S-34S.

27. Pirvu A, Gallet N, Perou S, Thony F, Magne JL. Midterm results of internal iliac artery aneurysm embolization. *J Med Vasc.* 2017;42(3):157-161.

28. Chaikof EL, Dalman RL, Eskandari MK, et al. The Society for Vascular Surgery practice guidelines on the care of patients with an abdominal aortic aneurysm. *J Vasc Surg.* 2018;67(1):2-77.e72.

Ashton Lee • Wei Zhou

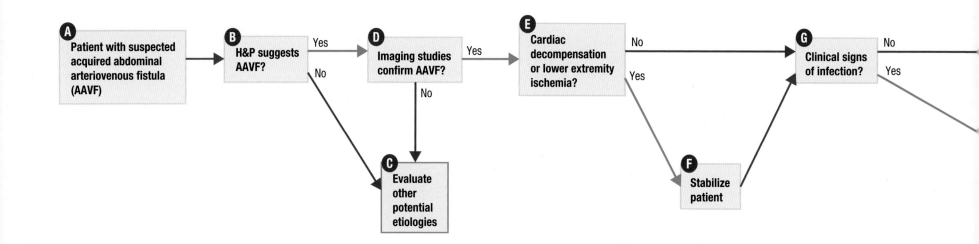

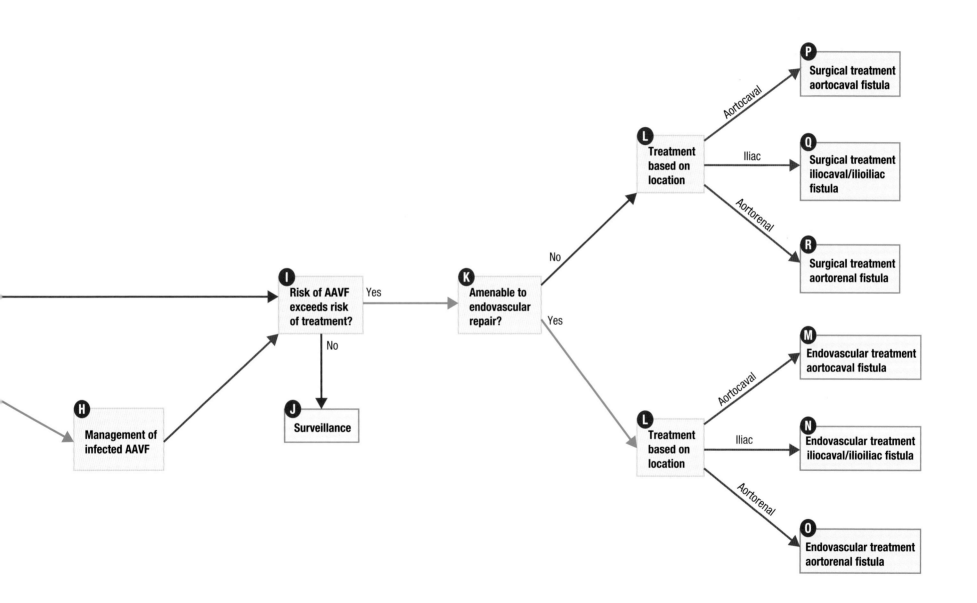

(A) Patient with suspected acquired abdominal arteriovenous fistula (AAVF)

Acquired abdominal arteriovenous fistula (AAVF) is a rare complication of abdominal aortic, iliac, or renal artery aneurysms or instrumentation/trauma. Incidence is estimated to be <1% in patients with AAA and 3% to 4% of AAAs that rupture.[1] It is estimated that 80% to 90% of AAVF are due to erosion of an aneurysm into the adjacent vein.[2,3] The remaining 10% to 20% are due to penetrating abdominal trauma, primarily related to lumbar instrumentation[4,5] and gunshot wounds.[6]

AAVFs have a wide variety of presenting symptoms that reflect differences in anatomy and sizes of the fistula. The "classic" presentation of an AVF associated with AAA is a pulsatile abdominal mass, abdominal bruit, and CHF.[7] However, this constellation of symptoms is rare, with most patients presenting with only one manifestation.[8] Common symptoms and signs, which may be seen independently or in combination, include abdominal bruit, pulsatile abdominal mass, abdominal or back pain, hematuria, hypotension, dyspnea, lower extremity edema, and rectal bleeding.[1,4,9,10] Rarely, an aortocaval fistula may be so large as to cause lower extremity ischemia, in addition to edema.

(B) H&P suggests AAVF?

Generally, patients with AAVF can present acutely or chronically. Patients who present acutely usually have symptoms of associated aneurysm rupture or impending rupture, including abdominal pain and hypotension.[1] In larger reviews and series, these patients constituted 25% to 45% of all patients with AAVF.[1,11] Patients with a component of aneurysm rupture (as evidenced by retroperitoneal hematoma) have increased associated mortality.[1,8] Conversely, patients who present chronically have symptoms of CHF including dyspnea, edema, and jugular venous distension. Chronic AAVF is often due to prior penetrating trauma, usually from gunshot wounds or lumbar instrumentation. Symptoms of CHF can develop slowly and present years or even decades after the original insult. Such patients are often younger than those with degenerative aneurysms, and are more able to have compensated for the gradually developing AAVF.[1,7] These patients often have been treated for heart failure for months or years before abdominal AAVF is diagnosed.[8] Ten percent to 35% of patients with AAVF present with symptoms of CHF.[1,8,11]

With respect to other abdominal AAVF, the combination of hematuria, abdominal pain, and AAA can indicate the presence of aortorenal fistula.[12] Iliac AVFs can be associated with CIA aneurysms as well as AAA; these patients may present with lower extremity edema as well as ischemia. Large fistulas often lead to CHF.[13]

(C) Evaluate other potential etiologies

Patients suspected of having AAVF may have alternative diagnoses. Owing to the variability of potential clinical presentation,

differential diagnosis can be extensive. Patients with pulmonary HTN, dyspnea, or lower extremity edema often have intrinsic cardiac disease and CHF. Patients who present with pulsatile mass, abdominal pain, or back pain more often have AAA or dissection than AAVF. Arterial occlusive disease should be considered in the rare patient initially suspected of having AAVF who presents with lower extremity ischemia. Patients who present with GI bleeding or hematuria are likely to have intrinsic causes that need evaluation.

(D) Imaging studies confirm AAVF?

Imaging of choice to confirm an AAVF is CTA or MRA. DSA is rarely required except as an adjunct to endovascular treatment. CTA or MRA is also used for preoperative surgical planning. Findings on contrast CT that lead to diagnosis of aortocaval fistula include enlarged IVC, passage of contrast from aorta to the IVC, and disappearance of normal fat planes between the IVC and the aorta. Sometimes direct communication between the two vessels is visualized.[14] Similarly, in fistulas involving the iliac vein (aortoiliac or ilioiliac), iliac vein dilation and early appearance of contrast in the vein suggest the presence of an AAVF.[13]

More difficult to diagnose is the aorto-left renal vein fistula, which sometimes cannot be well visualized using these modalities.[15] Abdominal DUS, in this situation, can provide valuable information. AAVF findings on DUS include enlarged renal vein or IVC, turbulent flow in the renal vein or IVC, and diastolic prolongation of flow.[16,17] DUS, however, is technician dependent, and, as such, should not be relied on for ruling out fistula or preoperative planning. DSA of the aorta and vena cava may be necessary to confirm the diagnosis in such cases. Accurate preoperative diagnosis has a significant impact on mortality.[11] Preoperative diagnosis of a fistula was associated with mortality of 24%, compared to a mortality of 33% in those without a preoperative diagnosis.[8]

(E) Cardiac decompensation or lower extremity ischemia?

Initial management depends on the clinical presentation. Patients who present with symptoms of chronic AAVF and hemodynamic dysfunction that lead to high-output heart failure should be worked up preoperatively with an ECHO and, if appropriate, right heart catheterization. ECHO may show preserved or elevated EF, as well as right heart chamber dilation with possible left heart chamber dilation.[16,17] This is due to blood flow from the high-pressure arterial system to the low-pressure venous system across the fistula, which leads to increased central venous pressure, decreased systemic venous resistance, and increased cardiac output. Hemodynamic studies have shown that cardiac output may be as high as 15 L/min in such patients.[17]

With excess blood flow being diverted to the low-pressure venous system, the patient may experience arterial insufficiency in the lower extremities, such as claudication or severe lower extremity ischemia. Symptoms can range from mild pain while walking

to ulceration in combination with lower extremity edema. Lower extremity DUS in patients with AAVF usually reveals low flow throughout the infrainguinal arterial tree.

(F) Stabilize patient

Diuresis, cardiac support, and careful fluid management may be required to obtain cardiovascular stability, and to achieve symptom (dyspnea, rales, edema) resolution. This should be done when possible in the stable patient to reduce surgical morbidity and mortality. However, medical management provides only temporary relief.[18,19] Lasting correction of abnormalities and spontaneous diuresis requires definitive repair of the AAVF.[5,19]

(G) Clinical signs of infection?

A special concern in AAVF, especially in those developing from aneurysmal aorta and external trauma, is the possibility of infection. Patients with concomitant mycotic aneurysm and AAVF may initially present with features of chronic CHF, with the only indication of infection being intermittent fevers.[20] Other findings that warrant consideration of an infectious component to the AAVF include rapid onset, generalized fatigue, leukocytosis, and elevated inflammatory markers (eg, CRP).[21]

(H) Management of infected AAVF

Infected AAVF is rare; however, infection, if present, must be treated aggressively. Patients with an infected AAVF should be treated in the same manner as those with chronic presentation (ICU admission, diuresis, and cardiac support as required) with the addition of IV antibiotics tailored to blood cultures.[20] If blood culture results are negative, broad-spectrum antibiotics can be used.[21] Case reports of this rare entity have described infection with Salmonella species and *Coxiella burnetii*, the causative agent of Q fever.[22-24]

(I) Risk of AAVF exceeds risk of treatment?

Without treatment, symptomatic AAVF is eventually fatal, and as such, repair should be offered to all patients with hemodynamically significant AAVF, unless the patient is either at excessively high surgical risk or refuses surgical intervention. Small AAVFs that might be discovered incidentally are rare, but could be initially followed in high-risk patients. Preoperative assessment of risk for open surgical and endovascular treatment must be performed to assess the risk–benefit ratio, and to help select open versus endovascular treatment in patients where both may be possible.

(J) Surveillance

Conservative management may be a reasonable option for asymptomatic patients with hemodynamically insignificant AAVFs. There are several reported cases of favorable outcomes for patients with a history of previous EVAR who presented with a type

II endoleak and aortocaval fistula including one instance where favorable remodeling of the aneurysm sac was observed.[25,26]

K Amenable to endovascular repair?

Similar to AAA repair, there are two broad interventional strategies for AAVF: open and endovascular repair. Open cases are associated with increased blood loss compared to endovascular cases, with average blood loss ranging from 4 to 6 L for aortocaval fistulas.[1] In a series of primarily stable, preoperatively diagnosed patients, those with aneurysmal disease had increased bleeding compared to those with a history of trauma.[1] Autotransfusion should be utilized in such cases.[1,11]

Endovascular intervention provides a less invasive alternative to open surgical repair when anatomic considerations allow placement of an arterial stent graft to close the AAVF. This approach may be preferred when the patient has a hostile abdomen from previous instrumentation, or has advanced CHF unresponsive to medical management.[27] However, for a patient to be considered for endovascular repair, anatomy must be suitable for treatment using available endografts. Large reviews of endovascular AAVF repair have focused on hemodynamically stable patients who meet anatomic criteria.[28] In general, the choice of endovascular versus open repair is similar to decision making for AAA repair (see Chapter 24).

L Treatment based on location

When open surgical of endovascular repair of AAVF is needed, the approach is based on the location of the lesion (aortocaval, iliac or renal).

M Endovascular treatment aortocaval fistula

Thoracic and abdominal aortic endoprosthesis can be used to treat aortocaval AAVF with suitable aortic anatomy. Aorto-uni-iliac devices with concomitant coiling embolization of the contralateral iliac artery have also been successfully used for selected patients.[18] In a review by Nakad et al., there was a 94% technical success in 50 cases, 74% of which involved endovascular repair of the aortocaval segment. Of patients with aortocaval fistula, 45% were treated with bifurcated aortic stent graft. A majority of patients in this review were hemodynamically stable, and mortality in this series was 21%.[28] However, in patients with severe cardiac decompensation, only one of four patients survived endovascular treatment despite technical success excluding the fistula.[29] The authors note that the outcome would likely not have been improved with open intervention.

N Endovascular treatment iliocaval/ilioiliac fistula

AAVF involving the iliac artery have been repaired successfully using aortic bifurcated stent grafts, straight stent grafts, and coiling, with overall success of 90% in cases involving the iliac segment.[28] The key is to select the appropriate endograft size. In one case of coiling, the iliocaval AAVF was a complication of previous EVAR.[30]

O Endovascular treatment aortorenal fistula

Case reports for endovascular repair of aortorenal fistula are limited. Successful repair has involved aortic bifurcated stent grafts, straight stent grafts, and vascular plugs.[28] Amplatzer vascular plugs have been utilized independently of stenting in cases of renal artery stump to IVC fistula.

P Surgical treatment aortocaval fistula

During open aortocaval fistula repair, the associated AAA is controlled and approached as in standard AAA repair. When opening the AAA, venous bleeding from the IVC can be controlled with digital compression or balloon occlusion catheter.[8,11] Owing to surrounding inflammation, it is best to avoid dissection of the vena cava for clamping, because of the high likelihood of venous injury. The fistula is then closed directly with polypropylene suture from within the aorta, incorporating the aortic back wall.[1] Great care needs to be taken to avoid air embolization by digital pressure and Trendelenburg positioning. Friable aortic wall that cannot be closed at the site of the fistula can be handled through the exclusion method, in which that section of the aorta is isolated by oversewing lumbar arteries and closing the aneurysm sac after proximal and distal ligation, allowing this segment to thrombose.[2] Large aortocaval fistulas (>3 cm) have been repaired with bovine patch angioplasty.[9] Aortic repair can be achieved with end-to-end anastomosis. Perioperative mortality rate of open surgical repair ranges from 12% to 30%.[8,11] In patients presenting with AAA rupture, mortality increases to 48%.[8]

Q Surgical treatment iliocaval/ilioiliac fistula

Much of the operative technique for aortocaval AAVF can be applied to AAVFs involving the iliac artery or vein, especially that associated with aortoiliac AAVF repair. Case reports have suggested predominance of aneurysmectomy and repair with ePTFE graft for open repair of ilioiliac fistula.[5,13] In the literature, there are very few reports of open iliocaval repair, most describing endovascular repair.

R Surgical treatment aortorenal fistula

Open repair of aortorenal vein fistula can be challenging in patients with AAA rupture, because the retroperitoneal tissues can become edematous and brittle owing to compression and hematoma.[31] Repair with Dacron bifurcated graft predominates in the literature. Renal vein ligation may be necessary. Transient hemodialysis may be required after repair of aortorenal AAVF.[10]

REFERENCES

1. Brewster DC, Cambria RP, Moncure AC, et al. Aortocaval and iliac arteriovenous fistulas: recognition and treatment. *J Vasc Surg.* 1991;13(2):253-265.
2. Kondo N, Takahashi K, Takeuchi S, Ito K. Surgical repair of arteriovenous fistula associated with iinfrarenal aorto-iliac aneurysm: report of two contrasting cases. *Ann Vasc Dis.* 2011;4(2):150-153.
3. Bednarkiewicz M, Pretre R, Kalangos A, Khatchatourian G, Bruschweiler I, Faidutti B. Aortocaval fistula associated with abdominal aortic aneurysm: a diagnostic challenge. *Ann Vasc Surg.* 1997;11(5):464-466.
4. Gallerani M, Maida G, Boari B, Galeotti R, Rocca T, Gasbarro V. High output heart failure due to an iatrogenic arterio-venous fistula after lumbar disc surgery. *Acta Neurochir (Wien).* 2007;149(12):1243-1247.
5. Machado-Atías I, Fornés O, González-Bello R, Machado-Hernández I. Iliac arteriovenous fistula due to spinal disk surgery. Causes severe hemodynamic repercussion with pulmonary hypertension. *Tex Heart Inst J.* 1993;20(1):60-65.
6. Spencer TA, Smyth SH, Wittich G, Hunter GC. Delayed presentation of traumatic aortocaval fistula: a report of two cases and a review of the associated compensatory hemodynamic and structural changes. *J Vasc Surg.* 2006;43(4):836-840.
7. Brightwell RE, Pegna V, Boyne N. Aortocaval fistula: current management strategies. *ANZ J Surg.* 2013;83(1-2):31-35.
8. Gilling-Smith GL, Mansfield AO. Spontaneous abdominal arteriovenous fistulae: report of eight cases and review of the literature. *Br J Surg.* 1991;78(4):421-425.
9. Takazawa A, Sakahashi H, Toyama A. Surgical repair of a concealed aortocaval fistula associated with an abdominal aortic aneurysm: report of two cases. *Surg Today.* 2001;31(9):842-844.
10. Tanaka H, Naito K, Murayama J, Ohteki H. Aorto-left renal vein fistula caused by a ruptured abdominal aortic aneurysm. *Ann Vasc Dis.* 2013;6(4):738-740.
11. Davidovic L, Dragas M, Cvetkovic S, Kostic D, Cinara I, Banzic I. Twenty years of experience in the treatment of spontaneous aorto-venous fistulas in a developing country. *World J Surg.* 2011;35(8):1829-1834.
12. Mansour MA, Rutherford RB, Metcalf RK, Pearce WH. Spontaneous aorto-left renal vein fistula: the "abdominal pain, hematuria, silent left kidney" syndrome. *Surgery.* 1991;109(1):101-106.
13. Iijima M, Kawasaki M, Ishibashi Y. Successful surgical repair of an ilio-iliac arteriovenous fistula associated with a ruptured common iliac artery aneurysm. *Int J Surg Case Rep.* 2015;13:55-57.
14. Kim H, Randolph S. Traumatic aortocaval fistula from gunshot wound, complicated by bullet embolization to the right ventricle. *Radiol Case Rep.* 2012;7(4):767.
15. Mansour MA, Russ PD, Subber SW, Pearce WH. Aorto-left renal vein fistula: diagnosis by duplex sonography. *AJR Am J Roentgenol.* 1989;152(5):1107-1108.
16. Abreo G, Lenihan DJ, Nguyen P, Runge MS. High-output heart failure resulting from a remote traumatic aorto-caval fistula: diagnosis by echocardiography. *Clin Cardiol.* 2000;23(4):304-306.
17. Lebon A, Agueznai M, Labombarda F. High-output heart failure resulting from chronic aortocaval fistula. *Circulation.* 2013;127(4):527-528.

18. Lau LL, O'Reilly MJ, Johnston LC, Lee B. Endovascular stent-graft repair of primary aortocaval fistula with an abdominal aortoiliac aneurysm. *J Vasc Surg*. 2001;33(2): 425-428.

19. Sata N, Hiramine K, Horinouchi T, et al. Progressive congestive heart failure due to common iliac arteriovenous fistula: a case report. *J Cardiol*. 2007;49(3):143-147.

20. Huang PL, Chua S, Guo GB, Fu M. Mycotic aneurysm leading to iliac arteriovenous fistula diagnosed by vascular duplex color scan. *J Ultrasound Med*. 1998;17(8):513-516.

21. Sasahashi N, Hamazaki M, Asada H, Kataoka T, Hamanaka K, Nishiyama K. Infected iliac artery aneurysm with aortocaval fistula. *Acute Med Surg*. 2016;3(4):400-403.

22. Karhof S, van Roeden SE, Oosterheert JJ, et al. Primary and secondary arterial fistulas during chronic Q fever. *J Vasc Surg*. 2018;68(6):1906-1913.e1.

23. Huang YK, Lin CC, Lin HS. Peritonitis as presentation of aorto-caval fistula with *Salmonella choleraesuis*-associated abdominal aortic aneurysm. *Surg Infect (Larchmt)*. 2015;16(1): 108-109.

24. Belyavskaya T, Baumann A. Ruptured aortic aneurysm complicated by aortocaval fistula due to *Salmonella* infection. *Eur J Vasc Endovasc Surg*. 2016;51(2):258.

25. Magnus S, Björn S, Timothy AR, Nuno VD, Jan H, Martin M. Aneurysm shrinkage is compatible with massive endoleak in the presence of an aortocaval fistula: potential therapeutic implications for endoleaks and spinal cord ischemia. *J Endovasc Ther*. 2016;23(3):529-532.

26. van de Luijtgaarden KM, Bastos Gonçalves F, Rouwet EV, Hendriks JM, Ten Raa S, Verhagen HJ. Conservative management of persistent aortocaval fistula after endovascular aortic repair. *J Vasc Surg*. 2013;58(4):1080-1083.

27. Rapacciuolo A, De Angelis MC, di Pietro E, et al. Percutaneous treatment of a aorto-caval fistula in a old high risk patient. *BMC Surg*. 2012;12(suppl 1):S32.

28. Nakad G, AbiChedid G, Osman R. Endovascular treatment of major abdominal arteriovenous fistulas. *Vasc Endovasc Surg*. 2014;48(5-6):388-395.

29. Akwei S, Altaf N, Tennant W, MacSweeney S, Braithwaite B. Emergency endovascular repair of aortocaval fistula—a single center experience. *Vasc Endovasc Surg*. 2011;45(5):442-446.

30. Laureys M, Tannouri F, Rommens J, Dussaussois L, Golzarian J. Percutaneous treatment of iatrogenic iliocaval fistula related to endograft placement for abdominal aortic aneurysm. *J Vasc Interv Radiol*. 2002;13(2, pt 1):211-213.

31. van Weel V, Watson A, Fioole B. Ruptured abdominal aortic aneurysm in a patient with an aorto-left renal vein fistula. *Ann Vasc Surg*. 2014;28(2):493.e11-e13.

Jill J. Colglazier • Thomas C. Bower

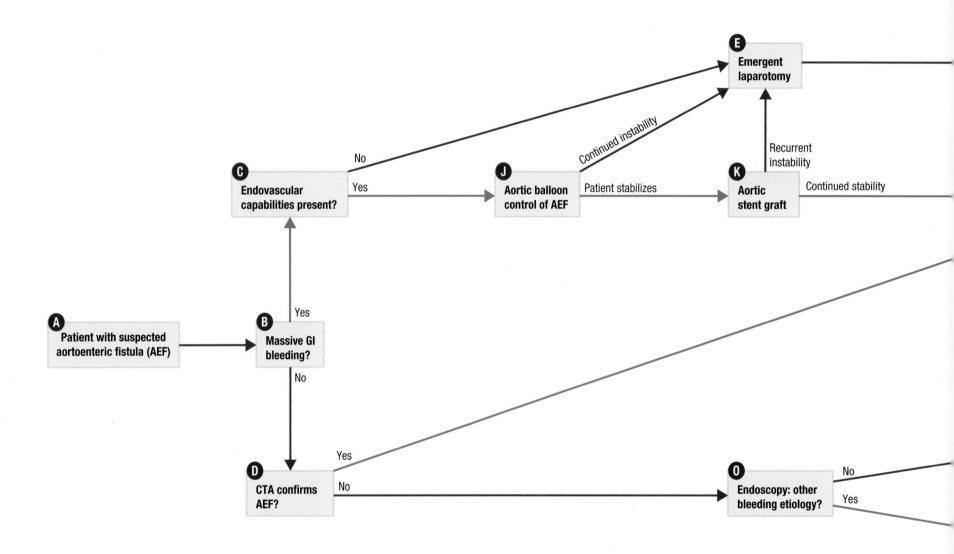

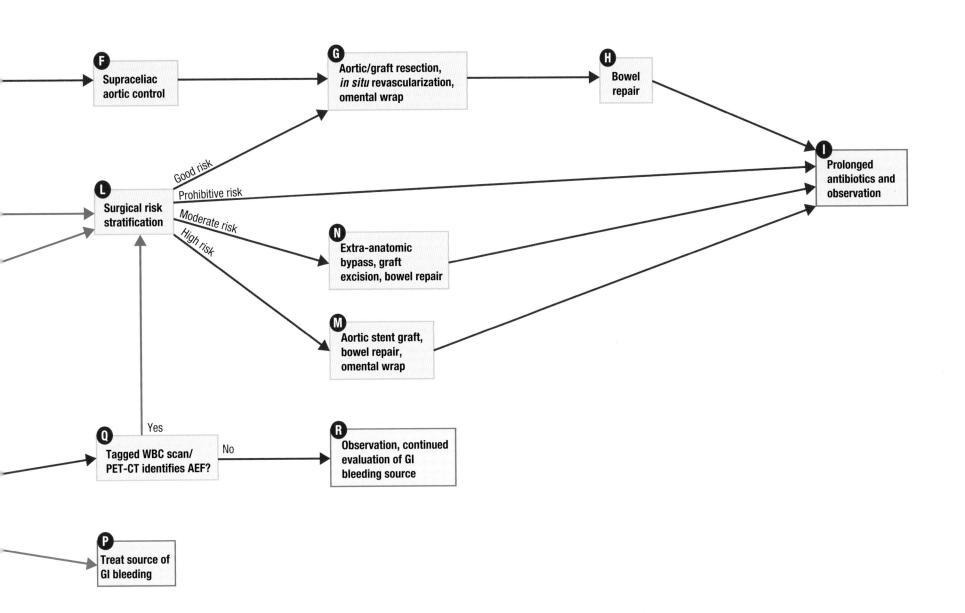

Ⓐ Patient with suspected aortoenteric fistula

A primary aortoenteric fistula (AEF) is a *de novo* connection between an AAA and the GI tract, most commonly the duodenum: It is very rare. A secondary AEF is the result of erosion of an aortic prosthetic graft anastomosis into the bowel: It occurs in 0.3% to 2% of patients with aortic grafts.[1-5] Both primary and secondary AEFs can result in GI bleeding. AAA and prior aortoiliac surgery or intervention are the most common risk factors for AEF. Less common risk factors include reflux esophagitis, peptic ulcer disease, malignancy, para-aortic radiation, aortitis, and aortic penetrating ulcer.[6-9] It is possible to develop a communication between the intestine and aortic prosthesis away from the anastomosis, which can present with sepsis without GI bleeding. Workup and treatment of such graft-enteric erosions (GEEs) follow the same algorithm as in patients with AEF.[10]

Ⓑ Massive GI bleeding?

Hematemesis, hematochezia, and melena are the most common presenting signs of an AEF. In a review of the literature, 94% of patients with AEF presented with a herald bleed, a brisk GI bleeding episode that spontaneously stops and can precede massive GI bleeding by hours to months.[11-14] If the patient presents with massive GI bleeding and is unstable, an emergent open or endovascular intervention is needed. If the patient has herald bleeding, and/or is hemodynamically stable, then abdominal-pelvic CTA is recommended. Other signs and symptoms of AEF include fever, malaise, weight loss, sepsis, abdominal/back pain, and polymicrobial bacteremia, which also characterize GEEs.[15,16]

Ⓒ Endovascular capabilities present?

In an unstable patient, control of hemorrhage is paramount. This requires an emergent laparotomy or endovascular aortic occlusion balloon depending on the capabilities of the hospital. The availability of a dedicated operating room with imaging capabilities, an inventory of wires, catheters, sheaths, compliant aortic balloons and stent grafts, and staff familiar with endovascular equipment are needed for emergency endovascular procedures. If these are available, endovascular treatment is preferred.

Ⓓ CTA confirms AEF?

Abdominal-pelvic CTA is the first study obtained to evaluate stable patients with suspected AEF or GEE. This imaging study has a sensitivity of 94% and a specificity of 84% for the diagnosis of AEF.[17] Findings on CTA that correlate strongly with AEF include extravasation of contrast material into the bowel wall lumen, ectopic gas adjacent to or within the aorta, focal bowel wall thickening next to the aorta, obliteration of the fat plane between the aorta and the bowel, and a retroperitoneal hematoma or hematoma within the bowel wall or lumen.[17-19] Delayed imaging helps visualize endoluminal contrast.[20] Findings on CTA associated with GEE include perigraft soft-tissue thickening, fluid, and loss of normal fat plane between the aorta and the adjacent bowel.[21]

Ⓔ Emergent laparotomy

Emergent intervention is required for a patient with life-threatening bleeding from an AEF. The goals of management include control of bleeding, stabilization of hemodynamics, control of infection, and maintenance of distal perfusion. If endovascular capabilities are not available, the patient requires open surgical treatment. The chest, abdomen, and bilateral lower extremities are prepared into the sterile field. A midline transperitoneal incision is made from the xiphoid to the pubis. Expedited exploration of the abdomen and retroperitoneum is conducted, especially if preoperative imaging is not obtained and the diagnosis of AEF is not confirmed.

Ⓕ Supraceliac aortic control

Expeditious control of the aorta proximal to the AEF is imperative. This is done either with intra-aortic balloon occlusion or isolation and clamping of the supraceliac aorta through the lesser sac. In rare circumstances, control is obtained through a limited thoracotomy. If intra-aortic balloon occlusion is used, we favor a percutaneous transfemoral approach, starting with a 6-French sheath for access, and then increasing the size to a 12-French, 70-cm-long sheath over a stiff wire. A large, compliant aortic balloon (32 mm Coda balloon, Cook Medical, Bloomington, IN) is placed over the stiff wire, positioned under fluoroscopic guidance in the supraceliac aorta, and inflated. The sheath is placed immediately caudal the inflated balloon to prevent downward displacement of the occlusion balloon.

Ⓖ Aortic/graft resection, *in situ* revascularization, omental wrap

Once the supraceliac aorta is clamped or balloon occluded, control of the iliac arteries or graft limbs is obtained. Mannitol and heparin are given depending on the clinical situation and hemodynamics. The juxtarenal aorta is dissected free, with care to protect the left renal vein. Alternatively, if there is scarring near the pararenal aorta, the aneurysm or graft can be opened to facilitate dissection and control of the suprarenal aortic segment. The bowel should not be dissected away from the infected aneurysm or graft. As soon as it is safe, the supraceliac clamp is transferred to an immediate suprarenal or infrarenal position to restore blood flow to the visceral and/or renal arteries. If balloon occlusion was used, the balloon is deflated and removed with the sheath as the aortic clamp is applied. The sheath is left in the femoral artery until the end of the operation when it can be removed and the femoral artery access site repaired.

For primary AEF, a piece of aortic wall is cut around the duodenal fistula, whereas with secondary AEF, a piece of graft is excised around the duodenal opening to maintain the integrity of the bowel. The bowel is packed out of the field with antibiotic-soaked laparotomy pads. Infected aortic tissue is resected for a primary AEF.

With a secondary AEF, the aortic graft anastomosis is taken down and the native aorta debrided. If possible, a piece of aortic tissue is sent to the pathologist for frozen section to evaluate for bacteria or micro abscesses. We prefer to resect only the infected part of the graft and save the incorporated limbs, because this avoids disruption of colonic and pelvic collateral blood flow that could result in bowel ischemia if the entire graft is removed. The periaortic tissue is debrided and the retroperitoneum irrigated with warm antibiotic solution. Gowns, gloves, and instruments are changed before placement of the new aortic graft. *In situ* reconstruction is done with either a cryopreserved aortoiliac allograft or Rifampin-soaked gelatin or collagen-coated polyester graft. The Rifampin-soaked graft is prepared using 600 mg of Rifampin powder solution (Merrell Dow Pharmaceuticals, Kansas City, MO) diluted in 250 mL of normal saline (2.4 mg/mL) for at least 30 minutes. Cryopreserved allograft requires a 45-minute thaw and preparation process. Blood type matching is not needed. Open side branches are closed as necessary, and ligated lumbar arteries are reinforced. The lumbar arteries are kept anterior when sewing the graft in place. These grafts may dilate and/or elongate by as much as 40%. Femoropopliteal vein is rarely used in emergent circumstances. The graft is wrapped circumferentially with one or more tongues of omentum, because this is associated with a lower reinfection rate.[13,22] The bowel is mobilized and the defect repaired, as described in H.

Management of GEE is similar to that of AEF, except that emergent operation is seldom required. Placement of ureteral stents before laparotomy helps avoid inadvertent ureteral injury during dissection in the inflamed periaortic retroperitoneum. *In situ* revascularization using a Rifampin-soaked, gelatin-coated polyester graft is done for patients with low-grade infections and without frank pus around the graft. Reinfection rates are higher when there is extensive perigraft purulence.[23] If the infective agent is methicillin-resistant *Staphylococcus aureus*, gram-negative species, or fungus or tuberculous species, an autogenous conduit is preferred. Partial versus total graft excision is based on the extent of infection. If the entire graft requires excision, new tunnels for the graft limbs should be created if safe to do. The bowel is repaired, as described in H.

Traditionally, axillobifemoral bypass, graft removal, and closure of the aortic stump in three layers was used to treat AEF or GEE, as described in N. In a large series of graft excision and extra-anatomic revascularization, however, the aortic stump blowout rate was 25%, the lower extremity amputation rate was 16%, and 1-year mortality was 73%.[24-26] *In situ* reconstruction using antibiotic-soaked prosthetic grafts eliminates the risk of aortic stump blowout and, in stable patients, is associated with mortality, limb salvage, and 10-year reinfection rates of 2.3%, 100%, and 4%, respectively. As such, it is preferred.[13,27]

H Bowel repair

The rim of native aortic tissue or graft fabric is excised around the bowel opening and the edges of the bowel mucosa freshened to healthy tissue. The defect in the bowel can usually be repaired primarily in two layers. Very rarely is an ostomy or bowel resection with primary anastomosis needed. A nasogastric tube is placed during the procedure and is used in the postoperative period until return of bowel function.

I Prolonged antibiotics and observation

Broad-spectrum IV antibiotics are administered initially, followed by organism-specific IV antibiotics for 4 to 8 weeks, depending on the infective organism. Thereafter, oral antibiotic suppression is used. The length of antibiotic treatment remains controversial, particularly after *in situ* reconstruction. If a prosthetic graft is used, oral antibiotic suppression is maintained lifelong. The current recommendations of the American Heart Association states that after an initial period of 6 weeks to 6 months of parenteral antibiotic therapy, lifelong antibiotic suppressive therapy may be considered given the risk of recurrent infection and associated high morbidity and mortality.[16,28]

J Aortic balloon control of AEF

If endovascular capabilities are available, the use of an aortic occlusion balloon, usually from a percutaneous transfemoral approach, allows rapid control of hemorrhage from an AEF. Aortography can be done to visualize both the aortic defect and presence of bleeding. If an aortic occlusion balloon fails to restore hemodynamic stability, the patient should undergo emergent laparotomy.

K Aortic stent graft

An aortic stent graft can be placed via a transfemoral approach to cover the aortic defect if anatomy allows, particularly in hemodynamically unstable, high-risk patients. Deployment of the stent graft should take less time than it does to perform a laparotomy, close the fistula, and repair the aorta. Endovascular repair serves as a bridge to more definitive reconstruction for most patients, with the exception of those at the highest risk or who are medically unfit.[29] In one multicenter study, the early advantage of endovascular repair of AEF was not maintained at follow-up of 2 years. Patients who have endovascular repair can develop fistula recurrence, recurrent sepsis, reoperation, and mortality rates of 49%, 72%, 50%, and 85% at 2 years, respectively. These outcomes suggest that stent grafts should be used for emergency treatment of AEF as a bridge to definitive open surgical repair whenever possible.[29] If after deployment of an aortic stent graft, the patient fails to regain hemodynamic stability, emergent laparotomy is required. However, if the patient stabilizes after endovascular repair, risk stratification is done to select the extent of more definitive treatment.

L Surgical risk stratification

Surgical risk stratification is important to determine the appropriate extent of treatment that can be performed to treat AEF or GEE in stable patients after bridging endovascular aortic stent-graft placement. Elderly deconditioned patients with multiple cardiac, pulmonary, and/or renal comorbidities may be at prohibitive risk to undergo even abdominal exploration. Unless the patient's risk can be reduced, the only option in this case is prolonged antibiotics, which may delay a fatal outcome (I).

M Aortic stent graft, bowel repair, omental wrap

High-risk patients with cardiopulmonary dysfunction, physical limitations, and/or stage 4 CKD may not be able to tolerate definitive open aortic repair, but may tolerate aortic stent grafting followed by abdominal exploration, repair of the bowel defect, washout of the retroperitoneum, and an omental flap placed around the aorta.

N Extra-anatomic bypass, graft excision, bowel repair

Moderate-risk patients should undergo interval resection of the infected aorta and/or the endovascular stent or graft, and extra-anatomic bypass. Repair of the bowel and omental wrap of the reconstructed aorta or aortic stump is necessary. The aortic stump is classically closed in three layers with monofilament suture. Fascia lata serves as a good buttress if necessary. In select emergency circumstances, this is done in one operation. In stable patients, extra-anatomic bypass can be performed initially, followed 1 to 2 days later by graft resection and bowel repair.

O Endoscopy: other bleeding etiology?

If findings on CTA are inconclusive, further testing is required to make the diagnosis. Upper endoscopy can be used in a hemodynamically stable patient to identify AEF or another source of GI bleeding. Findings indicative of AEF on endoscopy include fresh clot and/or graft material in third portion of the duodenum.[30]

P Treat source of GI bleeding

If an alternate source of GI bleeding is found, this condition is treated as appropriate.

Q Tagged WBC scan/PET-CT identifies AEF?

If endoscopy does not identify a source of GI bleeding or if GEF is suspected, tagged WBC scan or [18F]fluoro-2-deoxy-D-glucose PET/CT imaging can help identify localized infection. The anatomic location of uptake can accurately differentiate between infection of the aorta, aortic graft, or adjacent soft tissue.[31] PET-CT has a sensitivity of 96% and a specificity of 86% for the diagnosis of aortic graft infections.[32]

R Observation, continued evaluation of GI bleeding source

If CTA, upper endoscopy, and tagged WBC scan/PET-CT do not suggest AEF or GEE, then observation and continued evaluation of a GI bleeding source or infection is warranted. Colonoscopy and capsule endoscopy can be used to further evaluate a GI bleeding source.

REFERENCES

1. Thompson WM, Jackson DC, Johnsrude IS. Aortoenteric and paraprosthetic-enteric fistulas: radiologic findings. *Am J Roentgenol.* 1976;127:235-242.
2. Puglia E, Fry PD. Aortoenteric fistulas: a preventable problem? *Can J Surg.* 1980;23:74-76.
3. Champion MC, Sullivan SN, Coles JC, Goldbach M, Watson WC. Aortoenteric fistula. *Ann Surg.* 1982;195:314-317.
4. Hallett JW, Marshall DM, Petterson TM, et al. Graft-related complications after abdominal aortic aneurysm repair: reassurance from a 36-year population based experience. *J Vasc Surg.* 1997;25:277-284.
5. Menawat SS, Gloviczki P, Serry RD, Cherry KJ, Bower TC, Hallett JW. Management of aortic graft-enteric fistulae. *Eur J Vasc Endovasc Surg.* 1997;14(suppl 1):7481.
6. Calligaro KD, Bergen WS, Savarese RP, et al. Primary aortoduodenal fistula due to septic aortitis. *J Cardiovasc Surg.* 1992;33:192.
7. Podbielski FJ, Rodriguez HE, Zhu RY, et al. Aortoesophageal fistula secondary to reflux esophagitis. *Dig Surg.* 2007;24:66.
8. Odze RD, Begin LR. Peptic-ulcer-induced aortoenteric fistula. Report of a case and review of the literature. *J Clin Gastroenterol.* 1991;13:682.
9. Drognitz O, Pfeiffenberger J, Schareck W, et al. Primary duodenal fistula as late complication of para-aortic radiation therapy. *Chirug.* 2002;73:633.
10. O'Mara C, Imbembo AL. Paraprosthetic-enteric fistula. *Surgery.* 1977;81(5):556-566.
11. Reilly LM, Ehrenfeld WK, Goldstone J, Stoney RJ. Gastrointestinal tract involvement by prosthetic graft infection. The significance of gastrointestinal hemorrhage. *Ann Surg.* 1985;202:342.
12. O'Connor S, Andrew P, Batt M, Becquemin JP. A systematic review and meta-analysis of treatments for aortic graft infection. *J Vasc Surg.* 2006;44:38-45.
13. Oderich GS, Bower TC, Hofer J, et al. In situ rifampin-soaked grafts with omental coverage and antibiotic suppression are durable with low reinfection rates in patients with aortic graft enteric erosion or fistula. *J Vasc Surg.* 1997;25:277-284.
14. Saers S, Scheltinga M. Primary aortoenteric fistula. *Br J Surg.* 2005;92(2):143-152.
15. Swain TW, Calligaro KD, Dougherty MD. Management of infected aortic prosthetic grafts. *Vasc Endovascular Surg.* 2004;38:75-82.
16. Wilson WR, Bower TC, Creager MA, et al. Vascular graft infections, mycotic aneurysms and endovascular infections;

a scientific statement from the American Heart Association. *Circulation.* 2016;134:e412-e460.

17. Low RN, Wall SD, Jeffrey RB, et al. Aortoenteric fistula and perigraft infection: evaluation with CT. *Radiology.* 1990;175:157.

18. Hagspiel KD, Turba UC, Bolzar U, et al. Diagnosis of aortoenteric fistulas with CT angiography. *J Vasc Inter Radiol.* 2007;18:497.

19. Perks FJ, Gillespie I, Patel D. Multidetector computed tomography imaging of aortoenteric fistula. *J Comput Assist Tomogr.* 2004;28:343.

20. Odemis B, Basar O, Ertugrul I, et al. Detection of an aortoenteric fistula in a patient with intermittent bleeding. *Nat Clin Pract Gastroenterol Hepatol.* 2008;5:226.

21. Vu QD, Menias CO, Bhalla S, Peterson C, Wang LL, Balfe DM. Aortoenteric fistulas: CT features and potential mimics. *Radiographics.* 2009;29(1):197-209.

22. Noel AA, Gloviczki P, Cherry KJ, et al. United States Cryopreserved Aortic Allograft Registry. Abdominal aortic reconstruction in infected fields: early results of the United States cryopreserved aortic allograft registry. *J Vasc Surg.* 2002;35:847-852.

23. Oderich GS, Bower TC, Cherry KJ, et al. Evolution from axillofemoral to in situ prosthetic reconstruction for the treatment of aortic graft infections at a single center. *J Vasc Surg.* 2006;43(6):1166-1174.

24. Reilly LM, Stoney RJ, Goldstone J, Ehrenfeld WK. Improved management of aortic graft infection: the influence of operation sequence and staging. *J Vasc Surg.* 1987;5:421-431.

25. Kuestner LM, Reilly LM, Jicha DL, Ehrenfeld WK, Goldstone J, Stoney RJ. Secondary aortoenteric fistula: contemporary outcomes with use of extraanatomic bypass and infected graft excision. *J Vasc Surg.* 1995;21:184-195; discussion 195-196.

26. Armstrong PA, Back MR, Wilson JS, Shames ML, Johnson BL, Bandyk DF. Improved outcomes in the recent management of secondary aortoenteric fistula. *J Vasc Surg.* 2005;42:660-666.

27. Bandyk DF, Novotney ML, Johnson BL, Back MR, Roth SR. Use of rifampin-soaked gelatin-sealed polyester grafts for in situ treatment of primary aortic and vascular prosthetic infections. *J Surg Res.* 2001;95:44-49.

28. Setacci C, de Donato G, Setacci F. Endografts for the treatment of aortic infection. *Semin Vasc Surg.* 2011;24:242-249.

29. Kakkos SK, Antoniadis PN, Klonaris CN, et al. Open or endovascular repair of aortoenteric fistula? A multicenter comparative study. *Eur J Vasc Endovasc Surg.* 2011;41:625-634.

30. Delgado J, Jotkowitz AB, Delgado B. Primary aortoduodenal fistula: pitfalls and success in the endoscopic diagnosis. *Eur J Intern Med.* 2005;16:363.

31. Keidar Z, Nitecki S. FDG-PET in prosthetic graft infections. *Semin Nucl Med.* 2013;43(5):396-402.

32. Sah BR, Husmann L, Mayer D, et al.; VASGRA Chohort. Diagnostic performance of 18F-FDG-PET/CT in vascular graft infections. *Eur J Vasc Endovasc Surg.* 2015;49(4):455-461.

Edward J. Arous • Andres Schanzer

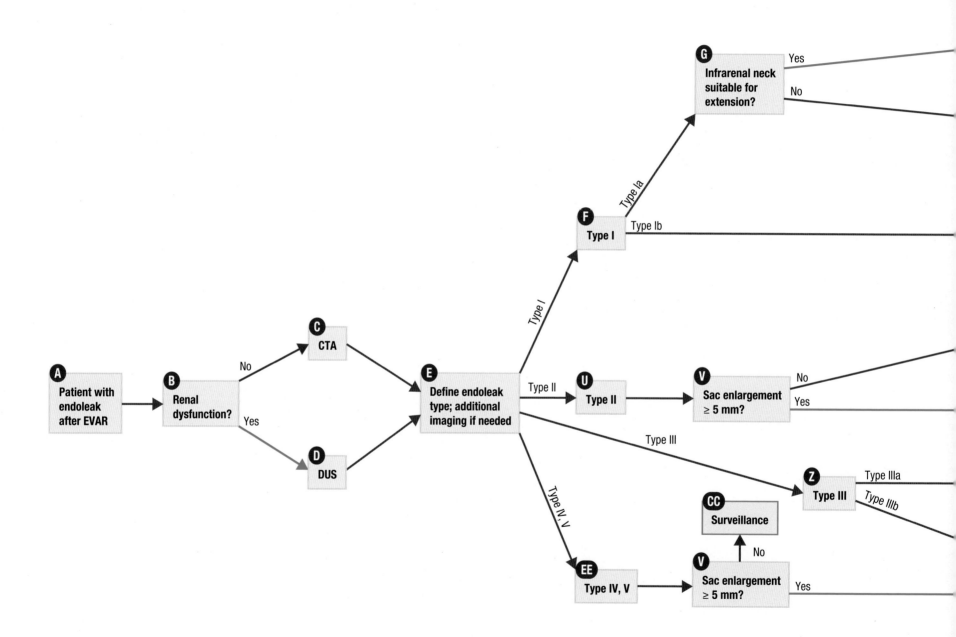

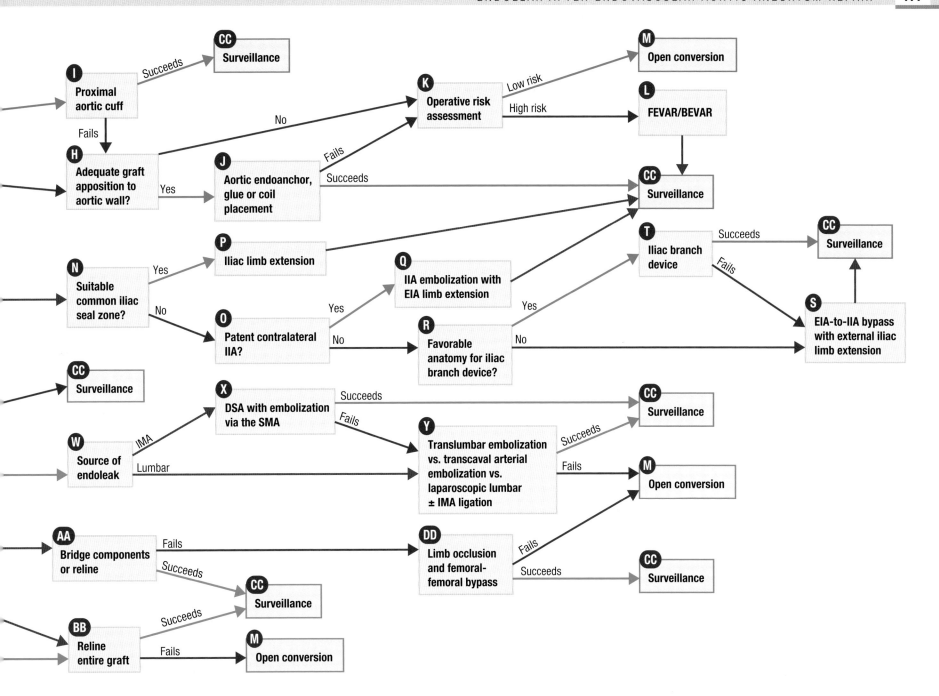

A Patient with endoleak after EVAR

A stable patient with a previous history of EVAR presents for evaluation of an endoleak. If the endoleak is associated with AAA rupture, see Chapter 25.

B Renal dysfunction?

The initial evaluation of a patient with an endoleak after EVAR should include an assessment of renal function. In patients with renal dysfunction, consider evaluation with DUS. If inconclusive, or if the patient has normal renal function, CTA is the preferred imaging modality for identification of the source of the endoleak.[1] In patients with compromised renal function, renal prehydration should be considered to minimize the risk of renal disease progression.

C CTA

CTA is the preferred imaging modality for evaluation of an endoleak after EVAR. Axial imaging provides critical information regarding aneurysm size change, angulation, seal zone characteristics, and identification of the types of endoleak.[2]

D DUS

DUS or contrast-enhanced ultrasound may provide an avenue for graft surveillance and endoleak detection in patients with renal dysfunction.[3] The Society for Vascular Surgery guidelines suggest that surveillance with ultrasound is safe for long-term surveillance if previous CT imaging demonstrates no evidence of endoleak and a stable aneurysm size.[2]

E Define endoleak type; additional imaging if needed

Endoleaks are classified as type I (seal zone), type II (side branch), type III (graft or junction), type IV (porosity), or type V (endotension). If the type is not clear on the basis of the initial imaging, further imaging with DSA, DUS, cone beam CT, or dynamic MRA[4] may identify the precise type(s) of endoleak.

F Type I

A type I endoleak occurs because of inadequate seal at the proximal (type Ia) or distal (type Ib) fixation sites of the graft. Type I endoleaks are associated with increased aneurysm sac pressure and have a higher risk of rupture.[5] (If the patient presents with an associated ruptured aneurysm, see Chapter 25.)

G Infrarenal neck suitable for extension?

For EVAR, anatomic parameters defining a suitable infrarenal neck remain controversial and device specific, but, in general, include an infrarenal aortic neck length ≥15 mm, diameter <32 mm, angulation <60°, <50% circumferential neck thrombus, <50% calcified neck, or nonconical neck.[6-9] Previous studies have demonstrated the importance of adhering to device IFU to minimize the risk of aneurysm sac enlargement and subsequent AAA rupture.[10] In addition to meeting these characteristics for use of an infrarenal endograft, it is critical to measure the distance from the preexisting endograft flow divider to the renal arteries to select the correct extension length. If an infrarenal extension is not possible, suprarenal extension with fenestrated grafts or renal chimney endografts can be considered.[11]

H Adequate graft apposition to aortic wall?

If it is not possible to extend the graft with a proximal cuff, but adequate current graft apposition to the aortic wall exists (with endoleak), circumferential aortic endoanchor placement can be considered.[12] Additional alternative options include coil[13] or glue[14] placement. If there is an unsuitable infrarenal aortic neck without graft apposition to the aortic wall, it is imperative to pursue open operative risk assessment.

I Proximal aortic cuff

In patients with a suitable infrarenal neck proximal to the edge of fabric associated with the EVAR device already in place, placement of a proximal aortic cuff may extend the seal zone to the level of the aorta just below the renal arteries and provide an adequate solution for treatment of a type Ia endoleak. Although inadequate data exist to define the exact anatomy appropriate for proximal aortic cuff placement, it is our belief and practice that a minimum of 10 mm of length is needed to consider endograft extension.

J Aortic endoanchor, glue, or coil placement

Despite limited early studies, endoanchors have demonstrated effectiveness in maintaining proximal fixation in patients with a hostile aortic neck anatomy. Similarly, they are useful in treating type Ia endoleaks after initial EVAR.[12] Embolization agents including ethylene-vinyl alcohol copolymer may be considered as an alternative for type Ia endoleaks, but they are only marginally effective in this setting.[15] Prior work has demonstrated that coil placement can provide 89% clinical success for select type I endoleaks, and 79% for type II endoleaks.[13]

K Operative risk assessment

An operative risk assessment, including a full cardiopulmonary evaluation, is necessary to characterize the patient's risks of general anesthesia and aortic cross-clamping. Significant risk factors include age, CKD, CHF, PAD, and liver disease.[16] Individual surgeon and hospital experience are also important determinants of operative outcome. Consider utilizing the model validated by the Vascular Quality Initiative (VQI) for patients under consideration for open surgery or EVAR (Tables 29-1 and 29-2).[17]

L FEVAR/BEVAR

In a patient with high operative risk, consider FEVAR/BEVAR for proximal extension to treat type Ia endoleak. A FEVAR/BEVAR will extend the proximal seal zone to the visceral aorta while maintaining patency of the visceral vessels through a combination of fenestrations or branches. The Cook Zenith Fenestrated device uses a modular proximal body graft with a distal bifurcated graft. In Europe, the Anaconda Fenestrated Stent graft uses an aortic endograft with two iliac limbs.[18] In addition, the Cook Zenith Pivot Branch (p-Branch) is available in Europe as an off-the-shelf device and it is currently being trialed in the United States.[19]

M Open conversion

In patients with low operative risk, open conversion will include explantation of the endograft with direct open repair. Careful assessment for the presence of suprarenal fixation of the initial EVAR device is important to determine location of aortic clamping (suprarenal vs. supraceliac). If the previous EVAR has slipped from its initial fixation site, without suprarenal fixation, then infrarenal clamping may also be possible. Similarly, the site for iliac artery clamping (CIA vs. EIA and IIA) is dependent on the location of previous iliac limb and the surgical plan. Depending on the

Table 29-1. VQI Point Scoring Model to Predict Risk of Mortality after EVAR and Open AAA Repair

Parameter	Points
Treatment	
EVAR	0
OAR (infrarenal)	2
OAR (suprarenal)	4
Aneurysm size, mm	
<65	0
≥65	2
Age, years	
≤75	0
>75	1
Gender	
Male	0
Female	1
Comorbidities	
Myocardial disease	1
Cerebrovascular disease	1
Chronic obstructive pulmonary disease	2
Laboratory value	
Creatinine, mg/dL	
<1.5	0
1.5 to <2	2
≥2	2

EVAR, endovascular aneurysm repair; OAR, open aneurysm repair. Reproduced from Eslami MH, Rybin D, Doros G, Kalish JA, Farber A. Comparison of a Vascular Study Group of New England risk prediction model with established risk prediction models of in-hospital mortality after elective abdominal aortic aneurysm repair. *J Vasc Surg*. 2015;62(5): 1125-1133.e2.

Table 29-2. Predicted Operative Mortality Based on Points

Points	Probability of Mortality (%)	Proposed Risk Designation
0	0.12	Low-risk group
1	0.20	
2	0.34	
3	0.59	
4	1.00	
5	1.71	Medium-risk group
6	2.91	
7	4.90	
8	8.14	High-risk group
9	13.2	
10	20.75	
11	31.05	Prohibitive high-risk group
12	43.63	
13	57.10	
14	69.59	

Reproduced from Eslami MH, Rybin D, Doros G, Kalish JA, Farber A. Comparison of a Vascular Study Group of New England risk prediction model with established risk prediction models of in-hospital mortality after elective abdominal aortic aneurysm repair. *J Vasc Surg.* 2015;62(5):1125-1133.e2.

situation, one can either remove the limbs or sew directly to the limbs if they are adequately sealed distally. Although explantation may be the best option, it is associated with significant morbidity and mortality.[20]

Ⓝ Suitable common iliac seal zone?

In patients with a type Ib endoleak, evaluation of the distal CIA for a suitable seal zone is necessary. The diameter of the distal CIA and the available length of the CIA are essential parameters to quantify whether a limb extension would provide a durable treatment option. Two centimeters of nonaneurysmal CIA proximal to the iliac bifurcation, measuring <20 mm in diameter, is preferred for safe and durable extension of the iliac limb without coverage of the IIA.

Ⓞ Patent contralateral IIA?

If there is no suitable CIA seal zone, it is important to determine the patency of the contralateral IIA. If it is patent, then we would embolize the ipsilateral IIA with extension of the iliac limb into the EIA, except in very active patients in whom any risk of buttock claudication would be intolerable. If the contralateral IIA is occluded, it is important to maintain patency of the ipsilateral IIA if at all possible.

Ⓟ Iliac limb extension

In patients with a suitable segment of CIA distal to the previous fixation site, and proximal to the iliac bifurcation, extension with an appropriately sized endograft limb provides durable treatment

for a type Ib endoleak. Generally speaking, limb extension can be performed with any commercial endograft limb regardless of the specific device type that is in place.

Ⓠ IIA embolization with EIA limb extension

Multiple studies have demonstrated that unilateral IIA embolization is typically tolerated without significant adverse events.[21,22] Although the rates of unilateral buttock claudication and erectile dysfunction may be as high as 40%, these typically improve over time.[23] Iliac extension limbs with distal diameters as low as 11 mm are available to accommodate the size discrepancy between CIA and EIA.

Ⓡ Favorable anatomy for iliac branch device?

An evaluation of the ipsilateral CIA, IIA, and EIA is important to determine feasibility for an iliac branch device. The CIA must be of adequate diameter at the bifurcation to accommodate both the branch stent graft and the external iliac stent graft. The EIA and the IIA diameters must be appropriate for creation of a seal: EIA diameter 6.5 to 25 mm; IIA diameter 6.5 to 13.5 mm. Early bifurcation of the IIA branch vessel will prohibit adequate seal of the iliac branch limb. In this scenario, we would perform an open EIA to IIA bypass with extension of the ipsilateral iliac limb into the EIA (see S).

Ⓢ EIA-to-IIA bypass with external iliac limb extension

There are multiple options to relocate the iliac artery bifurcation to facilitate a distal landing zone in the proximal EIA while maintaining IIA patency. This includes EIA to IIA bypass[24] or reimplantation of the IIA onto the more distal EIA.[25]

Ⓣ Iliac branch device

In patients with favorable anatomy, FDA-approved iliac branch grafts maintain antegrade perfusion to the IIA.[26] In patients with appropriate clinical scenarios, hypogastric-artery-sparing devices are preferred.[27] Ziegler et al. demonstrated 72% technical success rate of IIA preservation using branched devices with 87% 5-year patency.[28] The prospective, multicenter study of the Gore Iliac Branch Endoprosthesis demonstrated 95% limb patency and 95% freedom from type I or III endoleak.[29]

Ⓤ Type II

A type II endoleak is caused by persistent perfusion of the aneurysm sac from an aortic branch vessel. Most commonly, this occurs from a lumbar artery or the IMA, or rarely an accessory renal artery. The incidence of type II endoleaks after EVAR is 10% to 15%.[30] Type II endoleaks have varying effects on aneurysm sac progression.

Ⓥ Sac enlargement ≥ 5 mm?

Although AAA rupture from a type II endoleak is rare, it is more likely as sac enlargement occurs. Aneurysm sac expansion ≥5 mm warrants investigation and treatment of a type II endoleak, if one

exists. Although some previous studies suggest that a type II endoleak with ≥5 mm increase in sac diameter may be safe to observe,[31] we recommend treatment if possible. Less is known about the natural history of a type IV or V endoleak, but we also recommend pursuing treatment if the AAA sac expands by >5 mm and no other endoleak is identified. Careful continued surveillance is necessary to continue to monitor AAA sac expansion <5 mm.

Ⓦ Source of endoleak

It is imperative to identify the source of a type II endoleak. This may require further investigation using CTA, DSA, or DUS. DUS may provide critical information regarding direction of inflow and outflow from the aneurysm sac. For example, if the IMA provides inflow, and a lumbar artery outflow, treating the IMA would be important. In addition, CT imaging with aortic catheter contrast infusion may provide information to localize the source of the endoleak. If the source of the leak cannot be identified by DUS or CTA, DSA may be necessary to define the source.

Ⓧ DSA with embolization via the SMA

If the IMA is identified as the source of the type II endoleak, selective embolization may be attempted by accessing the SMA and advancing a catheter through the arc of Riolan or the marginal artery of Drummond. Single-center case series have demonstrated successful results at 2-year follow-up.[32]

Ⓨ Translumbar embolization vs. transcaval arterial embolization vs. laparoscopic lumbar ± IMA ligation

The CTA should be investigated to identify the source of endoleak. If the source of the endoleak is a lumbar artery, then consider several options for intervention including translumbar embolization,[33] transcaval arterial embolization,[34] or laparoscopic lumbar embolization possibly with IMA ligation.[35] Translumbar embolization is performed with CT and fluoroscopy. After accessing the aneurysm sac, a baseline pressure is recorded, before performing a diagnostic angiogram.[36] Transcaval arterial embolization is limited to type II endoleaks originating on the right side, or in close proximity to the inferior vena cava. Single-center studies have demonstrated 70% resolution of endoleaks with stability in aneurysm sac size.[34] A Cochrane review that examined 20 patients who underwent laparoscopic IMA ligation demonstrated a 90% technical success rate. All patients had regression or stability in aneurysm sac size.[37]

Ⓩ Type III

A type III endoleak describes a graft leak either at the junction of graft components (IIIa) or through a tear of the graft fabric (IIIb). It is important to identify the source of the endoleak on CTA, or DSA. An iliac branch junction endoleak (type IIIa) occurs at bridging points between limbs of the endograft. This is ideally treated with an additional bridging iliac limb across the area.

A type IIIa endoleak at the aortic cuff or bifurcation of the endograft signifies separation in the aortic component of the endograft. This is best treated by relining the entire stent graft with a new endograft. A type IIIb endoleak occurs from a tear within the graft fabric and is treated by relining the affected portion of the graft.

🅐🅐 Bridge components or reline

When the endoleak occurs across an iliac limb and its extension, treatment should include application of a bridging stent graft across the junction.[5,38] The selection of iliac limb extension should depend on the previous device type and size to match the diameter of the limb already in place. If there is overlap of the displaced limbs, crossing the defect may be facilitated by both femoral and brachial wire techniques. When the endoleak occurs at the aortic graft bifurcation or proximal cuff, relining of the entire stent graft with a new endograft is undertaken (see BB).

🅑🅑 Reline entire graft

In certain scenarios, relining the endograft may be necessary to fully exclude the endoleak. This entails reperforming the entire EVAR including the main body and iliac limbs. A careful assessment of the distance from the aneurysm to the renal arteries, as well as the distance from the flow divider to the renal arteries, is important to select the type of endograft. Any commercially available endograft can be used for relining as long as there is adequate length from the lowest renal to the previously placed endograft bifurcation to allow for opening of the contralateral gate above the flow divider.

🅒🅒 Surveillance

The Society for Vascular Surgery Guidelines recommend surveillance CT scan at 1 month and 12 months after initial EVAR. A 6-month CT scan should be considered If there are concerning findings identified at the 1-month interval. DUS is safe for long-term surveillance if previous CT imaging demonstrates no evidence of endoleak and a stable aneurysm size.[2] After repair of an endoleak, consider reinitiation of the initial surveillance regimen to confirm proper repair.

🅓🅓 Limb occlusion and femoral-femoral bypass

In scenarios where there is significant iliac tortuosity and distortion between the main body and iliac limb, the clinician may be unable to bridge the two segments of the vessel. In this scenario, we would embolize or plug occlude the proximal iliac limb, followed by concomitant crossover femoral-femoral bypass grafting.

🅔🅔 Type IV, V

A type IV endoleak results from a porous endograft and is seen immediately after placement and usually resolves within 30 days unless there is a graft defect. If a fabric-related endoleak persists beyond 30 days and the precise source cannot be determined, it should be considered an endoleak of undefined origin.[39] A type V endoleak (endotension) is defined as a continued expansion of the aneurysm sac without an identifiable endoleak. This may be secondary to sac perfusion that is undetected by the imaging modality, pressure transmission through the fabric, or accumulation of serous fluid across the endograft fabric.[40-42] The decision to proceed with intervention is contingent upon an increase in aortic sac diameter of at least 5 mm.

REFERENCES

1. Abraha I, Luchetta ML, De Florio R, et al. Ultrasonography for endoleak detection after endoluminal abdominal aortic aneurysm repair. *Cochrane Database Syst Rev.* 2017;6:CD010296.
2. Chaikof EL, Dalman RL, Eskandari MK, et al. The Society for Vascular Surgery practice guidelines on the care of patients with an abdominal aortic aneurysm. *J Vasc Surg.* 2018;67(1):2-77.e2.
3. Abbas A, Hansrani V, Sedgwick N, Ghosh J, McCollum CN. 3D contrast enhanced ultrasound for detecting endoleak following endovascular aneurysm repair (EVAR). *Eur J Vasc Endovasc Surg.* 2014;47(5):487-492.
4. van der Laan MJ, Bakker CJG, Blankensteijn JD, Bartels LW. Dynamic CE-MRA for endoleak classification after endovascular aneurysm repair. *Eur J Vasc Endovasc Surg.* 2006;31(2):130-135.
5. Buth J, Laheij RJF. Early complications and endoleaks after endovascular abdominal aortic aneurysm repair: report of a multicenter study. *J Vasc Surg.* 2000;31(1):134-146.
6. AbuRahma AF, Campbell J, Stone PA, et al. The correlation of aortic neck length to early and late outcomes in endovascular aneurysm repair patients. *J Vasc Surg.* 2009;50(4):738-748.
7. Hobo R, Kievit J, Leurs LJ, Buth J; EUROSTAR Collaborators. Influence of severe infrarenal aortic neck angulation on complications at the proximal neck following endovascular AAA repair: a EUROSTAR study. *J Endovasc Ther.* 2007;14(1):1-11.
8. Leurs LJ, Kievit J, Dagnelie PC, Nelemans PJ, Buth J; EUROSTAR Collaborators. Influence of infrarenal neck length on outcome of endovascular abdominal aortic aneurysm repair. *J Endovasc Ther.* 2006;13(5):640-648.
9. Albertini J, Kalliafas S, Travis S, et al. Anatomical risk factors for proximal perigraft endoleak and graft migration following endovascular repair of abdominal aortic aneurysms. *Eur J Vasc Endovasc Surg.* 2000;19(3):308-312.
10. Schanzer A, Greenberg RK, Hevelone N, et al. Predictors of abdominal aortic aneurysm sac enlargement after endovascular repair. *Circulation.* 2011;123(24):2848-2855.
11. Donas KP, Telve D, Torsello G, Pitoulias G, Schwindt A, Austermann M. Use of parallel grafts to save failed prior endovascular aortic aneurysm repair and type Ia endoleaks. *J Vasc Surg.* 2015;62(3):578-584.
12. de Vries JP, Ouriel K, Mehta M, et al. Analysis of EndoAnchors for endovascular aneurysm repair by indications for use. *J Vasc Surg.* 2014;60(6):1460-1467.e1.
13. Sheehan MK, Barbato J, Compton CN, et al. Effectiveness of coiling in the treatment of endoleaks after endovascular repair. *J Vasc Surg.* 2004;40(3):430-434.
14. Maldonado TS, Rosen RJ, Rockman CB, et al. Initial successful management of type I endoleak after endovascular aortic aneurysm repair with n-butyl cyanoacrylate adhesive. *J Vasc Surg.* 2003;38(4):664-670.
15. Ierardi AM, Franchin M, Fontana F, et al. The role of ethylene-vinyl alcohol copolymer in association with other embolic agents for the percutaneous and endovascular treatment of type Ia endoleak. *Radiol Med (Torino).* 2018;123:638–642.
16. Egorova N, Giacovelli JK, Gelijns A, et al. Defining high-risk patients for endovascular aneurysm repair. *J Vasc Surg.* 2009;50(6):1271-1279.e1.
17. Eslami MH, Rybin D, Doros G, Kalish JA, Farber A. Comparison of a Vascular Study Group of New England risk prediction model with established risk prediction models of in-hospital mortality after elective abdominal aortic aneurysm repair. *J Vasc Surg.* 2015;62(5):1125-1133.e2.
18. Graves HL, Jackson BM. The current state of fenestrated and branched devices for abdominal aortic aneurysm repair. *Semin Interv Radiol.* 2015;32(3):304-310.
19. Farber MA, Vallabhaneni R, Marston WA. "Off-the-shelf" devices for complex aortic aneurysm repair. *J Vasc Surg.* 2014;60(3):579-584.
20. Turney EJ, Steenberge SP, Lyden SP, et al. Late graft explants in endovascular aneurysm repair. *J Vasc Surg.* 2014;59(4):886-893.
21. Schoder M, Zaunbauer L, Hölzenbein T, et al. Internal iliac artery embolization before endovascular repair of abdominal aortic aneurysms: frequency, efficacy, and clinical results. *AJR Am J Roentgenol.* 2001;177(3):599-605.
22. Cynamon J, Lerer D, Veith FJ, et al. Hypogastric artery coil embolization prior to endoluminal repair of aneurysms and fistulas: buttock claudication, a recognized but possibly preventable complication. *J Vasc Interv Radiol.* 2000;11(5):573-577.
23. Farahmand P, Becquemin JP, Desgranges P, Allaire E, Marzelle J, Roudot-Thoraval F. Is hypogastric artery embolization during endovascular aortoiliac aneurysm repair (EVAR) innocuous and useful? *Eur J Vasc Endovasc Surg.* 2008;35(4):429-435.
24. Lee WA, Nelson PR, Berceli SA, Seeger JM, Huber TS. Outcome after hypogastric artery bypass and embolization

during endovascular aneurysm repair. *J Vasc Surg*. 2006;44(6):1162–1168; discussion 1168-1169.

25. Parodi JC, Ferreira M. Relocation of the iliac artery bifurcation to facilitate endoluminal treatment of abdominal aortic aneurysms. *J Endovasc Surg*. 1999;6(4):342-347.

26. Malina M, Dirven M, Sonesson B, Resch T, Dias N, Ivancev K. Feasibility of a branched stent-graft in common iliac artery aneurysms. *J Endovasc Ther*. 2006;13(4):496-500.

27. Serracino-Inglott F, Bray AE, Myers P. Endovascular abdominal aortic aneurysm repair in patients with common iliac artery aneurysms—initial experience with the Zenith bifurcated iliac side branch device. *J Vasc Surg*. 2007;46(2):211-217.

28. Ziegler P, Avgerinos ED, Umscheid T, Perdikides T, Erz K, Stelter WJ. Branched iliac bifurcation: 6 years experience with endovascular preservation of internal iliac artery flow. *J Vasc Surg*. 2007;46(2):204-210.

29. Schneider DB, Matsumura JS, Lee JT, Peterson BG, Chaer RA, Oderich GS. Prospective, multicenter study of endovascular repair of aortoiliac and iliac aneurysms using the Gore Iliac Branch Endoprosthesis. *J Vasc Surg*. 2017;66(3):775-785.

30. Kray J, Kirk S, Franko J, Chew DK. Role of type II endoleak in sac regression after endovascular repair of infrarenal abdominal aortic aneurysms. *J Vasc Surg*. 2015;61(4):869-874.

31. Sidloff DA, Gokani V, Stather PW, Choke E, Bown MJ, Sayers RD. Type II endoleak: conservative management is a safe strategy. *Eur J Vasc Endovasc Surg*. 2014;48(4):391-399.

32. Görich J, Rilinger N, Sokiranski R, et al. Embolization of type II endoleaks fed by the inferior mesenteric artery: using the superior mesenteric artery approach. *J Endovasc Ther*. 2000;7(4):297-301.

33. Lagios K, Karaolanis G, Bazinas T, Perdikides T, Bountouris I. Translumbar infusion of N-Butyl cyanoacrylate for the treatment of type II endoleaks. *J Vasc Interv Radiol*. 2018;29:826-839.

34. Giles KA, Fillinger MF, De Martino RR, Hoel AW, Powell RJ, Walsh DB. Results of transcaval embolization for sac expansion from type II endoleaks after endovascular aneurysm repair. *J Vasc Surg*. 2015;61(5):1129-1136.

35. Kuziez MS, Sanchez LA, Zayed MA. Abdominal aortic aneurysm type II endoleaks. *J Cardiovasc Dis Diagn*. 2016;4(5).

36. Bryce Y, Schiro B, Cooper K, et al. Type II endoleaks: diagnosis and treatment algorithm. *Cardiovasc Diagn Ther*. 2018;8(suppl 1):S131-S137.

37. Spanos K, Tsilimparis N, Larena-Avellaneda A, Giannoukas AD, Debus SE, Kölbel T. Systematic review of laparoscopic ligation of inferior mesenteric artery for the treatment of type II endoleak after endovascular aortic aneurysm repair. *J Vasc Surg*. 2017;66(6):1878-1884.

38. Harris PL, Vallabhaneni SR, Desgranges P, Becquemin JP, van Marrewijk C, Laheij RJ. Incidence and risk factors of late rupture, conversion, and death after endovascular repair of infrarenal aortic aneurysms: The EUROSTAR experience. *J Vasc Surg*. 2000;32(4):739-749.

39. Chaikof EL, Blankensteijn JD, Harris PL, et al. Reporting standards for endovascular aortic aneurysm repair. *J Vasc Surg*. 2002;35(5):1048-1060.

40. Gilling-Smith G, Brennan J, Harris P, Bakran A, Gould D, McWilliams R. Endotension after endovascular aneurysm repair: definition, classification, and strategies for surveillance and intervention. *J Endovasc Surg*. 1999;6(4):305-307.

41. van Sambeek MRHM, Hendriks JM, Tseng L, van Dijk LC, van Urk H. Sac enlargement without endoleak: when and how to convert and technical considerations. *Semin Vasc Surg*. 2004;17(4):284-287.

42. Peterson BG, Matsumura JS, Brewster DC, Makaroun MS. Five-year report of a multicenter controlled clinical trial of open versus endovascular treatment of abdominal aortic aneurysms. *J Vasc Surg*. 2007;45(5):885-890.

Misty D. Humphries

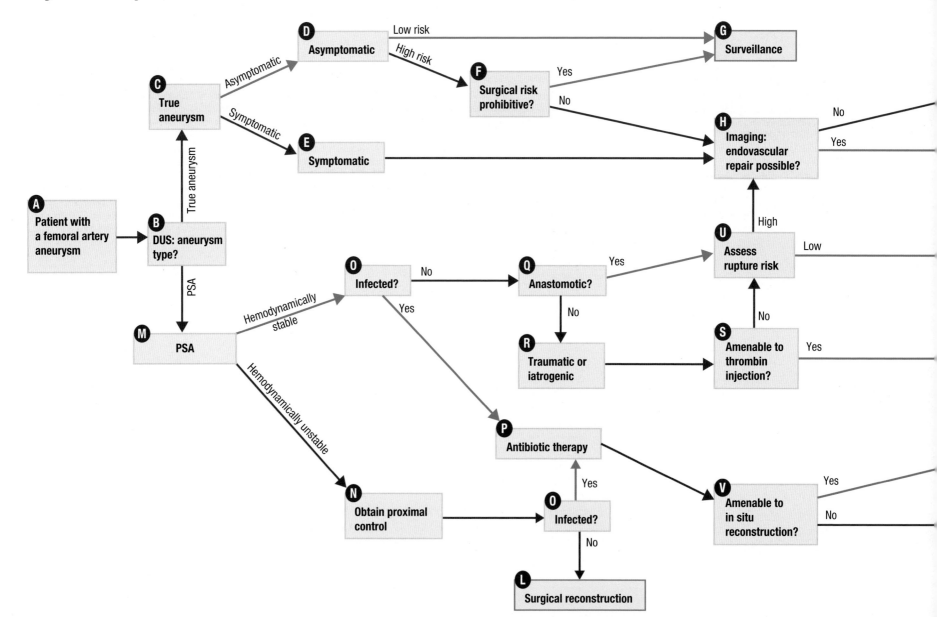

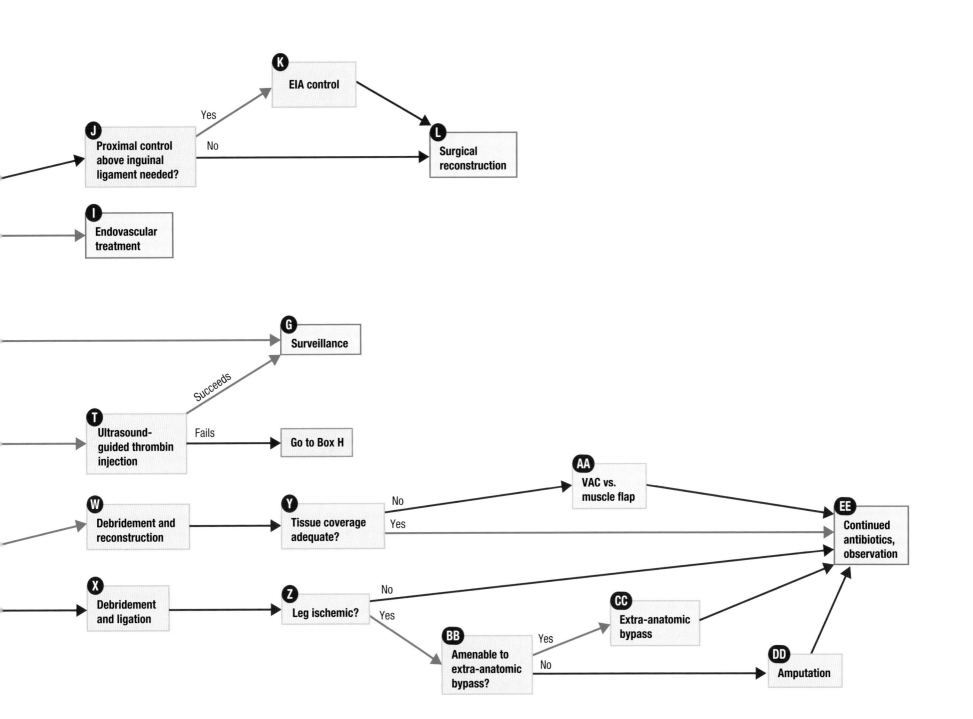

Ⓐ Patient with a femoral artery aneurysm

Patients with a femoral artery aneurysm (FAA) or PSA are often diagnosed by palpation of a prominent pulse in the inguinal area. True FAAs are rare and most commonly seen in elderly (>70 years old) men.[1] There is a 15:1 male to female predominance for true aneurysms.[1] The majority of these are asymptomatic (66%).[2] The most common symptom is pain from local compression followed by limb ischemia due to aneurysm thrombosis or distal embolism.[3] PSAs commonly result from iatrogenic injuries during angiography, intravenous drug abuse (IVDA), and trauma. Patients who present with groin pain or swelling after femoral access for angiography, have a history of femoral arterial graft placement, or who are IV drug users should immediately be suspected of having a femoral PSA. In addition to pain from expansion, PSAs can rupture causing an expanding hematoma that can lead to hemodynamic instability.

Ⓑ DUS: aneurysm type?

The screening test of choice to diagnose a true FAA or PSA is DUS which is fast, cost-effective, and highly accurate as a first-line imaging modality. DUS can differentiate a true aneurysm from a false aneurysm and be performed at the point of care in the emergency room, cardiac catheterization suite, or ICU by providers with basic ultrasound skills. When a FAA is diagnosed on DUS, the aneurysm etiology and morphology determines if further cross-sectional imaging is needed for preoperative repair planning and assessment of distal arterial perfusion.

Ⓒ True aneurysm

True FAAs are typically located in the CFA and are uncommon. The incidence in the general population is estimated at 7.4/100,000 in men and 1.0/100,000 in women.[4] Patients with a FAA should undergo workup for additional aneurysms because 95% of patients will have a second aneurysm either in the popliteal artery or the aortoiliac segment.[5] The reported incidence of bilateral femoral aneurysms is 59%.[6] For this reason, any patient who is diagnosed with FAA should undergo screening DUS to rule out aneurysms of popliteal artery and abdominal aorta.

Histologically, most true FAAs are degenerative, but in some cases they are associated with various connective tissue disorders.[7] These disorders include mutations in the *FBN1* gene causing Marfan syndrome, FBN2 mutations, Parks-Weber syndrome, Behçet disease, Ehlers-Danlos syndrome, and Wegener granulomatosis.[8,9] In 1973, Cutler and Darling developed a classification system for common femoral aneurysms based on involvement of the bifurcation. By their classification, type 1 FAAs are those confined to the common femoral segment and do not involve the femoral bifurcation, whereas type 2 FAAs are located at the bifurcation and involve the origin of the deep and superficial femoral arteries.[10] This classification was expanded in 2004 by Amer et al.

who defined type 3 FAAs as aneurysms that involve only the SFA, whereas type 4 involve only the deep femoral artery.[11] Although the classification is largely academic, it allows for uniform reporting and understanding of aneurysm location. Management of true FAAs depends on whether symptoms are present.

Ⓓ Asymptomatic

The majority of true FAAs are asymptomatic and discovered incidentally on CT imaging or as a nonpainful pulsatile groin mass. Their clinical significance is that they have potential to thrombose or embolize, which can lead to limb loss. In the largest reported study to date, Lawrence et al. found no episode of embolization or rupture in 156 asymptomatic true FAAs <3.5 cm in diameter.[2] Femoral aneurysms should be assessed for complication risk using size criteria and the presence of intraluminal thrombus. CFA aneurysms >3.5 cm or those with significant intraluminal thrombus are considered high risk and should be treated unless surgical risk is prohibitive.

Ⓔ Symptomatic

A minority of patients with true FAAs present with symptoms. A painful, tender, pulsatile mass caused by local compression is the most common presentation.[3] In 4% to 15 % of patients, rupture may be the presenting symptom, but this is most common in infected or anastomotic aneurysms. Thrombosis of FAAs is less common than for popliteal aneurysms and has been described to occur in 3% to 15% of symptomatic cases.[2,3] Similarly, distal embolization is less common but when present can cause severe ischemic symptoms. All patients with symptomatic FAAs should be considered for repair and therefore undergo additional imaging for preoperative planning.

Ⓕ Surgical risk prohibitive?

Because the mean age at presentation is 70 years, many patients with FAAs will have associated cardiovascular, cerebrovascular, renal disease, or other comorbidities that may, in some cases, make surgical risk prohibitive. All patients should undergo complete H&P as well as basic blood testing and ECG. In patients with limited functional capacity, further workup is indicated (see Chapter 1). The presence of severely depressed cardiac function can shift treatment away from open surgical options to endovascular repair or surveillance.

Ⓖ Surveillance

Surveillance is most appropriate for patients with asymptomatic true FAAs <3.5 cm in diameter and for patients whose perioperative risk is too high. Surveillance is performed using DUS because it avoids ionizing radiation and nephrotoxic agents and can delineate aneurysm size and presence of thrombus. There are no formal recommendations at this time on the frequency of reimaging; however, 50% of patients who undergo repair do so

within 2.5 years of the initial diagnosis.[2] For this reason, the authors recommend a surveillance strategy using DUS at intervals no longer than 1 year. It is reasonable to consider DUS every 6 months for aneurysms >2.0 cm and once a year for those with aneurysms <2 cm.

Ⓗ Imaging: endovascular repair possible?

When FAA repair is necessary, axial imaging with CTA is recommended for preoperative planning. CTA is fast, can completely delineate the involvement of arterial branches in the aneurysm, and provides valuable information about surrounding structures. In patients with an allergy to iodinated contrast, MRA with gadolinium can be used. Both imaging modalities can also provide valuable information regarding additional aneurysms in the abdomen or distal leg and rule out other potential etiologies of symptoms. In selective cases, lower extremity DSA may be needed to delineate the FAA and distal runoff.

Endovascular repair has limited utility in treatment of FAAs localized to the CFA because of external forces that the artery is subjected to from repeated flexion at the hip and the bifurcation of the artery. In cases of rupture and hemodynamic instability, endovascular treatment of CFA aneurysms has been described as a bridge to future definitive repair.[12] Endovascular therapy has mainly been used in treatment of SFA aneurysms or in cases of anastomotic PSA where outflow is limited to one vessel (eg, anastomotic PSA of an aortobifemoral bypass graft where the profunda femoris artery is the only outflow vessel).[13] Adequate seal zone above and below the aneurysm is required, and attention should be paid to ensuring that the stent graft will not extend into arterial segments with excessive bending.[14] It is also imperative to rule out a mycotic aneurysm before placement of a stentgraft.[14,15]

Ⓘ Endovascular treatment

When endovascular treatment is appropriate, stent sizing should be performed depending on the preoperative axial imaging. Contralateral femoral access is obtained, and an appropriately sized sheath is brought over the aortic bifurcation. DSA is performed to delineate the extent of the aneurysm and a self-expanding stent graft is placed with adequate seal zone proximally and distally within normal artery. Approximately 10% to 15% oversizing should be used. Postoperatively, patients should be placed on dual antiplatelet therapy and, when possible, this should be continued indefinitely to decrease the risk of stent thrombosis.[16]

Ⓙ Proximal control above inguinal ligament needed?

Proximal suprainguinal control may be necessary when the aneurysm or PSA extends above the inguinal ligament or when direct exposure of the aneurysm or PSA may be challenging, eg, active bleeding or in the setting of an infected artery.

K EIA control

In cases where EIA control is needed, either endovascular balloon occlusion or clamping via a retroperitoneal incision can be used. Balloon occlusion is less invasive and allows FAA repair through a limited incision below the inguinal ligament. This is done via a contralateral femoral approach in which a 6-French sheath of at least 40 cm is placed up and over the aortic bifurcation. A 7- or 8-mm balloon is inflated to profile in the ipsilateral EIA during the repair. If a contralateral approach is not possible, an ipsilateral approach can be used by puncturing the SFA to allow placement of a short 5-French sheath above the FAA repair zone for balloon occlusion. If the repair requires graft replacement of the femoral artery; however, an ipsilateral approach requires exchange of the occlusion balloon and potential blood loss. When balloon occlusion is not possible, open surgical exposure of the EIA via a retroperitoneal incision is required. This incision can be extended cephalad to gain control of the CIA or IIA if needed because of disease involving the EIA.

L Surgical reconstruction

Surgical reconstruction is the usual treatment of CFA aneurysms and varies depending on type of aneurysm (see C). For type 1, 3, and 4 femoral aneurysms, a simple interposition graft can be used. In the case of type 2 aneurysms, open surgical repair allows for reconstruction of the femoral bifurcation. This can be achieved by creating an end-to-end EIA or proximal CFA to deep femoral artery bypass with reimplantation of the SFA or a separate interposition graft to the SFA.

The choice of conduit for repair is based on the presence or absence of infection.[10] When infection is not present, either ePTFE or Dacron provides appropriate size matching and comparable long-term patency.[17] When infection is suspected, alternative conduits need to be considered. In situ reconstructions can be considered with specific criteria. The deep femoral vein has a better size match for the CFA, whereas the GSV can be used for deep femoral or SFA reconstructions. Cryopreserved allograft can be considered, although the long-term patency is worse than with autogenous vein. Rifampin-soaked Dacron can also be used. Extra-anatomic bypass with an axillo-SFA or popliteal or obturator bypass allows for utilization of prosthetic material and avoidance of the contaminated field.

For iatrogenic, post-angiography PSAs, a simple stitch repair of the arterial puncture site is often all that is needed after proximal and distal arterial control is obtained. In the rare case of severe arterial occlusive disease, a formal endarterectomy and patch repair may be required. Associated hematoma is removed and a surgical drain is placed as necessary.

M PSA

PSAs are contained hematomas that remain in communication with arterial blood flow after artery injury. Femoral PSAs are most often iatrogenic from access for angiography, with less common causes being arterial graft anastomotic disruption, trauma, or infection. Infection can be associated with any etiology and may be occult in some cases of arterial graft PSA (see Chapter 90). In patients who present with a PSA, hemodynamic stability dictates further evaluation versus emergent treatment.

N Obtain proximal control

If patients are hemodynamically unstable, urgent surgery should be planned. In these patients, proximal arterial control in the suprainguinal area is the key initial step. This can be achieved by a lower quadrant abdominal incision and retroperitoneal exposure of the EIA or inflow limb of the affected graft or endovascular balloon control (see J for details).

O Infected?

Infection is suspected when local erythema, swelling, pain, or fever is present, if fluid surrounding the aneurysm is seen on imaging, or in patients with recurrent systemic infections. A comprehensive infection workup should be performed, including complete blood count, blood cultures, and ECHO (if endocarditis is suspected). Coagulase negative Staphylococcus species are the most common cause of graft anastomotic PSAs.[18] MRSA and gram-negative organisms (Pseudomonas, *Escherichia coli*, Proteus, Klebsiella, Salmonella, Enterobacter) are more common in patients with aneurysms due to iatrogenic causes or IVDA. They are markedly virulent and more likely to lead to disruption of the arterial wall with rupture of the artery. Gram-negative organisms release alkaline proteinase and other elastases that lead to necrosis of the vascular wall.[19] Positive blood culture rates approach 78% in patients with infected aneurysms.[20]

P Antibiotic therapy

Although culture results should drive the choice of antibiotic therapy, initial treatment of PSA diagnosed or suspected of being infected begins with broad-spectrum antibiotics aimed at gram-positive and gram-negative bacteria. In patients recently hospitalized, initial antibiotics should cover more invasive organisms such as MRSA. In IV drug users, gram-negative and anaerobic bacteria need to be covered. The choice of specific antibiotic also depend on hospital antibiograms and practice patterns.

Q Anastomotic?

In patients who have had prior femoral arterial procedures, an anastomotic PSA should be suspected. Disruption of the anastomotic suture line or synthetic material itself, dilation of the graft fabric, and arterial wall degeneration are all possible. After many years, polyester (Dacron) graft dilation can occur, but graft failure with anastomotic disruption is seen mostly in the setting of infection or arterial wall degeneration. Once an anastomotic PSA is diagnosed, the patient should be considered for operative intervention.

R Traumatic or iatrogenic

Iatrogenic PSAs are seen after direct femoral artery instrumentation for angiography or arterial line placement. Procedures that require larger sheath sizes (eg, larger than 6 French), prolonged duration, use of closure devices, and the use of thrombolysis or anticoagulation increase the risk for PSA development.[21] DUS can delineate characteristics such as size, the presence of an AVF, or size/length of the PSA neck, which will help determine treatment.

Traumatic PSAs can result from blunt or penetrating injury. In the case of blunt trauma, the mechanism of injury is stretch of the artery with tearing of the wall. Although this can lead to arterial thrombosis, PSA formation has been reported.[22] Penetrating injury of the arterial wall leading to PSA formation can occur as the result of fractures of the femur with displacement of the bone, as well as direct injury by stabbing or gunshot.

S Amenable to thrombin Injection?

PSA size, anatomy of the feeding neck, presence of an AVF, and current anticoagulation or antiplatelet regimens will determine whether intervention is indicated. PSAs less than 2 cm and small AVF are likely to resolve on their own, provided the patient is not on anticoagulation, with a mean time to closure of 3 to 4 weeks.[23] Close observation with repeat DUS in 3 to 4 weeks is the best option in these cases. PSAs in patients on anticoagulation or multiple antiplatelet agents are not likely to close spontaneously.[24] For PSAs larger than 2 cm, intervention is indicated. Direct thrombin injection should be considered the first line of therapy given the ease of this intervention, Criteria that exclude thrombin injection for PSAs include a broad-based (>0.5 cm) or short (<0.2 cm) feeding neck and the presence of an AVF, because these anatomic features increase the risk of distal embolization. Femoral neuropathy, skin compromise, and distal ischemia warrant urgent surgical repair rather than thrombin injection. Another contraindication to thrombin injection is an allergy to bovine thrombin, if recombinant thrombin is not available. When the patient is not a candidate for thrombin injection, operative repair is indicated.

Ultrasound-guided compression to induce closure has been used when operative risk was considered prohibitive, although most practitioners have abandoned this modality because it is time consuming, painful for the patient, difficult for the technologist, and has a higher failure rate compared to thrombin injection. Successful thrombosis rates for ultrasound compression average only 73% but drop to as low as 40% in patients on anticoagulation.[25,26] In successful cases, the average time to thrombosis is 30 minutes, and ultrasound guidance does not increase the likelihood of success compared to direct manual compression over the PSA.[27]

T Ultrasound-guided thrombin injection

In appropriately selected patients, ultrasound-guided thrombin injection has several advantages in treating iatrogenic femoral PSAs. It is quick, can be performed with local anesthetic, and, aside from the ultrasound and thrombin, does not require specialized equipment. Ultrasound is essential to visualize the needle inside the PSA cavity and allow injection of thrombin away from the PSA neck. Once the needle is confirmed to be in the cavity, 500 to 1000 units of thrombin is slowly injected until color flow is no longer seen in the aneurysm sac. Success rates for ultrasound-guided thrombin injection are 97%, with patients occasionally requiring a second injection.[28] Repeat DUS is performed at 24 to 48 hours after injection to ensure aneurysm thrombosis.

U Assess rupture risk

If a femoral PSA is not amenable to thrombin injection, or is anastomotic, treatment versus surveillance is based on propensity of rupture. Iatrogenic PSAs < 2 cm are unlikely to rupture and given their propensity for spontaneous thrombosis, repeat DUS at 1- to 2-week intervals is appropriate. Anastomotic aneurysms and iatrogenic PSA > 2 cm not amenable to thrombin injection should undergo additional imaging to plan definitive treatment.

V Amenable to in situ reconstruction?

In situ reconstruction can be considered for infections without virulent bacteria (*E. coli*, Klebsiella, Pseudomonas), when the arterial wall is not severely diseased and will hold sutures for the new graft, and when there is adequate tissue coverage.

W Debridement and reconstruction

It is imperative that all infected arterial wall and prosthetic tissue be removed before reconstruction. Autologous vein reconstructions have the best long-term patency and are most resistant to infection. For deep femoral or SFA reconstructions, GSV is usually an appropriately sized conduit. For CFA reconstructions, the saphenous vein is too small and ipsilateral femoral vein can be used with limited morbidity.

If autologous vein is not available, antibiotic-treated prosthetic grafts can be used for infections with bacteria that form a low-grade biofilm, specifically coagulase-negative staphylococci, in grafts that have been in place for months or years, and where the patient does not have signs of systemic infection. A gel- or collagen-impregnated polyester graft is soaked in a solution of 600 mg or rifampin mixed with 250 mL of normal saline for 30 minutes.[29] Reinfection rates with antibiotic-soaked grafts when stringent selection criteria are used can be as low as 4%.

The final option for in situ reconstruction is the use of cryopreserved arterial or venous conduits. Although cryopreserved allografts have the advantage of being easier to handle and more resistant to infection than prosthetic grafts, low primary patency

and high reintervention rates have tempered the enthusiasm of many providers for their use outside of infected fields.[30]

X Debridement and ligation

When arterial ligation is needed, it is imperative that all infected arterial wall and prosthetic tissue be removed. The artery must be debrided to healthy tissue to prevent late rupture. Ligation is performed using a running nonabsorbable polypropylene suture.

Y Tissue coverage adequate?

When in situ repair is performed, it is important to provide adequate viable tissue coverage. Thin patients with large aneurysms that cause extensive tissue distortion may not have adequate tissue coverage. In the case of an infected aneurysm, debridement of the subcutaneous fat and surrounding tissue may lead to a large defect with minimal tissue left behind for coverage. In this case, a muscle flap or VAC coverage is indicated.

Z Leg ischemic?

Whether or not reconstruction is needed after arterial ligation is based on the degree of limb ischemia and can be tested intraoperatively by obtaining ankle pressures after ligation of the diseased artery. If perfusion is considered borderline, the patient can be observed. In cases where the initial indication for treatment was claudication, reconstruction may not be required. If perfusion is poor or worsens with observation, extra-anatomic bypass may be needed.

AA VAC versus muscle flap

If inadequate, healthy, well-vascularized tissue remains to cover an in situ reconstruction, VAC has shown good results and is now frequently used when there is concern for primary healing.[31] It allows for fluid removal from the wound, limits dressing changes, and can help close a large cavitary defect quicker than do standard dressing changes.

A sartorius rotational muscle flap can provide healthy tissue coverage of grafts with excellent long-term results.[32] The sartorius muscle is divided proximally from the iliac spine and rotated medially to cover the femoral vessels. The muscle is dissected along the lateral border to preserve blood flow to the flap. If the sartorius muscle is not on option because of prior use or patient frailty, alternatives include rectus abdominis, rectus femoris, tensor fasciae latae, and gracilis flaps.

BB Amenable to extra-anatomic bypass?

In cases not amenable to in situ reconstruction or if debridement and ligation lead to leg ischemia, extra-anatomic bypass with autogenous or synthetic material should be performed. In rare patients with multiple prior reconstructions, extensive infection, or radiation damage to tissue, extra-anatomic arterial targets can be

diminutive, thus removing bypass as a treatment option. These patients should be considered for primary amputation. Bypass should not be offered to patients who are nonambulatory, extremely frail, or have medical comorbidities that render them too high risk for surgery.

CC Extra-anatomic bypass

Extra-anatomic options include axillofemoral (common, superficial, or deep), axillopopliteal, femoral to femoral, and obturator bypasses with ringed PTFE tunneled through noninfected planes. Axillofemoral grafts have markedly better patency than do axillopopliteal grafts. Both the descending thoracic or ascending thoracic aorta are alternative inflow options and can be tunneled to the distal femoral or popliteal arteries. An obturator bypass from the iliac artery to the femoral or popliteal arteries is an excellent option when the distal aorta and iliac arteries are not involved in the infection and not diseased. Because of the significant distance between the inflow and target artery, autogenous vein conduits are not feasible to use. In special circumstances when the PSA is part of an infected aortobifemoral bypass graft, the neoaortoiliac system (NAIS) operation using bilateral femoral veins is an alternative option.

DD Amputation

When there is severe limb ischemia and extra-anatomic bypass is not an option, primary amputation should be considered after debridement of infected artery or graft and resection of the PSA. Amputation may also be the treatment offered to patients presenting with PSA rupture where arterial ligation is needed as a lifesaving treatment. The level of amputation is determined depending on potential for ambulation and available inflow to the limb (see Chapter 48).

EE Continued antibiotics, observation

In all patients presenting with infected PSA, long-term antibiotics are indicated. Duration of antibiotics is variable, and depends on the type of reconstruction, detected organisms, and possibility of residual infection. At a minimum, IV antibiotics should continue for 2 weeks. If a patient undergoes in situ replacement, then consideration for 4 to 6 weeks of IV antibiotics should be considered. Oral antibiotics such as linezolid or fluoroquinolones can be for used given their higher tissue levels for less invasive organisms. In some cases, indefinite oral antibiotic suppression has been used, because there is no precise evidence concerning the optimal duration of antibiotic treatment.

In the early period after discharge, patients should have frequent regular visits to ensure there is no recurrence of the infection or arterial breakdown. When there is skin and tissue coverage, this can be done with DUS. In cases where large cavitary defects exist, CT imaging may be necessary. Any signs of recurrence should prompt readmission and further evaluation.

REFERENCES

1. Graham LM, Zelenock GB, Whitehouse WM Jr, et al. Clinical significance of arteriosclerotic femoral artery aneurysms. *Arch Surg.* 1980;115(4):502-507.
2. Lawrence PF, Harlander-Locke MP, Oderich GS, et al. The current management of isolated degenerative femoral artery aneurysms is too aggressive for their natural history. *J Vasc Surg.* 2014;59(2):343-349.
3. Piffaretti G, Mariscalco G, Tozzi M, et al. Twenty-year experience of femoral artery aneurysms. *J Vasc Surg.* 2011;53(5):1230-1236.
4. Lawrence PF, Lorenzo-Rivero S, Lyon JL. The incidence of iliac, femoral, and popliteal artery aneurysms in hospitalized patients. *J Vasc Surg.* 1995;22(4):409-416.
5. Diwan A, Sarkar R, Stanley JC, et al. Incidence of femoral and popliteal artery aneurysms in patients with abdominal aortic aneurysms. *J Vasc Surg.* 2000;31(5):863-869.
6. Dent TL, Lindenauer SM, Ernst CB, Fry WJ. Multiple arteriosclerotic arterial aneurysms. *Arch Surg.* 1972;105(2): 338-344.
7. Adeoye PO, Adebola SO, Adesiyun OA, et al. Bilateral femoral artery aneurysm mimicking soft tissue sarcoma. *Ann Vasc Surg.* 2012;26(2):279.e1-e3.
8. Dolapoglu A, Ertugay S, Posacioglu H. Staged approach for surgical management of a true femoral artery aneurysm combined with bilateral iliac artery aneurysms. *SAGE Open Med Case Rep.* 2017;5:2050313x17726911.
9. Ratschiller T, Muller H, Schachner T, et al. Femoral artery aneurysm repair in a patient with a fibrillin-2 mutation. *Vasc Endovascular Surg.* 2018;52(7):583-586.
10. Cutler BS, Darling RC. Surgical management of arteriosclerotic femoral aneurysms. *Surgery.* 1973;74(5):764-773.
11. Amer N, Grocott E, Shami S. Time for a new classification of femoral artery aneurysm? *Vasa.* 2004;33(3):170-172.
12. Kasirajan K, Marek JM, Langsfeld M. Behcet's disease: endovascular management of a ruptured peripheral arterial aneurysm. *J Vasc Surg.* 2001;34(6):1127-1129.
13. Bakoyiannis CN, Tsekouras NS, Economopoulos KP, et al. A hybrid approach using a composite endovascular and open graft procedure for a symptomatic common femoral aneurysm extending well above the inguinal ligament. *J Vasc Surg.* 2008;48(2):461-464.
14. van Sambeek MR, Gussenhoven EJ, van der Lugt A, et al. Endovascular stent-grafts for aneurysms of the femoral and popliteal arteries. *Ann Vasc Surg.* 1999;13(3):247-253.
15. Lyazidi Y, Abissegue Y, Chtata H, et al. Endovascular treatment of 2 true degenerative aneurysms of superficial femoral arteries. *Ann Vasc Surg.* 2016;30:307.e1-e5.
16. Johnston PC, Vartanian SM, Runge SJ, et al. Risk factors for clinical failure after stent graft treatment for femoropopliteal occlusive disease. *J Vasc Surg.* 2012;56(4):998-1006, 1007.e1; discussion 1006-1007.
17. Sapienza P, Mingoli A, Feldhaus RJ, et al. Femoral artery aneurysms: long-term follow-up and results of surgical treatment. *Cardiovasc Surg.* 1996;4(2):181-184.
18. Ylonen K, Biancari F, Leo E, et al. Predictors of development of anastomotic femoral pseudoaneurysms after aortobifemoral reconstruction for abdominal aortic aneurysm. *Am J Surg.* 2004;187(1):83-87.
19. Geary KJ, Tomkiewicz ZM, Harrison HN, et al. Differential effects of a gram-negative and a gram-positive infection on autogenous and prosthetic grafts. *J Vasc Surg.* 1990;11(2):339-345; discussion 46-47.
20. Oderich GS, Panneton JM, Bower TC, et al. Infected aortic aneurysms: aggressive presentation, complicated early outcome, but durable results. *J Vasc Surg.* 2001;34(5):900-908.
21. Skillman JJ, Kim D, Baim DS. Vascular complications of percutaneous femoral cardiac interventions. Incidence and operative repair. *Arch Surg.* 1988;123(10):1207-1212.
22. Sharma S, Bhargava B, Mahapatra M, Malhotra R. Pseudoaneurysm of the superficial femoral artery following accidental trauma: result of treatment by percutaneous stent-graft placement. *Eur Radiol.* 1999;9(3):422-424.
23. Toursarkissian B, Allen BT, Petrinec D, et al. Spontaneous closure of selected iatrogenic pseudoaneurysms and arteriovenous fistulae. *J Vasc Surg.* 1997;25(5):803-808; discussion 808-809.
24. Kent KC, McArdle CR, Kennedy B, et al. A prospective study of the clinical outcome of femoral pseudoaneurysms and arteriovenous fistulas induced by arterial puncture. *J Vasc Surg.* 1993;17(1):125-131; discussion 31-33.
25. Eisenberg L, Paulson EK, Kliewer MA, et al. Sonographically guided compression repair of pseudoaneurysms: further experience from a single institution. *AJR Am J Roentgenol.* 1999;173(6):1567-1573.
26. Gorge G, Kunz T, Kirstein M. A prospective study on ultrasound-guided compression therapy or thrombin injection for treatment of iatrogenic false aneurysms in patients receiving full-dose anti-platelet therapy. *Z Kardiol.* 2003;92(7):564-570.
27. Paschalidis M, Theiss W, Kolling K, Busch R, Schömig A. Randomised comparison of manual compression repair versus ultrasound guided compression repair of postcatheterisation femoral pseudoaneurysms. *Heart.* 2006;92(2):251-252.
28. Schneider C, Malisius R, Kuchler R, et al. A prospective study on ultrasound-guided percutaneous thrombin injection for treatment of iatrogenic post-catheterisation femoral pseudoaneurysms. *Int J Cardiol.* 2009;131(3):356-361.
29. Oderich GS, Bower TC, Hofer J, et al. In situ rifampin-soaked grafts with omental coverage and antibiotic suppression are durable with low reinfection rates in patients with aortic graft enteric erosion or fistula. *J Vasc Surg.* 2011;53(1):99-106, 107.e1-7; discussion 106-107.
30. Lejay A, Delay C, Girsowicz E, et al. Cryopreserved cadaveric arterial allograft for arterial reconstruction in patients with prosthetic infection. *Eur J Vasc Endovasc Surg.* 2017;54(5):636-644.
31. Acosta S, Monsen C. Outcome after VAC® therapy for infected bypass grafts in the lower limb. *Eur J Vasc Endovasc Surg.* 2012;44(3):294-299.
32. Armstrong PA, Back MR, Bandyk DF, et al. Selective application of sartorius muscle flaps and aggressive staged surgical debridement can influence long-term outcomes of complex prosthetic graft infections. *J Vasc Surg.* 2007;46(1): 71-78.

Michael C. Madigan • Mohammad H. Eslami

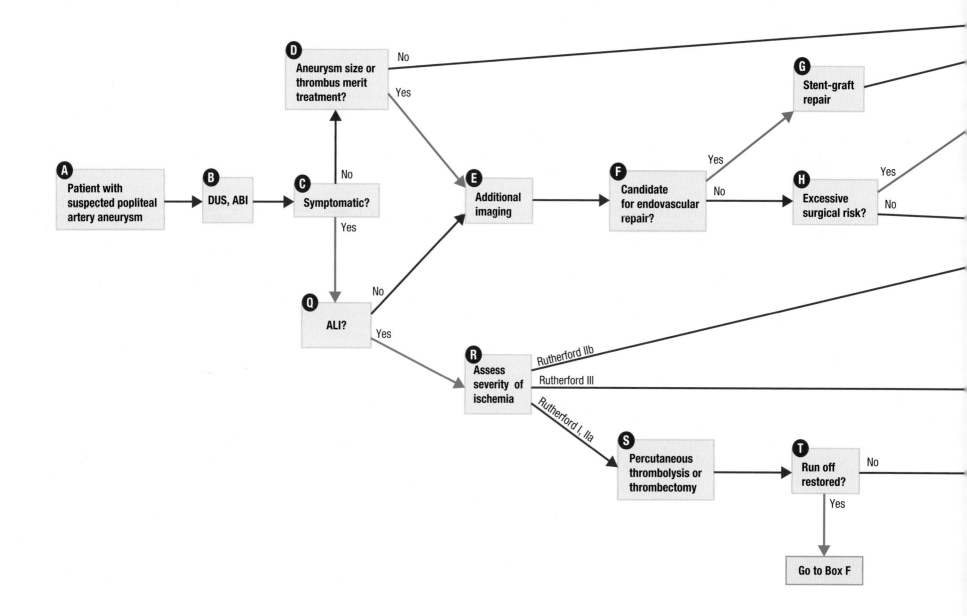

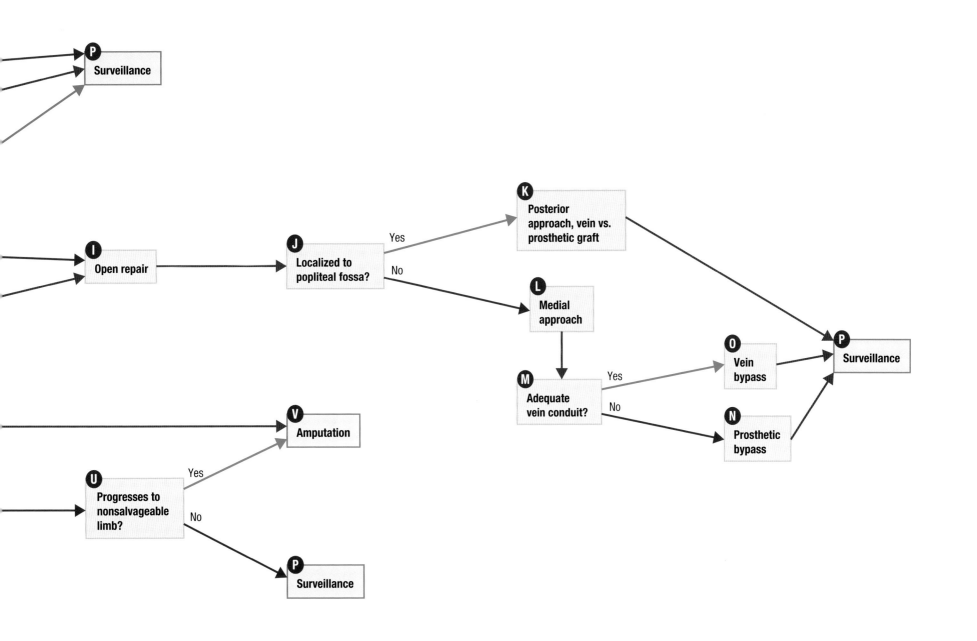

A Patient with suspected popliteal artery aneurysm

Popliteal artery aneurysms (PAAs) are the most common peripheral artery aneurysms.[1] They are found in 15% of patients with AAA and are bilateral 50% of the time.[2,3] PAAs nearly always occur in men >50 years of age.[1] They are usually identified on physical examination as an asymptomatic pulsatile mass behind the knee or incidentally on DUS, CTA, or MRA during a workup for lower extremity symptoms. The standard evaluation includes an H&P with a focused lower extremity pulse examination. Initial testing includes popliteal arterial DUS and ABIs to confirm the diagnosis and to define distal perfusion. Patients should also undergo DUS screening for AAA because these are found in >50% of people with PAAs.[2]

B DUS, ABI

DUS and ABIs are the initial, low-cost, noninvasive evaluation of PAAs. DUS can accurately measure the diameter and extent of the PAA above and below the knee. It can also identify presence of thrombus within the aneurysm, or evidence of occlusive disease in the proximal or distal arterial tree. The combination of the ABI and DUS is a sensitive first step to identify arterial insufficiency or distal embolization. In addition to DUS of the affected lower extremity, patients with a PAA should have a DUS of the contralateral extremity and abdominal aorta to rule out aneurysms in these locations.

C Symptomatic?

PAAs rarely rupture and therefore symptoms are most often related to thrombosis or embolization that result in acute or chronic lower extremity ischemia, with chronic ischemia resulting from repetitive embolization. Large PAAs may also cause local compression of the adjacent vein or nerve.[4] Thrombosis or embolization can cause claudication, ischemic rest pain, or tissue loss and ischemia can range from mild to severe. Local compression can cause leg swelling, DVT or neuropathy.[5] Although PAA rupture is rare even with large aneurysms, it is associated with a high rate of limb loss. All symptomatic aneurysms should be considered for intervention.

D Aneurysm size or thrombus merit treatment?

PAA ≥2 cm in diameter or those with significant thrombus burden have generally been recommended for repair given the concern for embolization or thrombosis.[6] However, natural history studies are not available to precisely define either optimal diameter or thrombus threshold for repair. In fact, some aneurysms <2 cm in diameter develop thrombosis. In general, treatment is recommended for PAAs ≥ 2 cm in patients who are relatively young and at good surgical risk, whereas for patients with advanced age or increased procedural risk, the intervention size threshold may be increased to >3 cm or more. In patients with concomitant asymptomatic large AAA and asymptomatic PAA, the "life-threatening" abdominal aneurysm, if of diameter that warrants repair, should be treated first.

E Additional imaging

CTA or MRA is usually the next step in the evaluation of patients who are considered for intervention. These studies better define the extent of the PAA and arterial runoff and allow for planning of optimal treatment. DSA may be used in combination with CTA or MRA to more clearly define runoff vessel patency and plan the course of open or endovascular therapy, but is usually not needed unless used as a part of endovascular treatment.

F Candidate for endovascular repair?

In patients with adequate runoff to the foot, endovascular stent-graft placement may be considered for both symptomatic and asymptomatic PAA, even though some studies suggest improved patency with open repair among asymptomatic patients.[7-9] Results of a meta-analysis suggest improved primary patency 79% (95% CI: 75%-84%) for open repair versus 68% (95% CI: 64%-73%) for an endovascular repair.[10] Either therapy, however, has similar secondary patency rates (87% [95% CI: 83%-90%] open versus 80% [95% CI: 74%-85%] endovascular) in patients followed up to 3 years post intervention.[10] Careful radiographic selection of these patients, including adequate landing zones and tibial runoff, leads to improved outcomes, because not every patient is a candidate for endovascular repair. CTA and MRA are often used to assess for potential endograft repair. DSA may be then used in conjunction with endovascular intervention to confirm adequate tibial vessel runoff. The SFA and popliteal arteries are measured above and below the aneurysm to plan for endograft size selection, where at least 1.5 cm length of normal artery is needed for the proximal and distal landing zones. The stent-graft diameter is selected depending on the diameter of the normal artery of the landing zones and often oversized by 10% to reduce the potential for type I endoleak. Data suggest that the best outcomes are achieved with ≥2 vessel runoff to the foot, although stent-graft placement in high operative risk patients with one vessel runoff may be considered.[11] In addition, one study suggested that young age and multiple stent grafts could lead to stent fracture and possible failure,[12] but a long-term follow-up study showed that the stent fracture by itself did not lead to graft failure and was not independently associated with failure.[13] Appreciating the limitations of these studies, it is perhaps prudent to avoid use of multiple stent grafts that can lead to fracture and possible failure. Currently available stent grafts (with lengths of up to 25 cm) may alleviate this concern. Significant size discrepancy of >3 mm between the proximal and distal landing zones may preclude endovascular repair. In the future, tapered stent grafts may overcome this shortcoming.

G Stent-graft repair

The placement of a self-expanding stent graft requires ≥1.5 cm normal artery landing zone above and below the aneurysm, absence of excessive tortuosity, and minimal size discrepancy between the proximal and distal landing zones. Endovascular repair begins with DSA of the affected extremity. CDT may precede endograft deployment if the PAA or runoff is acutely thrombosed. After the runoff is confirmed to be adequate and the aneurysm crossed with a wire, the patient is heparinized and the stent graft is deployed. If more than one stent graft needs to be deployed, then a minimum of 3 cm of graft overlap is recommended. If two stent grafts are required for coverage, the smaller diameter stent is always placed first to avoid endoleak. Post deployment PTA of the stent graft is needed, especially in atherosclerotic vessels. Completion DSA is performed to assess for the presence of appropriate seal and confirm distal runoff. Revascularization for severe ALI should prompt consideration of prophylactic fasciotomies to prevent potential compartment syndrome (see Chapter 51).

H Excessive surgical risk?

If the patient fails to meet criteria for endovascular intervention, then the surgical risk is assessed. Such assessment begins with an H&P to identify possible risk factors for surgery including evaluation for any cardiac, pulmonary, or renal contraindications. An ECG, chest x-ray, and baseline laboratory studies are typically obtained. On the basis of the patient's comorbidities, an ECHO or stress test may be completed for risk stratification. PFTs may be ordered in case of severe pulmonary disease, but these are rarely required. If the patient is deemed to be of prohibitive high risk by the preoperative workup, especially if the patient has minimal or no symptoms, then surveillance may be most appropriate.

I Open repair

In younger patients, those with only one runoff vessel, or patients who do not meet the anatomic criteria for endovascular repair, open repair using bypass should be considered. Also, in the patient with ALI and motor/sensory function loss, open popliteal or tibial thrombectomy through a below-the-knee popliteal exposure may be required to obtain immediate runoff to the foot. Open thrombectomy may also be needed if initiated CDT is unsuccessful or if the ischemic symptoms worsen during thrombolysis. In that clinical situation, bypass is performed following successful thrombectomy. Revascularization for ALI should prompt consideration of prophylactic fasciotomies to prevent potential compartment syndrome (see Chapter 51).

J Localized to popliteal fossa?

In planning open repair, the proximal and distal extent of PAA is an important consideration. The posterior approach is ideal for aneurysms that are confined to the popliteal fossa, whereas a medial approach is required for aneurysms that extend above or below the popliteal fossa.

K Posterior approach, vein vs. prosthetic graft

With the posterior approach, the aneurysm is controlled by proximal and distal clamping, and opened to expose branches that require ligation. Small aneurysms may be resected, whereas in large aneurysms, the back wall may be left in place. Either vein or prosthetic conduit may be used for bypass.

When the posterior approach is chosen, the choice of conduit is often a prosthetic graft to better match the size of the normal vessels and obviate the need to harvest GSV, which is challenging to do when the patient is positioned prone. The short saphenous vein, if of appropriate diameter and quality, can be harvested and utilized in that setting. A large prospective registry showed no difference in patency between vein (85%) and prosthetic (81%) graft using the posterior approach at 1-year follow-up ($P = 0.719$).[14] Better than 90% primary, primary-assisted, and secondary patency were demonstrated in one retrospective review of 30 patients treated using the posterior approach with either Dacron or ePTFE interposition grafts.[15] Arterial repair is performed by creating end-to-end anastomoses of the conduit and normal arteries proximal and distal to the aneurysm. One advantage of the posterior approach is that the aneurysm can be completely decompressed and, as such, obliterated. This approach is difficult if the PAA extends to the mid-thigh SFA or if bypass to the tibial arteries is required.

L Medial approach

If the medial approach is used, incisions are made in the distal thigh and proximal calf. The aneurysm is ligated proximally and distally for exclusion and a bypass from normal SFA or above-the-knee popliteal artery to a distal normal popliteal or tibial artery is created with vein or prosthetic graft. This approach is advantageous if the proximal anastomosis needs to be placed at or proximal to the mid-SFA or the target of the bypass is a tibial artery. One disadvantage of the medial approach is that it is difficult to decompress or fully obliterate the aneurysm and, as such, excluded aneurysms can continue to grow in size.

M Adequate vein conduit?

Adequacy of autogenous vein is usually evaluated using DUS. GSV should be the first choice of conduit, especially when a medial approach or tibial target is chosen. GSV grafts have been shown to have improved patency over prosthetic grafts.[16] In a large prospective registry, vein bypass grafts (90%) had superior patency at 1 year when compared to prosthetic grafts (72%) using the medial approach ($P < 0.001$).[14]

For best long-term results, the vein conduit used should be over 3 mm in diameter throughout and be without thickened walls or significant fibrosis.[17] In patients without adequate GSV, arm vein, prosthetic, or composite vein bypass may be considered.

N Prosthetic bypass

In some instances, when adequate vein is not available or is not preferred because of patient comorbidities or anticipated longer operative time, ePTFE or Dacron may be used. Some recommend reinforced ringed grafts to prevent kinking, but this benefit has not been proven.

O Vein bypass

Any autogenous vein that is of adequate size ($\geq$3 mm) and free of intraluminal defects can be used as conduit. However, single-segment GSV has been associated with best long-term outcomes and is preferred, if available.

P Surveillance

ABI and DUS are low-cost and widely accessible methods of ongoing surveillance for both small PAAs and after stent-graft or bypass intervention.[18] Because PAAs typically grow 1 mm or less per year,[19] nontreated aneurysms should be followed up every 6 to 18 months with physical examination, ABI, and DUS to observe for any signs or symptoms of embolization, increasing size, or thrombus burden. The follow-up interval may vary depending on the stability of the aneurysm and how close the aneurysm is to the threshold for repair.

After stent-graft or bypass intervention, a 1-month evaluation is usually performed, followed by 6- to 12-month evaluations. The ABI and DUS may be performed more frequently and up to every 3 months in patients at high risk for failure. A drop in ABI $\geq$ 0.15 and a stent-graft/bypass velocity elevation suggesting stenosis are indications for DSA and potential reintervention. Currently, there are no exact criteria to identify in-stent stenosis for popliteal stent grafts; however, PSV of >275 cm/s and prestenosis/stenosis velocity ratio of >3.5 have been correlated with $\geq$80% stenosis in SFA stents.[20]

Q ALI?

ALI caused by PAA thrombosis or distal embolization is more common than aneurysm rupture. Patients may present with worsening claudication, sensory deficits, motor loss, or a nonviable limb. The initial evaluation includes an H&P with a focus on the pulse examination, in combination with ABI and DUS assessment. Systemic heparinization with a bolus followed by a titrated IV heparin drip is initiated while awaiting further imaging or definitive intervention, depending on the degree of ischemia.

R Assess severity of ischemia

The severity of ischemia is assessed by clinical evaluation. The Rutherford ALI classification system is commonly used to help guide the timing and type of intervention.[21] Rutherford I and IIa ischemia is characterized by minimal to no sensory loss with normal motor function. A distal arterial Doppler signal is typically present. These patients have a marginally threatened limb and should undergo DSA to assess the adequacy of the tibial vessel runoff. If runoff is adequate, then the patient is a candidate for bypass of a thrombosed PAA without need for thrombolysis. However, if the outflow and PAA are thrombosed, CDT (or distal thrombectomy at the time of bypass) can be initiated to also allow better outflow for future endovascular or surgical repair.

Rutherford IIb ischemia is characterized by sensory loss with mild to moderate motor weakness. A Doppler signal may or may not be audible in the foot. These limbs are immediately threatened and require immediate revascularization for limb salvage. The patient should urgently proceed with operative repair with thrombectomy and bypass. Intraoperative DSA is used to assist with target assessment for bypass. Rutherford III ischemia is characterized by profound anesthesia, paralysis, and/or rigor. Such patients have nonsalvageable limbs and should undergo amputation rather than revascularization to avoid reperfusion injury, potential renal failure and a nonviable limb.

S Percutaneous thrombolysis or thrombectomy

CDT and/or percutaneous thrombectomy are used in attempt to establish runoff into the foot for either endovascular or open repair of PAA if thrombosis or significant distal embolization has occurred.[22] The patient must not have any contraindication to receiving thrombolytic therapy, an immediately threatened limb or nonsalvageable limb (see Chapter 53). The procedure begins with diagnostic DSA to evaluate the degree of thrombosis and potential distal revascularization targets. Usually, via contralateral femoral access, a sheath is placed in the proximal SFA. A wire is used to cross the thrombosed popliteal artery. With acute thrombosis, the wire should easily traverse the clot. Often, a distal perfusion wire or catheter can be placed into the tibial vessel to be lysed. A multiside hole catheter is then placed across the length of the thrombosed popliteal artery. A bolus of tissue plasminogen activator (tPA) (usually 2-4 mg) may be given through the infusion catheter. Thrombolysis is then continued in the ICU over the next 12 to 48 hours, with the patient brought back to the procedure suite every 12 to 24 hours depending on clinical improvement or deterioration. One milligram of tPA per hour is infused through the infusion catheter. Each institution should have a protocol in place to monitor for neurovascular changes, bleeding, and substantial drop in fibrinogen levels. Percutaneous mechanical thrombectomy using suction thrombectomy catheters and pulse-spray catheters may be used in conjunction with thrombolytics to help improve runoff.

T Runoff restored?

The distal bypass target may include the below-the-knee popliteal artery or any of the tibial arteries. The patient should have inline outflow from at least one vessel before proceeding with endovascular stent-graft repair or a surgical bypass. Thrombolysis may be continued or percutaneous thrombectomy attempted if, on the lysis check, the thrombus burden is improving but adequate flow to the foot is not established. The risk of bleeding complications for thrombolytic therapy increases above a cumulative dose of >30 mg of tPA. If the patient's leg ischemia worsens or significant bleeding is encountered, then lysis is aborted and either open thrombectomy is attempted or the patient is assessed for amputation.

Ⓤ Progresses to nonsalvageable limb?

On occasion, no distal target artery is identified despite CDT or open thrombectomy. The next step in management depends on the degree of ischemia. Patients with claudication or mild rest pain may be observed, whereas in those with persistent and severe rest pain, or tissue necrosis, amputation should be considered.

Ⓥ Amputation

If the patient presents with a nonsalvageable limb or attempts at revascularization fail, then the patient is considered for AKA or BKA depending on the extent of distal ischemia.[14] Preference is given for BKA in ambulatory patients as the potential to remain ambulatory after amputation is higher (see Chapter 48).

REFERENCES

1. Lawrence PF, Lorenzo-Rivero S, Lyon JL. The incidence of iliac, femoral, and popliteal artery aneurysms in hospitalized patients. *J Vasc Surg*. 1995;22(4):415-416.
2. Diwan A, Sarkar R, Stanley JC, Zelenock GB, Wakefield TW. Incidence of femoral and popliteal artery aneurysms in patients with abdominal aortic aneurysms. *J Vasc Surg*. 2000;31(5):863-869.
3. Huang Y, Gloviczki P, Noel AA, et al. Early complications and long-term outcome after open surgical treatment of popliteal artery aneurysms: is exclusion with saphenous vein bypass still the gold standard? *J Vasc Surg*. 2007;45(4):706-713.
4. Sie RB, Dawson I, van Baalen JM, Schultze Kool LJ, van Bockel JH. Ruptured popliteal aneurysms. An insidious complication. *Eur J Vasc Endovasc Surg*. 1997;13:432-438.
5. Dorigo W, Pulli R, Alessi Innocenti A, et al. A 33-year experience with surgical management of popliteal artery aneurysms. *J Vasc Surg*. 2015;62(5):1176-1182.
6. Lowell RC, Gloviczki P, Hallett WJ Jr, et al. Popliteal artery aneurysms: the risk of nonoperative management. *Ann Vasc Surg*. 1994;8(1):14-23.
7. Cervin A, Tjarnstrom J, Ravn H, et al. Treatment of popliteal aneurysm by open and endovascular surgery: a contemporary study of 592 procedures in Sweden. *Eur J Vasc Endovasc Surg*. 2015;50(3):342-350.
8. Eslami MH, Rybin D, Doros G, Farber A. Open repair of asymptomatic popliteal artery aneurysm is associated with better outcomes than endovascular repair. *J Vasc Surg*. 2015;61(3):663-669.
9. Leake AE, Avgerinos ED, Chaer RA, Singh MJ, Makaroun MS, Marone LK. Contemporary outcomes of open and endovascular popliteal artery aneurysm repair. *J Vasc Surg*. 2016;63(1):70-76.
10. Leake AE, Segal MA, Chaer RA, et al. Meta-analysis of open and endovascular repair of popliteal artery aneurysms. *J Vasc Surg*. 2017;65(1):246-256.
11. Garg K, Rockman CB, Kim BJ, et al. Outcome of endovascular repair of popliteal aneurysm using Viabahn endoprosthesis. *J Vasc Surg*. 2012;55(6):1647-1653.
12. Tielliu IF, Zeebregts CJ, Vourliotakis G, et al. Stent fractures in the Hemobhan/Viabahn stent graft after endovascular popliteal artery aneurysm repair. *J Vasc Surg*. 2010;51(6):1413-1418.
13. Golchehr B, Zeebregts CJ, Reijnen MMPJ, Tielliu IFJ. Long-term outcome of endovascular popliteal artery aneurysm repair. *J Vasc Surg*. 2018;67(6):1797-1804.
14. Ravn H, Wanhainen A, Bjorck M. Surgical technique and long-term results after popliteal artery aneurysm repair: results from 717 legs. *J Vasc Surg*. 2007;46(2):236-243.
15. Beseth BD, Moore WS. The posterior approach for repair of popliteal aneurysms. *J Vasc Surg*. 2006;43(5):940-945.
16. Serrano Hernando FJ, Martinez Lopez I, Hernandez Mateo MM, et al. Comparison of popliteal artery aneurysm therapies. *J Vasc Surg*. 2015;61(3):655-661.
17. Wengerter KR, Veith FJ, Gupta SK, Ascer E, Rivers SP. Influence of vein size (diameter) on infrapopliteal reversed vein graft patency. *J Vasc Surg*. 1990;11(4):525-531.
18. Stone PA, Armstrong PA, Bandyk DF, et al. The value of duplex surveillance after open and endovascular popliteal aneurysm repair. *J Vasc Surg*. 2005;41(6):936-941.
19. Magee R, Quigley F, McCann M, Buttner P, Golledge J. Growth and risk factors for expansion of dilated popliteal arteries. *Eur J Vasc Endovasc Surg*. 2010;39(5):606-611.
20. Baril DT, Rhee RY, Kim J, Makaroun MS, Chaer RA, Marone LK. Duplex criteria for determination of in-stent stenosis after angioplasty and stenting of the superficial femoral artery. *J Vasc Surg*. 2009;49(1):133-138.
21. Rutherford RB, Baker JD, Ernst C, et al. Recommended standards for reports dealing with lower extremity ischemia: revised version. *J Vasc Surg*. 1997;26(3):517-538.
22. Ravn H, Bjorck M. Popliteal artery aneurysm with acute ischemia in 229 patients. Outcome after thrombolytic and surgical therapy. *Eur J Vasc Endovasc Surg*. 2007;33(6):690-695.

Martyn Knowles • Carlos Timaran

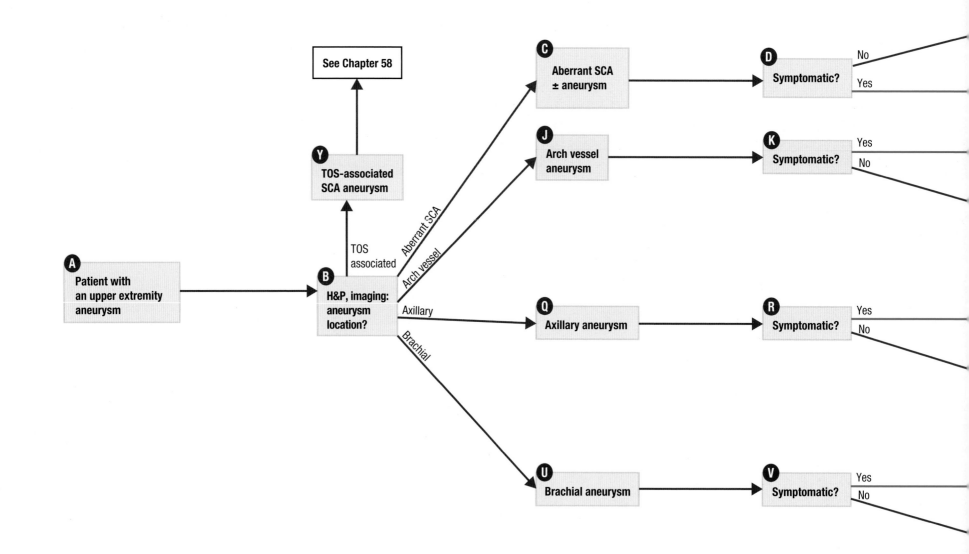

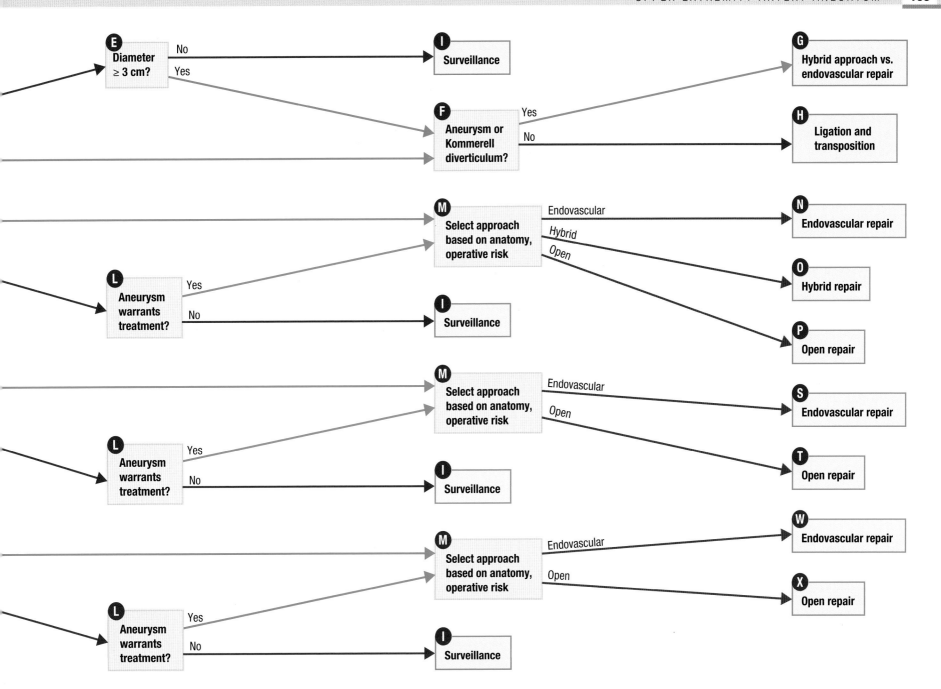

A Patient with an upper extremity aneurysm

Upper extremity (UE) aneurysms are relatively uncommon but can be life-threatening.[1] They can involve the brachial, axillary, subclavian, aberrant subclavian, and innominate arteries. These aneurysms can be asymptomatic or present with a variety of symptoms, including rupture, stroke, local nerve or esophageal compression, and thromboembolic symptoms. Most aneurysms involving the UE are degenerative in nature, but trauma, vasculitis, and other congenital conditions may be causative factors.

B H&P, imaging: aneurysm location?

Because of their location, UE aneurysms can cause compressive symptoms such as dysphagia, hoarseness, pain, and thromboembolic complications such as embolic stroke, and may rupture.[2] In current medical practice, given the frequency of axial imaging, the vast majority of UE aneurysms are found incidentally and therefore are asymptomatic. The patient with an UE aneurysm must first have a full H&P, with possible imaging evaluation of other possible sites of peripheral aneurysms because 30% to 50% of patients with nonspecific, degenerative arch vessel aneurysms have aortoiliac or other peripheral aneurysms. DUS, MRA, or CTA establishes the diagnosis; however, conventional arch and UE DSA may be required. Similarly, the competency of the contralateral vertebral circulation if the ipsilateral vertebral artery originates from an aneurysmal vessel and the anatomic suitability for endovascular repair can only be defined with CTA or MRA. Subsequent management depends on the location and etiology of the aneurysm: SCA associated with TOS, aberrant SCA, arch vessel, axillary, or brachial.

C Aberrant SCA ± aneurysm

An aberrant SCA is the most common congenital anomaly of the aortic arch, occurring in 0.5% to 1% of the population.[3] Its diagnosis is typically made from axial imaging such as CTA. An aberrant right SCA occurs when the right SCA arises from the descending thoracic aorta, usually distal to the left SCA. The artery then courses posterior to the arch typically between the esophagus and the spine, and rarely between the trachea and esophagus. This arterial anomaly can cause dysphagia secondary to impingement of the esophagus, usually secondary to aneurysmal degeneration known as a Kommerell diverticulum, or because of other less clear reasons related to aging, including arterial elongation, high aortic arch location, and HTN. An associated single common carotid trunk and esophageal dyskinesia may also result in the late onset of dysphagia. Of note, the right recurrent laryngeal nerve characteristically loops around the right SCA when in the normal location, and thus in this aberrant anatomy can be nonrecurrent and be prone to iatrogenic injury. Furthermore, a right-sided aortic arch can be associated with an aberrant left SCA. Most patients with this anomaly are asymptomatic unless they develop an aneurysm.

D Symptomatic?

Symptoms of aberrant SCA ± aneurysm include dysphagia known as "dysphagia lusoria," tracheal compression, dyspnea, coughing, chest pain, or UE ischemia from thromboembolism or, rarely, stenosis of the aberrant SCA.[2] Patients rarely may present emergently because of aneurysmal rupture. Symptoms, independent of the presence or size of an aneurysm, are usually an indication for treatment, unless very mild.

E Diameter ≥ 3 cm?

Patients without symptoms in whom an aberrant SCA is detected by imaging should be evaluated for potential prophylactic treatment depending on the presence and size of an aneurysm. Although there is a paucity of data, a size threshold of 3 cm has been suggested as a guideline for repair of an aneurysm of a standard or aberrant SCA in the absence of symptoms.[4]

F Aneurysm or Kommerell diverticulum?

Among patients with symptomatic aberrant SCA, the presence of an aneurysm or a Kommerell diverticulum dictates the type of repair that is required because its presence mandates resection or exclusion of the aneurysmal segment to avoid rupture. Conversely, a nonaneurysmal artery can just be divided to the left of the esophagus.

G Hybrid approach vs. endovascular repair

Patients with a Kommerell diverticulum should undergo treatment via a hybrid approach or endovascular repair. Owing to the high morbidity from an open repair secondary to neurologic complications, the hybrid combination of a thoracic aortic endograft to exclude the Kommerell diverticulum, combined with carotid-subclavian bypass/transposition is currently the treatment of choice. Endovascular stent coverage of the aberrant vessel origin alone is insufficient for most lesions, so distal ligation of the aberrant vessel and transposition to the carotid artery is the preferred technique.[5] With this approach, the SCA is dissected centrally to allow ligation as far proximally as possible. In patients with short, large necks in which this exposure is difficult, the aberrant SCA can be occluded near its origin with a vascular plug placed transfemorally or retrograde via the SCA.[6] Often, the left SCA and aberrant right SCA origins are closely situated, and may require coverage of both vessels by a thoracic aortic endograft being used to treat Kommerell diverticulum. Coverage of both vessels without revascularization of at least one is not recommended given the risk of spinal ischemia or stroke.[7] CTA is particularly helpful to identify the collateral circulation through the vertebral arteries to help with decision making and decrease morbidity. To reduce these complications, unilateral or bilateral subclavian transpositions or carotid-subclavian artery bypasses should be performed. The hybrid repair of the aberrant SCA with

an aneurysm appears to significantly decrease associated morbidity and mortality.[5]

H Ligation and transposition

Although simple ligation is possible, segmental replacement of the aorta is often required.[8] Most patients with dysphagia lusoria can be effectively treated via a right cervical approach that includes central ligation of the transected aberrant SCA combined with subclavian-carotid transposition. Finger dissection is used to expose the aberrant artery centrally, to allow ligation to the left of the esophagus if possible. Usually this relieves the symptoms of dysphagia, although there may be fibrotic bands that require attention. In patients with short/large necks where exposure is difficult, the aberrant SCA can be occluded near its origin with a vascular plug placed transfemorally or retrograde via the SCA.[6]

I Surveillance

Patients with asymptomatic UE aneurysms that do not meet criteria for treatment should be monitored for expansion or new symptoms that might warrant treatment. The natural history of these aneurysms is not well established, so the general approach is initial annual imaging, with potentially longer intervals if the aneurysm is stable. Imaging will be the least invasive type that provides sufficient information (usually DUS for peripheral and CTA for central aneurysms).

J Arch vessel aneurysm

Most UE arterial aneurysms arise from the arch vessels and are largely due to arterial degenerative disease. However, such aneurysms can also be caused by trauma, FMD, syphilis, cystic medial necrosis, vasculitis, tuberculosis, and idiopathic congenital causes.[9] In the distal SCA, external influence from thoracic outlet obstruction, cervical ribs, and other bony abnormalities can cause aneurysmal degeneration from repetitive trauma (see Z). Overall, only 1% of all peripheral aneurysms arise from the SCA and innominate arteries. Because up to 50% of patients with arch vessel aneurysms have aortoiliac or other peripheral artery aneurysms, evaluation of other possible sites is necessary.[10,11] True SCA aneurysms are degenerative in nature, although PSAs can be caused by trauma or iatrogenic injury from subclavian catheters. True innominate aneurysms account for 2% to 5% of arch vessel aneurysms, and iatrogenic injuries are less common than with subclavian aneurysms.[12] A true aneurysm of the CCA is very rare. Carotid PSAs are more frequent following carotid surgery, trauma, dissections, or infection. True common carotid aneurysms are mostly degenerative, with less frequent causes including FMD, Marfan syndrome, Behçet disease, Takayasu arteritis, and Cogan syndrome.[2]

K Symptomatic?

Most arch vessel aneurysms are asymptomatic and discovered on incidental imaging or occasionally by a pulsatile mass on physical examination. Symptoms can include pain in the chest, neck, and shoulder area from local compression or distally from thrombosis or embolization. Neurologic symptoms are possible from the proximity to the brachial plexus. Hoarseness, cough, respiratory insufficiency, TIAs, ischemic stroke, dysphagia, and hemoptysis are also possible depending on the location of the aneurysm.[2] Patients can have a supraclavicular mass or bruit, Horner syndrome, diminished pulses, ischemic fingers, or sensory/motor changes to the UE. DUS, MRA, or CTA establishes the diagnosis.

L Aneurysm warrants treatment?

Asymptomatic patients should be evaluated to determine whether the current diameter or rapid expansion of the UE aneurysm warrants treatment, when compared to the risk of intervention and the life expectancy of the patient. Unfortunately, the natural history of these aneurysms is poorly defined, so that criteria based on lower extremity aneurysms are usually applied. In general, we use 3 cm as a threshold for repair of central, and 2 to 2.5 cm for peripheral aneurysms, and modify this based on the health and life expectancy of the patient. Rapid expansion of aneurysms (>20% diameter per year) is generally considered an indication for repair.

M Select approach based on anatomy, operative risk

The options for repair depend on the anatomy and operative risk of the patient, and the proximity to branch vessels that may need to be covered with endovascular repair but could be preserved with open repair. In particular, vertebral circulation must be carefully evaluated preoperatively if treatment of adjacent aneurysms may compromise their circulation. The selection between endovascular, hybrid or open surgical repair must take into account many factors, including the urgency of the repair, anatomy, and patient risk. Endovascular repair has increasingly become a popular mechanism for repair of arch vessel pathology in those that are not good candidates for open repair. Hybrid repair of arch vessels using proximal endovascular occlusion and distal surgical reconstruction is often used to avoid the necessity for more complex direct arch reconstruction (See O). Careful evaluation of the anatomy is imperative for careful patient selection. The proximal SCA is most amenable to endovascular treatment. Often, appropriate landing zones are not available, and care must be taken to avoid vertebral artery coverage or embolization. Further care must be taken in patients with prior coronary bypass grafting. Extrinsic compression is an issue in the distal SCA from the first rib. Stroke is possible from embolization into the vertebral artery or coverage of the vessel, especially if the contralateral side is diminutive or diseased.

N Endovascular repair

Endovascular repair of arch vessel aneurysms is usually performed through a transbrachial or transfemoral approach; a transaxillary approach is occasionally necessary. Balloon-mounted and self-expandable stent-grafts are used. The more flexible stent grafts are preferred for arterial tortuosity and the discrepancy in proximal and distal landing zone diameters may require a combination of devices of different sizes. Frequently, balloon-mounted stent grafts are used for accurate proximal deployment at the origin of the vessel and extended with more flexible distal self-expanding stent grafts. Because of the relative rarity of arch vessel aneurysms, case series and case reports present the primary source of evidence for this repair. Overall, patency for subclavian stentgrafts is generally over 80% over 2 years. There are reports of stent fractures and stenosis associated with endovascular repair.[13]

O Hybrid repair

Hybrid repair typically involves embolization with coils or a vascular plug of a proximal SCA aneurysm combined with SCA transposition or carotid-subclavian bypass and proximal ligation. These procedures are typically staged. More frequently, placement of an aortic stent graft and coiling of the aneurysm before the vertebral takeoff is possible with selective revascularization of the SCA. The use of thoracic aortic endografts for hybrid repair of proximal aneurysms of the arch vessels entails exclusion of the origin of these vessels combined with extra-anatomic arch vessel revascularization (ie, carotid-carotid, subclavian transposition, and carotid-subclavian bypass).

P Open repair

Open repair is the standard technique for most arch vessel aneurysms. The general approach is resection or aneurysmorrhaphy and reestablishment of flow in an end-to-end manner. For the innominate and left CCA, a median sternotomy is used for exposure. After arterial control, the aneurysm is resected and a graft is either originated at the proximal innominate/CCA (if nonaneurysmal) or, more often, the ascending aorta proximal to the innominate/CCA origin. If the innominate aneurysm extends into the CCA and SCA, a bifurcated graft can be used, but care must be taken in graft placement to avoid compression after sternotomy closure. For proximal right SCA aneurysms, a median sternotomy is preferred, usually with extension into the supraclavicular fossa for more distal exposure. More distal subclavian aneurysms are approached via supra- or infraclavicular incisions. Partial medial clavicular resection is rarely necessary. In cases of proximal left SCA aneurysms, a left thoracotomy combined with supraclavicular exposure is used. Resection and interposition graft is then employed, most often with prosthetic conduit. Open repair has excellent durability, but has a high morbidity and mortality.[11,14]

Q Axillary aneurysm

Axillary artery aneurysms are rare and most are PSAs secondary to trauma, although congenital and degenerative aneurysms have been described.[15,16] Most traumatic injuries occur in young men from strenuous athletic activities. Repeated specific movements can cause external compression of the artery resulting in injury and subsequent aneurysm formation.

R Symptomatic?

The most common symptoms of an axillary artery aneurysm are shoulder pain or distal ischemia from embolization or thrombosis. Such symptoms usually warrant treatment unless mild, or in high-risk patients.

S Endovascular repair

Endovascular repair is a good option for traumatic axillary PSAs especially in the setting of instability. Most often, a single-covered stent-graft will suffice, but requires close follow-up and may be best considered a bridging therapy in young patients, given the unknown long-term results.[17,18] In a late elective setting, a more definitive repair can occur with surgical bypass of the stented area. On occasion, coil embolization of small side branches is also required.

T Open repair

Open repair often involves resection of the aneurysm and interposition grafting. GSV is the preferred conduit and has excellent results.[19] Prosthetic conduit is a reasonable alternative, but patency rates are not as high as with vein conduit. Great care must be taken during the exposure to avoid injury to the brachial plexus. Proximal control may be obtained by exposing the proximal axillary artery for more distal aneurysms, whereas exposure of the SCA using supraclavicular approach or transfemoral balloon occlusion may be required for more proximal aneurysms. A hybrid approach using transfemoral access and distal SCA balloon occlusion may be useful in large axillary aneurysms to avoid the need for an infraclavicular incision for subclavian control.

U Brachial aneurysm

The majority of brachial artery aneurysms are PSAs secondary to hemodialysis access or iatrogenic injury from brachial artery access.[20] IV drug use can cause infected brachial PSAs. Other uncommon causes of brachial artery aneurysms include dissection and congenital connective tissue abnormalities, such as type IV Ehlers-Danlos syndrome, Kawasaki syndrome, Buerger disease, Kaposi sarcoma, and cystic adventitial disease.[2]

V Symptomatic?

Owing to the close proximity of the median nerve, neurologic symptoms are commonly associated with brachial artery aneurysms. The median nerve distribution includes the thumb, index, and middle and half of the ring finger, and can cause sensory and motor deficits, which can be irreversible if not treated early. Other symptoms can include hand and digital ischemia from thrombosis or embolization.

W Endovascular repair

Endovascular repair is seldom used to treat a brachial artery aneurysm because of the ease of open repair under local or regional anesthesia, and common location in the antecubital fossa where stent grafts could kink with repeated arm flexion[21,22] Traumatic PSAs can be repaired with a stent graft in the setting of instability, even if as a bridging procedure.

X Open repair

Open surgical repair is the preferred method of treatment for brachial artery aneurysm or PSA. A patch repair, primary repair, suture repair, or an interposition vein graft is performed depending on the extent of injury. In the setting of a PSA from iatrogenic causes, thrombin injection usually cannot be performed because of the presence of a short neck. These cases are treated via an open suture or a patch repair.

Y TOS-associated SCA aneurysm

Although the majority of the subclavian artery aneurysms are due to degenerative causes, TOS may lead to SCA stenosis and post-stenotic aneurysm. These aneurysms are treated with interposition grafts after first rib resection as described in detail in Chapter 58.

REFERENCES

1. Dent TL, Lindenauer SM, Ernst CB, Fry WJ. Multiple arteriosclerotic arterial aneurysms. *Archiv Surg.* 1972;105(2):338-344.
2. Cronenwett JL, Johnston KW. *Rutherford's Vascular Surgery.* Philadelphia, PA: Saunders/Elsevier; 2014.
3. Austin EH, Wolfe WG. Aneurysm of aberrant subclavian artery with a review of the literature. *J Vasc Surg.* 1985;2(4):571-577.
4. Cina CS, Althani H, Pasenau J, Abouzahr L. Kommerell's diverticulum and right-sided aortic arch: a cohort study and review of the literature. *J Vasc Surg.* 2004;39(1):131-139.
5. Verzini F, Isernia G, Simonte G, De Rango P, Cao P; Italian AARSA Collaborative Group. Results of aberrant right subclavian artery aneurysm repair. *J Vasc Surg.* 2015;62(2):343-350.
6. Shennib H, Diethrich EB. Novel approaches for the treatment of the aberrant right subclavian artery and its aneurysms. *J Vasc Surg.* 2008;47(5):1066-1070.
7. Weinberger G, Randall PA, Parker FB, Kieffer SA. Involvement of an aberrant right subclavian artery in dissection of the thoracic aorta: diagnostic and therapeutic implications. *AJR Am J Roentgenol.* 1977;129(4):653-655.
8. Wooster M, Back M, Sutzko D, Gaeto H, Armstrong P, Shames M. A 10-year experience using a hybrid endovascular approach to treat aberrant subclavian arterial aneurysms. *Ann Vasc Surg.* 2018;46(1):60-64.
9. Cury M, Greenberg RK, Morales JP, Mohabbat W, Hernandez AV. Supra-aortic vessels aneurysms: diagnosis and prompt intervention. *J Vasc Surg.* 2009;49(1):4-10.
10. Pairolero PC, Walls JT, Payne WS, Hollier LH, Fairbairn JF. Subclavian-axillary artery aneurysms. *Surgery.* 1981;90(4):757-763.
11. McCollum CH, Da Gama AD, Noon GP, DeBakey ME. Aneurysm of the subclavian artery. *J Cardiovasc Surg (Torino).* 1979;20(2):159-164.
12. Bower TC, Pairolero PC, Hallett JW Jr, Toomey BJ, Gloviczki P, Cherry KJ Jr. Brachiocephalic aneurysm: the case for early recognition and repair. *Ann Vasc Surg.* 1991;5(2):125-132.
13. Hilfiker PR, Razavi MK, Kee ST, Sze DY, Semba CP, Dake MD. Stent-graft therapy for subclavian artery aneurysms and fistulas: single-center mid-term results. *J Vasc Interv Radiol.* 2000;11(5):578-584.
14. Naz I, Zia-ur-Rehman, Aziz M, Sophie Z. Subclavian artery aneurysms: management implications in a resource-limited setting. *Vascular.* 2012;20(6):301-305.
15. Ho PK, Weiland AJ, McClinton MA, Wilgis EF. Aneurysms of the upper extremity. *J Hand Surg Am.* 1987;12(1):39-46.
16. Perry SP, Massey CW. Bilateral aneurysms of the subclavian and axillary arteries; report of a case. *Radiology.* 1953;61(1):53-55.
17. Chopra A, Modrall JG, Knowles M, et al. Uncertain patency of covered stents placed for traumatic axillosubclavian artery injury. *J Am Coll Med.* 2016;223(1):174-183.
18. DuBose JJ, Rajani R, Gilani R, et al; Endovascular Skills for Trauma and Resuscitative Surgery Working Group. Endovascular management of axillo-subclavian arterial injury: a review of published experience. *Injury.* 2012;43(11):1785-1792.
19. McCarthy WJ, Flinn WR, Yao JS, Williams LR, Bergan JJ. Result of bypass grafting for upper limb ischemia. *J Vasc Surg.* 1986;3(5):741-746.
20. Fendri J, Palcau L, Cameliere L, Coffin O. True brachial artery aneurysm after arteriovenous fistula for hemodialysis: five cases and literature review. *Ann Vasc Surg.* 2017;39:228-235.
21. Klonaris C, Patelis N, Doulaptsis M, Katsargyris A. Hybrid treatment of large brachial artery pseudoaneurysms. *Ann Vasc Surg.* 2016;32:20-24.
22. Kurimoto Y, Tsuchida Y, Saito J, Yama N, Narimatsu E, Asai Y. Emergency endovascular stent-grafting for infected pseudoaneurysm of brachial artery. *Infection.* 2003;31(3):186-188.

Sung Ham • Fred A. Weaver

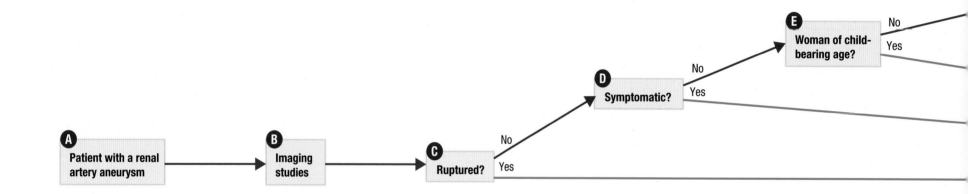

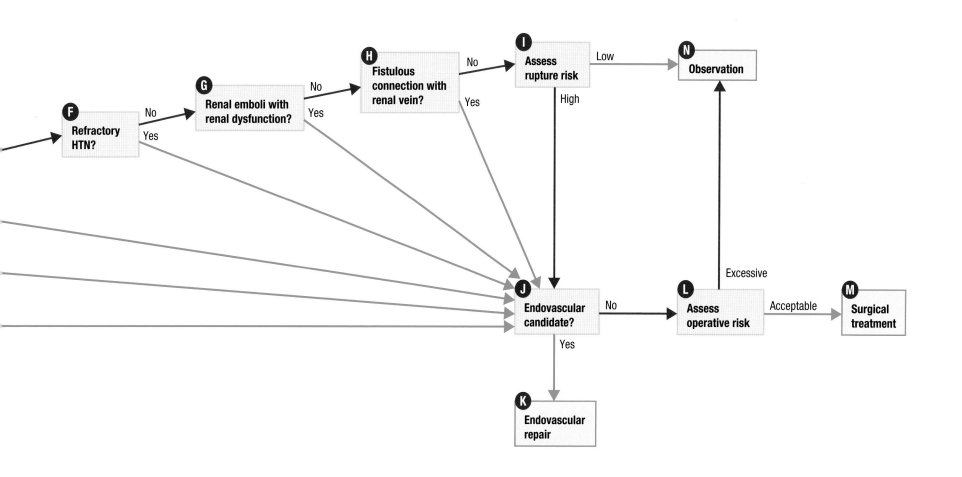

A   Patient with a renal artery aneurysm

Renal artery aneurysms (RAAs) often present asymptomatically and incidentally during a radiologic evaluation for other pathology. True degenerative RAAs are rare, with an estimated incidence of 0.01% to 0.09% based on autopsy studies.[1] The peak incidence occurs between 40 and 60 years of age and there is a female predominance. A more recent study reviewing abdominal CTA demonstrated a higher RAA incidence of 0.7%.[2] A variety of etiologies may lead to RAA formation and must undergo appropriate workup. These etiologies include atherosclerosis, fibrodysplasia, Takayasu arteritis, connective tissue disorders, trauma, and dissection. In particular, the association of arterial fibrodysplasia with aneurysm formation has been well documented.

More than 90% of true RAAs are extraparenchymal, with right-side laterality in 61%, and aneurysms are bilateral in 4% to 10% of patients.[2] The majority of RAAs are saccular and typically located at the primary or secondary order renal artery branch points. Isolated lesions to the main trunk of the renal artery are rare. Fusiform RAAs are less common, and because they are generally associated with atherosclerosis or ostial occlusive lesions, their extent is limited to the main renal artery.

B   Imaging studies

Most RAAs are found incidentally on CT, MRI, or DUS, and any one of these modalities are suitable in detecting the presence of an aneurysm. CTA with at least 1-mm cuts including an arterial and venous phase can further provide information regarding aneurysm size, morphology, extent in relation to branch vessels, and other associated pathology. Abdominal DSA with selective renal artery arteriograms in multiple views can provide anatomic detail with regard to underlying etiology, branch vessel involvement, and associated fistulous connection with the renal vein that may not be appreciated on CT imaging. DSA findings complement those from CT imaging and are critical for surgical planning, and, as such, both are recommended before treatment. MRA may be used as an alternative to CTA to limit radiation in pediatric patients or because of surgeon preference.

C   Ruptured?

Patients with a ruptured RAA can present with abdominal/flank pain, hypotension, shock, and macroscopic hematuria. Suspected rupture is most rapidly confirmed with CTA and requires emergent intervention. The incidence of RAA rupture varies in the literature between 1% and 14%; however, most relatively large series report a rupture rate of <3%.[2,3] RAA rupture is associated with a 10% mortality.[1,4] Initial treatment of these patients requires resuscitation and close hemodynamic observation before emergent surgical or endovascular intervention.

D   Symptomatic?

Although most RAAs are asymptomatic, 25% of patients can present with pain (abdominal or flank) or hematuria, which may reflect aneurysm expansion or pending rupture. Such symptoms are similar to those experienced by patients with symptomatic AAA. More common etiologies for abdominal or flank pain must be appropriately ruled out before attributing the symptoms to a RAA, particularly if the aneurysm is <2 cm. All patients with symptomatic RAAs should be evaluated for treatment.

E   Woman of child-bearing age?

The risk of RAA rupture during pregnancy is high and the available evidence justifies an aggressive surgical approach in this setting. The elevated risk of rupture is thought to be related to the physiologic changes in hemodynamics, increases in circulating blood volume, and hormonal effects on the aneurysm that accompany pregnancy. In a series of 18 patients who underwent repair of a RAA; rupture occurred in two patients, both of childbearing age, with aneurysms of only 1 cm.[5] In another series of 43 ruptured RAA repairs, 3 pregnant patients had aneurysms <2 cm.[6] RAA rupture in pregnancy is associated with 55% maternal mortality and 85% fetal mortality rate. Therefore, women of childbearing age with a RAA should be evaluated for repair regardless of size or symptomatic status.

F   Refractory HTN?

RAAs are associated with HTN in up to 82% of cases.[2] Various mechanisms to explain the pathophysiology of how RAAs cause renovascular HTN have been postulated. Embolization of aneurysmal thrombus can lead to chronic segmental ischemia with subsequent renin-angiotensin-mediated HTN.[7] Furthermore, the aneurysm may compress or kink the main renal artery or segmental branch vessels or demonstrate turbulent flow within the aneurysm itself. These events lead to local hypoperfusion with subsequent systemic vasoconstriction and fluid retention mediated by the renin-angiotensin system.

Refractory HTN is defined as blood pressure that remains above goal despite the use of three antihypertensive agents of different classes, one of which being a diuretic.[8] Refractory HTN in patients with a RAA is an indication for repair, if other etiologies have been excluded. Although a number of series have demonstrated the favorable impact of surgical repair of RAAs on HTN, a large multi-institutional study reported that 40% of patients had no improvement in blood pressure following repair for resistant HTN.[2,9-16] These findings underscore the importance of a thorough evaluation for other potential etiologies of refractory HTN before operative intervention is pursued.

G   Renal emboli with renal dysfunction?

Embolization of thrombus within a RAA is an indication for repair to prevent renal dysfunction. Chronic thromboembolism from a RAA can occur at a microscopic level, which over time can lead to not only renovascular HTN but also segmental renal parenchymal infarction and loss of renal mass and function. The normal aging process is associated with a steady decline in renal function, with GFR declining by about 8 mL/min/1.73 m[17] per decade starting at the fourth decade.[18] Furthermore, up to 10% of glomeruli may be sclerotic in the healthy person by the age of 40. Given the normal steady deterioration in renal function and mass with aging, and existing systemic diseases such as HTN and atherosclerosis, renal preservation becomes paramount in patients with a RAA, particularly in young patients with an otherwise normal life expectancy. The vast majority of patients included in published studies that specifically evaluated outcomes of surgical revascularization of a RAA are women 40 to 60 years old, in relative good health with a normal life expectancy.[2,9-16] The typical demographics of this patient population emphasizes the importance of renal preservation over their lifetime. Therefore, any evidence of embolization from a RAA warrants consideration for repair.

H   Fistulous connection with renal vein?

Fistulization of a RAA to the renal vein is extremely rare, but multiple cases have been reported in the literature. Their presentation can vary from no symptoms to frank rupture. Of the few reported cases, patients invariably had evidence of central high-output AVF continuous abdominal bruit, and heart failure. CTA may demonstrate a dilated renal vein with enhancement on the arterial phase. Aortogram with selective renal artery catheterization will clearly demonstrate AVF flow and confirm the diagnosis. Such a renal AVF is generally an indication for treatment.

I   Assess rupture risk

The decision to repair an asymptomatic RAA requires a careful evaluation of rupture risk. Although a diameter of >2 cm has traditionally been used as an indication for repair, there is still significant controversy regarding this threshold.[3] Furthermore, the natural history of RAAs has not been well defined because of their rarity. In the multi-institutional, Vascular-Low-Frequency Disease Consortium (VLFDC), a review of 865 RAAs in 760 patients reported only three ruptures. All three patients who presented with rupture had aneurysms >3 cm (mean 3.7 cm). Aneurysms that were treated with observation included 88 aneurysms >2 cm and 7 aneurysms >3 cm over a mean follow-up of 49 months with no ruptures. Calcification of the aneurysm was not protective. This large experience suggests that the risk of rupture for RAAs between 2 and 3 cm is very low and the traditional recommendation of repair for aneurysms >2 cm may be too aggressive.[2] Therefore, the indication for RAA repair should be based on rapid growth over time and consideration for repair should occur for asymptomatic RAAs >3 cm diameter.

J Endovascular candidate?

Numerous case series have demonstrated the technical feasibility of treating RAAs using endovascular techniques with embolization, stent grafts, or a combination of the two. Suitable anatomy amenable for endovascular repair will vary depending on the treating surgeon. Our criteria for endovascular repair mandate successful aneurysm exclusion using conventional endovascular tools without intentional sacrifice of branch vessels to maximize renal preservation. Fusiform aneurysms isolated to the main renal artery may be successfully excluded with a stent graft assuming there is adequate normal main renal artery for both proximal and distal seal. Some saccular aneurysms with a well-defined narrow neck originating from the main renal artery and up to the second-order branches can be treated with embolization using various liquid or metal agents without compromising the main renal artery or branch. Aneurysms located near the renal hilum in third-order branches have been treated successfully with endovascular embolization techniques, but partial renal infarcts can occur in up to 33%.[18,19] Although no immediate decline in renal function was observed in these reports, renal parenchymal preservation must be considered in young patients with an otherwise normal life expectancy. Therefore, a minimally invasive repair using endovascular techniques for RAAs should be considered for all patients but only offered if it can be executed without any renal parenchymal compromise, unless the patient cannot tolerate an open surgical procedure.

K Endovascular repair

Standard endovascular techniques from either femoral or brachial artery approach can be used to treat RAAs. Stent grafts or embolization with coils or liquid agents or a combination of the two can be utilized. Flow-diverting stents (FDSs) are currently used to treat intracranial aneurysms and reduce blood flow into the aneurysm sac while maintaining flow in the main artery and branch vessels. FDSs have been successfully used to treat extracranial aneurysms including those of the renal artery with satisfactory short-term results and may potentially serve as another tool for endovascular management of RAAs.[20] More experience with FDSs, however, is required.

L Assess operative risk

Patients who do not have suitable anatomy for an endovascular repair should be considered for surgical repair. A standard assessment of operative risk should be performed as with any abdominal vascular procedure requiring aortic cross-clamping. Operative risk should be weighed against risk of aneurysm rupture, with life expectancy considered equally important. If operative risk is deemed excessive and endovascular treatment is not possible, observation is the best option.

M Surgical treatment

A number of studies have demonstrated the safety, durability, and clinical benefits on blood pressure and renal function using open reconstructive and renal parenchymal protective techniques in the treatment of complex renal artery pathology.[9-16] Surgical techniques to manage RAAs include aneurysm excision with patch angioplasty or saphenous vein interposition graft, in situ or ex vivo renal artery reconstruction, and nephrectomy. Aortic inflow using hypogastric artery is the preferred configuration for reconstruction in pediatric patients to avoid later aneurysmal degeneration if vein grafts are used. Aneurysm morphology, location along the renal artery, and the extent of branch vessel involvement will dictate the type of repair. Aneurysms isolated to the main renal artery can be managed with excision and aortorenal bypass. Aneurysms located at the renal hilum can be managed using in situ repair ± cold preservation techniques depending on the complexity of branch vessel reconstruction. Alternatively, ex vivo repair with cold preservation provides excellent access to all segmental vessels allowing for exploration and complex branch vessel reconstruction in a bloodless field. Orthotopic replacement into the renal fossa or heterotopic autotransplantation to the pelvis depends on surgeon preference. For patients with infrarenal aortic occlusive disease, extra-anatomic bypass using the hepatic or splenic arteries can be used as alternative sources of inflow.[21]

Laparoscopic nephrectomy modeled after live-donor transplant techniques with back-table ex vivo reconstruction and heterotopic implantation in the pelvis have also been described. However, the putative advantage of the less incisional morbidity of this approach is tempered by the additional anastomosis between the ureter and bladder with the potential risk of stricture formation. Furthermore, the potential development and progression of atherosclerotic occlusive disease of the iliac vessels in the relatively young patients requiring RAA repair may compromise long-term durability. All surgical repairs should undergo periodic surveillance imaging indefinitely. Nephrectomy may occasionally be required in the setting of a RAA rupture, nonfunctioning kidney, or a nonreconstructible aneurysm.

N Observation

Clinical observation of a RAA includes imaging surveillance to monitor aneurysm growth, serial assessment of the hypertensive diathesis, and evaluation of renal function. Evidence of aneurysm expansion, development of resistant HTN, or a decline in renal function should prompt additional workup and, if appropriate, consideration of endovascular or open repair. The least invasive imaging modality should be used for monitoring, which could be DUS or CT, but may require CTA in some cases.

REFERENCES

1. Stanley JC, Rhodes EL, Gewertz BL, Chang CY, Walter JF, Fry WJ. Renal artery aneurysms. Significance of macroaneurysms exclusive of dissections and fibrodysplastic mural dilations. *Arch Surg.* 1975;110(11):1327-1333.
2. Klausner JQ, Lawrence PF, Harlander-Locke MP, et al. The contemporary management of renal artery aneurysms. *J Vasc Surg.* 2015;61(4):978-984.
3. Henke PK, Cardneau JD, Welling TH 3rd, et al. Renal artery aneurysms: a 35-year clinical experience with 252 aneurysms in 168 patients. *Ann Surg.* 2001;234(4):454-462; discussion 462-463.
4. Hageman JH, Smith RF, Szilagyi E, Elliott JP. Aneurysms of the renal artery: problems of prognosis and surgical management. *Surgery.* 1978;84(4):563-572.
5. Martin RS 3rd, Meacham PW, Ditesheim JA, Mulherin JL Jr, Edwards WH. Renal artery aneurysm: selective treatment for hypertension and prevention of rupture. *J Vasc Surg.* 1989;9(1):26-34.
6. Turpin S, Lambert R, Querin S, Soulez G, Leveille J, Taillefer R. Radionuclide captopril renography in postpartum renal artery aneurysms. *J Nucl Med.* 1996;37(8):1368-1371.
7. Calligaro KD, Dougherty MJ. Renovascular disease: aneurysms and arteriovenous fistulae. In: Sidawy AN, Perler BA, eds. *Rutherford's Vascular Surgery and Endovascular Therapy.* 9th ed. Philadelphia, PA: Elsevier; 2018:1696-1703.
8. Calhoun DA, Jones D, Textor S, et al. Resistant hypertension: diagnosis, evaluation, and treatment. A scientific statement from the American Heart Association Professional Education Committee of the Council for High Blood Pressure Research. *Hypertension.* 2008;51(6):1403-1419.
9. Anderson CA, Hansen KJ, Benjamin ME, Keith DR, Craven TE, Dean RH. Renal artery fibromuscular dysplasia: results of current surgical therapy. *J Vasc Surg.* 1995;22(3):207-215; discussion 15-16.
10. Barral X, Gournier JP, Frering V, Favre JP, Berthoux F. Dysplastic lesions of renal artery branches: late results of ex vivo repair. *Ann Vasc Surg.* 1992;6(3):225-231.
11. Crutchley TA, Pearce JD, Craven TE, Edwards MS, Dean RH, Hansen KJ. Branch renal artery repair with cold perfusion protection. *J Vasc Surg.* 2007;46(3):405-412; discussion 12.
12. Dean RH, Meacham PW, Weaver FA. Ex vivo renal artery reconstructions: indications and techniques. *J Vasc Surg.* 1986;4(6):546-552.
13. English WP, Pearce JD, Craven TE, et al. Surgical management of renal artery aneurysms. *J Vasc Surg.* 2004;40(1):53-60.
14. Ham SW, Weaver FA. Ex vivo renal artery reconstruction for complex renal artery disease. *J Vasc Surg.* 2014;60(1):143-150.
15. Murray SP, Kent C, Salvatierra O, Stoney RJ. Complex branch renovascular disease: management options and late results. *J Vasc Surg.* 1994;20(3):338-345; discussion 46.

16. Robinson WP 3rd, Bafford R, Belkin M, Menard MT. Favorable outcomes with in situ techniques for surgical repair of complex renal artery aneurysms. *J Vasc Surg.* 2011;53(3):684-691.

17. Davies DF, Shock NW. Age changes in glomerular filtration rate, effective renal plasma flow, and tubular excretory capacity in adult males. *J Clin Invest.* 1950;29(5):496-507.

18. Zhang Z, Yang M, Song L, Tong X, Zou Y. Endovascular treatment of renal artery aneurysms and renal arteriovenous fistulas. *J Vasc Surg.* 2013;57(3):765-770.

19. Tsilimparis N, Reeves JG, Dayama A, Perez SD, Debus ES, Ricotta JJ 2nd. Endovascular vs open repair of renal artery aneurysms: outcomes of repair and long-term renal function. *J Am Coll Surg.* 2013;217(2):263-269.

20. Sfyroeras GS, Dalainas I, Giannakopoulos TG, Antonopoulos K, Kakisis JD, Liapis CD. Flow-diverting stents for the treatment of arterial aneurysms. *J Vasc Surg.* 2012;56(3):839-846.

21. Ham SW, Weaver FA. Ex vivo renal artery reconstruction. In: Eskandari P, Pearce WH, Yao JST, eds. *Current Vascular Surgery: 2015, 40th Anniversary of the Northwestern Vascular Symposium.* Shelton, CT: People's Medical Publishing House; 2015.

Jonathan Kwong • Vikram S. Kashyap

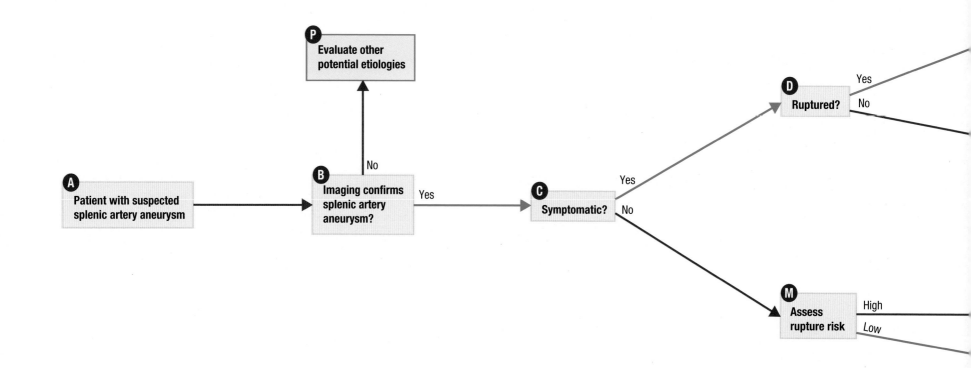

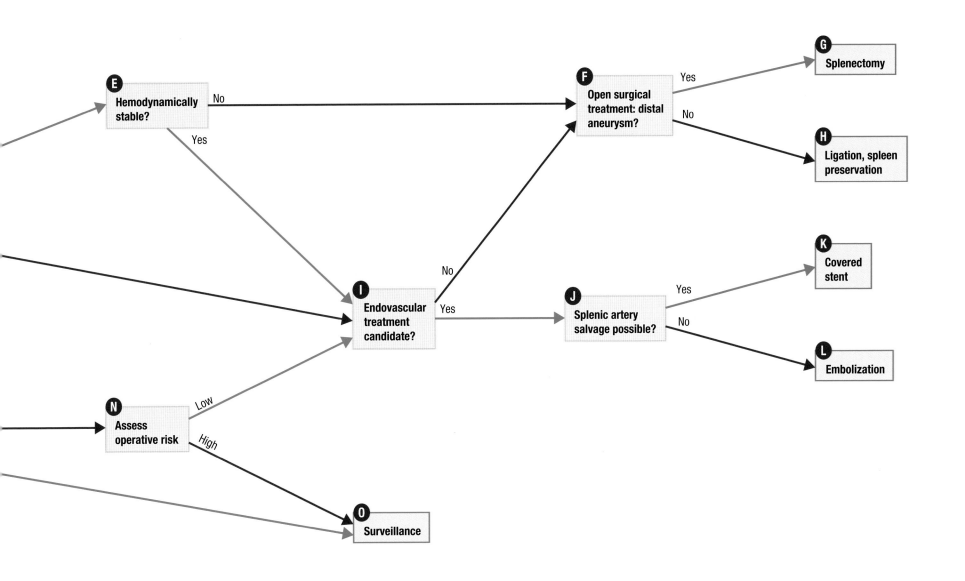

A Patient with suspected splenic artery aneurysm

Splenic artery aneurysms (SAAs) comprise approximately 60% of all splanchnic artery aneurysms, making them the most common type of visceral aneurysms. Their clinical significance arises from a potential risk for rupture. Overall incidence in the general population is relatively low (0.78%).[1] Diagnosis is most often made incidentally with a variety of imaging modalities. The overall rupture risk for patients with high-risk features is 3% to 10%; however, the rupture risk for patients without high-risk features is much lower, at 2%.[1] Most SAAs are discovered as incidental findings on abdominal imaging, but some patients present with abdominal symptoms (see Box C).

B Imaging confirms splenic artery aneurysm?

Although SAAs can be diagnosed using many imaging modalities, cross-sectional imaging has multiple advantages. CTA and MRA allow for an accurate determination of size and relevant anatomy for operative planning. Abdominal DUS is an attractive imaging modality for surveillance purposes because it spares the patient from radiation exposure, is readily available, and is generally well tolerated. DSA is usually reserved for therapeutic interventions.

C Symptomatic?

Most patients with SAA are asymptomatic at the time of diagnosis. Several large institutional studies have reported a 6% to 24% incidence of symptoms at the time of presentation.[2-4] Symptoms associated with a SAA are wide ranging and nonspecific. They can include epigastric abdominal pain, left upper quadrant abdominal pain, or pain radiating to the left shoulder. In cases of rupture, patients can present with hemodynamic collapse, syncope, peritonitis, or acute GI bleeding. Patients may develop a splenic artery PSA after pancreatitis or traumatic disruption of the artery. PSAs theoretically have a higher rupture risk.[2,3]

D Ruptured?

Ruptured SAAs represent a true surgical emergency. Mortality rates associated with SAA rupture average 25%,[5] with mortality rates for select populations being much higher (pregnancy, portal HTN, liver transplant). The "double-rupture phenomenon" has been described as rupture that is initially confined to the lesser sac before free rupture into the peritoneal cavity.[6] This can represent an important therapeutic window to intervene before the onset of intraperitoneal rupture and massive hemorrhage.

E Hemodynamically stable?

Any patient presenting with hemodynamic instability refractory to resuscitative efforts requires emergent operative exploration. Patients who present with free intraperitoneal rupture may even be taken to the operating room without definitive imaging or

diagnosis. The previously described "double-rupture phenomenon" represents the clinical scenario where patients can present with hemodynamic stability despite rupture. This may give the clinician a window to consider available endovascular treatment options.

F Open surgical treatment: distal aneurysm?

Before the advent of endovascular therapies, all SAAs were treated via an open surgical approach. Oftentimes, this was in the setting of intra-abdominal catastrophe with the diagnosis made during laparotomy without preoperative imaging. Open surgical treatment is established as an effective and durable standard to which other treatment options are compared. Anatomic location of the aneurysm, in relation to the spleen, is the main determinant of the type of open surgery performed. Aneurysms located in the proximal splenic artery are usually excluded by proximal and distal ligation, because the spleen can nearly always be preserved without splenic artery revascularization because of short gastric collaterals. Aneurysms in the distal splenic artery and hilum are usually treated with splenectomy because exposure requires sacrifice of collateral vessels.

Long-term results of surgical treatment of SAAs show an overall high survival and a low complication rate.[7] In comparing surgical and endovascular approaches, the former is associated with fewer long-term complications and reinterventions at the expense of slightly higher perioperative morbidity and mortality.[7] Splenic artery PSAs in the setting of pancreatitis or significant trauma can present the opportunity to use endovascular techniques as an adjunct to open repair. This can be done by obtaining proximal control of the splenic artery with an endovascular occlusion balloon before definitive open repair with splenectomy or proximal and distal ligation. Obtaining open proximal control in the setting of significant inflammation and/or infection can be particularly difficult and increases the risk of pancreatic and GI injury.

G Splenectomy

Distal SAAs, particularly those within the hilum of the spleen, are generally treated with splenectomy. The spleen is surgically approached in a variety of ways, with the general tenets involving mobilization of the splenocolic ligament and splenic flexure of the colon. The short gastric vessels as well as the splenic artery and vein require ligation and division. Laparoscopic splenectomy is an option for select patients. Vaccinations against encapsulated bacteria (*Streptococcus pneumoniae, Haemophilus influenzae,* and *Neisseria meningitides*) are required to prevent the rare, but devastating complication of overwhelming postsplenectomy sepsis. Vaccinations include the Pneumococcal, Meningococcal, and *H. influenza* type B vaccinations. On the basis of literature from the trauma population, these vaccinations should be administered within 14 days of splenectomy.[8,9]

H Ligation, spleen preservation

SAAs located in the proximal to mid splenic artery can be treated with proximal and distal ligation without revascularization given the collateral perfusion to the spleen via the short gastric vessels. Exposure to the proximal splenic artery is obtained by dividing the gastrohepatic ligament to enter the lesser sac. Aneurysmectomy is generally not necessary. In cases of SAA in the setting of pancreatitis, ligation of the splenic artery from within the aneurysm sac can be an option when isolation of the splenic artery from the surrounding peripancreatic inflammation is particularly challenging. Perioperative preparation is prudent with cell-saving suction, autotransfusion, and blood products available for challenging cases. Laparoscopic ligation of SAAs has also been described to reduce open surgical morbidity when endovascular treatment is not possible.[10]

I Endovascular treatment candidate?

Endovascular techniques to treat SAAs have become the preferred therapeutic option because of improved short-term outcomes including 30-day mortality and length of hospital stay as compared to open repair. Technical success rates with endovascular therapy have come to rival open repair as well.[7] Technical considerations for endovascular repair include access to the splenic artery, tortuosity, and ability to deliver embolic agents/devices. Risks associated with endovascular options include arterial access complications, postembolization syndrome, splenic infarction, delayed splenic rupture, splenic abscess formation, inconsistent and transient obliteration of the aneurysm, and migration/erosion.[2,3] Patients are candidates for endovascular treatment if appropriate access to the splenic artery can be obtained, and the splenic artery and aneurysm be crossed with wires and catheters. In some cases, severe tortuosity or a large SAA prevents access to the splenic artery distal to the aneurysm, in which case endovascular treatment may not be possible. These anatomic judgments are based on detailed preoperative images, but may not be determined until the endovascular treatment is attempted.

J Splenic artery salvage possible?

Preservation of the splenic artery offers the theoretical advantage of avoiding several of the complications associated with endovascular ablation namely, postembolization syndrome, splenic infarct, and splenic abscess formation, although these occur infrequently with splenic artery occlusion. Patients with a splenic artery able to accommodate a self-expanding stent graft, depending on size and tortuosity as well as with adequate proximal and distal seal zones, can be candidates for splenic artery salvage in the appropriate clinical scenario. In many cases, the tortuosity of the artery, combined with the relative rigidity of current stent grafts, will not allow this approach.

Ⓚ Covered stent

Covered stents offer an option for repair of SAAs located in the mid portion of the splenic artery because they allow for splenic preservation. Anatomic considerations based on size, tortuosity, and proximal and distal seal zones determine who would be a candidate for this procedure. However, given the usually adequate collateral circulation through the short gastric vessels, the benefit of preserving the splenic artery is unproven. As such, the literature on successful outcomes of this technique has been limited to case reports

Ⓛ Embolization

Percutaneous transcatheter embolization has become the preferred method of treatment for SAAs. Embolization has been employed using a variety of agents including coils, plugs, and cyanoacrylate glue. Cessation of antegrade and retrograde perfusion of the aneurysm is necessary for complete endovascular repair. Technically, the distal splenic artery is embolized first and thereafter the SAA and proximal splenic artery employing a technique called "sandwich embolization," where the splenic artery both proximal and distal to the aneurysm is occluded. Modified "sandwich embolization" techniques have also been described where Gelfoam or cyanoacrylate glue has been placed within the aneurysm sac between the two sets of coils or plugs. Success rates have been listed as high as 96%,[2] but potential complications include arterial access complications, postembolization syndrome, splenic infarction, delayed splenic rupture, splenic abscess formation, inconsistent and transient obliteration of the aneurysm, and late migration/erosion of plug or coils.

Ⓜ Assess rupture risk

In patients with asymptomatic or "bland" SAAs, several characteristics determine the overall risk for rupture. As with most fusiform aneurysms, size of the aneurysm remains very important. Most aneurysms are initially diagnosed at a size of about 2 cm; however, those patients who presented with rupture or symptoms had an average size of around 3 cm.[3] Given this fact, most authors advocate elective repair of "bland" SAAs in patients who are good surgical candidates once they are larger than 2 to 2.5 cm in diameter.[4] Apart from size criteria, there are several clinical scenarios that represent an increased risk for rupture and warrant close attention. It is generally agreed that women of child-bearing age and those who are pregnant should undergo SAA repair regardless of size because >50% of SAAs that present during pregnancy will go on to rupture, most often in the third trimester.[11] SAA rupture during pregnancy has a very high maternal and fetal mortality, approaching 75% and 95%,[12] respectively. Patients with SAAs undergoing liver transplantation should also be repaired because they are at a 2-fold increased risk for rupture in the posttransplant period with an associated 80% mortality.[13] The importance

of patient selection is particularly important given that the overall risk of rupture for patients with "bland" aneurysms is related to size and thought to be no higher than 2% for SAAs between 2 and 2.5 cm in diameter. Presence of thrombus or calcifications have not been shown to affect the risk of rupture for these "bland" aneurysms.[2]

Any PSA of the splenic artery, whether it is symptomatic or not, should be repaired if clinical circumstances allow.[14] Although rare, PSAs are associated with a substantial risk of rupture and associated morbidity and mortality. Trauma and pancreatitis-related manifestations are the most common etiology for PSA formation. Hemosuccus pancreaticus is a rare clinical scenario characterized by rupture of a SAA into the pancreatic duct causing upper GI hemorrhage.[14] In the setting of PSA caused by pancreatitis-related etiology, the rupture risk is approximately 20% with an associated 37% mortality.[15]

Ⓝ Assess operative risk

For "bland" SAAs, the reported overall rupture risk is quoted at approximately 2%.[1] Combining this with the approximately 25% mortality[5] associated with SAA rupture, elective repair of a "bland," asymptomatic SAA should be offered when the risk of perioperative death is less than 0.5%.

Ⓞ Surveillance

For those patients selected to undergo observation, surveillance generally entails yearly cross-sectional imaging. DUS is an attractive option because it avoids radiation exposure and is generally well tolerated; however, results can be operator dependent. Only approximately 10% of SAAs will grow in size during the corresponding surveillance period and very few will ultimately need intervention because of aneurysmal growth.[2-4]

Reevaluation of the risks versus benefits of SAA repair is critical in the surveillance period. Patients who become symptomatic warrant repair. Of the 10% of SAAs that enlarge in size during the surveillance period, the average rate of growth can be 0.2 to 0.6 mm/year.[2,3] In this scenario of minimal growth on serial imaging, it is important to have a detailed discussion of risks and benefits of intervention with the patient. In several large institutional studies, no patients undergoing surveillance went on to rupture during the surveillance period; however, a small percentage of patients did require intervention because of enlarging aneurysm size.[2-4]

Ⓟ Evaluate other potential etiologies

If a patient presents with abdominal symptoms suggesting a SAA, but this is not confirmed by imaging, other potential etiologies need to be evaluated. Because the abdominal symptoms associated with a SAA are very nonspecific, many other abdominal conditions could be responsible, and are often detected by the imaging done to evaluate the suspected SAA.

REFERENCES

1. Stanley JC, Fry WJ. Pathogenesis and clinical significance of splenic artery aneurysms. *Surgery.* 1974;76(6):898-909.
2. Lakin RO, Bena JF, Sarac TP, et al. The contemporary management of splenic artery aneurysms. *J Vasc Surg.* 2011; 53(4):958-964, discussion 965.
3. Abbas MA, Stone WM, Fowl RJ, et al. Splenic artery aneurysms: two decades experience at Mayo clinic. *Ann Vasc Surg.* 2002;16:442-449.
4. Corey MR, Ergul EA, Cambria RP, et al. The natural history of splanchnic artery aneurysms and outcomes after operative intervention. *J Vasc Surg.* 2016;63:949-957.
5. Stanley JC, Wakefield TW, Graham LM, Whitehouse WM Jr, Zelenock GB, Lindenauer SM. Clinical importance and management of splanchnic artery aneurysms. *J Vasc Surg.* 1986;3(5):836-840.
6. de Vries JE, Schattenkerk ME, Malt RA. Complications of splenic artery aneurysm other than intraperitoneal rupture. *Surgery.* 1982;91(2):200-204.
7. Hogendoorn W, Lavinda A, Hunink MG, et al. Open repair, endovascular repair, and conservative management of true splenic artery aneurysms. *J Vasc Surg.* 2014;60(6):1667-1676.
8. Shatz DV, Schinsky MF, Pais LB, Romero-Steiner S, Kirton OC, Carlone GM. Immune responses of splenectomized trauma patients to the 23-valent pneumococcal polysaccharide vaccine at 1 versus 7 versus 14 days after Splenectomy. *J Trauma.* 1998;44:765-766.
9. Shatz DV, Romero-Steiner S, Elie CM, Holder PF, Carlone GM. Antibody responses in postsplenectomy trauma patients receiving the 23-valent pneumococcal polysaccharide vaccine at 14 versus 28 days postoperatively. *J Trauma.* 2002;53:1037-1042.
10. Pietrabissa A, Ferrari M, Berchiolli R, et al. Laparoscopic treatment of splenic artery aneurysms. *J Vasc Surg.* 2009; 50(2):275-279.
11. Caillouette JC, Merchant EB. Ruptured splenic artery aneurysm in pregnancy: twelfth reported case with maternal and fetal survival. *Am J Obstet Gynecol.* 1993;168:1810-1813.
12. Ha JF, Phillips M, Faulkner K. Splenic artery aneurysm rupture in pregnancy. *Eur J Obstet Gynecol Reprod Biol.* 2009;146:133-137.
13. Bronsther O, Merhav H, Van Thiel D, Starzl TE. Splenic artery aneurysms occurring in liver transplant recipients. *Transplantation.* 1991;52(4):723-724.
14. Tessier DJ, Stone WM, Fowl RJ, et al. Clinical features and management of splenic artery pseudoaneurysm: case series and cumulative review of literature. *J Vasc Surg.* 2003; 38(5):969-974.
15. Stabile BE, Wilson SE, Debas HT. Reduced mortality from bleeding pseudocysts and pseudoaneurysms caused by pancreatitis. *Arch Surg.* 1983;118:45-51.

Timur P. Sarac

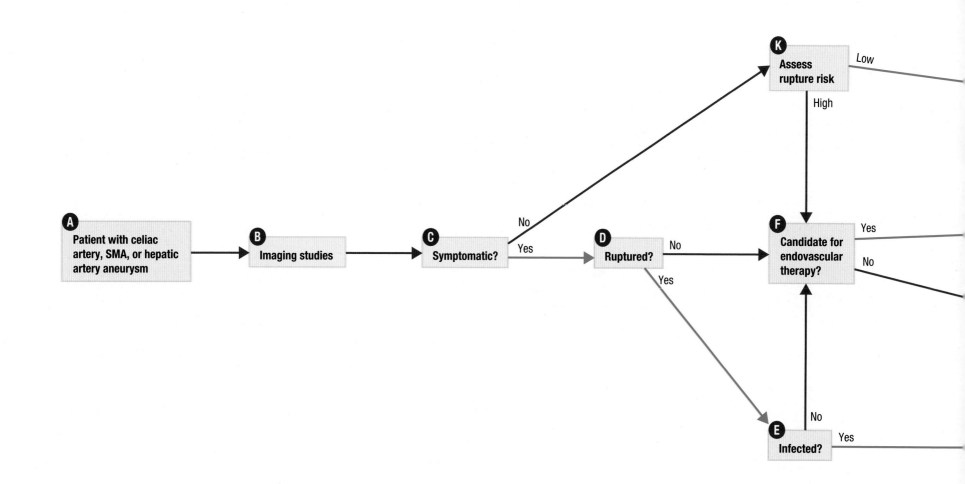

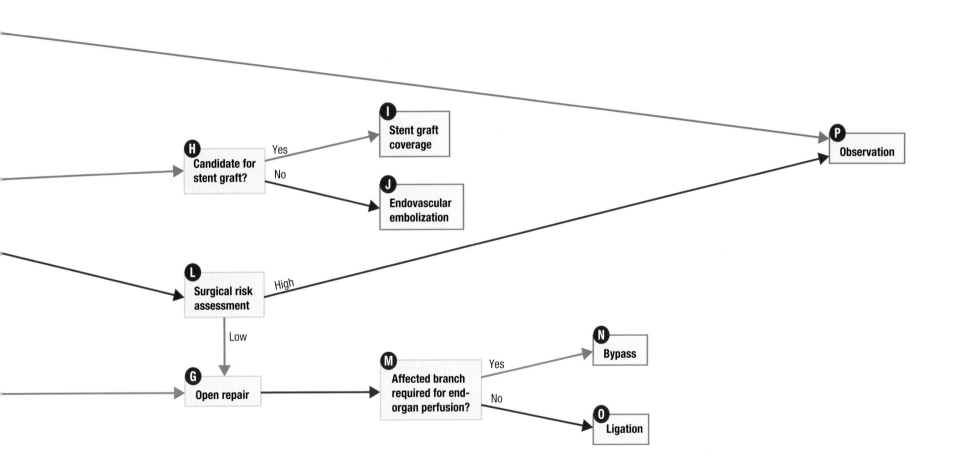

Ⓐ Patient with celiac, SMA, or hepatic artery aneurysm

Visceral, or splanchnic artery aneurysms (SAA), can involve the celiac, hepatic, splenic, superior mesenteric, inferior mesenteric arteries, and their branches. SAAs are rare with a reported incidence of <2% based on autopsy results; this rate increases in the elderly.[1-3] Up to 30% of patients with one SAA have other intra-abdominal aneurysms.[4]

Sixty percent of SAAs occur in the splenic artery, 20% in the hepatic artery, 8% in the SMA, 4% in the celiac artery, 4% in the gastric and gastroepiploic arteries, and 4% in the remaining splanchnic branches.[5] Splenic artery aneurysms are discussed in Chapter 34.

SAAs can be true or false (PSA). This distinction is important in identifying the etiology, considerations for repair, and follow-up. The majority are true aneurysms, with the most common etiology being degenerative. Other causes of SAAs include FMD, cystic medial necrosis, portal HTN, and multiparity.[6,7] Common causes of PSA development are inflammatory conditions (eg, pancreatitis), blunt and penetrating abdominal trauma, and iatrogenic injuries such as percutaneous biliary interventions.[8] The natural history of SAAs is not completely elucidated because of their low prevalence; however, rupture risk is reported to be high.[9]

Ⓑ Imaging studies

Although most SAAs are discovered incidentally on unrelated imaging studies, some are diagnosed during evaluation of abdominal or back pain. Abdominal CTA is the diagnostic imaging of choice, although both MRA and DUS can diagnose a SAA. Occasionally, the diagnosis is based on vascular calcifications, found on plain abdominal x-ray.

Ⓒ Symptomatic?

Most SAAs are asymptomatic before rupture.[10] If a patient develops sudden abdominal pain from a known or recently diagnosed SAA, rupture and/or acute expansion is the most likely cause. Rarely, epigastric or diffuse abdominal pain can be caused by compression of adjacent vessels or viscera.[11] Rarely, SAAs will present with upper GI bleeding, if the aneurysm erodes into intestine.[12,13] Such patients may present in shock of unclear etiology. Rarely, SAAs can rupture into the portal vein, creating acute portal HTN and bleeding gastroesophageal varices. Presence of symptoms in a patient with SAA requires urgent evaluation and emergent intervention if associated with rupture.

Ⓓ Ruptured?

Rupture occurs in 10% to 25% of patients with SAA and associated mortality ranges from 25% to 70%.[14,15] As such, ruptured SAAs require emergent repair. Hepatic artery aneurysms (HAAs) have the highest rupture rate of all SAAs.[16] Rupture rates and subsequent mortality rates for HAAs are 20% to 44% and 35% to 82%, respectively.[17,18]

Ⓔ Infected?

Infected SAAs represent a rare and distinct group of visceral aneurysms that most often involve the SMA and arise from hematogenous spread. Historically, infection involved Staphylococcus or Streptococcus species and originated from subacute bacterial endocarditis; however, more recently, varied and virulent organisms have been reported and are caused by an increasing rate of IV drug abuse. Patients with an infected SAA typically present with signs of infection, although these may be subtle. The diagnosis is usually made by CT scan and positive blood cultures; however in more occult cases, (18)F-fluorodeoxyglucose (FDG) PET/CT or WBC scans may aid in the diagnosis. Expeditious repair should be undertaken, usually with open surgery and autogenous interposition bypass graft or ligation, as necessary. However, in cases of extremis or prohibitive comorbidities, endovascular therapy can be a life-saving temporary measure.

Ⓕ Candidate for endovascular therapy?

The number of endovascular interventions for SAAs has continued to increase over the past decade.[19] Increased familiarity with endovascular techniques, improved technology, and low complication rates of endovascular therapy compared with open vascular repair have led to it becoming the treatment of choice when anatomically appropriate. To evaluate anatomic candidacy for endovascular intention, high-resolution CTA or visceral DSA is used. Anatomic requirements for stent graft placement to preserve distal flow include the usual adequate proximal and distal landing zones and adequate access without severe tortuosity to allow device delivery. If preserved arterial flow is not required, catheter-based embolization is performed. If flow preservation is required but a stent graft cannot be placed, the patient should be evaluated for open surgical repair.

Ⓖ Open repair

Although endovascular treatment of noninfected SAAs is the first line of therapy, when a patient is not an endovascular candidate, open surgical repair of SAA, in the elective or emergent setting, may be required. Open repair is preferred in the setting of infection. Open surgical repair requires transabdominal or retroperitoneal exposure of the aneurysm with or without arterial reconstruction and, possibly, end-organ resection (ie, partial hepatic or bowel resection). Autogenous vein is the preferred conduit when revascularization is performed.

Celiac: Approaching the celiac artery from a transabdominal approach can be quite tedious given the proximity of the artery to the pancreas. However, it does allow easy access for branch vessel revascularization. In addition, hybrid therapies have been described where supraceliac aorta to hepatic artery bypass is performed, with therapy completed with aortic stent graft coverage of the celiac orifice and aneurysm embolization. A retroperitoneal approach offers adequate exposure for ligation of the celiac orifice, aneurysm resection, and bypass.

SMA: Open repair of SMA aneurysms is usually conducted with an interposition graft. In the unusual case of an SMA orifice aneurysm, retroperitoneal exposure, anterior to the kidney, allows for adequate SMA exposure.

Other: HAAs are approached by exposure just medial to the porta hepatis and the aneurysm is repaired occurring at the IMA origin as part of an AAA; in this setting both aneurysms are repaired concomitantly. In the case of a distal branch aneurysm of a jejunal, ileal, or colic artery, excision of the mesentery and possible bowel resection should be considered.

Ⓗ Candidate for stent graft?

Maintaining in-line blood flow using a stent graft is the preferred endovascular option to treat SAAs,[15,20] but may not be feasible because of arterial tortuosity, discrepancy in the diameter of proximal and distal landing zones, or possible resultant exclusion of important collaterals. If stent graft exclusion is accomplished, small branches of the SAA can cause endoleaks. Thus, coil embolization of any large SAA branches should be performed before stent graft exclusion because subsequent endoleak treatment may be precluded.[21] In some cases, small arterial diameter or tortuosity may preclude stent graft delivery through larger sheaths that may be required. In addition, the size limitations of stent grafts (particularly for vessels <5 mm) can preclude their use. If stent graft SAA exclusion cannot be performed, embolization to achieve aneurysm thrombosis may be possible, if end-organ perfusion via the affected artery is not critical. Most celiac, hepatic, and IMA aneurysms can be treated with endovascular embolization without significant complications.[10] In most cases, proximal SMA aneurysm occlusion should be avoided, but coil embolization of a distal SMA branch aneurysm is usually tolerated albeit possibly requiring limited intestinal resection.

Ⓘ Stent graft coverage

Access to the SAA is accomplished through an antegrade approach from brachial or retrograde femoral artery access. Preferential use of balloon expandable stent grafts is ideal for orifical lesions where precise placement is mandatory, and there is no concern for kinking. Curved and tortuous arteries are better treated with more pliable self-expanding stent grafts.

Ⓙ Endovascular embolization

Endovascular options to occlude an SAA include percutaneous embolization using coils or plugs. Injection of glue (*N*-butyl cyanoacrolate or ethylene vinyl alcohol), endoluminal thrombin, polyvinyl alcohol, particles, and gelfoam have also been used.[22] Finally, hybrid procedures involving open bypass followed by endovascular coiling as well as direct open thrombin injection has been reported.[23] Coils or plugs usually provide adequate mechanical and thrombogenic surface to result in SAA thrombosis. However, sometimes, vessel tortuosity and location preclude coil or plug delivery, and, in such cases, liquid embolic agents may be used. This approach is less precise and has the risk of glue migrating to undesirable locations.

K Assess rupture risk

Most experts agree that main trunk true SAAs should be treated only if symptomatic or if diameter exceeds 2 cm.[24] In contrast, most PSAs merit treatment because their propensity to rupture is greater.[7,8,25] Although asymptomatic main trunk SAAs <2 cm in diameter can be observed, distal branch aneurysms and PSAs should be considered for repair, regardless of size, given their uncertain natural history and lethality of rupture. As with most aneurysms, elective repair should be considered after careful evaluation of both the risks and benefits of treatment. Risk factors for rupture of all SAAs include absolute size (>2 cm), HTN, tobacco use, pulmonary disease, saccular morphology, pain, and infection. If the patient has symptoms of pain, rupture may be imminent and urgent repair should be considered.[26]

L Surgical risk assessment

Among patients who are considered for SAA repair who are not endovascular candidates, open surgical risk assessment is required. Preoperative risk evaluation that places the patient in a high-risk category may prohibit such repair in asymptomatic patients. Preoperative risk evaluation is described in detail in Chapters 1 and 2.

M Affected branch ligation required for end-organ perfusion?

Most patients undergoing open SAA repair require arterial preservation. If the artery does not require preservation to maintain end-organ perfusion, simple ligation with aneurysm excision or exclusion can be performed. This is often considered in the open treatment of an infected SAA.

The liver derives 70% of its blood flow from the portal vein and 30% from the hepatic arteries. Although descriptions of hepatic artery ligation for trauma or rupture have been described, it is likely that some end-organ infarction will occur if the hepatic artery is ligated. In such cases, in patients with normal liver function, ligation with partial hepatectomy can be considered. However, preservation of hepatic artery flow with interposition grafting from the aorta, or extra-anatomic bypass from an aortic branch is preferred.[24,27]

For SMA aneurysm, distal flow preservation is almost always advisable unless the aneurysm solely involves a distal branch. Although celiac artery ligation without concomitant revascularization has been described, gastric necrosis following ligation has

been reported.[28,29] In general, peripheral branch SAAs can be ligated, but occasionally segmental intestinal resection is required. Therefore, selective DSA should be used to demonstrate adequate collateral circulation before performing ligation.[30-32]

N Bypass

Given that most SMA aneurysms are in the mid-portion of the artery, interposition grafting is usually required.[33] Occasionally, an aorto or iliac to SMA bypass might be performed. The celiac artery is usually short; therefore, an aorto to distal celiac bypass is usually required to treat a celiac aneurysm. Vein grafts are the best choice of conduit for an interposition graft, especially if there is evidence of infection or need for intestinal resection. In other cases, short prosthetic grafts can be used. The aorta is the most common inflow source for IMA aneurysm if these require flow preservation.

O Ligation

Location of SAA dictates whether the affected artery can be safely ligated or a bypass is required. When there is adequate collateral flow, ligation alone may suffice. In these circumstances, adequate collateralization should be demonstrated by both DSA and, more importantly, through direct intraoperative evaluation.[34]

P Observation

Asymptomatic patients with SAAs should be observed using CTA, MRA, or DUS. The frequency of surveillance studies is not clearly defined; however, most authors suggest annual or biannual imaging.

REFERENCES

1. Ailawadi G, Cowles RA, Stanley JC, et al. Common celiacomesenteric trunk: aneurysmal and occlusive disease. *J Vasc Surg.* 2004;40:1040-1043.
2. Detroux M, Anidjar S, Nottin R. Aneurysm of a common celiomesenteric trunk. *Ann Vasc Surg.* 1998;12:78-82.
3. Guntani A, Yamaoka T, Kyuragi R, et al. Successful treatment of a visceral artery aneurysm with a celiacomesenteric trunk: report of a case. *Surg Today.* 2011;41:115-119.
4. Carr SC, Mahvi DM, Hoch JR, et al. Visceral artery aneurysm rupture. *J Vasc Surg.* 2001;33:806.
5. Deterling RA. Aneurysms of the visceral arteries. *J Cardiovasc Surg.* 1971;12:309.
6. Gehlen JM, Heeren PA, Verhagen PF, et al. Visceral artery aneurysms. *Vasc Endovasc Surg.* 2011;45:681-687.
7. Stanley CJ, Shah NL, Messina LM. Common splanchnic artery aneurysms: splenic, hepatic, and celiac. *Ann Vasc Surg.* 1996;10:315-322.
8. Boudghène F, L'Hermine C, Bigot JM. Arterial complications of pancreatitis: diagnostic and therapeutic aspects in 104 cases. *J Vasc Interv Radiol.* 1993;4:551-558.
9. Stanley JC, Wakefield TW, Graham LM, et al. Clinical importance and management of splanchnic artery aneurysms. *J Vasc Surg.* 1986;3:836-840.
10. Tulsyan N, Kashyap V, Greenberg R, et al. The endovascular management of visceral artery aneurysms and pseudoaneurysms. *J Vasc Surg.* 2007;45:276-283.
11. Zachary K, Geier S, Pellecchia C, et al. Jaundice secondary to hepatic artery aneurysm: radiological appearance and clinical features. *Am J Gastroenterol.* 1986;81:295-298.
12. Lambert CJ, Williamson JW. Splenic artery aneurysm. A rare cause of upper gastrointestinal bleeding. *Am Surg.* 1990;56:543-545.
13. Eckhauser FE, Stanley JC, Zelenock GB. Gastroduodenal and pancreaticoduodenal artery aneurysms: a complication of pancreatitis causing spontaneous gastrointestinal hemorrhage. *Surgery.* 1980;88:335-344.
14. Saltzberg SS, Maldonado TS, Lamparello PJ, et al. Is endovascular therapy the preferred treatment for all visceral artery aneurysms? *Ann Vasc Surg.* 2005;19:507-515.
15. Reil TD, Gevorgyan A, Jimenez JC, et al. Endovascular treatment of visceral artery aneurysms. In: Moore WS, Ahn SS, eds. *Endovascular Surgery.* 4th ed. St. Louis, MO: Saunders; 2010:521-527.
16. Salo JA, Aarnio PT, Jarvinen AA, Kivilaakso EO. Aneurysms of the hepatic arteries. *Am Surg.* 1989;5:705.
17. Stanley JC, Thompson NW, Fry WJ. Splanchnic artery aneurysms. *Arch Surg.* 1971;101:689-697.
18. Reiter DA, Fischman AM, Shy BD. Hepatic artery psedudoaneurysm rupture: a case report and review of the literature. *J Emerg Med.* 2013;44:100-103.
19. Chin JA, Heib A, Ochoa Chaar CI, Cardella JA, Orion KC, Sarac TP. Trends and outcomes in endovascular and open surgical treatment of visceral aneurysms. *J Vasc Surg.* 2017;66(1):195-201.
20. Cochennec F, Riga CV, Allaire E, et al. Contemporary management of splanchnic and renal artery aneurysms: results of endovascular compared with open surgery from two European vascular centers. *Eur J Vasc Endovasc Surg.* 2011;42:340-346.
21. Nosher JL, Chung J, Brevetti LS, et al. Visceral and renal artery aneurysms: a pictorial essay on endovascular therapy. *Radiographics.* 2006;26:1687-1704.
22. Hemp JH, Sabri SS. Endovascular management of visceral arterial aneurysms. *Techn Vasc Interv Radiol.* 2015;18(1):14-23.
23. McIntyre TP, Simone ST, Stahlfeld KR. Intraoperative thrombin occlusion of a visceral artery aneurysm. *J Vasc Surg.* 2002;36:393-395.
24. Abbas MA, Fowl RJ, Stone WM, et al. Hepatic artery aneurysm: factors that predict complications. *J Vasc Surg.* 2003;38:41-45.
25. Sharma G, Semel ME, McGillicuddy EA, Ho KJ, Menard MT, Gates JD. Ruptured and unruptured mycotic superior mesenteric artery aneurysms. *Ann Vasc Surg.* 2014;28(8):1931.

26. Sarac TP, Gates L. Endovascular repair of splanchnic artery aneurysms. In: Hans S, Shepard AD, Weaver MR, Bove P, Long GW, eds. *Practical Endovascular and Open Vascular Reconstruction.* Boca Raton, FL: CRC Press; 2016.

27. Berceli SA. Hepatic and splenic artery aneurysms. *Semin Vasc Surg.* 2005;18:196-201.

28. Graham LM, Stanley JC, Whitehouse WM, et al. Celiac artery aneurysms: historic (1745-1949) versus contemporary (1950-1984) differences in etiology and clinical importance. *J Vasc Surg.* 1985;2:757-764.

29. Stone WM, Abbas MA, Gloviczki PP, et al. Celiac arterial aneurysms: a critical reappraisal of a rare entity. *Arch Surg.* 2002;137:670-674.

30. Moore E, Matthews MR, Minion DJ, et al. Surgical management of peripancreatic arterial aneurysms. *J Vasc Surg.* 2004;40:247-253.

31. Manazer JR, Monzon JR, Dietz PA, et al. Treatment of pancreatic pseudoaneurysm with percutaneous transabdominal thrombin injection. *J Vasc Surg.* 2003;38:600-602.

32. Tessier DJ, Abbas MA, Fowl RJ, et al. Management of rare mesenteric arterial branch aneurysms. *Ann Vasc Surg.* 2002;16:586-590.

33. Lorelli DR, Cambria RA, Seabrook GR, et al. Diagnosis and management of aneurysms involving the superior mesenteric artery and its branches—a report of four cases. *Vasc Endovasc Surg.* 2003;37:59-66.

34. Sachdev-Ost U. Visceral artery aneurysms: review of current management options. *Mt Sinai J Med.* 2010;77:296-303.

Patric Liang • Mark C. Wyers

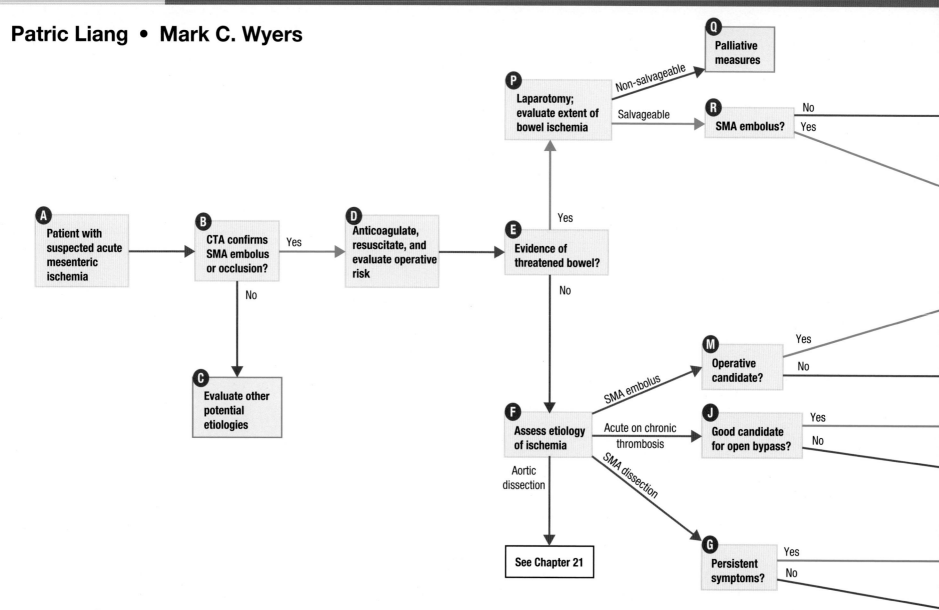

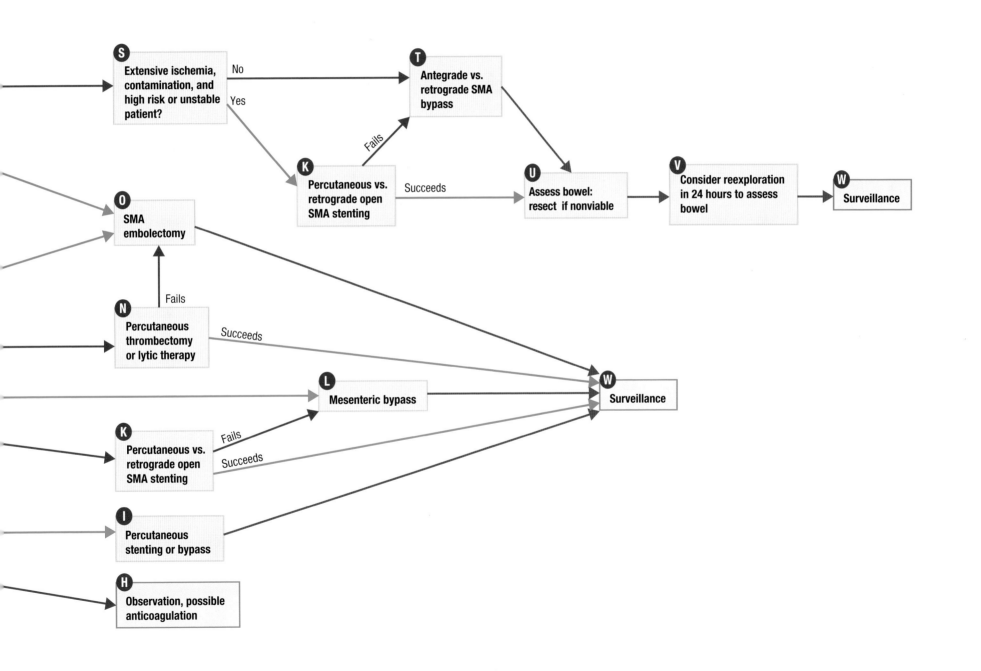

A **Patient with suspected acute mesenteric ischemia**

Despite advancements in treatment options, mortality and morbidity rates for patients presenting with acute mesenteric ischemia (AMI) remain high. The reported postoperative mortality following revascularization ranges from 28% to 50%, depending on the presentation severity and type of intervention performed.[1,2] Early diagnosis and treatment is critical in the management of AMI because of the limited time to salvage the acutely threatened bowel and the rapid progression of AMI to a catastrophic, nonsalvageable abdominal event. Unfortunately, the diagnosis of AMI is elusive and delayed diagnosis is common. The classic presentation of AMI with abdominal pain that is out of proportion to physical examination is absent in up to a quarter of patients.[3] This is further complicated by the rarity of the disease and the large differential in the workup of generalized abdominal pain.

Symptoms and factors more associated with AMI than with other causes of abdominal pain include rapid progression of pain, atrial fibrillation, and longstanding chronic mesenteric ischemia. Physical examination of the abdomen in early stages of AMI may not elicit significant tenderness to palpation. In later stages, patients with transmural bowel necrosis ± bowel perforation will develop peritonitis. Other symptoms such as abdominal distension, diarrhea, metabolic acidosis, sepsis, and GI bleeding can aid in diagnosis, but are neither specific nor sensitive findings.

B **CTA confirms SMA embolus or occlusion?**

Patients with high suspicion of AMI should undergo abdominal CTA with arterial and early venous phase without oral contrast. CTA not only evaluates mesenteric vessels but can also help identify related signs of bowel ischemia or other sources of abdominal pain if the mesenteric arteries are patent. In addition, thrombotic versus embolic causes of AMI can be differentiated. Patients with acute on chronic mesenteric ischemia will have significant calcification and stenosis at the ostia of the mesenteric arteries with intraluminal thrombosis of the remaining vessel lumen. Patients with embolic disease typically lack evidence of significant atherosclerosis of the mesenteric arteries with an embolus found lodged beyond the origin of the SMA. Even in patients with nonanaphylactic contrast allergies and renal insufficiency, quality imaging outweighs the potential risks to avoid delay in diagnosis.

DUS and MRA, although useful for chronic disease, have lesser roles in the diagnosis of AMI. Mesenteric DUS imaging in the acute setting can be limited by off-hour availability, patient pain, bowel gas, and inability to evaluate alternative causes of abdominal pain. Plain abdominal x-ray findings are often normal and nonspecific. However, findings of ileus may indicate early intestinal ischemia. Bowel edema, pneumatosis, or free abdominal air can be seen with more advanced intestinal ischemia as well as with bowel perforation. MRA imaging is suboptimal in the acute

setting because of limited availability and long acquisition times. MRA imaging also does not demonstrate vessel calcification and fails to provide adequate resolution to assess for emboli in smaller mesenteric branches.

C **Evaluate other potential etiologies**

Other common etiologies of acute abdominal pain include bowel perforation, bowel obstruction, volvulus, appendicitis, biliary colic, acute cholecystitis, pancreatitis, diverticulitis, gastric ulcers, incarcerated or strangulated hernia, nephrolithiasis, and gastroenteritis.

D **Anticoagulate, resuscitate, and evaluate operative risk**

Initial resuscitation for all patients begins with administration of isotonic crystalloid solution and correction of electrolyte imbalances. Large amounts of crystalloid resuscitation may be necessary given ongoing fluid sequestration, especially in patients who have progressed to bowel necrosis or sepsis. Broad-spectrum antibiotics covering commensal gut flora are administered. Patients should be assessed for bleeding risks before initiating anticoagulation. If no contraindications exist, therapeutic anticoagulation should be started immediately to hinder thrombus progression. IV heparin is administered with an appropriate loading bolus (80 U/kg) and maintenance (18 U/kg) rate with a PTT goal of 60 to 80 seconds. In general, vasopressors, especially pure α-adrenergic agents, should be avoided given risk of worsening intestinal ischemia from vasoconstriction in the presence of marginally viable bowel. Patients presenting with AMI are typically older and have multiple comorbidities; however, optimization of preoperative comorbidities is difficult because of the emergent treatment required. Although it is important to gauge operative risk, this evaluation should not delay revascularization.

E **Evidence of threatened bowel?**

The presence or absence of threatened bowel heavily influences the decision between immediate exploration and further etiologic workup. On the venous-phase portion of the CTA, bowel wall nonenhancement, thickening, pneumatosis, and portal venous gas are signs suggesting need for bowel resection. However, absence of these radiographic findings does not rule out threatened bowel, so other clinical parameters in addition to experienced surgeon judgment are needed to determine the need for immediate laparotomy. Helpful physical examination findings include fever, tachycardia, tachypnea, and focal abdominal tenderness. Leukocytosis is the most specific indicator of threatened bowel. Lactic acidosis may support the diagnosis but is not sensitive or specific for bowel ischemia. Short of laparotomy in patients with concern for threatened bowel, other methods of bowel evaluation such as diagnostic laparoscopy are likely inadequate. Laparoscopy may have a role in the hands of advanced laparoscopists; however, we recommend a low threshold for a definitive exploratory

laparotomy when threatened bowel is suspected, given the lack of data to support diagnostic laparoscopy in AMI.[4,5]

F **Assess etiology of ischemia**

In a stable patient without clinical or radiographic evidence of threatened bowel, treatment options are determined by the etiology of AMI.

Spontaneous isolated symptomatic mesenteric dissections are rare and are more often discovered incidentally on CT imaging. Mesenteric dissections as an extension of aortic dissection are discussed in Chapter 21. Isolated SMA dissection can involve proximal or distal branches of the SMA and can vary in size and extent. Although uncontrolled hypertension is seen in aortic dissection, patients with isolated SMA dissections are often normotensive and these dissections typically occur at the anterior surface.[6] Symptomatic patients can present with abdominal, back, or flank pain secondary to the dissection itself or from intestinal ischemia.

An acute thrombotic event secondary to progression of chronic mesenteric ischemia accounts for 25% to 30% of AMI cases.[7] History of postprandial abdominal pain, food fear, or weight loss, suggestive of chronic mesenteric ischemia, can often be elicited. Typically, a 3- to 6-cm segment of calcified and stenotic SMA involving the vessel origin is found to be the culprit lesion. Less commonly, the SMA may have been chronically occluded, but progression of celiac or IMA disease can reduce collateral flow and cause AMI. Some patients may present with occlusion of visceral stents or bypasses if they have had prior interventions for chronic mesenteric ischemia. Patients with chronic mesenteric ischemia often develop collateral mesenteric circulation during the slow progression of their mesenteric disease. Therefore, compared to patients suffering from embolic AMI, those with acute on chronic SMA thrombosis typically have slower progression to irreversible bowel ischemia. In fact, some patients may present with multiple days to weeks of vague abdominal pain, diarrhea, or GI bleeding without frank bowel necrosis. Nevertheless, without proper treatment, transmural bowel ischemia can occur. Given the proximal location of the SMA occlusion, the majority of the bowel is affected and there is no sparing of the proximal jejunum or transverse colon, as seen in embolic disease.

Arterial embolism, typically from a cardiac source, is the most common cause of AMI and accounts for 40% to 50% of cases.[7-9] The downward angle of the SMA from the abdominal aorta predisposes this visceral artery to thromboembolism. Predisposing cardiac factors include atrial fibrillation, decompensated heart failure, and recent MI. Alternatively, other sources of emboli include valvular vegetations and aortic thrombus. Therefore, following successful treatment of AMI, it is important to investigate the source of emboli via ECHO and thoracic aortic cross-sectional imaging to identify culprit lesions and prevent future embolic events.

Emboli typically lodge distal to the middle colic artery; however, proximal occlusion can also occur in 15% of cases.[10] The pattern of bowel ischemia with an SMA embolus just distal to the middle colic artery characteristically spares the proximal jejunum and transverse colon. This contrasts with a proximal occlusion of the SMA, which results in more diffuse bowel ischemia and necrosis. Because of the lack of preexisting mesenteric collaterals, the risk of rapid progression to bowel threat is much higher in this subset of AMI patients.

G Persistent symptoms?

Management of isolated SMA dissection is based on the patient's symptom status, extent of dissection, and presence of bowel ischemia.[11] The majority of patients with isolated spontaneous SMA dissection can be managed medically unless symptoms develop. Patients with concern for secondary mesenteric ischemia may benefit from DSA. Surgical management is rarely required.[12,13]

H Observation, possible anticoagulation

In asymptomatic patients with isolated mesenteric dissections, first-line therapy is observation with serial abdominal exams, blood pressure control, and medical management. Medical therapy should include statin and a single antiplatelet therapy for all patients. Anticoagulation with IV heparin is used selectively in patients with severe flow limitation to prevent vessel occlusion. Repeat CTA imaging is performed in the setting of persistent or worsening abdominal pain. Predischarge CTA imaging can be used to determine the long-term antiplatelet or anticoagulation plan. For patients with minimal symptoms but with evidence of severe flow limitation, anticoagulation therapy is continued for 6 to 12 months. If the dissection is stable or resolving, then antiplatelet therapy alone is likely adequate.

I Percutaneous stenting or bypass

Pain from SMA dissection itself is common and needs to be distinguished from intestinal malperfusion. In cases of abdominal pain secondary to intestinal ischemia, percutaneous endovascular SMA stenting or open repair is performed. The goal of either endovascular or open approach is to repair the initial entry tear and restore flow to the true lumen. Focal dissections can be stented. Percutaneous stenting can be performed either via transfemoral or brachial approach. Given the downward angle of the SMA, a brachial approach may allow for easier cannulation of the SMA. However, with development of steerable sheaths, the transfemoral approach has become more technically feasible with a lower risk of access site complications. Unlike orificial lesions associated with atherosclerosis, SMA dissections more often start beyond the SMA origin and involve the more distal aspects of the artery. Typically, a self-expanding nitinol stent is used to cover the dissection origin and reexpand the true lumen. It may be necessary to cross some jejunal branches, but only if necessary to establish flow to the main ileocolic branches. More complex dissections or occlusions may require surgical intimectomy with patch angioplasty or surgical bypass.

J Good candidate for open bypass?

Treatment options for acute on chronic thrombosis with evidence of bowel ischemia are based on anatomic considerations and medical comorbidities. Short-segment occlusions may be worth an initial aortogram and percutaneous endovascular recanalization. More extensive occlusion may better be treated with bypass. Bypass requires adequate inflow either from the iliac, infrarenal, or supraceliac aorta, although, in the urgent setting, iliac inflow is preferred because it can be rapidly established and avoids hemodynamic stress of an aortic clamp. In the absence of adequate inflow arteries due to severe aortic or iliac calcification, a hybrid approach with retrograde open mesenteric stenting (ROMS) can be used to recanalize even extensive occlusions. Patients with severe pulmonary or cardiac disease may not tolerate bypass and may also benefit from a percutaneous or hybrid approach.

K Percutaneous vs. retrograde open SMA stenting

Endovascular management with PTA and stenting can be an option for patients who do not require immediate laparotomy out of concern for bowel compromise. Transfemoral SMA intervention can be facilitated with a steerable tip sheath. Brachial access can also be helpful given the downward angle of the SMA. Success rates with percutaneous intervention are higher if the SMA origin is still visible on lateral aortography. In general, percutaneous interventions with long-segment flush occlusions are technically challenging and time consuming.

ROMS has a higher rate of technical success for more difficult SMA lesions and is a good alternative to the percutaneous approach, especially in patients who require bowel exploration.[14] Compared to open bypass, ROMS offers a less invasive method of revascularization and avoids the time needed for vein harvest, the concern for prosthetic graft infection and kinking, and the need for aortic clamping. ROMS is performed through an upper midline incision. A local thromboendarterectomy of the distal SMA is initially performed with patch angioplasty. Wires, catheters, and sheaths are then advanced via this site in a retrograde manner into the aorta, after which the SMA stenosis is treated with one or occasionally overlapping balloon-expandable stents. Both bare-metal and covered stents are appropriate for mesenteric stenting; however, some retrospective studies have shown better patency rates and less symptom recurrences with stent grafts.[15]

L Mesenteric bypass

For patients with extensive SMA occlusive disease with favorable inflow arteries, open bypass provides a more durable definitive revascularization. Open bypass for thrombotic mesenteric occlusions is analogous to bypass grafting for chronic mesenteric ischemia with a bias toward single-vessel retrograde bypass to the SMA. This often takes the form of a prosthetic graft oriented in a "lazy C" configuration from the right CIA to the SMA immediately below the pancreas. Antegrade bypass from the supraceliac aorta is not ideal for patients with poor cardiac function, patients with a calcified supraceliac aorta, or in the emergent setting. Although there is concern for graft infection in the setting of compromised bowel, use of vein conduit is plagued by higher risk of graft kinking and revascularization delays because of additional vein harvest time. With limited contamination, prosthetic grafts can be covered with an omental flap to reduce the chance of prosthetic graft infection.[16] In the setting of feculent peritonitis, vein conduit is preferred.

M Operative candidate?

For almost all patients with an SMA embolus, SMA embolectomy is the preferred method given the shorter time to definitive revascularization and the ability to assess the bowel for viability. However, in very select patients who are not immediately threatened by bowel ischemia and who have other baseline comorbidities that make them high risk for laparotomy, percutaneous thrombectomy ± lytic therapy has been used with varying degrees of success.[17,18] Patients who may be too high risk for laparotomy include patients with decompensated heart failure, oxygen-dependent pulmonary disease, prior complex abdominal wall reconstructions, or extensive adhesions.

N Percutaneous thrombectomy or lytic therapy

Percutaneous treatment using mechanical and chemical thrombectomy is achieved by selective cannulation of the SMA via brachial or femoral access, placement of a lytic catheter, and infusion tPA lysis. Adjunct treatments with rheolytics, suction, and other mechanical thrombectomy devices are frequently needed to restore flow within the mesenteric lumen. However, mature, well-organized cardiac emboli may not respond to any of these treatments. Failure to restore flow carries a high morbidity/mortality in this patient group. Prolonged attempts at lysis are therefore inadvisable.

O SMA embolectomy

Open SMA embolectomy is performed via laparotomy and transverse incision of the SMA between the middle and right colic branches. Sometimes, opening the outflow expels proximal clot given high systemic aortic pressure. If this does not occur, a 3- to 4-Fr Fogarty balloon catheter is passed retrograde from the SMA incision to remove the embolus and establish inflow. Distal clot can be sometimes be manually milked from smaller branches. Occasionally, 2-Fr Fogarty balloon catheters can be carefully passed distally to remove any remaining clot. The transverse incision can usually be closed primarily, but in some cases, a small patch may be required to prevent narrowing.

P Laparotomy; evaluate extent of bowel ischemia

Exploratory laparotomy is performed for any patient with evidence of threatened bowel to prevent irreversible ischemia or perforation. Systematic exploration from the ligament of Treitz to the sigmoid colon is performed with attention to color, peristalsis, and pattern of ischemia (see U for adjuncts to determine bowel viability). At initial exploration, resection is limited to areas of frank necrosis and perforation in an effort to preserve the critical length for absorption and survival. After revascularization, the bowel is again reevaluated for further potential resection. After resecting a segment of bowel, the remaining bowel is often left in discontinuity with plans for a second-look evaluation in the ensuing 24 to 48 hours after there has been time for reperfusion and demarcation. This is done to reduce the likelihood of failure due to ischemia at the site of bowel anastomosis.

Q Palliative measures

In critically ill patients with extensive bowel necrosis, a decision not to revascularize is sometimes made when the chance of survival is negligible. In other cases, it may be reasonable to perform revascularization and bowel resection with the understanding that short gut syndrome may occur. Patients with less than 200 cm of combined jejunum-ilium are at risk for developing short gut syndrome. During subsequent operations, further bowel resection is often necessary, contributing to further malabsorption and malnutrition, and, ultimately, death. In these dire circumstances, further exploration and revascularization is abandoned in favor of palliative care measures.

R SMA embolus?

Treatment options are determined by the etiology of AMI. Patients with SMA embolus should undergo immediate open embolectomy. Patients with acute on chronic thrombosis can either undergo retrograde or antegrade mesenteric bypass or ROMS.

S Extensive ischemia, contamination, and high-risk or unstable patient?

ROMS is the preferred treatment modality in the setting of extensive bowel ischemia or bowel perforation, and for high-risk or unstable patients. Compared to open bypass, ROMS offers a quicker, less invasive method of revascularization by avoiding the need for conduit harvest and dissection and clamping of the iliac or aortic inflow vessels. In addition, ROMS eliminates the potential for graft kinking from the difficult orientation associated with retrograde bypass grafts. Finally, in the setting of peritoneal sepsis, ROMS avoids placement of a prosthetic graft in a contaminated field. Open bypass is preferred in patients with extensive SMA occlusive disease with favorable inflow arteries and for patients who fail ROMS (see K for description of ROMS technique).

T Antegrade vs. retrograde SMA bypass

In the emergent setting, retrograde bypass is preferred over antegrade bypasses to avoid the additional physiologic insult associated with supraceliac aortic clamping. Antegrade bypass is occasionally necessary if there is no available iliac inflow vessel and may avoid problems with graft kinking because of a more direct orientation. With either approach, limiting the revascularization to the SMA is adequate and advisable (see L for description of technique for mesenteric bypass).

U Assess bowel; resect if nonviable

Signs of successful reperfusion include a palpable SMA pulse, Doppler signals throughout the mesenteric arcade, and return of normal appearing bowel serosa ± peristalsis. Other adjuncts such as fluorescein injection and laser Doppler flowmeters have been used; however, none of these modalities have been shown to be superior to good surgical judgment.[19-21] Following reperfusion, 20 to 30 minutes should be allowed before declaring and resecting a segment of irreversibly threatened bowel. Glucagon (1 mg IV) can be given to reduce splanchnic vasoconstriction.[22,23] Typically, a staged second-look operation is performed to allow questionably viable segments of bowel time to recover. However, in select patients with early presentation, minimal metabolic derangement, and clearly viable bowel, the abdomen can be closed without plans for reexploration.

V Consider reexploration in 24 hours to assess bowel

For most patients in whom bowel viability is unclear after the initial exploration and revascularization, an obligate plan for a second-look operation should be made. The intestine is left in discontinuity if a resection was performed and the abdomen left open with a vacuum dressing. The timing of a second-look operation is typically 12 to 48 hours after continued aggressive resuscitation in the intensive care unit. At the second-look operation, having allowed time for bowel demarcation, further resection is frequently needed.[24] If bowel viability is clear at this time without significant bowel edema, bowel anastomoses are performed and the abdomen is closed. If the abdomen cannot be closed, a third operation may be necessary.

W Surveillance

Restenosis of mesenteric stents is seen in one-third of patients within the first year. Close surveillance and reintervention with percutaneous treatments is important to avoid mesenteric stent thrombosis. Mesenteric bypass grafts are also prone to restenosis or occlusion and must be followed up closely. DUS is the most cost-effective modality to follow mesenteric stent or bypass patency. After index revascularization, we recommend DUS three times in the first year followed by twice yearly indefinitely. Standard mesenteric DUS criteria or symptoms are used to evaluate

the need for further imaging or reintervention. However, there is no current consensus regarding the absolute velocity threshold for reintervention because it is recognized that mesenteric stents without stenoses can falsely elevate velocities. DUS to evaluate anastomotic stenoses is analogous to other bypass graft surveillance, but because of the variability of graft configurations, communication with the vascular ultrasound technologist is important. CTA imaging can be used selectively to confirm findings from DUS and help evaluate the need for reintervention.

REFERENCES

1. Arthurs ZM, Titus J, Bannazadeh M, et al. A comparison of endovascular revascularization with traditional therapy for the treatment of acute mesenteric ischemia. *J Vasc Surg.* 2011;53(3):698-704.
2. Schermerhorn ML, Giles KA, Hamdan AD, Wyers MC, Pomposelli FB. Mesenteric revascularization: management and outcomes in the United States, 1988-2006. *J Vasc Surg.* 2009;50(2):341-348.e1.
3. Howard TJ, Plaskon LA, Wiebke EA, Wilcox MG, Madura JA. Nonocclusive mesenteric ischemia remains a diagnostic dilemma. *Am J Surg.* 1996;171(4):405-408.
4. Cudnik MT, Darbha S, Jones J, Macedo J, Stockton SW, Hiestand BC. The diagnosis of acute mesenteric ischemia: a systematic review and meta-analysis. *Acad Emerg Med.* 2013;20(11):1087-1100.
5. Stefanidis D, Richardson WS, Chang L, Earle DB, Fanelli RD. The role of diagnostic laparoscopy for acute abdominal conditions: an evidence-based review. *Surg Endosc.* 2009;23(1):16-23.
6. Park YJ, Park CW, Park KB, Roh YN, Kim DI, Kim YW. Inference from clinical and fluid dynamic studies about underlying cause of spontaneous isolated superior mesenteric artery dissection. *J Vasc Surg.* 2011;53(1):80-86.
7. Lock G. Acute intestinal ischaemia. *Best Pract Res Clin Gastroenterol.* 2001;15(1):83-98.
8. Acosta S, Ögren M, Sternby NH, Bergqvist D, Björck M. Clinical implications for the management of acute thromboembolic occlusion of the superior mesenteric artery: Autopsy findings in 213 patients. *Ann Surg.* 2005;241(3):516-522.
9. Zettervall SL, Lo RC, Soden PA, et al. Trends in treatment and mortality for mesenteric ischemia in the United States from 2000 to 2012. *Ann Vasc Surg.* 2017;42:111-119.
10. Boley SJ, Feinstein FR, Sammartano R, Brandt LJ, Sprayregen S. New concepts in the management of emboli of the superior mesenteric artery. *Surg Gynecol Obstet.* 1981;153(4):561-569.
11. Min S Il, Yoon KC, Min SK, et al. Current strategy for the treatment of symptomatic spontaneous isolated dissection of superior mesenteric artery. *J Vasc Surg.* 2011;54(2):461-466.

12. Heo SH, Kim YW, Woo SY, Park YJ, Park KB, Kim DK. Treatment strategy based on the natural course for patients with spontaneous isolated superior mesenteric artery dissection. *J Vasc Surg.* 2017;65(4):1142-1151.

13. Zettervall SL, Karthaus EG, Soden PA, et al. Clinical presentation, management, follow-up, and outcomes of isolated celiac and superior mesenteric artery dissections. *J Vasc Surg.* 2017;65(1):91-98.

14. Wyers MC, Powell RJ, Nolan BW, Cronenwett JL. Retrograde mesenteric stenting during laparotomy for acute occlusive mesenteric ischemia. *J Vasc Surg.* 2007;45(2):269-275.

15. Oderich GS, Erdoes LS, Lesar C, et al. Comparison of covered stents versus bare metal stents for treatment of chronic atherosclerotic mesenteric arterial disease. *J Vasc Surg.* 2013; 58(5):1316-1323.

16. Kazmers A. Operative management of acute mesenteric ischemia. *Ann Vasc Surg.* 1998;12(2):187-197.

17. Brountzos EN, Critselis A, Magoulas D, Kagianni E, Kelekis DA. Emergency endovascular treatment of a superior mesenteric artery occlusion. *Cardiovasc Intervent Radiol.* 2001; 24(1):57-60.

18. Gartenschlaeger S, Bender S, Maeurer J, Schroeder RJ. Successful percutaneous transluminal angioplasty and stenting in acute mesenteric ischemia. *Cardiovasc Intervent Radiol.* 2008;31(2):398-400.

19. Whitehill TA, Pearce WH, Rosales C, Yano T, Van Way CW, Rutherford RB. Detection thresholds of nonocclusive intestinal hypoperfusion by Doppler ultrasound, photoplethysmography, and fluorescein. *J Vasc Surg.* 1988; 8(1):28-32.

20. Wright CB, Hobson RW. Prediction of intestinal viability using Doppler ultrasound technics. *Am J Surg.* 1975; 129(6):642-645.

21. Carter MS, Fantinl GA, Sammartano RJ, Mttsudo S, Silverman DG, Boley SJ. Qualitative and quantitative fluorescein fluorescence in determining intestinal viability. *Am J Surg.* 1984;147(1):472-481.

22. Kazmers A, Zwolak R, Appelman HD, et al. Pharmacologic interventions in acute mesenteric ischemia. Improved survival with intravenous glucagon, methylprednisolone, and prostacyclin. *J Vasc Surg.* 1984;1(3):472-481.

23. Gangadharan SP, Wagner RJ, Cronenwett JL. Effect of intravenous glucagon on intestinal viability after segmental mesenteric ischemia. *J Vasc Surg.* 1995;21(6):900-907; discussion 907-908.

24. Kougias P, Lau D, El Sayed HF, Zhou W, Huynh TT, Lin PH. Determinants of mortality and treatment outcome following surgical interventions for acute mesenteric ischemia. *J Vasc Surg.* 2007;46(3):467-474.

Nicholas J. Swerdlow • Marc L. Schermerhorn

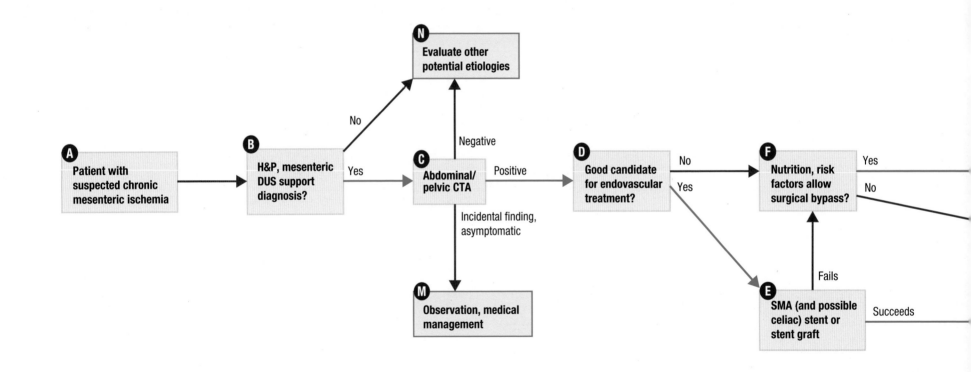

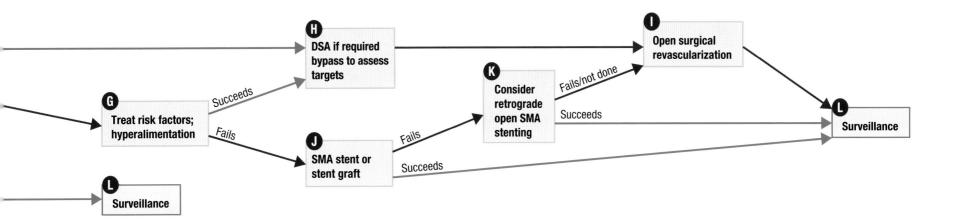

A Patient with suspected chronic mesenteric ischemia

Chronic mesenteric ischemia (CMI) typically presents in patients in their sixties. Unlike PAD or aneurysmal disease in which men predominate, women comprise 70% to 80% of patients. Most patients with CMI have a history of smoking and cardiovascular comorbidities including HTN, CAD, and PAD.[1,2] Because of the rich collateral circulation of the gut, patients with CMI usually have "three-vessel" disease involving the celiac artery (CA), SMA, and IMA, although two- or even one-vessel involvement can occasionally cause symptoms if collateral circulation is inadequate.

B H&P, mesenteric DUS support diagnosis?

The most common presenting symptoms of CMI are abdominal pain, present in more than 90% of patients, and weight loss, present in more than 70% of patients. Although this pain is typically postprandial, occurs 10 to 15 minutes after eating, and lasts 1 to 4 hours, overall presentation may be more vague. Another frequent symptom is "food fear," a fear of eating caused by postprandial severe pain, eventually leading to weight loss, which can be substantial if diagnosis is delayed. Diarrhea, nausea, or vomiting can often be seen in patients with CMI.[1,3] The classic triad of symptoms (postprandial pain, "food-fear," and weight loss), is seldom observed. Physical examination findings in CMI are nonspecific, although signs of recent weight loss and an abdominal bruit can be suggestive. The diagnosis of CMI is often delayed given the nonspecific nature of presenting symptoms, and many patients undergo significant workup of their abdominal pain before vascular surgery evaluation. This is in part because other causes of abdominal pain, such as gastroesophageal reflux disease or symptomatic cholelithiasis, are much more common than CMI.

Mesenteric DUS is an excellent screening tool for patients for whom a diagnosis of CMI is suspected. Although limited by overlying bowel gas and body habitus in some cases, fasting DUS assessment of the CA and SMA is technically successful in most patients. Diagnostic criteria for the diagnosis of CA and SMA stenosis have been published and subsequently validated.[4-6] A PSV $\geq$275 cm/s or no flow predicts $\geq$70% SMA stenosis with 89% sensitivity and 92% specificity and a PSV $\geq$200 or no flow predicts $\geq$70% CA stenosis with 75% sensitivity and 89% sensitivity. An end-diastolic velocity (EDV) >55 cm/s predicts $\geq$70% SMA stenosis with 88% sensitivity and 94% specificity and predicts $\geq$70% CA stenosis with 58% sensitivity and 77% specificity.[5] Retrograde flow in the common hepatic artery is 100% predictive of high-grade CA stenosis or CA occlusion.[6]

C Abdominal/pelvic CTA

Patients with symptoms suggestive of CMI with a negative, equivocal, or nondiagnostic DUS warrant further evaluation with CTA or MRA, if CTA is contraindicated. Such studies are obtained in all patients before any intervention. A high-quality CTA allows for identification of lesions of the CA, SMA, and IMA, as well as providing detailed characterization of each lesion, specifically severity, length, and degree of calcification, which aid in planning intervention. A CTA also evaluates for alternative abdominal pathology and can aid in the assessment of bowel viability in acute or acute-on-CMI (see Chapter 36). Gadolinium-enhanced MRA provides a similar evaluation and preference of CTA or MRA is largely center dependent. However, it is important to note that MRA lacks the evaluation of calcification provided by CTA, which is an important factor in the decision to proceed with endovascular or open repair and for clamp placement with open revascularization.

Because the use of CTA for the diagnosis of abdominal pathology has increased, so has the incidence of asymptomatic mesenteric arterial disease diagnosed as an incidental finding. Patients referred to a vascular surgeon with an incidental finding of mesenteric arterial disease should undergo a thorough evaluation for the signs and symptoms of CMI and patients with symptoms suggestive of CMI should undergo continued workup and subsequent treatment.

The natural history of asymptomatic mesenteric arterial disease, however, is generally benign, requiring only risk factor management and observation. Among 553 asymptomatic elderly patients, 18% had at least single-vessel mesenteric arterial disease; however, at 6 years, no patients became symptomatic and there were no deaths attributed to mesenteric ischemia.[7] In another review of 980 aortograms not done for mesenteric disease, 8% had at least CA, SMA, or IMA stenosis. Over mean follow-up of 2.6 years, four patients developed symptomatic CMI, all of whom had three-vessel disease initially. Thus, in the rare patient incidentally found to have asymptomatic, but diseased CA, SMA and IMA, prophylactic treatment is rarely needed.

D Good candidate for endovascular treatment?

Consistent with trends nationwide, the authors have adopted an endovascular-first approach to CMI treatment. Nearly all mesenteric arteries can be successfully treated via femoral access if a deflecting tip sheath is used. Brachial access can be employed when a femoral approach is unsuccessful because of steep downward angulation of the mesenteric vessels. Patients with severely calcific three-vessel disease and patients with chronic occlusions are less amenable to endovascular revascularization, and open bypass should be considered if the patient is a surgical candidate.

There have been no randomized, controlled trials comparing open and endovascular treatment of CMI, but large observational studies have found endovascular intervention to be associated with lower perioperative mortality, despite an older cohort with more medical comorbidities.[2,8-10] In contrast, smaller single-center series and meta-analyses have not demonstrated a difference in mortality between the two approaches, although open surgery is consistently associated with a higher rate of perioperative complications.[1,11-13]

Despite excellent rates of technical success at the index procedure, recurrent stenosis and symptom recurrence are common after endovascular treatment of CMI. At 5 years, primary patency has been reported as low as 41% with close to 50% of patients experiencing a recurrence of symptoms.[11,14] When reintervening after prior mesenteric artery stenting, the authors use an endovascular-first approach with repeat angioplasty $\pm$ stenting as needed. However, if endovascular intervention is unsuccessful, patients deemed at appropriate operative risk may require mesenteric bypass to restore adequate flow.

E SMA (and possible celiac) stent or stent graft

Most patients with CMI have multivessel involvement, most commonly SMA disease with concurrent CA and/or IMA disease.[14,15] The decision to pursue single-vessel versus multiple-vessel revascularization in these patients remains controversial. For patients undergoing open mesenteric bypass, single-center series of patients undergoing SMA revascularization alone demonstrate excellent durability with 4-year patency approaching 90%.[16,17] However, there are data suggesting that multivessel revascularization is associated with higher long-term patency.[18] Similar data are more limited for patients undergoing endovascular intervention. However, in a series from the Mayo Clinic, SMA and CA stenting did not appear to impart an advantage over SMA stenting alone in patients with multivessel disease, although there is likely substantial selection bias in this cohort, because the decision to pursue multivessel stenting was partially dependent on the outcome of the first intervention.[15]

In patients undergoing both single- or multiple-vessel revascularization with either an open or endovascular approach, the success of the revascularization relies heavily on the SMA. Therefore, the SMA should be the primary target for revascularization in all patients with multivessel disease and SMA involvement. Isolated CA endovascular revascularization is associated with high rates of reintervention and should be avoided if possible.[15-17,19,20] Although the data are limited and stent choice depends largely on lesion characteristics, there is evidence that use of balloon-expandable stent grafts is associated with higher long-term patency than with balloon-expandable bare-metal stents.[21]

Although most patients presenting with CMI, over 90% in most series, have two- or three-vessel disease, a small proportion of patients with CMI will have SMA disease alone.[14,15,17] These patients warrant reevaluation of the diagnosis of CMI and further workup of other possible causes if their prior workup was incomplete. Attention should also be paid to collateral flow between the SMA and CA. Patients with a small or absent gastroduodenal artery, whether congenitally or due to previous abdominal surgery, are prone to single-vessel SMA disease because of lack of collateral flow from the CA. If there is high suspicion for CMI, patients with isolated SMA disease should undergo revascularization.

A patient presenting with signs/symptoms of CMI and isolated CA disease should raise suspicion for celiac artery compression syndrome (discussed separately in Chapter 39).

The authors do not intervene on the IMA unless the SMA and CA are not amenable to revascularization.

F Nutrition, risk factors allow surgical bypass?

Patients with mesenteric atherosclerotic disease likely have atherosclerotic disease in coronary, peripheral, and carotid arterial; vascular beds. The rate of CAD in patients undergoing revascularization for CMI has been reported to be as high as 69%. Other common comorbid conditions include HTN, hypercholesterolemia, COPD, and diabetes.[1,10,22,23] Therefore, a thorough preoperative evaluation is required to determine whether the patient is a candidate for open mesenteric bypass. On the basis of the patient's history, this workup may include a cardiac stress test, PFTs, carotid DUS, and lower extremity noninvasive arterial studies.

Malnutrition is common in patients presenting with CMI. Therefore, an evaluation of nutritional status must be performed before open surgical revascularization including iron, albumin, and vitamin levels.

G Treat risk factors; hyperalimentation

Patients who are not endovascular candidates and are at high risk for open surgery with modifiable risk factors should undergo treatment to optimize them for surgery. For example, patients with treatable CAD should undergo coronary revascularization before mesenteric bypass. In addition, all patients should undergo medical management to slow the progression of their atherosclerotic disease. This consists primarily of smoking cessation (see Chapter 3) and management of hyperlipidemia (see Chapter 4). Finally, patients with CMI should be on antiplatelet and statin therapy (regardless of lipid levels).

Some patients with symptomatic CMI may not be surgical candidates because of their nutritional status. The symptoms of CMI can lead to a dramatic decrease in caloric intake and subsequent weight loss and malnutrition. Patients with malnutrition at diagnosis should undergo oral nutritional supplementation. If this cannot be tolerated because of the severity of symptoms, patients should undergo IV hyperalimentation to improve their nutrition before bypass. To the extent that these measures are successful, open surgical bypass can be undertaken. If not, endovascular treatment can be attempted even if anatomic features are not ideal.

H DSA if required to assess bypass targets

Historically the gold standard in the diagnosis of mesenteric artery stenosis, the role of diagnostic mesenteric angiography has largely been replaced by CTA. If there are specific anatomic concerns, or the quality of preoperative CTA is limited, such as in patients with streak artifact from a metal implant, a preoperative DSA may be needed.

When performing mesenteric arteriography, CA and SMA lesions are best visualized in a lateral projection. The AP projection, on the other hand, will demonstrate the full arborization of the SMA, identify distal disease, and demonstrate collaterals between the SMA, CA, and IMA. In many cases, multiple projections will be needed to visualize the full extent of a lesion. DSA is an important adjunct to improve visualization of detailed anatomic features of the mesenteric lesions.

I Open surgical revascularization

Although no randomized controlled trials have compared open to endovascular treatment of CMI, evidence from observational studies suggest that open repair is associated with higher perioperative morbidity and possibly higher perioperative mortality.[9,10] However, mesenteric bypass is associated with higher long-term durability than mesenteric stenting with 3-year primary patency rates as high as 93%.[12,13,17,23,24] Mesenteric bypass for the treatment of CMI in the endovascular era is used primarily for patients with a pattern of disease not amenable to an endovascular approach or who failed initial endovascular intervention, in addition to those with restenosis or occlusion after prior endovascular intervention(s).

The three primary technical considerations when performing mesenteric bypass for CMI are target vessel(s), graft configuration, and conduit. Most patients undergoing revascularization for CMI have multivessel disease. In single-center series of patients undergoing open revascularization, most patients underwent multivessel bypass. However, these studies failed to demonstrate a benefit to multivessel revascularization compared to single-vessel revascularization, and isolated SMA bypass has comparable long-term durability in most series. Regardless of target vessel, bypass grafts can be configured in an antegrade manner from the supraceliac aorta or in a retrograde manner from the infrarenal aorta or CIA. There is no evidence clearly demonstrating superiority of one approach over the other. Therefore, the choice of inflow should be made on a case-by-case basis depending on surgeon preference and patient anatomy. Finally, both prosthetic graft and vein can be used as conduit for mesenteric revascularization. A mesenteric bypass is generally a relatively short, high-flow graft and thus a prosthetic graft is more commonly used, although there is limited evidence comparing prosthetic and vein conduits for mesenteric bypass.[16,17,22,23,25]

The authors prefer antegrade two-vessel bypass when feasible, because the additional bypass adds little morbidity, but may be helpful if one graft later fails. If there is no healthy aorta for a supraceliac anastomosis, a single-vessel retrograde bypass from the right CIA is used, ideally to the SMA if there is an adequate target. The left CIA and infrarenal aorta can also be used for inflow. The authors' practice is to use a prosthetic graft, either Dacron or ringed ePTFE. However, in cases of acute ischemia with necrotic bowel requiring bowel resection, the risk of graft infection is elevated and the use of a vein graft should be considered (see Chapter 36).

J SMA stent or stent graft

In patients who are poor endovascular candidates or have failed prior endovascular intervention but are unsuitable for open revascularization despite medical treatment of comorbidities and adequate nutritional support, endovascular intervention remains an option. When repeating an intervention after a prior technical failure, better equipment should be used (eg, a deflecting tip sheath, wire, and catheters designed to cross difficult lesions), a different approach should be considered (eg, brachial access if femoral access was used originally), and a different vessel could be targeted. A detailed discussion with the patient explaining the possibility of treatment failure or incomplete treatment is necessary, along with a discussion balancing the risks and benefits of attempted treatment. During treatment, a suboptimal plan may be necessary, including isolated CA stenting if the SMA cannot be treated. IMA intervention is also an option if no other treatment options exist.

K Consider retrograde open SMA stenting

Retrograde open mesenteric artery stenting (ROMS) involves direct access to the SMA distal to the lesion via a laparotomy, and has been successfully used to cross and treat lesions that could not be treated in an antegrade manner. It is a less extensive open procedure than is mesenteric bypass. Although primarily used for acute ischemia, this technique has also been described in the treatment of CMI, and is an option for patients who fail an antegrade approach and are suboptimal candidates for open bypass either due to calcification of the aortoiliac vessels or medical comorbidity.[26]

L Surveillance

Restenosis is common after both open and especially endovascular treatment of CMI. Given that a proportion of patients will develop significant restenosis before recurrence of symptoms, follow-up based purely on symptom status is insufficient and periodic imaging is indicated. Mesenteric DUS is the mainstay of follow-up evaluation following mesenteric revascularization. In the authors' practice, patients are evaluated at 1 month, 6 months, 1 year, and then annually. However, follow-up is repeated more frequently if there is evidence of at least moderate restenosis. In addition, prompt diagnostic imaging with DUS or CTA is indicated on symptom recurrence. Patients with stenosis following primary endovascular intervention are at high risk for restenosis after repeat endovascular intervention and mesenteric bypass should be considered if the patient is of appropriate operative risk. However, repeat endovascular intervention may be beneficial before planned bypass to prevent further progression of disease and subsequent preoperative malnutrition. Patients who have undergone both open and endovascular revascularization for CMI remain at risk for acute mesenteric ischemia, and if their presentation is consistent with acute ischemia, emergent workup and treatment is indicated (see Chapter 36).

Importantly, DUS criteria for native mesenteric arteries may not apply in the follow-up period for patients treated with mesenteric artery stenting because these criteria may overestimate in-stent restenosis. For instance, most patients with an SMA stent will have a PSV of ≥275 cm/s, the cutoff for >70% stenosis in a native SMA, immediately following technically successful SMA stenting. Although there are no clearly defined criteria, Soult et al. found that a PSV threshold of ≥445 cm/s was predictive of ≥70% SMA in-stent restenosis with a sensitivity and specificity of 83%. A PSV threshold of ≥289 was predictive of ≥70% CA stenosis with 100% sensitivity and 57% specificity.[27,28] Although, "normal" PSV post stenting may be higher than in unstented arteries, it is important to note that an initial high posttreatment PSV may also be the result of a poor initial technical result.

Ⓜ Observation, medical management

Patients with asymptomatic CMI should be counseled on risk factor management, especially smoking cessation (see Chapter 3) and management of hyperlipidemia (see Chapter 4). All patients with CMI should be on antiplatelet therapy in the absence of contraindication. They should also be counseled on the symptoms of CMI and be instructed to return to clinic if they develop any concerning symptoms. Finally, in select circumstances, patients with asymptomatic mesenteric arterial disease may benefit from mesenteric revascularization if undergoing concomitant aortic surgery.[29]

Ⓝ Evaluate other potential etiologies

Patients with abdominal pain, weight loss, and/or other GI symptoms who do not have CMI require a further diagnostic workup. A variety of GI conditions, including malignancies, can mimic CMI.

REFERENCES

1. Tallarita T, Oderich GS, Gloviczki P, et al. Patient survival after open and endovascular mesenteric revascularization for chronic mesenteric ischemia. *J Vasc Surg.* 2013;57(3):747-755.
2. Schermerhorn ML, Giles KA, Hamdan AD, Wyers MC, Pomposelli FB. Mesenteric revascularization: management and outcomes in the United States, 1988-2006. *J Vasc Surg.* 2009;50(2):341-348.
3. Ryer EJ, Oderich GS, Bower TC, et al. Differences in anatomy and outcomes in patients treated with open mesenteric revascularization before and after the endovascular era. *J Vasc Surg.* 2011;53(6):1611-1618.e2.
4. Bowersox JC, Zwolak RM, Walsh DB, et al. Duplex ultrasonography in the diagnosis of celiac and mesenteric artery occlusive disease. *J Vasc Surg.* 1991;14(6):780-786; discussion 786-788.
5. Moneta GL, Yeager RA, Dalman R, Antonovic R, Hall LD, Porter JM. Duplex ultrasound criteria for diagnosis of splanchnic artery stenosis or occlusion. *J Vasc Surg.* 1991;14(4):511-520.
6. Zwolak RM, Fillinger MF, Walsh DB, et al. Mesenteric and celiac duplex scanning: a validation study. *J Vasc Surg.* 1998;27(6):1078-1088.
7. Wilson DB, Mostafavi K, Craven TE, Ayerdi J, Edwards MS, Hansen KJ. Clinical course of mesenteric artery stenosis in elderly Americans. *Arch Intern Med.* 2006;166(19):2095-2100.
8. Zettervall SL, Lo RC, Soden PA, et al. Trends in treatment and mortality for mesenteric ischemia in the United States from 2000 to 2012. *Ann Vasc Surg.* 2017;42:111-119.
9. Erben Y, Jean RA, Protack CD, et al. Improved mortality in treatment of patients with endovascular interventions for chronic mesenteric ischemia. *J Vasc Surg.* 2018;67(6):1805-1812.
10. Lima FV, Kolte D, Kennedy KF, et al. Endovascular versus surgical revascularization for chronic mesenteric ischemia. *JACC Cardiovasc Interv.* 2017;10(23):2440-2447.
11. Gupta PK, Horan SM, Turaga KK, Miller WJ, Pipinos II. Chronic mesenteric ischemia: endovascular versus open revascularization. *J Endovasc Ther.* 2010;17(4):540-549.
12. Cai W, Li X, Shu C, et al. Comparison of clinical outcomes of endovascular versus open revascularization for chronic mesenteric ischemia: a meta-analysis. *Ann Vasc Surg.* 2015;29(5):934-940.
13. Alahdab F, Arwani R, Pasha AK, et al. A systematic review and meta-analysis of endovascular versus open surgical revascularization for chronic mesenteric ischemia. *J Vasc Surg.* 2018;67(5):1598-1605.
14. Oderich GS, Bower TC, Sullivan TM, Bjarnason H, Cha S, Gloviczki P. Open versus endovascular revascularization for chronic mesenteric ischemia: risk-stratified outcomes. *J Vasc Surg.* 2009;49(6):1472-1479.e3.
15. Malgor RD, Oderich GS, McKusick MA, et al. Results of single- and two-vessel mesenteric artery stents for chronic mesenteric ischemia. *Ann Vasc Surg.* 2010;24(8):1094-1101.
16. Gentile AT, Moneta GL, Taylor LM, Park TC, McConnell DB, Porter JM. Isolated Bypass to the Superior Mesenteric Artery for Intestinal Ischemia. *Arch Surg.* 1994;129(9):926-932.
17. Foley MI, Moneta GL, Abou-zamzam AM, et al. Revascularization of the superior mesenteric artery alone for treatment of intestinal ischemia. *J Vasc Surg.* 2000;32(1):37-47.
18. McAfee MK, Cherry KJ, Naessens JM, et al. Influence of complete revascularization on chronic mesenteric ischemia. *Am J Surg.* 1992;164(3):220-224.
19. Cho JS, Carr JA, Jacobsen G, Shepard AD, Nypaver TJ, Reddy DJ. Long-term outcome after mesenteric artery reconstruction: a 37-year experience. *J Vasc Surg.* 2002;35(3):453-460.
20. Goldman MP, Reeve TE, Craven TE, et al. Endovascular treatment of chronic mesenteric ischemia in the setting of occlusive superior mesenteric artery lesions. *Ann Vasc Surg.* 2017;38:29-35.
21. Oderich GS, Erdoes LS, Lesar C, et al. Comparison of covered stents versus bare metal stents for treatment of chronic atherosclerotic mesenteric arterial disease. *J Vasc Surg.* 2013;58(5):1316-1323.
22. Kruger AJ, Walker PJ, Foster WJ, Jenkins JS, Boyne NS, Jenkins J. Open surgery for atherosclerotic chronic mesenteric ischemia. *J Vasc Surg.* 2007;46(5):941-945.
23. McMillan WD, McCarthy WJ, Bresticker MR, et al. Mesenteric artery bypass: objective patency determination. *J Vasc Surg.* 1995;21(5):729-741.
24. Zacharias N, Eghbalieh SD, Chang BB, et al. Chronic mesenteric ischemia outcome analysis and predictors of endovascular failure. *J Vasc Surg.* 2016;63(6):1582-1587.
25. Park WM, Cherry KJ, Chua HK, et al. Current results of open revascularization for chronic mesenteric ischemia: a standard for comparison. *J Vasc Surg.* 2002;35(5):853-859.
26. Oderich GS, Macedo R, Stone DH, et al. Multicenter study of retrograde open mesenteric artery stenting through laparotomy for treatment of acute and chronic mesenteric ischemia. *J Vasc Surg.* 2018;68(2):470-480.
27. Soult MC, Wuamett JC, Ahanchi SS, Stout CL, Larion S, Panneton JM. Duplex ultrasound criteria for in-stent restenosis of mesenteric arteries. *J Vasc Surg.* 2016;64(5):1366-1372.
28. Mitchell EL, Chang EY, Landry GJ, Liem TK, Keller FS, Moneta GL. Duplex criteria for native superior mesenteric artery stenosis overestimate stenosis in stented superior mesenteric arteries. *J Vasc Surg.* 2009;50(2):335-340.
29. Thomas JH, Blake K, Pierce GE, Hermreck AS, Seigel E, Gerwertz BL. The clinical course of asymptomatic mesenteric arterial stenosis. *J Vasc Surg.* 1998;27(5):840-844.

Stefan Acosta

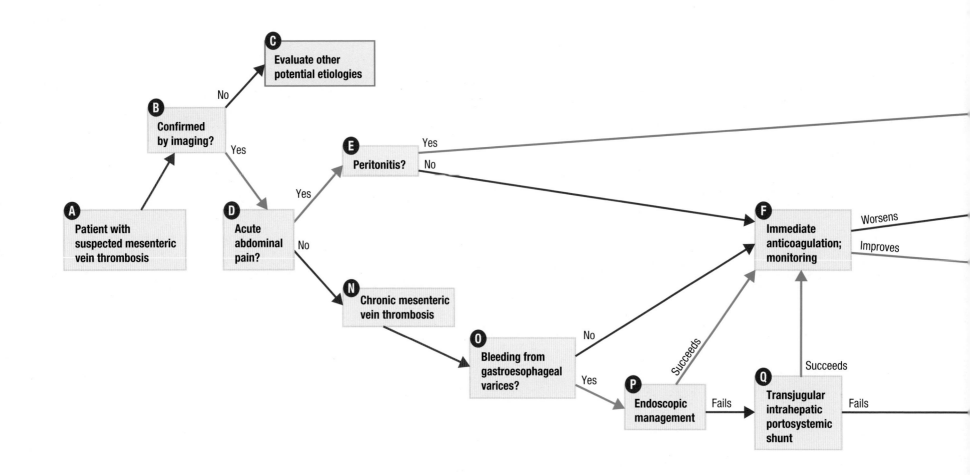

C
Evaluate other
potential etiologies

B
Confirmed
by imaging?

No

Yes

E
Peritonitis?

Yes

No

A
Patient with
suspected mesenteric
vein thrombosis

D
Acute
abdominal
pain?

Yes

No

F
Immediate
anticoagulation;
monitoring

Worsens

Improves

N
Chronic mesenteric
vein thrombosis

O
Bleeding from
gastroesophageal
varices?

No

Yes

P
Endoscopic
management

Succeeds

Fails

Q
Transjugular
intrahepatic
portosystemic
shunt

Succeeds

Fails

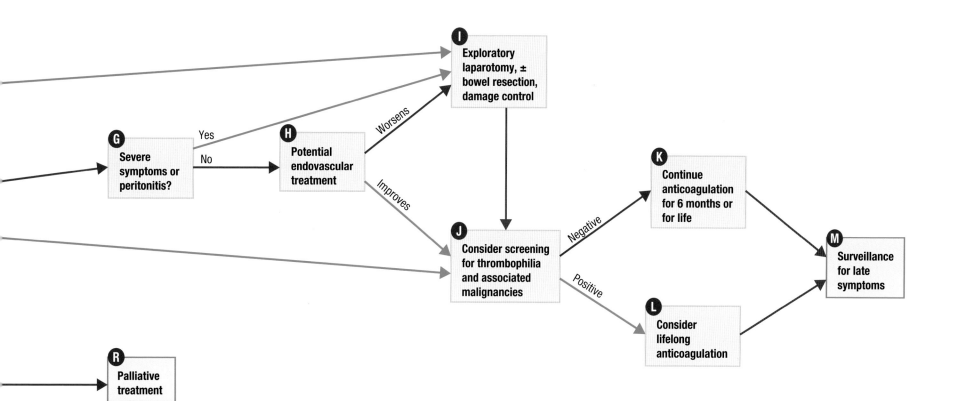

A Patient with suspected mesenteric vein thrombosis

Mesenteric vein thrombosis (MVT) occurs in middle- and older-age patients with equal sex distribution. Approximately 10% of cases are idiopathic, whereas 90% are associated with an underlying condition predisposing to thrombosis, including venous congestion, thrombophilia, and trauma. Symptoms usually consist of nonspecific abdominal pain in the early stage of the disease, whereas localized abdominal pain develops later. Melena, hematemesis, or hematochezia occurs in only 15%, but occult blood in the stool may be present in 50% of cases.[1] Fever and signs of peritonitis suggest progression of ischemia to intestinal infarction, which combined with hypotension (SBP < 90 mm Hg) are associated with poor prognosis.[2] As MVT is rarely diagnosed on clinical grounds,[3] CTA with imaging in the portal phase has become the most important, reliable, and accurate method for diagnosis.[4,5] CTA can accurately image the extent of thrombosis within the portomesenteric venous system and intestinal lesions secondary to MVT. Thrombosis within the superior mesenteric vein, in strong contrast with isolated portal vein thrombosis, is associated with symptoms related to intestinal ischemia in the overwhelming majority (92%) and often results in intestinal infarction if untreated.[6,7] A low percentage of patients with MVT will be asymptomatic and diagnosed incidentally on unrelated imaging.

B Confirmed by imaging?

The protocol for urgent CTA of the abdomen varies with the clinical history provided by the referring physician, and sometimes a second CTA with an optimized protocol for imaging may be needed. Diagnosis of portal vein thrombosis with DUS alone is not sufficient to evaluate the extent of thrombosis and cannot evaluate secondary intestinal findings, although it can suggest the diagnosis.

The responsible physicians should scrutinize CT images, as intestinal findings secondary to MVT have an impact on the need for bowel resection and mortality. CT findings such as complete thrombosis of the superior mesenteric vein and portal vein, small bowel wall thickening suggesting edema, enhancement defects of the bowel wall, and ascites are factors that increase the risk of bowel infarction.[8]

C Evaluate other potential etiologies

If CTA does not confirm presence of MVT, a myriad of alternative diagnoses must be pursued, some of which may be discovered by the CT imaging.

D Acute abdominal pain?

Acute MVT is defined by the acute onset of symptoms (within 4 weeks) of presentation and the majority of patients in a series of MVT have acute MVT.[9] The duration of symptoms, usually abdominal pain, ranges from hours to weeks;[10] however, most often these patients present within a few days to 1 week.

E Peritonitis?

A small proportion of patients with MVT will have developed peritonitis on presentation. Signs of peritonitis may not, however, correlate with the severity of intestinal ischemia. Repeated physical examination of the abdomen, laboratory testing of CRP and leucocyte count levels, and/or repeated CT examinations for evaluation of changes in intestinal abnormalities form the basis of clinical decision making.[11]

F Immediate anticoagulation; monitoring

The mainstay for treatment of MVT is anticoagulation. In the absence of major contraindications, such as bleeding esophageal varices or intracranial hemorrhage, anticoagulant therapy is recommended for all patients with acute, symptomatic MVT. In patients with chronic MVT, including incidental MVT, recommendation for anticoagulation therapy is much weaker, but may be considered in addition to further diagnostic laboratory workup. Systemic anticoagulation should be initiated immediately after confirmed diagnosis by using unfractionated or LMWH followed by vitamin K antagonists (VKAs) or direct oral anticoagulants (DOACs) to reduce the risk of thrombus propagation, intestinal infarction, portal HTN, recurrence of VTE, and overall mortality.[12] In the early phase, unfractionated heparin has the advantage of being reversible with protamine if laparotomy for intestinal infarction or GI bleeding from intestinal ischemia becomes necessary. It has been shown that early anticoagulation results in recanalization in >80% of patients and complete recanalization is associated with less extensive thrombotic disease at diagnosis.[13]

G Severe symptoms or peritonitis?

A small proportion of patients with MVT will fail with anticoagulation therapy alone.[14] Patients with persisting or recurrent symptoms, or worsening abdominal pain after initiation of anticoagulation, may be considered for either exploratory laparotomy or endovascular therapy based on severity of symptom progression. It is safer to proceed directly to laparotomy in the setting of peritonitis as it allows for direct visualization of the affected bowel and possible resection if necessary.

H Potential endovascular treatment

There are a number of endovascular techniques available,[15] including transjugular intrahepatic portosystemic shunt (TIPS) with mechanical aspiration thrombectomy, direct thrombolysis followed by angioplasty if necessary, percutaneous transhepatic mechanical thrombectomy, percutaneous transhepatic thrombolysis, and thrombolysis via the SMA. Endovascular techniques have been reported to yield favorable survival and patency of the portomesenteric veins, low rates of portal HTN and complications, and prevention of bowel resection.[16] In contrast, in a study of 16 MVT patients treated with thrombolysis via the

transhepatic route or SMA, clearance of thrombus was often only partially achieved, and treatment was associated with significant bleeding complications requiring blood transfusion in 60% of patients.[17] Currently, individual practitioner experience guides the selection of these different endovascular options if this strategy is pursued. Careful monitoring after endovascular intervention is required because laparotomy and bowel resection may still be needed.

I Exploratory laparotomy, ± bowel resection, damage control

Surgical resection of necrotic bowel with bowel anastomosis is standard in this setting. However, intraoperative distinction between irreversibly ischemic and viable bowel can be difficult. The length of the ischemic intestinal segment is often confined to the jejunum and/or ileum, and rarely involves the large bowel.[18] Every attempt is made to limit the extent of bowel resection. A damage control approach to mesenteric ischemia[15] implies immediate laparotomy with eventual resection of infarcted bowel, no attempt to restore GI continuity, a skin-only closure, or an open abdominal dressing in lieu of abdominal fascial closure. The patient is returned to the ICU to be stabilized with full anticoagulation prior to a planned subsequent second-look procedure to define the viability of the ischemic bowel and to perform a bowel anastomosis of less edematous bowel.

J Consider screening for thrombophilia and associated malignancies

Most thromboses in the superior mesenteric vein are secondary[19] to the presence of one or more predisposing conditions, either local or systemic, favoring venous thrombosis. Family history of VTE should be evaluated. Inherited thrombophilia has been identified in 36% to 55%[9,19,20] of patients with MVT. Although factor V Leiden mutation is a genetic defect, peripheral venous thrombotic manifestations are frequently delayed until adulthood. If there is no local cause for the venous thrombosis, a myeloproliferative neoplasm should be considered and screening for JAK-2 V617 (Janus-activated kinase gain of function substitute of valine to phenylalanine at position 617) mutation, an acquired disorder, is indicated. The high rate of prothrombotic factors in patients with MVT may justify routine screening, especially for factor V Leiden, prothrombin gene G20210A, and JAK-2 mutation.[21]

JAK-2 mutation–positive patients with MVT should be referred to a hematologist for evaluation of a myeloproliferative disorder. MVT is a common first clinical manifestation in patients with newly diagnosed myeloproliferative disorders such as polycythemia vera or essential thrombocytosis and often occurs before a rise in peripheral blood counts.

A significant proportion of MVT patients will have a concomitant abdominal cancer, with metastatic and pancreatic cancer commonly found.[21] Patients with cancer, particularly mucin-producing adenocarcinomas, have an increased risk of VTE. Because concomitant intra-abdominal cancer is a strong trigger for MVT, there is no reason to test for thrombophilia in such patients.[22]

K Continue anticoagulation for 6 months or for life

Anticoagulation should be given for at least 3 to 6 months, or indefinitely, if underlying, persistent prothrombotic factors are identified. Oral anticoagulation (VKA or DOAC) can be started after the acute phase of venous mesenteric ischemia (usually after 2-3 weeks) when the phase of acute ischemic injury has passed. In a multicenter, prospective registry of 604 patients with MVT,[23] anticoagulation prevented thrombotic events, but at the expense of increased major bleeding. Treatment discontinuation doubled the incidence of thrombotic events and lowered the major bleeding rate substantially.

In patients with MVT provoked by strong triggers and reversible causes such as trauma, infection, and pancreatitis, anticoagulation for 6 months is recommended.[15] Secondary prevention with LMWH in the first 3 to 6 months may be considered as an alternative to VKA or NOAC in patients with cancer.[12] The duration of anticoagulation therapy in patients with cancer is determined on the basis of the continued presence of cancer or ongoing treatment.

L Consider lifelong anticoagulation

Patients with the newly detected JAK-2 mutation should be considered for indefinite treatment. In patients with inherited thrombophilia such as factor V Leiden and prothrombin gene G20210A, especially with unprovoked MVT, lifelong anticoagulation therapy should be considered.[15]

M Surveillance for late symptoms

Patients managed conservatively with full anticoagulation should not be discharged until the possibility of intestinal infarction is ruled out. Patients should be closely followed up after discharge if the in-hospital stay was long and complicated by persistence of abdominal pain or bowel symptoms, findings of intestinal ischemia on CT at admission, and no convincing resolution of pain. A small proportion of patients will be readmitted within a few weeks of discharge with intestinal infarction or within weeks or months with severe intestinal stricture and ileus and will require emergent bowel surgery.[14]

Bleeding is commonly reported during follow-up and may be related to underlying diseases, gastroesophageal varices, and/or anticoagulation treatment. In the presence of GI bleeding, anticoagulation treatment should only be initiated after the bleeding source has been successfully treated and the patient is hemodynamically stable. The decision to start anticoagulation therapy is based on the presence of major risk factors for recurrence and/or progression of thrombosis, extent of thrombosis in the portomesenteric venous system, and the ability to address the underlying cause for bleeding.[24]

N Chronic mesenteric vein thrombosis

Patients with MVT and mild symptoms lasting 4 weeks or longer, or those without a recent onset of abdominal complaints where MVT was an incidental finding on CT, have chronic MVT. On CTA, features of a cavernoma (cavernous transformation of the portal vein) and presence of numerous collateral veins around a thrombosed portomesenteric vein system suggest chronicity. A substantial proportion of patients with MVT will develop radiologic features of chronic MVT after anticoagulation therapy,[25] whereas a minor, but not insignificant, proportion of patients will develop clinical features of portal HTN and bleeding from esophageal or gastric varices at the time of presentation,[26] or later.

O Bleeding from gastroesophageal varices?

There is a 50% incidence of radiographically noted long-term sequelae from MVT related to portal venous HTN, defined as esophageal varices, portal vein cavernous transformation, splenomegaly, or hepatic atrophy. These features were more often noted in cases of initial complete thrombosis of the superior mesenteric vein.[26] The use of anticoagulant medications in chronic MVT, for patients presenting with variceal bleeding and hypersplenism but without signs of recent occlusion, should not be considered. Acute esophageal variceal hemorrhage is a dreaded complication of portal HTN and is associated with significant mortality.

P Endoscopic management

Placement of a balloon tamponade device in the management of acute variceal hemorrhage before, or after failed, endoscopic therapy may be used as a bridge to more definitive therapy.[27] Endoscopic therapy is used to arrest bleeding varices and prevent early rebleeding. The combination of vasoconstrictor and endoscopic therapy is superior to vasoconstrictor or endoscopic therapy alone for control of acute esophageal variceal hemorrhage.[28]

Q Transjugular intrahepatic portosystemic shunt

TIPS creation is a well-established therapy for refractory variceal bleeding. Experience and technical improvements, including covered stents, have led to improved TIPS outcomes that have encouraged expanded applications such as in portomesenteric venous thrombosis.[29] Emergency TIPS should be considered early to decompress the portal venous HTN in patients with refractory variceal bleeding once endoscopic sclerotherapy and medical treatment fail, before the clinical condition worsens.[30]

R Palliative treatment

For patients with MVT and bleeding gastroesophageal varices who have failed endoscopic therapy and TIPS, palliative treatment may be necessary. Multidisciplinary discussion with the interventional radiology, gastroenterology, and hepatology teams can help drive further therapy for these patients.

REFERENCES

1. Kumar S, Sarr MG, Kamath PS. Mesenteric venous thrombosis. *N Engl J Med*. 2001;345:1683-1688.
2. Hamoud B, Singal AK, Kamath PS. Mesenteric venous thrombosis. *J Clin Exp Hepatol*. 2014;4:257-263.
3. Salim S, Ekberg O, Elf J, Zarrouk M, Gottsäter A, Acosta S. Clinical implications of CT findings in mesenteric venous thrombosis at admission. *Emerg Radiol*. 2018;25:407-413.
4. Oliva IB, Davarpanah AH, Rybicki FJ, et al. ACR Appropriateness Criteria® imaging of mesenteric ischaemia. *Abdom Imaging*. 2013;38:714-719.
5. Rajesh S, Mukund A, Arora A. Imaging diagnosis of splanchnic venous thrombosis. *Gastroenterol Res Pract*. 2015;2015: 101029.
6. Acosta S. Epidemiology of mesenteric vascular disease: clinical implications. *Semin Vasc Surg*. 2010;23:4-8.
7. Amitrano L, Guardascione MA, Scaglione M, et al. Prognostic factors in noncirrhotic patients with splanchnic vein thromboses. *Am J Gastroenterol*. 2007;102:2464-2470.
8. Kim HK, Hwang D, Park S, Lee JM, Huh S. Treatment outcomes and risk factors for bowel infarction in patients with acute superior mesenteric venous thrombosis. *J Vasc Surg Venous Lymphat Disorder*. 2017;5:638-646.
9. Acosta S, Alhadad A, Svensson P, Ekberg O. Epidemiology, risk and prognostic factors in mesenteric venous thrombosis. *Br J Surg*. 2008;95:1245-1251.
10. Singal AK, Kamath PS, Tefferi A. Mesenteric venous thrombosis. *Mayo Clin Proc*. 2013;88:285-294.
11. Brunaud L, Antunes L, Collinet-Adler S, et al. Acute mesenteric venous thrombosis: case for nonoperative management. *J Vasc Surg*. 2001;34:673-679.
12. Kearon C, Akl EA, Comerota AJ, et al. Antithrombotic therapy and prevention of thrombosis, 9th ed: American College of chest physicians evidence-based clinical practice guidelines. *Chest*. 2012;141:e419S-e494S.
13. Condat B, Pessione FF, Helene Denninger M, Hillaire S, Valla D. Recent portal or mesenteric venous thrombosis: increased recognition and frequent recanalization on anticoagulant therapy. *Hepatology*. 2000;32:466-470.
14. Salim S, Zarrouk M, Elf J, Gottsäter A, Ekberg O, Acosta S. Improved prognosis and low failure rate with anticoagulation as first line therapy in mesenteric venous thrombosis. *World J Surg*. 2018;42:3803-3811.

15. Björck M, Koelemay M, Acosta S, et al. Editor's choice—management of the diseases of mesenteric arteries and veins: clinical practice guidelines of the European Society of Vascular Surgery (ESVS). *Eur J Vasc Endovasc Surg.* 2017;53:460-510.

16. Di Minno MN, Milone F, Milone M, et al. Endovascular thrombolysis in acute mesenteric vein thrombosis: a 3-year follow-up with the rate of short and long-term sequaelae in 32 patients. *Thromb Res.* 2010;126:295-298.

17. Hollingshead M, Burke CT, Mauro MA, Weeks SM, Dixon RG, Jaques PF. Transcatheter thrombolytic therapy for acute mesenteric and portal vein thrombosis. *J Vasc Interv Radiol.* 2005;16:651-661.

18. Acosta S, Ögren M, Sternby NH, Bergqvist D, Björck M. Mesenteric venous thrombosis with transmural intestinal infarction: a population-based study. *J Vasc Surg.* 2005;41:59-63.

19. Thatipelli MR, McBane RD, Hodge DO, Wysokinski WE. Survival and recurrence in patients with splanchnic vein thromboses. *Clin Gastroenterol Hepatol.* 2010;8:200-205.

20. Morasch MD, Ebaugh JL, Chiou AC, Matsumura JS, Pearce WH, Yao JS. Mesenteric venous thrombosis: a changing clinical entity. *J Vasc Surg.* 2001;34:680-684.

21. Zarrouk M, Salim S, Elf J, Gottsäter A, Acosta S. Testing for thrombophilia in mesenteric venous thrombosis—Retrospective original study and systematic review. *Best Pract Res Clin.* 2017;31:39-48.

22. Connors JM. Thrombophilia testing and venous thrombosis. *N England J Med.* 2017;377:1177-1187.

23. Ageno W, Riva N, Schulman S, et al. Long-term clinical outcomes of splanchnic vein thrombosis: results of an International Registry. *JAMA Intern Med.* 2015;175:1474-1480.

24. Ageno W, Beyer-Westendorf J, Garcia D, Lazo-Langner A, McBane R, Paciaroni M. Guidance for the management of venous thrombosis in unusual sites. *J Thromb Thrombolysis.* 2016;41:129-143.

25. Vietti Violi N, Fournier N, Duran R, et al. Acute mesenteric vein thrombosis: factors associated with evolution to chronic mesenteric vein thrombosis. *Am J Roentg.* 2014;203:54-61.

26. Maldonado TS, Blumberg SN, Sheth SU, et al. Mesenteric vein thrombosis can be safely treated with anticoagulation but is associated with significant sequelae of portal hypertension. *J Vasc Surg Venous Lymphat Disord.* 2016;4:400-406.

27. Nadler J, Stankovic N, Uber A, et al. Outcomes in variceal hemorrhage following the use of a balloon tamponade device. *Am J Emerg Med.* 2017;35:1500-1502.

28. Lo GH. Endoscopic treatments for portal hypertension. *Hepatol Int.* 2018;12:91-101.

29. Smith M, Durham J. Evolving indications for TIPS. *Tech Vasc Interv Radiol.* 2016;19:36-41.

30. Loffroy R, Favelier S, Pottecher P, et al. Transjugular intrahepatic portosystemic shunt for acute variceal gastrointestinal bleeding: indications, techniques and outcomes. *Diagn Interv Imaging.* 2015;96:745-755.

Richard J. Powell

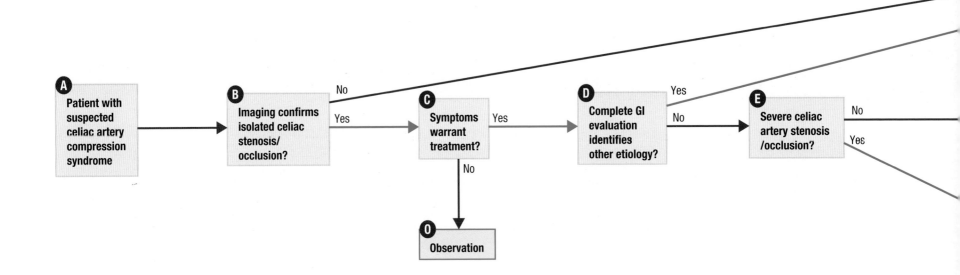

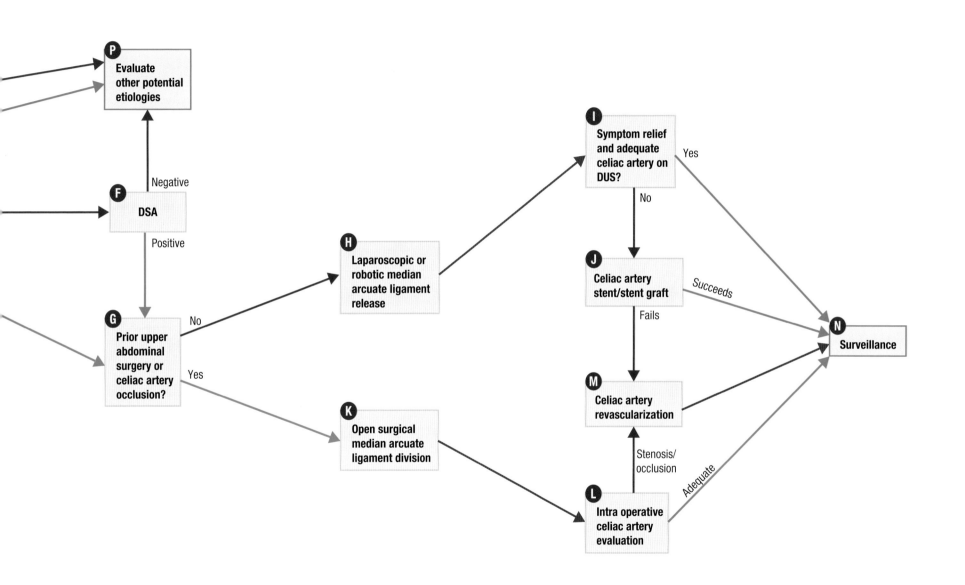

A Patient with suspected celiac artery compression syndrome

The existence of celiac artery compression syndrome (CACS), comprised of compression of the celiac artery and the celiac ganglion by the median arcuate ligament (MAL), that is associated with chronic abdominal symptoms is controversial.[1,2] Patients with CACS present with celiac artery stenosis and a wide array of symptoms that can be difficult to differentiate from other GI pathologies. These include chronic abdominal pain, weight loss, nausea, and vomiting. As such, most patients have had extensive GI evaluations prior to the diagnosis of CACS, and the diagnosis is one of exclusion.

B Imaging confirms isolated celiac stenosis/occlusion?

Patients evaluated for CACS must have a significant stenosis or occlusion of the celiac artery on imaging to consider this diagnosis. Imaging needs to be performed both at end inspiration and expiration to confirm a stenosis that may not be initially apparent on routine study. This is most easily accomplished with DUS, but can also be performed with CTA, MRA, or DSA. At end expiration, the peak systolic velocities and the severity of the stenosis will be the most severe. If imaging does not confirm celiac artery stenosis, other possible etiologies should be evaluated (see D).

C Symptoms warrant treatment?

Asymptomatic stenosis of the celiac artery is a common incidental finding in 4% to 21% of patients undergoing CTA and DUS. In patients without other causes, celiac artery stenosis can be due to compression by the MAL.[3,4] In the absence of symptoms, no further diagnostic evaluation or treatment of CACS is warranted. Usually, there is sufficient collateral circulation from the SMA even in the presence of celiac artery occlusion. If patients experience sufficient pain, weight loss, or other GI symptoms, further evaluation and potential treatment of the celiac artery stenosis is indicated. If not, they are observed and advised to return if symptoms worsen.

D Complete GI evaluation identifies other etiology?

Patients with symptoms suggestive of CACS should have completed a full GI workup, including upper endoscopy, assessment for cholelithiasis, evaluation for gastroesophageal reflux, impaired gastric emptying, and malabsorption syndrome. These etiologies are more common than CACS, should be excluded in pursuing a diagnosis of CACS, and treated if confirmed, prior to consideration of any potential CACS treatment.

E Severe celiac artery stenosis/occlusion?

Patients with a severe celiac artery stenosis or occlusion, symptoms severe enough to warrant treatment, and a negative GI

evaluation should be considered for MAL release. Certain clinical factors are associated with a higher likelihood of successful outcome after CACS treatment. Patients presenting with chronic epigastric abdominal pain that is worsened with eating or exertion tend to have better functional outcomes following MAL release than patients presenting with unprovoked abdominal pain or nausea and vomiting.[5] In addition, younger patients and those who have experienced weight loss tend to have better outcomes. If the clinical suspicion for CACS is strong, but the celiac stenosis does not appear severe on imaging, DSA and pressure measurements across the stenosis can help confirm the diagnosis.

F DSA

Patients with suspected CACS but less than severe celiac artery stenosis on DUS or CTA can be considered for arteriography to more precisely define the severity of stenosis. End-expiration aortography in a lateral projection and pressure measurements to confirm the existence of a hemodynamically significant stenosis should be performed. A systolic pressure gradient of >20 mm Hg is considered significant. If this supports the diagnosis of CACS, treatment is recommended.

G Prior upper abdominal surgery or celiac artery occlusion?

Treatment of CACS begins with surgical division of the MAL. This can be performed via laparoscopic, robotic, or open surgical approaches. Patients with total occlusion of the celiac artery or poststenotic aneurysmal degeneration require celiac revascularization after MAL division. Patients with previous upper abdominal surgery may not be candidates for laparoscopic or robotic MAL release due to adhesions.

H Laparoscopic or robotic median arcuate ligament release

Laparoscopic ligament release for CACS can be performed safely with a low complication rate assuming sufficient clinical experience with the technique.[6-9] The celiac artery should be completely released from the MAL and the celiac ganglion should be resected (neurolysis), because it is hypothesized that pain may arise from MAL stimulation of this ganglion, independent of arterial compression.[10] This procedure is commonly performed using a 5-port laparoscopic technique. The lesser sac is entered, and once the celiac artery is identified, the MAL and muscular fibers of the diaphragmatic crus are divided with hook electrocautery. Ganglionic tissue surrounding the celiac artery is then removed.

Early reports suggested a high 9% conversion rate to open surgery due to intraoperative hemorrhage. A much lower rate of conversion was noted in more recent reports, including our series of 22 patients with no instances of open conversion during laparoscopic MALS release.[9] Among these patients, we found that 81% had improved and reported weight gain. The average

hospital length of stay required after surgery was 1 to 2 days. In a large meta-analysis, 85% of patients reported immediate symptom relief following surgery and 5.7% of patients developed late symptom recurrence.[5]

I Symptom relief and adequate celiac artery on DUS?

After MAL release, patients should be observed for symptom improvement and reevaluated with DUS or CTA. The celiac artery stenosis may not resolve after decompression. In general, we allow at least 1 month to assess symptoms before deciding whether celiac artery stenosis warrants treatment after MAL release.

J Celiac artery stent/stent graft

Patients with persistent symptoms following laparoscopic or robotic MALS release and a residual celiac artery stenosis on DUS or CTA can be treated with celiac artery balloon-expandable stent or stent-graft placement. This procedure is typically performed through a femoral approach. Bare metal stent placement can be performed through a small 5-Fr introducer sheath or a 6-Fr guide catheter. Stent graft placement may be more resistant to in-stent restenosis but requires a larger introducer sheath to deliver the device. Occasionally, the proximal celiac artery may have such a significant downward angle that it is not possible to deliver the device via a transfemoral approach in which case a brachial or transradial approach can be used. Stent or stent-graft placement was required in 33% of our patients following laparoscopic treatment alone and was performed at an average 49 days after initial MAL release.[9]

K Open surgical median arcuate ligament division

Open surgical division of the MAL and resection of the celiac ganglion is performed through an upper midline incision.[6,10] The patient is positioned supine and a nasogastric tube is placed. The left lobe of the liver is mobilized to the patient's right, the lesser sac is entered, and the stomach is retracted inferiorly. A self-retaining retractor system is used to maintain exposure. The esophagus can be identified by palpating the nasogastric tube and, if needed, mobilized to the patient's left. The tissue anterior to the aorta is divided with the electrocautery and the celiac artery is identified. The MAL and crus of the diagram are divided with the electrocautery. The nerve tissue surrounding the celiac artery is excised. Once this is completed, the celiac artery is inspected visually and with DUS to assess for residual stenosis. If residual stenosis is present, then the celiac artery stenosis can be repaired either by patch angioplasty or bypass grafting.

L Intraoperative celiac artery evaluation

After MAL release during open surgery, the celiac artery should be evaluated for periarterial fibrosis or residual stenosis by intraoperative DUS and visual inspection. If stenosis that cannot be remedied by additional periarterial dissection is found, celiac revascularization should be performed. In a large meta-analysis, surgical bypass was required in conjunction with open MALS release in 25% of cases.[5] In a single-center report by Reilly et al., celiac artery bypass in conjunction with MALS release was associated with a 50% decrease in late symptom recurrence (22% vs. 44%).[10]

Ⓜ Celiac artery revascularization

Residual celiac artery stenosis after open MAL release is treated by either patch angioplasty or bypass grafting. If the proximal celiac artery is not involved, then patch angioplasty can be performed with proximal control provided with a side-biting aortic clamp. If the celiac artery is diffusely diseased or there is aneurysmal degeneration, then bypass grafting originating from the supraceliac aorta using a prosthetic bypass can be performed. We typically use a 7-mm polyester graft although autogenous saphenous vein can also be used.

Ⓝ Surveillance

Following treatment of CACS, patients should be followed up at 1 month with clinical evaluation and DUS of the celiac artery or bypass. In patients with symptom improvement following laparoscopic release with or without endovascular intervention who subsequently develop recurrent celiac stenosis or occlusion, celiac artery bypass is appropriate (see K).

Ⓞ Observation

Patients with significant CACS and no significant bothersome symptoms are followed expectantly. If symptoms develop, then further evaluation is undertaken.

Ⓟ Evaluate other potential etiologies

If CACS is not confirmed, the many other etiologies of abdominal pain need to be evaluated and treated, as appropriate.

REFERENCES

1. Plate G, Eklof B, Vang J. The celiac compression syndrome: myth or reality? *Acta Chir Scand*. 1981;147:201-203.
2. Lindner HH, Kemprud E. A clinic-anatomical study of the arcuate ligament of the diagram. *Arch Surg*.1971;103:600-605.
3. Derrick JR, Pollard HS, Moore RM. The pattern of arteriosclerotic narrowing of the celiac and superior mesenteric arteries. *Ann Surg*. 1959;149:684-689.
4. Baskan O, Kaya E, Gungoren FZ, Erol C. Compression of the celiac artery by the median arcuate ligament: multi-detector computed tomographic findings and characteristics. *Can Assoc Radiol J*. 2015;66;272-276.
5. Jimenez JC, Harlander-Locke M, Dutson EP. Open and laparoscopic treatment of median arcuate ligament syndrome. *J Vasc Surg*. 2012;56:869-873.
6. Tulloch AW, Jimenez JC, Lawrence PF, et al. Laparoscopic versus open celiac ganglionectomy in patients with median arcuate ligament syndrome. *J Vasc Surg*. 2010;52:1283-1289.
7. Fajer S, Cornateanu R, Ghinea R, Inbar R, Avital S. Laparoscopic repair of median arcuate ligament syndrome: a new approach. *J Am Coll Surg*. 2014;219(6):e75-e78. doi:10.1016/j.jamcollsurg.2014.08.009.
8. Berard X, Cau J, Déglise S, et al. Laparoscopic surgery for coeliac artery compression syndrome: current management and technical aspects. *Eur J Vasc Endovasc Surg*. 2012;43:38-42.
9. Columbo JA, Trus T, Nolan B, et al. Contemporary management of median arcuate ligament syndrome provides early symptom improvement. *J Vasc Surg*. 2015;62(1):151-156.
10. Reilly LM, Ammar AD, Stoney RJ, Ehrenfeld WK. Late results following operative repair for celiac artery compression syndrome. *J Vasc Surg*. 1985;2:79-91.

Matthew S. Edwards

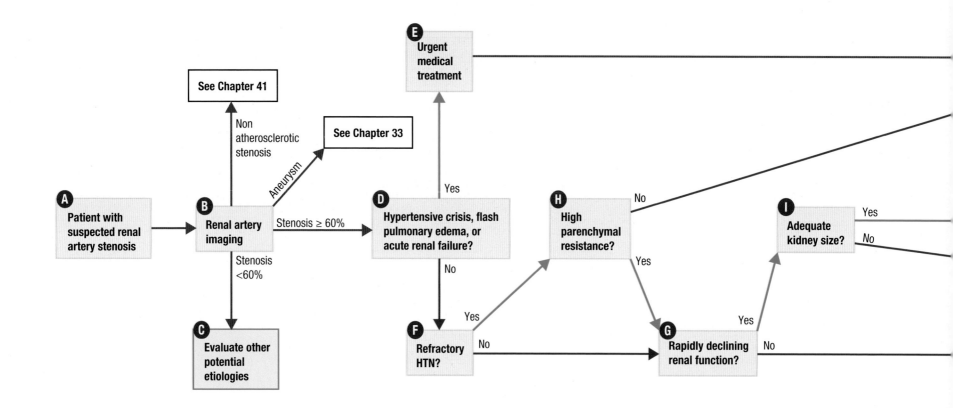

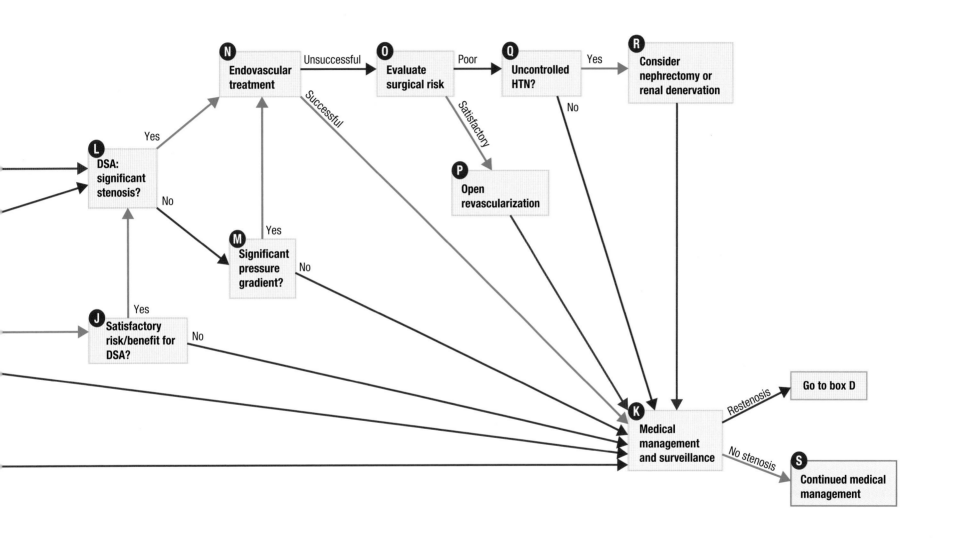

A Patient with suspected renal artery stenosis

Atherosclerotic renal artery stenosis (RAS) is a known potential cause of secondary HTN and excretory renal insufficiency. Other causes include FMD, dissections, and aneurysms—topics are covered elsewhere in this text. RAS has been associated with increased cardiovascular morbidity and mortality. The prevalence of RAS independent of associated HTN or renal failure has been demonstrated to be approximately 7% in adults 65 years or older.[1] Factors that increase the prevalence of disease include advanced age, CKD, HTN, PAD, and CAD.[2] Approximately 90% of RAS lesions are atherosclerotic, and the disease is typically located at the ostium or within the proximal renal artery. RAS may be accompanied by an abdominal bruit, but this is not a specific or sensitive finding. Severe HTN often raises suspicion, which leads to imaging to confirm the diagnosis. Renal function is assessed with creatinine measurement in all such patients.

B Renal artery imaging

Renal DUS is a valuable screening test to identify suspected atherosclerotic RAS.[3] The study should include measurements of a proximal aortic velocity at the level of the SMA to calculate the renal–aortic ratio (RAR); spectral waveform analysis of the proximal, mid, and distal renal artery noting the highest PSV and any distal flow disturbance; kidney length pole to pole; and a parenchymal renal resistive index (RRI). The normal renal artery spectral waveform has low-resistance forward flow throughout the cardiac cycle, a rapid systolic upstroke, and a PSV < 180 cm/s. Accepted criteria for establishing $\geq 60\%$ stenosis include PSV ≥ 180 cm/s and RAR ≥ 3.5.[4] If renal DUS is not available or if it is nondiagnostic and clinical suspicion remains high, then CTA and/or MRA are alternative imaging modalities. Arteriography is rarely needed to establish the diagnosis of RAS, and is usually only used as a confirmatory study during planned renal artery intervention. If RAS is excluded by imaging or if RAS is $<60\%$, other etiologies for HTN or renal dysfunction should be evaluated and treated. For DUS findings of renal artery aneurysm or nonatherosclerotic stenosis, please see Chapters 33 and 41, respectively.

C Evaluate other potential etiologies

A RAS $< 60\%$ is not functionally significant and such patients do not benefit from revascularization. In patients with significant HTN and/or renal insufficiency without RAS, other etiologies for secondary HTN and/or excretory renal insufficiency should be evaluated and treated.

D Hypertensive crisis, flash pulmonary edema, or acute renal failure?

After diagnosing $>60\%$ RAS, it is important to identify patients who are likely to benefit from renal artery revascularization.

Currently there is no level I evidence from randomized trials that has demonstrated a benefit from renal revascularization in the general treatment of HTN and renal insufficiency. Indications for treatment in more highly selected patients should consider consensus guidelines.[5,6] For patients presenting with flash pulmonary edema, hypertensive crisis (HTN that leads to end-organ damage), and/or acute renal failure, the general recommendations are to stabilize the patient and allow their renal function to return to baseline prior to intervention, if possible. Once stabilization of the patient's clinical status and renal function has occurred, revascularization can proceed on an elective basis. If this approach fails and the patient's condition remains tenuous, revascularization can be performed in a subacute setting.

E Urgent medical treatment

Patients who present with high-grade RAS and a hypertensive crisis, flash pulmonary edema, or acute renal failure should be aggressively managed as inpatients because their condition can deteriorate rapidly. These patients have to be medically optimized prior to procedural intervention, if possible. Medical optimization includes aggressive, closely monitored blood pressure control, establishment of euvolemia, management of any hypertensive demand-induced cardiac ischemia, and attention to any specific end-organ damage. If acute kidney injury or renal failure is present, temporary cessation of ACE inhibitors and angiotensin receptor antagonists is indicated; additional nephrotoxic exposures (iodine-based contrast, etc.) are strictly avoided.

F Refractory HTN?

The efficacy of modern medical therapy alone for RAS was demonstrated in the CORAL trial, which randomized 947 patients to best medical management versus renal artery stenting for high-grade atherosclerotic RAS. Patients were required to have persistent systolic HTN despite taking two or more antihypertensive medications or to have renal insufficiency with eGFR < 60 mL/min/1.73 m^2 of body surface area. Stenting showed no benefit at a median follow-up of 43 months over optimal medical management alone in reducing the composite endpoint of renal and cardiovascular events (cardiovascular or renal cause of death, stroke, MI, hospitalization for CHF, progressive renal insufficiency, or dialysis).[7] During follow-up, there was a modest difference in SBP that favored the stent group (-2.3 mm Hg). The results of this trial stress the importance of optimizing medical therapy.

The lack of any demonstrated benefit for revascularization in CORAL remains controversial. High volume centers treating patients with severe HTN and renal function issues have demonstrated potential benefits for selected patients in numerous published series. The major conundrum in treating RAS today is identifying those patients who have significant likelihood to benefit. Prior work from our group and others, combined with the results of CORAL, would

suggest that patients most likely to benefit from intervention are those who have failed optimal medical therapy with continued severe HTN refractory to medical management, observed decline in renal function, or the presence of the previously mentioned cardiac disturbance syndromes (ie, flash pulmonary edema). To attempt to identify patients in whom revascularization may provide benefit, we recommend further evaluation of kidney characteristics (ie, kidney size, kidney volume, resistive index, proteinuria).

G Rapidly declining renal function?

RAS can cause ischemic nephropathy that ultimately leads to impaired glomerular filtration and is likely caused by a complex interaction of hypoperfusion and circulating angiotensin II levels. There are no randomized trials to clearly guide the management of patients with RAS and declining renal function. Prior work by our group and others have demonstrated that improved renal function is the strongest predictor of improved adverse event-free survival after renal revascularization.[8-10] Patients with normal renal function treated with renal artery stenting have no potential for renal function recovery and are instead exposed to the risks of the procedure, including contrast nephropathy, in hopes of uncertain blood pressure response and cardiovascular benefit. One of the more common predictors of renal function response to stenting is rapid preoperative decline in baseline renal function (measured as a rapid decline in baseline GFR).[11] We favor considering revascularization for a patient with an observed decline in preoperative kidney function with an identified high-grade RAS, especially if it affects the entirety of the functional renal mass (bilateral RAS or RAS to a solitary kidney). Patients with either stable renal disease or one with a slow decline over the years are less likely to benefit from revascularization; in most cases, such patients should be treated medically.

H High parenchymal resistance?

There are a number of additional methods to assess the functional impact of RAS. The first includes the RRI, which is used to measure resistance within the renal parenchyma. RRI is defined as follows: $(PSV - EDV)/PSV$ in the main renal artery. A normal RRI is 0.6 to 0.8 and an abnormal RRI > 0.8 suggests intrinsic renal disease (nephrosclerosis). An abnormally high RRI has demonstrated an association with impaired blood pressure response, continued renal function decline, and higher mortality following renal revascularization.[12] For these reasons, our group generally avoids renal revascularization in patients with RRI > 0.8. Renal vein renin analysis has also been used to assess the functional significance of RAS. Renal vein renin sampling is an extremely complicated endeavor that is poorly tolerated by patients and it is only useful in delineating the functional significance of unilateral RAS as the comparisons are made relative to the functioning contralateral kidney. We no longer employ renal vein renin analysis in our current management strategy given the controversy over treatment for HTN alone and the efficacy of newer antihypertensive agents in the management of renin-based HTN.

Ⓘ Adequate kidney size?

Kidney length is also an important consideration in determining whether renal artery revascularization is likely to improve renal function. The normal adult kidney length is 10 to 12 cm, so a short kidney length (<7 cm) is suggestive of an atrophic kidney that may have irreversible sclerotic damage due to ischemic nephropathy. Kidney length is therefore a surrogate for functional kidney mass. The likelihood of improved renal function after revascularization of an atrophic kidney is low. If additional information is needed, nuclear renography can be used to assess residual renal function in the affected kidney. A normal-sized kidney with a normal RRI and evidence of declining excretory function would all be deemed favorable criteria for revascularization. In small kidneys, we will attempt revascularization if the smaller kidney continues to provide more than 20% of the total renal function.

Ⓙ Satisfactory risk/benefit for DSA?

Catheter-based DSA is the gold standard for renal artery imaging and offers an opportunity for intervention. Although the risk of DSA is low, potential complications include bleeding and PSAs related to arterial puncture. The reported incidence of femoral artery PSAs varies widely from <0.2% to 3.8%.[13] In rare instances, access-related complications can lead to limb-threatening ischemia, retroperitoneal hemorrhage, or arterial occlusion. Other complications include contrast nephropathy, exposure to ionizing radiation, allergic reaction to iodinated contrast, plaque (or cholesterol) embolization, contrast-induced renal insufficiency, and distal renal artery/parenchymal injury from guidewires. These risks must be weighed individually with each patient prior to proceeding with an invasive intervention. The periprocedural mortality of renal artery angioplasty and stent placement is 0% to 2%.[14]

Ⓚ Medical management and surveillance

All patients with renal artery disease require cardiovascular risk reduction pharmacotherapy and individualized medical management. Medical management of both HTN and CKD should be optimized before consideration is given to procedural intervention. The primary goals of medical management are the prevention of adverse cardiovascular events and renal function decline. Risk reduction pharmacotherapy includes smoking cessation, institution of antiplatelet therapy, use of a statin medication unless intolerant, control of diabetes, and blood pressure control. Evidence suggests that statins may may induce stabilization or regression of the renal sequelae of atherosclerotic renovascular disease.[15] ACE inhibitors and angiotensin receptor blockers are first-line therapy for blood pressure control. These medications

should be used with appropriate monitoring of potential renal function decline in patients with known bilateral critical RAS because acute renal failure has been reported after initiation of therapy.[16] Most patients with significant RAS will require more than one class of blood pressure medication for adequate control. Beta blockers, diuretics (useful in patients with bilateral disease), calcium channel blockers, and clonidine are frequently used.

Patients who have been treated with revascularization for RAS should continue taking a statin long term, given the demonstrated benefits of reduction in risk for restenosis. We also advise patients to take clopidogrel (in addition to aspirin unless contraindicated for other reasons) for at least 4 weeks after intervention. Patients should undergo surveillance with a renal artery DUS immediately following the intervention (to establish baseline) and every 12 months thereafter. Restenosis remains the primary failure after intervention. Patients should be monitored for the development of declining renal function, medically refractory HTN, or cardiac disturbance syndromes during follow-up. Predictors of restenosis include small renal artery caliber, residual stenosis after previous revascularization, a history of prior restenosis, smoking, and lack of statin therapy. Estimated risk of restenosis after renal artery stenting has been estimated at 50% at 12 months and 60% at 18 months.[17] DUS is accurate for identifying restenosis after renal artery stenting but uses a higher PSV threshold (245-295 cm/s) to identify a 60% stenosis, compared with de novo stenoses.[18,19] Repeated intervention should be reserved for patients with recurrent HTN or renal function decline. Reintervention should not be performed for asymptomatic recurrent RAS.

Given the relative slow progression of RAS in patients with no history of intervention, annual surveillance is not justified for patients with <60% RAS, unless clinical symptoms develop. Prospective population-based studies of elderly men and women >65 years of age in the United States have demonstrated a significant change in baseline renovascular disease in only 14% of kidneys on follow-up at 8 years (annualized rate 1.3% per year) with progression to significant renovascular disease in only 4% and no progression to occlusion.[20]

Ⓛ DSA: significant stenosis?

Patients with DUS evidence of >60% RAS and clinical criteria for revascularization should undergo renal artery DSA to confirm the severity of stenosis and to allow simultaneous endovascular treatment when indicated. Because many of these patients have CKD, procedural contrast should be minimized. CO_2 aortography and preintervention IV hydration with normal saline are adjuncts for periprocedural renal protection. Focused imaging of the renal arteries can be obtained with dilute contrast (1/2-1/3 strength). Oblique imaging is usually required to adequately delineate the renal artery orifices and/or stenoses; the appropriate angle can be determined from preoperative cross-sectional imaging, if available.

Ⓜ Significant pressure gradient?

In equivocal cases, pressure gradients can be used to determine the hemodynamic significance of RAS. We prefer using the minimal contact technique (described in N) to engage the renal artery ostium and use an end-hole catheter to measure the gradient in a pull-back fashion. The catheter is advanced to the distal main renal artery prior to its bifurcating branches and pressures are recorded as the catheter is pulled back through the renal artery into the aorta. In cases where a pull-back pressure gradient is considered hazardous for losing access, pressure sensing wires or the Medtronic Export™ catheter can be used to avoid losing wire access while measuring pressures. A systolic gradient >10 mm Hg across any lesion in the renal artery is considered significant. It is important to minimize manipulation of the renal artery ostium and avoid measuring a pressure gradient (given the associated risk of atheroembolization) if DSA alone clearly demonstrates high-grade stenosis.[21]

Ⓝ Endovascular treatment

Primary renal artery stenting is the preferred mode of intervention for revascularization in atherosclerotic RAS. Stenting ostial lesions has proved superior in randomized studies to balloon PTA alone, with higher rates of technical success and primary patency at 6 months.[22] The procedure is typically performed using either percutaneous femoral or brachial access. We prefer femoral access contralateral to the side of the renal artery to be treated because this provides easier ostial cannulation as the catheter tends to track along the aortic wall contralateral to the site of femoral access. Renal artery cannulation should be performed using minimal contact technique with ostial engagement by an angled guide catheter. A guidewire is then passed across the lesion after the orifice of the renal artery is engaged. Stenting is typically performed with balloon-expandable bare-metal stents that are sized to match the diameter of the distal normal renal artery. The stent should be positioned to completely cover the stenotic lesion and extend 1 to 2 mm into the aortic lumen. Lesion predilation before stent placement is sometimes necessary and usually performed with a 2- to 3-mm diameter balloon. Technical success requires no significant residual diameter-reducing stenosis (<30%) on completion angiography and no evidence of iatrogenic dissection or other trauma. Pressure measurement confirming resolution of the translesion gradient can be performed.

Interventions for in-stent restenosis are usually performed using PTA alone. For refractory in-stent stenosis, technical success has been described using a cutting balloon. Small series have also been reported for treatment of restenotic lesions with covered stents.[23] Recent promising data have also been reported regarding the use of drug-eluting stents in RAS for prevention of restenosis.[24]

Ⓞ Evaluate surgical risk

Endovascular intervention is the mainstay of therapy for RAS and has largely replaced open revascularization. Open reconstruction, however, remains an important treatment modality for situations in which endovascular treatment is contraindicated. Anatomic contraindications include RAS extending into the terminal portion of the main renal artery, disease involving a short main renal artery, disease in multiple small arteries, branch-level disease, or the presence of adjacent aortic pathology requiring surgical treatment. Because open revascularization is associated with a higher incidence of mortality and major morbidity than endovascular treatment, the benefits of an open procedure must outweigh its risks to the patient.

P Open revascularization

Open surgery remains a reasonable option in highly selected patients, including those undergoing concomitant aortic reconstruction for aneurysms, patients with disease in multiple ipsilateral renal arteries or branch vessels, patients who have failed endovascular therapy, and children (see Chapter 41). Aortorenal bypass and renal artery thromboendarterectomy are the two most commonly used techniques for surgical renal artery revascularization. Alternative methods include renal artery reimplantation, extra-anatomic bypass such as hepatorenal or splenorenal bypass, and *ex vivo* branch vessel reconstruction. Common intraoperative steps for all reconstructions involve administration of IV mannitol (12.5-25 mg) and heparin (100 U/kg with ACT monitoring). For adult patients, prosthetic or saphenous vein grafts are acceptable for main renal artery bypass. The distal anastomosis can be end to end or end to side and should be performed with the arteriotomy at least three times the diameter of the renal artery to prevent late suture line stenosis.[25] Thromboendarterectomy usually involves a transaortic technique and is an excellent option for disease in multiple renal arteries and in cases where avoidance of prosthetic conduit is preferred. A more proximal level of aortic control is required and a longitudinal or transverse aortotomy is made with endarterectomy of the aorta and eversion endarterectomy of the renal arteries.[25] The aortotomy is usually closed with a running suture. A patch may be used for closure as well. *Ex vivo* reconstruction is reserved for complex repair of branch-level and distal main renal artery pathology. This technique is rarely required for RAS and is used more frequently for renal artery aneurysms (see Chapter 33). Descriptions of this technique have been previously published.[26]

Selected retrospective cohort analyses of renal artery revascularization have demonstrated a perioperative mortality rate between 3% and 8%, with perioperative complications occurring in 7% to 30% of patients.[14] Surgical renal revascularization was followed by early improvement in postoperative renal function in 26% to 58% of patients and worsened renal function in 3% to 27%.[14] The addition of renal artery revascularization to aortic aneurysm repair has demonstrated increased perioperative mortality and a lower rate of favorable blood pressure response relative to renal artery revascularization performed in isolation.[27]

Q Uncontrolled HTN?

Patients with severe RAS who have failed an attempt at endovascular treatment and are poor surgical candidates for open revascularization can be managed medically as previously discussed. For such patients with ongoing uncontrolled HTN despite maximal medical therapy, renal denervation or nephrectomy can be considered.

R Consider nephrectomy or renal denervation

Alternative treatment strategies have been explored for patients with multidrug-resistant HTN not amenable to or not responsive to renal revascularization. Nephrectomy has been advocated to treat renovascular HTN in atrophic kidneys when there are no options for reconstruction and the patient has limited residual excretory function in the affected kidney. Nephrectomy eliminates the high levels of circulating renin and angiotensin that are the underlying drivers of HTN. Consideration of nephrectomy is the only situation in which our group currently performs lateralizing tests such as renal vein renin sampling. In this instance, confirmation of hyperactive renin secretion to the atrophic kidney in question is desirable prior to incurring the risks of surgery and anesthesia.

More recently, endovascular catheter techniques have been developed to enable adventitial denervation of the kidney using radiofrequency energy. Successful treatment is designed to reduce sympathetic activity and renin release. Trials of renal denervation versus nephrectomy to treat uncontrolled HTN have yielded conflicting results and there is currently no level I evidence supporting either treatment strategy for managing RAS. However, new devices continue to be developed for renal denervation, so continued analysis of potential progress is warranted.

S Continued medical management

Continued medical management to minimize the risk of incident or recurrent cardiovascular events is vital in the management of patients with successfully treated RAS. Many of these therapies are useful in preventing renal function decline and restenosis in stented renal arteries. As previously discussed, therapy will include blood pressure control (including an ACE or ARB), statin therapy, antiplatelet agent administration, smoking cessation, diabetes control, and regular exercise.

REFERENCES

1. Hansen KJ, Edwards MS, Craven TE, et al. Prevalence of renovascular disease in the elderly: a population-based study. *J Vasc Surg*. 2002;36:443-451.
2. Kalra PA, Guo H, Kausz AT, et al. Atherosclerotic renovascular disease in the United States patients aged 67 years or older: risk factors, revascularization, and prognosis. *Kidney Int*. 2005;68:293-301.
3. Hansen KJ, Tribble RW, Reavis SW, et al. Renal duplex sonography: evaluation of clinical utility. *J Vasc Surg*. 1990; 12:227-236.
4. Hoffmann U, Edwards J, Carter S, et al. Role of duplex scanning for the detection of atherosclerotic renal artery disease. *Kidney Int*. 1991;39:1232-1239.
5. Aboyans V, Björck M, Brodmann M; ESC Scientific Document Group, et al. Questions and answers on diagnosis and management of patients with peripheral arterial diseases: a companion document of the 2017 ESC guidelines for the diagnosis and treatment of peripheral arterial diseases, in collaboration with the European Society for Vascular Surgery (ESVS). *Eur J Vasc Endovasc Surg*. 2018;55(4):457-464. doi:10.1016/j.ejvs.2017.08.014.
6. Corriere MA, Edwards MS. Results of the major randomized clinical trials of renal stenting and implications for future treatment strategies. *Semin Vasc Surg*. 2013;26(4): 161-164.
7. Cooper CJ, Murphy TP, Cutlip DE, et al. Stenting and medical therapy for atherosclerotic renal-artery stenosis. *N Engl J Med*. 2014;370(1):13-22.
8. Cherr GS, Hansen KJ, Craven TE, et al. Surgical management of atherosclerotic renovascular disease. *J Vasc Surg*. 2002;35(2):236-245.
9. Kennedy DJ, Colyer WR, Brewster PS, et al. Renal insufficiency as a predictor of adverse events and mortality after renal artery stent placement. *Am J Kidney Dis*. 2003; 42:926-935.
10. Zeller T, Frank U, Müller C, et al. Stent-supported angioplasty of severe atherosclerotic renal artery stenosis: long-term results of a prospective registry with 456 lesions. *Eur Heart J*. 2003;24:698.
11. Kashyap VS, Sepulveda RN, Bena JF, et al. The management of renal artery atherosclerosis for renal salvage: does stenting help? *J Vasc Surg*. 2007;45(1):101-108.
12. Crutchley TA, Pearce JD, Craven TE, Stafford JM, Edwards MS, Hansen KJ. Clinical utility of the resistive index in atherosclerotic renovascular disease. *J Vasc Surg*. 2009;49:148-155.
13. Stone P, Campbell J, AbuRahma A. Femoral pseudoaneurysms after percutaneous access. *J Vasc Surg*. 2014;60(5):1359-1366.
14. Edwards MS, Corriere MA. Contemporary management of atherosclerotic renovascular disease. *J Vasc Surg*. 2009; 50(5):1197-1210.
15. Cheung CM, Patel A, Shaheen N, et al. The effects of statins on the progression of atherosclerotic renovascular disease. *Nephron Clin Pract*. 2007;107:35-42.
16. Johansen TL, Kjaer A. Reversible renal impairment induced by treatment with the angiotensin II receptor antagonist candesartan in a patient with bilateral renal artery stenosis. *BMC Nephrol*. 2001;2:1.

17. Corriere M, Edwards M, Pearce J, Andrews J, Geary R, Hansen K. Restenosis after renal artery angioplasty and stenting: Incidence and risk factors. *J Vasc Surg.* 2009;50(4):813-819.

18. Cain BC, Wuamett JC, Soult M, Larion S, Ahanchi S, Panneton JM. Duplex ultrasound criteria for renal artery in-stent restenosis. *J Vasc Surg.* 2016;64(5):1548.

19. Del Conde I, Galin I, Trost B, et al. Renal artery duplex ultrasound criteria for the detection of significant in-stent restenosis. *Catheter Cardiovasc Interv.* 2014;83:612-618.

20. Pearce JD, Craven BL, Craven TE, et al. Progression of atherosclerotic renovascular disease: a prospective population-based study. *J Vasc Surg.* 2006;44(5):955-962.

21. Hiramoto J, Hansen KJ, Pan XM, Edwards MS, Sawhney R, Rapp JH. Atheroemboli during renal artery angioplasty: an ex vivo study. *J Vasc Surg.* 2005;41(6):1026-1030.

22. van de Ven PJ, Kaatee R, Beutler JJ, et al. Arterial stenting and balloon angioplasty in ostial atherosclerotic renovascular disease: a randomized trial. *Lancet.* 1999;353(9149):282-286.

23. Giles H, Lesar C, Erdoes L, Sprouse R, Myers S. Balloon-expandable covered stent therapy of complex endovascular pathology. *Ann Vasc Surg.* 2008;22(6):762-768. doi:10.1016/j.avsg.2008.09.001.

24. Bradaric C, Eser K, Preuss S, et al. Drug-eluting stents versus bare metal stents for the prevention of restenosis in patients with renovascular disease. *EuroIntervention.* 2017;13(2):e248-e255. doi:10.4244/EIJ-D-16-00697.

25. Benjamin ME, Dean RH. Techniques in renal artery reconstruction: part I. *Ann Vasc Surg.* 1996;10:306-314.

26. Crutchley TA, Pearce JD, Craven TE, Edwards MS, Dean RH, Hansen KJ. Branch renal artery repair with cold perfusion protection. *J Vasc Surg.* 2007;46(3):405-412; discussion 412.

27. Benjamin ME, Hansen KJ, Craven TE, et al. Combined aortic and renal artery surgery. A contemporary experience. *Ann Surg.* 1996;223(5):555-565.

Dawn M. Coleman

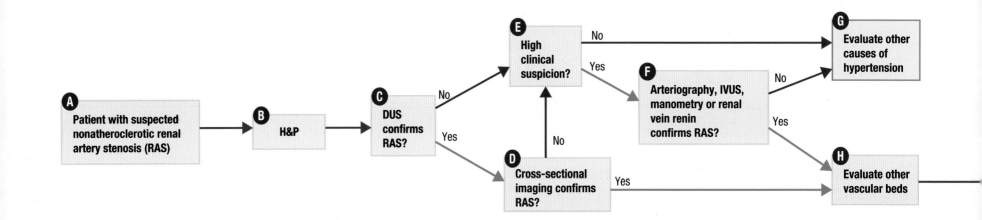

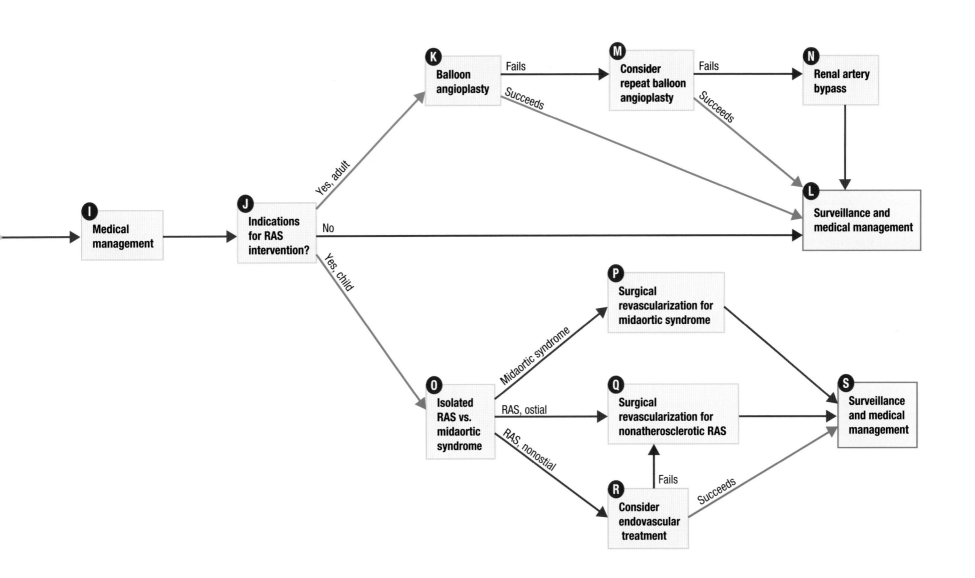

A Patient with suspected nonatherosclerotic RAS

Renal artery occlusive disease is a common and correctable cause of HTN in adults and the third most common cause of HTN in children. Renovascular HTN (RVH) is classically refractory to medical management and should be considered as a potential etiology for childhood HTN, severe HTN in women <45 years of age, acute and rapid escalation of mild HTN in older patients (>50 years), initial diastolic BP > 115 mm Hg, and rapid deterioration in renal function following the administration of antihypertensive therapy (especially with angiotensin-converting enzyme inhibitors [ACEi] or angiotensin receptor antagonists [ARBs]). Although RAS is usually due to atherosclerosis, FMD causes approximately 5% to 10% of RVH in adults. RVH secondary to RAS and abdominal aortic coarctation is the third most common cause of pediatric HTN, following thoracic aortic coarctation and parenchymal renal disease.[1,2] FMD is defined as a nonatherosclerotic, noninflammatory vascular disease that may result in arterial stenosis, occlusion, aneurysm, or dissection that affects primarily younger women.[3] The prevalence of FMD in the general population is unknown, although renal involvement is the most common phenotype comprising 58% to 75% of all FMD cases.[4,5] This chapter describes decision making for renal FMD and midaortic syndrome.

B H&P

Clinical history should elicit constitutional symptoms concerning for vasculitis, endocrine dysfunction, flank pain, and hematuria. Additional symptoms of carotid (tinnitus, dizziness, neck pain, amaurosis fugax, stroke), mesenteric (flank/abdominal pain, postprandial abdominal pain), and lower extremity (claudication) FMD should also be considered. Clinical examination should assess for abdominal bruit, abdominal mass, pulse abnormalities, Horner syndrome (suggesting carotid dissection), neurologic deficit, and a complete cardiopulmonary examination that considers hypertrophic cardiomyopathy. Laboratory evaluation should include assessment of renal function (BUN, creatinine), vasculitis (CRP), and electrolytes. Increased plasma renin activity supports the diagnosis of RVH, whereas aldosterone, thyroid, and catecholamine levels are useful screens for alternative diagnoses related to endocrine dysfunction.

C DUS confirms RAS?

Renal DUS remains the first-line imaging modality to assess patients with suspected RVH. An elevated PSV (>180 or >200 cm/s) or elevated renal aortic ratio >3.5 detects RAS with a sensitivity and specificity of 84% and 97%, respectively.[6] DUS also includes renal length measurement and may identify aneurysms of the main renal artery or pathology of adjacent structures (ie, obstruction, masses, aortic aneurysm). DUS can also provide insight into parenchymal disease based on the resistive index. Limitations of renal artery DUS include imaging difficulty related to obesity or bowel gas and relatively limited assessment of branch or parenchymal renal arteries.

D Cross-sectional imaging confirms RAS?

If DUS detects RAS, cross-sectional imaging is used to confirm this diagnosis. Both CTA and MRA have received a class I indication (evidence level B) as tests to confirm the diagnosis of RAS.[7] CTA offers excellent resolution and three-dimensional multiplanar images that can assist with treatment planning, but carries the risk of contrast-induced nephropathy and may not detect subtle FMD lesions or definitively characterize branch vessel disease. Sensitivity and specificity range from 86% to 93% and 90% to 100%, respectively.[8] MRA has diagnostic sensitivity and specificity for RAS of 97% and 93%, respectively, and is often favored in younger patients because it avoids radiation exposure.[9] Although gadolinium is less nephrotoxic than iodinated contrast and may be advantageous for those patients with mild renal insufficiency, the risk of nephrogenic systemic fibrosis prohibits its use in those patients with a GFR $\leq$ 30 mL/min/1.73 m^2. If cross sectional imaging does not confirm RAS, it may disclose other pathology that requires further evaluation. If no RAS is detected, but there is high clinical suspicion, additional testing may be indicated.

E High clinical suspicion?

Patients with early-onset hypertension (ie, <40 years of age), accelerated HTN, medically resistant HTN, malignant HTN, HTN with unexplained unilateral small kidney, and HTN with intolerance to medication should be considered "high clinical suspicion" for RVH in the absence of another hypertensive etiology. If this is the case, additional diagnostic studies are indicated even in the absence of a confirmed RAS by DUS.

F Arteriography, IVUS, pressure measurement, or renal vein renin confirms RAS?

If cross-sectional imaging is nondiagnostic for RAS despite a high level of suspicion, catheter arteriography should be considered. Arteriography remains the gold standard imaging modality for the diagnosis of RAS offering unrivaled spatial resolution and the capacity to reliably detect branch vessel and parenchymal involvement. Additionally, catheter manometry during arteriography can assess pressure gradients across a stenosis (a systolic pressure gradient >10 mm Hg is considered abnormal). IVUS may be used to further characterize the renal artery, especially in patients with FMD.[10] Indicated therapeutic interventions based on arteriography results can be performed in the same clinical setting.

Selective renal vein renin sampling permits calculation of renal vein ratios and may be helpful in scenarios of diagnostic uncertainty or equivocal results from routine tests. With unilateral RAS, the renal vein renin ratio (RVRR) is calculated by dividing the renin activity in venous blood from the affected kidney by that from the (normal) contralateral kidney. An RVRR > 1.48 supports a functionally relevant RAS.[11,12] In patients with bilateral RAS, a systemic renin index (RSRI) is calculated by subtracting systemic renin activity from individual renal vein renin activity and dividing the remainder by systemic renin activity; this index reflects individual kidney renin release.[11] There is a steady state of normal renal renin release; normal renal vein renin activity from each kidney is approximately 24% higher than systemic activity (with the total of both kidneys being then 48% higher than systemic activity). Documentation of renin hypersecretion (RSRI > 0.48) associated with contralateral kidney renin suppression (RSRI 0-0.24) provides a method to differentiate those patients who will be cured or improved of RVH following renal revascularization or nephrectomy.[11,13]

G Evaluate other causes of hypertension

If clinical suspicion for RAS is low after initial evaluation, or if catheter-based angiography with adjuncts fails to reveal RAS, ongoing evaluation for other causes of HTN should ensue. The differential diagnosis in this scenario includes essential HTN, endocrine dysfunction (pheochromocytoma, hyperaldosteronism, and hyperthyroidism), renal parenchymal disease, toxins/drugs (steroid, sympathomimetic drug, and cocaine use), and central nervous system pathology.

H Evaluate other vascular beds

If renal FMD is confirmed by imaging, further imaging should be performed (one-time head-to-toe CTA or MRA) to assess for concurrent arterial dysplasia and related occlusive or aneurysmal disease.[4]

I Medical management

Medical therapy is the mainstay of treatment for RVH. Clinical guidelines support the use of ACEi, ARBs, calcium channel blockers, and beta-blockers with a class I indication.[7] Although beta-blockers are often utilized first-line, ACEi and ARBs are often central to antihypertensive regimens offering 86% to 92% efficacy.[2] Renal function must be monitored closely as these agents modulate the renin–angiotensin system in cases of RAS affecting a solitary functioning kidney, severe bilateral RAS, or advanced chronic kidney disease risking acute renal injury.[14-16]

J Indications for RAS intervention?

Patients may fail medical management, despite an appropriate regimen of antihypertensive agents. Although randomized, controlled trials assessing renal revascularization for renal artery FMD are lacking, current guidelines support the following indications for renal revascularization in this patient cohort: (1) resistant HTN despite an appropriate three-drug regimen, (2) HTN of short duration with a curative goal, (3) renal artery dissection, (4) renal artery aneurysm, and (5) preservation of renal function in patients with severe stenosis.[4,17] Current guidelines support renal revascularization for hemodynamically significant RAS in several clinical scenarios[7]:

1. Asymptomatic bilateral or solitary viable kidney disease
2. Accelerated HTN, resistant HTN, malignant HTN, HTN with unexplained unilateral small kidney, and HTN with intolerance to medication
3. Progressive kidney disease with bilateral RAS or a RAS to a solitary functioning kidney
4. Chronic renal insufficiency with unilateral RAS
5. Recurrent unexplained CHF or sudden, unexplained pulmonary edema
6. Unstable angina

Subsequent steps depend on whether the patient is adult or pediatric.

Balloon angioplasty

PTA of the renal artery is the procedure of choice for adults with RAS secondary to FMD offering hypertension cure rates that approach 50%, with improvement rates of 86%, and a 20% to 30% risk of reintervention, and low risk of minor complications.[4] Complete imaging should include an aortogram and selective catheterization with evaluation of the ostia, main renal artery, branch renal arteries, and parenchyma of each kidney from multiple projections. A translesion pressure gradient evaluation should quantify the hemodynamic significance of a radiographic stenosis. Additionally, there is growing enthusiasm for the role of IVUS in the evaluation of renal FMD as it may help identify minor angiographic irregularities and intraluminal webs.[10] Hemodynamic significance (>10 mm Hg gradient) should be documented by manometry prior to any intervention in these patients and success defined by resolution of this gradient post angioplasty. Stenting should only be utilized selectively for treatment of FMD (PTA complicated by flow-limited dissection) given high rates of in-stent stenosis. Because most FMD patients are younger than those with atherosclerotic RAS, they demonstrate pronounced vasoreactivity and vasospasm of the renal vasculature is common. Patients may benefit from premedication with short-acting dihydropyridines (nifedipine) if not already receiving treatment with calcium channel blockers and catheter-directed infusion of nitroglycerin to minimize vasospasm. Although dissection and arterial rupture are rare with rates approaching 2% to 6%, care should be taken not to over-size balloons. Cutting, scoring, and thermal balloons are not recommended as first-line balloons for angioplasty. Technical success rates for balloon angioplasty of adult renal FMD approach 100%. Although HTN cure is as low as 6%, HTN is improved in two-third of patients.[18] Freedom from worsening HTN is 75% at 5 years, and while primary patency is 95% and 71% at 1 and 5 years, respectively, primary-assisted patency approaches 100% at 9 years.

Ⓛ Surveillance and medical management

Patients with RAS managed medically or after intervention or surgery should receive antiplatelet therapy, ideally implemented preoperatively, as well as their antihypertensive regimen. Because RAS and RVH can recur after intervention and worsen under medical management, judicious surveillance is imperative and recurrent HTN should prompt repeat arteriography and intervention as clinically indicated. Annual surveillance should reconcile home blood pressure logs, office-based blood pressure measurements and trends, renal function (eGFR), and renal DUS to screen for recurrent RAS or renal atrophy.

Ⓜ Consider repeat balloon angioplasty

Recurrent medically refractory HTN after prior renal artery angioplasty should prompt repeat arteriography with catheter manometry. Stenosis secondary to neointimal hyperplasia is best treated with repeat balloon angioplasty. Cutting or scoring balloon angioplasty may be considered in this setting, with selective utilization of stenting for flow-limiting residual stenosis or dissection. Although data regarding the benefit of secondary renal artery angioplasty for FMD are lacking, renal artery angioplasty to maintain primary-assisted patency is reported with good technical success; experience with failed operative repairs suggests that secondary procedures may be associated with beneficial blood pressure response.[18-21]

Ⓝ Renal artery bypass

For recurrent and recalcitrant cases, open revascularization with aorto-renal bypass should be considered for appropriate-risk patients. Surgical exposure can be approached through a vertical midline incision, whereas an extended subcostal incision may be appropriate for unilateral renal revascularization and enhances distal renal exposure. Typically, renal veins lie anterior to the arteries and, as such, venous retraction facilitates arterial exposure; this is enhanced with the ligation and division of renal venous branches (ie, lumbar, gonadal, and adrenal veins). For complex and distal revascularization, medial visceral rotation can facilitate exposure of the distal renal artery and first-/second-order branches. Autogenous saphenous vein is the preferred conduit for revascularization of nonatherosclerotic RAS.[22,23] Thin-walled ePTFE and hypogastric artery are reasonable alternatives, the former requiring target renal artery diameter of >4 mm. The end-to-side aortic anastomosis is performed, removing an ellipse of the anterolateral aortic wall. Partial aortic occlusion can be considered if the aorta is soft. The distal end-to-end renal artery anastomosis can be performed with continuous or interrupted sutures of fine monofilament. Care must be taken to avoid redundancy in length due to the risk of kinking and thrombosis. *Ex vivo* reconstruction can be considered for patients with extensive branch disease.

Patients with anatomy not amenable to PTA (aneurysms or branch vessel involvement) or those who have had a prior balloon angioplasty should be considered for open surgical operation with very good surgical outcomes at high-volume centers. HTN benefits occur in up to 90% of patients postoperatively; cure rates can approach 30%.[22-25] These results are better than those seen for patients treated for atherosclerosis and likely reflecting younger age, improved renal function, and few cardiovascular risk factors. Surgical revascularization also offers good durability, with patency rates of 80% to 90% at 5 years.

Isolated RAS vs. midaortic syndrome

RVH secondary to RAS and abdominal aortic coarctation (midaortic syndrome) are important causes of pediatric HTN, the natural history of which risks failure to thrive, heart failure, hypertensive encephalopathy, impaired mental development, hemorrhagic stroke, and early mortality.[26] It is estimated that 5% to 10% of pediatric HTN may be explained by RVH resulting from RAS and/or midaortic syndrome.[26]

Ⓟ Surgical revascularization for midaortic syndrome

Surgical revascularization remains the gold standard for children with midaortic syndrome.[26] Options for revascularization include aorto-aortic bypass around the narrowed aortic segment, aortic patch aortoplasty and, less commonly, interposition grafting of the aortic segment. Revascularization of renal artery or mesenteric stenosis are performed concomitantly as indicated. The proximal extent of the coarctation and severity of such will often determine the optimal surgical approach. If renal revascularization is intended, a transverse laparotomy will facilitate renal exposure for mobilization. Exposure of the suprarenal aorta typically requires medial visceral rotation. Patch aortoplasty is preferred when the coarctation segment maintains adequate diameter to allow completion of an anastomosis without an overlap of sutures from the opposing side. An ePTFE patch is sized to not be constrictive with growth into adulthood, yet not so generous as to risk development of unstable laminar thrombus. Aorto-aortic bypass is favored for those patients whose coarctation precludes patch aortoplasty secondary to diminutive caliber and in certain complex cases that require concomitant renal and splanchnic reconstruction. The ePTFE conduit should be sized at least 60% to 70% the size of the adult aorta to prevent it from becoming an energy-consuming constriction as the aorta matures. This translates into an 8- to 12-mm graft in young children, a 12- to 16-mm graft in early adolescents, and a 14- to 20-mm graft in late adolescents and adults. Graft length should be slightly more redundant in younger children to allow for stretch with axial growth; however, there is minimal axial growth from the diaphragm to the pelvis after 9 to 10 years of age. Rarely, interposition aortic grafts may be considered to treat short-segment coarctations in the absence of branch vessel involvement.

This often permits a more limited exposure. In the clinical setting of RVH, any RAS warrants simultaneous revascularization at the time of aortic reconstruction, with the exception being the child at the extremes of youth (<3 years of age). Surgical revascularization of pediatric RVH is associated with HTN cure rates that approach 70%, improvement rates of approximately 25%, and failure rates ≤10% across several large series.[26-29]

Q Surgical revascularization for nonatherosclerotic RAS

For nonatherosclerotic RAS in the pediatric population, technical options for open renal artery revascularization include renal artery reimplantation onto the aorta for ostial stenosis or aorto-renal bypass using autogenous conduit for distal renal and branch disease. The internal iliac artery is the preferred conduit as saphenous vein is prone to aneurysmal degeneration and prosthetic conduits are more predisposed to anastomotic restenosis. Surgical exposure is similar to bypass in adults (see N). Surgical revascularization of pediatric RVH is associated with HTN cure rates that approach 70%, improvement rates of approximately 25%, and failure rates ≤10% across several large series.[26-29]

R Consider endovascular treatment

There may be a role for angioplasty for select cases of pediatric RAS. This is supported by the HTN improvement rates that mainly average 50% to 60% across larger series of pediatric RAS treated with PTA.[30-33] Early and late failures of balloon angioplasty for pediatric patients with RAS often result from significant recoil of lesions that are often hypoplastic and associated with highly fibrotic aortic narrowing. Renal PTA for the treatment of pediatric RVH due to ostial disease may be complicated by failures requiring technically complex remedial revascularization procedures or nephrectomy.[34] Renal artery stenting in children should be avoided. Moreover, HTN cure is less likely following remedial operation (24% in comparison to 70% as referenced above).

S Surveillance and medical management

Ongoing surveillance of pediatric patients treated for RAS or midaortic syndrome is imperative. Recurrent HTN should prompt repeat arteriography and intervention as clinically indicated. Annual surveillance should reconcile home blood pressure logs, office-based blood pressure measurements and trends, ambulatory BP measurements, urinalysis (for protein), renal function (eGFR), and renal DUS for renal size/mass and arterial waveforms/velocities. Additional considerations following open revascularization for midaortic syndrome include annual surveillance of lower extremity blood flow with exercise ankle-brachial indices. Serial MRA/CTA is often performed at 2-year intervals during periods of robust growth and is also indicated to assess for changes in surveillance ABIs and acute escalations of blood pressure. Reintervention is infrequent but may be required for anastomotic narrowing or if a patient outgrows the adequacy of the primary procedure.

REFERENCES

1. Stanley JC. The evolution of surgery for renovascular occlusive disease. *Cardiovasc Surg.* 1994;2(2):195-202.
2. Safian RD, Textor SC. Renal-artery stenosis. *N Engl J Med.* 2001;344(6):431-442.
3. Olin JW, Froehlich J, Gu X, et al. The United States Registry for fibromuscular dysplasia: results in the first 447 patients. *Circulation.* 2012;125(25):3182-3190.
4. Olin JW, Gornik HL, Bacharach JM, et al. Fibromuscular dysplasia: state of the science and critical unanswered questions: a scientific statement from the American Heart Association. *Circulation.* 2014;129(9):1048-1078.
5. Cragg AH, Smith TP, Thompson BH, et al. Incidental fibromuscular dysplasia in potential renal donors: long-term clinical follow-up. *Radiology.* 1989;172(1):145-147.
6. Taylor DC, Kettler MD, Moneta GL, et al. Duplex ultrasound scanning in the diagnosis of renal artery stenosis: a prospective evaluation. *J Vasc Surg.* 1988;7(2):363-369.
7. Hirsch AT, Haskal ZJ, Hertzer NR, et al. ACC/AHA 2005 Practice Guidelines for the management of patients with peripheral arterial disease (lower extremity, renal, mesenteric, and abdominal aortic): a collaborative report from the American Association for Vascular Surgery/Society for Vascular Surgery, Society for Cardiovascular Angiography and Interventions, Society for Vascular Medicine and Biology, Society of Interventional Radiology, and the ACC/AHA Task Force on Practice Guidelines (Writing Committee to Develop Guidelines for the Management of Patients With Peripheral Arterial Disease): endorsed by the American Association of Cardiovascular and Pulmonary Rehabilitation; National Heart, Lung, and Blood Institute; Society for Vascular Nursing; TransAtlantic Inter-Society Consensus; and Vascular Disease Foundation. *Circulation.* 2006;113(11):e463-654.
8. Willmann JK, Wildermuth S, Pfammatter T, et al. Aortoiliac and renal arteries: prospective intraindividual comparison of contrast-enhanced three-dimensional MR angiography and multi-detector row CT angiography. *Radiology.* 2003; 226(3):798-811.
9. Tan KT, van Beek EJ, Brown PW, van Delden OM, Tijssen J, Ramsay LE. Magnetic resonance angiography for the diagnosis of renal artery stenosis: a meta-analysis. *Clin Radiol.* 2002;57(7):617-624.
10. Gowda MS, Loeb AL, Crouse LJ, Kramer PH. Complementary roles of color-flow duplex imaging and intravascular ultrasound in the diagnosis of renal artery fibromuscular dysplasia: should renal arteriography serve as the "gold standard"? *J Am Coll Cardiol.* 2003;41(8):1305-1311.
11. Stanley JC, Gewertz BL, Fry WJ. Renal: systemic renin indices and renal vein renin ratios as prognostic indicators in remedial renovascular hypertension. *J Surg Res.* 1976;20(3): 149-55.
12. Vaughan ED Jr., Buhler FR, Laragh JH, Sealey JE, Baer L, Bard RH. Renovascular hypertension: renin measurements to indicate hypersecretion and contralateral suppression, estimate renal plasma flow, and score for surgical curability. *Am J Med.* 1973;55(3):402-414.
13. Stanley JC, Fry WJ. Surgical treatment of renovascular hypertension. *Arch Surg.* 1977;112(11):1291-1297.
14. Hannedouche T, Godin M, Fries D, Fillastre JP. Acute renal thrombosis induced by angiotensin-converting enzyme inhibitors in patients with renovascular hypertension. *Nephron.* 1991;57(2):230-231.
15. Wynckel A, Ebikili B, Melin JP, Randoux C, Lavaud S, Chanard J. Long-term follow-up of acute renal failure caused by angiotensin converting enzyme inhibitors. *Am J Hypertens.* 1998;11(9):1080-1086.
16. Johansen TL, Kjaer A. Reversible renal impairment induced by treatment with the angiotensin II receptor antagonist candesartan in a patient with bilateral renal artery stenosis. *BMC Nephrol.* 2001;2:1.
17. Chobanian AV, Bakris GL, Black HR, et al. The Seventh Report of the Joint National Committee on Prevention, Detection, Evaluation, and Treatment of High Blood Pressure: the JNC 7 report. *JAMA.* 2003;289(19):2560-2572.
18. Mousa AY, Campbell JE, Stone PA, Broce M, Bates MC, AbuRahma AF. Short- and long-term outcomes of percutaneous transluminal angioplasty/stenting of renal fibromuscular dysplasia over a ten-year period. *J Vasc Surg.* 2012; 55(2):421-427.
19. Christie JW, Conlee TD, Craven TE, et al. Early duplex predicts restenosis after renal artery angioplasty and stenting. *J Vasc Surg.* 2012;56(5):1373-1380; discussion 80.
20. Hansen KJ, Deitch JS, Oskin TC, Ligush J Jr, Craven TE, Dean RH. Renal artery repair: consequence of operative failures. *Ann Surg.* 1998;227(5):678-689; discussion 89-90.
21. Davies MG, Saad WE, Peden EK, Mohiuddin IT, Naoum JJ, Lumsden AB. The long-term outcomes of percutaneous therapy for renal artery fibromuscular dysplasia. *J Vasc Surg.* 2008;48(4):865-871.
22. Ham SW, Kumar SR, Wang BR, Rowe VL, Weaver FA. Late outcomes of endovascular and open revascularization for nonatherosclerotic renal artery disease. *Arch Surg.* 2010; 145(9):832-839.
23. Carmo M, Bower TC, Mozes G, et al. Surgical management of renal fibromuscular dysplasia: challenges in the endovascular era. *Ann Vasc Surg.* 2005;19(2):208-217.
24. Marekovic Z, Mokos I, Krhen I, Goreta NR, Roncevic T. Long-term outcome after surgical kidney revascularization for fibromuscular dysplasia and atherosclerotic renal artery stenosis. *J Urol.* 2004;171(3):1043-1045.
25. Anderson CA, Hansen KJ, Benjamin ME, Keith DR, Craven TE, Dean RH. Renal artery fibromuscular dysplasia: results

of current surgical therapy. *J Vasc Surg*. 1995;22(3):207-215; discussion 15-16.

26. Stanley JC, Criado E, Upchurch GR Jr, et al. Pediatric renovascular hypertension: 132 primary and 30 secondary operations in 97 children. *J Vasc Surg*. 2006;44(6):1219-28; discussion 28-29.

27. Martinez A, Novick AC, Cunningham R, Goormastic M. Improved results of vascular reconstruction in pediatric and young adult patients with renovascular hypertension. *J Urol*. 1990;144(3):717-720.

28. O'Neill JA Jr. Long-term outcome with surgical treatment of renovascular hypertension. *J Pediatr Surg*. 1998;33(1): 106-111.

29. Lacombe M. Surgical treatment of renovascular hypertension in children. *Eur J Vasc Endovasc Surg*. 2011;41(6):770-777.

30. Shroff R, Roebuck DJ, Gordon I, et al. Angioplasty for renovascular hypertension in children: 20-year experience. *Pediatrics*. 2006;118(1):268-275.

31. Courtel JV, Soto B, Niaudet P, et al. Percutaneous transluminal angioplasty of renal artery stenosis in children. *Pediatr Radiol*. 1998;28(1):59-63.

32. Casalini E, Sfondrini MS, Fossali E. Two-year clinical follow-up of children and adolescents after percutaneous transluminal angioplasty for renovascular hypertension. *Invest Radiol*. 1995;30(1):40-3.

33. Srinivasan A, Krishnamurthy G, Fontalvo-Herazo L, et al. Angioplasty for renal artery stenosis in pediatric patients: an 11-year retrospective experience. *J Vasc Interv Radiol*. 2010;21:1672-1680.

34. Eliason JL, Coleman DM, Criado E, et al. Remedial operations for failed endovascular therapy of 32 renal artery stenoses in 24 children. *Pediatr Nephrol*. 2016;31(5):809-817.

Jonathan R. Thompson • Matthew A. Corriere

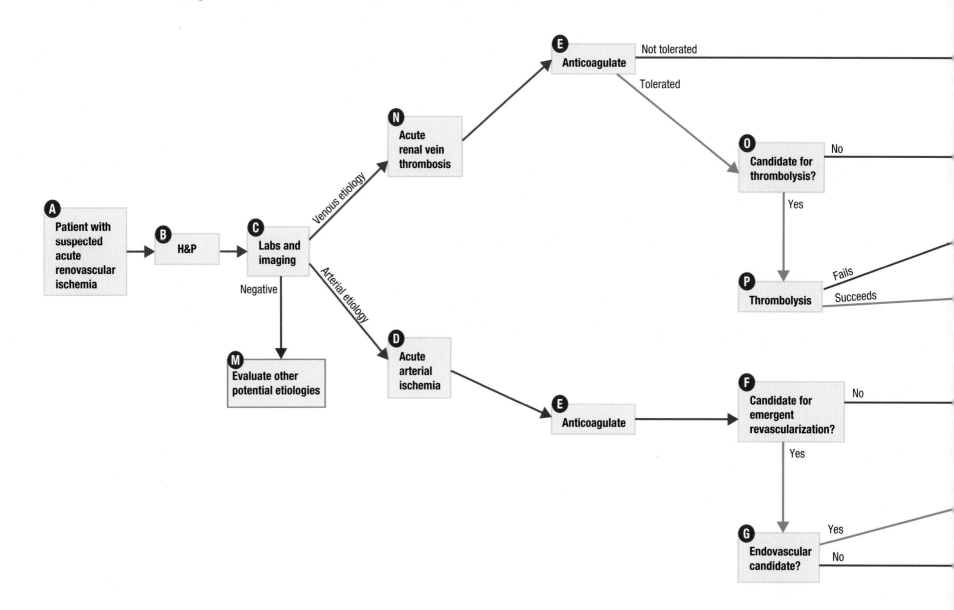

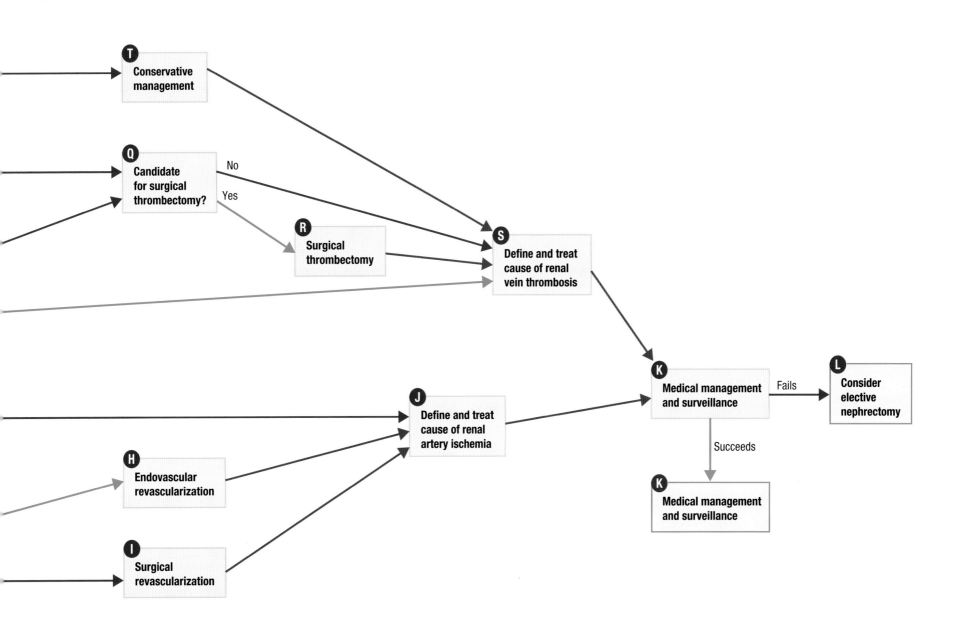

A Patient with suspected acute renovascular ischemia

Acute renal ischemia is rare, with an incidence of <1% among patients hospitalized for renal embolism,[1] <1% for renal artery injury in the setting of blunt abdominal trauma,[2] and <1 case per million adults per year for renal vein thrombosis.[3] Other causes with unknown incidence and prevalence include dissection of the aorta and/or renal arteries and iatrogenic renal vascular injury or coverage.

B H&P

Acute renal ischemia usually presents with lateralized flank, back, or abdominal pain. Many patients present >24 hours after symptom onset.[4] Pain is often constant rather than colicky, which may be useful in distinguishing acute renal ischemia from other diagnoses such as appendicitis and kidney stones.[1,4] Accompanying symptoms may include hematuria, dark urine, and dysuria. Arterial ischemia is usually acute in onset, with most patients able to define the hour when their symptoms began. Ischemia from renal vein thrombosis is usually associated with more gradual onset. Suspicion of embolic renal artery ischemia should be heightened when patients present with a history of atrial fibrillation, valvular heart disease, or a hypercoagulable disorder. Patients with descending thoracic aortic dissection and associated renal involvement usually present with tearing or ripping back pain, HTN, and pulse deficits. Physical examination should include assessment of heart rate and rhythm (accompanied by electrocardiogram), a thorough pulse, genitourinary and abdominal examination, noting any flank tenderness.[5]

C Labs and imaging

Laboratory findings associated with acute renal ischemia include leukocytosis, elevated LDH, elevated D-dimer, eosinophilia, proteinuria, and either gross or microscopic hematuria.[4] Although these findings are nonspecific, the triad of elevated LDH, proteinuria, and flank or abdominal pain is present in most patients with acute renal arterial ischemia.[4] Abnormal serum creatinine, however, is present in only half of patients at initial presentation.

CTA is the preferred imaging test for acute renal ischemia, with a sensitivity of 80% for arterial ischemia and 100% for acute renal vein thrombosis.[1,6] CTA is capable of easily distinguishing between arterial and venous ischemia, and also provides soft-tissue imaging to rule out alternative diagnoses. Inclusion of a noncontrast phase can identify kidney stones (a common alternative diagnosis), and some have proposed that a negative noncontrast CT performed for suspected kidney stones should be followed by a CTA to exclude acute renal ischemia.[1,7]

Although DSA is also highly sensitive for acute arterial ischemia and permits endovascular treatment, it should only be used when the index of suspicion is high (such as concern for intraoperative ischemia) or ischemia develops during a procedure where DSA is already being utilized.

Nuclear isotope scanning is also highly sensitive for acute renal ischemia, but the time-consuming nature of this test makes it better suited for confirming functional renal mass in the setting of main renal artery occlusion with collateral perfusion, rather than for diagnosing suspected acute ischemia.

D Acute arterial ischemia

Acute arterial renal ischemia can be caused by embolism or thrombosis.[5] Acute thrombosis may occur within native vascular disease or be a consequence of traumatic vascular injury. Key considerations for management include the duration of ischemia, the likely etiology, and whether ischemia involves one or both kidneys. The time-sensitive nature of acute arterial ischemia makes immediate recognition critical for potential salvage of renal function.

E Anticoagulate

All patients with acute renal ischemia (arterial or venous) should be therapeutically anticoagulated in the absence of contraindications as soon as this diagnosis is suspected.[5,8] Anticoagulation with unfractionated heparin does not require dosage adjustment in the setting of acute renal failure, prevents repeat thromboembolism, and can prevent thrombus propagation that may threaten important renal artery collaterals (lumbar, gonadal, adrenal, and periureteral collaterals).[1,9] If anticoagulation is contraindicated or not tolerated, medical management alone is undertaken, although judicious intra-procedural anticoagulation is often possible.

F Candidate for emergent revascularization?

The duration of warm renal ischemia is a key factor in determining whether a patient with acute renal ischemia is a candidate for revascularization.[10] Two hours of warm renal ischemia decreases long-term potential for functional recovery to <50% of baseline, and ischemia becomes irreversible at 3 to 4 hours.[11-13] Severe baseline chronic kidney disease further reduces the potential benefit of emergent revascularization. Patients with acute renal ischemia resulting from in situ thrombosis of chronic renal artery stenosis (RAS) may have developed arterial collaterals, which preserve parenchymal perfusion after main renal artery thrombosis.[9] In such patients, treatment after longer intervals of ischemia may be considered. Functional renal salvage in the setting of renal artery trauma is rare because these patients often have prolonged warm ischemia, contraindications to anticoagulation, and may have associated injuries to the renal parenchyma or upper urinary tract.[14]

G Endovascular candidate?

Patients presenting with acute renal artery ischemia caused by thrombosis of a critical main RAS or thrombosis affecting renal artery branches are candidates for endovascular therapy. Endovascular therapy can be employed as a bridge to definitive surgical therapy for patients with acute arterial thrombosis and anatomy not suitable for endovascular therapy. Patients who are not ideal endovascular candidates may include those requiring open surgical management of associated injuries or disease (ie, acute renal ischemia during open aortic surgery, urologic procedures, or discovered during exploration for abdominal trauma) where open surgical revascularization may result in less warm ischemia time.

H Endovascular revascularization

Renal artery stenting is useful for treatment of acute renal artery ischemia caused by thrombosis of a critical main RAS, ± catheter aspiration thrombectomy and/or catheter-directed thrombolysis to clear distal thrombus. For thrombosis affecting renal branch arteries (ie, embolism or renal artery aneurysm thrombosis), thrombolysis or aspiration alone can be used.[15,16] Thrombolysis may also be used to salvage renal artery patency before staged surgical revascularization when anatomy is suboptimal for definitive endovascular treatment.

I Surgical revascularization

Surgical treatment of acute renal ischemia includes renal artery thrombectomy or bypass. Distal reconstitution of the main or branch renal arteries through collaterals has been suggested as a predictor of functional recovery after surgical revascularization for main renal artery thrombosis.[17] Because renal artery exposure and reconstruction take considerably longer than does endovascular treatment, surgical reconstruction is often contraindicated depending on the duration of warm renal ischemia. Situations where surgical reconstruction may be preferred include iatrogenic thrombosis that is recognized during a procedure (eg, renal artery thrombosis resulting from intraoperative endograft coverage or thrombosis during surgical manipulation of the kidney or pararenal aorta). Renal artery dissections frequently extend into the distal main renal artery and branches; surgical reconstruction can therefore be technically challenging and should be used conservatively for this diagnosis. Renal artery bypass for acute ischemia should be performed with prosthetic conduit in the absence contamination to minimize warm ischemia time. Aortorenal endarterectomy with patch angioplasty is usually performed for chronic disease rather than for acute ischemia.

J Define and treat cause of renal artery ischemia

Acute arterial renal ischemia can be caused by embolism or thrombosis.[5] Renal artery embolism may occur secondary to chronic atrial fibrillation, valvular heart disease, cardiac tumor, aortic disease (including mural thrombus, aneurysm, or atherosclerosis), or paradoxical embolism (ie, embolism from a venous source in the setting of patent foramen ovale or other cardiac septal defect).[1] In situ renal artery thrombosis may occur in association with preexisting critical main RAS from atherosclerosis or FMD (including in-stent thrombosis), acute dissection of the aorta or renal artery, arteritis, thrombosis of a renal artery aneurysm, or hypercoagulable state. Iatrogenic acute renal artery thrombosis may be caused by coverage of the renal artery, ligation or injury during aortic reconstruction, or renal artery manipulation during nonvascular procedures (such as partial nephrectomy or retroperitoneal tumor excision). The underlying etiology should be treated when possible to prevent recurrent ischemia.

K Medical management and surveillance

Post-revascularization anticoagulation is indicated in the majority of patients with acute renal arterial ischemia regardless of whether revascularization is performed. Anticoagulation reduces risk of recurrent arterial embolism (to the renal arteries and elsewhere) in patients with chronic atrial fibrillation. Anticoagulation is also the definitive management for the majority of patients with acute renal ischemia resulting from renal vein thrombosis.[8] For patients with modifiable risk factors, a 3- to 6-month course of anticoagulation is suggested. Although recurrent thrombosis is uncommon following acute renal vein thrombosis (one episode per 100 patient-years of follow-up), chronic anticoagulation is associated with survival advantage.[18] Hemodialysis is seldom required for patients with acute renal vein thrombosis.[19] Renal DUS is usually satisfactory for long-term surveillance, with selective cross-sectional imaging usually reserved for scenarios where DUS is technically inadequate or raises concerns for restenosis or recurrent thrombosis. If medical management of persisting hypertension or pain due to an ischemic, nonfunctional kidney is not successful, nephrectomy may be required.

L Consider elective nephrectomy

Nephrectomy can have a palliative role in patients with an ischemic, nonfunctional kidney who experience severe pain or HTN that cannot be managed medically.[6] These patients often have significant renal atrophy. Palliative nephrectomy is supported by the absence of nuclear scan perfusion combined with high renal vein renin levels that lateralize to the nonfunctional kidney. Elective nephrectomy performed using laparoscopic or robotic techniques is associated with lower risk than is surgical revascularization. Nephrectomy also allows for definitive management of postinfarction hemorrhage in patients who require chronic anticoagulation.

M Evaluate other potential etiologies

Signs and symptoms of acute renal ischemia include flank, abdominal, or back pain; hematuria; anuria; and HTN. Alternative diagnoses consistent with these signs and symptoms include kidney stones, urinary tract infection, appendicitis, cholecystitis, mesenteric ischemia, splenic infarct, MI, PE, ectopic pregnancy, pelvic inflammatory disease, incarcerated hernia, and testicular torsion.[1,5]

N Acute renal vein thrombosis

Risk factors for acute renal vein thrombosis include hypercoagulable disorders (particularly nephrotic syndrome), renal cell carcinoma, retroperitoneal tumors, oral contraceptive use, infection, history of DVT, history of IVC filter or central venous catheter, and recent surgery.[8,18] Central venous catheters and critical illness are the most common risk factors in neonates.[20]

O Candidate for thrombolysis?

Thrombolysis can be considered for appropriate-risk candidates with renal vein thrombosis who experience failure of anticoagulation (ie, thrombus propagation or new venous thromboembolism while therapeutically anticoagulated), bilateral thrombosis, thrombosis affecting a solitary kidney, or acute renal failure.[21,22] Contraindications to thrombolysis include history of GI bleeding, recent stroke, history of intracranial bleeding, recent major surgery (especially intracranial or spine surgery), recent trauma, uncontrolled HTN, and renal vein thrombosis associated with a renal cell carcinoma.[22] Thrombolysis should not be performed if renal ischemia is likely irreversible.

P Thrombolysis

Thrombolysis for renal vein thrombosis is performed through percutaneous femoral vein access. The affected renal vein is selected with a guide catheter for selective venography. Carbon dioxide can be used instead of iodinated contrast in patients with acute renal failure.[22] Thrombectomy can be performed using mechanical rheolytic thrombectomy or aspiration catheters. Results may be improved when thrombectomy is preceded by pulsed bolus of alteplase into the thrombosed segment. When residual thrombus is identified following these measures, a multiple side-hole infusion catheter can be positioned within the renal vein for continuous alteplase infusion. Repeat venography should be performed within 24 hours to assess for interval improvement, with cessation of thrombolysis once anatomic resolution is achieved or if no improvement is identified within 24 to 48 hours.

Q Candidate for surgical thrombectomy?

Surgical renal vein thrombectomy is rarely necessary but should be considered for renal vein thrombosis in the setting of failure of thrombolysis to reestablish patency, thrombosis associated with renal malignancy (particularly when nephrectomy or partial nephrectomy is planned), or thrombosis with contraindication to anticoagulation.[6] Thrombectomy may also be considered when extrinsic compression (eg, from a retroperitoneal mass) is the suspected etiology and is being treated surgically.

R Surgical thrombectomy

Surgical thrombectomy is seldom utilized for acute ischemia; the technique, however, has been described for patients with renal malignancy and chronic renal vein thrombosis extending into the vena cava.[23,24] The proximal extent of the thrombus is a key consideration for planning, and echocardiography should be considered if CT venography suggests involvement of the vena cava near or proximal to the hepatic veins. Cardiopulmonary bypass may be required when thrombus extends to the retrohepatic vena cava or right atrium.

S Define and treat cause of renal vein thrombosis

Acute renal vein thrombosis is commonly caused by hypercoagulable states, mechanical obstruction, or foreign bodies (such as central venous catheters or IVC filters located adjacent to the renal veins).[6,8] In the absence of modifiable risk factors (eg, oral contraceptive use and malignancy), life-long anticoagulation is usually recommended if no contraindications exist because of lack of evidence supporting safety and duration of temporary anticoagulation.[18]

T Conservative management

Patients with renal vein thrombosis who cannot be safely anticoagulated have limited options other than supportive management. Placement of a suprarenal IVC filter can be considered to prevent PE, but limited evidence exists to guide use of any specific management strategy under these circumstances. Thrombectomy should be avoided if anticoagulation is contraindicated because of risk of procedure-related embolization and recurrent thrombosis.

REFERENCES

1. Hazanov N, Somin M, Attali M, et al. Acute renal embolism. Forty-four cases of renal infarction in patients with atrial fibrillation. *Medicine (Baltimore)*. 2004;83(5):292-299.
2. Sangthong B, Demetriades D, Martin M, et al. Management and hospital outcomes of blunt renal artery injuries: analysis of 517 patients from the National Trauma Data Bank. *J Am Coll Surg*. 2006;203(5):612-617.
3. Zoller B, Li X, Sundquist J, Sundquist K. Familial risks of unusual forms of venous thrombosis: a nationwide epidemiological study in Sweden. *J Intern Med*. 2011;270(2):158-165.
4. Huang CC, Lo HC, Huang HH, et al. ED presentations of acute renal infarction. *Am J Emerg Med*. 2007;25(2):164-169.
5. Velazquez-Ramirez G, Corriere MA. Renovascular disease: acute ischemia. In: Sidawy AN, Perler BA, eds. *Rutherford's Vascular Surgery and Endovascular Therapy*. Philadelphia, PA: Elsevier; 2019:1704-1713.
6. Asghar M, Ahmed K, Shah SS, Siddique MK, Dasgupta P, Khan MS. Renal vein thrombosis. *Eur J Vasc Endovasc Surg*. 2007;34(2):217-223.
7. Krinsky G. Unenhanced helical CT in patients with acute flank pain and renal infarction: the need for contrast material in selected cases. *AJR Am J Roentgenol*. 1996;167(1):282-283.
8. De Stefano V, Martinelli I. Abdominal thromboses of splanchnic, renal and ovarian veins. *Best Pract Res Clin Haematol*. 2012;25(3):253-264.

9. Flye MW, Anderson RW, Fish JC, Silver D. Successful surgical treatment of anuria caused by renal artery occlusion. *Ann Surg.* 1982;195(3):346-353.

10. Navaravong L, Ali RG, Giugliano GR. Acute renal artery occlusion: making the case for renal artery revascularization. *Cardiovasc Revasc Med.* 2011;12(6):399-402.

11. Lohse JR, Shore RM, Belzer FO. Acute renal artery occlusion: the role of collateral circulation. *Arch Surg.* 1982;117(6):801-804.

12. Hamilton PB, Phillips RA, Hiller A. Duration of renal ischemia required to produce uremia. *Am J Physiol.* 1948;152(3):517-522.

13. Semb C. Partial resection of the kidney: anatomical, physiological and clinical aspects. *Ann R Coll Surg Engl.* 1956;19(3):137-155.

14. Knudson MM, Harrison PB, Hoyt DB, et al. Outcome after major renovascular injuries: a Western trauma association multicenter report. *J Trauma.* 2000;49(6):1116-1122.

15. Blum U, Billmann P, Krause T, et al. Effect of local low-dose thrombolysis on clinical outcome in acute embolic renal artery occlusion. *Radiology.* 1993;189(2):549-554.

16. Syed MI, Shaikh A, Ullah A, et al. Acute renal artery thrombosis treated with t-PA power-pulse spray rheolytic thrombectomy. *Cardiovasc Revasc Med.* 2010;11(4):264.e1-264.e7.

17. Ouriel K, Andrus CH, Ricotta JJ, DeWeese JA, Green RM. Acute renal artery occlusion: when is revascularization justified? *J Vasc Surg.* 1987;5(2):348-355.

18. Wysokinski WE, Gosk-Bierska I, Greene EL, Grill D, Wiste H, McBane RD. Clinical characteristics and long-term follow-up of patients with renal vein thrombosis. *Am J Kidney Dis.* 2008;51(2):224-232.

19. Zigman A, Yazbeck S, Emil S, Nguyen L. Renal vein thrombosis: a 10-year review. *J Pediatr Surg.* 2000;35(11):1540-1542.

20. Brandao LR, Simpson EA, Lau KK. Neonatal renal vein thrombosis. *Semin Fetal Neonatal Med.* 2011;16(6):323-328.

21. Lam KK, Lui CC. Successful treatment of acute inferior vena cava and unilateral renal vein thrombosis by local infusion of recombinant tissue plasminogen activator. *Am J Kidney Dis.* 1998;32(6):1075-1079.

22. Kim HS, Fine DM, Atta MG. Catheter-directed thrombectomy and thrombolysis for acute renal vein thrombosis. *J Vasc Interv Radiol.* 2006;17(5):815-822.

23. Calero A, Armstrong PA. Renal cell carcinoma accompanied by venous invasion and inferior vena cava thrombus: classification and operative strategies for the vascular surgeon. *Semin Vasc Surg.* 2013;26(4):219-225.

24. Haidar GM, Hicks TD, El-Sayed HF, Davies MG. Treatment options and outcomes for caval thrombectomy and resection for renal cell carcinoma. *J Vasc Surg Venous Lymphat Disord.* 2017;5(3):430-436.

Christine Lotto • Matthew T. Menard

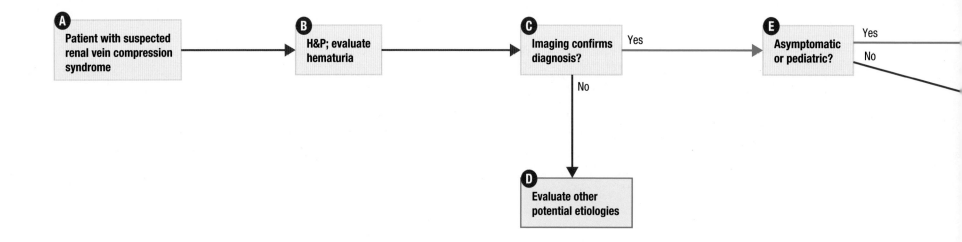

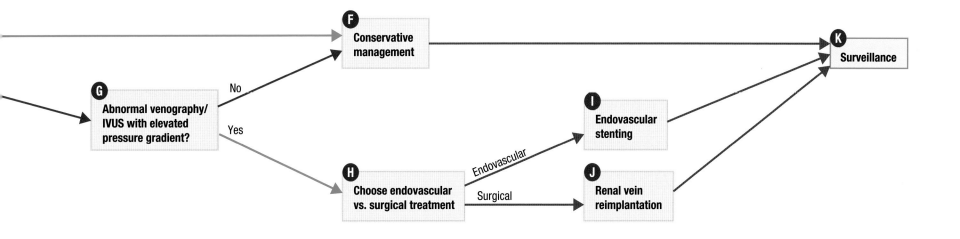

A Patient with suspected renal vein compression syndrome

Renal vein compression syndrome, one of several referred to as "nutcracker" syndrome, is caused by compression of the left renal vein between the SMA and the aorta, resulting in left renal, and sometimes pelvic, venous congestion. Patients are often referred for incidental CTA or MRA findings of renal vein compression or when they manifest left-sided flank pain with either gross or microscopic hematuria. The hematuria has been postulated to be due to microvascular rupture of thin-walled renal pelvic and periureteral varices and may be intermittent. Additional symptoms are attributable to pelvic congestion from left renal vein hypertension and resultant elevated pressure in the gonadal venous circuit, leading to left-sided varicocele formation in men and chronic pelvic pain, left lateral vaginal tenderness, dyspareunia, or dysmenorrhea in women (so-called pelvic congestion syndrome).[1] Exacerbation of symptoms with sitting or standing has also been noted.[2] The majority of patients with renal vein compression syndrome are young or middle aged, but cases have been reported in children. Often patients have a thin body habitus. The lack of retroperitoneal fat may contribute to the narrow aortomesenteric angle in these patients and result in left renal vein compression.[3] Any constellation of the abovementioned symptomatology may warrant further investigation into left renal vein compression.

B H&P; evaluate hematuria

A comprehensive H&P should be performed to exclude multiple other diagnostic possibilities, because the differential diagnosis for abdominal or left-sided flank pain and hematuria may be broad. Imaging is required to establish the diagnosis of renal vein compression syndrome.

For patients presenting with hematuria, a urologic workup for other causes of hematuria should be done, because other etiologies are more likely. Cystoscopic evaluation can localize bleeding to the left ureteral orifice, thereby strengthening the diagnosis of renal vein compression syndrome (particularly when gross hematuria is a presenting symptom). Given the intermittent and often microscopic nature of the hematuria, however, a negative cystoscopy does not rule out renal vein compression.[1]

C Imaging confirms diagnosis?

Confirmation with imaging is essential to making the diagnosis of renal vein compression syndrome. Cross-sectional imaging with either CTA or MRA can accurately delineate the relationship of the left renal vein to the surrounding structures and rule out other causes of pelvic pain and hematuria. Relative supportive findings include proximal dilation of the left renal vein and the presence of enlarged pelvic venous collaterals. Abrupt narrowing of the left renal vein with an acute angle (beak sign) was the most accurate CT diagnostic finding in one study.[15] DUS can also be useful in making the diagnosis, although not with as much precision as does

CTA or MRA. In addition to left renal vein enlargement, the examiner should look for collateral veins and for reflux into the left gonadal vein on DUS. Stenosis of the left renal vein is considered significant if the anteroposterior diameter of the left renal vein on the left side of the aorta is more than five times the diameter at the level of stenosis. Peak velocity measurements also suggest a significant stenosis when the peak velocity measured at the stenosis is more than five times that measured at the renal hilum.[4] The sensitivity and specificity of duplex scanning for renal vein compression syndrome have been reported as 78% and 100%, respectively.[5] If imaging does not show renal vein compression, other diagnoses should be pursued.

D Evaluate other potential etiologies

Given the wide differential diagnosis of pain of the abdomen or left flank, alternative diagnoses need to be considered when confirmatory imaging studies for renal vein compression return inconclusive or negative findings. If hematuria is present, a full urologic workup is indicated to delineate the cause. Compression of the left renal vein can lead to pelvic congestion, but it is important to recognize that pelvic congestion syndrome is a separate entity, characterized by pelvic pain that worsens with standing, lasting more than 6 months, and is associated with pelvic vein dilatation and reflux. On physical examination, male patients may have a left-sided varicocele, whereas women may have vulvar varices.[6]

E Asymptomatic or pediatric?

Because renal vein compression can be a harmless variant, asymptomatic patients referred because of radiographic findings of compression can be observed. This is especially true for pediatric patients, of whom up to 75% present with asymptomatic hematuria but experience complete resolution over 24 months with conservative management alone.[4,5]

F Conservative management

Conservative treatment is generally advocated for children with suspected renal vein compression syndrome because resolution of venous compression can occur with growth and weight gain.[7] Careful observation is also appropriate for adults with negative confirmatory studies or uncertainty of the diagnosis. Notably, some authors have described spontaneous resolution of symptoms in adult patients as well.[8] Thus, in asymptomatic or minimally symptomatic patients, conservative management with surveillance is recommended.

G Abnormal venography/IVUS with elevated pressure gradient?

The definitive test to confirm the diagnosis of renal vein compression syndrome remains venocavography. This study allows one to demonstrate both a renocaval pressure gradient and angiographic

findings of a collateral venous network. Normal individuals have a renocaval pressure gradient of <3 mm Hg, with most patients having a gradient of ≤1 mm Hg.[9] Patients with symptomatic renal vein compression typically have an elevated gradient ≥3 mm Hg.[10] IVUS can be especially helpful in confirming renal vein compression, especially for patients with equivocal imaging. It has a reported specificity as high as 90%.[6] If appropriate anatomy is found in a symptomatic patient, treatment can be recommended.

H Choose endovascular vs. surgical treatment

Patients with significant symptoms and confirmatory imaging should be considered for treatment. Endovenous stenting has risen in popularity because of its less invasive nature and acceptable short- and midterm outcomes. However, lack of long-term data plus reporting of complications of stent migration, in-stent restenosis, and thrombosis[6] have prevented this treatment from becoming the gold standard. Stenting is preferred for patients who are poor open surgical candidates, those with a hostile abdomen, and for those patients with renal vein restenosis after open repair. In good-risk patients, however, renal vein reimplantation surgery may offer more durability, at the cost of increased initial morbidity. As in all cases of endovascular versus surgical treatment, patient preference will have a strong impact on the ultimate choice.

I Endovascular stenting

The largest study comparing endovascular treatment to open treatment for renal vein compression syndrome compared 15 patients treated with stenting to five patients treated surgically.[8] After 6 years of follow-up, all stented patients were pain-free, although two patients had persistent hematuria. The authors favored self-expanding, uncovered stents, because they conform better to the renal vein anatomy; they also recommend 20% stent oversizing relative to renal vein diameter (on initial venography), and most commonly used a 14-mm-diameter stent. Standard intraprocedural use of heparin and postprocedural initiation of antiplatelet therapy are recommended.

J Renal vein reimplantation

The authors share Gloviczki et al.'s view[11] that left renal vein transposition is the surgical method of choice for renal vein compression syndrome. In their series of 11 patients who underwent this technique, and were followed up for 11 years, hematuria resolved in all patients. Flank pain also resolved or improved in 8 of 10 patients, and at a mean follow-up of 70 months, all reimplanted left renal veins were confirmed to be widely patent.[12] Technically, the procedure involves a laparotomy and division of the left renal vein from its insertion into the IVC. Mobilization of the adrenal or other tethering collateral branches may be necessary for sufficient mobilization. After oversewing the renal vein stump, the renal vein is transposed more caudally onto the IVC at a distance sufficient to relieve the SMA compression. Bower et al. have advocated for the use of a saphenous vein patch to alleviate overstretching or tension on the reimplanted renal vein and as a means to prevent restenosis[13]; this has not been the authors' practice.

Others have more recently favored left gonadal vein transposition as a simplified alternative to left renal vein transposition, arguing that in patients in whom the gonadal vein is substantially enlarged, the procedure is equally efficacious and avoids the morbidity of manipulating the renal vein.[12] Although good functional outcomes have also been reported with external stenting of the left renal vein with a ringed PTFE graft,[14] a procedure analogous to but potentially more morbid than internal venous stenting, this treatment option is not frequently performed in the current era. Other strategies that more directly decompress the hypertensive circuit include left renocaval and left gonadocaval bypass. The more extreme techniques of autotransplantation of the kidney or nephrectomy have also demonstrated effective and durable symptomatic relief but are typically reserved as bailout or last-resort options. Among these many surgical options, the simplest and most recommended procedure is left renal vein reimplantation onto the IVC.

🄚 Surveillance

Periodic surveillance with DUS or cross sectional imaging is recommended following treatment or conservative management. New symptoms or restenoses associated with symptoms should be reevaluated for potential treatment. In the absence of good evidence to define optimal surveillance intervals, initial annual surveillance progressing to longer intervals, if stable, seems appropriate.

REFERENCES

1. Menard MT, McPhee J. Current management approach to the left renal vein entrapment syndrome (the so-called Nutcracker syndrome). *Intervent Cardiol*. 2011;3(5).
2. Rudloff U, Holmes R, Prem J, Faust G, Moldwin R, Seigel D. Mesoaortic compression of the left renal vein (nutcracker syndrome): case reports and review of the literature. *Ann Vasc Surg*. 2006;20:120-129.
3. Menard MT. Nutcracker syndrome: when should it be treated and how? *Perspect Vasc Surg Endovasc Ther*. 2009;21(2):117-124.
4. Alimi Y, Hartung O. Iliocaval venous obstruction: surgical treatment. In: *Rutherford's Vascular Surgery*. Philadelphia, PA: Elsevier; 2014:928-954.
5. Takebayashi S, Ueki T, Ikeda N, Fujikawa A. Diagnosis of the nutcracker syndrome with color doppler sonography: correlation with flow patterns on retrograde left renal venography. *Am J Roentgenol*. 1999;172:39-43.
6. Ananthan K, Onida S, Davies AH. Nutcracker syndrome: an update on current diagnostic criteria and management guidelines. *Eur J Vasc Endovasc Surg*. 2017;53:886-894.
7. Genc G, Ozkaya O, Bek K, Acikgoz Y, Danaci M. A rare cause of recurrent hematuria in children: nutcracker syndrome. *J Trop Pediat*. 2010;56:275-277.
8. Zhang H, Li M, Jin W, San P, Xu P, Pan S. The left renal entrapment syndrome: diagnosis and treatment. *Ann Vasc Surg*. 2007;21:198-203.
9. Beinart C, Sniderman K, Tamura S, Vaughan E, Sos T. Left renal vein to inferior vena cava pressure relationship in humans. *J Urol*. 1982;127:1070-1071.
10. Nishimura Y, Fushiki M, Yoshida M, et al. Left renal vein hypertension in patients with left renal bleeding of unknown origin. *Radiology*. 1986;160(3):663-667.
11. Reed N, Kalra M, Bower T, Vrtiska T, Ricotta J, Gloviczki P. Left renal vein transposition for nutcracker syndrome. *J Vasc Surg*. 2009;49:386-393
12. Benrashid E, Turley R, Shortell C. Nutcracker syndrome. In: *Rutherford's Vascular Surgery and Endovascular Therapy*. Philadelphia, PA: Elsevier; 2018:2166-2173.
13. Said S, Gloviczki P, Kalra M, et al. Renal nutcracker syndrome: surgical options. *Semin Vasc Surg*. 2013;26:35-42
14. Scultetus A, Villavicencio J, Gillespie D. The nutcracker syndrome: its role in the pelvic venous disorders. *J Vasc Surg*. 2001;34:812-819.
15. Kim K, Cho J, Kim S, et al. Diagnostic value of computed tomographic findings of nutracker syndrome: correlation with renal venography and renocaval pressure gradients. *Eur J Radiol*. 2011;80:648-654.

Philip Goodney

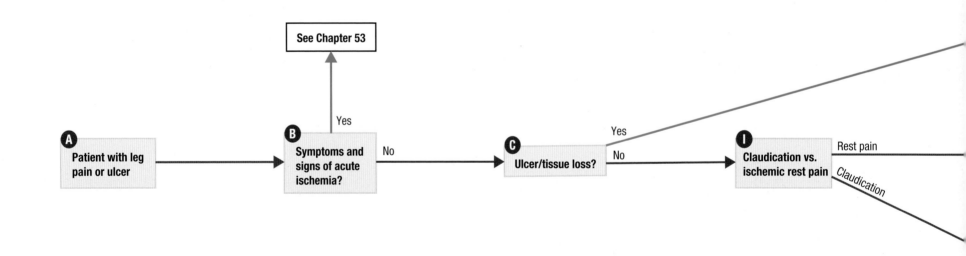

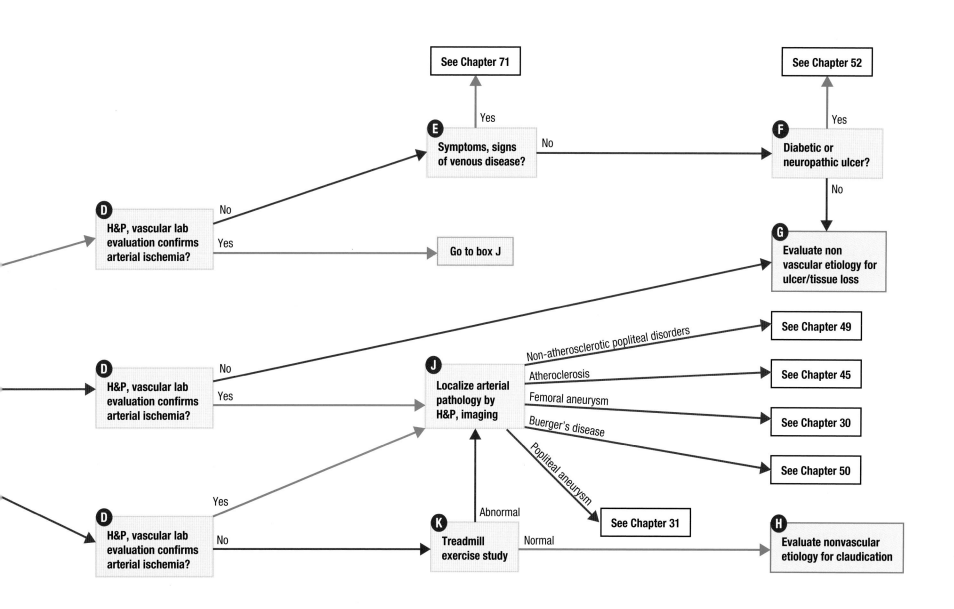

Ⓐ Patient with leg pain or ulcer

Vascular physicians and their teams are often asked to provide consultation for patients with leg pain or ulceration. This request can occur as an elective, office-based visit for a long-standing ulceration or as an urgent emergency room visit for a patient with a cold, painful, acutely ischemic limb. Although leg pain or ulceration is often related to vascular disease, it can have a nonvascular etiology. Having a clear algorithm to evaluate a patient with leg pain or ulceration is a key skill set for vascular physicians.

Ⓑ Symptoms and signs of acute ischemia?

In patients presenting with acute-onset pain, numbness, and weakness, attention should be turned to elucidating the time and rapidity of onset. The well-known "rule of 6 Ps" provides a framework to evaluate signs and symptoms of acute ischemia—pain, pallor, paresis, pulselessness, paresthesia, and poikilothermia (altered temperature). Physical examination follows this framework and makes comparison with the opposite extremity to classify the severity of ALI. In acute ischemia, sensory nerves are impacted earliest, resulting in loss of sensation. Motor nerves are next impacted, resulting in muscle weakness, and, finally, progression to skin necrosis or muscle tenderness is indicative of advanced ischemia.[1]

Ⓒ Ulcer/tissue loss?

In patients without evidence of acute ischemia, the presence and characteristics of tissue ulceration can provide further insight into the etiology of leg pain and tissue loss. Specifically, the chronicity and progression of the ulceration as well as the location of the wounds can prove useful in differentiating different vascular etiologies of tissue loss.[2,3]

Ⓓ H&P, vascular lab evaluation confirms arterial ischemia?

Complete history should be obtained with a focus on predisposing risk factors for atherosclerotic disease, because this is the most common cause of lower extremity ischemia. Specifically, HTN, hyperlipidemia, diabetes mellitus, CKD, and tobacco use are often present in these patients. Comorbid conditions such as CAD, cerebrovascular disease, and COPD should be identified. The history should also focus on the chronicity and localization of ischemic pain. Muscle pain with walking (intermittent claudication) is an early sign of PAD, whereas pain at rest or tissue loss represents CLI and more advanced disease. Intermittent claudication usually occurs in the calf, but may involve the thigh or buttock if iliac or proximal femoral artery disease is present. CLI usually requires multilevel arterial involvement, typically involving two of the three segments (aortoiliac, femoral-popliteal, and tibial).

Physical examination begins with visual inspection of the extremity. Arterial insufficiency can manifest with muscular atrophy of the calf, loss of hair over the lower leg, foot, and toes, as well as thickening of nails. Progression of chronic arterial ischemia results in loss of subcutaneous tissue resulting in thin, shiny skin. Dependent limb rubor can also develop and is replaced with pallor when the limb is elevated.[4,5] Ischemic ulcers can develop secondary to repetitive, minor soft-tissue trauma, and impaired tissue healing because of inadequate perfusion to allow for cellular replication necessary for healing. These ulcers develop primarily on the distal aspects of the toes or on the heels. Ulcers can develop more proximally but tend to result from more obvious trauma.[5]

Vascular laboratory evaluation begins with the measurement of segmental arterial pressures and the calculation of ABI. ABI < 0.90 is indicative of arterial insufficiency. Patients with ischemic ulceration or tissue loss typically have ABIs < 0.3. In individuals with diabetes or on hemodialysis, extensive vessel calcification can result in noncompressible arteries with resultant falsely normal or elevated ABIs. In such cases, adjuncts such as toe pressure measurements, PVRs, and Doppler waveform analyses are used to confirm arterial ischemia.[5-7] DUS, DSA, CTA, and MRA can be employed to further localize arterial occlusive disease and plan further intervention.[4,5,7-9]

Ⓔ Symptoms, signs of venous disease?

Venous disease is manifested by a spectrum of symptoms ranging from mild to severe. The most common symptoms are leg swelling, pain, and ulceration. Patients typically describe pain that worsens with prolonged standing and associated swelling beginning in the foot and ankle and progressing proximally. Venous stasis skin changes also can occur and tend to first manifest in the perimalleolar region of the ankle. These changes range from hyperpigmentation due to hemosiderin deposition to lipodermatosclerosis (fibrotic changes to skin and subcutaneous tissues) to chronic ulceration. Like venous skin changes, ulceration typically develops in the gaiter region of the lower calf and ankle. Although unilateral symptoms are suggestive of venous disease, bilateral presentation does not exclude the diagnosis of venous disease.[2,10,11]

Ⓕ Diabetic or neuropathic ulcer?

Diabetic neuropathic ulcers develop because of the complex interplay of decreased sensation, impaired biomechanics, repetitive trauma, and impaired wound healing. These types of ulcers are typically located at weight-bearing locations on the foot, such as the metatarsal heads, as opposed to isolated ischemic ulcers, which are located at the very distal ends of the toes. Diabetic ulcers arise from the effects of chronic hyperglycemia. Impaired sensory neuron function leaves the patient without protective sensation and allows for repetitive tissue injury to occur. Furthermore, motor neuropathy allows for the development of foot deformities resulting in pathologic pressure distribution. The combination of impaired biomechanics and sensation results in ulceration overlying the areas of the foot exposed to repetitive high pressures.[2,3,8]

Ⓖ Evaluate nonvascular etiology for ulcer/tissue loss

Arterial, venous, and diabetic diseases cause the majority of ulcers in patients who present for vascular surgery evaluation. Ulceration in patients without these conditions warrants further evaluation and consideration. The differential diagnoses for nonvascular ulcerations include autoimmune inflammatory diseases such as pyoderma gangrenosum, endocrine disorders, blood dyscrasias, dermatologic diseases, and malignancy (Marjolin ulcer). These ulcers are usually located in the calf, and form "punched-out" lesions without the typical stigmata of venous or arterial disease. Even less common causes of such types of ulcerations can be diseases such as Kaposi sarcoma, sickle cell anemia, and rheumatoid arthritis. A multidisciplinary approach is usually required for the optimal diagnosis and management of these causes of ulceration.[2,4]

Ⓗ Evaluate nonvascular etiology for claudication

Those patients who do not have an arterial or venous cause for their pain on ambulation should be evaluated for nonvascular causes for claudication, which include neurogenic claudication, arthritis, regional pain syndromes or chronic compartment syndrome (see Chapter 51).

Ⓘ Claudication vs. ischemic rest pain

Chronic arterial ischemia can present as pain varying from claudication to ischemic rest pain. Claudication results from insufficient arterial perfusion to meet the metabolic demands of skeletal muscle. It presents as burning, aching, cramping, fatigue, or numbness in the calves, thighs, or buttocks (depending on the level of arterial disease) with ambulation or exercise and is quickly and completely relieved by rest. Ischemic rest pain stems from chronic sensory nerve ischemia and occurs because of inadequate perfusion of the distal extremity at rest. It presents as a diffuse burning or aching pain in the foot, usually in the forefoot. In most patients, this pain is worsened with elevation of the extremity and somewhat improved with dependent positioning of the limb.[5,8] Venous claudication, an uncommon condition, is a similar manifestation of leg pain with ambulation that is caused by chronic deep venous occlusion and concomitant venous HTN. It is often described as a bursting pain sensation that can begin abruptly after a certain amount of walking. Neurogenic claudication, referred to as pseudoclaudication, occurs when patients with spinal stenosis or other low back pathology experience referred pain with ambulation. Physical examination differences—normal arterial pulses but evidence of venous disease or back pain—should alert the examiner to the potential for these disorders.

ⓙ Localize arterial pathology by H&P, imaging

Although atherosclerosis affects most patients with arterial ischemia, other less common etiologies must be considered, appropriately diagnosed, and treated.

Buerger disease is a nonatherosclerotic chronic, inflammatory, thrombotic, obliterative tobacco-associated vasculopathy that involves the infrapopliteal and infrabrachial arteries with resultant distal extremity ischemia. More proximal arteries are usually unaffected. Buerger disease is a clinical diagnosis and most often impacts males <50 years of age with heavy tobacco use history. Imaging such as DSA, CTA, and MRA, when performed, may demonstrate segmental occlusions and normal proximal arteries[12,13] (see Chapter 50).

Lower extremity arterial ischemia is the most common presenting symptom of femoral and popliteal aneurysms as a result of thrombosis or distal embolization. Less frequently, patients may present with compressive symptoms such as lower extremity swelling due to vein compression or neuropathic pain due to nerve compression. Thorough physical examination may allow for palpation of these aneurysms. Imaging modalities such as DUS, CTA, or MRA are useful in identifying and assessing femoral and popliteal aneurysms[5,14-16] (see Chapters 30 and 31).

Popliteal artery entrapment occurs because of anatomic variations in the popliteal artery and the muscles within the popliteal fossa, resulting in compression of the popliteal artery. This manifests most frequently as calf claudication in young, healthy individuals. Rarely do patients present with more advanced ischemia such as rest pain or tissue loss. Physical examination often demonstrates palpable pedal pulses that disappear with passive dorsiflexion or active plantar flexion of the foot. The absence of pedal pulses without the abovementioned maneuvers is indicative of popliteal artery occlusion. Although DUS can be performed, imaging modalities such as DSA, CTA, and MRA more reliably diagnose popliteal artery entrapment[17,18] (see Chapter 49).

Popliteal adventitial cystic disease occurs because of arterial compression by a mucoid adventitial cyst. The etiology of these cysts is thought to stem from the embryologic development of arteries and neighboring joints with resultant mesenchymal mucin-secreting cells from the embryologic joints becoming included in the embryologic adventitia. Similar to popliteal artery entrapment, adventitial cystic disease manifests most frequently as calf claudication in young, healthy individuals. DUS can be used to identify the cysts and visualize compression of arterial lumen, but cross-sectional imaging modalities such as CTA and MRA yield more information about the cyst and associated arterial anatomy[18,19] (see Chapter 49).

ⓚ Treadmill exercise study

Some patients with vascular claudication may have normal resting leg pressures, because the stenosis only causes a pressure gradient during the high blood flow associated with exercise. In such cases, a treadmill exercise study is performed, in which the patient ambulates on the treadmill at a set speed for 10 minutes or until ischemic symptoms arise, such as evidence of claudication. Segmental pressures are obtained every 2 minutes for 10 minutes thereafter or until pressures return to baseline. The lowest systolic ankle pressure after exercise is compared to the baseline pressure and expressed as a ratio. A drop in the resting ABI by more than 20% after exercise indicates a significant arterial stenosis.[7] Conversely, if there is no significant pressure decrease, arterial etiology for the symptoms is ruled out, and other causes, such as neurogenic claudication, should be evaluated.

REFERENCES

1. Earnshaw JJ. Acute ischemia: evaluation and decision making. In: Cronenwett JL, Johnston KW, eds. *Rutherford's Vascular Surgery*. 8th ed. Philadelphia, PA: Elsevier; 2014:2518-2527.
2. Marston WA. Wound care. In: Cronenwett JL, Johnston KW, eds. *Rutherford's Vascular Surgery*. 8th ed. Philadelphia, PA: Elsevier; 2014:1221-1240.
3. Nouvong A, Armstrong DG. Diabetic foot ulcers. In: Cronenwett JL, Johnston KW, eds. *Rutherford's Vascular Surgery*. 8th ed. Philadelphia, PA: Elsevier; 2014:1816-1835.
4. Goodney PP. Patient clinical evaluation. In: Cronenwett JL, Johnston KW, eds. *Rutherford's Vascular Surgery*. 8th ed. Philadelphia, PA: Elsevier; 2014:202-213.
5. Dosluoglu HH. Lower extremity arterial disease: general considerations. In: Cronenwett JL, Johnston KW, eds. *Rutherford's Vascular Surgery*. 8th ed. Philadelphia, PA: Elsevier; 2014:1660-1674.
6. Al-Qaisi M, Nott DM, King DH, Kaddoura S. Ankle brachial pressure index (ABPI): an update for practitioners. *Vasc Health Risk Manag*. 2009;5:833-841. http://www.ncbi.nlm.nih.gov/pubmed/19851521
7. Kohler TR, Sumner DS. Vascular laboratory: arterial physiologic assessment. In: Cronenwett JL, Johnston KW, eds. *Rutherford's Vascular Surgery*. 8th ed. Philadelphia, PA: Elsevier; 2014:214-229.
8. Liapis C, Kakisis J. Atherosclerotic risk factors: general considerations. In: Cronenwett JL, Johnston KW, eds. *Rutherford's Vascular Surgery*. 8th ed. Philadelphia, PA: Elsevier; 2014:400-415.
9. Gerhard-Herman MD, Gornik HL, Barrett C, et al. 2016 AHA/ACC Guideline on the Management of Patients With Lower Extremity Peripheral Artery Disease: A Report of the American College of Cardiology/American Heart Association Task Force on Clinical Practice Guidelines. *Circulation*. 2017;135(12):e726-e779. http://www.ncbi.nlm.nih.gov/pubmed/27840333
10. Eberhardt RT, Raffetto JD. Chronic venous insufficiency. *Circulation*. 2005;111(18):2398-2409. http://www.ncbi.nlm.nih.gov/pubmed/15883226
11. Raffetto JD, Eberhardt RT. Chronic venous disorders: general considerations. In: Cronenwett JL, Johnston KW, eds. *Rutherford's Vascular Surgery*. 8th ed. Philadelphia, PA: Elsevier; 2014:842-857.
12. Piazza G, Creager MA. Thromboangiitis obliterans. *Circulation*. 2010;121(16):1858-1861. http://www.ncbi.nlm.nih.gov/pubmed/20421527
13. Akar AR, Durdu S. Thromboangiitis obliterans (Buerger's disease). In: Cronenwett JL, Johnston KW, eds. *Rutherford's Vascular Surgery*. 8th ed. Philadelphia, PA: Elsevier; 2014:1167-1186.
14. Varga ZA, Locke-Edmunds JC, Baird RN. A multicenter study of popliteal aneurysms. Joint Vascular Research Group. *J Vasc Surg*. 1994;20(2):171-177. http://www.ncbi.nlm.nih.gov/pubmed/8040939
15. Piffaretti G, Mariscalco G, Tozzi M, Rivolta N, Annoni M, Castelli P. Twenty-year experience of femoral artery aneurysms. *J Vasc Surg*. 2011;53(5):1230-1236. http://www.ncbi.nlm.nih.gov/pubmed/21215583
16. Jacobowitz G, Cayne NS. Lower extremity aneurysms. In: Cronenwett JL, Johnston KW, eds. *Rutherford's Vascular Surgery*. 8th ed. Philadelphia, PA: Elsevier; 2014:2190-2205.
17. Sinha S, Houghton J, Holt PJ, Thompson MM, Loftus IM, Hinchliffe RJ. Popliteal entrapment syndrome. *J Vasc Surg*. 2012;55(1):252-262.e30. http://www.ncbi.nlm.nih.gov/pubmed/22116047
18. Forbes TL. Nonatheromatous popliteal artery disease. In: Cronenwett JL, Johnston KW, eds. *Rutherford's Vascular Surgery*. 8th ed. Philadelphia, PA: Elsevier; 2014:1801-1815.
19. Paravastu SC, Regi JM, Turner DR, Gaines PA. A contemporary review of cystic adventitial disease. *Vasc Endovascular Surg*. 2012;46(1):5-14. http://www.ncbi.nlm.nih.gov/pubmed/22169114

Jeffrey Siracuse • Alik Farber

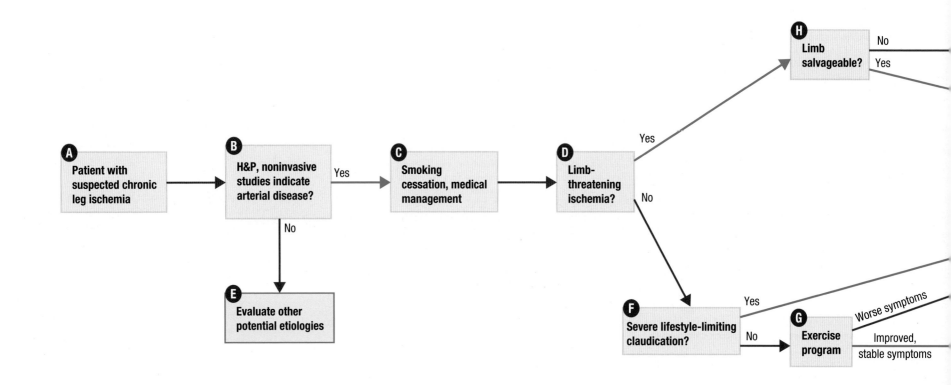

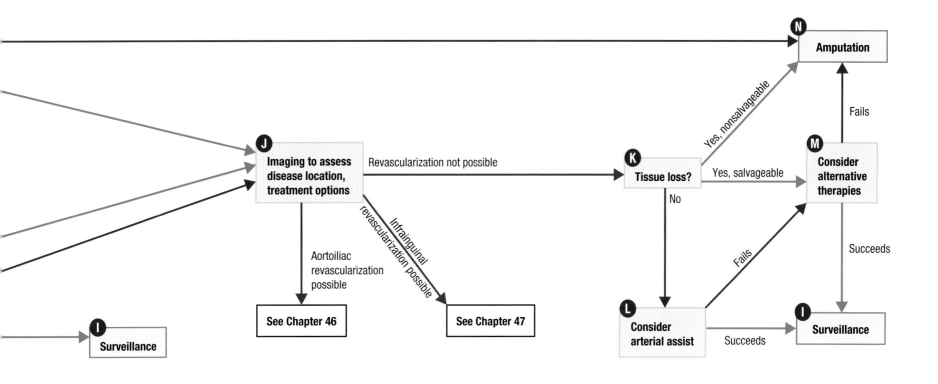

(A) Patient with suspected chronic leg ischemia

Chronic limb ischemia can present as intermittent claudication or limb threat and is usually caused by PAD, an obliterative process that limits blood flow to the extremities. Although a number of etiologies can lead to chronic ischemia, atherosclerosis is the most common. Arterial stenoses and occlusions in the limb reduce distal perfusion such that metabolic requirements of the distal limb exceed its supply.[1] Although collaterals form, via angiogenesis, to improve perfusion, arterial flow in the limb is often inadequate to maintain adequate distal perfusion, leading to symptoms.[1]

Intermittent claudication is manifested by inadequate tissue perfusion of working skeletal muscles and is characterized by pain or weakness in leg muscle groups with activity. It has a prevalence of 1% to 2% in patients older than 55 years. CLI is manifested by chronic, inadequate limb perfusion at rest. It is characterized by ischemic rest pain, ulcers, or gangrene in the presence of objective hemodynamic evidence of arterial insufficiency. The estimated incidence of CLI is 220 to 2500 cases per million and its prevalence is between 1% and 2%. It is estimated that over a 5-year period, 5% to 10% of patients with asymptomatic PAD or intermittent claudication will develop CLI.[1-4]

(B) H&P, noninvasive vascular studies indicate arterial disease?

History of present illness should focus on leg symptoms, duration and factors that improve or worsen them. Risk factors for atherosclerosis such as smoking, HTN, diabetes, hyperlipidemia, and family history of cardiovascular disease should be evaluated. Past medical and surgical history as well as current medication regimen is assessed. Physical examination of the lower extremity should include evaluation of skin quality, tissue loss, neurologic function, and pulse assessment. Although patients with intermittent claudication may have a completely normal limb examination, evaluation of those with CLI may be notable for absence of pulses, dependent rubor, thin or shiny skin, an absence of hair, and increased capillary refill time. Tissue loss usually affects the toes, although the heel, ankle, and even the calf may be involved. Erythema that persists with foot elevation may represent infection that can range from minor cellulitis to abscess or sepsis. Plantar tenderness suggests the presence of a foot abscess.[1-3,5] To confirm the diagnosis of chronic ischemia, a battery of noninvasive vascular tests, including ankle pressures, toe pressures, PVR, and Doppler waveforms, can be performed. The ABI, a ratio of the highest ankle pressure divided by the highest brachial pressure, is the most common test for confirming the presence of PAD. ABI ≤0.9 has been shown to have a high sensitivity and specificity to identify malperfusion to the extremity.[1-5] ABI with and without exercise is used to confirm diagnosis of intermittent claudication in patients with normal resting ABI. Because there are many causes of leg pain and ulceration, if the initial evaluation does not support the diagnosis of PAD, other etiologies should be evaluated.

(C) Smoking cessation, medical management

The initial treatment for PAD includes smoking cessation if the patient is an active smoker (see Chapter 3). Other medical therapy includes aspirin and statin plus treatment of hyperlipidemia (see Chapter 4), HTN, and diabetes, as applicable.[5] A decrease in systemic cardiovascular events has been shown in patients with known atherosclerotic disease treated with antiplatelet medications, statin therapy, blood pressure control, glucose control, and smoking cessation.[6-10] Cilostazol, 100 mg two times daily, can be started in patients with intermittent claudication because it has been shown to improve walking in a subset of claudicants.[5,11] A multicenter randomized, placebo controlled, prospective study of cilostazol in 516 claudicants noted a >50% increase in total walking distance and pain-free walking distance after 24 weeks.[12] Another prospective randomized trial of cilostazol showed a 35% increase in pain-free and a 41% increase in total walking distance.[13] Half of the patients identified as being "better" or "much better" and half were unchanged in the cilostazol arm compared to only 19% "better" or "much better" and 63% unchanged in the placebo group.[13] A 3-month trial is prescribed to those who do not have CHF or other contraindications, and continued if beneficial. Recently, rivaroxaban, a selective, direct Factor Xa Inhibitor and a member of a larger family of direct oral anticoagulants, has been evaluated in PAD. In the VOAYGER PAD trial, patients with symptomatic PAD treated with rivaroxaban gained a 15% risk reduction in the composite primary efficacy endpoint of ALI, major amputation for vascular cause, MI, ischemic stroke or cardiovascular death. This benefit was observed early and was enduring.[14]

(D) Limb-threatening ischemia?

An assessment for CLI, as manifested by ischemic rest pain or tissue loss, should be made. Ischemic pain occurs at rest and usually affects the forefoot. Some patients have numbness rather than pain.[1,3,15] The pain is worse with elevation and lessens with dependency. Tissue loss (wounds, ulcers, gangrene), particularly in the distal limb, suggests limb threat. Presentation should be correlated with noninvasive vascular tests.[1,3,12] The ABI may be falsely elevated because of calcified arteries and digital artery pressures may be more accurate. These may be correlated with PVRs, monophasic Doppler waveforms, and transcutaneous oxygen measurements, which are useful in confirming severe ischemia.[1] Ankle pressures of <70 mm Hg, toe pressures <60 mm Hg, monophasic Doppler tibial waveforms, low-amplitude calf PVRs, or $TcPO_2$ < 30 mm Hg strongly support the diagnosis of CLI.[1]

(E) Evaluate other potential etiologies

If H&P and noninvasive imaging data do not support the diagnosis of PAD, then alternate causes should be worked up. These include neurologic or musculoskeletal etiologies of symptoms.[5,16]

Others include venous claudication, chronic compartment syndrome (see Chapter 51), nerve root compression, Baker cyst, spinal stenosis, and arthritis.[5]

(F) Severe lifestyle-limiting claudication?

Claudication is initially managed conservatively, unless it is severely lifestyle limiting, such that it prevents work or essential life activities.[5] The definition of "severely lifestyle limiting" varies according to individual activity level and goals and is assessed in the context of current ambulatory status, overall health, patient preference, and lifestyle. Patients with mild claudication are often successfully treated with an exercise program. In patients with severe claudication in whom rapid or substantial improvement is needed, imaging can be performed to determine the nature of possible revascularization.

(G) Exercise program

Initial conservative therapy for claudication involves supervised exercise therapy and risk factor reduction. A supervised exercise program of at least 12 weeks, 3 days per week, for 30 to 60 minutes/d is recommended.[5,17-19] Unsupervised exercise programs are theoretically also beneficial, but studies have shown poor patient compliance without supervision.[19] Supervised exercise therapy has been shown to increase total walking distance and pain-free walking distance by 37% and 50%, respectively, compared to home-based exercise therapy.[19] Recent decisions by payers to reimburse exercise therapy for claudication will allow increased access to this treatment modality for more patients. An assessment needs to be made during and after exercise therapy for symptomatic improvement, stability, or deterioration.

(H) Limb salvageable?

For patients with CLI, a determination of whether the limb is salvageable needs to be made. This is based on the extent of tissue loss, the degree of limb ischemia, and presence of concomitant infection.[1,3] The Society for Vascular Surgery Wound, Ischemia, and foot Infection (WIfI) classification system has been developed to help assess limb salvageability among these three domains (wound, ischemia, and foot infection) and has been shown to predict amputation risk and wound healing after revascularization in patients with CLI.[20-22] Each domain is graded from 0 to 3 (none, mild, moderate, severe) and on the basis of these scores, amputation risk is staged from 1 to 4. Stage 1 is low risk, stages 2 and 3 are intermediate risk, and stage 4 is high risk for amputation (see also Chapter 52).

(I) Surveillance

Surveillance of patients with intermittent claudication occurs at regular intervals to assess for improvement or worsening of leg pain and walking distance. Progression to worse claudication or CLI is an indication for imaging to assess treatment options. Smoking cessation is critical for those continuing to smoke (see Chapter 3), and risk factor optimization with medical therapy is continued. Response to cilostazol, if taken, is assessed. The interval for surveillance is individualized depending on stability of symptoms and the patient is cautioned to request reevaluation if symptoms progress. Surveillance in patients with successfully treated CLI is also important because their disease often progresses, and prompt detection may allow additional treatment.

Ⓙ Imaging to assess disease location, treatment options

When a decision is made for potential interventional or surgical treatment of PAD, imaging should be performed to assess for location and extent of occlusive disease.[23] Noninvasive imaging including MRA, CTA, and DUS can be used.[1,5,21-23] Both MRA and CTA can be particularly helpful for assessment of inflow aortoiliac lesions but have limited value in infrapopliteal vessels. MRA quality is highly dependent on MR scanner hardware and local radiology expertise. MRA may be helpful in cases of high calcium burden that obscures CTA findings. Arterial DUS is least invasive imaging but requires an experienced vascular technologist. DSA has traditionally been used to define arterial anatomy[1,21] and allows for immediate endovascular intervention. However, it is also associated with a higher risk of complications. Imaging is pursued until sufficient information is obtained to determine whether revascularization is possible. Revascularization for aortoiliac disease is discussed in Chapter 46 and that for infrainguinal disease in Chapter 47.

Ⓚ Tissue loss?

If revascularization is not possible, the presence and extent of tissue loss dictates optimal management. Extensive tissue loss that renders the limb nonsalvageable is treated by amputation. Patients with rest pain or severe claudication, but without tissue loss, can be considered for arterial assist therapy. In patients without diabetes who have small ulcers, a variety of treatments, including cell-based dressings, gene therapy, and hyperbaric oxygen (HBO) have been used. Management of patients with tissue loss and diabetes is discussed in Chapter 52.

Ⓛ Consider arterial assist

For those patients with severe claudication or ischemic rest pain but no revascularization options, an arterial assist device such as ArtAssist (ACI Medical, San Marcos, CA) may be considered. This is a garment that provides high-pressure sequential compression to the foot, ankle, and calf in an effort to improve distal arterial flow. This form of pneumatic compression therapy has been shown to be associated with improved walking distances and quality-of-life measures in patients with claudication; however, studies are limited to small numbers of patients. It has been also associated with improvement of symptoms and increased quality

of life for those with ischemic rest pain. However, its benefit for wound healing and amputation prevention is not established.[24-26]

Ⓜ Consider alternative therapies

As an additional option for tissue loss in a limb that cannot be revascularized, HBO, cell-based dressings, and gene therapy can be considered, although there are limited data in nondiabetic patients to support these therapies. Overall, HBO therapy has been shown to have some short-term benefit in wound healing in diabetics; however, it has not been associated with improved long-term wound healing; Notably, many of the supporting studies have been hampered by flawed methodology.[27-29] Randomized data comparing HBO with standard of care alone showed no difference in healing outcomes.[27]

Bone marrow stem cell therapy has been shown to have good potential in both diabetic and nondiabetic patients with revascularization options; however, larger and more controlled studies are needed.[30] Other gene therapy options include hepatocyte growth factor; however, again, definitive controlled data is needed.[31]

Ⓝ Amputation

Although the frequency of amputation is decreasing,[32] it is still required for patients who present with advanced disease and unsalvagable limbs. Although contemporary techniques allow revascularization in most ischemic limbs, this is not always possible, in which case, amputation may be the only available option. In diabetic patients with minimal tissue loss, additional options may be available as discussed in Chapter 52. Amputation is considered in detail in Chapter 48.

REFERENCES

1. Farber A. Chronic limb-threatening ischemia. *N Engl J Med.* 2018;379(2):171-180.
2. Alahdab F, Wang AT, Elraiyah TA, et al. A systematic review for the screening for peripheral arterial disease in asymptomatic patients. *J Vasc Surg.* 2015;61(3 suppl):42S-53S.
3. Farber A, Eberhardt RT. The current state of critical limb ischemia: a systematic review. *JAMA Surg.* 2016; 151(11):1070-1077.
4. Nehler MR, Duval S, Diao L, et al. Epidemiology of peripheral arterial disease and critical limb ischemia in an insured national population. *J Vasc Surg.* 2014;60(3): 686-695.e2.
5. Society for Vascular Surgery Lower Extremity Guidelines Writing Group, Conte MS, Pomposelli FB, Clair DG, et al. Society for Vascular Surgery Society for Vascular Surgery practice guidelines for atherosclerotic occlusive disease of the lower extremities: management of asymptomatic disease and claudication. *J Vasc Surg.* 2015;61(3 Suppl):2S-41S.
6. Armstrong EJ, Wu J, Singh GD, et al. Smoking cessation is associated with decreased mortality and improved amputation-free survival among patients with symptomatic peripheral artery disease. *J Vasc Surg.* 2014;60(6):1565-1571.
7. Antithrombotic Trialists' Collaboration. Collaborative meta-analysis of randomised trials of antiplatelet therapy for prevention of death, myocardial infarction, and stroke in high risk patients. *BMJ.* 2002;324(7329):71-86.
8. Squizzato A, Bellesini M, Takeda A, Middeldorp S, Donadini MP. Clopidogrel plus aspirin versus aspirin alone for preventing cardiovascular events. *Cochrane Database Syst Rev.* 2017;12:CD005158.
9. Chou R, Dana T, Blazina I, et al. *Statin use for the Prevention of Cardiovascular Disease in Adults: A Systematic Review for the U.S. Preventive Services Task Force.* Rockville, MD: Agency for Healthcare Research and Quality (US); 2016.
10. Saiz L, Gorricho J, Garjón J, et al. Blood pressure targets for the treatment of people with hypertension and cardiovascular disease. *Cochrane Database Syst Rev.* 2017;10:CD010315.
11. Bedenis R, Stewart M, Cleanthis M, Robless P, Mikhailidis DP, Stansby G. Cilostazol for intermittent claudication. *Cochrane Database Syst Rev.* 2014;(10):CD003748.
12. Beebe HG, Dawson DL, Cutler BS, et al. A new pharmacological treatment for intermittent claudication: results of a randomized, multicenter trial. *Arch Intern Med.* 1999;159(17):2041-2050.
13. Dawson DL, Cutler BS, Meissner MH, Strandness DE Jr. Cilostazol has beneficial effects in treatment of intermittent claudication: results from a multicenter, randomized, prospective, double-blind trial. *Circulation.* 1998;98(7):678-686.
14. Bonaca MP, Bauersachs RM, Anand SS, et al. Rivaroxaban in peripheral artery disease after revascularization. *N Engl J Med.* 2020. doi:10.1056/NEJMoa2000052.
15. Menard MT, Farber A, Assmann SF, et al. Design and rationale of the best endovascular versus best surgical therapy for patients with critical limb ischemia (BEST-CLI) trial. *J Am Heart Assoc.* 2016;5(7).
16. Haig AJ, Park P, Henke PK, et al. Reliability of the clinical examination in the diagnosis of neurogenic versus vascular claudication. *Spine J.* 2013;13(12):1826-1834.
17. Gardner AW, Poehlman ET. Exercise rehabilitation programs for the treatment of claudication pain. A meta-analysis. *JAMA.* 1995;274(12):975-980.
18. Gardner A, Katzel LI, Sorkin JD, et al. Exercise rehabilitation improves functional outcomes and peripheral circulation in patients with intermittent claudication: a randomized controlled trial. *J Am Geriatr Soc.* 2001;49(6):755-762.
19. Hageman D, Fokkenrood HJ, Gommans LN, van den Houten MM, Teijink JA. Supervised exercise therapy versus home-based exercise therapy versus walking advice

for intermittent claudication. *Cochrane Database Syst Rev.* 2018;4:CD005263.

20. Zhan LX, Branco BC, Armstrong DG, Mills JL Sr. The Society for Vascular Surgery lower extremity threatened limb classification system based on Wound, Ischemia, and foot Infection (WIfI) correlates with risk of major amputation and time to wound healing. *J Vasc Surg.* 2015;61(4):939-944.

21. Weaver M, Hicks C, Canner J, et al. The Society for Vascular Surgery Wound, Ischemia, and foot Infection (WIfI) classification system predicts wound healing better than direct angiosome perfusion in diabetic foot wounds. *J Vasc Surg.* 2018;68(5):1473-1481.

22. van Haelst STW, Teraa M, Moll FL, de Borst GJ, Verhaar MC, Conte MS. Prognostic value of the Society for Vascular Surgery Wound, Ischemia, and foot Infection (WIfI) classification in patients with no-option chronic limb-threatening ischemia. *J Vasc Surg.* 2018;68(4):1104-1113.

23. Hingorani A, Ascher E, Markevich N, et al. Magnetic resonance angiography versus duplex arteriography in patients undergoing lower extremity revascularization: which is the best replacement for contrast arteriography? *J Vasc Surg.* 2004;39(4):717-722.

24. Zaki M, Elsherif M, Tawfick W, El Sharkawy M, Hynes N, Sultan S. The role of sequential pneumatic compression in limb salvage in non-reconstructable critical limb ischemia. *Eur J Vasc Endovasc Surg.* 2016;51(4):565-571.

25. Kavros SJ, Delis KT, Turner NS, et al. Improving limb salvage in critical ischemia with intermittent pneumatic compression: a controlled study with 18-month follow-up. *J Vasc Surg.* 2008;47(3):543-549.

26. Chang ST, Hsu JT, Chu CM, et al. Using intermittent pneumatic compression therapy to improve quality of life for symptomatic patients with infrapopliteal diffuse peripheral obstructive disease. *Circ J.* 2012;76(4):971-976.

27. Santema KTB, Stoekenbroek RM, Koelemay MJW, et al.; DAMO2CLES Study Group. Hyperbaric oxygen therapy in the treatment of ischemic lower-extremity ulcers in patients with diabetes: results of the DAMO2CLES multicenter randomized clinical trial. *Diabetes Care.* 2018;41(1):112-119.

28. Kranke P, Bennett MH, Martyn-St James M, Schnabel A, Debus SE, Weibel S. Hyperbaric oxygen therapy for chronic wounds. *Cochrane Database Syst Rev.* 2015;(6):CD004123.

29. Stoekenbroek R, Santema T, Legemate DA, Ubbink DT, van den Brink A, Koelemay MJ. Hyperbaric oxygen for the treatment of diabetic foot ulcers: a systematic review. *Eur J Vasc Endovasc Surg.* 2014;47(6):647-655.

30. Giles KA, Rzucidlo EM, Goodney PP, Walsh DB, Powell RJ. Bone marrow aspirate injection for treatment of critical limb ischemia with comparison to patients undergoing high-risk bypass grafts. *J Vasc Surg.* 2015;61(1):134-137.

31. Cui S, Guo L, Li X, et al. Clinical safety and preliminary efficacy of plasmid pUDK-HGF expressing human hepatocyte growth factor (HGF) in patients with critical limb ischemia. *Eur J Vasc Endovasc Surg.* 2015;50(4):494-501.

32. Goodney PP, Tarulli M, Faerber AE, Schanzer A, Zwolak RM. Fifteen-year trends in lower limb amputation, revascularization, and preventive measures among Medicare patients. *JAMA Surg.* 2015;150(1):84-86.

Derek de Grijs • William P. Robinson III

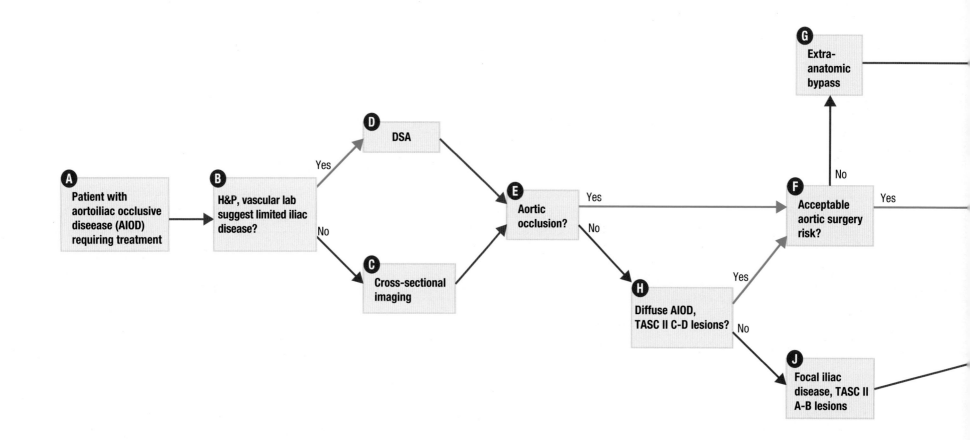

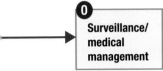

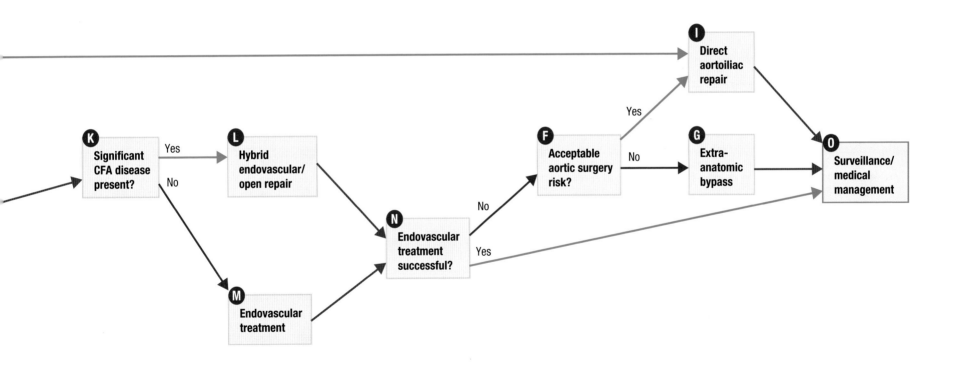

A Patient with aortoiliac occlusive disease requiring treatment

Indications for treatment of aortoiliac occlusive disease (AIOD) include lifestyle-limiting claudication, ischemic rest pain, tissue loss, and distal atheroembolism from aortoiliac plaque. Regardless of presentation, given that atherosclerosis is the most common cause of PAD, patients with symptomatic AIOD should be treated with optimal medical therapy including antiplatelet agents, statins, smoking cessation, blood pressure, and diabetes control. Such treatment has been shown to improve cardiovascular outcomes and minimize periprocedural risk.[1-3] Claudication is initially treated using conservative measures including medical optimization, structured exercise, and smoking cessation. In patients who failed conservative therapy and have lifestyle-limiting symptoms, revascularization is recommended.[4] Because less invasive endovascular techniques have become more successful and durable, a lower threshold for intervention in the claudicant is often justified.[5]

B H&P, vascular lab suggest limited iliac disease?

Patients with the typical H&P and arterial DUS findings consistent with limited or focal iliac disease may be considered for DSA followed by planned endovascular intervention during the same procedure without any preoperative cross-sectional imaging. Leg claudication and a reduced unilateral femoral pulse are most consistent with limited iliac disease. Bilateral hip claudication, buttock atrophy, and erectile dysfunction are generally indicative of more extensive bilateral disease, or disease involving the IIAs. In limited iliac disease, resting ABI may be higher than is expected for the presenting symptoms. In these instances, postexercise ABI may be necessary to indicate the presence of a hemodynamically significant inflow lesion. Evidence also suggests that postexercise CFA Doppler waveforms can be more sensitive than postexercise ABIs in detecting inflow disease. A normal postexercise common femoral waveform has high predictive value in excluding significant aortoiliac disease.[6]

C Cross-sectional imaging

In patients who appear to have more extensive iliac occlusive disease, CTA is usually the preferred imaging modality for planning intervention because it allows for detailed visualization of the aorta and inflow vessels, outflow vessels, and runoff to the lower extremities. Alternatively, MRA can be used, and is favored over CTA in some institutions with substantial MRA expertise. We prefer CTA because of rapid acquisition times, improved spatial resolution allowing for more accurate preoperative planning, and the ability to thoroughly evaluate previously placed stents. MRA may be favored when avoidance of radiation or iodinated contrast is desired, although MRA has been shown to overestimate degree of stenosis in a higher percentage of cases compared to CTA.[7] CTA and MRA are generally well tolerated in patients with normal renal function; however, both modalities carry some risk of contrast-induced nephropathy or gadolinium-induced nephrogenic systemic fibrosis, respectively. Patients' kidney function should be evaluated before and after undergoing these studies.

D DSA

When limited aortoiliac disease is suspected, DSA provides definitive diagnosis and anatomic evaluation with a single radiographic study while simultaneously providing the potential for endovascular treatment. In the absence of preoperative cross-sectional imaging, the presence of a palpable contralateral femoral pulse is essential to ensure ease of retrograde femoral access when performing aortography and bilateral iliac angiography. This generally indicates that catheterization of the infrarenal aorta from the contralateral CFA will be possible without crossing a high-grade iliac stenosis.

Despite advances in acquisition times and clarity of cross-sectional imaging studies, invasive DSA remains the "gold standard" imaging modality for AIOD. Complete aortoiliac arteriography should be undertaken if cross-sectional imaging was not obtained before the procedure. This includes anterior-posterior (AP) projections of the infrarenal aorta and iliac arteries and oblique views (generally 30° anterior-oblique in each direction). Both projections are necessary because ubiquitous posterior plaque is often underestimated in an AP projection and oblique views are helpful in visualization of the iliac bifurcation.

DSA is also utilized if questions remain regarding anatomic considerations in planning intervention despite cross-sectional imaging. If endovascular therapy is pursued, DSA is strategically utilized to conduct the revascularization and evaluate the result. When the decision is made to perform angiography for AIOD without preoperative cross-sectional imaging, it is expected that endovascular interventions will not be feasible in all cases. In cases where disease is more extensive than expected, or the ipsilateral CFA and/or profunda femoris arteries are found to have flow-limiting stenoses, the arteriogram may serve as a detailed roadmap for further planning for an open or combined open/endovascular (hybrid) reconstruction.

When DSA cannot definitively determine whether a lesion is hemodynamically significant, pullback arterial pressures across the lesion using a soft end-hole catheter via retrograde femoral access can be obtained as the catheter is withdrawn from proximal to distal across the area of interest. A hemodynamic gradient of 10 mm Hg at rest or a fall in pressure >15% when limb-reactive hyperemia is pharmacologically induced (using nitroglycerin or papaverine) is diagnostic of a hemodynamically significant inflow lesion.

E Aortic occlusion?

One of the most important considerations in the treatment of AIOD is the presence of aortic occlusion, constituting a TASC II D (most severe) lesion.[8] Although nearly all AIOD is considered appropriate for endovascular repair, the presence of aortic occlusion poses both technical and durability issues. Although short-length occlusion can be treated using endovascular techniques, extensive or long-segment aortic occlusion is best treated using open reconstruction. Aortic occlusion immediately below the renal arteries almost always requires an open operation, because endovascular therapy may risk occlusive complications to the renal arteries and subintimal reentry in the pararenal aorta is hazardous, owing to the potential for vessel occlusion or perforation.

F Acceptable aortic surgery risk?

A careful assessment of a patient's comorbidities, functional limitations, and life expectancy should be taken into consideration when planning an intervention for aortic occlusion. A variety of operative risk stratification/predictive models have been developed to aid in the process of assessing surgical risk. These include guidelines by the American College of Cardiology/American Heart Association[1] (ACC/AHA), the Revised Cardiac Risk Index (RCRI),[9] and the American College of Surgery/National Surgical Quality Improvement Program (ACS/NSQIP) Universal Surgical Risk Calculator.[10] In addition, the Vascular Quality Initiative Cardiac Risk Index (VQI-CRI)[11] and the Vascular Study Group of New England (VSG-CRI)[12] have developed cardiac risk predictive models based specifically on outcomes in patients having undergone major vascular surgery, and may be most applicable for this patient population. Commonly used criteria for evaluation in these models include type of surgery, ASA classification, functional status, and the presence of CAD, abnormal renal function, diabetes, or advanced age. MI is the leading perioperative complication of open surgery for AIOD and carries significant long-term risk.[6] Patients with mild or stable CAD can ordinarily undergo open direct in-line aortoiliac reconstruction without great risk, whereas patients with severe or nonreconstructable CAD are best treated with procedures of lesser magnitude such as extra-anatomic bypass or endovascular interventions when feasible. In addition, older patients with severe cardiopulmonary disease (FEV_1 < 75% of expected, EF < 35%) are considered poor candidates for direct reconstruction, and should similarly be treated with lesser invasive procedures or endovascular interventions (see Chapter 1 for further information about cardiac risk assessment). In patients with aortic occlusion, open, direct aortofemoral bypass is preferred if they are at acceptable risk for this procedure; otherwise, extra-anatomic bypass is selected.

G Extra-anatomic bypass

Extra-anatomic bypass should be considered in patients with AIOD who are at high risk for direct aortic repair, those with a "hostile" abdomen, or a history of intra-abdominal infection. Femoral-femoral (FFB), ilio-contralateral-femoral and axillo-femoral bypass (AxFB) have been used most commonly. Patency of extra-anatomic bypass has been described to be less than for direct in-line reconstruction using aortobifemoral (ABF) bypass.[13]

The expected patency of ABF is 88% to 97% at 5 years, and 81% to 90% at 10 years.[14,15] In contrast, the primary and secondary patency of FFB are approximately 60% and 70% at 3 to 5 years, although primary patency rates in excess of 82% at 3 years have been reported.[16] Reported primary patency rates for AxFB are more variable, generally ranging between 40% and 74% at 3 to 5 years.[17] Traditional dogma has held that the patency of unilateral axillofemoral grafting is inferior to that of a bifemoral configuration because of reduced flow rates,[18] although other authors have found no differences in patency rates.[19] In many instances, lower patency rates of extra-anatomic bypass are acceptable given the decreased cardiopulmonary complications in higher risk patients. Increasingly, hybrid-type repairs utilizing endovascular iliac artery treatment angioplasty/stenting in conjunction with FFB are being performed in lieu of AxFB grafting, because of decreased operative morbidity and higher rates of long-term primary patency of FFB compared to AxFB (71% vs. 63% at 3 years).[20,21]

H Diffuse AIOD, TASC II C-D lesions?

Advanced AIOD, manifesting as extensive, diffuse disease involving the distal aorta and iliac arteries, is classified as TASC II C or D[8] (Figure 46-1). Although the TASC II classification system has generally been accepted as a means to broadly classify AIOD severity, it is not widely accepted as a guideline to dictate therapy. Advanced AIOD has traditionally been treated primarily with direct surgical repair, which provides excellent long-term patency, but is associated with significant morbidity. Owing to advancements in endovascular therapies, most AIOD can now be considered for endovascular repair. Increasingly, even TASC C- and D-type lesions can be successfully treated with an endovascular approach.[22]

Endovascular intervention should be considered for diffuse AIOD in patients who are poor open surgical candidates. Long-term data on the durability of endovascular therapy for TASC C and D lesions are lacking, however, and this approach is likely to be less durable, albeit with less morbidity than is open surgery. Kashyap et al. showed significantly lower rates of postoperative respiratory failure and wound infection with endovascular aortoiliac reconstructions, while noting decreased primary patency compared to ABF at 3 years (74% vs. 93%), although secondary patency was comparable (97% vs. 95%).[23]

I Direct aortoiliac repair

In patients with advanced AIOD who are at acceptable surgical risk, open anatomic, direct repair in the form of ABF, aortoiliac, or iliofemoral bypass remains the treatment of choice. Bypass to the femoral level is generally recommended for treatment of AIOD because of the tendency of occlusive disease to progress in the EIA over time. Aortobi-iliac bypass may be appropriate for combined aneurysmal and occlusive disease, or in patients in whom significant iliac disease is limited to the CIAs and there are substantial risks for performing a groin incision. Direct anatomic reconstructions carry low perioperative mortality (2.4%-4%),[24,25] and have excellent long-term patency (88%-97% at 5 years, 81%-90% at 10 years),[14,15] which is superior to that reported for extra-anatomic bypass or endovascular intervention. However, the superior long-term outcomes of these procedures must be balanced against the higher risk of perioperative morbidity. It is estimated that approximately 20% of patients undergoing direct aortic reconstruction experience major complications. Pulmonary (10%) and cardiac (6%) complications are most common, with bleeding (2%), graft occlusion (1.9%), renal failure (1.8%), mesenteric ischemia (1.6%), and stroke (1%) occurring less frequently. Minor and major incision-related complications are also significant, occurring in 13% of cases.[24]

Thoracobifemoral bypass can be safely utilized in patients with a severely diseased infrarenal aorta who have failed infrarenal aortic replacement, have severe circumferential abdominal aortic calcification, and in those with infected abdominal aortic prostheses. Morbidity and long-term patency are comparable to that reported for aortofemoral grafting.[26,27]

J Focal iliac disease, TASC II A-B lesions

In general, endovascular intervention is indicated for more focal iliac disease (TASC A and B) and increasingly for TASC C lesions (Figure 46-1).[8] Short, focal, stenotic lesions of the distal

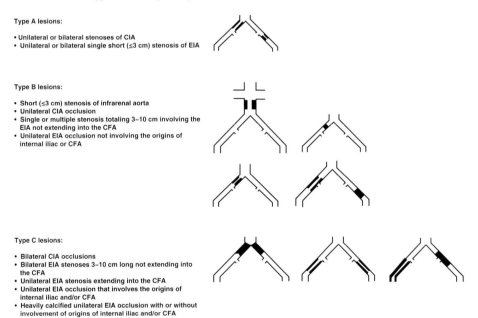

Type A lesions:
• Unilateral or bilateral stenoses of CIA
• Unilateral or bilateral single short (≤3 cm) stenosis of EIA

Type B lesions:
• Short (≤3 cm) stenosis of infrarenal aorta
• Unilateral CIA occlusion
• Single or multiple stenosis totaling 3–10 cm involving the EIA not extending into the CFA
• Unilateral EIA occlusion not involving the origins of internal iliac or CFA

Type C lesions:
• Bilateral CIA occlusions
• Bilateral EIA stenoses 3–10 cm long not extending into the CFA
• Unilateral EIA stenosis extending into the CFA
• Unilateral EIA occlusion that involves the origins of internal iliac and/or CFA
• Heavily calcified unilateral EIA occlusion with or without involvement of origins of internal iliac and/or CFA

Type D lesions:
• Infra-renal aortoiliac occlusion
• Diffuse disease involving the aorta and both iliac arteries requiring treatment
• Diffuse multiple stenoses involving the unilateral CIA, EIA, and CFA
• Unilateral occlusions of both CIA and EIA
• Bilateral occlusions of EIA
• Iliac stenoses in patients with AAA requiring treatment and not amenable to endograft placement or other lesions requiring open aortic or iliac surgery

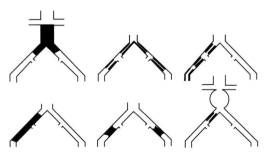

Figure 46-1. Aortoiliac TASC II classification.

aorta and iliac arteries are treated via an endovascular approach with excellent results. Galaria et al. examined 10-year patency of TASC A/B AIOD lesions treated endovascularly and observed 71% primary assisted patency at 10 years.[28] Although advanced AIOD has long been thought best approached via open surgical repair, advances in endovascular surgery have proved that endovascular treatment of extensive AIOD can be successfully performed by experienced interventionalists in selected patients. Although primary patency rates at 5 years are lower than those reported for surgical revascularization (open: 88%-97% vs. endo: 66%-86%), reinterventions can often be performed percutaneously, with secondary patency of endovascular repair comparable to surgical repair (80%-98%).[29]

K Significant CFA disease present?

All patients with AIOD should be evaluated for the presence of concomitant CFA disease using DUS, cross-sectional imaging, or DSA with ipsilateral anterior oblique views to best visualize CFA and profunda femoral artery. Without patent CFA and either profunda femoral or SFA outflow, revascularization of the iliac arteries is unlikely to relieve symptoms. In addition, patency of iliac endovascular intervention in the face of outflow obstruction is invariably limited. Therefore, the importance of the CFA and the profunda femoral artery cannot be overemphasized.

Patients with AIOD often present with either coexistent SFA disease or develop SFA disease in the future. Even in the presence of an SFA occlusion, a patent aortoiliac segment in conjunction with patent outflow via the CFA and profunda femoral artery can adequately perfuse the leg. Although such patients may have leg claudication, progression to critical ischemia and limb loss is rare. The treatment of choice for flow-limiting CFA and profunda femoral disease remains surgical endarterectomy with patch angioplasty and profundaplasty as needed.

L Hybrid endovascular/open repair

When CFA disease is present in conjunction with ipsilateral iliac disease, a hybrid open/endovascular approach utilizing endovascular treatment of the iliac disease in conjunction with open femoral endarterectomy and patch angioplasty is recommended. This is best undertaken in a hybrid operating room with a modern fixed imaging system. The CFA, SFA, and profunda femoral arteries are first dissected and controlled to allow for the required endarterectomy. Endovascular iliac intervention can then be undertaken in a retrograde manner either before or after the femoral endarterectomy and patch angioplasty. Many surgeons ensure the ability to traverse the diseased iliac segment with a wire placed through the exposed CFA before committing to femoral endarterectomy and patch angioplasty that is subsequently performed around the wire. Concomitant treatment of the EIA often necessitates extending the stent or stent graft into the patch to ensure complete treatment of the diseased segment.

This hybrid approach to the treatment of concomitant iliac and CFA disease has yielded excellent clinical results, with reported 3-year primary patency of 91%[30] and 5-year assisted primary patency of 97%.[31]

M Endovascular treatment

A wide array of endovascular strategies for treating AIOD exists, and a full discussion of these techniques is beyond the scope of this text. For focal lesions, most advocate PTA ± stenting. When stenting is desired, balloon-expandable and self-expandable stents or stent grafts are utilized. The Covered versus Balloon Expandable Stent Trial (COBEST) demonstrated superior performance in both long-term patency and clinical outcomes of stent grafts in more advanced (TASC C/D) aortoiliac lesions.[32] Generally, balloon-expandable stents are used for placement precision and radial strength in the CIAs, whereas the flexibility and conformability of self-expanding stents make them more useful for treating the EIA. Flow-limiting disease of the aortic bifurcation and the origin of the CIAs is best treated with bilateral or "kissing" balloon-expandable stents to prevent hazardous plaque shift into the contralateral CIA, which could result from unilateral treatment.[33] For severe combined infrarenal aortic and proximal CIA disease, covered aortic stent grafting may be used with acceptable results in patients otherwise not candidates for more invasive reconstruction.[34] In cases with long-segment occlusions and high calcific burden, advanced endovascular techniques including subintimal crossing with subsequent intraluminal reentry may be warranted. Iliac atherectomy has been used in highly calcific arteries that may be resistant to PTA ± stenting, although these devices are not approved for use in the iliac arteries at this time. Emerging technology such as intravascular lithotripsy in conjunction with PTA and/or stenting may prove to be beneficial for highly calcific, bulky aortoiliac disease.

N Endovascular treatment successful?

Immediate technical success of an endovascular intervention is defined as achieving <30% residual stenosis without flow-limiting dissection or complication. Clinical success is defined by a physiologic increase in perfusion and/or resolution of symptoms. When targeted disease cannot be traversed either with a wire to allow endovascular therapy or the endovascular result is suboptimal, the treatment algorithm shifts toward open surgical reconstruction. In some instances, approaching the iliac lesions from a different access point (ie, brachial artery) may be helpful if the iliac lesion could not be crossed from femoral access. Additional adjuncts such as reentry devices may also be employed. As noted previously, a patient's preoperative risk should always be assessed before advancing to open surgery because some patients with unsuccessful endovascular treatment may not be good surgical candidates.

O Surveillance/medical management

The goal of surveillance and medical management is to maintain the durable patency of the reconstruction, be it surgical or endovascular. Regular follow-up should include measurement of ABI, TBI, and/or PVRs at 1, 6, and 12 months postintervention, and annually thereafter. DUS interrogation of an inflow bypass or implanted aortoiliac stents may also be beneficial at these intervals to detect significant stenosis that may be present before a substantial drop in ABI or return of symptoms is appreciated. A step-up in peak systolic velocity of 3-4:1 in comparison to the preceding normal arterial segment generally indicates a >60% to 70% stenosis. Such a lesion, unexplained recurrence, or progression of symptoms should prompt additional cross-sectional imaging or DSA with the expectation that reinterventions may be needed. Optimal medical management includes smoking cessation, management of diabetes, and antiplatelet, statin, and antihypertensive therapy. The literature supports benefit with the use of dual antiplatelet therapy (DAPT) medications, in the form of aspirin and clopidogrel, for 1 to 6 months postprocedure, because DAPT has been shown to reduce peri-interventional platelet activation with no risk of increased bleeding.[35]

REFERENCES

1. Fleisher LA, Fleischmann KE, Auerbach AD, et al. 2014 ACC/AHA guideline on perioperative cardiovascular evaluation and management of patients undergoing noncardiac surgery: executive summary: a report of the American College of Cardiology/American Heart Association Task Force on Practice Guidelines. *Circulation.* 2014;130:2215-2245.
2. O'Neil-Callahan K, Katsimaglis G, Tepper MR, et al. Statins decrease perioperative cardiac complications in patients undergoing noncardiac vascular surgery. *J Am Coll Card.* 2005;45(3):336-342.
3. Durazzo AE, Machado FS, Ikeoka DT, et al. Reduction in cardiovascular events after vascular surgery with atorvastatin: a randomized trial. *J Vasc Surg.* 2004;39(5):967-975.
4. Society for Vascular Surgery Lower Extremity Guidelines Writing Group, Conte MS, Pomposelli FB, Clair DG, et al. Society for Vascular Surgery practice guidelines for atherosclerotic occlusive disease of the lower extremities: management of asymptomatic disease and claudication. *J Vasc Surg.* 2015;61(3 suppl):2S-41S.
5. Belch JJF, Topol EJ, Agnelli G, et al. Critical issues in peripheral arterial disease detection and management: a call to action. *Arch Intern Med.* 2003;163(8):884-892. doi:10.1001/archinte.163.8.884.
6. Kalish J, Nguyen T, Hamburg N, Eberhardt R, Farber A. The postexercise common femoral artery doppler waveform: a powerful noninvasive vascular laboratory test to exclude aortoiliac disease. *J Vasc Ultrasound.* 2012;36(4):1-5.

7. Pollak AW, Norton P, Kramer CM. Multimodality imaging of lower extremity peripheral arterial disease: current role and future directions. *Circ Cardiovasc Imaging.* 2012;5(6):797-807. doi:10.1161/CIRCIMAGING.111.970814.

8. Norgren L, Hiatt WR, Dormandy JA, et al. Inter-society consensus for the management of peripheral arterial disease (TASC II). *J Vasc Surg.* 2007;45(suppl S):S5-S7.

9. Lee TH, Marcantonio ER, Mangione CM, et al. Derivation and prospective validation of a simple index for prediction of cardiac risk of major noncardiac surgery. *Circulation.* 1999;100:1043-1049.

10. Bilimoria KY, Liu Y, Paruch JL, et al. Development and evaluation of the universal ACS NSQIP surgical risk calculator: a decision aid and informed consent tool for patients and surgeons. *J Am Coll Surg.* 2013;217:833-842. e831-e833.

11. Bertges DJ, Neal D, Schanzer A, et al. The Vascular Quality Initiative Cardiac Risk Index for prediction of myocardial infarction after vascular surgery. *J Vasc Surg.* 2016;64(5):1411-1421.e4.

12. Bertges DJ, Goodney PP, Zhao Y, et al. The Vascular Study Group of New England Cardiac Risk Index (VSG-CRI) predicts cardiac complications more accurately than the Revised Cardiac Risk Index in vascular surgery patients. *J Vasc Surg.* 2010;52:674-683, 683.e1-683.e3.

13. Ricco JB, Probst H; French University Surgeons Association. Long-term results of a multicenter randomized study on direct versus crossover bypass for unilateral iliac artery occlusive disease. *J Vasc Surg.* 2008;47:45-54.

14. Hertzer NR, Bena JF, Karafa MT. A personal experience with direct reconstruction and extra-anatomic bypass for aortobifemoral occlusive disease. *J Vasc Surg.* 2007;45:527.

15. Chiesa R, Marone EM, Tshomba Y, Logaldo D, Castellano R, Melissano G. Aortobifemoral bypass grafting using expanded polytetrafluoroethylene stretch grafts in patients with occlusive atherosclerotic disease. *Ann Vasc Surg.* 2009;23:764-769.

16. Rinckenbach S, Guelle N, Lillaz J, Al Sayed M, Ritucci V, Camelot G. Femorofemoral bypass as an alternative to a direct aortic approach in daily practice: appraisal of its current indications and midterm results. *Ann Vasc Surg.* 2012;26:359-364.

17. Passman MA, Taylor LM, Moneta GL, et al. Comparison of axillofemoral and aortofemoral bypass for aortoiliac occlusive disease. *J Vasc Surg.* 1996;23:263-271.

18. LoGerfo FW, Johnson WC, Corson JD, et al. A comparison of the late patency rates of axillobilateral femoral and axillounilateral femoral grafts. *Surgery.* 1977;81:33-40.

19. Ascer E, Veith FJ, Gupta SK, et al. Comparison of axillounifemoral and axillobifemoral bypass operations. *Surgery.* 1985;97(2):169-175.

20. Schneider JR, McDaniel MD, Walsh DB, Zwolak RM, Cronenwett JL. Axillofemoral bypass: outcome and hemodynamic results in high-risk patients. *J Vasc Surg.* 1992;15:952-963.

21. Criado E, Burnham SJ, Tinsley EA Jr, Johnson G Jr, Keagy BA. Femorofemoral bypass graft: analysis of patency and factors influencing long term outcome. *J Vasc Surg.* 1993;18:495-504.

22. Leville CD, Kashyap VS, Clair DG, et al. Endovascular management of iliac artery occlusions: extending treatment to transatlantic inter-society consensus class C and D patients. *J Vasc Surg.* 2006;43:32-39.

23. Kashyap VS, Pavkov ML, Bena JF, et al. The management of severe aortoiliac occlusive disease: endovascular therapy rivals open reconstruction. *J Vasc Surg.* 2008;48:1451-1457.

24. Bredahl K, Jensen LP, Schroeder TV, Sillesen H, Nielsen H, Eiberg JP. Mortality and complications after aortic bifurcated bypass procedures for chronic aortoiliac occlusive disease. *J Vasc Surg.* 2015;62:75-82.

25. Kakkos SK, Haurani MJ, Shepard AD, et al. Patterns and outcomes of aortofemoral bypass grafting in the era of endovascular interventions. *Eur J Vasc Endovasc Surg.* 2011;42:658-666.

26. McCarthy WJ, Mesh, CL, McMillan WD, Flinn WR, Pearce WH, Yao JS. Descending thoracic aorta-to-femoral artery bypass: Ten years' experience with a durable procedure. *J Vasc Surg.* 1993;17:336-348.

27. Passman MA, Farber MA, Criado E, Marston WA, Burnham SJ, Keagy BA. Descending thoracic aorta to iliofemoral artery bypass grafting: a role for primary revascularization for aortoiliac occlusive disease? *J Vasc Surg.* 1999;29:249-258.

28. Galaria II, Davies MG. Percutaneous transluminal revascularization for iliac occlusive disease: long-term outcomes in transatlantic inter-society consensus A and B lesions. *Ann Vasc Surg.* 2005;19:352-360.

29. Jongkind V, Akkersdijk GJ, Yeung KK, Wisselink W. A systematic review of endovascular treatment of extensive aortoiliac occlusive disease. *J Vasc Surg.* 2010;52:1376-1383.

30. Piazza M, Ricotta JJ 2nd, Bower TC, et al. Iliac artery stenting combined with open femoral endarterectomy is as effective as open surgical reconstruction for severe iliac and common femoral occlusive disease. *J Vasc Surg.* 2011;54(2):402-411.

31. Chang RW, Goodney PP, Baek JH. Long-term results of combined common femoral endarterectomy and iliac stenting/stent grafting for occlusive disease. *J Vasc Surg.* 2008;48:362-367.

32. Mwipatayi BP, Thomas S, Wong J, et al. A comparison of covered vs bare expandable stents for the treatment of aortoiliac occlusive disease. *J Vasc Surg.* 2011;54:1561-1570.

33. Pulli R, Dorigo W, Fargion A, et al. Early and long-term comparison of endovascular treatment of iliac artery occlusions and stenosis. *J Vasc Surg.* 2011;53:92-98.

34. Ali AT, Modrall JG, Lopez J, et al. Emerging role of endovascular grafts in complex aortoiliac occlusive disease. *J Vasc Surg.* 2003;38:486-491.

35. Tepe G, Bantleon R, Brechtel K, et al. Management of peripheral arterial interventions with mono or dual antiplatelet therapy—the MIRROR study: a randomised and double-blinded clinical trial. *Eur Radiol.* 2012;22:1998-2006.

Sikandar Z. Khan • Hasan H. Dosluoglu

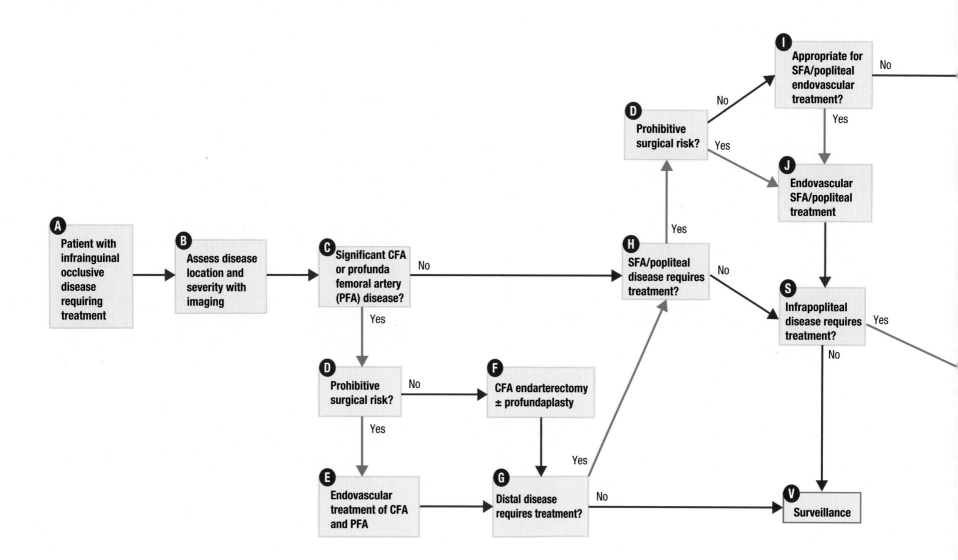

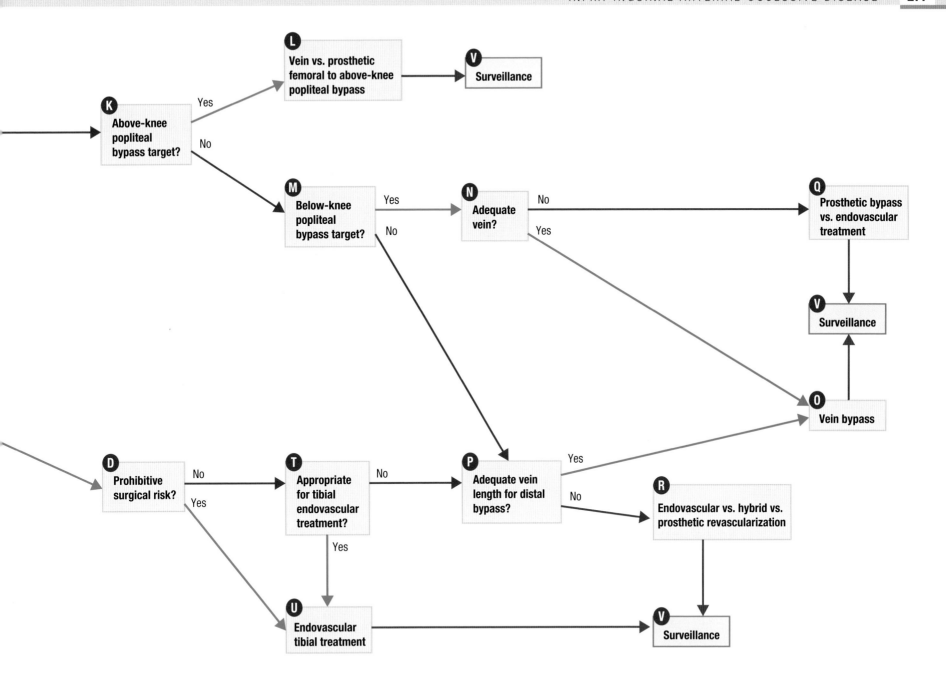

(A) Patient with infrainguinal occlusive disease requiring treatment

Patients with symptomatic infrainguinal PAD requiring treatment (see Chapter 45) present with intermittent claudication or CLI. The goal of intervention in patients with claudication is to improve ambulatory function and quality of life. In CLI, the goal is to relieve pain, heal wounds, preserve a functional limb, avoid major amputation, and maintain ambulatory function.

(B) Assess disease location and severity with imaging

After a decision is made for revascularization, appropriate imaging is needed to assess the extent and severity of occlusive disease. DSA remains the gold standard for infrainguinal imaging, particularly for infrapopliteal arteries. However, other noninvasive techniques are widely used as the initial imaging modality. For patients with normal renal function, and reduced femoral pulses on examination, suggesting iliac and/or aortic disease, CTA is preferred. CTA is very accurate in defining femoropopliteal disease and allows visualization of prior stents, bypasses, and concomitant aneurysms. However, CTA is limited in assessment of tibial vessels in the setting of severe calcification or concomitant proximal stenosis, which limits distal contrast.[1] For patients with severe tibial disease, DSA is the best initial study. It is important to emphasize that pedal anatomy should be clearly demonstrated in patients with CLI, because this influences outcomes and treatment required.

MRA can be considered, especially in patients with mild to moderate CKD. Its specificity and sensitivity to detect lower extremity stenosis and occlusion is >90%[2]; however, it tends to overestimate the degree of stenosis. MRA cannot visualize arterial calcifications but it is useful in assessing the degree of stenosis in highly calcified lesions. It is limited by motion artifact and cannot be performed in patients with pacemakers, incompatible implants, and claustrophobia. DUS has also been used to evaluate peripheral arteries with good correlation with DSA. However, it is operator dependent and limited in assessing multilevel disease.

(C) Significant CFA or profunda femoral artery (PFA) disease?

CFA and PFA disease is usually associated with concomitant aortoiliac or infrainguinal disease, but may be isolated. Because of hip flexion, stenting of CFA is avoided in favor of endarterectomy when possible. Therefore, presence of significant CFA disease plays a central role in planning of endovascular (EV), surgical, and hybrid revascularization. CTA and DUS are accurate for quantitating CFA disease severity, whereas DSA often underestimates stenosis unless oblique views are obtained.

(D) Prohibitive surgical risk?

Patients who require surgical or interventional treatment require risk assessment to determine whether they can safely undergo the required procedure. Because EV treatment is less invasive, it is chosen when surgical risk is prohibitive. Risk assessment mainly focuses on cardiopulmonary morbidity (see Chapters 1 and 2), but also risks for surgical site infection, including severe obesity, which leads to significant morbidity after infrainguinal surgery.

Patients who present with CLI have a much higher operative risk than do patients with claudication. Prediction models such as Finnvasc reported 30-day limb loss or mortality rates ranging from 8% to 27% in patients with CLI undergoing infrainguinal bypass, depending on the presence of diabetes, CAD, foot gangrene, and urgent operation.[3] Similarly, a PREVENT III-trial-based assessment tool stratified patients undergoing infrainguinal bypass into low-, medium-, and high-risk categories depending on dialysis-dependence, tissue loss, age ≥75, advanced CAD, and low hematocrit (<30%).[4] In this system, high-risk patients had <45% amputation-free survival at 1 year, suggesting that bypass surgery should not be preferred in this population. Even after isolated femoral endarterectomy, mortality can be significant in patients with advanced age, poor functional status, dialysis-dependence, sepsis, emergency surgery, and ASA classes 4 to 5. In a risk prediction model, 30-day mortality was as high as 32% in patients with many risk factors.[5] Thus, prediction models and clinical experience must be used to determine whether patients with infrainguinal disease are at prohibitive risk for surgery, such that EV or medical treatment alone can be considered.

(E) Endovascular treatment of CFA and PFA

Patients with CFA or PFA disease who are at prohibitive risk for surgery can be considered for EV intervention. Stenting is not preferred in this location because of the likelihood of stent kinking and thrombosis. However, some studies have reported 1-year primary patency rates of 73% to 81% after angioplasty with provisional stenting.[6] Furthermore, a randomized trial comparing femoral endarterectomy with nitinol stenting in patients with CFA stenoses (no occlusions) showed that 30-day morbidity and mortality were less (26% vs. 12.5%, $P = 0.05$) in the stented group with similar 2-year patency.[7] Atherectomy has also been used in patients with CFA stenoses with improved patency rates reported when used in combination with angioplasty.[8] Thus, CFA and PFA disease can be treated with EV techniques, depending on individual operator experience and preference, in patients who are at prohibitive surgical risk. If such patients also have severe SFA, popliteal, or tibial disease, these may also require EV treatment (see K and V), although it is often prudent to treat the proximal disease alone initially, before determining whether more distal treatment is required.

(F) CFA endarterectomy ± profundaplasty

In patients with isolated CFA occlusive disease, endarterectomy and patch angioplasty or eversion endarterectomy is the preferred treatment.[6] It is associated with limited morbidity and is well tolerated by the majority of patients. A critical component of CFA endarterectomy is to remove adjacent plaque extending into the PFA and the proximal SFA if this is patent. Excellent patency rates following femoral endarterectomy have been reported with 5-year primary patency of 91%, and secondary patency reaching 100%.[9,10] Perioperative morbidity and mortality of isolated femoral endarterectomy were 15% and 3.4%, respectively, in a recent study, with 8% perioperative wound complications.[5]

(G) Distal disease requires treatment?

Isolated CFA lesions without distal disease requiring treatment are uncommon. However, in high-risk patients or in those with inadequate conduit for distal bypass, CFA combined with PFA endarterectomy is sometimes performed as an initial step. If distal disease requires treatment, it is done in combination with femoral endarterectomy, either as a bypass or as a hybrid interventional procedure.

(H) SFA/popliteal disease requires treatment?

SFA or popliteal disease causing claudication or CLI can be treated with surgical bypass or EV techniques. If the patient is a good anatomic candidate for EV treatment or has high surgical risk, less invasive EV treatment is selected, as described later.

(I) Appropriate for SFA/popliteal endovascular treatment?

Owing to advances in EV techniques with availability of special catheters, wires, reentry devices, intraluminal and subintimal crossing techniques, antegrade and retrograde crossing, including popliteal and pedal access, the majority of SFA-popliteal lesions can be treated using EV means. Initial success and patency rates vary, depending on certain anatomic features. Lesion length, occlusion versus stenosis, and location have been considered in the TASC recommendations.[11] Although EV treatment of lesions up to 15 cm (corresponding to TASC II C) was initially recommended,[12] lesions up to 20 cm can now be treated with good outcomes, whereas EV treatment of >20 cm occlusions (TASC II D) have significantly worse patency. However, in the most recently published European Society for Vascular Surgery guidelines,[13] EV treatment has been proposed for SFA lesions up to 25 cm. In the latest proposed Global Anatomic Staging System (GLASS),[14] the most severe grade 4 includes either >20-cm SFA occlusion, >5-cm popliteal disease, disease extending into trifurcation, or any popliteal occlusion. These lesions have high expected EV failure rates but this grading system is yet to be validated.

In addition to lesion length, SFA-popliteal calcification is a significant factor that reduces the patency rate after EV intervention. Technical success rates of EV treatment of severely calcified SFA-popliteal lesions are significantly worse, mainly due to the inability to cross the lesions or reenter into the true lumen after subintimal crossing. The second failure mode is the inability to adequately expand these lesions with angioplasty or stenting. For this reason, atherectomy is more often applied in calcified lesions. However, current evidence has failed to show superiority of atherectomy over plain balloon angioplasty (PBA) or bare-metal stents (BMS) for treating SFA-popliteal disease.[15-17]

In patients with flush SFA origin occlusions or single-vessel tibial runoff with high risk of embolization (occlusions with soft organized clot component, exophytic lesions, aneurysms), EV interventions should only be considered in those with prohibitive risk for open revascularization.

When considering the relative suitability of SFA-popliteal lesions for EV treatment, one needs to balance the adequacy of conduits for bypass and surgical risk.

Life expectancy should also be considered when selecting EV versus surgical femoral-popliteal revascularization. In the BASIL trial, among patients who survived more than 2 years, the bypass-first group had better amputation-free survival and reduced all-cause mortality compared to the angioplasty-first group.[18]

BASIL remains the only randomized controlled trial comparing the EV-first (N = 224) to the bypass-first (N = 228) approach.[19] One- and 3-year amputation-free survival were comparable, although the morbidity and cost were higher in the surgery-first group during the first year.[19] In patients who survived more than 2 years, bypass-first was associated with a significant increase in mean overall survival of 7.3 months (P = 0.02) and a nonsignificant increase in mean amputation-free survival of 5.9 months (P = 0.06) as compared to angioplasty-first.[20] Patients who underwent a bypass after a failed angioplasty did worse than those who had bypass as their initial procedure.

J Endovascular SFA/popliteal treatment

The choice of EV intervention for femoral-popliteal disease depends primarily on lesion length, occlusion versus stenosis, and calcification. For short lesions (TASC II A & B and GLASS 1), PBA is recommended, with provisional BMS placement for flow-limiting dissection or >30% residual stenosis. In a meta-analysis of SFA PBA, primary patency (61% at 3 years) was best in patients with claudication with <10-cm stenotic lesions and progressively worsened in patients with CLI and occlusions (30% at 3 years).[21] The adjunctive use of self-expanding nitinol stents has led to improved patency in long-segment SFA-popliteal disease, providing more durable results than do balloon-expandable stainless steel stents or PBA alone. Primary stent placement is recommended for lesions >10 cm (TASC II B and C, GLASS 2). In the DURABILITY II trial,[22] self-expanding nitinol stents were used to treat lesions with a mean length of 8.9 cm (range 7-20 mm) with a 3-year primary patency rate of 60%.

For patients with long-segment lesions (>20 cm, TASC II C, GLASS 3), especially with >20-cm occlusions (TASC II D, GLASS 4), angioplasty with nitinol stent placement should be the primary EV treatment modality. The STELLA registry[23] reported primary patency of 62% among patients with mean SFA lesion length of 26 cm. Studies on CLI patients with long-segment SFA-popliteal occlusions have shown acceptable limb salvage rates (67%-75% at 5 years).[24,25]

Another option to treat long-segment SFA-popliteal lesions is heparin-bonded ePTFE stent grafts because recent trials have shown improved midterm patency compared with BMS.[26] However, more data are required before the primary use of covered stents can be recommended, and caution is warranted over the failure mode of covered stents with higher rates of ALI as compared to BMS, especially if large collaterals are covered.

Plaque debulking with various atherectomy devices has also been proposed, both as an alternative or adjunct treatment, especially in calcified lesions.[15-17] Various atherectomy devices including directional, orbital, rotational, and laser atherectomy have shown good procedural success and midterm outcomes.[15-17] However, concerns for long-term durability remain, along with the risk of dissection, perforation, and distal embolization.[27] Atherectomy is recommended to treat short-to-medium-length calcified SFA-popliteal lesions, ideally with distal protection. In a series including 800 patients with claudication or CLI and SFA-popliteal lesions up to 20 cm treated with directional atherectomy,[15] primary patency was 78% at 12 months, and the rate of freedom from major unplanned amputation in CLI subjects was 95%.

Antiproliferative drug-coated balloons (DCBs) can be used as adjuncts or alternatives to PBA in medium- to long-length SFA-popliteal lesions, with studies showing improved patency. In the IN.PACT SFA trial,[28] paclitaxel DCB treatment of SFA and proximal popliteal arteries was associated with 69% primary patency compared to 45% with PBA at 3 years. DCBs have improved patency after angioplasty without requiring placement of a permanent endoprosthesis. This is especially important when treating arteries crossing joints that are more likely to cause stent kinking and thrombosis. However, there is concern regarding the limited efficacy of DCB in heavily calcified lesions.[29] In these cases, vessel preparation with atherectomy to debulk the plaque before treating with DCB may lead to improved results.[30]

Another option to treat medium- to long-segment SFA-popliteal lesions is drug-eluting stents (DESs), with studies showing improved outcomes. The 5-year results of the Zilver PTX randomized trial showed sustained superiority of DES over PBA with provisional BMS.[31] Because both drug delivery mechanisms (DCB and DES) have shown similar promising results in longer lesions, preferential use of one technology over the other remains unclear. A recent meta-analysis showed that DESs had superior primary patency as compared to other treatment modalities

for femoral artery disease including BMS, DCB, stent grafts, and PBA.[32]

More recently, a meta-analysis of 28 randomized trials demonstrated an increase in 2- and 5-year mortality with the use of paclitaxel-coated devices in the femoropopliteal arteries.[33] In response, the FDA convened a panel of experts and their findings confirmed the increased mortality risk with paclitaxel-coated devices (1.57, 95% CI, 1.16-2.13). The panel also determined that additional clinical study data are needed to evaluate the late mortality signal. Although these devices continue to be available, the FDA recommends considering alternative treatment options that may have a more favorable benefit-risk profile based on currently available information. The FDA also recommends discussing the increased mortality risk with paclitaxel-coated devices in the informed consent process.[34]

Other SFA-popliteal EV treatment modalities include cutting and scoring balloon angioplasty, which are designed for fibrocalcific lesions, and cryoplasty, but evidence to support their use is lacking. The choice of EV treatment type is often based on individual operator experience because techniques are constantly evolving and rigorous comparison trials are usually not available.

K Above-knee popliteal bypass target?

Patients with SFA disease will typically have reconstitution of the popliteal artery via PFA branches, either above or below knee. Although bypass to an above-knee target is preferred, it is noteworthy that reported patency rates of below-knee popliteal GSV bypass average 77% at 4 years, which compares favorably to above-knee bypass with vein (69%).[35] This is likely a reflection of overlooked popliteal disease distal to the above-knee popliteal segment, leading to higher than anticipated failure rates. Hence, if the P1 and P2 (proximal 2/3) segments of the popliteal artery are mildly diseased and the P3 (distal third) segment is normal, a below-knee popliteal bypass may be preferable to above-knee bypass provided there is adequate vein.

The number of runoff vessels is a significant determinant of outcomes after above-knee popliteal prosthetic bypass procedures, with significantly lower patency rates in those with 0 to 1 patent tibial arteries. In contrast, patency rates of above-knee popliteal bypass in patients with two- to three-vessel runoff were noted to be comparable with prosthetic and autogenous conduit.[36]

L Vein vs. prosthetic femoral to above-knee popliteal bypass

Although synthetic grafts (ePTFE or polyester [Dacron]) have been used extensively because of perceived equivalency with vein bypass, autologous bypass performs better in this location, with 5-year primary patency rates ranging from 61% to 76%, compared to ePTFE ranging from 37% to 52%, and Dacron ranging from 43% to 46%.[35] Even in studies showing similar primary patency of vein and ePTFE in patients with two- to three-vessel runoff, assisted primary patency rates were still better after vein bypass.[36] Thus, single-segment GSV (SSGSV) is the preferred conduit for femoral—above-knee popliteal bypass, if available. In patients without suitable vein, heparin-bonded ePTFE grafts can be used with reported 5-year primary patency of 64% and secondary patency of 75%.[37] A randomized trial has shown that heparin-bonded ePTFE grafts had 1-year primary patency of 80% versus 70% (P = 0.03) for standard ePTFE above-knee popliteal grafts.[38] Dacron and ePTFE grafts have comparable patency, with larger (8 mm) grafts performing better.[39] Distal anastomotic adjuncts are typically not used for above-knee prosthetic bypass.

Bypass to isolated popliteal segment is rarely performed, but can be considered if the femoral popliteal segment is not amenable to EV recanalization and there is no tibial or pedal artery target. Five-year patency rates between 50% and 74% have been reported for such constructs.

Ⓜ Below-knee popliteal bypass target?

The below-knee popliteal artery is often preserved in patients with infrainguinal disease and is used as a bypass target when the proximal popliteal artery is diseased. To serve as a bypass target, the below-knee popliteal artery must have minimal disease and be associated with adequate tibial artery runoff to assure good distal perfusion and patency. The choice of below-knee popliteal versus more distal target artery is predicated on the location and amount of tissue loss, available vein length, pedal circulation, and the quality of the target arteries. In the absence of tissue loss, the best distal target with the shortest distance from the proximal anastomosis should be used. For patients with tissue loss, the most proximal target that provides in-line flow to the angiosome containing the tissue loss is selected.

Ⓝ Adequate vein?

Availability of autologous vein for infrainguinal bypass should be evaluated before DSA, because this will impact decision making for potential concomitant EV treatment. DUS is used to evaluate the GSV, followed by the small saphenous vein (SSV) and arm veins if the GSV is not adequate. Optimal vein is >3 mm in diameter without sclerosis and calcification. If segments of GSV appear small (2-3 mm) but not sclerotic on DUS, the vein can be reassessed intraoperatively because it may dilate adequately. In patients without an ipsilateral GSV, the contralateral GSV can be used if there is low likelihood of future bypass in that leg.[40] SSGSV is the best conduit for bypass. In the PREVENT III trial involving 1404 CLI patients, who underwent bypass with autologous veins, vein diameter <3.5 mm and composite vein configuration was associated with early (30-day) graft failure. In addition, factors negatively impacting 1-year patency rates in a multivariate analysis included non-GSV conduit, vein length >50 cm, and diameter <3.5 mm.[41] However, in the absence of an adequate-length

SSGSV (ipsilateral or contralateral), alternative veins can be used, with two-piece GSV splicing associated with the most favorable outcomes.[42] GSV bypass to below-knee popliteal target has superior patency compared to prosthetic conduits. In some patients with inadequate vein length, proximal SFA endarterectomy can be performed, so that the proximal anastomosis is more distal in the endarterectomized SFA; this may obviate harvest of additional veins and creation of a composite bypass. If adequate vein is not available for a femoral popliteal bypass, prosthetic graft (or medical management in patients with claudication) is selected.

Ⓞ Vein bypass

GSV bypass to the below-knee popliteal artery has superior patency compared to prosthetic bypass. GSV bypass can be performed in either reversed or in situ manner, based on the preference of the surgeon, with similar 5-year patency rates of 68% to 77% and limb salvage rates in CLI of 83%.[35] When the ipsilateral GSV is not available, contralateral GSV or good-quality alternative autogenous veins (SSV and arm veins) can be used.

Femoral-distal bypass with GSV (reversed, nonreversed, or in situ) is the gold standard for revascularization in patients with multilevel disease and CLI. The overall reported 5-year primary patency for reversed GSV and in situ bypasses are 62% and 68%, and secondary patency rates are 76% and 81%, respectively.[35] Limb salvage rates are 82% and 83%, respectively, approaching 90% in some series.

At the completion of the vein bypass, the graft is inspected for kinks and twists, and the pulse should be palpable in the operative field distal to the anastomosis, and at the pedal level, depending on the runoff vessel(s). In a cold, vasoconstricted leg, it may be difficult to obtain palpable pedal pulses immediately after completion; however, capillary refill and Doppler signals should be noticeably improved. A completion DUS is used by some and can detect abnormalities in up to 12% of cases.[43,44] If found, lesions associated with an increase in PSV are repaired.

Completion angiography has been reported to detect correctable abnormalities in 8% to 27% of leg vein grafts,[45] resulting in improvement of early patency rates. However, DSA is not necessarily good enough to assess the adequacy of valve disruption in nonreversed or in situ vein grafts and either DUS or angioscopy can be used for this purpose, particularly when the graft flow is inadequate.

The GSV is usually harvested via a continuous long incision or skip incisions along the length of the vein. This can be associated with significant harvest site wound complications such as infection and dehiscence, with studies reporting rates of 10% to 30%.[46,47] Endoscopic vein harvest (EVH) has been proposed to reduce the morbidity associated with traditional harvest techniques; however, there is concern regarding poor patency of endoscopically harvested veins,[46] presumably due to injury during harvest, although some authors have shown comparable outcomes.[47]

Ⓟ Adequate vein length for distal bypass?

If bypass distal to the popliteal artery is required, adequacy of vein conduit and its length must be assessed (see O). If adequate vein conduit is not available, a prosthetic graft or aggressive EV treatment is selected.

Ⓠ Prosthetic bypass vs. endovascular treatment

In patients who require a below-knee popliteal bypass but do not have adequate autologous veins, an aggressive attempt at EV recanalization should be considered before proceeding with prosthetic bypass, even in patients with complex disease (see K). In addition, prosthetic bypass is not desirable in patients with infection. The primary patency of below-knee femoral popliteal ePTFE grafts has been reported to be 40% to 54% at 4 years.[35] The addition of vein cuffs at the distal anastomosis has been shown to improve patency rates.[48] A randomized trial showed that vein-cuffed ePTFE grafts had better primary patency (52%) than noncuffed grafts (29%, P = 0.03) for below-knee popliteal bypass (with no difference in above-knee popliteal bypass).[49]

In the BASIL trial, amputation-free and overall survival were significantly better in the PBA group than in those who had prosthetic bypass,[50] and the currently ongoing BEST-CLI trial has a subgroup being randomized to non-SSGSV conduit bypass, which will compare prosthetic bypass and EV-first revascularization. Other single-center series have also reported superior limb salvage and amputation-free survival in EV-treated patients as compared to those undergoing prosthetic bypass.[51] Hence, aggressive EV attempts should be made in patients without autologous conduit including subintimal crossing with the help of reentry devices, if reentry into the true lumen is unsuccessful using guidewires and supporting catheters. If reentry devices are unsuccessful, retrograde crossing via popliteal, tibial, or pedal artery access can be attempted. ePTFE bypass can be used if EV options are unsuccessful, with some studies showing acceptable secondary patency (68% vs. 57%, P = 0.1) and limb salvage rates (80% vs. 77%, P = 0.3) as compared to autologous veins.[52]

Heparin-bonded ePTFE grafts have been increasingly used for below-knee popliteal bypass, although the 4-year primary patency was lower (45%) compared to autologous vein grafts (61%, P = 0.004), However, secondary patency (68% vs. 57%, P = 0.1) and limb salvage rates (80% vs. 77%, P = 0.3) were similar.[52]

Ⓡ Endovascular vs. hybrid vs. prosthetic revascularization

In patients who require distal revascularization without adequate venous conduit, less effective EV, hybrid, or prosthetic bypass treatment must be selected. For tibial bypass, even disadvantaged vein conduit has better outcome than prosthetic grafts.[42]

In general, a hybrid approach is preferred to a long prosthetic bypass, if possible. In patients with short-to-medium-length SFA disease (<20 cm) and limited vein length, the proximal disease can be addressed by EV means (see K) and the distal disease addressed by a short vein bypass from distal SFA or popliteal artery. Alternatively, if tibial disease is amenable to EV intervention, a femoral popliteal bypass can be performed. EV can be either performed before the planned bypass, at the time of the initial angiogram, or intraoperatively in a staged or simultaneous hybrid manner.[53] In patients who are not candidates for a hybrid approach, a composite-sequential bypass is an option. This involves a prosthetic femoral popliteal bypass to an isolated popliteal segment and a jump graft to the distal target using autologous vein. The patency and limb salvage rates using this technique were reported to be 80% and 85%, respectively, at 3 years.[48]

If a hybrid or sequential graft approach is not possible, aggressive EV recanalization should be considered before proceeding with a prosthetic tibial bypass, because the latter has 1-year secondary patency of only 46% and is much more invasive.[35]

If a tibial prosthetic bypass is performed, a variety of distal vein patches and cuffs (Miller cuff, Wolfe cuff, Taylor patch, and Linton patch) have been suggested. A prospective randomized trial comparing the Miller cuff to standard anastomosis did not show any difference at the above-knee level; however, the patency rates were significantly better at the below-knee level.[49] In a more recent retrospective analysis of 270 patients (94% tibial) undergoing distal ePTFE bypass with vein patch, the 2-year and 4-year primary patency rates were 76% and 51% with corresponding limb salvage rates of 78% and 68%.[54]

Biologic grafts (cryopreserved venous or arterial allografts, bovine heterografts) are considered in patients who do not have an autologous conduit or EV option and in whom ePTFE is precluded because of close proximity to an infected field or inadequate tissue coverage over the graft (as in dorsalis pedis, perimalleolar posterior tibial). However, in a recent report, primary patency of cryopreserved vein graft to tibial arteries was only 35% at 1 year.[19]

⑤ Infrapopliteal disease requires treatment?

Infrapopliteal disease is common in patients with diabetes and CKD and usually manifests as CLI. The small size of the vessels and frequent diffuse calcifications make tibial interventions challenging. There is frequently concomitant involvement of femoral popliteal segments and the goal of intervention is to restore in-line flow to the angiosome of interest. In GLASS,[14] the femoropopliteal and tibial segments are graded separately according to increasing severity of disease from grade 1 to 4. However, they are combined into infrainguinal GLASS stages (I-III; average-intermediate-high complexity), according to expected technical failure rate (<10%, 10%-50% vs. >50%) and 12-month limb-based patency (>70%, 50%-70%, and <50%).[14] This system is developed to define the infrainguinal target artery path (TAP), which needs to be treated to achieve in-line flow to the foot. The type of revascularization is decided depending on patient's risk estimation (periprocedural risk, 2-year life expectancy, and candidacy for limb salvage), severity of limb threat (WIfI Staging System[55]), as well as the anatomic complexity (PLAN).[14]

⑥ Appropriate for tibial endovascular treatment?

Typically, short tibial lesions are treated with EV interventions, whereas long-segment occlusions are treated with surgical bypass. In the updated TASC II guidelines,[52] focal TASC A and B infrapopliteal lesions were defined as <5-cm stenosis (A), and multiple stenoses each <5 cm, not exceeding a total of 10 cm, or single occlusions <3 cm in length (B). The most recently proposed GLASS[14] classifies infrapopliteal lesions into four grades. Grade 0 is defined as mild or no significant disease; grade 1 is <3-cm focal stenosis; grade 2 is defined as stenosis involving one-third of the tibial vessel length or <3-cm occlusion not involving the tibioperoneal trunk or the origin of the target arteries; grade 3 is defined as disease involving up to two-thirds of the vessel length or occlusion up to one-third of the vessel length, which may involve the vessel origin but not the tibioperoneal trunk; and grade 4 is diffuse stenoses involving more than two-thirds or occlusion involving more than one-third of the vessel length or any occlusion involving the tibioperoneal trunk if anterior tibial is not the target artery. EV treatment is recommended for short-segment stenoses and occlusions (TASC A, B, GLASS 1 and 2).

Data from the currently ongoing multicenter randomized trials (BEST-CLI, BASIL-2) will provide needed information about whether open or EV strategy has best clinical, functional, and cost outcomes for patients with CLI and tibial disease.

⑦ Endovascular tibial treatment

PBA is the mainstay for tibial EV intervention, and although previously it was only used in patients with focal tibial disease (GLASS 1 and 2) or high-risk patients, it is being increasingly used in more complex patients (GLASS 3 and 4). Tibial interventions are usually reserved for CLI patients with goals to improve blood flow, to promote wound and ulcer healing and ensure limb salvage. In a study of 1023 patients,[56] tibial PBA was associated with similar limb salvage (75% vs. 76%) and amputation-free survival (37% vs. 37%) as surgical bypass. Other studies have also shown that PBA is associated with similar limb salvage rates; however, durability is limited.[57] There are no randomized data comparing isolated tibial EV intervention with distal surgical bypass. BEST-CLI and BASIL 2 promise to contribute needed data to clarify whether surgical or EV option is best in these patients.

Angioplasty with DCB is also an option for tibial artery treatment; however, in a recent meta-analysis of four randomized trials, DCBs had similar outcomes to PBA in terms of restenosis, TLR, and amputation rates.[58]

Self-expanding and balloon-expandable BMS and DESs have also been used to treat tibial disease, both as adjunct to PBA as well as primary treatment. Although primary BMS placement has not been shown to be superior to PBA alone, DESs have been shown to be associated with lower rates of restenosis, TLR, and amputation.[59,60] It is to be noted that most such trials included short focal lesions, whereas most tibial lesions are diffuse. Given the limitations of current evidence, PBA with bailout stenting for focal residual stenosis is a reasonable approach. DES probably has better outcomes as compared to BMS.[60]

Atherectomy has also been used to treat tibial disease; however, it has not been found to be superior to PBA.[61] In addition, there is concern for embolization.[27] However, studies have shown decrease in bailout stenting rate after atherectomy as compared to PBA.[17] Additional trials are needed to clarify the best EV options for tibial-level disease.

Although surgical revascularization involves choosing the best outflow vessel, EV techniques allow treatment of more than one artery at a single setting. Proponents of this approach suggest that this leads to higher tissue perfusion and improved wound healing.[62] However, some argue that patients with CLI have extensive collaterals due to chronic disease and that multivessel recanalization is not needed.[63] If tissue loss is extensive, involves more than one angiosome, and the pedal arch and collaterals are not intact, multivessel intervention should be considered to increase flow to the site of tissue loss.

⑧ Surveillance

Post-procedural surveillance recommendations depend on the status of the patient and the procedure type. Patients with wounds should be followed up closely until healing. ABIs (or other noninvasive tests) should be obtained during each visit, with a decrease in the ABI > 0.15 warranting further investigation.

For vein grafts, regular DUS surveillance has been shown to improve patency by detecting stenoses that occur in up to 30% to 40% of patients, most commonly within the first 18 months.[64] The highest risk group for graft occlusion (>70% stenosis with low graft flow, category I) have either significantly increased DUS PSV (>300 cm/s and velocity ratio >3.5) or very low PSV (<40 cm/s) and a decrease in ABI > 0.15. Such patients should undergo a prompt DSA and possible reintervention even in the absence of symptoms or other clinical signs, to confirm and potentially treat stenosis before graft thrombosis. Patients with high risk for graft failure (category II, >70% stenosis, normal graft flow) also have increased PSV and velocity ratio; however, graft flow is >45 cm/s, and ABI decrease is <0.15. They should undergo DSA for possible revision/intervention within 1 to 2 weeks.

DUS surveillance of prosthetic grafts is not routinely performed and was not recommended in TASC II; however, PSV >300 cm/s and midgraft flow <45 cm/s have been proposed to be predictive of graft thrombosis. Initiation of Coumadin in patients with midgraft PSV < 60 cm/s has been proposed to decrease graft thrombosis.[43]

Routine surveillance is recommended after EV interventions,[65] although there is lack of strong data to support these recommendations. PSV > 300 cm/s or velocity ratio >2.0, with a decrease in ABI > 0.15 should prompt an angiogram. Patients with failing EV interventions are typically not treated in the absence of symptoms; however, those with recurrent symptoms and nonhealing or recurrent ulcers should undergo DSA with possible intervention.

For patients who experience graft or stent thrombosis despite surveillance, management is discussed in detail in Chapters 87 and 89.

REFERENCES

1. Met R, Bipat S, Legemate DA, Reekers JA, Koelemay MJ. Diagnostic performance of computed tomography angiography in peripheral arterial disease: a systematic review and meta-analysis. *JAMA*. 2009;301:415-424.
2. Menke J, Larsen J. Meta-analysis: accuracy of contrast enhanced magnetic resonance angiography for assessing steno-occlusions in peripheral arterial disease. *Ann Intern*. 2010;53:325-334.
3. Biancari F, Salenius JP, Heikkinen M, Luther M, Ylönen K, Lepäntalo M. Risk-scoring method for prediction of 30-day postoperative outcome after infrainguinal surgical revascularization for critical lower-limb ischemia: a Finnvasc registry study. *World J Surg*. 2007;31:217-225.
4. Schanzer A, Mega J, Meadows J, Samson RH, Bandyk DF, Conte MS. Risk stratification in critical limb ischemia: derivation and validation of a model to predict amputation-free survival using multicenter surgical outcomes data. *J Vasc Surg*. 2008;48:1464-1471.
5. Nguyen BN, Amdur RL, Abugideiri M, Rahbar R, Neville RF, Sidawy AN. Postoperative complications after common femoral endarterectomy. *J Vasc Surg*. 2015;61:1489-1494. e1481.
6. Halpin D, Erben Y, Jayasuriya S, Cua B, Jhamnani S, Mena-Hurtado C. Management of isolated atherosclerotic stenosis of the common femoral artery: a review of the literature. *Vasc Endovascular Surg*. 2017;51:220-227.
7. Gouëffic Y, Della Schiava N, Thaveau F, et al. Stenting or surgery for De Novo common femoral artery stenosis. *JACC Cardiovasc Interv*. 2017;10:1344-1354.
8. Mehta M, Zhou Y, Paty PS, et al. Percutaneous common femoral artery interventions using angioplasty, atherectomy, and stenting. *J Vasc Surg*. 2016;64:369-379.
9. Kang JL, Patel VI, Conrad MF, Lamuraglia GM, Chung TK, Cambria RP. Common femoral artery occlusive disease: contemporary results following surgical endarterectomy. *J Vasc Surg*. 2008;48(4):872-877.
10. Ballotta E, Gruppo M, Mazzalai F, Da Giau G. Common femoral artery endarterectomy for occlusive disease:an 8-year single center prospective study. *Surgery*. 2010;147: 268-274.
11. Norgren L, Hiatt WR, Dormandy JA, et al. Inter-Society Consensus for the Management of Peripheral Arterial Disease (TASC II). *J Vasc Surg*. 2007;45(suppl S):S5-S67.
12. Setacci C, de Donato G, Teraa M, et al. Chapter IV: Treatment of critical limb ischaemia. *Eur J Vasc Endovasc Surg*. 2011;42(suppl 2):S43-S59.
13. Aboyans V, Ricco JB, Bartelink MEL, et al. Editor's Choice—2017 ESC Guidelines on the Diagnosis and Treatment of Peripheral Arterial Diseases, in collaboration with the European Society for Vascular Surgery (ESVS). *Eur J Vasc Endovasc Surg*. 2018;55:305-368.
14. Conte MS, Bradbury AW, Kolh P, et al. Global vascular guidelines on the management of chronic limb-threatening ischemia. *J Vasc Surg*. 2019;69(6S):3S-125S.
15. McKinsey JF, Zeller T, Rocha-Singh KJ, Jaff MR, Garcia LA; DEFINITIVE LE Investigators. Lower extremity revascularization using directional atherectomy: 12-month prospective results of the DEFINITIVE LE study. *JACC Cardiovasc Interv*. 2014;7(8):923-933.
16. Shammas NW, Lam R, Mustapha J, et al. Comparison of orbital atherectomy plus balloon angioplasty vs. balloon angioplasty alone in patients with critical limb ischemia: results of the CALCIUM 360 randomized pilot trial. *J Endovasc Ther*. 2012;19(4):480-488.
17. Ambler GK, Radwan R, Hayes PD, et al. Atherectomy for peripheral arterial disease. *Cochrane Database Syst Rev*. 2014;(3):CD006680.
18. Bradbury AW, Adam DJ, Bell J, et al. Bypass versus Angioplasty in Severe Ischaemia of the Leg (BASIL) trial: a survival prediction model to facilitate clinical decision making. *J Vasc Surg*. 2010;51(5 suppl):52S-68S.
19. O'Banion LA, Wu B, Eichler CM, Reilly LM, Conte MS, Hiramoto JS. Cryopreserved saphenous vein as a last-ditch conduit for limb salvage. *J Vasc Surg*. 2017;66:844-849.
20. Jaff MR, White CJ, Hiatt WR, et al. An update on methods for revascularization and expansion of the TASC lesion classification to include below-the-knee arteries: a supplement to the inter-society consensus for the management of peripheral arterial disease (TASC II). *J Endovasc Ther*. 2015;22(5):663-677.
21. Muradin GS, Bosch JL, Stijnen T, Hunink MG. Balloon dilation and stent implantation for treatment of femoropopliteal arterial disease: meta-analysis. *Radiology*. 2001;221(1):137-145.
22. Matsumura JS, Yamanouchi D, Goldstein JA, et al. The United States StuDy for EvalUating EndovasculaR TreAtments of Lesions in the Superficial Femoral Artery and Proximal Popliteal By usIng the Protégé EverfLex NitInol STent SYstem II (DURABILITY II). *J Vasc Surg*. 2013;58(1):73-83.
23. Davaine JM, Quérat J, Guyomarch B, et al. Primary stenting of TASC C and D femoropopliteal lesions: results of the STELLA register at 30 months. *Ann Vasc Surg*. 2014;28(7):1686-1696.
24. Ihnat DM, Duong ST, Taylor ZC, et al. Contemporary outcomes after superficial femoral artery angioplasty and stenting: the influence of TASC classification and runoff score. *J Vasc Surg*. 2008;47(5):967-974.
25. Surowiec SM, Davies MG, Eberly SW, et al. Percutaneous angioplasty and stenting of the superficial femoral artery. *J Vasc Surg*. 2005;41(2):269-278.
26. Lammer J, Zeller T, Hausegger KA, et al. Sustained benefit at 2 years for covered stents versus bare-metal stents in long SFA lesions: the VIASTAR trial. *Cardiovasc Intervent Radiol*. 2015;38(1):25-32.
27. Shrikhande GV, Khan SZ, Hussain HG, et al. Lesion types and device characteristics that predict distal embolization during percutaneous lower extremity interventions. *J Vasc Surg*. 2011;53(2):347-352.
28. Schneider PA, Laird JR, Tepe G, et al. Treatment effect of drug-coated balloons is durable to 3 years in the femoropopliteal arteries: long-term results of the IN.PACT SFA randomized trial. *Circ Cardiovasc Interv*. 2018;11(1):e005891.
29. Fanelli F, Cannavale A, Gazzetti M, et al. Calcium burden assessment and impact on drug-eluting balloons in peripheral arterial disease. *Cardiovasc Intervent Radiol*. 2014;37(4):898-907.
30. Zeller T, Langhoff R, Rocha-Singh KJ, et al. Directional atherectomy followed by a paclitaxel-coated balloon to inhibit restenosis and maintain vessel patency: twelve-month results of the DEFINITIVE AR study. *Circ Cardiovasc Interv*. 2017;10(9).
31. Dake MD, Ansel GM, Jaff MR, et al. Durable clinical effectiveness with paclitaxel-eluting stents in the femoropopliteal artery: 5-year results of the zilver PTX randomized trial. *Circulation*. 2016;133(15):1472-1483.
32. Antonopoulos CN, Mylonas SN, Moulakakis KG, et al. A network meta-analysis of randomized controlled trials comparing treatment modalities for de novo superficial femoral artery occlusive lesions. *J Vasc Surg*. 2017;65(1): 234-245.
33. Katsanos K, Spiliopoulos S, Kitrou P, Krokidis M, Karnabatidis D. Risk of Death following application of paclitaxel-coated balloons and stents in the femoropopliteal artery of the leg: a systematic review and meta-analysis of randomized controlled trials. *J Am Heart Assoc*. 2018;7(24):e011245.
34. Hydromer. Best-in-class technology for your medical devices. https://www.fda.gov/medical-devices/letters-health-care-providers/august-7-2019-update-treatment-peripheral-arterial-disease-paclitaxel-coated-balloons-and-paclitaxel Accessed September 8, 2019.

35. Mills JL. Infrainguinal disease: surgical treatment. In: Perler B, Sidawy A, eds. *Rutherford's Vascular Surgery and Endovascular Therapy*. 9th ed. Philadelphia, PA: Elsevier; 2019.

36. Aburahma AF, Robinson PA, Holt SM. Prospective controlled study of polytetrafluoroethylene versus saphenous vein in claudicant patients with bilateral above-knee peripheral bypasses. *Surgery*. 1999;126:594-601.

37. Piffaretti G, Dorigo W, Castelli P, Pratesi C, Pulli R; PROPATEN Italian Registry Group. Results from a multicenter registry of heparin-bonded expanded polytetrafluoroethylene graft for above-the-knee femoropopliteal bypass. *J Vasc Surg*. 2018;67:1463-1471.

38. Lindholt JS, Gottschalksen B, Johannesen N, et al. The Scandinavian Propaten(®) trial—1-year patency of PTFE vascular prostheses with heparin-bonded luminal surfaces compared to ordinary pure PTFE vascular prostheses—a randomised clinical controlled multi-centre trial. *Eur J Vasc Endovasc Surg*. 2011;41:668-673.

39. Abbott WM, Green RM, Matsumoto T, et al. Prosthetic above-knee femoropopliteal bypass grafting: results of a multicenter randomized prospective trial. *J Vasc Surg*. 1997;25:19-28.

40. Robin C, Lermusiaux P, Bleuet F, Martinez R. Distal bypass for limb salvage: should the contralateral great saphenous vein be harvested? *Ann Vasc Surg*. 2006;20:761-766.

41. Schanzer A, Hevelone N, Owens CD, et al. Technical factors affecting autogenous vein graft failure: observations from a large multicenter trial. *J Vasc Surg*. 2007;46:1180-1190.

42. Albers M, Romiti M, Brochato-Neto FC, Pereira CA. Meta-analysis of alternate autologous vein bypass grafts to infrapopliteal arteries. *J Vasc Surg*. 2005;42:449-455.

43. Johnson BL, Bandyk DF, Back MR, Avino AJ, Roth SM. Intraoperative duplex monitoring of infrainguinal vein bypass procedures. *J Vasc Surg*. 2000;31(4):678-690.

44. Bandyk DF, Mills JL, Gahtan V, Esses GE. Intraoperative duplex scanning of arterial reconstructions: fate of repaired and unrepaired defects. *J Vasc Surg*. 1994;20:426-432.

45. Mills JL, Fujitani RM, Taylor SM. Contribution of routine intraoperative completion arteriography to early infrainguinal bypass patency. *Am J Surg*. 1992;164:506-510.

46. Teixeira PG, Woo K, Weaver FA, Rowe VL. Vein harvesting technique for infrainguinal arterial bypass with great saphenous vein and its association with surgical site infection and graft patency. *J Vasc Surg*. 2015;61(5):1264-1271.

47. Khan SZ, Rivero M, McCraith B, Harris LM, Dryjski ML, Dosluoglu HH. Endoscopic vein harvest does not negatively affect patency of great saphenous vein lower extremity bypass. *J Vasc Surg*. 2016;63(6):1546-1554.

48. Gargiulo NJ 3rd, Veith FJ, O'Connor DJ, Lipsitz EC, Suggs WD, Scher LA. Experience with a modified composite sequential bypass technique for limb-threatening ischemia. *Ann Vasc Surg*. 2010;24(8):1000-1004.

49. Stonebridge PA, Prescott RJ, Ruckley CV. Randomized trial comparing infrainguinal polytetrafluoroethylene bypass grafting with and without vein interposition cuff at the distal anastomosis. The Joint Vascular Research Group. *J Vasc Surg*. 1997;26:543-550.

50. Bradbury AW, Adam DJ, Bell J, et al. Bypass versus Angioplasty in Severe Ischaemia of the Leg (BASIL) trial: analysis of amputation free and overall survival by treatment received. *J Vasc Surg*. 2010;51(5 suppl):18S-31S.

51. Dosluoglu HH, Lall P, Harris LM, Dryjski ML. Long-term limb salvage and survival after endovascular and open revascularization for critical limb ischemia after adoption of endovascular-first approach by vascular surgeons. *J Vasc Surg*. 2012;56:361-371.

52. Dorigo W, Pulli R, Piffaretti G, et al. Results from an Italian multicentric registry comparing heparin-bonded ePTFE graft and autologous saphenous vein in below-knee femoro-popliteal bypasses. *J Cardiovasc Surg (Torino)*. 2012;53:187-194.

53. Schneider PA, Caps MT, Ogawa DY, Hayman ES. Intraoperative superficial femoral artery balloon angioplasty and popliteal to distal bypass graft: an option for combined open and endovascular treatment of diabetic gangrene. *J Vasc Surg*. 2001;33:955-962.

54. Neville RF, Lidsky M, Capone A, Babrowicz J, Rahbar R, Sidawy AN. An expanded series of distal bypass using the distal vein patch technique to improve prosthetic graft performance in critical limb ischemia. *Eur J Vasc Endovasc Surg*. 2012;44:177-182.

55. Mills JL Sr, Conte MS, Armstrong DG, et al; Society for Vascular Surgery Lower Extremity Guidelines Committee. The Society for Vascular Surgery Lower Extremity Threatened Limb Classification System: risk stratification based on wounds, ischemia, and foot infection (WIfI). *J Vasc Surg*. 2014;59:220-234.e1-2.

56. Söderström MI, Arvela EM, Korhonen M, et al. Infrapopliteal percutaneous transluminal angioplasty versus bypass surgery as first-line strategies in critical leg ischemia: a propensity score analysis. *Ann Surg*. 2010;252(5):765-773.

57. Romiti M, Albers M, Brochado-Neto FC, Durazzo AE, Pereira CA, De Luccia N. Meta-analysis of infrapopliteal angioplasty for chronic critical limb ischemia. *J Vasc Surg*. 2008;47(5):975-981.

58. Wu R, Tang S, Wang M, Li Z, Yao C, Wang S. Drug-eluting balloon versus standard percutaneous transluminal angioplasty in infrapopliteal arterial disease: a meta-analysis of randomized trials. *Int J Surg*. 2016;35:88-94.

59. Zhang J, Xu X, Kong J, et al. Systematic review and meta-analysis of drug-eluting balloon and stent for infrapopliteal artery revascularization. *Vasc Endovascular Surg*. 2017;51(2):72-83.

60. Katsanos K, Kitrou P, Spiliopoulos S, Diamantopoulos A, Karnabatidis D. Comparative effectiveness of plain balloon angioplasty, bare metal stents, drug-coated balloons, and drug-eluting stents for the treatment of infrapopliteal artery disease: systematic review and Bayesian network meta-analysis of randomized controlled trials. *J Endovasc Ther*. 2016;23(6):851-863.

61. McKinsey JF, Goldstein L, Khan HU, et al. Novel treatment of patients with lower extremity ischemia: use of percutaneous atherectomy in 579 lesions. *Ann Surg*. 2008;248(4):519-528.

62. Biagioni RB, Biagioni LC, Nasser F, et al. Infrapopliteal angioplasty of one or more than one artery for critical limb ischaemia: a randomised clinical trial. *Eur J Vasc Endovasc Surg*. 2018;55(4):518-527.

63. Darling JD, McCallum JC, Soden PA, et al. Clinical results of single-vessel versus multiple-vessel infrapopliteal intervention. *J Vasc Surg*. 2016;64(6):1675-1681.

64. Tinder CN, Chavanpun JP, Bandyk DF, et al. Efficacy of duplex ultrasound surveillance after infrainguinal vein bypass may be enhanced by identification of characteristics predictive of graft stenosis development. *J Vasc Surg*. 2008;48:613-618.

65. Mohler ER, Gornik HL, Gerhard-Herman M, Misra S, Olin JW, Zierler RE. ACCF/ACR/AIUM/ASE/ASN/ICAVL/SCAI/SCCT/SIR/SVM/SVS 2012 appropriate use criteria for peripheral vascular ultrasound and physiological testing part 1: arterial ultrasound and physiological testing. *J Am Coll Cardiol*. 2012;60:242-276.

Cassra N. Arbabi • Ahmed M. Abou-Zamzam

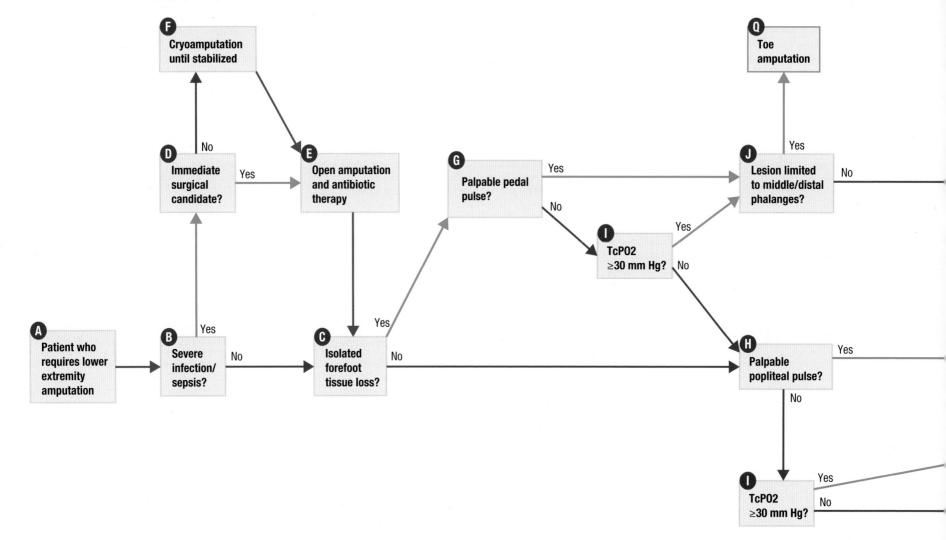

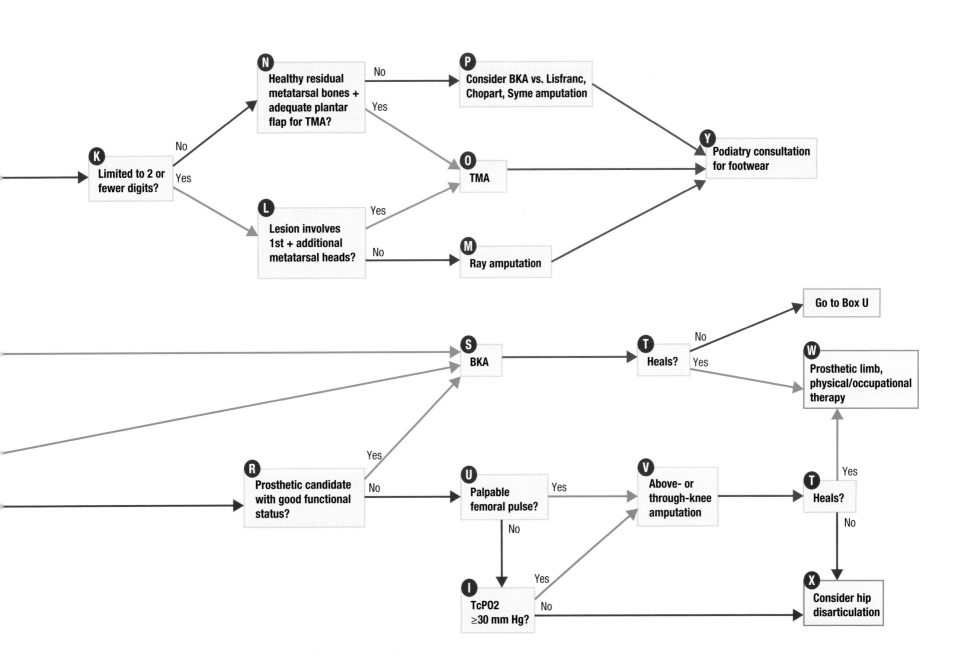

Ⓐ Patient who requires lower extremity amputation

Lower extremity amputation (LEA) remains an essential part of every vascular surgeon's armamentarium. Uncontrolled infection and PAD continue to be the leading indications for LEA, and result in significant morbidity, health care costs, and mortality.[1-3] Recent data from the Vascular Quality Initiative (VQI) reported that a major LEA carries an overall 30-day mortality of 5%, and that patients undergoing AKA have more than double the mortality risk (7% vs. 3%) compared with BKA.[2] The objective of an amputation is to eliminate infected, necrotic, or painful tissue so as to achieve uncomplicated wound healing and maximize the patient's potential to remain ambulatory. Amputations above the level of the ankle are deemed "major," whereas those within the foot are "minor." For determination of proper amputation level in this chapter, it is assumed that lower extremity circulation has been optimized by revascularization when possible.

Ⓑ Severe infection/sepsis?

Patients presenting with infected lower extremity tissue loss that is responsible for systemic sepsis require immediate intervention. Early initiation of fluid resuscitation, broad-spectrum IV antibiotics, and prompt infection source control improve mortality.[4] On initial assessment, the surgeon should determine both the viability of the limb and whether the patient is in suitable health to tolerate a LEA. In these patients, the level of amputation is primarily determined by the extent of infection or tissue loss. If the limb is nonsalvageable, then urgent guillotine amputation should be performed to eliminate the infection source. However, if the patient is a poor surgical candidate, then cryoamputation is the preferred method of source control.[5,6] Patients without systemic sepsis do not require immediate surgical intervention, allowing more time to further evaluate the complete clinical picture so as to determine the optimal level of amputation.

Ⓒ Isolated forefoot tissue loss?

Over the past decade, there has been a decrease in major LEA, whereas the number of minor foot amputations has increased.[7,8] This trend may be a result of better endovascular technologies and techniques, leading to an increase in overall interventions, and better limb salvage rates.[8,9] Lesions that are limited to the forefoot should undergo further evaluation for the prospect of a minor foot amputation. Options for minor foot amputations include digital (partial or metatarsophalangeal [MTP] disarticulation), ray, TMA, and midfoot amputations. Careful consideration should be made with regard to the different functional outcomes for each type of amputation. Operative mortality for minor amputations is approximately 2% to 4%.[7] Physical examination findings, including a thorough pulse examination, and noninvasive studies such as ABI, toe pressures, or TcPO₂ should also be performed to evaluate the healing potential of a minor foot amputation. Lesions

of the hindfoot are difficult to manage because of the lack of skin and subcutaneous tissue available for coverage. If the tissue loss involves the hindfoot or ankle, and debridement is not feasible, then a major amputation should be considered, as partial hindfoot amputations carry a significant failure rate with high rate of revision to BKA.[10]

Ⓓ Immediate surgical candidate?

When a patient presents with systemic sepsis related to lower extremity tissue loss, early recognition and prompt initiation of treatment is critical (see C). If the patient is unstable from sepsis or other reversible causes, such that immediate amputation is not possible, cryoamputation can be used to control the infection source until the patient is stabilized and can undergo amputation.[5,6] In most patients, immediate open (guillotine) amputation can be performed above the infection source.

Ⓔ Open amputation and antibiotic therapy

Patients who present with tissue loss and associated systemic sepsis should be taken to the operating room immediately for open (guillotine) amputation. This allows for rapid source control and can be lifesaving. The primary objective is to eliminate the source of sepsis and potential ascending infection, while preserving the maximal length of the residual limb. Thus, the level of amputation depends on the extent and location of gangrene. A patient with a nonsalvageable foot should undergo a guillotine amputation at or just proximal to the ankle. If the infection extends beyond the ankle, and into the proximal portion of the leg precluding a BKA, then a guillotine through the knee or a more proximal level is required. Intraoperative cultures should be taken from deep tissues to avoid contaminants, and the patient should be continued on broad-spectrum antibiotics until speciation is determined and antibiotics can be narrowed. The Infectious Diseases Society of America (IDSA) recommends continuation of antibiotics until, but not beyond, resolution of findings of infection, but *not* through complete healing of the wound.[11] Guillotine amputation requires a subsequent, more proximal closed amputation that results in lower wound complication rates and shorter hospital stays when compared to the single-stage approach.[12] Although this comes at the expense of an additional operation, data have shown significantly higher primary healing rates after guillotine ankle amputation followed by later closed BKA (97% vs. 78%) when compared to primary closed BKA at initial foot infection presentation. Furthermore, rates of BKA revision to AKA were significantly lower (0% vs. 11%) in the two-stage approach.[12,13]

Ⓕ Cryoamputation until stabilized

If the patient is too unstable for an operation, cryoamputation should be considered. Cryoamputation is a temporizing measure that can be done at the bedside. Also known as a "physiologic amputation," cryoamputation ultimately controls the infectious

source, and limits the dissemination of toxic metabolites, inflammatory cytokines, and myoglobin, while allowing time to continue resuscitation of the patient and potentially correct any hemodynamic and metabolic derangements. In the frail and elderly population, cryoamputation has been shown to improve mortality, when compared to emergency surgical amputation. A recent study showed that for patients presenting with severe lower extremity infection and septic shock, all were eventually stabilized following cryoamputation and later underwent amputation, with median time to definitive operation of 3 days.[5] Cryoamputation is cost-effective and easy to set up, requiring only a large Styrofoam container, dry ice, towels, and a heating pad. The container is prepared by cutting a circular opening on one end, to a diameter that will seal the proximal extent of the amputation. A heating pad is then placed circumferentially over a protective towel just proximal to the frost line and the extremity is placed inside the container. Adequate analgesia is essential and should be started just before the procedure. The container is then filled with dry ice, surrounding the entire extremity and initiating the process of physiologic amputation. The status of the limb should be assessed frequently, because migration of the frost line is a known complication and can lead to the need for a more proximal ultimate amputation.[6] Definitive amputation is then performed when hemodynamic and metabolic derangements are resolved.

Ⓖ Palpable pedal pulse?

When the patient presents with isolated forefoot tissue loss requiring an amputation, the surgeon should first ascertain the potential for wound healing. Prediction of adequate wound healing depends on nutritional status, tobacco use, glycemic control, compliance with offloading, and, most notably, the presence of adequate blood supply. A thorough physical examination focused on the presence or absence of a pedal pulse can aid in the decision-making process; palpable pulses indicate adequate healing potential for a minor forefoot amputation.[14] Presence of a palpable dorsalis pedis or posterior tibial pulse nearly always represents sufficient blood flow to the foot to allow for healing. In the absence of palpable pedal pulses, a forefoot TcPO₂ ≥ 30 mm Hg has been shown to accurately predict wound healing[15-17]; in that setting the surgeon can proceed with a minor foot amputation.

Ⓗ Palpable popliteal pulse?

Proper amputation level selection requires good clinical judgment and physical examination findings. An experienced vascular surgeon can typically achieve high primary amputation healing rates, with some studies reporting 80% in BKA and 90% to 95% in AKA.[7,14,15] The presence of a palpable pulse immediately proximal to a proposed amputation predicts successful healing in nearly 100% of patients undergoing either major or minor amputation.[14] When evaluating a patient for BKA versus AKA, the presence of a palpable popliteal pulse is a reliable indication that the patient will successfully heal a BKA. Conversely, the absence of a popliteal pulse may not preclude the patient from BKA, and additional measures such as Doppler examination and TcPO$_2$ should be performed to assist in the decision making (see I). In certain situations, an AKA may be the best option despite a palpable popliteal pulse.[18] A nonambulatory patient with a knee contracture, or a patient who is bedridden with very poor functional status, benefits more from an AKA because healing is more likely.

Ⓘ TcPO$_2$ ≥ 30 mm Hg?

TcPO$_2$ is an effective tool that can be used to predict amputation healing and thus aid in amputation level selection. It can be measured just above the planned level of amputation. TcPO$_2$ is non-invasive, reproducible, and reliable, with some studies showing an 87% to 100% accuracy in predicting amputation healing.[15-17,19] A threshold value of 30 mm Hg is often recommended; however, this value should be used in combination with clinical judgment and physical examination findings when determining amputation level.[17] There are limitations to the accuracy of TcPO$_2$, because results are unreliable in patients with extensive lower extremity edema, inflammation, or infection. Other objective testing methods such as skin temperature measurements, toe pressures, and skin perfusion pressure (SPP) can be used; however, TcPO$_2$ is the authors' preferred objective testing method.

Ⓙ Lesion limited to middle/distal phalanges?

Lesions limited to the middle or distal phalanges can be treated with a partial toe amputation or metatarsophalangeal (MTP) joint disarticulation. Preservation of the proximal phalanx and metatarsal head will provide a mechanical advantage and prevent the migration of adjacent toes that can occur after an MTP disarticulation. Because the first metatarsal head is crucial for balance and foot mechanics it should be preserved if possible when performing a first toe amputation. If the lesion involves the entire digit, including the proximal phalanx or metatarsal head, then a more extensive amputation such as a single or multiple ray (which includes the toe and metatarsal head), or full TMA may be necessary.

Ⓚ Limited to 2 or fewer digits?

Amputation of multiple digits can typically be well tolerated when the tissue loss is limited to the middle or distal phalanges. However, if it is necessary to amputate three rays, a TMA is preferred instead. Loss of the first ray results in poor foot balance and transferred pressure under the lesser metatarsals leads to further ulcerations.[20] In such cases, podiatry consultation for proper custom offloading footwear is helpful.

Ⓛ Lesion involves first + additional metatarsal heads?

Lesions involving the first metatarsal head plus additional metatarsal heads should be treated with full TMA. The two main complications of the resection of one or more rays are delayed or poor

wound healing and a functionally compromised residual foot. The latter problem results because the foot bears weight unevenly, and recurrent pressure ulcers develop under the residual metatarsal heads. In both cases, the best salvage is revision to a more proximal level, usually a full TMA.[20]

Ⓜ Ray amputation

Ray amputation should be performed when the extent of the wound requires amputation of the entire digit along with all or part of the metatarsal head; it is especially useful in the treatment of malperforans ulcers. Ray amputation has more morbidity than does toe amputation, because removal of the metatarsal head leads to a distinct change in gait and ambulation, potentially leading to further tissue destruction. Narrowing of the foot can create problems of increased pressure under the forefoot or side-to-side movement within the shoe, but this usually can be accommodated by the use of an insole.[20] Recurrent ulceration has been reported in up to 60% of patients following first ray amputation.[21] Reamputation rates after partial first ray amputations have been reported as high as 20%.

Ⓝ Healthy residual metatarsal bones + adequate plantar flap for TMA?

The fundamental objective of a full TMA (involving all toes) is to achieve a stable plantigrade foot that allows for ambulation, while decreasing the risks of further ulceration. The decision to perform a TMA is largely influenced by the health of the metatarsal bones and the quality of the plantar tissue flap. Unhealthy plantar tissue and/or inadequate flap length, resulting in excessive tension, will likely result in failure of the incision to heal and subsequent revision or reamputation. Healing rates for a TMA range from 40% to 70%, and are dependent on various factors such as proper footwear, abstinence from smoking, tight glycemic control, adequate nutrition, and tissue oxygen delivery.[22]

Ⓞ TMA

TMA is the preferred operation in the following clinical scenarios: lesions involving greater than three metatarsal heads; lesions involving the first metatarsal head plus any number of additional metatarsal heads; or lesions involving the entire forefoot. In cases of infection, the surgeon should leave the TMA wound open and treat these patients with appropriate antibiotics and serial debridement before closure. Generally, it is beneficial to maintain as much length of the metatarsals as possible while having adequate soft-tissue coverage upon closure. An advantage of the TMA over more proximal amputations is the preservation of the tibialis anterior and peroneus brevis tendon insertions, which are essential for active dorsiflexion during ambulation. TMA is considered preferable to isolated first ray amputation because of better healing rates and improved foot mechanics (see L). Equinus contracture, or the inability to bring the foot up to a neutral position, can occur

because of unopposed tightness of the muscles and/or tendons of the calf, and is a cause of failure of a TMA. Achilles tendon lengthening at the time of TMA has been shown to lower the risk of equinus contracture, as well as the development of future ulcerations in neuropathic patients.[20] Other complications after TMA include recurrent and recalcitrant stump ulceration, flap ischemia/necrosis, and wound infection. TMA carries a 20% to 40% risk of revision or reamputation that should not be overlooked because approximately one-third of TMAs will result in a major amputation.[22]

Ⓟ Consider BKA vs. Lisfranc, Chopart, Syme amputation

When patients present with foot tissue loss too extensive for a TMA, a more proximal amputation is required. In this scenario, a BKA is usually performed because of the superior functional outcomes and wound-healing results, when compared to midfoot amputations. Midfoot amputations (Lisfranc, Chopart, and Syme) are performed on occasion. They could be considered in young healthy patients in the setting of trauma, patients who would be unable to ambulate with a BKA amputation prosthesis, or patients with a strong opposition to a BKA. Usually, however, in cases of chronic ischemia requiring more than TMA, the hindfoot circulation is also inadequate to support healing of a midfoot amputation.

The Lisfranc amputation involves tarsometatarsal disarticulation, combined with Achilles or gastrocnemius tendon lengthening and reimplantation of the tibialis anterior and peroneus brevis tendons. A Chopart amputation is a disarticulation through the transtarsal joints of the talonavicular and calcaneocuboid joints combined. The Chopart has some advantages over the Syme amputation, including more preservation of limb length, the ability to wear an ankle foot orthosis (AFO) rather than a knee-high prosthesis, and it is a technically easier operation to perform.[10] A Syme amputation, or ankle disarticulation, is generally performed in the setting of trauma, acute infection, or gangrene, when a staged operation with subsequent BKA is necessary; it can also be performed in a single stage as a definitive operation. The advantages of these operations are limb length preservation, at the expense of durability and more difficult ambulation with prostheses.

Ⓠ Toe amputation

Toe amputation is appropriate for treatment of wounds limited to the middle/distal phalanx and not involving the skin over the metatarsal head. Lesions limited to the distal phalanx can be treated with either a terminal amputation of the distal phalanx and nail plate or an MTP joint disarticulation. When the lesion involves the distal phalanx of the great toe, another approach is amputation through the base of the proximal phalanx. The benefit of performing an MTP disarticulation of the hallux is that it is a technically easier and faster operation. However, there are advantages of preserving the base of the proximal phalanx, including maximizing the weight-bearing function of the first metatarsal, altering the plantar pressures, and reducing the pressure on the second and third metatarsal heads. It is recommended to preserve at least 1 cm of the base of the proximal first phalanx, and with preservation of the attachments of the plantar fascia and flexor hallucis brevis tendon, the independent plantar flexion mechanism of the hallux is maintained.[20] When performing an amputation of the lesser toes, the advantage of a partial amputation versus MTP disarticulation is that the residual portion of the digit blocks migration of the adjacent toes toward each other. Before closure, the surgeon should carefully inspect the tissue flaps, confirming a tension-free closure with healthy viable tissue. Postoperatively, the patient should not place direct weight on the affected digit to prevent shearing and/or pressure-related wound complications such as dehiscence or necrosis. Heel touch, or hindfoot weight-bearing should be recommended, and the use of forefoot offloading shoes can aid in this process. Approximately 25% of toe amputations fail to heal and require additional amputation at a higher level, and of these approximately 40% require BKA.[23,24]

R Prosthetic candidate with good functional status?

Patients with a nonpalpable popliteal pulse *and* below-knee TcPO$_2$ < 30 mm Hg are much less likely to heal a BKA; however, special considerations can be made in a patient with good functional status who is a good BKA prosthesis candidate. In this circumstance, the decision should be based on the clinical judgment of the surgeon and preferences of the patient, with the understanding that failure of the BKA to heal may occur and an additional, more proximal amputation may be necessary.

S BKA

A transtibial amputation or BKA is the most common major LEA performed, with a BKA:AKA ratio of nearly 1.3:1.[2] There are various techniques for performing a BKA, each of which is named for the origin of the flap used to cover the tibia. There are five types of flaps: posterior flap, sagittal flap, skew flap, fish-mouth flap, and medial flap. The posterior flap is the most frequent technique used and is preferred if adequate healthy tissue exists. Before the development of the posterior flap, the fish-mouth flap was the most common technique performed. Fish-mouth flap is used in the setting of significant lower leg edema and chronic venous insufficiency. The sagittal, medial, and skew flaps are seldom used; they may be beneficial if there is inadequate skin or tissue available to successfully perform a long posterior flap. Following BKA, the residual limb should be placed in a knee immobilizer to prevent contractures, which can be devastating to the patient's rehabilitation potential. A stump shrinker should be placed after the incision has healed, to compress the stump and reduce edema. The patient should have adequate pain control, and be placed on thromboprophylaxis medication. The risk of DVT and

PE is quite significant in patients following major LEA. Without proper prophylactic medication, DVT has been reported in up to 50% of patients, and data have shown that one out of every six amputation-related deaths are caused by PE.[7,25] Our recommendation is to use LMWH, because it can be dosed once per day (40 mg/d), and is equally effective in reducing the incidence of postoperative DVT when compared to unfractionated heparin (UFH).[26] Approximately 20% to 30% of BKAs fail to heal properly, and about half of these failures can be salvaged at the same level, with one study showing only a 10% BKA to AKA conversion rate. Overall survival following BKA is about 70% and 35% at 1 and 5 years, respectively, and is significantly worse for patients with diabetes mellitus and ESRD.[25,27] Early involvement of multidisciplinary care teams and prosthetics evaluation is vital to the outcome of the patient; and screening for depression should strongly be considered, because amputees with depression can lose motivation to eat, and/or participate in rehabilitation.[7]

T Heals?

Inadequate healing is evidenced by dehiscence, tissue necrosis, infection, or recurrent ulceration. Failure of the incision to heal can be due to ischemic/infectious complications, from trauma or pressure ulceration from bony prominences. If the wound is not salvageable with minor debridement and/or local wound care, a revision or more proximal amputation is indicated. When the incision successfully heals, the patient should be referred to physical therapy and evaluated for a potential prosthesis. Psychiatry evaluation may also be considered if the patient is exhibiting depressive symptoms or inability to cope with the limb loss. Social work involvement may also be beneficial depending on the patient's support system and living situation. Durable medical equipment (DME) may be required and, with the help of case management staff, can be provided to the patient upon discharge, if necessary.

U Palpable femoral pulse?

The presence of a palpable femoral pulse can accurately predict wound healing in most patients undergoing an AKA. In the absence of a palpable femoral pulse, an above-knee TcPO$_2$ ≥ 30 mm Hg has been shown to accurately predict wound healing at that level and the surgeon should proceed with AKA (or consider through-knee amputation [TKA]).

V Above- or through-knee amputation

Patients undergoing AKA are less likely to have postoperative complications but have double the mortality risk when compared to those undergoing BKA. However, the reoperation rates (3% vs. 10%) and revision to a higher level (<1% vs. 5%) are significantly less for AKA.[2] Similar to BKA, patients undergoing AKA should be placed on DVT prophylaxis (see S) with early involvement of multidisciplinary care teams and depression screening. Postoperative dressings should aim to prevent fecal and urine

contamination, while providing adequate compression to mitigate edema. Patients undergoing AKA require a significantly higher energy expenditure (63% above baseline) to ambulate with a prosthesis, and therefore have a much lower reported rate of prosthetic use.[28] A TKA is an alternative to an AKA in select patients; however, it is a technically more demanding operation when compared to AKA, and should be reserved for patients with good rehabilitation potential. A TKA results in a longer lever arm and uses a simple end-weight-bearing prosthesis as opposed to an ischial weight–bearing AKA prosthesis. If done properly, TKA can preserve more limb length and lead to less energy expenditure during ambulation, albeit at the cost of more wound complications than does AKA. Migration or nonunion of the patella may occur in 3% of patients, and reamputation at a higher level occurs in 10% to 15% of patients after TKA.[25]

W Prosthetic limb, physical/occupational therapy

The main objective after major or minor LEA is to achieve successful wound healing and prepare the patient for rehabilitation and prosthesis use if feasible. The likelihood of achieving ambulation depends largely on the level of amputation, with 80% of BKA and 38% to 50% of AKA patients achieving ambulation once their incisions have healed. Patients who underwent AKA require 63% more than their baseline energy expenditure to ambulate with a prosthesis, whereas BKA patients require 10% to 40% more, depending on the length of the stump.[29] It is for this reason that appropriate amputation level selection is critical, because the prospect of achieving ambulation with a prosthesis is substantially different when comparing BKA to AKA. Prosthetic use has been reported to be 50% to 100% following BKA; however, only 10% to 30% following AKA.[28] Age, comorbidities, mental status, and preoperative ambulation status also play a significant role. Patients <60 years, who were ambulating preoperatively, can anticipate a 70% ambulatory rate, whereas patients with poor preoperative functional status, dementia, ESRD, and advanced CAD have much worse functional outcomes post amputation.[30] Each patient should be evaluated by a multidisciplinary team, including physical therapy, occupational therapy, rehabilitation, prosthetics, nutrition, and psychology. Data have shown that centers with dedicated multidisciplinary teams have much more successful rehabilitation outcomes.[7]

X Consider hip disarticulation

In most cases, arterial revascularization can be done to allow for successful AKA. In the rare instance that an AKA fails to heal properly, or when there is absence of a palpable femoral pulse coupled with above-knee TcPO$_2$ < 30 mm Hg (which cannot be improved with revascularization), the surgeon should consider hip disarticulation. This extremely morbid operation results in high morbidity, a very high (82% above baseline) energy expenditure, and very low ambulation rates (0%-10%).[7] Thus, palliative care is also an option, depending on patient status and preference.

Ⓨ Podiatry consultation for footwear

Following partial foot or even toe amputation, podiatry evaluation for appropriate footwear is important, and may need to include shoe inserts to avoid subsequent injury of preserved tissue.

REFERENCES

1. Armstrong EJ, Ryan MP, Baker ER, et al. Risk of major amputation or death among patients with critical limb ischemia initially treated with endovascular intervention, surgical bypass, minor amputation, or conservative management. *J Med Econ.* 2017;20(11):1148-1154.
2. Gabel J, Jabo B, Patel S, et al. Descriptive analysis of patients going major lower extremity amputation in the Vascular Quality Initiative. *Ann Vasc Surg.* 2018;47:75-82.
3. HCUP Nationwide Inpatient Sample (NIS). *Healthcare Cost and Utilization Project (HCUP).* Rockville, MD: Agency for Healthcare Research and Quality; 2009.
4. Nguyen HB, Jaehne AK, Jayaprakash N, et al. Early goal directed therapy in severe sepsis and septic shock: insights and comparisons to process, promise, and arise. *Critical Care.* 2016;20(1):160.
5. Chen SL, Kuo IJ, Kabuty NK, et al. Physiologic cryoamputation in managing critically ill patients with septic, advanced acute limb ischemia. *Ann Vasc Surg.* 2017;42:50-55.
6. Hunsaker RH, Schwartz JA, Keagy BA, et al. Dry ice cryo-amputation: a twelve-year experience. *J Vasc Surg.* 1985;2(6):812-816.
7. Bianchi C, Abou-Zamzam AM Jr. Lower extremity amputation: epidemiology, procedure selection and rehabilitation outcome. In: Sidawy AN, Perler BA, eds. *Rutherford's Vascular Surgery.* 9th ed. Philadelphia, PA: Elsevier Saunders; 2018.
8. Goodney PP, Beck AW, Nagle J, et al. National trends in lower extremity bypass surgery, endovascular interventions, and major amputations. *J Vasc Surg.* 2009;50(1):54-60.
9. Ziegler-Graham K, MacKenzie EJ, Ephraim PL, et al. Estimating the prevalence of limb loss in the United States: 2005 to 2050. *Arch Phys Med Rehabil.* 2008;89(3):422-429.
10. Johnson JE, Klein SE, Brodsky JW. Diabetes. In: Coughlin M, Saltzman C, Anderson RB, eds. *Mann's Surgery of the Foot and Ankle.* 9th ed. Philadelphia, PA: Elsevier Saunders; 2014:1385-1480.
11. Lipsky BA, Berendt AR, Cornia PB, et al. 2012 Infectious diseases society of America clinical practice guideline for the diagnosis and treatment of diabetic foot infections. *Clin Infect Dis.* 2012;54(12):132-173.
12. Fisher DF Jr, Clagett GP, Fry RE, et al. One-stage versus two-stage amputation for wet gangrene of the lower extremity: a randomized study. *J Vasc Surg.* 1988;8(4):428-433.
13. McIntyre KE Jr, Bailey SA, Malone JM, et al. Guillotine amputation in the treatment of nonsalvageable lower-extremity infections. *Arch Surg.* 1984;119(4):450-453.
14. Dwars BJ, van den Broek TA, Rauwerda JA, et al. Criteria for reliable selection of the lowest level of amputation in peripheral vascular disease. *J Vasc Surg.* 1992;15(3):536-542.
15. Malone JM, Anderson GG, Lalka SG, et al. Prospective comparison of noninvasive techniques for amputation level selection. *Am J Surg.* 1987;154(2):179-184.
16. Bunt TJ, Holloway GA. TcPO$_2$ as an accurate predictor of therapy in limb salvage. *Ann Vasc Surg.* 1996;10(3):224-227.
17. Ballard JL, Bianchi C. Transcutaneous oxygen tension: principles and application. In: Abu-Rhama AF, Bergan JJ, eds. *Noninvasive Vascular Diagnosis.* New York, NY: Springer; 2000:403.
18. Abou-Zamzam AM Jr, Teruya TH, Killeen JE, et al. Major lower extremity amputation in an academic vascular center. *Ann Vasc Surg.* 2003;17(1):86-90.
19. DeFrang RD, Taylor LM Jr, Porter JM. Basic data related to amputations. *Ann Vasc Surg.* 1991;5(2):202-207.
20. Brodsky JW, Saltzman CL. Amputations of the foot and ankle. In: Coughlin M, Saltzman C, Anderson RB, eds. *Mann's Surgery of the Foot and Ankle.* 9th ed. Elsevier Saunders; 2014:1481-1506.
21. Murdoch D, Armstrong DG, Dacus JB, et al. The natural history of great toe amputations. *J Foot Ankle Surg.* 1997;36(3):204-208.
22. Iosue H, Rosenblum B. Transmetatarsal amputation: predictors of success and failure. *Podiatry Today.* 2017;30(8):42-47.
23. Izumi Y, Satterfield K, Lee S, et al. Risk of reamputation in diabetic patients stratified by limb and level of amputation: a 10 year observation. *Diabetes Care.* 2006:29(3):566-570.
24. Dillingham TR, Pezzin LE, Shore AD. Reamputation, mortality, and health care costs among persons with dysvascular lower limb amputations. *Arch Phys Med Rehabil.* 2005;86(3):480-486.
25. Eidt JF, Kalapatapu VR. Lower extremity amputation: techniques and results. In: Cronenwett J, Johnston KW, eds. *Rutherford's Vascular Surgery.* 8th ed. Philadelphia, PA: Elsevier Saunders; 2014:1848-1866.
26. Lastoria S, Rollo HA, Yoshida WB, et al. Prophylaxis of deep-vein thrombosis after lower extremity amputation: comparison of low molecular weight heparin with unfractionated heparin. *Acta Cirurgica Brasileira.* 2006;21(3):184-186.
27. Aulivola B, Hile CN, Hamdan AD, et al. Major lower extremity amputation: outcome of a modern series. *Arch Surg.* 2004;139(4):395-399.
28. Nehler MR, Coll JR, Hiatt WR, et al. Functional outcome in a contemporary series of major lower extremity amputations. *J Vasc Surg.* 2003;38(1):7-14.
29. Tang PC, Ravji K, Key JJ, et al. Let them walk! Current prosthesis options for leg and foot amputees. *J Am Coll Surg.* 2008;206(3):548-560.
30. Taylor SM, Kalbaugh CA, Blackhurst DW, et al. Preoperative clinical factors predict postoperative functional outcomes after major lower limb amputation: an analysis of 553 consecutive patients. *J Vasc Surg.* 2005;42(2):227-235.

Jake F. Hemingway • Niten Singh

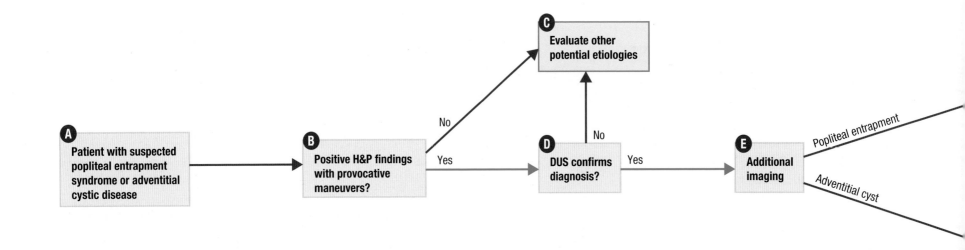

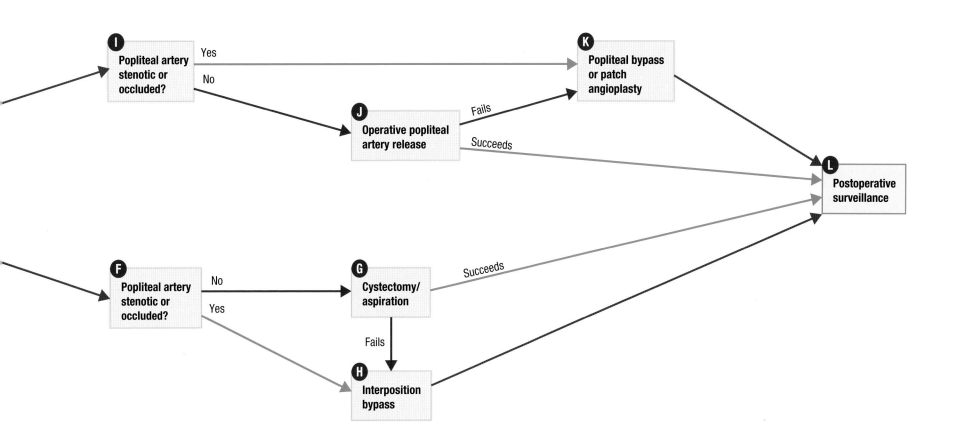

A Patient with suspected popliteal entrapment syndrome or adventitial cystic disease

Popliteal entrapment syndrome (PES) is a rare condition that results from the compression of the popliteal artery. It has an estimated clinical incidence of 0.17% in a large screening study of Greek military men. Approximately 90% of affected patients are male, with more than half presenting before 30 years of age. PES is divided into six anatomic types depending on the embryologic underpinnings. Type I involves displacement of the popliteal artery medial to the medial head of the gastrocnemius. Type II PES involves compression of a normally placed popliteal artery by an abnormally lateral attachment of the medial head. Type III PES results from an abnormal gastrocnemius muscle slip that compresses a normally placed popliteal artery. Type IV involves a persistent fetal axial artery that lies deep to and is compressed by the popliteus muscle. Type V includes any type of PES when concomitant popliteal vein involvement is present. Type VI is considered functional PES and is caused by popliteal artery compression between hypertrophied heads of the gastrocnemius. The majority of described patients have type I or II PES. PES should be suspected in a young patient who presents with exertional calf pain or progressive claudication in the absence of usual atherosclerotic risk factors or comorbidities. Bilateral symptoms are present in 20% of patients.[1-4]

Adventitial cystic disease (ACD) is another rare cause of intermittent claudication in young adults (ages 20-50), characterized by arterial lumen compression by a gelatinous collection of mucoproteins and mucopolysaccharides that form between the media and adventitia. ACD most commonly affects men (5:1), and generally involves the popliteal artery, although 15% of cases are extrapopliteal. Typically, patients present with progressive intermittent claudication in the absence of usual atherosclerotic risk factors or comorbidities.[5,6] Symptoms associated with PES and ACD usually justify intervention in these typically younger, healthy patients.

B Positive H&P findings with provocative maneuvers?

A thorough H&P is essential to make the diagnosis of PES or ACD. A history of an active lifestyle and claudication symptoms while performing strenuous or long-distance running is often seen in patients with PES and/or ACD; this active lifestyle differentiates patients with more common atherosclerotic disease who are usually less active. When examining a patient with suspected PES or ACD, the popliteal fossa should be auscultated for the presence of a popliteal bruit.[7,8] ABI may be abnormal in these patients if popliteal occlusion or severe stenosis is present. A baseline ABI is helpful as a comparative preoperative study if surgery is later performed; however, a normal ABI does not exclude nonocclusive or functional PES.[9] Any diminution of pedal pulses or Doppler signals with provocative maneuvers, which include active and passive plantar and dorsiflexion of the foot and flexion of the knee, offer further evidence of PES or ACD.[10]

C Evaluate other potential etiologies

Young patients who present with claudication symptoms and have normal physical examination findings with provocative maneuvers likely do not have PES or ACD. Therefore, alternative diagnoses such as chronic exertional compartment syndrome (see Chapter 51) or tibial stress syndrome should be considered in this patient population.

D DUS confirms diagnosis?

Patients with clinical H&P findings suggestive of PES or ACD should undergo DUS and treadmill ABIs. In the evaluation of PES, DUS and ABIs during provocation maneuvers (see B) have a sensitivity of 83% and 90%, respectively.[3] DUS allows for visualization of arterial flow patterns during provocative maneuvers and remains the most sensitive test in diagnosing ACD.[11,12] In both PES and ACD, compression of the popliteal artery will be noted with provocative DUS; however, in the case of ACD, an ovoid cystic structure without calcifications that narrows the arterial lumen can be observed. In advanced cases, DUS may show occlusion of the popliteal artery.

E Additional imaging

Axial imaging, with CTA or MRA, provides high spatial resolution information regarding the anatomic relationship of the popliteal artery to surrounding structures. The high soft-tissue resolution in both modalities allows for differentiation of vessel, muscle, fat, and bone within the popliteal space. Popliteal artery stenosis and/or occlusion is also well visualized. By providing information regarding abnormalities in anatomic relationships among these structures, axial imaging assists in both the diagnosis of PES or ACD and in operative planning. Very high correlation exists between MRA or CTA and DSA.[13-16] In some cases, DSA may be required to plan treatment, especially if popliteal occlusion has occurred and outflow arteries are poorly visualized by CTA or MRA. When performed in patients with ACD, arteriography will demonstrate a smooth curvilinear stenosis in the popliteal artery. This angiographic finding is commonly referred to as the "scimitar sign," and can also be appreciated on CTA or MRA in reformatted plane views. CTA or MRA may not demonstrate clear muscular anomalies for types III, V, and VI PES; therefore, if the clinical suspicion is high, DSA should be performed in such cases. Evidence of popliteal artery compression on DSA with provocative maneuvers is diagnostic for PES; concurrent use of IVUS allows for intimal changes within the popliteal artery to be evaluated to determine whether bypass is needed for treatment.[5]

F Popliteal artery stenotic or occluded?

Once confirmed, ACD usually requires surgical repair in patients with sufficient symptoms to justify treatment. The natural history of ACD is not well established, because most young patients who develop symptoms request treatment. A few case reports of spontaneous resolution exist.[17] The treatment approach depends on whether the popliteal artery is stenotic or occluded by the associated cyst.

G Cystectomy/aspiration

For patients with ACD and a patent popliteal artery, cystectomy or aspiration may be considered. Because of the rare nature of this condition, the long-term success of aspiration is not clear. Techniques such as open surgical aspiration and ultrasound-guided aspiration have been described in case reports with resolution of symptoms. Reported treatment success rates are similar for evacuation and aspiration of the cyst alone (85%) compared with cyst resection and bypass (93%).[18,19]

H Interposition bypass

For patients with ACD causing popliteal artery stenosis or occlusion, interposition bypass grafting is preferred. A posterior surgical approach to the popliteal artery is ideal for this pathology, because the disease process is focal and can be better visualized via this approach than via the standard medial approach. GSV, or if it is adequate in size, the small saphenous vein, can be utilized for conduit. Resection of the cystic portion of the artery may allow more anatomic bypass placement. In cases of focal popliteal stenosis, cystectomy and vein patch angioplasty can be performed. Among patients undergoing bypass, vein grafts have a higher success rates (96%) than do synthetic grafts (75%). Endovascular interventions have been attempted but have been associated with very high failure rates and, as such, are not recommended.[19,20]

I Popliteal artery stenotic or occluded?

Once the diagnosis and type of PES has been confirmed with imaging, the patient should be counseled regarding treatment options. If the patient declines operative repair, then popliteal artery surveillance is mandatory because repetitive arterial compression can lead to stenosis or occlusion and subsequent limb ischemia.[21-30] In the presence of a healthy, patent popliteal artery, open surgical release of the compressing muscle is the appropriate treatment. In contrast, an occluded popliteal artery should be treated with an interposition bypass, and muscle release if required for anatomic placement of the graft. In cases of popliteal stenosis, the artery should be evaluated with DUS or DSA in the operating room after surgical release of the compressing muscle. In some cases, this release may correct the stenosis, whereas in other cases, vein patch angioplasty or bypass can be required. Endovascular treatment of popliteal artery disease for patients with PES does not address the underlying cause, subjects the patient to future arterial restenosis and, as such, is not recommended.[31]

J Operative popliteal artery release

Popliteal artery release is recommended for patients with PES without stenotic or occluded popliteal artery. Either a medial or posterior approach is utilized for popliteal artery release.[32] The posterior approach allows for excellent visualization of structures and adequate muscular release. The medial approach is often preferred because of surgeon familiarity. Adequate artery release can be obtained via this approach; however, complete exposure of the popliteal artery and its relationship to the muscular structures can be challenging. We recommend a posterior approach with confirmation of adequate release via intraoperative DUS. Surgical options include musculotendinous resection for functional PES and selective myomectomy of a portion of the medial head of the gastrocnemius, causing compression and anatomic entrapment. Intraoperative DUS or DSA allows for the evaluation of intimal arterial damage and residual stenosis after decompression.[5] If operative release fails to restore a nonstenotic popliteal artery, additional arterial treatment is required.

🄺 Popliteal bypass or patch angioplasty

In the presence of popliteal artery stenosis or occlusion, arterial reconstruction with a saphenous interposition vein graft is recommended. Vein grafts are preferable to synthetic grafts given their higher patency for below-knee bypass. For patients with functional popliteal stenosis, vein patch angioplasty or bypass should be performed if the stenosis is not adequately treated with arterial release. Nearly all surgically treated patients will have complete resolution of their symptoms and a full return to their prior level of activity.[9] A 15% postoperative complication rate has been observed, with the majority being seroma, hematoma, and surgical site infection.[9]

🄻 Postoperative surveillance

Although no guidelines for postoperative surveillance exist, a reasonable surveillance approach is to study the popliteal artery repair with DUS at 4 weeks, 6 months, and 12 months postoperatively, followed by decreasing frequency if no recurrence is demonstrated. The need for DUS surveillance is not established in the literature; however, patients should be counseled to return if claudication symptoms recur. One of the complexities of managing these patients is that long-term follow up can be difficult because patients are young and typically relocate.

REFERENCES

1. di Marzo L, Venturini L. Contemporary treatment of popliteal artery entrapment syndrome. *Rev Vasc Med.* 2014;2(2):73-76. doi:10.1016/j.rvm.2014.01.001.
2. Landry GJ, Edwards JM. Popliteal entrapment syndrome. In: Moore WS, ed. *Vascular and Endovascular Surgery: A Comprehensive Review.* 8th ed. Philadelphia, PA: Elsevier, Inc.; 2013:123-124.
3. Sinha S, Houghton J, Holt PJ, Thompson MM, Loftus IM, Hinchliffe RJ. Popliteal entrapment syndrome. *J Vasc Surg.* 2012;55(1):252-262.e30. doi:10.1016/j.jvs.2011.08.050.
4. Causey MW, Singh N, Miller S, Quan R, Curry T, Andersen C. Intraoperative duplex and functional popliteal entrapment syndrome: strategy for effective treatment. *Ann Vasc Surg.* 2010;24(4):556-561. doi:10.1016/j.avsg.2009.07.036.
5. Ricci P, Panzetti C, Mastantuono M, et al. Cross-sectional imaging in a case of adventitial cystic disease of the popliteal artery. *Cardiovasc Intervent Radiol.* 1999;22(1):71-74. doi:10.1007/s002709900333.
6. Steffen CM, Ruddle A, Shaw JF. Adventitial cystic disease: multiple cysts causing common femoral artery occlusion. *Eur J Vasc Endovasc Surg.* 1995;9:118-119. https://core.ac.uk/download/pdf/82314577.pdf. Accessed July 8, 2018.
7. Eastcott H. Cystic myxomatous degeneration of the popliteal artery. *Br Med J.* 1963;2(5367):1270. http://www.ncbi.nlm.nih.gov/pubmed/14056916. Accessed July 8, 2018.
8. Pham TT, Kapur R, Harwood MI. Exertional leg pain: teasing out arterial entrapments. *Curr Sports Med Rep.* 2007;6(6):371-375. doi:10.1007/s11932-007-0054-3.
9. Heneghan RE, Singh N. In patients with popliteal entrapment syndrome, does surgery improve quality of life? In: Skelly CL, Milner R, eds. *Difficult Decisions in Vascular Surgery: An Evidence-Based Approach.* Cham: Springer International Publishing; 2017:207-218.
10. Tsolakis IA, Walvatne CS, Caldwell MD. Cystic adventitial disease of the popliteal artery: diagnosis and treatment. *Eur J Vasc Endovasc Surg.* 1998;15(3):188-194. doi:10.1016/S1078-5884(98)80175-5.
11. Roche-Nagle G, Wong K, Oreopoulos G. Vascular claudication in a young patient: popliteal entrapment syndrome. *Hong Kong Med J.* 2009;15(5):388-390. www.hkmj.org. Accessed July 8, 2018.
12. Brodmann M, Stark G, Pabst E, et al. Cystic adventitial degeneration of the popliteal artery—the diagnostic value of duplex sonography. *Eur J Radiol.* 2001;38(3):209-212. doi:10.1016/S0720-048X(00)00302-8.
13. Hai Z, Guangrui S, Yuan Z, et al. CT angiography and MRI in patients with popliteal artery entrapment syndrome. *Am J Roentgenol.* 2008;191(6):1760-1766. doi:10.2214/AJR.07.4012.
14. Atilla S, Ilgit ET, Akpek S, Yucel C, Tali ET, Isik S. MR imaging and MR angiography in popliteal artery entrapment syndrome. *Eur Radiol.* 1998;8(6):1025-1029. http://www.ncbi.nlm.nih.gov/pubmed/9683714. Accessed July 7, 2018.
15. Müller N, Morris DC, Nichols DM. Popliteal artery entrapment demonstrated by CT. *Radiology.* 1984;151(1):157-158. doi:10.1148/radiology.151.1.6701307.
16. Fujiwara H, Sugano T, Fujii N. Popliteal artery entrapment syndrome: accurate morphological diagnosis utilizing MRI. *J Cardiovasc Surg (Torino).* 1992;33(2):160-162. http://www.ncbi.nlm.nih.gov/pubmed/1572871. Accessed July 7, 2018.
17. Pursell R, Torrie EP, Gibson M, Galland RB. Spontaneous and permanent resolution of cystic adventitial disease of the popliteal artery. *J R Soc Med.* 2004;97(2):77-78. http://journals.sagepub.com/doi/pdf/10.1177/014107680409700208. Accessed July 8, 2018.
18. Baxter AR, Garg K, Lamparello PJ, Mussa FF, Cayne NS, Berland T. Cystic adventitial disease of the popliteal artery: is there a consensus in management? *Vascular.* 2011;19(3):163-166. doi:10.1258/vasc.2010.cr0233.
19. van Rutte PW, Rouwet EV, Belgers EH, Lim RF, Teijink JA. In treatment of popliteal artery cystic adventitial disease, primary bypass graft not always first choice: two cases reports and review of the literature. *Eur J Vasc Surg.* 2011;42(3):347-354.
20. Rai S, Davies RS, Vohra RK. Failure of endovascular stenting for popliteal cystic disease. *Ann Vasc Surg.* 2009;23(3):410.e1-e5. doi:10.1016/j.avsg.2008.01.014.
21. Liu Y, Sun Y, He X, et al. Imaging diagnosis and surgical treatment of popliteal artery entrapment syndrome: a single-center experience. *Ann Vasc Surg.* 2014;28(2):330-337. doi:10.1016/j.avsg.2013.01.021.
22. Lane R, Nguyen T, Cuzzilla M, Oomens D, Mohabbat W, Hazelton S. Functional popliteal entrapment syndrome in the sportsperson. *Eur J Vasc Endovasc Surg.* 2012;43(1):81-87. doi:10.1016/j.ejvs.2011.10.013.
23. Levien LJ, Veller MG. Popliteal artery entrapment syndrome: more common than previously recognized. *J Vasc Surg.* 1999;30(4):587-598. doi:10.1016/S0741-5214(99)70098-4.
24. di Marzo L, Cavallaro A, Mingoli A, Sapienza P, Tedesco M, Stipa S. Popliteal artery entrapment syndrome: the role of early diagnosis and treatment. *Surgery.* 1997;122(1):26-31. doi:10.1016/S0039-6060(97)90260-9.
25. Turnipseed WD. Functional popliteal artery entrapment syndrome: a poorly understood and often missed diagnosis that is frequently mistreated. *J Vasc Surg.* 2009;49(5):1189-1195. doi:10.1016/j.jvs.2008.12.005.
26. Radowsky J, Patel B, Fox CJ. Delayed presentations of popliteal artery entrapment syndrome in a middle-aged military population. *Ann Vasc Surg.* 2013;27(8):1184.e1-e6. doi:10.1016/j.avsg.2012.11.012.
27. Kim SY, Min SK, Ahn S, Min SI, Ha J, Kim SJ. Long-term outcomes after revascularization for advanced popliteal artery entrapment syndrome with segmental arterial occlusion. *J Vasc Surg.* 2012;55(1):90-97. doi:10.1016/j.jvs.2011.06.107.
28. Bustabad MR, Ysa A, Pérez E, et al. Popliteal artery entrapment: eight years experience. *EJVES Extra.* 2006;12(4):43-51. doi:10.1016/j.ejvsextra.2006.05.003.
29. Turnipseed WD. Popliteal entrapment syndrome. *J Vasc Surg.* 2002;35(5):910-915. doi:10.1067/mva.2002.123752.
30. Pillai J. A current interpretation of popliteal vascular entrapment. *J Vasc Surg.* 2008;48(6):61S-65S. doi:10.1016/j.jvs.2008.09.049.
31. di Marzo L, Cavallaro A, O'Donnell SD, Shigematsu H, Levien LJ, Rich NM. Endovascular stenting for popliteal vascular entrapment is not recommended. *Ann Vasc Surg.* 2010;24(8):1135.e1-e3. doi:10.1016/j.avsg.2010.03.010.
32. Gourgiotis S, Aggelakas J, Salemis N, Elias C, Georgiou C. Diagnosis and surgical approach of popliteal artery entrapment syndrome: a retrospective study. *Vasc Health Risk Manag.* 2008;4(1):83-88.

Gregory J. Landry

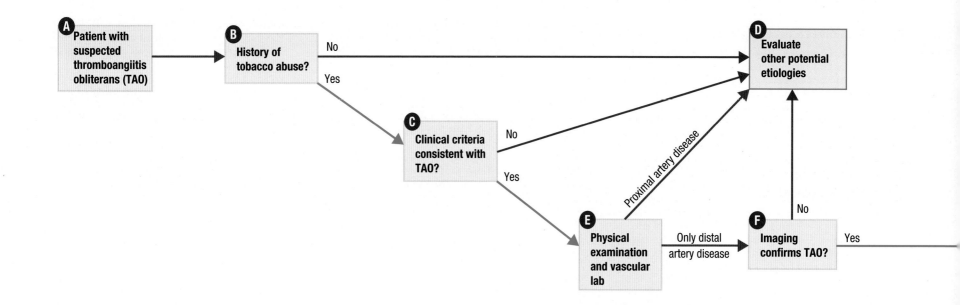

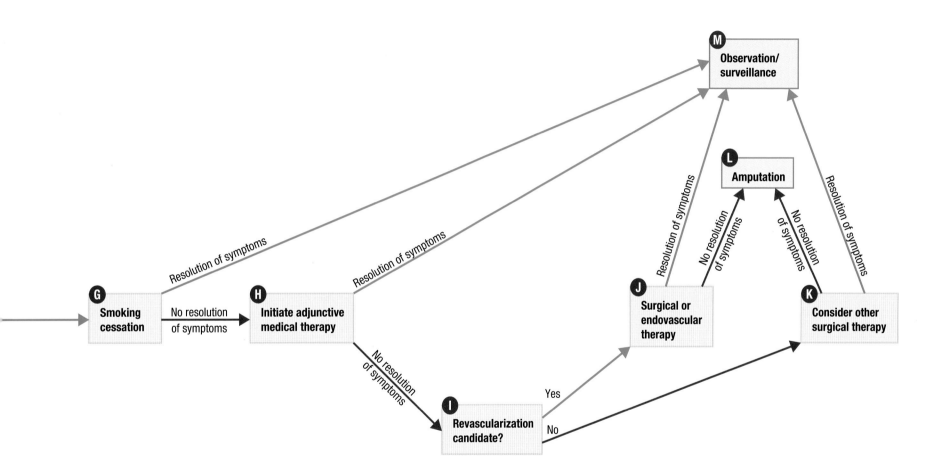

A Patient with suspected thromboangiitis obliterans (TAO)

Thromboangiitis obliterans (TAO), often referred to as Buerger's disease (after the physician who first described it), is a non-atherosclerotic, segmental, inflammatory disease of small and medium-sized arteries of the distal extremities of tobacco users, distinct from either atherosclerosis or immune arteritis. TAO typically affects young male smokers (<50 years of age); however, there is an increasing prevalence in women. It is more prevalent in the Middle and Far East than in North America and Western Europe.[1] Patients may present with early findings of pain or coldness in the fingers or toes. Involvement is upper extremity alone in approximately 30%, lower extremity alone in 45%, and both in 25%.[2] Multiple extremity involvement is also common, with 16% having two extremities, 41% three extremities, and 43% four extremities involved.[3] Late findings include rest pain, skin ulcers, and gangrene. Approximately 40% of patients with TAO will have a history of Raynaud syndrome, superficial migratory thrombophlebitis, or both.[2]

B History of tobacco abuse?

TAO is universally associated with tobacco use. In a young patient with digital ischemia (<50 years of age) with a heavy smoking history, the diagnosis of TAO should be strongly considered. Absent tobacco use, other etiologies should be evaluated.

C Clinical criteria consistent with TAO?

Although other etiologies such as atherosclerosis can lead to digital ischemia, utilizing the Shionoya clinical diagnostic criteria can assist in the diagnosis of Buerger disease. These clinical diagnostic criteria include the following:

1. Smoking history
2. Onset before the age of 50 years
3. Infrapopliteal arterial occlusions
4. Upper limb involvement or phlebitis migrans
5. Absence of atherosclerotic risk factors other than smoking[3]

A wider set of major criteria, all of which must be met to establish the diagnosis of TAO, has been suggested by Mills and Porter.[4] These include the following:

1. Onset of symptoms before age 45
2. Tobacco use
3. Distal occlusive disease documented by plethysmography, histopathology, or arteriography
4. No arterial disease proximal to the popliteal or distal brachial artery
5. Exclusion of other disease processes, including a proximal embolic source, trauma, popliteal entrapment or cystic disease, autoimmune disease, hypercoagulable state, and atherosclerosis or atherosclerotic risk factors

D Evaluate other potential etiologies

An important aspect of clinical evaluation is to rule out other possible causes of digital ischemia. These include ruling out a proximal embolic source, trauma and local lesions (eg, popliteal entrapment or cystic adventitial disease), autoimmune disease, hypercoagulable states, and atherosclerosis.

E Physical examination and vascular lab

Physical examination findings in patients with TAO are consistent with distal but not proximal arterial disease. Brachial and popliteal pulses are typically palpable with reduced or absent pulses at the wrist and/or ankle. Digital ischemia manifesting as cyanosis, ulcers, or gangrene of the fingers and/or toes is often present, and bilateral involvement is usual. Vascular laboratory findings reflect a similar distribution, with normal DUS or PVR findings to the level of the popliteal or brachial arteries, but severe occlusive disease distal to this with markedly dampened or completely flattened PPG waveforms and reduced digital pressures (digital:brachial index <0.6) in the fingers and/or toes. If pulse and vascular laboratory studies confirm isolated distal arterial disease, additional imaging should be performed to confirm the diagnosis of TAO. If proximal arterial disease is present, other etiologies should be evaluated, except for the rare young patient who could have premature atherosclerosis and TAO simultaneously.

F Imaging confirms TAO?

DSA in a patient with TAO typically demonstrates distal arterial occlusion with the presence of characteristic corkscrew collateral arteries. The same findings may be visible on CTA or MRA. Depending on the likelihood of the diagnosis (see C), DSA versus CTA may be selected as the optimal imaging modality to confirm or exclude the diagnosis of TAO.

G Smoking cessation

Total tobacco cessation is the only treatment that improves symptoms and reduces the risk of amputation if achieved before the onset of gangrene or tissue loss.[5] Over 90% of patients who quit smoking avoid amputations.[2] Patients who cannot stop smoking have relentless disease progression, often leading to major amputation in 20% to 40% over a follow-up period of 7 to 10 years.[2,5] Refer to smoking cessation management as outlined in Chapter 3.

H Initiate adjunctive medical therapy

If smoking cessation does not result in gradual resolution of symptoms and healing of tissue loss, adjunctive medical therapy is initiated, even though this is not curative in patients with TAO. Many medications have been recommended including antiplatelet agents, immunomodulators,[6] prostacyclin analogs,[7-10] vasodilators,[11,12] hemorheologic agents, and anticoagulants. Results of adjunctive medical therapy are mixed, with some studies showing improvement in pain and ulcer healing, although most publications are uncontrolled case series.[6,7,9-12] Randomized controlled trials are lacking, and no therapies have been shown to be effective in the absence of smoking cessation. An emerging area of research is gene and stem cell therapy in patients with "no option" CLI. In most such studies, autologous bone marrow cells were injected into distal leg muscle, which is rich in endothelial progenitor cells.[13-19] Although promising, there are currently no FDA-approved gene or stem cell therapies, and outside of clinical trials, these agents are not available to most patients.

I Revascularization candidate?

If smoking cessation and adjunctive medical treatment are not successful, endovascular intervention or surgical bypass can be considered, but is rarely possible in patients with TAO because distal target arteries are often occluded. Occasionally, arteriography will reveal a distal tibial or inframalleolar target artery that can serve as outflow for a distal bypass or endovascular recanalization.

J Surgical or endovascular therapy

Autogenous vein bypass in patients with TAO has not proved to be durable, with 5-year patency rates of 30% to 60% in several series.[5,20-23] Given the very distal arterial occlusion in TAO, with limited outflow, endovascular treatment is typically not feasible; however, two small case series have shown acceptable short-term patency and amputation-free survival in selected patients.[24,25]

K Consider other surgical therapy

In patients with progressive symptoms who are not candidates for revascularization, other surgical treatments can be considered. Sympathectomy has been used to treat TAO but is of unproven benefit. Case series demonstrate short-term benefits for pain relief and ulcer healing for both upper extremity[26] and lumbar sympathectomy,[27] but long-term data are lacking. Electrical stimulation of the spinal cord has also been performed in small uncontrolled case series with some evidence of pain relief and ulcer healing, although further confirmatory testing is needed.[28] Likewise, surgical series from India have reported improved ulcer healing with pedicled omental flaps to the lower extremities, although this technique has not been widely adopted.[29,30] All these treatment modalities are unproved, and none have been shown to be effective in the absence of smoking cessation; hence, they should only be considered in refractory cases.

L Amputation

For patients with TAO and finger ulcers, the ulcers will often heal with conservative local management including debridement, nail removal as needed, and rongeur removal of exposed phalangeal bone. Partial or complete finger amputations are reported in approximately 30% to 40% of patients followed up longer than 5 years, although hand amputations are extremely rare.[1,5,19] In contrast, patients with lower extremity TAO often require digital amputations; major amputation rates of 12% to 40% have been reported in patients followed up over 5 to 10 years.[2,5,31,32]

Ⓜ Observation/surveillance

For patients who improve after smoking cessation, observation is recommended, with emphasis on the critical importance of avoiding tobacco. For less responsive patients, more frequent follow-up is likely needed to monitor ulcer healing and pain control. For the rare patient who undergoes surgical or endovascular revascularization, standard graft surveillance is needed (see Chapters 47 and 54).

REFERENCES

1. Mills JL. Buerger's disease in the 21st century: diagnosis, clinical features, and therapy. *Semin Vasc Surg*. 2003;16:179-189.
2. Olin JW. Thromboangiitis obliterans (Buerger's disease). *N Engl J Med*. 2000;343:864-869.
3. Shionoya S. Diagnostic criteria of Buerger's disease. *Int J Cardiol*. 1998;66(suppl 1):S243-S245.
4. Mills JL, Porter JM. Buerger's disease: a review and update. *Semin Vasc Surg*. 1993;6:14-23.
5. Ohta T, Ishioashi H, Hosaka M, Sugimoto I. Clinical and social consequences of Buerger disease. *J Vasc Surg*. 2004;39:176-180.
6. Saha K, Chabra N, Gulati SM. Treatment of patients with thromboangiitis obliterans with cyclophosphamide. *Angiology*. 2001;52:399-407.
7. Fiessinger JN, Schafer M. Trial of iloprost versus aspirin treatment for critical limb ischaemia of thromboangiitis obliterans. The TAO Study. *Lancet*. 1990;335:555-557.
8. The European TAO Study Group. Oral iloprost in the treatment of thromboangiitis obliterans (Buerger's disease): a double-blind, randomized, placebo-controlled trial. *Eur J Vasc Endovasc Surg*. 1998;15:300-307.
9. Fernandez B, Strootman D. The prostacyclin analog, treprostinil sodium, provides symptom relief in severe Buerger's disease—a case report and review of literature. *Angiology*. 2006;57:99-102.
10. Bozkurt AK, Cengiz K, Arslan C, et al. A stable prostacyclin analogue (iloprost) in the treatment of Buerger's disease: a prospective analysis of 150 patients. *Ann Thorac Cardiovasc Surg*. 2013;19:120-125.
11. Narvaez J, Garcia-Gomez C, Alvarez L, et al. Efficacy of bosentan in patients with refractory thromboangiitis obliterans (Buerger disease): a case series and review of the literature. *Medicine (Baltimore)*. 2016;95:e5511.
12. De Haro J, Acin F, Bleda S, et al. Treatment of thromboangiitis obliterans (Buerger's disease) with bosentan. *BMC Cardiovasc Disord*. 2012;12:5.
13. Isner JM, Baumgartner I, Rauh G, et al. Treatment of thromboangiitis obliterans (Buerger's disease) by intramuscular gene transfer of vascular endothelial growth factor: preliminary clinical results. *J Vasc Surg*. 1998;28:964-973.
14. Miyamoto K, Nishigami K, Nagaya N. Unblinded pilot study of autologous transplantation of bone marrow mononuclear cells in patients with thromboangiitis obliterans. *Circulation*. 2006;114:2679-2684.
15. Kim DI, Kim MJ, Joh JH, et al. Angiogenesis facilitated by autologous whole bone marrow stem cell transplantation for Buerger's disease. *Stem Cells*. 2006;24:1194-1200.
16. Durdu S, Akar AR, Arat M, Sancak T, Eren NT, Ozyurda U. Autologous bone-marrow mononuclear cell implantation for patients with Rutherford grade II-III thromboangiitis obliterans. *J Vasc Surg*. 2006;44:732-739.
17. Saito Y, Sasaki K, Katsuda Y, et al. Effect of autologous bone-marrow cell transplantation on ischemic ulcer in patients with Buerger's disease. *Circ J*. 2007;71:1187-1192.
18. Motukuru V, Suresh KR, Vivekanand V, Raj S, Girija KR. Therapeutic angiogenesis in Buerger's disease (thromboangiitis obliterans) patients with critical limb ischemia by autologous transplantation of bone marrow mononuclear cells. *J Vasc Surg*. 2008;48:53S-60S.
19. Idei N, Soga J, Hata T, et al. Autologous bone-marrow mononuclear cell implantation reduces long-term major amputation risk in patients with critical limb ischemia: a comparison of atherosclerotic peripheral arterial disease and Buerger disease. *Circ Cardiovasc Interv*. 2011;4:15-25.
20. Sasajima T, Kubo Y, Inaba M, Goh K, Azuma N. Role of infrainguinal bypass in Buerger's disease: an eighteen-year experience. *Eur J Vasc Endovasc Surg*. 1997;13:186-192.
21. Shindo S, Matsumoto H, Ogata K, et al. Arterial reconstruction in Buerger's disease: by-pass to disease-free collaterals. *Int Angiol*. 2002;21:228-232.
22. Dilege S, Aksoy M, Kayabali M, Genc FA, Senturk M, Baktiroglu S. Vascular reconstruction in Buerger's disease: is it feasible? *Surg Today*. 2002;32:1042-1047.
23. Ates A, Yekeler I, Ceviz M, et al. One of the most frequent vascular disease in northeastern of Turkey: thromboangiitis obliterans or Buerger's disease (experience with 344 cases). *Int J Cardiol*. 2006;111:147-153.
24. Kim DH, Ko YG, Ahn CM, et al. Immediate and late outcomes of endovascular therapy for lower extremity arteries in Buerger disease. *J Vasc Surg*. 2018;67:1769-1777.
25. Graziani L, Morelli L, Parini F, et al. Clinical outcome after extended endovascular recanalization in Buerger's disease in 20 consecutive patients. *Ann Vasc Surg*. 2012;26:387-395.
26. Kothari R, Sharma D, Thakur DS, Kumar V, Somashekar U. Thoracoscopic dorsal sympathectomy for upper limb Buerger's disease. *J Soc Laparoendo Surg*. 2014;18:273-276.
27. Bozkurt AK, Koksal C, Demirbas MY, et al. A randomized trial of intravenous iloprost (a stable prostacyclin analogue) versus lumbar sympathectomy in the management Buerger's disease. *Int Angiol*. 2006;25:162-168.
28. Donas KP, Schulte S, Ktenidis K, Horsch S. The role of epidural spinal cord stimulation in the treatment of Buerger's disease. *J Vasc Surg*. 2005;41:830-836.
29. Singh L, Ramteke VK. The role of omental transfer in Buerger's disease: New Delhi's experience. *Aust N Z J Surg*. 1996;66:372-376.
30. Talwar S, Jain S, Porwal R, Laddha BL, Prasad P. Pedicled omental transfer for limb salvage in Buerger's disease. *Int J Cardiol*. 2000;72:127-132.
31. Borner C, Heidrich H. Long-term follow-up of thromboangiitis obliterans. *Vasa*. 1998;27:80-86.
32. Cooper LT, Tse TS, Mikhail MA, McBane RD, Stanson AW, Ballman KV. Long-term survival and amputation risk in thromboangiitis obliterans (Buerger's disease). *J Am Coll Cardiol*. 2004;44:2410-2411.

Fatemeh Malekpour • J. Gregory Modrall

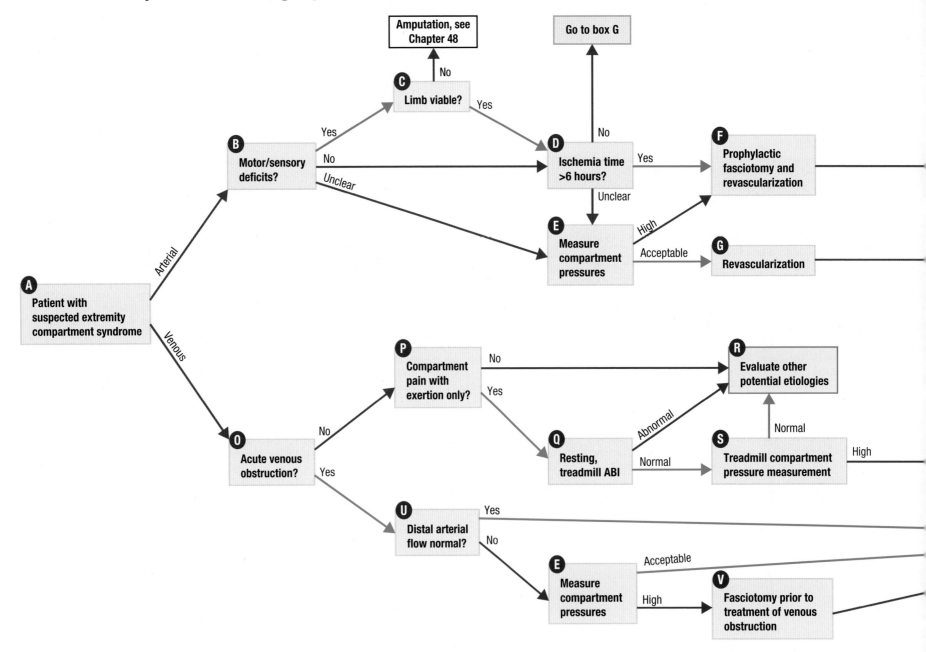

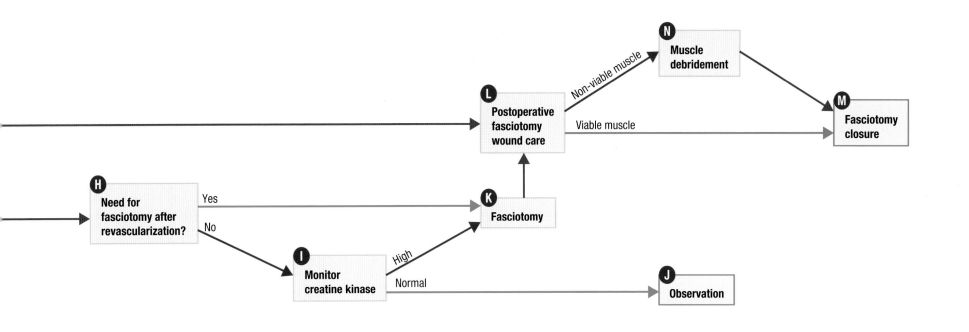

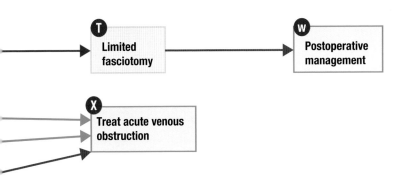

Ⓐ Patient with suspected extremity compartment syndrome

Extremity compartment syndrome as a pathologic entity is managed by orthopedic, vascular, and general surgeons. The concepts discussed in this chapter relate to vascular etiologies of extremity compartment syndrome, recognizing that long bone fractures are the cause of 75% of all extremity compartment syndromes.[1]

Acute extremity compartment syndrome is a clinical condition caused by compartmental hypertension, leading to malperfusion of neurovascular structures in confined myofascial spaces.[2] Potential clinical findings of acute compartment syndrome include extremity pain out of proportion to examination findings, tense muscle compartments, pain with passive movements of muscles in the affected compartment, numbness in the extremity distal to the compartment, and paresis or paralysis of muscles traversing the affected compartments.[3] Distal acute limb ischemia can occur.

Reperfusion following treatment of acute arterial ischemia is one of the main causes of extremity compartment syndromes encountered by vascular surgeons. Increased duration and extent of ischemia cause increase microvascular permeability, plasma protein efflux, and interstitial edema; reperfusion causes oxygen radical generation, cell wall lipid peroxidation, and further augmentation of microvascular permeability and interstitial edema.[2] Ischemia can be caused by different etiologies, including arterial embolism, thrombosis, or even decreased distal perfusion because of large occlusive sheaths used in arterial interventions. The latter category is becoming more common in the era of advanced endovascular aortic and cardiac interventions.[4,5]

We have divided compartment syndrome of the lower extremity into three broad etiologies for ease of decision making: acute arterial, venous, and chronic exertional. Venous compartment syndrome mainly results from acute proximal extensive venous outflow obstruction, resulting in high compartment pressures. Chronic exertional compartment syndrome is caused by exercise-induced increased intracompartmental pressures that lead to reversible ischemia. Extremity compartment syndromes can also occur following long bone fractures, soft-tissue crush injury, burns, or extrinsic muscle compression and are beyond the scope of this chapter.

Ⓑ Motor/sensory deficits?

The earliest symptom of compartment syndrome is pain out of proportion to the severity of injury. With increased duration of ischemia and increased tissue pressure, patients will experience sensory and/or motor deficits.[2] The most sensitive finding for calf compartment syndrome is paresthesia between the first and second digits, signifying an anterior compartment syndrome affecting the deep peroneal nerve. More advanced ischemia can present with motor dysfunction. Persistent long-term neurologic dysfunction is common in patients who develop neurovascular deficits before compartment syndrome.[6]

The most common findings on physical examination include the presence of a tense, swollen compartment and pain elicited by passive movements of muscles traversing the affected compartment. A careful neurologic examination based on the involved compartment is essential. The anterior compartment of the lower leg is the most commonly affected. Anatomic knowledge is necessary to correlate neurologic symptoms and signs with specific compartments. The anterior compartment contains the anterior tibial artery and the deep peroneal nerve. The superficial posterior compartment contains the sural nerve. The deep posterior compartment contains the posterior tibial nerve, artery, and veins, and the peroneal artery and veins. Lastly, the lateral compartment contains the superficial peroneal nerve. When symptoms and signs consistent with compartment syndrome accompany an ischemic event, such as an embolus or thrombosis, further testing may confuse or delay the diagnosis. In general, the presence of a turgid compartment with either of the two criteria—pain with passive muscle movements or neurologic changes—is sufficient to warrant fasciotomy.[2]

Ⓒ Limb viable?

If an extremity is nonviable because multiple injuries or severe irreversible ischemia (Rutherford class III ischemia), the limb is cold, demonstrates a complete absence of neurologic function in the relevant anatomic distribution, and has no distal arterial or venous Doppler signals. Nonviable limbs are best managed by urgent amputation because revascularization is futile and may provoke a massive washout of muscle breakdown products, including potassium, that may be life-threatening. The level and type of amputation are determined by the arterial anatomy, concurrent injuries, and the patient's physiologic status and comorbidities. Amputation is discussed in detail in Chapter 48.

Ⓓ Ischemia time >6 hours?

Compartment syndrome caused by ischemia-reperfusion usually arises if revascularization occurs after more than 6 hours of total ischemia time, although this time threshold is highly dependent on the severity of ischemia and the extent of preexisting collateral circulation.[2] The longer the ischemic time, the more likely is a compartment syndrome to develop. This dictum guides the decision to perform prophylactic fasciotomies in patients with prolonged ischemia times.

Ⓔ Measure compartment pressures

Diagnosing compartment syndrome in patients who are confused, comatose, or intubated poses a challenge because sensorimotor deficits cannot be accurately assessed. In such cases, or whenever the clinical diagnosis is unclear, compartment pressures should be measured.

Compartment pressure can be measured in three different ways: a handheld device (eg, Stryker® manometer), wick/slit catheter technique, and a simple needle manometer system. The most

frequently used technique is the handheld manometer, because of its portability, simplicity, and relative accuracy.[2,7] Normal tissue pressure at rest is <10 to 12 mm Hg. Systemic blood pressure and, more specifically, diastolic blood pressure have an important role in setting the threshold for the need to intervene. Although hypertensive patients can tolerate higher compartment pressure before developing permanent nerve damage, patients with PAD or hypovolemic shock may have a lower compartment pressure threshold. Compartment syndrome should be suspected if the difference between diastolic blood pressure and the compartment pressure ("delta pressure") is ≥20 to 30 mm Hg.[6] A delta pressure below 20 mm Hg is acceptable. Delta pressures between 20 and 30 mm Hg should be interpreted in the clinical setting, and a delta pressure above 30 mm Hg is considered high.

Ⓕ Prophylactic fasciotomy and revascularization

When the ischemic time is over 6 hours, and/or the compartment delta pressure is >20 to 30 mm Hg, fasciotomy should be performed before revascularization. This approach decompresses the compartments and improves the perfusion pressure. Fasciotomies are relatively simple and quick to perform and preclude the development of a subsequent compartment syndrome secondary to reperfusion, which is a common finding following revascularization in the setting of prolonged ischemia (see K and Chapter 53).

Ⓖ Revascularization

Revascularization for acute arterial ischemia is discussed in Chapter 53.

Ⓗ Need for fasciotomy after revascularization?

It is not uncommon to start a revascularization procedure on an ischemic limb within the 6-hour ischemia time window; however, time to revascularization may extend beyond 6 hours. Such patients, along with those who develop turgid compartments upon revascularization or have severe motor sensory loss preoperatively despite shorter ischemic time, require postrevascularization fasciotomy. Under general or regional anesthesia, motor-sensory function cannot be assessed after revascularization. Thus, the vascular surgeon should determine need for fasciotomy before and immediately after revascularization; if a decision is made not to perform fasciotomies after revascularization, continued monitoring for compartment syndrome is essential.

Ⓘ Monitor creatine kinase

As the pressure in the extremity increases and muscle breakdown starts, serum creatine kinase (CK) levels may increase. If myonecrosis occurs, myoglobinuria may ensue as well. In patients with baseline normal neurologic examination and acceptable compartment pressures, the intracompartmental pressure may start to rise upon revascularization. This may increase slowly and not reach a level requiring fasciotomy. Serum CK and myoglobinuria should be followed up for patients at risk for postrevascularization compartment syndrome. The level of CK that reflects severe muscle injury/death to be concerned about is often in thousands.[8]

J Observation

Patients with normalizing postoperative CK levels can be safely observed. Aside from monitoring CK in this group, the clinician may opt to follow the compartment pressure with serial measurements. Venous DUS, focusing on changes in augmentation and spontaneous respiratory variation, is another noninvasive test that may be helpful in defining the need for fasciotomy.

K Fasciotomy

Acute compartment syndrome occurs most commonly in the lower leg. Lower leg four-compartment fasciotomy techniques include double incision and single incision with fibulectomy. The double-incision fasciotomy technique is the most commonly used and includes a longitudinal incision on the anterolateral lower leg to decompress the anterior and the lateral compartments and a separate longitudinal incision on medial lower leg to decompress the deep and superficial posterior compartments. The fascia of each compartment is opened using a long Metzenbaum scissors along the entire length of the compartment. Incomplete fasciotomies caused by incomplete fascial or skin incisions may lead to secondary compartment syndrome as the underlying muscles swell.

Acute compartment syndrome affecting the thigh muscles is uncommon and usually results from crush injury or high-velocity vehicle accidents. Thigh fasciotomy is performed via a lateral incision, releasing both the anterior and posterior compartment muscles. The medial compartment of the thigh rarely requires decompression.[9] Buttock[10] and foot[11] compartment syndromes have been described and may require distinct fasciotomies; orthopedic and podiatry support may be needed for such cases.

In the upper extremity, the median and ulnar nerve and flexor muscles of the hand and forearm occupy the volar compartment of forearm. The dorsal compartment contains the extensor muscles of the wrist and fingers. Acute compartment syndrome of the upper extremity most commonly occurs in the context of comminuted fractures, supracondylar fractures, and crush injuries. Upper extremity compartment syndrome may also accompany vascular (arterial or venous) events. Forearm fasciotomy is performed using a curvilinear volar incision from medial epicondyle to midpalm, and a straight dorsal incision. The hand has 10 compartments, and fasciotomy incisions in the hand should be tailored to the involved compartment groups; hand surgery support may be needed for such cases.[2]

L Postoperative fasciotomy wound care

After fasciotomy for acute compartment syndrome, skin and subcutaneous tissue are usually left open to accommodate further muscle edema. The fasciotomy wound requires dressing changes during the recovery period and the frequency of dressing changes depends on the fluid egress. Vacuum-assisted dressings are ideal for decreasing the frequency of dressing changes and mitigating pain associated with ongoing wound care. During dressing changes, muscle viability is carefully monitored to determine if debridement is necessary.

M Fasciotomy closure

When muscle edema has resolved, fasciotomy wounds should be closed. Closure can be performed via delayed primary closure (reapproximation of skin edges using stitches), closure by secondary intention (no approximation), gradual apposition, skin grafts, or myocutaneous flaps. Delayed primary closure is reserved for cases with minimal muscle swelling. Secondary intention closure is safer in critically ill patients with nutritional deficits and other accompanying problems, but requires a much longer time to heal. Vacuum-assisted closure and different gradual dermal apposition devices can accelerate this method of closure.[12] Split-thickness skin grafting has been proposed by most authors as the preferred method of closure, whereas myocutaneous flaps are reserved for patients with exposed bone or neurovascular bundles.[2] An important component of the postoperative care of patients with acute compartment syndrome is early and aggressive physical therapy to optimize functional outcomes and prevent muscle shortening.

N Muscle debridement

Muscle debridement is rarely required during the index fasciotomy procedure. At a later stage, debridement may be necessary to remove nonviable and necrotic muscle.

O Acute venous obstruction?

Venous compartment syndrome can occur in patients who develop acute, severe venous outflow obstruction. When there is sufficiently increased venous and interstitial pressure, compartment syndrome can result. If venous hypertension is sufficient to prohibit small arterial and arteriolar flow, distal arterial ischemia may occur (phlegmasia cerulea dolens).[13] Extensive DVT usually involving iliofemoral veins is the most common cause of venous compartment syndrome. Surgical harvest of the femoral vein may also result in this syndrome.

Examination findings of acute venous compartment syndrome include severe limb edema and tense compartments. Similar to arterial compartment syndrome, pain out of proportion to the physical examination finding and neurologic findings are diagnostic. Measurement of compartment pressures may be necessary to confirm the diagnosis.

P Compartment pain with exertion only?

In chronic exertional compartment syndrome (CECS), exercise-induced venous hypertension and muscle swelling can cause a transient increase in compartment pressure and reversible ischemia. CECS usually occurs in well-conditioned runners or in the active military population.[14,15] Symptoms are most prevalent in the anterolateral, deep posterior, and superficial posterior compartments of the lower leg. Symptoms abate with rest, but quickly return on exercising. Anti-inflammatory medications and physical therapy do not improve the symptoms. When compared with intermittent claudication caused by PAD, these patients experience symptoms only after a longer duration and distance of exertion and have symptoms isolated to a muscle group typical for CECS. There are no associated findings of arterial or venous insufficiency. Bilateral symptoms are common and CECS rarely causes permanent neuromuscular damage, because discomfort restricts ongoing activity.[6]

Q Resting, treadmill ABI

After measuring resting ABI (assessed in the supine position after 20 minutes of rest), ABIs are remeasured after treadmill testing, performed with the patient walking at 2 mph and a 12° incline for 5 minutes or until symptoms occur. If the patient has normal resting ABI and abnormal exertional ABI, vascular etiologies other than CECS should be ruled out.

R Evaluate other potential etiologies

The differential diagnosis for CECS includes atherosclerotic disease, popliteal entrapment syndrome, adventitial cystic disease of the popliteal artery, and endofibrosis of external iliac artery. These diagnoses can be made on the basis of further physiologic studies and imaging.

S Treadmill compartment pressure measurement

The diagnosis of CECS requires the exclusion of more common causes of claudication. If no other diagnoses are apparent, and treadmill ABI is normal, compartment pressure measurements are indicated.

The diagnostic criteria published by Pedowitz et al.[16] include the following:

- Resting compartment pressure ≥15 mm Hg
- Compartment pressure ≥30 mm Hg, 1 to 2 minutes after completion of exercise sufficient to cause compartment pain
- Compartment pressure ≥20 mm Hg, 5 minutes after completion of such exercise

One or more of these criteria along with typical pain with exercise are sufficient for diagnosis of CECS.[16] Patients can exercise on a treadmill or run outside the office until symptoms occur. Pressures should be measured in the affected compartment; the anterior and lateral leg compartments are most commonly affected.

T Limited fasciotomy

Unlike patients with acute compartment syndrome, fasciotomy for CECS does not require decompression of all compartments, and only the involved compartments should be decompressed. The surgical technique for compartment decompression also differs between acute compartment syndrome and CECS. Both fasciotomy and fasciectomy are options in the management of CECS.[2] For fasciotomy, two small transverse skin incisions are made in either ends of the compartment and the fascia is incised, while the overlaying skin is left intact. Transverse incisions are placed over the intermuscular septum between the anterior and lateral compartments, so that both compartments can be decompressed using the same incision. For fasciectomy, a single longitudinal incision over the intermuscular septum is used to perform longitudinal fascial incisions in the anterior and lateral compartments, followed by excision of an ellipse of fascia measuring 2×6 cm from each compartment.[2]

U Distal arterial flow normal?

It is important to ensure that distal extremity perfusion is normal. Presence of distal pulses, Doppler signals, normal capillary refill, and skin color are all reassuring signs. Neurologic examination should also be taken into consideration, because the presence of sensory or motor deficits is an ominous sign that requires emergent management.

V Fasciotomy prior to treatment of venous obstruction

In patients without normal distal arterial flow, whose compartment pressures are high, performing fasciotomies should precede the management of acute venous outflow obstruction. Releasing the closed compartment spaces will improve perfusion in the involved extremity. In this setting, fasciotomies should not be delayed until definitive treatment of venous outflow obstruction. Some endovascular options in management of acute DVT require an indwelling lysis catheter and return to the operating room for a second stage. These options are not appropriate in acute DVT cases with compartment syndrome.

W Postoperative management

Patients with CECS generally do not have large wounds and their postoperative management is more focused on early mobilization and physical therapy. After 48 hours of rest, these patients are encouraged to ambulate. When the surgical wounds have healed, patients with CECS can begin nonimpact training exercises, such as swimming and stationary biking. After 1 month, they may begin a sports rehabilitation program.[6,14]

X Treat acute venous obstruction

Acute venous obstruction causing compartment syndrome is usually due to extensive iliofemoral DVT, the treatment of which is discussed in detail in Chapter 79. Other causes of acute venous obstruction, such as tumor compression or femoral vein harvest, require specific associated treatment that is beyond the scope of this chapter.

REFERENCES

1. Elliott KG, Johnstone AJ. Diagnosing acute compartment syndrome. *J Bone Joint Surg Br*. 2003;85:625.
2. Chung J, Modrall JG. Compartment syndrome. In: Cronenwett JL, Johnston KW, eds. *Rutherford's Vascular Surgery*. 8th ed. Philadelphia, PA: Elsevier Saunders; 2014:2544-2553.
3. Olson SA, Glasgow RR. Acute compartment syndrome in lower extremity musculoskeletal trauma. *J Am Acad Orthop Surg*. 2005;13:436.
4. Kreibich M, Czerny M, Benk C, et al. Thigh compartment syndrome during extracorporeal life support. *J Vasc Surg Venous Lymphat Dis*. 2017;5:859-863.
5. Charitable JF, Maldonado TS. Lower extremity compartment syndrome after elective percutaneous fenestrated endovascular repair of an abdominal aortic aneurysm. *J Vasc Surg Cases Innov Tech*. 2017;3:41-43.
6. Turnipseed WD. Compartment syndrome. In: Cronenwett JL, Rutherford RB, eds. *Decision Making in Vascular Surgery*. Philadelphia, PA: W.B. Saunders; 2001:222-226.
7. Shadgan B, Menon M, O'Brien PJ, et al. Diagnostic techniques in acute compartment syndrome of the leg. *J Orthop Trauma*. 2008;22(8):581-577. doi:10.1097/BOT.0b013e318183136d.
8. Valdez C, Schroeder E, Amdur R, et al. Serum creatine kinase levels are associated with extremity compartment syndrome. *J Trauma Acute Care Surg*. 2013;74(2):441-445; discussion 445-447. doi:10.1097/TA.0b013e31827a0a36
9. Ojike NI, Roberts CS, Giannoudis PV. Compartment syndrome of the thigh: a systematic review. *Injury*. 2010;41:133-136.
10. MacLean J, Wustrack R, Kandemir U. Gluteal compartment syndrome. *Tech Orthopaedics*. 2012;27(1):43-46.
11. Myerson M. Experimental decompression of the fascial compartments of the foot—the basis for fasciotomy in acute compartment syndromes. *Foot Ankle*. 1988;8:308-314.
12. Zannis J, Angobaldo J, Marks M, et al. Comparison of fasciotomy wound closures using traditional dressing changes and the vacuum-assisted closure device. *Ann Plast Surg*. 2009;62:407.
13. Warkentin TE. Ischemic limb gangrene with pulses. *N Engl J Med*. 2015;373:642-655.
14. Turnipseed WD. Clinical review of patients treated for atypical claudication: a 28-year experience. *J Vasc Surg*. 2004;40:79-85.
15. Waterman BR, Liu J, Newcomb R, Schoenfeld AJ, Orr JD, Belmont PJ Jr. Risk factors for chronic exertional compartment syndrome in a physically active military population. *Am J Sport Med*. 2013;41:2545-2549.
16. Pedowitz RA, Hargens AR, Mubarak SJ, Gershuni DH. Modified criteria for the objective diagnosis of chronic compartment syndrome of the leg. *Am J Sports Med*. 1990;18:35-40.

Laura Shin • David G. Armstrong

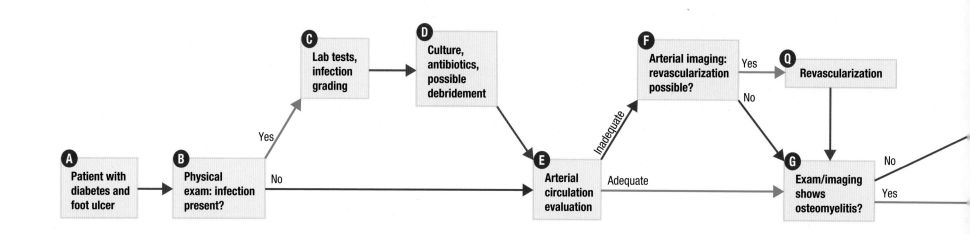

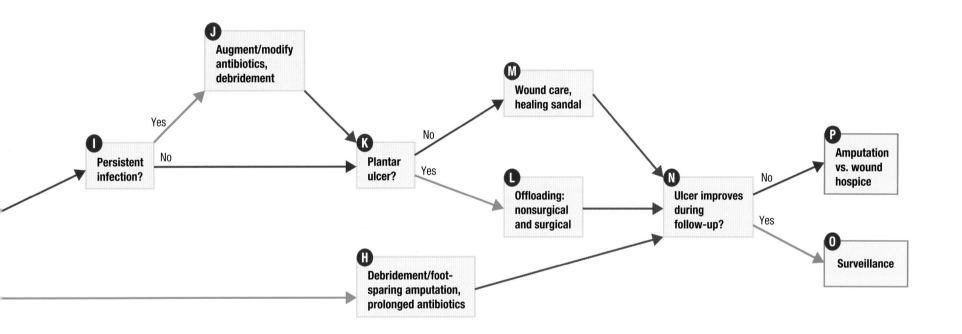

Table 52-1. Points Assigned by WIfI Limb Threat Classification System

A. Wound
    0. No ulcer and no gangrene
    1. Small ulcer and no gangrene
    2. Deep ulcer or gangrene limited to toes
    3. Extensive ulcer or gangrene
B. Ischemia: toe pressure or $TCPO_2$
    0. ≥60 mm Hg
    1. 40 to 59 mm Hg
    2. 30 to 39 mm Hg
    3. <30 mm Hg
C. Infection
    0. No infection
    1. Mild, ≤2 cm cellulitis
    2. Moderate, >2 cm cellulitis/purulence
    3. Severe, systemic response/sepsis

Data from Lazzarini PA, Pacella RE, Armstrong DG, van Netten JJ. Diabetes-related lower-extremity complications are a leading cause of the global burden of disability. *Diabet Med.* 2018. doi:10.1111/dme.13680.

A Patient with diabetes and foot ulcer

Of the 435 million people with diabetes, worldwide, up to 34% (148 million) will develop a diabetic foot ulcer in their lifetime.[1,2] Lower extremity complications of diabetes are a leading cause of infection and hospitalization and are now a major source of global disability.[2] Optimal treatment in this population requires a team approach. Core participation of vascular and podiatric surgery along with physical therapy, diabetology, infectious disease, and nursing appear to reduce time to treatment and thereby the risk for high-level amputation.[3-5] When patients with diabetes present with tissue loss, they should be assessed for overall limb threat. This should be done systematically using the wound, ischemia, and foot infection (WIfI) score. By assessing whether a wound, degree of ischemia, or infection is "none, mild, moderate, or severe" (0,1,2,3), one can rapidly communicate the degree of limb threat to the patient and other members of the interdisciplinary team (Table 52-1).[6,7]

B Physical exam: infection present?

Patients with diabetes presenting with foot ulcers should undergo a comprehensive dermatologic, neurologic, musculoskeletal, and vascular examination.[8] The diagnosis of a diabetic foot infection is a clinical one. Importantly, bacteria in the wound are not a qualifier of active infection because all wounds have microorganism colonization. The examination should include an evaluation for soft-tissue erythema, wound size, depth, associated drainage, and tissue/bone exposure. Infection can be identified by erythema, calor, drainage, and/or malodor, with inflammation and purulence identifying active infection. Because patients with diabetes have neuropathy, they may not have the painful feedback or other local/regional symptoms otherwise associated with inflammation.

Infections should be classified as mild (superficial and limited in size and depth), moderate (deeper or more extensive), or severe (accompanied by systemic signs or metabolic perturbations).[8] Patients with active infection require specific management. The first examination should include an assessment of the degree of tissue loss, graded by the WIfI system.[7]

C Lab tests, infection grading

Patients who present with a diabetic foot infection require basic blood testing including a CBC, serum chemistries, and inflammatory markers (erythrocyte sedimentation rate and/or CRP).[9] The overall grade of infection is scored by the systemic inflammatory response syndrome (SIRS) score, with one point for each of the following potential findings:

- Temperature >38°C or <36°C
- Heart rate >90 beats/min
- Respiratory rate >20 breaths/min or $PaCO_2$ < 32 mm Hg
- WBC > 12,000 or <4000 cells/μL or ≥10% immature (band) form[10]

Patients with SIRS score >2 require more urgent resuscitation and intravenous antibiotics.

People diagnosed with SIRS and WIfI foot infection grade 3 require more intensive medical and surgical intervention than do those in lower infection grades. It is critical to also correct associated hyperglycemia and other electrolyte or metabolic disorders.

D Culture, antibiotics, possible debridement

Patients with diabetes and an infected foot ulcer should have their wound cultured before or concomitant with the administration of antibiotics. Blood and deep tissue (obtained during debridement) cultures can help select appropriate antibiotics.[11] Although superficial cultures are often obtained in these patients, they have limited utility because most wounds have superficial skin flora contamination that does not necessarily identify the organism responsible for the infection. After culture findings are obtained and diabetic infection is confirmed, empiric antibiotic therapy should be initiated and subsequently be narrowed down as much as possible after bacterial speciation and drug sensitivities are available. Empiric treatment should be based on severity of infection by the suspected organism, and detailed recommendations have been published by the Infectious Diseases Society of America.[8] If infection is severe enough to require hospitalization, intravenous antibiotics are used. Undrained purulence or nonviable tissue should be surgically debrided in as expeditious a manner as possible. Generally, advancing infection should take precedence over revascularization.[12]

E Arterial circulation evaluation

Because of the frequent association of ischemia with diabetic foot ulcers, all patients should undergo an evaluation of the arterial circulation to the foot, starting with pulse examination. Noninvasive

vascular laboratory assessment should be performed in all patients with reduced pulses or examination findings of digital ischemia. ABIs are obtained initially but may be falsely elevated or normal in patients with diabetes because the medial calcification of tibial arteries makes them noncompressible. Because digital arteries are often spared, the toe-brachial index may provide a more accurate representation of distal foot perfusion than do the ABIs.[13] Low-amplitude pulse-volume recordings and monophasic Doppler waveforms support the diagnosis of severe ischemia in such patients. Although there is no absolute threshold, ABI > 0.8, TBI > 0.6, or absolute toe pressure >60 mm Hg is generally adequate for ulcer healing, recognizing that the more extensive the tissue loss, the better the circulation must be to allow healing. Conversely, if ABI < 0.5, TBI < 0.3 or toe pressure is <30 mm Hg, healing is unlikely. Individual decision making is needed for each patient to determine whether arterial revascularization is needed to allow ulcer healing, and sometimes this is determined by the course of ulcer healing during the treatment program (see I). If there is any doubt about the adequacy of arterial evaluation, further imaging is warranted to assess the potential for healing or the need for revascularization.

F Arterial imaging: revascularization possible?

Patients presenting with PAD and tissue loss have up to a 40% chance of progressing to major amputation within 6 months. Unfortunately, limb loss is far more likely if revascularization is not performed in patients with severe arterial disease. DUS, CTA, or MRA can provide minimally invasive imaging to define the location and severity of arterial disease, and usually allows a decision to be made about whether revascularization is possible. In some cases, arteriography may be required to define detailed anatomy of distal arteries and may be done for surgical bypass planning or as part of an endovascular intervention. In most patients, when arterial circulation is inadequate to allow ulcer healing, endovascular or surgical revascularization is possible and should be attempted in all but the highest risk patients.[14,15]

G Exam/imaging shows osteomyelitis?

Likelihood of bone infection is significantly increased if it is possible to manually probe to the bone through the ulcer. This is especially true when this examination is performed in an inpatient setting where the pretest probability is high.[16] Radiographs can also be helpful if they show obvious bone destruction. In equivocal cases, MRI can be utilized to confirm the diagnosis.[17] It is important to determine whether osteomyelitis is present because bone debridement and prolonged antibiotics will likely be required to allow wound healing, even in patients with adequate circulation.

H Debridement/foot-sparing amputation, prolonged antibiotics

For patients with diabetic foot infection involving bone, definitive surgical treatment may be required to eradicate the infection.[18]

In this case, all devitalized tissue and bone should be surgically removed. In some cases, soft-tissue and partial bone excision may be adequate, but in many cases, especially with forefoot osteomyelitis, transmetatarsal amputation or panmetatarsal head excision may be required. Recent data also suggest that for some patients, suppressive antimicrobial therapy may be clinically successful.[19]

I Persistent infection?

During the course of treatment, foot ulcers should be carefully monitored for new or worsening infection versus improvement of infection, and treatment altered if infection is persistent and not improving.

J Augment/modify antibiotics, debridement

If patients have adequate circulation, and absence of underlying osteomyelitis, but do not respond to the initial treatment with oral antibiotics, the route or type of antimicrobial should be reconsidered. Repeat wound cultures of deep tissue and consultation with infectious disease colleagues may also be helpful at this stage. The ulcer should be carefully inspected for nonviable tissue, and additional local debridement performed at any stage where this is necessary.

K Plantar ulcer?

Autonomic neuropathy can lead to decreased capillary bed perfusion and resultant dry and cracked skin. Disruption of the skin's protective barrier can increase the risk of bacterial infection at this site. *Motor neuropathy* can result in claw-toe deformity, intrinsic muscle wasting, and distortion of the foot's normal weight-bearing surface, which predisposes the foot pressure necrosis and ulceration. *Sensory neuropathy* impairs proprioception and decreases the foot's ability to adapt to repetitive local stresses. This can result in injury or ulcerations that go unnoticed by the patient. Unfortunately, neuropathy sets the stage for ulcer recurrences, treatment failures, and the Charcot foot. Neuropathic ulcers typically develop in areas of increased plantar pressure, especially under the metatarsal heads, on the plantar surface, and on the distal and dorsal ends of deformed digits.[1,20,21] When a plantar ulcer is present, an offloading strategy at the site of the ulcer is needed.

L Offloading: nonsurgical and surgical

The gold standard for offloading remains the total contact cast (TCC).[20-22] This device works best for plantar wounds without uncontrolled infection or severe ischemia. Other offloading devices such as the removable cast walker, instant TCC, and depth inlay shoes are also prescribed to relieve external foot pressure and enhance wound healing and may be used when the TCC is not.[23]

The presence of structural foot deformities increases the risk for ulcerations because of the increased pressure to the area of deformity. Although offloading and, ultimately, appropriate shoe gear are essential for wound healing in these patients, surgical reconstruction of the deformity may be required to prevent recurrent foot ulcerations This may involve an osteotomy/arthroplasty to allow a metatarsal or digit to be less prominent, an Achilles tendon lengthening to reduce plantar pressure in the forefoot, or a midfoot or hindfoot reconstruction for patients with Charcot arthropathy.[22,24]

Specifically, for patients with severe foot deformities such as a rocker bottom foot resulting from Charcot neuropathy, if nonsurgical means of offloading (total contact casting Charcot restraint orthotic walkers) are ineffective or inadequate to get a patient to a postacute stage where they are shoe-able, surgical reconstruction with external fixation is used to correct the foot deformity and allow the wounds to heal. A staged approach, with internal fixation, may also be utilized when ulcerations are in remission.

M Wound care, healing sandal

Choosing an appropriate offloading device or shoe is essential for ulcer healing and to prevent ulcer recurrence. Wounds that are not on the plantar aspect of the foot may require a less complex strategy such as a healing sandal that protects the margins or distal ends of digits.

N Ulcer improves during follow-up?

Ulcer size should ideally be measured at each visit to assess the healing trajectory. If an ulcer has healed by 50% at 4 weeks, it is likely to heal entirely over the subsequent 3 to 4 months. However, the converse is also true.[25-27] Wounds that do not progress should be reassessed for (a) possible progression of ischemia, (b) development or persistence of occult infection, or (c) adequacy of debridement and offloading strategies.

O Surveillance

After ulcer healing, 40% of patients will have a recurrence at 1 year and nearly two-thirds at 3 years. Recurrence is not only common, but likely. Therefore, when an ulcer is healed, the term "remission" should be used to communicate this to the patient and other members of the team.[28] Patients should be enrolled into a program designed around remission management including frequent (every 2-3 months) visits, shoe gear and insole modifications, and reconstructive surgery as necessary to treat deformities that progress or develop. Furthermore, this program can and should be synchronized for the patient with concomitant vascular noninvasive surveillance of endovascular or open vascular reconstruction as appropriate.[29-31]

P Amputation vs. wound hospice

Despite optimal care, some diabetic foot ulcers either ultimately require or are best treated with foot amputation.[32,33] Amputation is covered in detail in Chapter 48. In other patients where mobility is limited or where aggressive therapy is not ideal, the goals may change from wound healing to "wound hospice." In other words, the goals may be to keep the wound uncomplicated and uninfected so as to increase hospital-free days as much as possible.[34]

Q Revascularization

Revascularization in diabetic patients usually involves below the knee arteries which in contemporary practice can be accomplished with both endovascular and open surgical techniques as discussed in detail in Chapters 45 to 47. Revascularization of ischemic feet is necessary for ulcer healing and resolution of infection. In cases of severe infection, debridement or even distal amputation must precede revascularization, while in less severely infected cases, revascularization is often required to resolve infection even with aggressive antibiotic treatment. After revascularization, wound care and infection treatment continues as outlined in the decision tree.

REFERENCES

1. Armstrong DG, Boulton AJM, Bus SA. Diabetic foot ulcers and their recurrence. *N Engl J Med*. 2017;376(24):2367-2375.
2. Lazzarini PA, Pacella RE, Armstrong DG, van Netten JJ. Diabetes-related lower-extremity complications are a leading cause of the global burden of disability. *Diabet Med*. 2018. doi:10.1111/dme.13680.
3. Rogers LC, Andros G, Caporusso J, Harkless LB, Mills JL Sr, Armstrong DG. Toe and flow: essential components and structure of the amputation prevention team. *J Vasc Surg*. 2010;52(3 suppl):23S-27S.
4. Skrepnek GH, Mills JL, Armstrong DG. Foot-in-wallet disease: tripped up by "cost-saving" reductions? *Diabetes Care*. 2014;37(9):e196-e197. doi:10.2337/dc14-0079.
5. Driver VR, Fabbi M, Lavery LA, Gibbons G. The costs of diabetic foot: the economic case for the limb salvage team. *J Vasc Surg*. 2010;52(3 suppl):17S-22S.
6. Armstrong DG, Mills JL. Juggling risk to reduce amputations: the three-ring circus of infection, ischemia and tissue loss-dominant conditions. *Wound Med*. 2013;1:13-14.
7. Mills JL Sr, Conte MS, Armstrong DG, et al. The Society for Vascular Surgery Lower Extremity Threatened Limb Classification System: risk stratification based on wound, ischemia, and foot infection (WIfI). *J Vasc Surg*. 2014; 59(1):220-234.e1-e2.
8. Lipsky BA, Berendt AR, Cornia PB, et al. 2012 Infectious Diseases Society of America clinical practice guideline for the diagnosis and treatment of diabetic foot infections. *Clin Infect Dis*. 2012;54(12):1679-1684.
9. Wukich DK, Armstrong DG, Attinger CE, et al. Inpatient management of diabetic foot disorders: a clinical guide. *Diabetes Care*. 2013;36(9):2862-2871.
10. Lipsky BA, Silverman MH, Joseph WS. A proposed new classification of skin and soft tissue infections modeled on

the subset of diabetic foot infection. *Open Forum Infect Dis.* 2017;4(1):ofw255.

11. Malone M, Bowling FL, Gannass A, Jude EB, Boulton AJM. Deep wound cultures correlate well with bone biopsy culture in diabetic foot osteomyelitis. *Diabetes Metab Res Rev.* 2013;29(7):546-550.

12. Fisher TK, Scimeca CL, Bharara M, Mills JL Sr, Armstrong DG. A step-wise approach for surgical management of diabetic foot infections. *J Vasc Surg.* 2010;52(3 suppl):72S-75S.

13. Tehan PE, Bray A, Chuter VH. Non-invasive vascular assessment in the foot with diabetes: sensitivity and specificity of the ankle brachial index, toe brachial index and continuous wave Doppler for detecting peripheral arterial disease. *J Diabetes Complications.* 2016;30(1):155-160.

14. Woo K, Palmer OP, Weaver FA, Rowe VL; Society for Vascular Surgery Vascular Quality Initiative. Outcomes of completion imaging for lower extremity bypass in the Vascular Quality Initiative. *J Vasc Surg.* 2015;62(2):412-416.

15. El-Sayed HF. Bypass surgery for lower extremity limb salvage: vein bypass. *Methodist Debakey Cardiovasc J.* 2012;8(4):37-42.

16. Lavery LA, Armstrong DG, Peters EJG, Lipsky BA. Probe-to-bone test for diagnosing diabetic foot osteomyelitis: reliable or relic? *Diabetes Care.* 2007;30(2):270-274.

17. Lam K, van Asten SAV, Nguyen T, La Fontaine J, Lavery LA. Diagnostic accuracy of probe to bone to detect osteomyelitis in the diabetic foot: a systematic review. *Clin Infect Dis.* 2016;63(7):944-948.

18. Armstrong DG, Lipsky BA. Diabetic foot infections: stepwise medical and surgical management. *Int Wound J.* 2004;1(2):123-132.

19. Tone A, Nguyen S, Devemy F, et al. Six-week versus twelve-week antibiotic therapy for nonsurgically treated diabetic foot osteomyelitis: a multicenter open-label controlled randomized study. *Diabetes Care.* 2015;38(2):302-307.

20. Armstrong DG, Nguyen HC, Lavery LA, van Schie CH, Boulton AJ, Harkless LB. Off-loading the diabetic foot wound: a randomized clinical trial. *Diabetes Care.* 2001;24(6):1019-1022.

21. Bus SA, Valk GD, van Deursen RW, et al. The effectiveness of footwear and offloading interventions to prevent and heal foot ulcers and reduce plantar pressure in diabetes: a systematic review. *Diabetes Metab Res Rev.* 2008;24(suppl 1):S162-S180.

22. Bus SA, Armstrong DG, van Deursen RW, et al. IWGDF guidance on footwear and offloading interventions to prevent and heal foot ulcers in patients with diabetes. *Diabetes Metab Res Rev.* 2016;32(suppl 1):25-36.

23. Boghossian JA, Miller JD, Armstrong DG. Offloading the diabetic foot: toward healing wounds and extending ulcer-free days in remission. *Chronic Wound Care Manag Res.* 2017;4:83-88.

24. van Schie C, Slim FJ. Biomechanics of the diabetic foot: the road to foot ulceration. In: Boulton AJM, ed. *The Diabetic Foot.* 2012:203-216.

25. Lavery LA, Barnes SA, Keith MS, Seaman JW Jr, Armstrong DG. Prediction of healing for postoperative diabetic foot wounds based on early wound area progression. *Diabetes Care.* 2008;31(1):26-29.

26. Robson MC, Hill DP, Woodske ME, Steed DL. Wound healing trajectories as predictors of effectiveness of therapeutic agents. *Arch Surg.* 2000;135(7):773-777.

27. Sheehan P, Jones P, Caselli A, Giurini JM, Veves A. Percent change in wound area of diabetic foot ulcers over a 4-week period is a robust predictor of complete healing in a 12-week prospective trial. *Diabetes Care.* 2003;26(6):1879-1882.

28. Boghossian JA, Miller JD, Armstrong DG. Towards extending ulcer-free days in remission in the diabetic foot syndrome. *Front Diabet.* 2017;26:210-218.

29. Boulton AJ, Armstrong DG, Albert SF, et al. Comprehensive foot examination and risk assessment: a report of the task force of the foot care interest group of the American Diabetes Association, with endorsement by the American Association of Clinical Endocrinologists. *Diabetes Care.* 2008;31(8):1679-1685.

30. Khan T, Shin L, Woelfel S, Rowe V, Wilson BL, Armstrong DG. Building a scalable diabetic limb preservation program: four steps to success. *Diabet Foot Ankle.* 2018;9(1):1452513.

31. Khan T, Armstrong DG. Ulcer-free, hospital-free and activity-rich days: three key metrics for the diabetic foot in remission. *J Wound Care.* 2018;27(suppl 4):S3-S4.

32. Armstrong DG, Fiorito JL, Leykum BJ, Mills JL. Clinical efficacy of the pan metatarsal head resection as a curative procedure in patients with diabetes mellitus and neuropathic forefoot wounds. *Foot Ankle Spec.* 2012;5(4):235-240.

33. Fiorito J, Trinidad-Hernandez M, Leykum B, Smith D, Mills JL, Armstrong DG. A tale of two soles: sociomechanical and biomechanical considerations in diabetic limb salvage and amputation decision-making in the worst of times. *Diabet Foot Ankle.* 2012;3. doi:10.3402/dfa.v3i0.18633.

34. Mills JL, Armstrong DG. The concept and proposed definition of "wound simplification." *Wound Med.* 2013;2-3:9-10.

James D. Brooks • Murray L. Shames

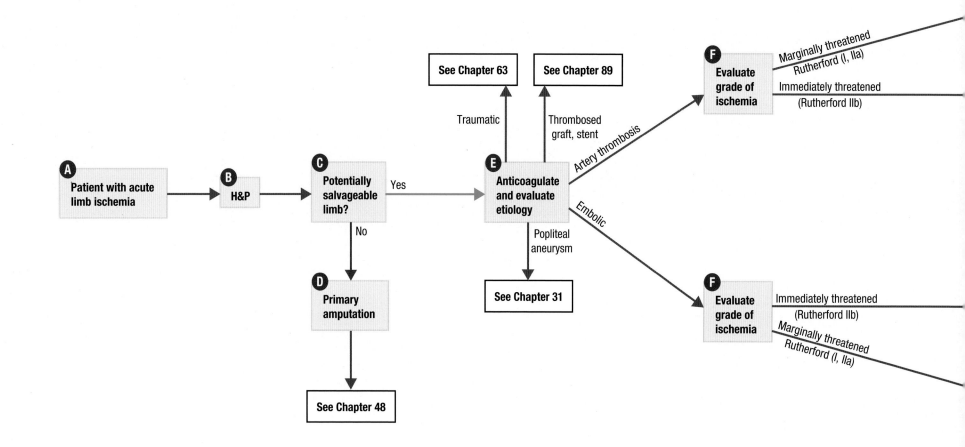

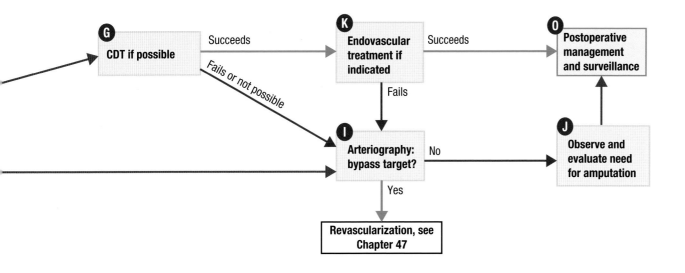

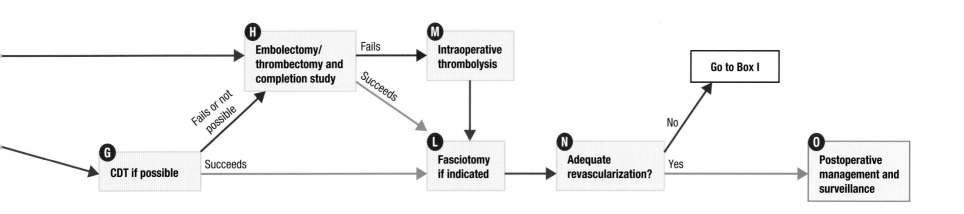

(A) Patient with acute limb ischemia

Acute limb ischemia (ALI) is caused by a sudden loss of arterial flow to an extremity and represents a limb-threatening condition associated with high risk of amputation and mortality.[1,2] It has a variety of local and anatomically remote causes and is associated with severe local and systemic complications.[1,3] Early recognition and appropriate treatment according to etiology and severity of clinical presentation are paramount in maximizing the rate of functional limb salvage. The duration of acute ischemia that leads to limb loss is variable, depending on the severity and location of the occlusive lesion and the amount of collateral circulation. Although a maximum of 6 hours ischemic time to avoid limb loss is often quoted, this duration can be shorter or longer depending on these factors.

(B) H&P

Patients with ALI usually present within hours of developing symptoms. Attempts should be made to ascertain the exact time of symptom onset because the duration of ischemia affects outcomes.[4] A thorough medical history should be obtained including vascular risk factors (smoking, HTN, diabetes mellitus, hyperlipidemia, CKD), CAD, prior MI, CHF, arrhythmias, stroke, preexisting PAD, history of any prior vascular interventions (bypass and/or stenting) in the extremities, and an active list of medications.[1,4]

A number of non-ischemic causes of extremity pain can mimic ALI. These include neuropathy, minor soft-tissue trauma, gout, acute spinal cord ischemia, and DVT (most notably phlegmasia cerulea dolens).[1,3,5] Presence of any of these conditions should not hinder the accurate diagnosis of ALI, however, which reinforces the crucial role of the meticulous physical examination in this setting.

Although a full cardiopulmonary and vascular examination should be performed,[4] the focused physical examination of a patient with ALI is directed toward assessment of the affected extremity. The limb should be inspected for evidence of the 6 P's[1,3] of ALI: pain, pallor, poikilothermia (coolness of the limb), pulselessness, paresthesia, and paresis/paralysis. Assessment of palpable pulses should be supplemented with a careful examination using a continuous-wave Doppler.[1] This examination should also be repeated in the contralateral extremity for comparison.

(C) Potentially salvageable limb?

ALI causes potentially irreversible damage to muscle, nerve, and skin.[1] The combination of physical examination findings used to assess the acutely ischemic limb is also used to determine salvageability.[1] After the initial report by Blaisdell et al.,[6] which outlined the selective approach to treatment of ALI based on time since symptom onset and limb status, the Society for Vascular Surgery (SVS)[7] has defined standards for assessment and reporting of ALI. A limb with profound sensory loss and motor dysfunction (paralysis/rigor) and inaudible arterial and venous Doppler signals

is considered to be irreversibly damaged (Rutherford grade III). Such a limb should be considered for primary amputation with the understanding that revascularization in this setting will result in a viable, yet nonfunctional limb. Lesser forms of ischemia ranging from no motor or sensory loss in the presence of audible Doppler signals to minimal/moderate sensory and/or motor loss in the absence of audible Doppler signals warrant attempts at revascularization for limb salvage.[1,4,7]

(D) Primary amputation

The nonsalvageable, acutely ischemic limb should be considered for primary amputation in most patients. In a small subgroup of patients with advanced age, limiting cardiac/pulmonary comorbidities, and immobility, palliative care without amputation is considered.[8] On the basis of the results of one historical longitudinal study,[9] up to 22% of patients will present needing primary amputation. Furthermore, more contemporary data suggest that despite revascularization attempts, patients with advanced ischemia, thrombosed bypass, and failure of the initial revascularization procedure have a 9%, 18%, and 28% rates of 30-day, 1-year, and 5-year amputation rates, respectively.[10] Amputation is discussed in detail in Chapter 48.

(E) Anticoagulate and evaluate etiology

Initial steps in the management of ALI include anticoagulation with intravenous weight-based heparin infusion (bolus and continuous rate dosing).[1,4] The causes of ALI are variable, however, and most commonly result from arterial embolism or thrombosis. Embolism can be cardiac or noncardiac in origin. Cardiac embolism can result from atrial fibrillation, MI, or valvular disease. Noncardiac embolism can be caused by atherosclerotic disease or mural thrombus of upstream arteries, aneurysms (see Chapter 31) or DVT (paradoxical embolism). Thrombosis can occur in a native artery, bypass, or stent (see Chapter 89). It can also occur within an aneurysm (see Chapter 31), can be caused by phlegmasia cerulea dolens, and can be triggered by a hypercoagulable state. ALI can less commonly be caused by extremity trauma (see Chapter 63), aortic dissection (see Chapter 21), and hemodynamic states (shock, vasopressor use, cocaine).[1,4,11,12] An etiology should be immediately sought because it influences choice of limb revascularization strategy. A potential hypercoagulable state should be evaluated as discussed in Chapter 5.

(F) Evaluate grade of ischemia

Determining the grade of ischemia is critical for timing and choice of initial intervention for the salvageable limb. The SVS has promoted the classification put forth by Rutherford et al.[7] in selecting optimal management depending on physical examination alone. The patient with a viable limb (audible arterial Doppler signals and no sensory or motor loss) is considered to be Rutherford grade I. Patients with inaudible Doppler signals and evidence of *any* sensory (Rutherford grade IIa) and/or motor

dysfunction (Rutherford grade IIb) are considered to have a marginally or immediately threatened limb, respectively.

In patients with Rutherford grade I or IIa ischemia (when the limb is not immediately threatened), catheter-directed thrombolysis (CDT) (when not contraindicated) is often recommended because it is less invasive than is open surgical treatment, and there is time to perform lysis without risking limb loss due to excessive ischemic time. This especially applies for idiopathic thrombosis or one related to a clotting abnormality, such that no additional treatment besides lysis is likely required. In other cases, where an underlying arterial or graft stenosis that requires open surgical treatment is known to be present, direct thrombectomy is more expeditious. In some cases, such as a thrombosed popliteal aneurysm, thrombolysis may be required to clear outflow arteries, even though surgical treatment is planned. For embolic disease, surgical embolectomy is usually more expeditious, but in high-risk patients, those with very distal emboli, or only Rutherford grade I ischemia, thrombolysis may be preferred. Clinical experience and local expertise significantly influence decision making for ALI treatment. In patients with Rutherford grade I or IIa acute ischemia, when the presenting etiology or level of arterial occlusion is unclear, or further delineation of the arterial anatomy is warranted for operative planning, there is usually time to obtain expedited arterial DUS or CTA/MRA. Obtaining imaging, however, should never delay emergency revascularization.[1]

In patients with Rutherford grade IIb ischemia (an immediately threatened limb) or in patients with a marginally threatened limb in whom CDT is not appropriate or feasible, embolectomy/thrombectomy or surgical bypass should be performed.[1,3,4,7]

(G) CDT if possible

CDT is considered appropriate for patients with low-grade (Rutherford grades I or IIa) ischemia and absence of any contraindication to receiving a fibrinolytic agent. Absolute contraindications include major surgery within 2 weeks, recent stroke or neurosurgery within 2 months, and patients with significant risk of bleeding (eg, recent gastrointestinal bleed or known bleeding diathesis).[13] The most commonly used agent for thrombolysis is currently alteplase, a recombinant form of tissue plasminogen activator (tPA).

The established role of arteriography and CDT comes from three randomized controlled clinical trials comparing this technique to open surgical revascularization: the University of Rochester study, the STILE trial, and the TOPAS trial.[13] The University of Rochester study demonstrated improved survival in the CDT arm likely due to fewer in-hospital cardiopulmonary complications.[14] Analysis of the results of the STILE trial found that patients receiving CDT within 14 days of ischemia onset had a lower rate of amputation; conversely, patients with duration of ischemia longer than 14 days treated with CDT had better outcomes with surgery.[4,15,16] The TOPAS study evaluated patients with ALI duration of less than 14 days receiving open surgery versus CDT with urokinase, an older fibrinolytic agent.[16,17] Results revealed an increased rate of hemorrhagic complications in the CDT group; however, the use of CDT allowed for some patients to avoid open surgical intervention altogether and reduced the number of open surgical procedures needed without a significant increase in mortality, amputation rate, or hospital length of stay.[17] The high rate of hemorrhage prompted the search for fibrinolytic agents with more favorable safety profiles.[16] Contemporary series report reduced rates of hemorrhage and acceptable rates of limb loss and mortality with recombinant tPA.[18]

The use of adjunctive techniques in thrombolysis has been reported for ALI,[18-21] specifically the use of rheolytic/pharmacomechanical thrombolysis, with promising results; however, there are no current randomized controlled trials comparing pharmacomechanical thrombolysis to conventional CDT or open surgical techniques in this clinical setting.

ⓗ Embolectomy/thrombectomy and completion study

In patients with an immediately threatened limb (Rutherford grade IIb) and/or in whom etiology, duration of ischemia or contraindication to fibrinolytic therapy precludes use of CDT, surgical embolectomy/thrombectomy is the appropriate next step in management.[17,22,23] The use of a Fogarty embolectomy catheter[1] has long been proved to be the indispensable instrument of choice for the removal of emboli/thrombi. A useful improvement upon the original embolectomy catheter is the development of an over-the-wire form of this device,[1] which can allow selective fluoroscopic guidance into a target vessel. Depending on the etiology (embolic vs. thrombotic), the patient may need adjunctive endovascular or surgical intervention following successful thrombus extraction.[1,22,23]

ⓘ Arteriography: bypass target?

DSA is an essential adjunct to revascularization in ALI. Aside from its use in guiding endovascular intervention following successful thrombolysis and/or thromboembolectomy, it serves a vital role in planning surgical bypass. Alternatively, it may reveal that a patient has no suitable bypass targets. If these cannot be improved with CDT, the patient is observed and considered for possible future amputation, if necessary. DSA is also useful as a completion study to evaluate the success of open, endovascular, or hybrid revascularization strategies.

In patients with embolic or thrombotic ALI in whom endovascular techniques are contraindicated or fail to restore inflow, or in whom embolectomy/thrombectomy fails to restore inflow, surgical bypass should be considered. DSA should be performed to identify the appropriate inflow artery and an adequate bypass target. Details of surgical bypass are discussed in Chapter 47. On the basis of the Vascular Study Group of New England data, bypass performed in this setting accounted for 5.7% of all lower

extremity bypasses between 2003 and 2011.[2] These patients were found to have higher rates of cardiac, pulmonary, and renal complications. Furthermore, bypass for ALI compared to CLI was associated with higher rates of major amputation and mortality, with ALI being an independent predictor for both of these end points.[2] A smaller, single-center retrospective review of European data revealed similar findings with respect to these outcomes; no difference was found in patency and reintervention rates between bypasses performed for ALI versus CLI with follow-up to 24 months.[24]

ⓙ Observe and evaluate need for amputation

In patients without a bypass target and Rutherford grade IIb ischemia, a period of close observation is advised to allow for the determination of amputation level. In this scenario, if the patient becomes systemically ill from ischemic tissue (rising serum creatine kinase, myoglobinuria, or renal impairment), then an emergent amputation must be performed.

ⓚ Endovascular treatment if indicated

Following successful restoration of inflow to the limb with CDT or embolectomy/thrombectomy, lesions amenable to endovascular repair may be treated with PTA and/or stenting where appropriate. In one large retrospective series[18] examining CDT outcomes, 89% of patients required adjunctive revascularization procedures performed after successful CDT; of these, 68.8% of were able to be performed with endovascular techniques alone. In case of failure of endovascular therapy, assessment for bypass surgery is done.

ⓛ Fasciotomy if indicated

Reperfusion of the limb may cause profound increased cellular edema, which increases the pressure within the muscular compartments of the leg.[1,3] Four-compartment fasciotomy[25] via medial and lateral leg incisions can prevent permanent nerve and muscle damage in that setting. In patients with ischemic time >6 hours,[26] prophylactic four-compartment fasciotomy is recommended. In patients with postoperative severe calf pain, tenderness, decreased sensation, and weakness of the revascularized limb, the possibility of compartment syndrome should be immediately evaluated. The primary diagnosis of extremity compartment syndrome centers on the physical examination; however, a measured compartment pressure >30 mm Hg can confirm this diagnosis. Increased serum creatine kinase levels and myoglobinuria support diagnosis of compartment syndrome as well.[1,3] Compartment syndrome is much less common after treatment of ALI of the upper extremity, primarily because collateral circulation is usually better in the arm, so the ischemic injury is less severe. However, compartment syndrome can occur in the upper extremity and is treated with forearm fasciotomy. This involves release of the volar and dorsal compartments of the forearm including the "mobile wad" and can

be accomplished via several approaches including two-incision techniques or a single incision in a gentle S-shaped curve along the volar aspect of the forearm.[27,28] If tissue swelling extends into the hand, a hand specialist will be required for additional carpal tunnel release and/or hand compartment fasciotomies.

ⓜ Intraoperative thrombolysis

It is not uncommon to visualize thrombus in the distal tibial, pedal, or forearm arteries after thrombectomy or embolectomy. Repeated attempts at removal may be unsuccessful and can injure these vessels. In this setting, administering 2 to 4 mg of tPA into the distal artery may allow for thrombus resolution after the inflow has been restored. Following embolectomy, an objective assessment of procedural success should be performed. This includes evaluation for restoration of a palpable pedal pulse, audible Doppler signals, and signs of improved perfusion such as increased temperature and normal capillary refill.[1] The use of imaging modalities such as intraoperative DUS or, more commonly, intraoperative completion DSA will provide definitive evidence of the efficacy of the revascularization procedure. If a marginal but partially successful result is obtained, close observation with anticoagulation is needed. Vasospasm identified on arteriography can be with vasodilators such as nitroglycerin or papaverine.[1] If revascularization is inadequate, distal bypass may be required, if adequate distal target arteries exist (see Chapter 47).

ⓝ Adequate revascularization

Adequate revascularization, determined by objective assessment, includes restoration of a palpable pedal pulse, audible and improved Doppler signals, and evidence of improved tissue perfusion such as increased temperature and normal capillary refill.1 Intraoperative DUS or completion angiography can provide definitive evidence of the adequacy of the revascularization procedure. If embolectomy/thrombolysis does not provide adequate revascularization, the potential for distal bypass should be evaluated.

ⓞ Postoperative management and surveillance

The immediate postoperative management of patients with ALI includes continued anticoagulation with frequent neurovascular examination of the extremity. Patients who do not undergo prophylactic fasciotomy should be monitored for development of compartment syndrome. Among the common medical complications of interventions for ALI are MI, CHF exacerbation, pulmonary complications, and acute kidney injury.[2] The ischemia-reperfusion syndrome is associated with rhabdomyolysis, intracellular potassium leak, and hydrogen ion release. These factors, in addition to risks inherent to the revascularization procedure, contribute to possible metabolic acidosis, hyperkalemia, and acute kidney injury in the perioperative period.[3]

Patients with ALI due to thrombotic arterial occlusion may have an inherited or acquired hypercoagulable syndrome.[29] Long-term anticoagulation is associated with reduced risk of amputation and recurrence of ALI,[30] although the need for chronic anticoagulation and choice of anticoagulant will be etiology- and patient dependent.

In patients with embolic ALI, the embolic source should be sought via ECG; echocardiography (ideally transesophageal); CTA of the chest, abdomen, and pelvis; and lower extremity venous DUS in patients identified on echocardiography to have a patent foramen ovale. These studies may identify atrial fibrillation, cardiac thrombus, popliteal and/or aortic aneurysm, mobile aortic atheroma/thrombus, or paradoxical emboli, all of which may be sources of peripheral embolism.[4]

It has also been reported that patients with ALI are less likely to be optimally medically managed compared to patients with chronic ischemia; specifically, the use of aspirin and statin therapy is significantly lower in this cohort.[2] These therapies should be implemented in addition to standard risk-reduction therapies for atherosclerosis such as smoking cessation, antihypertensive therapy, and diabetes control.[4,31]

All adjunctive vascular interventions performed during revascularization including bypass or stenting have particular modes of failure and should be monitored accordingly. The SVS[32] has published recommendations to guide the frequency and type of monitoring after lower extremity intervention; this generally involves at minimum an ABI and DUS within the first month of intervention, at 3 and/or 6 months, 12 months, and annually thereafter following intervention depending on the procedure and location.

REFERENCES

1. Creager MA, Kaufman JA, Conte MS. Clinical practice. Acute limb ischemia. *N Engl J Med.* 2012;366(23):2198-2206.
2. Baril DT, Patel VI, Judelson DR, et al.; Vascular Study Group of New England. Outcomes of lower extremity bypass performed for acute limb ischemia. *J Vasc Surg.* 2013;58(4):949-956.
3. Fukuda I, Chiyoya M, Taniguchi S, Fukuda W. Acute limb ischemia: contemporary approach. *Gen Thorac Cardiovasc Surg.* 2015;63(10):540-548.
4. Vemulapalli S, Patel MR, Jones WS. Limb ischemia: cardiovascular diagnosis and management from head to toe. *Curr Cardiol Rep.* 2015;17(7):611.
5. Sontheimer DL. Peripheral vascular disease: diagnosis and treatment. *Am Fam Physician.* 2006;73(11):1971-1976.
6. Blaisdell FW, Steele M, Allen RE. Management of acute lower extremity arterial ischaemia due to embolism and thrombosis. *Surgery.* 1978;84:822-834.
7. Rutherford RB, Baker JD, Ernst C, et al. Recommended standards for reports dealing with lower extremity ischemia: revised version. *J Vasc Surg.* 1997;26(3):517-538.
8. Campbell WB, Verfaillie P, Ridler BM, Thompson JF. Non-operative treatment of advanced limb ischaemia: the decision for palliative care. *Eur J Vasc Endovasc Surg.* 2000;19(3):246-249.
9. Ljüngman C, Holmberg L, Bergqvist D, Bergström R, Adami HO. Amputation risk and survival after embolectomy for acute arterial ischaemia. Time trends in a defined Swedish population. *Eur J Vasc Endovasc Surg.* 1996;11(2):176-182.
10. Genovese EA, Chaer RA, Taha AG, et al. Risk factors for long-term mortality and amputation after open and endovascular treatment of acute limb ischemia. *Ann Vasc Surg.* 2016;30:82-92.
11. Kim KH, Choi JB, Kuh JH. Simultaneous relief of acute visceral and limb ischemia in complicated type B aortic dissection by axillobifemoral bypass. *J Thorac Cardiovasc Surg.* 2014;147(1):524-525.
12. Kovacević M, Boroe M, Medved I, Kovacić S, Primc D, Sokolić J. Successful treatment of acute aortic dissection type stanford a presenting as limb ischemia, successfully treated with operative and endovascular procedures. *Coll Antropol.* 2015;39(4):953-956.
13. Lukasiewicz A. Treatment of acute lower limb ischemia. *Vasa.* 2016;45(3):213-221.
14. Ouriel K, Shortell CK, DeWeese JA, et al. A comparison of thrombolytic therapy with operative revascularization in the initial treatment of acute peripheral arterial ischemia. *J Vasc Surg.* 1994;19(6):1021-1030.
15. Results of a prospective randomized trial evaluating surgery versus thrombolysis for ischemia of the lower extremity. The STILE Trial. *Ann Surg.* 1994;220:251-266.
16. Wicky S, Guedes Pinto E, Oklu R. Catheter-directed thrombolysis of arterial thrombosis. *Semin Thromb Hemost.* 2013;39:441-445.
17. Ouriel K, Veith FJ, Sasahara AA. A comparison of recombinant urokinase with vascular surgery as initial treatment for acute arterial occlusion of the legs. Thrombolysis or Peripheral Arterial Surgery (TOPAS) Investigators. *N Engl J Med.* 1998;338:1105-1111.
18. Byrne RM, Taha AG, Avgerinos ED, Marone LK, Makaroun MS, Chaer RA. Contemporary outcomes of endovascular interventions for acute limb ischemia. *J Vasc Surg.* 2014;59(4):988-995.
19. Silva JA, Ramee SR, Collins TJ, et al. Rheolytic thrombectomy in the treatment of acute limb-threatening ischemia: immediate results and six-month follow-up of the multicenter AngioJet registry. Possis Peripheral AngioJet Study AngioJet Investigators. *Cathet Cardiovasc Diagn.* 1998;45(4):386-393.
20. Kasirajan K, Gray B, Beavers FP, et al. Rheolytic thrombectomy in the management of acute and subacute limb-threatening ischemia. *J Vasc Interv Radiol.* 2001;12(4):413-421.
21. Taha AG, Byrne RM, Avgerinos ED, Marone LK, Makaroun MS, Chaer RA. Comparative effectiveness of endovascular versus surgical revascularization for acute lower extremity ischemia. *J Vasc Surg.* 2015;61(1):147-154.
22. Kempe K, Starr B, Stafford JM, et al. Results of surgical management of acute thromboembolic lower extremity ischemia. *J Vasc Surg.* 2014;60(3):702-707.
23. de Donato G, Setacci F, Sirignano P, Galzerano G, Massaroni R, Setacci C. The combination of surgical embolectomy and endovascular techniques may improve outcomes of patients with acute lower limb ischemia. *J Vasc Surg.* 2014;59(3):729-736.
24. Marqués de Marino P, Martínez López I, Revuelta Suero S, et al. Results of infrainguinal bypass in acute limb ischaemia. *Eur J Vasc Endovasc Surg.* 2016;51(6):824-830.
25. Murbarak SJ, Owen CA. Double-incision fasciotomy of the leg for decompression in compartment syndromes. *J Bone Joint Surg.* 1977;59:184-187.
26. Papalambros EL, Panayiotopoulos YP, Bastounis E, Zavos G, Balas P. Prophylactic fasciotomy of the legs following acute arterial occlusion procedures. *Int Angiol.* 1989;8(3): 120-124.
27. Ojike NI, Alla SR, Battista CT, Roberts CS. A single volar incision fasciotomy will decompress all three forearm compartments: a cadaver study. *Injury.* 2012;43(11): 1949-1952.
28. Benamran L, Masquelet AC. A cadaver study into the number of fasciotomies required to decompress the anterior compartment in forearm compartment syndrome. *Surg Radiol Anat.* 2018;40(3):281-287.
29. Deitcher SR, Carman TL, Sheikh MA, Gomes M. Hypercoagulable syndromes: evaluation and management strategies for acute limb ischemia. *Semin Vasc Surg.* 2001;14(2): 74-85.
30. Campbell WB, Ridler BM, Szymanska TH. Two year follow-up after acute thromboembolic limb ischaemia: the importance of anticoagulation. *Eur J Vasc Endovasc Surg.* 2000;19:169-173.
31. Gossage JA, Ali T, Chambers J, Burnand KG. Peripheral arterial embolism: prevalence, outcome, and the role of echocardiography in management. *Vasc Endovascular Surg.* 2006;40(4):280-286.
32. Zierler RE, Jordan WD, Lal BK, et al. The Society for Vascular Surgery practice guidelines on follow-up after vascular surgery arterial procedures. *J Vasc Surg.* 2018;68(1): 256-284.

Sean P. Roddy

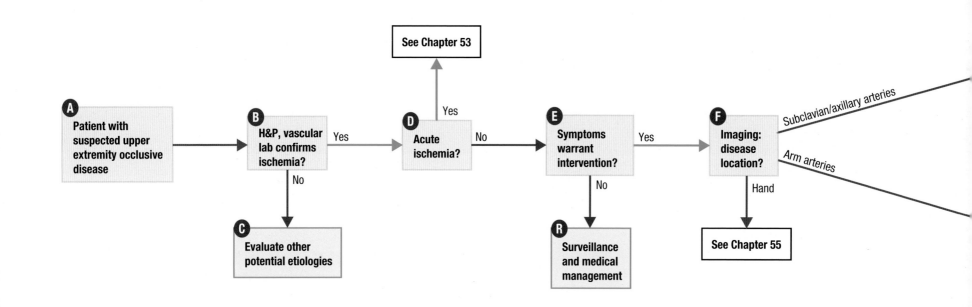

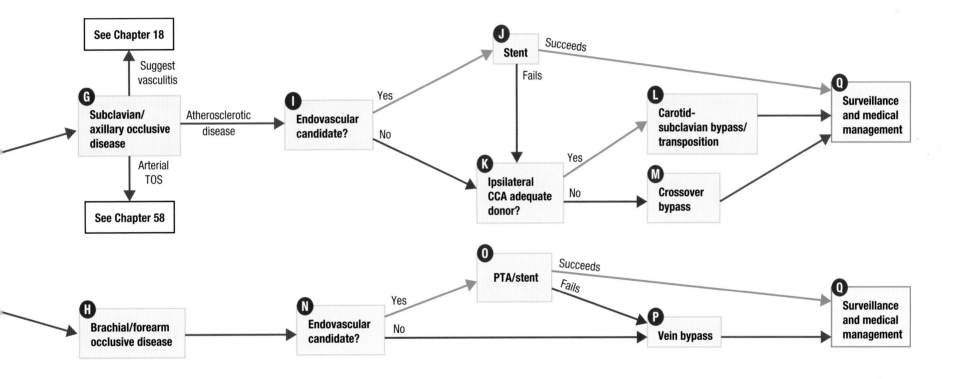

A Patient with suspected upper extremity occlusive disease

Occlusive arterial disease of the upper extremity is much less frequent than is lower extremity disease, representing <5% of patients with limb ischemia.[1] Unlike lower extremity occlusive disease, which is mainly caused by atherosclerosis, upper extremity occlusive disease can be caused by atherosclerosis and disparate disease processes such as autoimmune disorders, vasculitides, ESRD, trauma, Raynaud phenomenon, and aneurysms (upper extremity aneurysms are discussed separately in Chapter 31).

B H&P, vascular lab confirms ischemia?

H&P is important to establish the severity of ischemia and determine its underlying etiology. Patient age, onset, duration or concurrence of symptoms, presence of constitutional symptoms, extent of physical activity, work history, family history, and comorbidities can provide insight into the cause of ischemia. Medical history should include vascular risk factors (smoking, HTN, diabetes mellitus, hyperlipidemia, CKD), CAD or prior MI, CHF, arrhythmia, stroke, carotid or chronic lower extremity PAD, prior vascular interventions, and active list of medications. On PE, signs of ischemia should be evaluated, including skin changes, tissue loss, diminished or absent pulses, and poor capillary refill. Diminished or asymmetric pulses can suggest an inflow problem, whereas augmented pulses may imply presence of an aneurysm.

Noninvasive vascular laboratory studies including brachial, forearm, and finger pressure measurements, Doppler waveform or PVR analysis, and DUS imaging are used to confirm the diagnosis and severity of upper extremity occlusive disease.

C Evaluate other potential etiologies

If ischemia is not found, other etiologies for the presenting symptoms should be evaluated. Several disease processes can cause upper extremity symptoms and may initially be mistaken for upper extremity occlusive disease, including stroke, cervical radiculopathy, and neurogenic TOS. Patients with neurogenic TOS may complain of arm/hand pain, paresthesias, and finger discoloration (see Chapter 56).

D Acute ischemia?

Patients may present with acute or chronic ischemia. Acute symptoms usually occur abruptly and are more intense in nature. By convention, symptoms occurring within 14 days are deemed acute, whereas those older than 14 days are defined as chronic. Patients with acute ischemia present with some or all of the "6 P's," that is, pain, pallor, poikilothermia (coolness of the limb), pulselessness, paresthesia, and paresis/paralysis. Acute ischemia with symptoms of motor loss, numbness, or pain requires urgent

intervention because if untreated, patients ultimately experience poor functional outcomes.[2] Treatment of ALI is discussed in Chapter 53. Because of the extensive collateral system found in the upper extremity, acute ischemia tends to be not as severe as is lower limb ischemia, so that limb loss is a relatively rare event. However, if ischemia is left uncorrected, patients can experience long-term disability.

E Symptoms warrant intervention?

Symptoms of chronic upper extremity ischemia that warrant intervention include exertion-induced pain (similar to claudication in the lower extremities), rest pain, numbness, and ulcerations or gangrene of the digits. Some patients may have less severe ischemia that merits surveillance and medical management of the underlying problem rather than intervention.

F Imaging: disease location?

If a patient has chronic upper extremity ischemia that warrants intervention, arterial imaging studies are performed to delineate the location and extent of the underlying disease process, and to confirm its etiology. Imaging is guided by H&P and vascular laboratory findings, and often begins with DUS. In most cases where proximal arm arteries are diseased, CTA rather than DSA can be utilized to evaluate disease location, because it is less invasive and provides sufficient anatomic detail to plan treatment. However, for forearm and hand pathology, diagnostic DSA is usually indicated to provide sufficient anatomic detail to plan treatment. Subsequent management depends on the location and etiology of the occlusive lesions. Subclavian, axillary, and arm lesions are discussed in this chapter, whereas distal disease is discussed in Chapter 55.

G Subclavian/axillary occlusive disease

Atherosclerosis is the most common cause of subclavian/axillary occlusive disease, which can present with arm/hand ischemia or neurologic symptoms due to subclavian-vertebral steal. The left SCA is more frequently involved than is the right, whereas the axillary artery is less often the culprit. Because there is considerable collateral circulation to the arm, pain with exertion may be mild, even with subclavian occlusion. More severe hand or finger ischemia can result from subclavian/axillary atheroemboli, but this is uncommon.

With proximal subclavian stenosis or occlusion, collateral circulation to the arm is recruited in part from the vertebral artery, causing vertebral flow reversal on the affected side. If the contralateral vertebral artery is normal, or if there are good anterior to posterior brain collaterals via posterior communicating arteries, this vertebral flow reversal may cause no symptoms. As such, asymptomatic subclavian stenosis with associated reversed vertebral artery flow is not an indication for treatment. However, if collateral circulation to the posterior fossa is not

adequate, subclavian steal can cause posterior neurologic symptoms including light headedness, drop attacks, and imbalance (see Chapter 6). In some cases, these symptoms may be provoked by upper extremity exercise, but this is often not the case. Rarely, subclavian occlusive disease can cause vertebral atheroemboli that can cause TIAs or stroke. Severe subclavian occlusive disease may also result in posterior fossa low-flow symptom TIAs or, less commonly, stroke. Subclavian occlusive disease that results in neurologic deficits is usually an indication for interventional or surgical treatment.

Less common causes of subclavian/axillary occlusive disease include Takayasu disease and giant cell arteritis. Takayasu disease tends to affect a younger population and is characterized by an acute inflammatory phase, followed by a sclerotic phase that leads to fibrosis. It is often bilateral and leads to diffuse arterial stenosis and occlusions. Giant cell arteritis affects the older population and usually involves axillary rather than subclavian arteries. Acute inflammatory phase, if present, is treated medically before surgical intervention is considered (see Chapter 18).

Another potential cause of more distal subclavian/proximal axillary occlusive disease is arterial TOS, which can cause stenosis that sometimes results in formation of a poststenotic aneurysm that can either thrombose or embolize (see Chapter 58).

H Brachial/forearm occlusive disease

The most common cause of brachial artery occlusion is a cardiac origin embolus, which causes acute ischemia (see Chapter 53). Atherosclerosis uncommonly affects the brachial artery. Distal axillary, proximal brachial stenosis due to repetitive trauma caused by crutch use has been reported.

Forearm artery occlusive disease is most often seen in patients with ESRD or advanced diabetes that can result in diffuse and often severely calcific atherosclerosis of the radial and ulnar arteries. Although such disease does not often lead to severe ischemia, it can be very difficult to treat if this occurs, because of its diffuse nature and limited outflow targets for bypass. Another cause of upper extremity ischemia in patients with AV access is steal syndrome (see Chapter 69).

Less common causes of forearm arterial disease include Buerger disease, which presents as distal extremity ischemia in a smoker >50 years. Such patients can present with hand pain, cyanosis, rubor, Raynaud phenomenon, and tissue loss (see Chapter 50).

I Endovascular candidate?

Endovascular treatment of occlusive disease in the lower extremities has become first-line therapy in many cases and has proved to be an alternative to open surgery. The same is not true for upper extremity occlusive disease, except for management of first-order aortic arch branch vessels for certain pathologies. SCA occlusive disease is now frequently treated with stenting. In general, subclavian stenoses or short occlusions are more amenable to stenting than are long occlusions. In addition, lesions in close proximity to a patent vertebral artery make endovascular treatment less optimal because of the potential risk for vertebral-artery-related stroke. The ability to cross an occluded or complex lesion during arteriography can determine whether the patient is a potential endovascular candidate.

ⓙ Stent

The use of stents in arch vessels has become a primary treatment modality. Stent patency rates range between 77% and 100% at 2 years, making endovascular treatment a feasible approach.[3,4] Balloon-expandable stents are commonly used for ostial lesions because of placement precision. Stent grafts have been used with excellent success and may also be considered.

The method of vascular access, via the groin or arm, is determined by patient anatomy. Care must be taken in patients with small brachial arteries, however, given the increased risk of thrombosis. If a brachial approach is considered in a patient with a small artery, cutdown for arterial access may be needed.

From a groin approach, the left SCA is usually the easiest to access. Once access is achieved, a long 6F sheath can be advanced over a wire and positioned at the origin of the vessel. The lesion is crossed using a crossing wire/catheter combination. After predilatation is performed, a stent can be advanced across the lesion. The stent should not extend beyond the origin of the vertebral artery.

Patients with difficult aortic arches (eg, type 3), or those with subclavian arterial occlusions (particularly flush occlusions), are best approached using retrograde access from the brachial artery. Once access is obtained, a long 5F or 6F sheath is placed, and a crossing wire in conjunction with a catheter is used to cross the lesion. Care must be taken to ensure that reentry into the aorta occurs, to avoid dissection of the aortic arch. A stent is advanced over the wire and, for ostial lesions, should be deployed 1 to 2 mm into the aorta.

ⓚ Ipsilateral CCA adequate donor?

For patients with SCA occlusive disease who are not endovascular candidates, open surgery remains the standard for revascularization. Although direct bypass from the aortic arch through a median sternotomy is possible, it is associated with significant morbidity and mortality. Therefore, extra-anatomic reconstruction is more commonly used for subclavian occlusive disease unless multiple arch vessels are also diseased (see Chapter 13). The preferred inflow artery for subclavian revascularization is the ipsilateral CCA. Evaluation of its adequacy as a donor vessel can include DUS, CTA, and/or angiography if warranted. If the ipsilateral CCA has a stenosis approaching 50% or has a resting pressure gradient, it is likely that adding additional outflow through a revascularized SCA would aggregate the existing pressure gradient and therefore

not provide adequate inflow. In this circumstance, the contralateral CCA or the subclavian, if normal, can be used as donor vessels in a crossover extra-anatomic bypass. If all arch vessels have significant stenoses, interventional or hybrid treatment of the least diseased vessel can be considered to create an adequate donor artery (see Chapter 13).

ⓛ Carotid-subclavian bypass/transposition

When a patient is not an endovascular candidate, or has failed endovascular intervention, a carotid-subclavian bypass or subclavian to carotid transposition can be performed. The decision to perform either a bypass or a transposition is influenced by various factors. Subclavian to carotid transposition has the advantage of obviating a prosthetic conduit. However, this approach requires more operative dissection that includes the vertebral artery. Significant occlusive disease at the origin of the vertebral artery or presence of a patent mammary-coronary artery bypass should preclude a subclavian to carotid transposition. Both procedures have comparable patency rates: 5-year patency of 88% to 96%[5-7] and 100% for carotid-subclavian bypass and subclavian to carotid transposition, respectively.[8]

For subclavian to carotid transposition, a transverse supraclavicular incision is made between the two heads of the sternocleidomastoid muscle. The CCA is dissected and retracted medially, while the internal jugular vein and vagus nerve are retracted laterally. The vertebral vein is identified and divided, and the proximal SCA is exposed and dissected, along with the proximal vertebral artery and internal mammary arteries. Once heparin is administered and the arteries are clamped, the proximal SCA is transected and the stump oversewn. An end-to-side anastomosis is then performed to the CCA.

A carotid-subclavian bypass does not require as extensive a dissection and therefore is performed more frequently. A transverse supraclavicular incision is made, although this incision is more lateral than that needed for a transposition. The SCA is exposed after dividing the insertion of the anterior scalene muscle onto the first rib. The CCA is also dissected and a tunnel space for the graft is created behind the internal jugular vein. An 8-mm ePTFE or polyester graft is used as a conduit. Once systemic heparin is administered, the proximal and distal anastomoses are performed in an end-side manner. Generally, the more challenging distal anastomosis is performed first.

ⓜ Crossover bypass

If the ipsilateral CCA is not an adequate inflow vessel because of proximal stenosis/occlusion, a crossover bypass can be considered. If the contralateral CCA is normal, a bypass crossing the midline posterior to the sternocleidomastoid muscles to the ipsilateral SCA can be created. Alternatively, if the ipsilateral CCA is diseased, and also requires revascularization, a crossover CCA

to CCA bypass (anterior or retroesophageal) with extension to the SCA can be performed. If the contralateral CCA is not an adequate donor, but the contralateral subclavian is adequate, either a crossover subclavian-subclavian or axillary-axillary bypass is a viable alternative (see Chapter 13 for more details on treating multiarch vessel disease).

ⓝ Endovascular candidate?

Endovascular therapy is not used often in the treatment of forearm occlusive disease because of the diffuse nature of such atherosclerotic disease in most patients. The most common endovascular treatment of forearm disease is for revascularization in patients with ESRD. Revascularization for this patient population is usually palliative, for pain control, rather than for limb salvage per se, because the mortality of ESRD patients with hand tissue loss is very high at 1 year. Endovascular options are considered in those patients who are either at high surgical risk, lack conduit, or have no outflow targets for distal bypass.

ⓞ PTA/stent

Experience with PTA to treat lesions of the distal arm and hand is anecdotal, so outcomes are not well defined. When performed, small diameter balloons are used; stents are generally reserved for lesions unresponsive to PTA or for dissection following angioplasty.

ⓟ Vein bypass

Vein bypass in the arm for occlusive disease remains the standard for revascularization. Bypasses as distal as the superficial or deep palmar arch have good patency rates and functional results.[9,10] Autogenous vein is the conduit of choice and can be evaluated with preoperative DUS. As with lower extremity bypasses, the GSV is preferable, although cephalic or basilic vein can also be used. Most bypasses are tunneled subcutaneously, although bypasses originating from the axillary artery are tunneled anatomically, if possible, to reduce kinking with shoulder movement. Bypasses to the distal ulnar or the superficial palmar arch are tunneled subcutaneously, whereas bypasses to the distal radial artery are tunneled over the anatomic snuffbox to the dorsum of the hand.

ⓠ Surveillance and medical management

Patients who have undergone revascularization for upper extremity occlusive disease, whether endovascular or surgical, require surveillance of the repair. Vascular laboratory testing performed periodically to assess hemodynamic flow in the arm, and in the case of vein bypass, a graft DUS are performed to detect potential stenosis.

Because upper occlusive disease is associated with systemic disease, medical treatment is warranted in these patients. Medical treatment should be directed toward the underlying pathology.

REFERENCES

1. McCarthy WJ, Flinn WR, Yao JS, et al. Result of bypass grafting for upper limb ischemia. *J Vasc Surg.* 1986;3:741-747.
2. Galbraith K, Collin J, Morris PJ, Wood RF. Recent experience with arterial embolism of the limbs in a vascular unit. *Ann R Coll Surg Engl.* 1985;67:30-33.
3. Brountzos EN, Petersen B, Binkert C, et al. Primary stenting of subclavian and innominate artery occlusive disease: a single center's experience. *Cardiovasc Intervent Radiol.* 2004;27:616-623.
4. Przewlocki T, Kablack-Ziembicka A, Pieniazek P, et al. Determinants of immediate and long-term results of subclavian and innominate artery angioplasty. *Catheter Cardiovasc Interv.* 2006;67:519-526.
5. Vitti MJ, Thompson BW, Read RC, et al. Carotid-subclavian bypass: a twenty-two-year experience. *J Vasc Surg.* 1994;20:411-417.
6. Law MM, Colburn MD, Moore WS, et al. Carotid-subclavian bypass for brachiocephalic occlusive disease choice of conduit and long-term follow-up. *Stroke.* 1995;26:1565-1571.
7. AbuRahma AF, Robinson PA, Jennings TG. Carotid-subclavian bypass grafting with polytetrafluoroethylene grafts for symptomatic subclavian artery stenosis or occlusion: a 20-year experience. *J Vasc Surg.* 2000;32:411-419.
8. Schardy HM, Meyer G, Rau HG, et al. Subclavian carotid transposition: an analysis of a clinical series and a review of the literature. *Eur J Vasc Endovasc Surg.* 1996;12:431-436.
9. Chang BB, Roddy SP, Darling RC 3rd, et al. Upper extremity bypass grafting for limb salvage in end-stage renal failure. *J Vasc Surg.* 2003;38:1313-1315.
10. Roddy SP, Darling RC 3rd, Chang BB, et al. Brachial artery reconstruction for occlusive disease: a 12-year experience. *J Vasc Surg.* 2001;33:802-805.

Amani D. Politano • Erica L. Mitchell

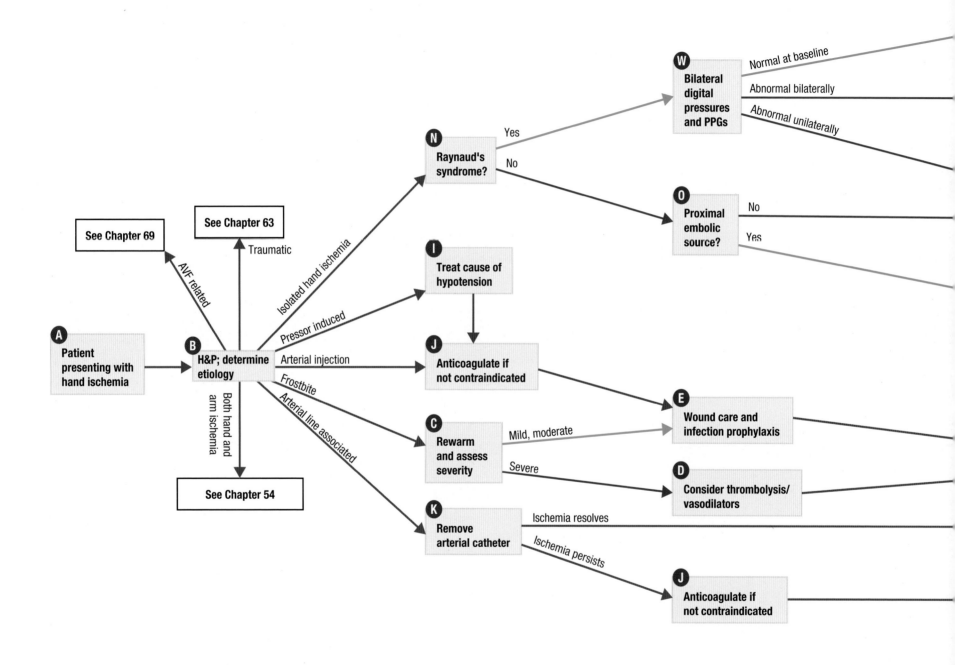

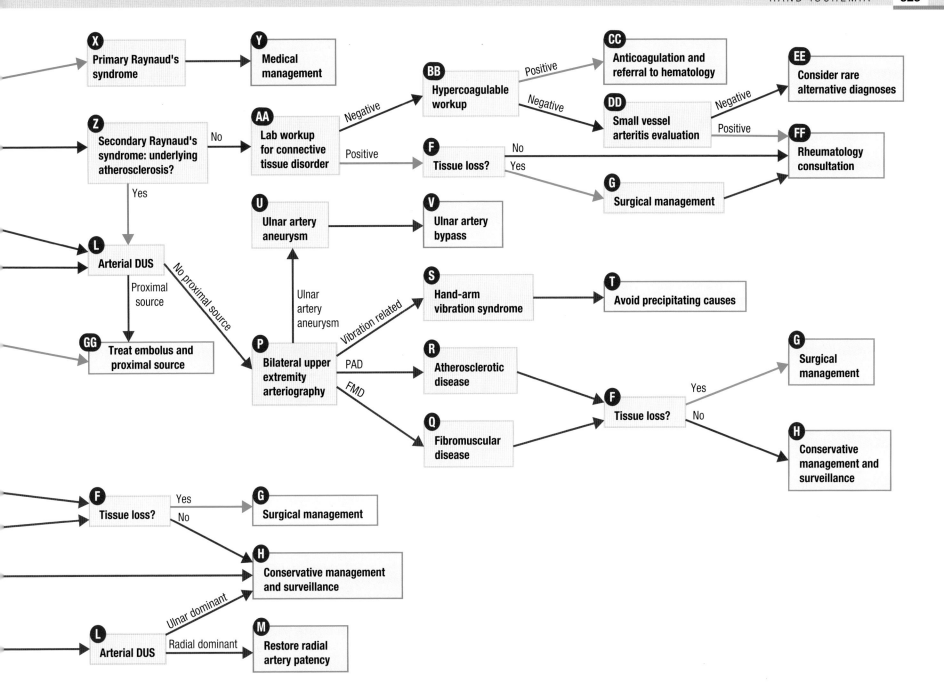

A Patient presenting with hand ischemia

Hand ischemia results when arterial perfusion to the hand is compromised by arterial vasospasm, constriction, obstruction, or trauma. Decreased or absent perfusion to the hand occurs as a result of five main pathophysiologic mechanisms including embolism, thrombosis, occlusive disease, vasospasm, and low-flow states.[1] Regardless of the cause, ischemia of the hand is manifested by color and temperature changes, pallor, numbness, cold intolerance, digital ulcerations, and/or gangrenous changes.

Hand ischemia has many potential etiologies that can be acute or chronic. Conditions resulting in acute arterial obstruction with markedly diminished perfusion to the hand usually present with acute hand ischemia. Systemic, congenital, and genetic diseases typically result in chronic ischemic conditions to the hand.

B H&P; determine etiology

Management of hand ischemia depends on the etiology, which can usually be determined by the H&P. This chapter addresses the treatment algorithms for patients presenting with isolated hand ischemia associated with atherosclerosis, local trauma (hypothenar hammer syndrome, hand-arm vibration syndrome), iatrogenic trauma (pressor induced, arterial injection, arterial line associated), embolism, connective tissue disorders, myeloproliferative and immunologic disorders, and toxins. H&P will immediately differentiate and drive management for traumatic, frostbite, pressor-induced, arterial injection, arterial-line-associated, and AVF-related hand ischemia. Chapter 54 addresses the workup and management for patients presenting with both arm and hand ischemia.

For patients presenting with either acute or chronic hand ischemia, the history should assess for Raynaud's syndrome (RS) (see N), history of cold intolerance, and frequency of ischemic pain. It is important to elicit a smoking history; occupation involving repetitive injury or vibration trauma; and systemic diseases including cardiac disease, diabetes, and ESRD; and the presence of an AV fistula, drug use, sepsis, blood dyscrasias, and peripheral neurologic abnormalities. Unilateral RS symptoms are especially suspicious and are usually indicative of arterial occlusive disease on the affected side. Physical examination should assess laterality and whether the ischemia is isolated to the hand or includes both the hand and upper extremity. It should include Doppler auscultation of the radial and ulnar arteries if a pulse is not present, as well as the palmar arch.

C Rewarm and assess severity

Frostbite is defined as severe, cold-induced localized tissue injury that results from the freezing of tissue. It is most frequently seen in patients with prolonged exposure to outdoor winter conditions including mountaineers, soldiers, those who work in the cold, the homeless, and individuals stranded outdoors in the winter. The tissue destruction of frostbite results from both the immediate cold-induced cell death as well as subsequent reperfusion-related tissue injury associated with rewarming of affected tissues.

Treatment can be divided into prehospital care and definitive treatment. Prehospital care includes moving the patient into a warm environment, removing wet clothing, rewarming the tissue with warm (not hot) water, and avoiding further injury to the ischemic tissue (not rubbing frostbitten areas in an attempt to rewarm them).[2,3] Once in the hospital, definitive care consists of rapid rewarming of frostbitten tissue, determination of injury severity, wound care, and adjunctive measures to enhance tissue viability. Rewarming consists of immersing the affected area(s) in a water bath (ideally in a whirlpool to maintain a steady temperature) heated to 37°C to 39°C (98.6-102.2°F) until the tissue is red/purplish in color and the tissue soft to touch.[3] Higher warming temperatures are not recommended and may result in more tissue injury and/or localized pain.

The next step in treatment is to define the extent of tissue injury and determine the need for adjunctive treatment protocols. The extent of severe cyanosis assessed after rewarming is predictive of the potential need for amputation and determines subsequent management. Patients with minimal-moderate cyanosis isolated to the distal phalanges do well with conservative management or debridement. Those with intermediate and proximal phalangeal cyanosis will require amputation of digits, whereas those with cyanosis extending to carpal or tarsal bones are at risk for partial or complete hand amputation.[2] Because frostbite is associated with microvascular thrombosis of affected tissue, administration of IV or intra-arterial heparin, enoxaparin, or tPA is recommended for patients at high risk for life-altering amputation (multiple digits or proximal amputation).

D Consider thrombolysis/vasodilators

For patients with severe frostbite (cyanosis proximal to the interphalangeal joints) who are at high risk for life-altering amputation, evidence supports treatment with intra-arterial tPA and intra-arterial heparin (provided treatment is initiated within 24 hours of the injury), unless contraindications exist.[4,5] IV tPA and heparin or subcutaneous LMWH are suitable treatment options for patients being treated in facilities not capable of using intra-arterial therapy. Intra-arterial treatment starts with arteriography of the affected limb(s), administration of 2 to 4 mg tPA bolus to the area of concern, followed by an infusion of 0.5 to 1 mg/h of tPA via the arterial catheter and 400 to 500 units/h of heparin via the arterial sheath. Arteriography should be repeated every 8 to 12 hours, with treatment continued until perfusion is restored or maximum treatment time limit of 48 hours is met. After treatment with tPA is completed, we recommend a 14-day course of subcutaneous enoxaparin, 1 mg/kg twice daily. Administration of tPA is associated with higher digit salvage rates compared to similar cohorts not treated with tPA.[4,5]

Patients appropriate for treatment with tPA are also appropriate for treatment with intra-arterial vasodilators. The administration of papaverine followed by tPA has been associated with good outcomes.[6] Prostacyclin (eg, iloprost) therapy has also shown promise for the treatment of frostbite, even in patients with contraindications for tPA.[7] It is used, with or without tPA, for patients presenting with severe frostbite if it can be provided within 48 hours of injury. When used without tPA, administration of iloprost does not require an ICU setting or angiographic imaging to confirm therapeutic effect. Dosing infusion starts at 0.5 ng/kg/min increased every 30 minutes by 0.5 ng/kg/min to a maximum dose of 2 ng/kg/min. Dosing should be decreased for headache or hypotension. The infusion is given for 6 hours/d and continued for 5 days at the maximum tolerable dose.[7]

E Wound care and infection prophylaxis

Injured tissue should be treated with appropriate wound care and close surveillance. Wound care includes protection of the extremities from any additional injury, keeping any open wounds clean and dry with nonadhesive dressings, and hydrotherapy to improve range of motion. Limited drainage of blisters may be required, with debridement applied to necrotic, infected tissue. Amputation should be delayed until tissue demarcation occurs. Topical aloe, analgesia, and anti-inflammatory medications (aspirin or ibuprofen) can be used to control pain and limit associated inflammation. Tetanus prophylaxis is recommended.[8] Prophylactic antibiotics are controversial, and little evidence supports its routine use.[2,7]

F Tissue loss?

The surgeon should evaluate for and treat any tissue loss as necessary. Lesions without evidence of deep infection may be amenable to conservative treatment, especially if there is a targeted treatment for the identified underlying condition. Treatment of ulceration includes antibiotics if there is concern for infection, assessment of tissue status, and serial debridement or amputation.

G Surgical management

Surgical debridement may be required for patients with severe tissue loss, compartment syndrome, infection, or persistent pain. Surgical therapy may include repeated tissue debridement, escharotomy, fasciotomy, sympathectomy, and potentially delayed amputation. Allowing marginal tissue time to demarcate may reduce the amount of tissue resection required and allow preservation of finger length and function. If tissue deeper than the subcutaneous layer requires resection, it may be wise to include a hand specialist to aid with preservation of function. Debridement of digital ulcers can be performed under general anesthesia or with a regional block. Limited debridement of the ulcer base should suffice, and the debridement should not be targeted to reach tissue that bleeds normally, because this will result in more tissue loss than is necessary. Ulcers that occur in the setting of concomitant underlying atherosclerotic disease may have prolonged healing times.

Cervical sympathectomy was used routinely in the past to alleviate pain. Although cervical sympathectomy provides some short-term improvement, studies now demonstrate recurrent symptoms within 6 to 9 months; this adjuvant therapy is no longer recommended.[9] Chemical digital or regional (wrist) sympathectomy can reverse vasoconstriction and associated Raynaud's phenomena. Digital or regional block with lidocaine or bupivacaine (without epinephrine) or botulinum toxin A can be temporarily effective in reversing digital vasospasm and associated digital pain, and is more effective than is cervical sympathectomy.[10,11]

Amputation should be reserved for patients refractory to other interventions. Distal tissue loss may autoamputate with minimal pain. If this is not the case, formal amputation may provide relief. A focus on length and functional preservation is necessary and involvement of a hand specialist is recommended.

Ⓗ Conservative management and surveillance

The principal management of hand ischemia without tissue loss is conservative therapy. In the absence of significant tissue loss or infection, which may require debridement or amputation, careful wound care and expectant management provide the best opportunity for preservation of tissue and function. Antiplatelet medications are often prescribed for patients with Raynaud's phenomenon, although there is no direct evidence for this intervention. Statins may be beneficial for their pleomorphic effects, although direct evidence for this is lacking. Patients with radial arterial-line-associated persistent ischemia with ulnar artery dominance can usually be treated conservatively. If the underlying disorder is identified and treated either medically or surgically, the tissues may recover without need for resection; however, surveillance is required to ensure that there is no development of infection or progression to gangrene.

Ⓘ Treat cause of hypotension

Excessive vasoconstriction in response to hypotension and vasopressor use can result in inadequate perfusion to the extremities, kidneys, and the viscera. Excessive vasoconstriction with insufficient end-organ perfusion (usually with systemic vascular resistance (SVR) > 1330 dynes × sec/cm[5]) commonly occurs in the setting of inadequate volume resuscitation and insufficient cardiac output.

Finger ischemia in the ICU is frequently associated with the presence of arterial lines and the use of vasopressor medications, of which phenylephrine and norepinephrine are most frequent.[12] This is usually seen bilaterally and affects both upper and lower extremities. Treating the underlying cause of hypotension so that the vasopressors can be discontinued is essential to prevent or mitigate digital ischemia. Progression to amputation is rare, whereas patients with finger ischemia in the ICU have a high rate of mortality, particularly in the presence of cancer. Finger amputations are seldom required for these patients (5%), unlike non-ICU patients hospitalized with finger ischemia who more frequently have underlying connective tissue disorders.[12]

Ⓙ Anticoagulate if not contraindicated

Patients with *vasopressor-induced digital ischemia* benefit from antiplatelet therapy or systemic anticoagulation if not otherwise contraindicated, although treating the source of hypotension remains paramount. Therapeutic anticoagulation should be administered (assuming no contraindications) if ischemic symptoms do not resolve after arterial catheter removal, or if the catheter cannot be removed due to the severity of the patient's medical condition.

Unintentional *intra-arterial injections* are rare but may have devastating consequences. Intra-arterial injection of drugs (medical or recreational) may cause acute, severe extremity ischemia, and gangrene by inducing arterial vasoconstriction, thrombosis, or direct tissue destruction and death, depending on the inciting substance. Patients most at risk include hypotensive patients, morbidly obese patients, and those with darkly pigmented skin.[13] Early symptoms include discomfort and pain on injection, which may not be evident in sedated patients or trauma patients with distracting injuries. Pallor, paresthesia, hyperemia, and cyanosis of the affected limb quickly develop, with severe cases progressing to profound edema and gangrene. Most cases of accidental intra-arterial cannulation involve radial artery branches of the forearm and hand and most often result from vascular anomalies.[13] Drugs that cause the most severe injury are barbiturates.[13]

No consensus on treatment has been established owing to the wide variety of possible injected agents, incomplete understanding of the underlying pathophysiology, and the absence of case-controlled, prospective human studies. Prompt, appropriate management will minimize subsequent injury. The affected extremity should be elevated to improve lymphatic and venous drainage. Analgesia is a priority. Therapeutic levels of anticoagulation, if not contraindicated, are recommended for hand ischemia associated with *vasopressor-induced digital ischemia*, *intra-arterial injection*, and *arterial-line-associated hand ischemia* to prevent progression of microvascular thrombosis. Other pharmacologic agents that have been used in addition to anticoagulation include thromboxane inhibitors (aspirin, methylprednisolone), which may help reverse the tissue ischemia, vasodilators (papaverine, iloprost) to facilitate vascular smooth muscle relaxation, or locally applied topical nitroglycerin patches.[13]

Ⓚ Remove arterial catheter

Significant complications of arterial catheterization are uncommon. Most complications occur at the insertion site and include local and systemic infection, bleeding, hematoma, arterial PSA, bruising, pain, swelling, compartment syndrome, nerve injury, and arterial thrombosis and/or embolization. *Arterial thrombosis* can be detected in 25% of patients who have an arterial catheter, although clinically it is only evident in <1% of such patients.[14] Risk factors for arterial catheter thrombosis include duration of catheterization >72 hours, larger catheters, smaller arteries, low-flow states, PAD, and vasospastic disorders. Thrombosis prevention includes flushing the catheter routinely with heparin or sodium citrate in the case of heparin-induced thrombocytopenia. Extremity ischemia can also result from *arterial embolization* of

thrombus associated with the arterial catheter. Symptoms depend on the presence (or absence) of collaterals and size of the embolized debris. Digital ischemia is the presentation most typical of emboli related to indwelling catheters; more proximal limb ischemia occurs when the access site itself thromboses. Treatment of both conditions starts with removal of the arterial catheter, which often leads to symptomatic improvement.

Ⓛ Arterial DUS

Upper extremity arterial DUS, PVR, and wrist and digital pressure measurement are used to rule out proximal arterial obstruction and provide valuable information to guide therapy in the setting of upper extremity ischemia. If ischemia persists following radial arterial catheter removal and anticoagulation, arterial DUS can assess patency of the radial and ulnar arteries and can establish dominance of one or the other artery. If the ulnar artery is dominant, no further treatment should be required, but if the radial artery is dominant, restoring patency may be needed. Similarly, if a patient with isolated hand ischemia does not have concurrent Raynaud's phenomenon and there is no obvious thrombotic or embolic source, upper extremity wrist-brachial indices and arterial DUS may identify a stenosis, aneurysm, or vessel occlusion suggestive of embolic phenomenon. If a proximal embolic source is identified, treatment follows the algorithm described in Chapters 32, 54, and 58. For patients with brachial artery catheters and associated hand/forearm ischemia, the catheter should be removed and anticoagulation initiated if otherwise not contraindicated. For persistent hand/forearm ischemia despite catheter removal, surgical intervention is warranted. This may require brachial arterial repair and/or distal arterial thromboembolectomy.

Ⓜ Restore radial artery patency

The radial artery gives off a volar carpal branch at the wrist that joins the ulnar artery and then courses over the dorsum of the first web space forming the deep palmar arch. The radial artery contributes the principal circulation of the thumb and index finger as well as the skin over the thenar region. Radial artery thrombosis, in the absence of a complete superficial palmar arch, will cause ischemia to the first two digits and the thenar region and can result in loss of the thumb and index finger. In 80% of patients, the superficial arch is complete with the predominant blood supply from the ulnar artery. The remaining 20% of patients have variant anatomy that could potentially put them at risk for volar hand ischemia with *radial artery thrombosis*.[15]

An essential but occluded radial artery in the setting of persistent ischemia after removal of a radial artery catheter warrants revascularization. Arterial thrombosis can be confirmed on DUS. Arteriography to evaluate extent of the injury and arterial perfusion to and within the hand can be helpful. Operative intervention may be required to remove thrombus from an occluded radial artery, repair a lacerated radial artery, or perform a reversed vein bypass to the very distal radial artery.[15]

N Raynaud's syndrome?

RS, first described by the French physician Maurice Raynaud's in 1862, describes the characteristic tricolor change featuring pallor (ischemic phase), cyanosis (deoxygenation phase), and erythema (reperfusion phase) induced by cold or stress.[16] Patients who present with isolated hand or digital ischemia and who do not have one of the conditions identified should be evaluated for RS: the symptom complex of digital color change (white to blue to red) with numbness or cold sensation in response to cold exposure or emotional stimuli.[17] Although it can affect the lower extremities or even other tissues, it is most common in the upper extremities. RS presents clinically either as primary RS, formerly referred to as Raynaud's disease, where this condition is isolated, or as secondary RS, formerly known as Raynaud's phenomenon, where it is associated with other illnesses, usually connective tissue disorders.[16] The estimated prevalence of RS in the general population is 3% to 5%, and it is more common among young women, younger age groups, and family members of patients with RS.[16]

The diagnosis is mainly clinical, based on patient descriptions of skin changes. Initial evaluation of patients who present with the classic triad of color change and symptoms of RS should include detailed H&P. Patient history should document the presence or history of ulcers, digital pitting, gangrene, symptoms of connective tissue diseases, symmetry of symptoms, medications, potential occupational exposure, family history, and risk factors for atherosclerosis. Physical examination includes assessment of peripheral pulses, bruits, tissue loss, and evaluation of nailfold capillaries. Once a diagnosis of RS is made, it must be further classified as either primary or secondary RS, because the implications and treatments vary.[18]

O Proximal embolic source?

In the absence of classic RS tricolor skin changes, or in the setting of acute hand ischemia, a search for a proximal embolic source should ensue. Echocardiography (transthoracic or transesophageal) can identify atrial or ventricular thrombus, especially in patients with a history of atrial fibrillation or recent MI. A CTA or MRA of the chest and upper extremities can identify aneurysmal, ulcerative, or thrombotic disease of the arch or arm arteries.

P Bilateral upper extremity arteriography

If no other cause of hand ischemia is identified within the H&P, or noninvasive imaging studies, bilateral upper extremity arteriography should be performed. Arteriography can detect lesions not seen on previous studies, including subtle aneurysmal dilation, stenosis, or vessel compression with positional changes. It is also superior for assessing digital arteries, and can detect small vessel occlusion, aneurysms, or other abnormalities. Finally, it can help

discern between fibromuscular disease, atherosclerosis, vasculitis, Buerger disease, and vibration-induced occlusion.

Q Fibromuscular disease

Fibromuscular dysplasia (FMD) is demonstrated by the tell-tale "beads on a string" appearance on arteriography. In the upper extremity, it is most commonly seen in the brachial artery (90%), followed by the subclavian/axillary arteries (7%) and the radial/ulnar arteries (3%). FMD is often multifocal and predominantly bilateral.[19] When symptomatic, hand or digit ischemia is the most common presentation (31%), followed by arm pain with exertion (27%) and RS triad of finger discoloration (7%).[19] Treatment includes angioplasty, antiplatelet medication, and/or anticoagulation, and avoidance of stent placement. Arterial occlusion may require surgical bypass, providing there is a suitable distal target.[19]

R Atherosclerotic disease

Atherosclerotic disease is evidenced by either focal or diffuse vessel stenosis without the typical pattern of FMD on arteriography. Treatment includes revascularization using endovascular therapy or surgical bypass (see Chapter 54) and optimal medical management including smoking cessation, antiplatelet agents, statins, and control of diabetes, HTN, and renal disease.

S Hand-arm vibration syndrome

Hand-arm vibration syndrome (HAVS) aka "vibration white finger" or vibration-induced digital ischemia is related to repetitive trauma in workers who frequently use drills, jackhammers, and chainsaws. Although the exact mechanism is unknown, high-frequency vibration can cause endothelial injury and sympathetic hyperreactivity to cold.[20] Patients with occupational exposure to vibrating tools may develop digital numbness, paresthesias, classic tricolor skin changes, and hand/arm pain. First symptoms are usually neurologic and include numbness and tingling; vascular manifestations usually present later with the classic RS triad of finger discoloration.[21] Occupational exposure history is key to the diagnosis. The vascular abnormalities result from arterial spasm, stenosis, and occlusion; injury to the intima leads to thrombosis while injury to the media can result in aneurysm formation.[21] Differentiating HAVS and hypothenar hammer syndrome (HHS) is crucial because the treatment modalities widely differ and arteriography can help differentiate these syndromes. Typical radiographic findings for HAVS include distal radial and/or ulnar arterial segmental occlusion, corkscrew collaterals arising from the interosseous arteries, and an incomplete palmar arch.[20] Although symptoms may be unilateral, arteriographic changes can be seen in bilateral extremities. HHS may be amenable to surgical therapy (see U), whereas little evidence supports surgical reconstruction for HAVS.

T Avoid precipitating causes

Initial treatment of HAVS is to discontinue use of the vibrational instruments. If eliminating the offending equipment is not feasible, use of gloves to prevent cold digits or reduce vibratory impact may lessen symptoms. Medical adjuncts for advanced vasospastic disease are those described for medical management of RS, including smoking cessation, calcium channel blockers, and locally applied nitro paste.[21] Nitro paste is thought to recruit localized capillary beds and increase oxygen delivery to the affected area.[21] HAVS can lead to occupational difficulties, disability, and poor quality of life. Disability can extend beyond the workplace with the patient unable to perform normal activities of daily living such as writing, opening lids, and buttoning clothing. Prompt recognition of HAVS is important so that the exposure to vibration can be limited to prevent further damage to the hand and arm vasculature.[21]

U Ulnar artery aneurysm

Arteriography can reveal the presence of an ulnar artery aneurysm. This finding may be consistent with HHS, an uncommon cause of secondary RS occurring mainly in patients who use the hypothenar part of their hand as a hammer. Because of its anatomic configuration within the Guyon canal, the ulnar artery is vulnerable to mechanical injury. Specifically, owing to repetitive trauma, the hook of the hamate bone pressing against the superficial palmar branch of the ulnar artery leads to the development of progressive periadventitial injury and scarring, damage to the media, disruption of the internal elastic lamina, and subintimal hematoma. Arterial changes include segmental occlusion, corkscrew-appearing degeneration, and aneurysm formation, which can lead to embolization or thrombosis.[22] Bilateral arteriographic abnormalities are often seen despite unilateral symptomatic presentation, suggesting that there may be an associated and underlying FMD condition, although this relationship has not been proved.[22,23] Conservative treatment options include smoking cessation, elimination of repetitive trauma, calcium channel blockers, and antiplatelet agents. Anticoagulation is reserved for patients with tissue loss, and in severe cases, surgical intervention may be required. Thenar hammer syndrome (THS) has also been described. THS is caused by local damage to the radial artery at the wrist and presents similarly to HHS except in the thenar distribution. Treatment is similar to that for HHS, except as applied to the radial artery.[21]

V Ulnar artery bypass

If conservative treatment does not relieve ischemia, surgical treatment can be performed. Intervention for ulnar artery aneurysm can include ligation (in the setting of appropriate collateral flow), aneurysm resection with primary end-end anastomosis, or inter-position vein bypass.[22,24]

Ⓦ Bilateral digital pressures and PPGs

The differentiation between vasospastic and obstructive mechanisms of RS is made using digital pressures and PPG. As such, patients presenting with RS should undergo bilateral digital pressure measurement and PPGs to further characterize the disease pattern. Normal patients will have normal digital pressures and a homogeneous pattern of digital waveforms with normal amplitude across all fingers. Patients with primary RS will have the same findings at room temperature. However, when exposed to cold by immersion of the hand into cold water, waveforms with dampened amplitude and reduced finger pressures across all digits are likely to be appreciated. Cold challenge testing, such as ice water immersion with temperature recovery, is highly sensitive but lacks specificity.[16] Secondary RS is manifest by variation in PPG findings among fingers at room temperature. Waveforms with variably decreased amplitude and abnormal digital pressures may be noted in both hands, and in some fingers; these changes are indicative of arterial occlusion.[25] An abnormal finding limited to one extremity should prompt evaluation for a proximal or large-vessel cause.

Ⓧ Primary Raynaud's syndrome

Primary or idiopathic RS (formerly known as Raynaud's disease) usually has an age of onset between 15 and 40 years of age, is more common in women, and may occur in multiple family members.[16] Although patients with primary RS are generally healthy, comorbid conditions including HTN, cardiovascular disease, and diabetes may aggravate attacks.

Diagnostic criteria for primary RS include typical episodic and transient attacks of digital ischemia, cyanosis, and reperfusion (triad discoloration of digits) triggered by exposure to cold temperature or stress. On physical examination, the peripheral pulses are normal, and there is no evidence of digital pitting, ulcers, or gangrene. Laboratory evaluation findings including complete blood count, antinuclear antibody (ANA), rheumatoid factor (RF), and erythrocyte sediment rate are usually normal. Noninvasive vascular laboratory study (digit pressures and PPGs) findings are normal at room temperature. Nailfold capillary microscopy, a method most commonly used in clinical practice to differentiate between primary and secondary RS, returns normal findings in patients with primary RS. This study examines the nailfold capillary loops at high magnification, and is performed by dropping oil on the periungual surface and examining it with an ophthalmoscope (set at diopter 40). Enlarged or distorted capillary loops and/or dropout or loss of loops suggest an underlying autoimmune rheumatic disease.[16] Normal findings for these diagnostic criteria support a diagnosis of primary RS.[26]

Ⓨ Medical management

Conservative treatment of primary RS begins with cold avoidance and appropriate climate preparation (eg, gloves, socks, hats). Smoking cessation is critical.[27] Calcium channel blockers (nifedipine 10-40 mg twice daily or amlodipine 5-10 mg once daily) are considered first-line therapy as long as side effects (headache, flushing, hypotension) are tolerable.[16,27] Gradual titration may mitigate these effects. Alternative medications in the setting of intolerance or persistent symptoms include angiotensin II receptor blockers (losartan 12.5-100 mg once daily) or angiotensin-converting enzyme inhibitors (captopril 12.5-25 mg twice to three times a day or enalapril 20 mg daily), α-blockers (prazosin 0.5-2 mg twice daily), or selective serotonin reuptake inhibitors (fluoxetine 20-40 mg once daily).[16,27] Phosphodiesterase inhibitors (sildenafil 25-50 mg three times daily or tadalafil 10-20 mg every other day or daily) have also been used with benefit.[27-29] Local application of topical nitrates has been proposed but has frequent systemic side effects and is not available in a commercially available preparation for RS.[30] Combined medications may have synergistic effects but should be monitored for side effects. IV prostanoid therapy can be used for very severe cases, usually when CLTI is present.[29]

Careful follow-up is necessary for all patients diagnosed with primary RS to ensure that secondary causes of RS do not emerge. Transition to defined secondary autoimmune rheumatic disease usually occurs within 2 to 3 years of presentation with RS phenomenon. Among those initially diagnosed with primary RS, the presence of abnormalities on nailfold capillary microscopy or presence of autoantibodies may predict the development of secondary RS.[16]

Ⓩ Secondary Raynaud's syndrome: underlying atherosclerosis?

Secondary RS (formerly known as Raynaud's phenomenon) refers to those patients with RS in whom an associated disease may underlie the hand syndrome. Diseases commonly associated with secondary RS include autoimmune rheumatic diseases such as systemic lupus erythematous, systemic sclerosis (scleroderma), mixed connective tissue disease, Sjögren syndrome, Wegener granulomatous, and dermatomyositis/polymyositis. Hematologic abnormalities associated with secondary RS include cryoglobulinemia, cold agglutinin disease, cryofibrinogenemia, paraproteinemia, and POEMS (*p*olyneuropathy, *o*rganomegaly, *e*ndocrinopathy, *m*onoclonal gammopathy, and *s*kin changes). Occupational causes include HHS and HAVS, as well as carpal tunnel syndrome and frostbite. Drugs or toxins that precipitate or exacerbate RS symptoms include some chemotherapeutic agents (ie, cisplatin and bleomycin) and drugs (amphetamines).

Secondary RS requires an evaluation to identify the underlying systemic disorder. Patient history should evaluate the many causes of secondary RS including connective tissue diseases (systemic sclerosis is the most common), hand-arm vibration syndrome, extrinsic compression (cervical rib), large artery disease, certain medications, chemical or occupational exposures, or other rare associated diseases (hypothyroidism).[27]

In patients with abnormal PPGs bilaterally, and concomitant atherosclerotic or vascular risk factors (prior smoking history, diabetes, renal disease), arterial DUS should be employed to rule out primary arterial pathology. Medical management should proceed as indicated for the inciting cause, differing by disease state.[29]

ⒶⒶ Lab workup for connective tissue disorder

Serologic screening is advocated in patients with secondary RS to rule out associated connective tissue disorders. This involves multiple laboratory tests, often coordinated with a rheumatology specialist, including complete blood count, ANA test, ESR, RF and, in some settings, thyroid function tests.[31,32] Additional laboratory investigation includes anticentromere and antitopoisomerase (anti-Scl-70) antibodies.[31-33] Because RS may be the first manifestation of an underlying connective tissue disorder, full evaluation is often necessary as it substantially influences treatment.

ⒷⒷ Hypercoagulable workup

If the laboratory investigation result for systemic connective tissue disorders is negative, a hypercoagulable workup is indicated. This includes laboratory tests for antithrombin III, protein C and protein S deficiencies, factor V Leiden and prothrombin gene mutations, and antiphospholipid antibody.[34] In addition, factor VIII, IX, and XI activity, fasting homocysteine levels, CRP, ESR, lupus anticoagulant level, β-2-glycoprotein-1 IgM and IgG, cardiolipin antibodies, and lipoprotein (a) levels can be checked. Age-appropriate cancer screening should be performed in appropriate clinical settings[35] (see Chapter 5 for details).

ⒸⒸ Anticoagulation and referral to hematology

Patients with a hypercoagulable syndrome associated with secondary RS should be started on anticoagulation and be referred to a hematologist. It should be noted that many tests comprising the hypercoagulable workup are not reliable when performed in the setting of acute thrombosis or during warfarin/heparin therapy.[34] In that setting, the acute episode should be treated, and after resolution, anticoagulation can be halted to allow for more definitive testing. The implication of such testing can influence lifelong anticoagulation as well as provide information for relatives.

ⒹⒹ Small vessel arteritis evaluation

If connective tissue disease and hypercoagulable evaluation results are negative in patients with secondary RS, small vessel vasculitis such as granulomatosis with polyangiitis (Wegener granulomatosis), eosinophilic granulomatosis with polyangiitis (Churg-Strauss syndrome), or microscopic polyangiitis should be considered. Constitutional symptoms are often present with these diseases and should be assessed in the history. Antineutrophil cytoplasmic antibodies (ANCA) can be tested and are often positive in small vessel vasculitis. In addition, ESR, CRP, liver and renal function tests, ANAs, complement, cryoglobulins, hepatitis serology, rheumatoid factor, and a urinalysis (due to frequent renal involvement) should be ordered. Biopsy of the affected tissue can be useful because it allows for pathologic diagnosis of vasculitis.[36]

Although these vasculitides frequently present with constitutional symptoms and pulmonary, renal, intestinal, and cutaneous involvement, digital ischemia has also been reported.[37,38] If small vessel vasculitis is suspected, a rheumatology consultation should be requested.

EE Consider rare alternative diagnoses

If assessments for small artery vasculitis are negative, a search for rare entities should be considered. Behçet disease (venous and arterial thrombosis, aneurysms), lupus vasculitis (leukocytoclastic vasculitis, thrombosis), rheumatoid vasculitis (cutaneous vasculitis, digital infarctions), and relapsing polychondritis (cutaneous vasculitis, aneurysms) can present with extremity involvement. Radiation arteritis can present in any vascular bed that had been exposed. Pseudoxanthoma elasticum, medication-induced arteriopathy, neurofibromatosis type 1, and cryoglobulinemic vasculitis should also be considered.[39]

FF Rheumatology consultation

Positive assays for connective tissue disorders or vasculitis should prompt referral to a rheumatologist for further targeted treatment of the underlying disease. Treatment of the ANCA-associated vasculitides is with anti-inflammatory medications such as corticosteroids and immunosuppressing agents.[36] However, accurate diagnosis is critical, because the treatment for vasculitis is different from that for systemic sclerosis, and therefore a specialist should guide this level of therapy.[18]

GG Treat embolus and proximal source

Hand ischemia due to a proximal source is usually associated with a distal embolus, which requires treatment by balloon catheter embolectomy or sometimes thrombolytic therapy, as discussed in detail in Chapter 53. In addition, the proximal embolic source needs treatment to avoid recurrence. Embolization from a proximal upper extremity arterial aneurysm is discussed in detail in Chapter 32 while embolization due to arterial TOS is discussed in Chapter 58. More common cardiac origin emboli are usually large enough that they lodge in arteries proximal to the hand, but

cause hand ischemia, usually associated with arm ischemia. Atrial fibrillation is the most common associated cardiac disease, and is treated with chronic anticogulation, but other cardiac sources are possible, and are managed individually.

REFERENCES

1. Jones NF. Acute and chronic ischemia of the hand: pathophysiology, treatment, and prognosis. *J Hand Surg Am.* 1991;16(6):1074-1083.
2. Petrone P, Kuncir EJ, Asensio JA. Surgical management and strategies in the treatment of hypothermia and cold injury. *Emerg Med Clin North Am.* 2003;21(4):1165-1178.
3. McIntosh SE, Hamonko M, Freer L, et al. Wilderness Medical Society practice guidelines for the prevention and treatment of frostbite. *Wilderness Environ Med.* 2011;22(2):156-166.
4. Bruen KJ, Ballard JR, Morris SE, Cochran A, Edelman LS, Saffle JR. Reduction of the incidence of amputation in frostbite injury with thrombolytic therapy. *Arch Surg.* 2007;142(6):546-551.
5. Gonzaga T, Jenabzadeh K, Anderson CP, Mohr WJ, Endorf FW, Ahrenholz DH. Use of intra-arterial thrombolytic therapy for acute treatment of frostbite in 62 patients with review of thrombolytic therapy in frostbite. *J Burn Care Res.* 2016;37(4):e323-e334.
6. Saemi AM, Johnson JM, Morris CS. Treatment of bilateral hand frostbite using transcatheter arterial thrombolysis after papaverine infusion. *Cardiovasc Intervent Radiol.* 2009;32(6):1280-1283.
7. Handford C, Buxton P, Russell K, et al. Frostbite: a practical approach to hospital management. *Extrem Physiol Med.* 2014;3:7.
8. Chan TY, Smedley FH. Tetanus complicating frostbite. *Injury.* 1990;21(4):245.
9. Claes G, Drott C, Göthberg G. Thoracoscopic sympathicotomy for arterial insufficiency. *Eur J Surg Suppl.* 1994;(572):63-64.
10. Balogh B, Mayer W, Vesely M, Mayer S, Partsch H, Piza-Katzer H. Adventitial stripping of the radial and ulnar arteries in Raynaud's disease. *J Hand Surg Am.* 2002;27(6):1073-1080.
11. Neumeister MW. Botulinum toxin type A in the treatment of Raynaud's phenomenon. *J Hand Surg Am.* 2010;35(12):2085-2092.
12. Landry GJ, Mostul CJ, Ahn DS, et al. Causes and outcomes of finger ischemia in hospitalized patients in the intensive care unit. *J Vasc Surg.* 2018;68(5):1499-1504.
13. Lake C, Beecroft CL. Extravasation injuries and accidental intra-arterial injection. *Contin Educ Anaesth Crit Care Pain.* 2010;10(4):109-113.
14. Sen S, Chini EN, Brown MJ. Complications after unintentional intra-arterial injection of drugs: risks, outcomes, and management strategies. *Mayo Clin Proc.* 2005;80(6):783-795.
15. Wallach SH. Cannulation injury of the radial artery: diagnosis and treatment algorithm. *Am J Crit Care.* 2004;13:315-319.
16. Valdovinos T, Landry GJ. Raynaud syndrome. *Tech Vasc Interv Radiol.* 2014;17(4):241-246.
17. LeRoy EC, Medsger TA Jr. Raynaud's phenomenon: a proposal for classification. *Clin Exp Rheumatol.* 1992;10(5):485-488.
18. Herrick AL. The pathogenesis, diagnosis and treatment of Raynaud phenomenon. *Nat Rev Rheumatol.* 2012;8(8):469-479.
19. Nguyen N, Sharma A, West JK, et al. Presentation, clinical features, and results of intervention in upper extremity fibromuscular dysplasia. *J Vasc Surg.* 2017;66(2):554-563.
20. Thompson A, House R. Hand-arm vibration syndrome with concomitant arterial thrombosis in the hands. *Occup Med (Lond).* 2006;56(5):317-321.
21. Campbell RA, Janko MR, Hacker RI. Hand-arm vibration syndrome: a rarely seen diagnosis. *J Vasc Surg Cases Innov Tech.* 2017;3:60-62.
22. Ferris BL, Taylor LM Jr, Oyama K, et al. Hypothenar hammer syndrome: proposed etiology. *J Vasc Surg.* 2000;31(1, pt 1):104-113.
23. Larsen BT, Edwards WD, Jensen MH, et al. Surgical pathology of hypothenar hammer syndrome with new pathogenetic insights: a 25-year institutional experience with clinical and pathologic review of 67 cases. *Am J Surg Pathol.* 2013;37(11):1700-1708.
24. Lifchez SD, Higgins JP. Long-term results of surgical treatment for hypothenar hammer syndrome. *Plast Reconstr Surg.* 2009;124(1):210-216.
25. Rosato E, Rossi C, Borghese F, Molinaro I, Pisarri S, Salsano F. The different photoplethysmographic patterns can help to distinguish patients with primary and sclerodermic Raynaud phenomenon. *Am J Med Sci.* 2010;340(6):457-461.
26. Maverakis E, Patel F, Kronenberg DG, et al. International consensus criteria for the diagnosis of Raynaud's phenomenon. *J Autoimmun.* 2014;48-49:60-65.
27. Herrick AL. Evidence-based management of Raynaud's phenomenon. *Ther Adv Musculoskelet Dis.* 2017;9(12):317-329.
28. Roustit M, Blaise S, Allanore Y, Carpentier PH, Caglayan E, Cracowski JL. Phosphodiesterase-5 inhibitors for the treatment of secondary Raynaud's phenomenon: systematic review and meta-analysis of randomised trials. *Ann Rheum Dis.* 2013;72(10):1696-1699.
29. Kowal-Bielecka O, Fransen J, Avouac J, et al; EUSTAR Coauthors. Update of EULAR recommendations for the treatment of systemic sclerosis. *Ann Rheum Dis.* 2017;76(8):1327-1339.
30. Teh LS, Manning J, Moore T, et al. *Br J Rheumatol.* 1995;34(7):636-641.
31. Landry GJ, Edwards JM, McLafferty RB, Taylor LM Jr, Porter JM. Long-term outcome of Raynaud's syndrome

in a prospectively analyzed patient cohort. *J Vasc Surg.* 1996;23(1):76-85.

32. Koenig M, Joyal F, Fritzler MJ, et al. Autoantibodies and microvascular damage are independentpredictive factors for the progression of Raynaud's phenomenon to systemic sclerosis: a twenty-year prospective study of 586 patients, with validation of proposed criteria for early systemicsclerosis. *Arthritis Rheum.* 2008;58(12):3902-3912.

33. Wigley FM. Clinical practice. Raynaud's phenomenon. *N Engl J Med.* 2002;347(13):1001-1008.

34. Graham N, Rashiq H, Hunt BJ. Testing for thrombophilia: clinical update. *Br J Gen Pract.* 2014;64(619):e120-e122.

35. Orfanakis A, Deloughery T. Patients with disorders of thrombosis and hemostasis. *Med Clin North Am.* 2013;97(6):1161-1180.

36. Jennette JC, Falk RJ. Small-vessel vasculitis. *N Engl J Med.* 1997;337(21):1512-1523.

37. Leung A, Sung CB, Kothari G, Mack C, Fong C. Utilisation of plasma exchange in the treatment of digital infarcts in Wegener's granulomatosis. *Int J Rheum Dis.* 2010;13(4):e59-e61.

38. Jandus P, Bianda N, Alerci M, Gallino A, Marone C. Eosinophilic vasculitis: an inhabitual and resistant manifestation of a vasculitis. *Vasa.* 2010;39(4):344-348.

39. Pipitone N, Holl-Ulrich K, Gross WL, Lamprecht P. Unclassified vasculitis with acral ischemic lesions: "forme fruste" or idiopathic vasculitis? *Clin Exp Rheumatol.* 2008;26(3 suppl 49):S41-S46.

Hugh A. Gelabert

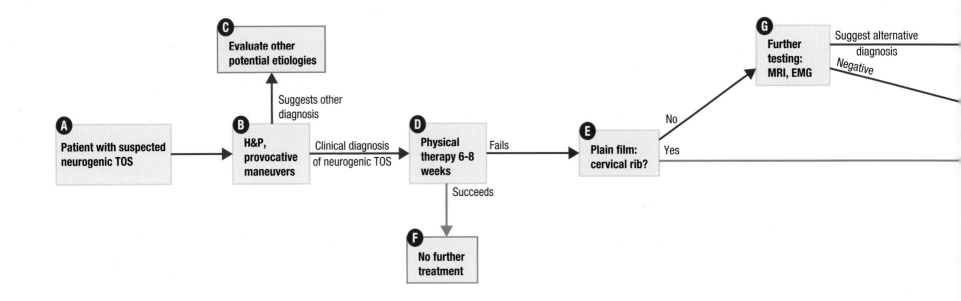

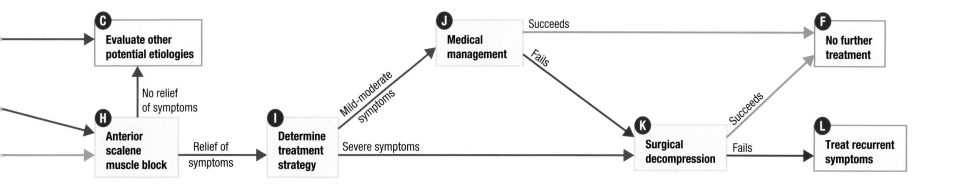

Ⓐ Patient with suspected neurogenic TOS

Neurogenic TOS (nTOS) is a condition that affects a wide variety of patients. Although ages of presentation range from preteen to septuagenarian, the most commonly affected patients are in the late 20s to mid-40s. Incidence of this disorder is uncertain and is estimated to range from 3 to 80 per 1000 patient years. Between 2000 and 2500 nTOS decompression operations are performed yearly in the United States.[1]

Ⓑ H&P, provocative maneuvers

Patient history should enquire into core presenting symptoms including pain, numbness, and tingling (PNT), which typically extend from the base of the neck to the fingers. Absent these symptoms, the diagnosis should be questioned. Presentation with symptoms limited to the neck or shoulder should also be questioned because isolated neck pain is not typical of nTOS. Additional history should be congruent with the development of nTOS, including whiplash injury, repetitive motion injury, or a distraction injury of the arm.

On physical examination, palpation and Tinel testing may result in irritability of the nerves at the thoracic outlet. Provocative maneuvers include (1) abduction with external rotation (AER), a maneuver where the arm is abducted, deep breath is held while turning the head to the side, and loss of pulse or development of bruit is assessed; (2) elevated arm stress test (EAST) performed by having the patient elevate arms and open and close hands repeatedly while reproduction of nTOS symptoms are sought; and (3) upper extremity limb tension test (UELTT) where the patient's arms are extended laterally, hands fully extended dorsally, and neck tilted to right and left while radiation of symptoms down the arm are evaluated for. These provocative maneuvers often elicit positional exacerbation of symptoms.[2,3]

Ⓒ Evaluate other potential etiologies

For patients not presenting with classic nTOS symptoms, the differential diagnosis includes a shoulder disorder, cervical spine compression, or peripheral nerve compression (carpal or cubital tunnel syndrome). These diagnoses would be suggested by a history of PNT limited to the neck and shoulder or limited to the forearm and hand. Pain which is focused on the shoulder alone is not consistent with TOS.[2,3]

Ⓓ Physical therapy 6-8 weeks

For patients with clinical diagnosis of nTOS, based on appropriate symptoms and physical examination findings, physical therapy (PT) (posture correction, stretching exercises for scalene muscles, for opening chest, and strengthening of upper back musculature) is the first step in treatment. It is anticipated that up to 85% of patients will benefit from PT. Simultaneous evaluation of causation, ergonomic assessment of work place, and resting of the limb are

important adjuncts. Unfortunately, cessation of PT can lead to recurrence of symptoms. If symptoms persist or recur after PT cessation, further evaluation is indicated. If symptoms resolve, then no further intervention is necessary.[2,3]

Ⓔ Plain film: cervical rib?

When considering treatment of nTOS after failed PT, evaluation should start with plain x-ray imaging (chest or neck films) to assess for the presence of a cervical rib. The presence of a cervical rib is a strong predictor of nTOS as the etiology of the patient's symptoms.[4] Furthermore, if present and surgical decompression is undertaken, the cervical rib must be excised.

Ⓕ No further treatment

If PT or medical management succeeds in eliminating or sufficiently reducing symptoms, patients are advised to implement lifelong PT exercises to help manage nTOS symptoms. No routine surveillance is required; rather, patients are advised to return if symptoms recur. Recurrence of symptoms may be initially managed with PT and evaluation of precipitating cause of recurrence. Persistence after an initial course of PT would warrant reassessment of other possible causes.

Ⓖ Further testing: MRI, EMG

MRI of the cervical spine, upper extremity EMG, and nerve conduction velocities (NCVs) are helpful in excluding other diagnoses that may present similarly to nTOS. Specifically, these tests can differentiate cervical spine degenerative disease as well as carpal and cubital tunnel syndromes. If these test results are positive for a diagnosis alternative to nTOS, then formal consultation with a spine or hand surgeon is warranted.[2-4]

Ⓗ Anterior scalene muscle block

Anterior scalene muscle block (ASMB) using lidocaine injection into the scalene muscle is the most specific and sensitive diagnostic test for nTOS. A positive response results in a significant (at least 50%) reduction in nTOS symptoms, with symptom relief lasting the duration of the block. When lidocaine is used for the block, the symptoms will typically recur within 4 to 6 hours.

It is important to differentiate between an ASMB and an interscalene or brachial plexus block. ASMB is diagnostic for nTOS, whereas the interscalene block is not. ASMB should allow normal use of the arm with normal sensation in the arm and hand. An interscalene block may result from inadvertent injection of lidocaine outside of the desired location and can result in paralysis, weakness, and/or anesthesia of the limb. An interscalene block is not useful for making the diagnosis of TOS.

A positive ASMB confirms the diagnosis of nTOS and indicates that scalene muscle spasm is a fundamental element in the presentation of nTOS. A positive study also suggests that

botulinus toxin (onabotulinumtoxin A, usually referred to by the brand name "Botox") may be useful for medical management of this condition. Botox produces longer term (3-4 months) relaxation of the scalene muscles than does the local anesthetic. Repeated injections may be used as an alternative to surgical decompression. A positive ASMB block is predictive that 90% to 95% of patients with nTOS will significantly improve after surgical decompression.[5-8]

Ⓘ Determine treatment strategy

Severity of symptoms will dictate the course of treatment. Mild to moderate TOS may be managed with PT, work adjustments, and NSAIDs. More severe presentations are more successfully managed with periodic Botox injections. Severe, disabling presentations are best managed with surgical decompression.

Symptom severity can be objectively assessed by reviewing the impact of the condition or the patient's ability to work and perform activities of daily living. Objective data obtained using disability scores like the Somatic Pain Score, QUICK DASH (disability of arm, shoulder, and hand), Cervicobrachial score, SF12, or SF36 can also be helpful.[6,10,11]

Ⓙ Medical management

Patients with mild to moderate symptoms may be treated with PT or Botox. Long-term ongoing PT is limited by cost and/or insurance reimbursement. Ideally, patients manage the condition through a home exercise PT program. Scalene muscle Botox injection may provide relief of nTOS symptoms for a period of 3 to 4 months. Symptom resumption tends to be gradual, so that it may be possible to manage mild to moderately severe nTOS symptoms with Botox injections alone every 6 months. The primary limitation to this treatment is financial, because insurance companies rarely will allow this form of treatment indefinitely, and ultimately the cost is shifted to the patient. It should also be noted that Botox is slightly less effective than is lidocaine, with only 80% to 85% of patients responding to Botox therapy.[8] Thus, although lidocaine injections potentially identify those who could benefit from Botox, a number of patients who try scalene muscle Botox injections do not respond to this form of treatment. This cohort of patients is then faced with the decision of living with their symptoms or electing for surgical decompression. Because of its short duration of action, lidocaine is not practical for treating TOS long term, even though it is temporally more likely to relieve nTOS symptoms than is Botox.

Ⓚ Surgical decompression

Surgical decompression is indicated for those patients with positive examination findings, positive ASMB, and moderately severe to severe nTOS symptoms. First rib (and cervical rib, if present) resection results in significant improvement in 90% to 95% of such patients. This statistic is specifically associated with transaxillary first rib resection.[6] Other surgical options include resection of the scalene muscles alone and supraclavicular resection of first rib and scalene muscles. Rib resection (transaxillary or supraclavicular) is associated with slightly better outcomes than with scalene muscle resection alone.[4,6,9-11] In most cases, the surgical approach is selected depending on the training and experience of the surgeon, and all surgical approaches have similar results. In his personal series, Sanders noted similar 5-year outcomes for both transaxillary and supraclavicular rib resections (71% vs. 69%).[12]

Ⓛ Treat recurrent symptoms

Recurrent symptoms can develop after initially successful surgical treatment, or if initial surgery is not successful. Management depends on the original operation performed. If the original operation involved scalenectomy without rib resection, then a first rib resection would be indicated. If the original operation included first rib resection, then adequacy of the rib resection should be ensured via chest x-ray. If an inadequate rib resection was initially performed (ie, insufficient rib resected), then redo/completion rib resection is indicated. If the original operation included partial scalenectomy and an adequate rib resection via a transaxillary approach, then these patients should undergo supraclavicular completion scalenectomy.[13]

REFERENCES

1. Lee JT, Dua MM, Chandra V, Hernandez-Boussard TM, Illig KA. Surgery for thoracic outlet syndrome: a nationwide perspective. *J Vasc Surg*. 2011;53(6):100s-101s.
2. Sanders RJ, Hammond SL, Rao NM. Diagnosis of thoracic outlet syndrome. *J Vasc Surg*. 2007;46(3):601-604.
3. Balderman J, Holzem K, Field BJ, et al. Associations between clinical diagnostic criteria and pretreatment patient-reported outcomes measures in a prospective observational cohort of patients with neurogenic thoracic outlet syndrome. *J Vasc Surg*. 2017;66(2):533-544.e2.
4. Gelabert HA, Rigberg DA, O'Connell JB, Jabori S, Jimenez JC, Farley S. Transaxillary decompression of thoracic outlet syndrome patients presenting with cervical ribs. *J Vasc Surg*. 2018;68(4):1143-1149.
5. Jordan SE, Ahn SS, Gelabert HA. Differentiation of thoracic outlet syndrome from treatment-resistant cervical brachial pain syndromes: development and utilization of a questionnaire, clinical examination and ultrasound evaluation. *Pain Physician*. 2007;10(3):441-452. Erratum in: *Pain Physician*. 2007;10(4):599.
6. Jordan SE, Machleder HI. Diagnosis of thoracic outlet syndrome using electrophysiologically guided anterior scalene blocks. *Ann Vasc Surg*. 1998;12(3):260-264.
7. Jordan S, Machleder HI. Electrodiagnostic evaluation of patients with painful syndromes affecting the upper extremity. In: Machleder HI, eds. *Vascular Disorders of the Upper Extremity*. 3rd ed. Armonk, NY: Futura Publishing; 1998:137-153.
8. Jordan SE, Ahn SS, Gelabert HA. Combining ultrasonography and electromyography for botulinum chemodenervation treatment of thoracic outlet syndrome: comparison with fluoroscopy and electromyography guidance. *Pain Physician*. 2007;10:541-546.
9. Sanders RJ, Monsour JW, Gerber WF, Adams WR, Thompson N. Scalenectomy versus first rib resection for treatment of the thoracic outlet syndrome. *Surgery*. 1979;85(1):109-121.
10. Sanders RJ. Outcomes after surgery for thoracic outlet syndrome. *J Vasc Surg*. 2001;33:1220-1225.
11. Sanders RJ, Pearce WH. The treatment of thoracic outlet syndrome: a comparison of different operations. *J Vasc Surg*. 1989;10:626-634.
12. Sanders RJ. *Result of Treatment and Comments in Thoracic Outlet Syndrome—A Common Sequela of Neck Injuries*. Philadelphia, PA: J.P Lippincott and Co; 1991:171-191.
13. Likes K, Dapash T, Rochlin DH, Freischlag JA. Remaining or residual first ribs are the cause of recurrent thoracic outlet syndrome. *Ann Vasc Surg*. 2014;28(4):939-945.

Rameen S. Moridzadeh • David Rigberg

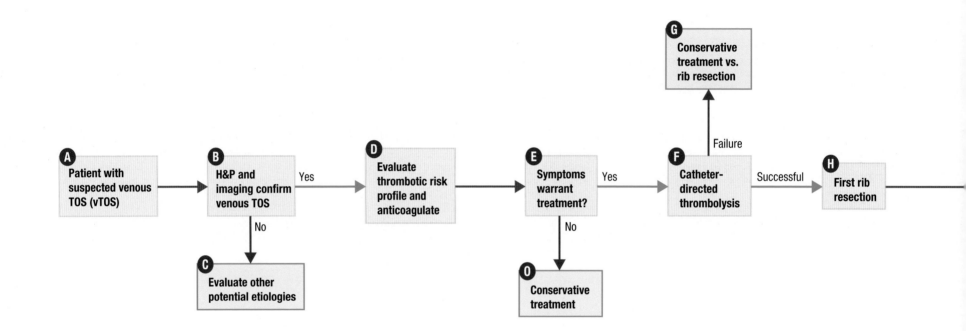

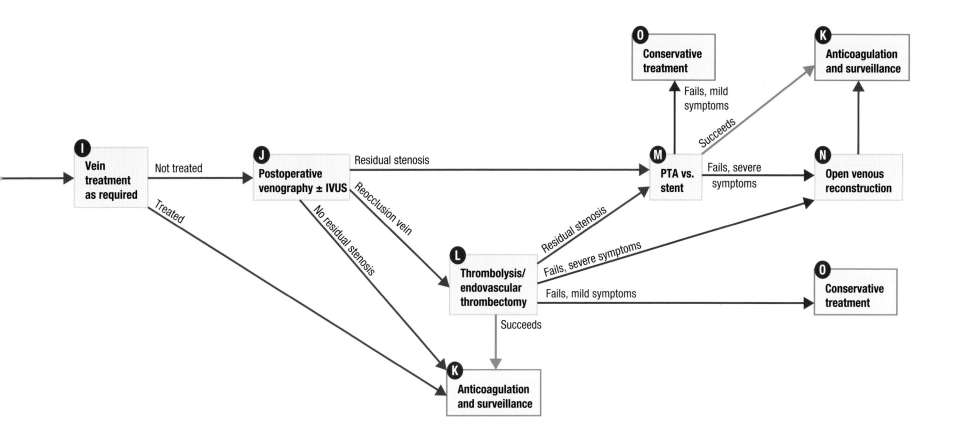

A Patient with suspected venous TOS

TOS is a general term used to describe the various disorders that arise from compression of neurologic or vascular structures that exit the thorax to enter the upper extremity. The thoracic outlet comprises the narrow aperture created by the first rib, surrounding musculature, and the clavicle. Together, these structures surround the subclavian vein, artery, and brachial plexus as they travel distally to the upper extremity. These disorders, as a whole, are rare. The three main forms are, in decreasing prevalence, neurogenic, venous (vTOS, also known as Paget Schroetter syndrome), and arterial. Although uncommon, these disorders are encountered by most vascular surgeons at some point, and it is imperative to at least be able to diagnose, if not treat, vTOS.

The symptoms of vTOS result from axillosubclavian vein thrombosis due to compression at the thoracic outlet, and, as such, typically present suddenly in an otherwise healthy person. Often symptoms occur after rigorous upper body exercise, leading to the term "effort" thrombosis. Commonly involved athletes include weight lifters, swimmers, volleyball players, and baseball players, although the disorder can also occur in nonathletes. Incidence is estimated at about 2.01/100,000 patients per year and there is roughly a 2:1 male to female ratio.[1,2]

B H&P and imaging confirm vTOS?

Patients with axillosubclavian vein thrombosis due to vTOS report a history of arm swelling, congestion, and/or discoloration/cyanosis. Symptoms are usually exacerbated during arm exercise. Clinical examination often reveals arm edema and/or dilated collateral veins of the arm or chest wall.[3] Other causes of axillosubclavian vein thrombosis in addition to vTOS should be considered, including hypercoagulable states, prior/current catheter or pacemaker use, and local trauma or surgery. These causes of axillosubclavian DVT should be entertained when there is an atypical location of thrombosis (not at the thoracic outlet). Therapy in these cases does not require decompression of the thoracic outlet.

Patients should undergo imaging to support the clinical diagnosis of vTOS. DUS is ideal to detect the presence of axillosubclavian DVT with a sensitivity and specificity ranging from 81% to 100%.[4,5] This modality is preferred because it is readily available, does not require nephrotoxic agents, and avoids radiation. Other modalities to facilitate diagnosis include CT and MR venogram and catheter-based venography. These modalities allow for confirmation of axillosubclavian DVT and underlying subclavian vein compression, if present. Images should be obtained with the arm in the neutral and stress positions (arm abducted and externally rotated). Cervical ribs commonly associated with neurogenic TOS are more posterior structures, and rarely associated with vTOS. Additional workup might include CTA of the chest to evaluate for PE if the patient has appropriate symptoms, but this occurs in <10% of patients with subclavian DVT from all causes.[6,7] As stated previously,

if vTOS is not confirmed as the cause of the axillosubclavian DVT, alternative diagnoses should be sought.

C Evaluate other potential etiologies

Other possible causes may be readily apparent (venous catheter or pacemaker-lead-associated axillosubclavian DVT). Axillosubclavian DVT is also associated with trauma, particularly orthopedic injuries and the treatment of these injuries. Patients with a history of ESRD and upper extremity catheter use or fistula/graft placement are at risk for thrombosis secondary to central venous stenosis. Finally, patients with hypercoagulable conditions can present with axillosubclavian DVT and no identifiable anatomic causes of thrombosis.

D Evaluate thrombotic risk profile and anticoagulate

Once the diagnosis of axillosubclavian DVT is confirmed, patients with a prior DVT or a family history of VTE should undergo an assessment of their thrombotic risk profile and testing for hypercoagulable disorders (see Chapter 5). These include genetic tests (most commonly for factor V Leiden and the prothrombin gene mutation), functional tests (protein C and S function, antithrombin III activity), and tests for the presence of antibodies (anticardiolipin, antiphospholipid antibodies, or heparin antibodies).

Therapeutic anticoagulation for DVT should be initiated on making the diagnosis. There are a range of options now available. Previous protocols required continuous intravenous heparin, typically while oral anticoagulation with Coumadin (warfarin) was established. Newer agents, including Lovenox (enoxaparin) injections as well as the new oral anticoagulants—Pradaxa (dabigatran), Xarelto (rivaroxaban), and Eliquis (apixaban)—allow for more flexibility in care plans. It is important to remember that some hypercoagulable studies and assays are difficult to interpret while patients are anticoagulated, so ideally these laboratory evaluations should be drawn before initiating anticoagulation therapy.

E Symptoms warrant treatment?

Most patients with acute-onset axillosubclavian vein DVT caused by vTOS will have symptoms sufficient to warrant treatment, especially because delay in treatment will make thrombolysis less successful. However, a very delayed presentation and development of adequate venous collateral circulation may result in mild symptoms requiring only conservative management. In addition, if there are contraindications to thrombolysis or surgery, conservative management is appropriate.

F Catheter-directed thrombolysis

For patients presenting with less than 2 weeks of vTOS symptoms, venography via the basilic vein should be performed and recanalization of the axillosubclavian vein with catheter-directed thrombolysis (CDT) and potential venoplasty should be attempted. Aspiration thrombectomy can be used as an adjunct,

particularly if residual thrombus is found on follow-up venograms during lysis. Venoplasty is added to CDT if severe stenosis that will likely lead to rethrombosis before rib resection can be performed exists. Venoplasty will not restore the vein to normal caliber because of the ongoing external compression. Short-term patency results after CDT plus venoplasty are favorable, but if the extrinsic compression from the first rib is not addressed, the long-term durability of endovascular intervention alone is poor.[8] It should be noted that stenting of the subclavian vein before surgical decompression results in high rates of stent thrombosis and/or fracture because of extrinsic compression of the stent from the first rib. As such, stenting of the vein before decompression is not recommended.[9,10]

Some practitioners draw a distinction between patients who present within 2 weeks of symptom onset versus those who do not. This distinction is predicated on the evidence of poor lysis results for thrombus present for more than 2 weeks. Studies have reported success rates for CDT of 85% to 100% when performed within 2 weeks of symptom onset but almost no success when CDT is started thereafter.[11,12] From a practical standpoint, some practitioners will not initiate lysis after this 14-day point, but rather will proceed to rib resection with a plan to either perform an endovascular recanalization of the vein after decompression or to perform an open reconstruction of the vein at the time of reconstruction.[13] Finally, it is worth noting that there is some controversy regarding the need for any lysis before rib resection, with some authors citing equivalent results simply anticoagulating patients until rib resection and then proceeding with vein repair. These data are limited to institutional series,[14] however, with most practitioners recommending CDT followed by interval first rib resection for vTOS.

G Conservative treatment vs. rib resection

As stated in F, lysis failure is unusual for patients treated within 2 weeks of symptoms. If lysis fails, a decision is made whether to pursue rib resection or to treat the patient conservatively. Most favor rib resection, because there is evidence (see E) that this can lead to improved outcomes. For a chronically occluded vein with good collateralization, conservative treatment with anticoagulation may be considered.

H First rib resection

Following successful CDT (flow restored, although some residual thrombus may remain), first rib resection should be performed. Transaxillary, supraclavicular, infraclavicular, or combined infra/supra clavicular approaches can be used. The choice of surgical approach depends on both surgeon experience/preference and patient preference. Good outcomes can be anticipated with any of these techniques.

Advocates of the transaxillary approach emphasize the ability to remove the entire first rib with good visualization of the vein and the rib from the subclavius muscle/tendon all the way posterior to the nerve roots. The incision is hidden, and many structures encountered in an anterior approach (lymphatics, phrenic nerve) are avoided. Those who use this approach do not plan on an open vein repair at the same setting. They, rather, reimage the vein, usually within a few weeks of surgery, and perform endovascular venous treatment if required.[15]

Some surgeons plan on performing imaging at the time of surgery so that endovascular or open repair of the vein can be performed concurrently, if needed. The exposure for open vein reconstruction is best afforded by an infraclavicular approach, which may require the addition of a supraclavicular incision for adequate exposure during vein repair. Generally, advocates of this approach cite the ability to reconstruct the vein (usually with patch venoplasty of a residual stricture at the site of compression) during one operation and decreased risk of brachial plexus injury.

I. Vein treatment as required

Some practitioners routinely perform venography at the time of first rib resection and treat significant residual stenosis with venoplasty ± stenting or open venoplasty. Advocates cite the patient benefit of a single intervention and obviation of the risk of vein rethrombosis that can occur in the acute postsurgical recovery period.[16] Transaxillary advocates prefer not to stent a vein in a fresh surgical field. Details of angioplasty, stenting, and open venous reconstruction are described in sections K through N. If the vein is not treated during the rib resection procedure, it should be evaluated with venography approximately 2 weeks following rib resection to determine whether endovascular or surgical treatment is indicated.

J. Postoperative venography ± IVUS

If the underlying venous stenosis/synechia from vTOS is not treated at the time of first rib resection, venography should be performed to assess the status of the axillosubclavian vein following surgery. This is typically timed 2 weeks postoperatively.[13,14] This study will reveal any residual subclavian vein stenosis or intraluminal thrombus. Ideally, access should be obtained via the basilic vein because venography via the cephalic vein limits complete imaging of the axillary vein. Adding IVUS to the evaluation allows for more accurate measurement of any residual axillosubclavian vein stenosis.[17] Subsequent steps depend on whether there is significant residual stenosis or reocclusion of the vein.

K. Anticoagulation and surveillance

Following venoplasty, stenting, or open reconstruction, patients should be continued on anticoagulation to prevent rethrombosis. The ideal duration for treatment has not been defined; however, most practitioners recommend 3 to 6 months of anticoagulation following definitive therapy.[18] Imaging protocols also vary, although DUS examinations are typically performed at 30 days, 6 months, and yearly thereafter. Recurrence of symptoms mandates reevaluation.

L. Thrombolysis/endovascular thrombectomy

For patients with axillosubclavian vein rethrombosis after first rib resection, endovascular recanalization with CDT should be attempted. CDT may be combined with aspiration thrombectomy if required. If residual stenosis persists, balloon venoplasty and possible stenting can be performed. Patients typically respond favorably to this treatment after the thoracic outlet has been decompressed, with reported 1-year primary and secondary patency rates of 92% and 96%, respectively.[19] If axillosubclavian vein patency cannot be restored, symptoms must be evaluated, and, if severe, open venous reconstruction considered.

M. PTA vs. stent

Patients who have significant residual axillosubclavian stenosis after first rib resection should undergo endovascular intervention at the time of venography. PTA may relieve the stenosis, and excellent patency rates can be expected.[20] Stenting may be considered for patients who do not achieve satisfactory results with angioplasty after first rib resection, although available data demonstrate worse patency when stents are placed than with venoplasty alone.[18] It is as yet unclear whether this is related to the presence of the stent or the venographic findings leading to the placement of the stent. If the residual stenosis cannot be successfully treated with an endovascular approach, open venous reconstruction is considered if severe symptoms warrant more aggressive treatment. Mild symptoms are managed conservatively.

N. Open venous reconstruction

Following rib resection, reasonable surgical risk patients with severe symptoms and residual venous stenosis or occlusion after failed endovascular therapy should be offered open reconstruction. It should be noted that axillosubclavian rethrombosis may result from inadequate resection of the anterior section of the first rib or subclavius muscle tendon. This should be investigated and addressed at the time of open venous reconstruction.

As noted previously, open reconstruction is performed via an anterior infraclavicular and/or supraclavicular approach, and this is the case for both repair at the time of rib excision and if done as a subsequent operation. Decision regarding the extent of the incision is based on surgeon preference and the needed exposure for safe clamping of the vein. A saphenous vein patch venoplasty is performed, although there is usually also a requirement for removal of residual thrombus and fibrin within the vein. If central control of healthy vein cannot be attained with this exposure, the incision can be extended medially to the sternum and then angled cephalad toward the sternal notch.[18] This can add significant morbidity to the operation. For patients with a vein that is chronically occluded/obliterated, some authors advocate jugular turndown as an option, but there are limited data to support this in the setting of vTOS.[21]

O. Conservative treatment

For patients failing venous reconstruction, continued anticoagulation for 3 to 12 months may be indicated while additional venous collaterals circulation develop and to prevent rare PE, although there are not good data to resolve this question. Decisions regarding further treatment should be made depending on the degree to which the patient is compensating for the venous occlusion.

REFERENCES

1. Lindblad B, Tengborn L, Bergqvist D. Deep vein thrombosis of the axillary-subclavian veins: epidemiologic data, effects of different types of treatment and late sequelae. *Eur J Vasc Surg*. 1988;2:161-165.
2. Horattas MC, Wright DJ, Fenton AH, et al. Changing concepts of deep venous thrombosis of the upper extremity—report of a series and review of the literature. *Surgery*. 1988;104:561-567.
3. Schneider DB, Azakie A, Messina LM. Management of vascular thoracic outlet syndrome. *Chest Surg Clin N Am*. 1999;9:781-802.
4. Mustafa BO, Rathbun SW, Whitsett TL, Raskob GE. Sensitivity and specificity of ultrasonography in the diagnosis of upper extremity deep vein thrombosis: a systematic review. *Arch Intern Med*. 2002;162(4):401-404.
5. Zucker EJ, Ganguli S, Ghoshhajra BB, Gupta R, Prabhakar AM. Imaging of venous compression syndromes. *Cardiovasc Diagn Ther*. 2016;6(6):519-532.
6. Kommareddy A, Zaroukian MH, Hassouna HI. Upper extremity deep venous thrombosis. *Semin Thromb Hemost*. 2002;28(1):89-99.
7. Kaczynski J, Sathiananthan J. Paget-Schroetter syndrome complicated by an incidental pulmonary embolism. *BMJ Case Rep*. 2017 2;2017.
8. Urschel HC Jr, Razzuk MA. Paget-Schroetter syndrome: what is the best management? *Ann Thorac Surg*. 2000;69:1663-1668; discussion 1668-1669.
9. Meier GH, Pollak JS, Rosenblatt M, Dickey KW, Gusberg RJ. Initial experience with venous stents in exertional axillary-subclavian vein thrombosis. *J Vasc Surg*. 1996;24(6):974-981.
10. Mallios A, Taubman K, Claiborne P, Blebea J. Subclavian vein stent fracture and venous motion. *Ann Vasc Surg*. 2015;29(7):1451.e1-e4.
11. Doyle A, Wolford HY, Davies MG, et al. Management of effort thrombosis of the subclavian vein: today's treatment. *Ann Vasc Surg*. 2007;21:723-729.

12. Adelman MA, Stone DH, Riles TS, Lamparello PJ, Giangola G, Rosen RJ. A multidisciplinary approach to the treatment of Paget-Schroetter syndrome. *Ann Vasc Surg*. 1997;11:149-154.

13. Archie M, Rigberg D. Vascular TOS-creating a protocol and sticking to it. *Diagnostics (Basel)*. 2017;7(2). pii: E34. doi:10.3390/diagnostics7020034.

14. Guzzo JL, Chang K, Demos J, Black JH, Freischlag JA. Preoperative thrombolysis and venoplasty affords no benefit in patency following first rib resection and scalenectomy for subacute and chronic subclavian vein thrombosis. *J Vasc Surg*. 2010;52(3):658-662; discussion 662-663. doi:10.1016/j.jvs.2010.04.050.

15. Chang KZ, Likes K, Demos J, Black JH 3rd, Freischlag JA. Routine venography following transaxillary first rib resection and scalenectomy (FRRS) for chronic subclavian vein thrombosis ensures excellent outcomes and vein patency. *Vasc Endovascular Surg*. 2012;46(1):15-20. doi:10.1177/1538574411423982.

16. Molina JE, Hunter DW, Dietz CA. Paget-Schroetter syndrome treated with thrombolytics and immediate surgery. *J Vasc Surg*. 2007;45:328-334.

17. Archie MM, Rollo JC, Gelabert HA. Surgical missteps in the management of venous thoracic outlet syndrome which lead to reoperation. *Ann Vasc Surg*. 2018;49:261-267. doi:10.1016/j.avsg.2018.01.067.

18. Illig KA, Doyle AJ. A comprehensive review of Paget-Schroetter syndrome. *J Vasc Surg*. 2010;51(6):1538-1547. doi:10.1016/j.jvs.2009.12.022.

19. Schneider DB, Dimuzio PJ, Martin ND, et al. Combination treatment of venous thoracic outlet syndrome: open surgical decompression and intraoperative angioplasty. *J Vasc Surg*. 2004;40(4):599-603.

20. Kreienberg PB, Chang BB, Darling RC 3rd, et al. Long-term results in patients treated with thrombolysis, thoracic inlet decompression, and subclavian vein stenting for Paget-Schroetter syndrome. *J Vasc Surg*. 2001;33:s100-s105.

21. Wooster M, Fernandez B, Summers KL, Illig KA. Surgical and endovascular central venous reconstruction combined with thoracic outletdecompression in highly symptomatic patients. *J Vasc Surg Venous Lymphat Disord*. 2019;7(1): 106-112.e3.

Anahita Dua • Jason T. Lee

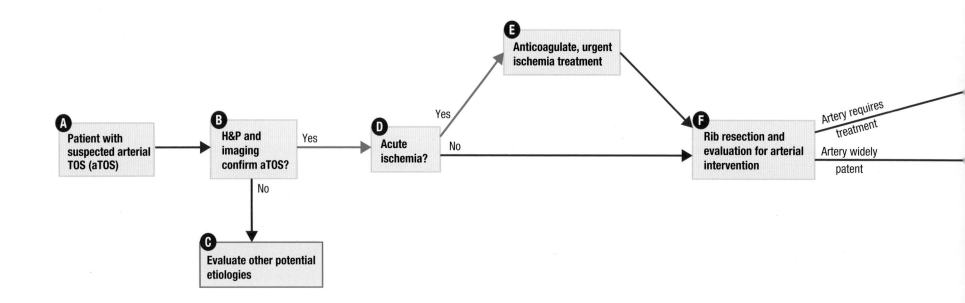

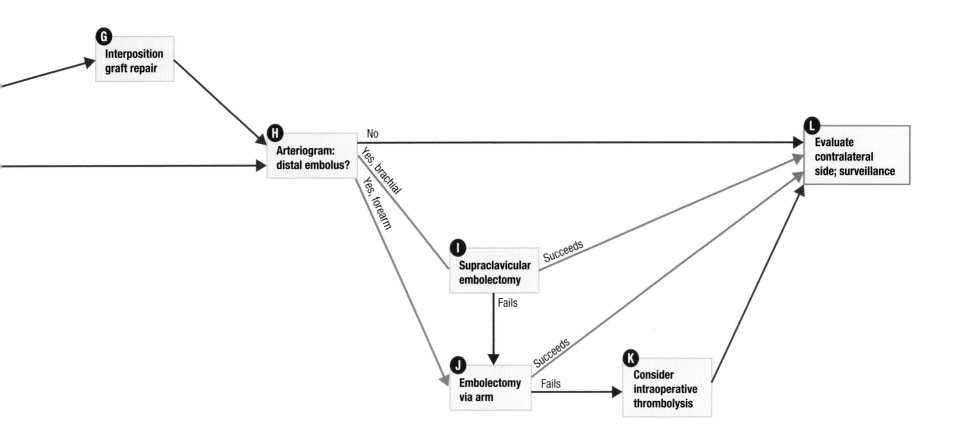

A   Patient with suspected arterial TOS

Diagnosing TOS can be challenging because of variations in presentations and symptoms. Most patients with TOS who undergo operations in the United States present with neurogenic (95%), followed by venous (4%) and arterial (aTOS) (<1%) symptoms.[1] Most commonly, aTOS results from compression of the subclavian artery by an associated cervical or anomalous first rib. This external compression can cause stenosis and intimal damage with resultant thrombosis or embolization. Compression can also cause poststenotic dilation of the subclavian artery that may progress to aneurysm formation with thrombus accumulation that can embolize to the distal extremity. Depending on the pathology described earlier, clinical presentation, with regard to onset of ischemia, can be acute or gradual. Most patients are young adults with a mean age of 37 years, with equal proportion of men and women.[1-3]

B   H&P and imaging confirm aTOS?

The most common presentation of aTOS is gradual and intermittent hand ischemia caused by distal embolization, which initially may be mild (splinter hemorrhages) and difficult to diagnose. Exertional arm pain or Raynaud syndrome can result from stenosis without embolization. Larger emboli may cause ALI. Physical examination may reveal reduced ipsilateral arm blood pressure, supraclavicular bruit or pulsatile mass, reduced or absent distal pulses, or signs of hand ischemia. Provocative shoulder maneuvers (Adson and Wright tests) that result in diminution of distal pulses can be observed in patients with aTOS, although pulse diminution has been described in normal individuals (false positive). Imaging is required for definitive diagnosis. Plain radiographs can detect a cervical rib or other bony abnormality such as protruding callus at a prior clavicular fracture. DUS can detect elevated velocities consistent with subclavian stenosis and may visualize aneurysmal changes, although the clavicle can interfere with imaging. CTA is most useful in delineating subclavian stenosis or aneurysm formation, and with 3D reconstruction and more distal arm imaging, can accurately identify the site of compression and any distal arterial compromise. MRA is preferred in some centers but has been less precise in establishing the diagnosis. DSA is rarely needed as a pure diagnostic tool but can be helpful in documenting digital emboli or confirming subclavian intimal pathology if this is not revealed on CTA.[2-5]

C   Evaluate other potential etiologies

If the diagnosis of aTOS is ruled out with imaging, other potential etiologies should be considered. These include nonatherosclerotic vascular disease, systemic lupus erythematosus, CREST syndrome (calcinosis, Raynaud phenomenon, esophageal dysmotility, sclerodactyly, and telangiectasia), scleroderma, Buerger

disease, FMD, vasculitis, giant cell arteritis, Takayasu disease, leukofibrinogenemia, trauma, subclavian stenosis from other causes, cardiac embolism, and iatrogenic pathology.

D   Acute ischemia?

The majority of patients with aTOS present with mild, subacute to chronic arm/hand ischemia, and, as such, can undergo a thorough evaluation without increasing the ischemic risk to the limb.[1,2] These symptoms may be similar to that in patients with neurogenic TOS and include numbness, weakness, tingling, arm fatigue, pallor, coolness, and/or pain throughout the extremity to the finger tips. Chronic ulceration or nonhealing wounds may also be present in the more advanced or untreated patients with long-standing symptoms.[1] Patients presenting with acute ischemia from subclavian thrombosis or larger embolization complain of more rapid or severe symptoms and require expedited workup and treatment.[1,2]

E   Anticoagulate, urgent ischemia treatment

Patients presenting with limb-threatening ALI should be immediately anticoagulated with IV heparin and prepared for urgent surgical treatment. In cases with acute limb threat due to ischemia (Rutherford IIb) from distal embolization, but with a patent subclavian artery, attention is first directed to treating the distal embolus, as outlined in Chapter 53. This most likely would require transbrachial embolectomy, potential intraoperative adjunctive thrombolysis, and fasciotomy. After this is accomplished, the subclavian artery pathology from aTOS would be treated as outlined in this decision tree. In cases of severe acute ischemia associated with subclavian artery thrombosis, distal embolectomy would need to be combined with proximal thrombectomy to restore adequate circulation. In some cases, this might require first rib resection and subclavian graft interposition, as outlined in this decision tree.

F   Rib resection and evaluation for arterial intervention

Treatment of aTOS requires thoracic outlet decompression, as well as arterial repair and restoration of distal circulation, if needed.[2-9] Intervention must include operative exposure of the compressed arterial region and removal of the inciting bony abnormality, which is most often a cervical rib. Most recommend also excising the first rib to reduce the potential for recurrence. Intraoperatively, if other bony abnormalities or fibrous tissue bands are found to be compressive of the subclavian artery, they must be excised. Surgical decompression is usually performed via a supraclavicular approach, which is our preferred approach because it allows excellent visualization of arterial structures involved. General exposure includes transection of the clavicular head of the sternocleidomastoid and mobilization of the underlying scalene fat pad, taking care to preserve the phrenic nerve.

The anterior scalene muscle attachments to the cervical and first rib are then transected to expose the underlying subclavian artery. Lateral and inferior intercostal muscle attachments are also divided to allow cervical and first rib excision.

After the mechanical thoracic outlet decompression, the underlying arterial pathology must be explored and repaired, if necessary. If the extent of arterial damage is not obvious on inspection or preoperatively on CTA, intraoperative DSA, via a femoral artery or ipsilateral brachial artery approach, can be used to confirm or rule out arterial pathology and/or distal embolization. Intraoperative DUS or IVUS can also be helpful to examine the artery if the defect is not obvious. In cases of mild poststenotic dilatation, arterial repair may not be required, because aneurysmal resolution after decompression has been described. Similarly, mild intimal injury may heal after decompression. However, in most cases, especially when there has been distal embolization, surgical replacement of the diseased subclavian artery is indicated. In a recent series, 70% of patients undergoing surgery for aTOS required subclavian artery repair. If there is only mild stenosis or intimal injury, patch angioplasty may suffice. However, in cases of aneurysm or stenosis/occlusion, with associated arterial scarring/fibrosis, arterial resection and graft interposition is required.

G   Interposition graft repair

Endovascular treatments such as thrombolysis alone or stenting of stenosis or aneurysmal lesions are not able to successfully treat aTOS because they do not treat the underlying compressive pathology.[2,3,5,6] An interposition graft using ePTFE or Dacron is the most commonly employed treatment after thoracic outlet decompression and resection of the pathologic segment of subclavian artery. Vein grafts can be used, but usually result in a size mismatch and their patency is not superior to prosthetic grafts for short interposition replacement. If the subclavian aneurysm is large, more distal control and anastomosis may require further exposure of axillosubclavian artery with an additional infraclavicular incision. Outcomes of interposition graft repair have been excellent, with a recent series of 40 patients treated for aTOS reporting graft patency of 92% at 5 years, with no further stenosis or embolism, although chronic post-ischemic symptoms were present in six patients, emphasizing the importance of early diagnosis and treatment.[1]

H   Arteriogram: distal embolus?

Completion DSA should be performed after thoracic outlet decompression and primary treatment of the affected subclavian artery to determine the need for further intervention on the affected limb unless this has already been planned on preoperative evaluation.[2] Distal embolization is a well-described sequela of aTOS, especially in the setting of post-stenotic dilatation of the subclavian artery. Emboli tend to occlude arteries at branch points (brachial bifurcation and digital arteries). Further treatment depends on whether distal emboli exist and whether they can be extracted from the subclavian artery or require brachial or more distal exposure for extraction.

Supraclavicular embolectomy

For isolated brachial artery emboli, balloon catheter embolectomy via the exposed subclavian artery may be successful in removing emboli, and if successful avoids the need for brachial exposure. Thromboembolectomy is usually performed via a 3- or 4-Fogarty balloon catheter. Completion angiography of the affected limb should be performed via the exposed artery to confirm complete thromboembolus extraction. If the brachial or more distal radial/ulnar thrombus cannot be extracted via this approach, brachial exposure will be necessary to clear the obstructing distal lesions.

Embolectomy via arm

For more distal forearm emboli, exposure of the brachial bifurcation facilitates direct radial and ulnar embolectomy. Thromboembolism to the brachial bifurcation and ulnar and/or radial arteries is best treated via exposure of the brachial bifurcation.[3,7] Fogarty balloon thrombectomy (2 or 3) catheters should be utilized for these smaller vessels.

Cut down of the radial and ulnar arteries, at the wrist crease, may be required to remove emboli (2-Fogarty balloons) obstructing the palmar arch vessels. For digital emboli, not amenable to catheter embolectomy, thrombolysis may be considered. Adjunctive infusion of a vasodilator (200 mcg nitroglycerine) into the distal arteries may reverse vasospasm that can develop during and after thromboembolectomy.

K Consider intraoperative thrombolysis

If the patient has thromboembolism to the palmar arch and digital arteries, intra-arterial tissue plasminogen activator (tPA, 2–4 mg) can be injected into the distal radial/ulnar or palmar arch vessels. Alternatively, or in addition, postoperative IV heparin infusion can be initiated to prevent further thrombosis and allow time for intrinsic thrombolysis or improved collateral circulation to develop. Typically, an IV infusion of 500 to 700 units/heparin/hour for 48 hours is recommended after arterial thromboembolectomy. Heparin is started 4 hours after completion of the operation to avoid immediate postoperative hematoma formation. Given the rarity of these cases, there is not good evidence to support either approach. Our decision-making protocol is extrapolated from other similar conditions. The usual contraindications and precautions for thrombolytic agents should obviously be evaluated as part of the decision-making process.

L Evaluate contralateral side; surveillance

Patients with aTOS may have bilateral cervical ribs but be asymptomatic on the other arm. If so, they should be followed up with DUS or CTA evaluation to ensure that aneurysmal or stenotic changes do not develop. After aTOS treatment, patients should undergo routine periodic surveillance graft with DUS and arm pressure measurements. Because the patency of these reconstructions is quite high, surveillance may be discontinued after several years, if no issues arise.

REFERENCES

1. Vemuri C, McLaughlin LN, Abuirqeba AA, Thompson RW. Clinical presentation and management of arterial thoracic outlet syndrome. *J Vasc Surg.* 2017;65(5):1429-1439. doi:10.1016/j.jvs.2016.11.039.
2. Urschel HC Jr. Management of the thoracic-outlet syndrome. *N Engl J Med.* 1972;286(21):1140-1143.
3. Qaja E, Honari S, Rhee R. Arterial thoracic outlet syndrome secondary to hypertrophy of the anterior scalene muscle. *J Surg Case Rep.* 2017;2017(8):rjx158.
4. Davidovic LB, Kostic DM, Jakovljevic NS, Kuzmanovic IL, Simic TM. Vascular thoracic outlet syndrome. *World J Surg.* 2003;27(5):545-550.
5. Mitsos S, Patrini D, Velo S, et al. Arterial thoracic outlet syndrome treated successfully with totally endoscopic first rib resection. *Case Rep Pulmonol.* 2017;2017:9350735. doi:10.1155/2017/9350735.
6. Nejim B, Alshaikh HN, Arhuidese I, et al. Perioperative outcomes of thoracic outlet syndrome surgical repair in a nationally validated database. *Angiology.* 2017;68(6):502-507. doi:10.1177/0003319716677666.
7. Archie M, Rigberg D. Vascular TOS-creating a protocol and sticking to it. *Diagnostics (Basel).* 2017;7(2). pii: E34. doi:10.3390/diagnostics7020034.
8. Klaassen Z, Sorenson E, Tubbs RS, et al. Thoracic outlet syndrome: a neurological and vascular disorder. *Clin Anat.* 2014;27(5):724-732. doi:10.1002/ca.22271.
9. Hussain MA, Aljabri B, Al-Omran M. Vascular thoracic outlet syndrome. *Semin Thorac Cardiovasc Surg.* 2016;28(1):151-157. doi:10.1053/j.semtcvs.2015.10.008.

Paul W. White • Todd E. Rasmussen

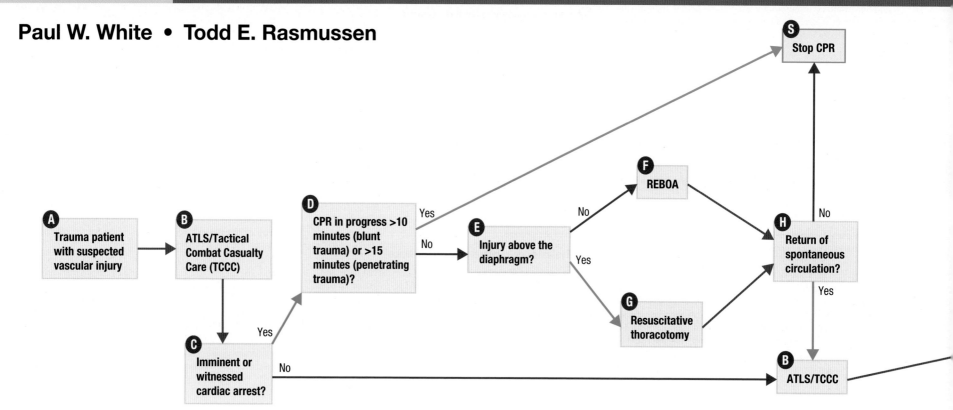

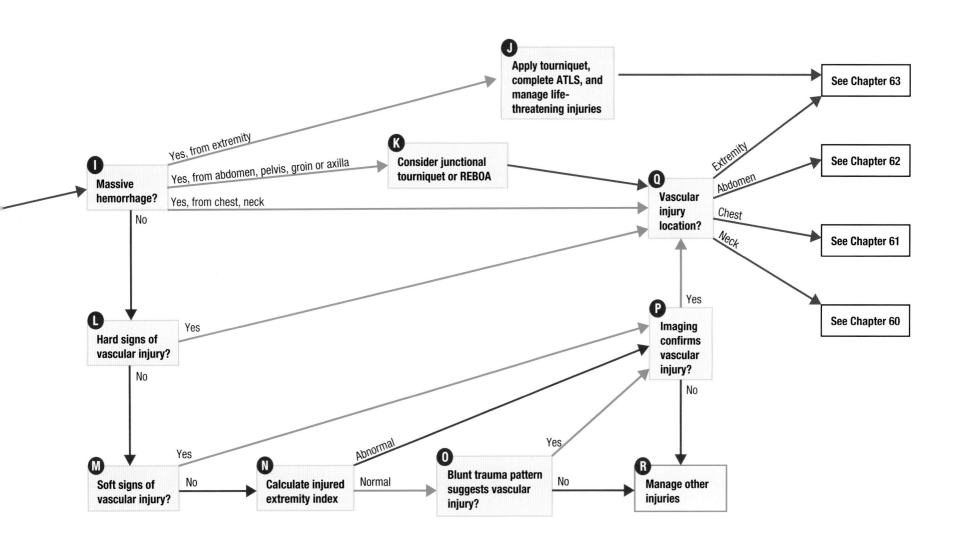

A Trauma patient with suspected vascular injury

Patients often present with hemorrhagic shock after traumatic injury. Although this may be the result of an injury to a large, named vessel, bleeding and shock can also result from severe injury to the solid organs (eg, grade IV or V injury to the liver, kidney, or spleen), the bony structure of the pelvis, or the lung parenchyma. An algorithmic approach to the severely injured patient allows for immediate life-saving measures regardless of the exact source of bleeding, until a more definitive diagnosis can be made and definitive treatments rendered.

The epidemiology of vascular trauma is complex and varies according to the population studied. Because military casualties represent a discrete population within a well-circumscribed time frame, epidemiologic studies of wartime vascular injury provide a reasonably accurate and comprehensive picture of the prevalence and impact of vascular injuries. The U.S. military has seen a steady increase in the incidence of vascular injuries since World War I.[1,2] Civilian populations pose a more difficult challenge. A 2010 review of the National Trauma Databank (NTBD) found a 1.6% prevalence of vascular trauma in all patients in the NTDB. Although extremity injuries are most common in both military and civilian populations, torso injuries comprise a higher fraction of vascular injuries in civilian populations.[3]

B ATLS/Tactical Combat Casualty Care (TCCC)

ATLS was developed by the American College of Surgeons Committee on Trauma (ACS-COT) and is updated on a regular basis. ATLS provides a concise algorithm for the assessment and treatment of injured patients who often present with complex and difficult problems.[4] TCCC was developed by the special operations medical community in the U.S. military to adapt similar principles of immediate trauma care for medics and first responders in the prehospital setting.[5] ATLS/TCCC should form the framework for the initial treatment of severely injured patients. Returning to this algorithm as the clinical picture changes and as diagnoses are made or excluded is essential.

Both ATLS and TCCC use a stepwise algorithm that emphasizes treating life-threatening pathologies as they are identified. ATLS begins with a primary survey based on the ABCDEs. (A) irway, (B)reathing, (C)irculation, (D)isability, and (E)xposure/Environmental Control are quickly assessed and life-threatening injuries treated in this sequence. Once a primary survey is complete, a secondary survey consisting of a thorough head-to-toe physical examination, a brief history, and indicated radiologic studies and laboratory studies is completed. TCCC uses a similar alphabetic mnemonic "MARCH." (M)assive hemorrhage, (A)irway, (R)espiration, (C)irculation, and (H)ypothermia are assessed and treated in a manner similar to that of the ABCDEs of ATLS.[4,5] Massive

hemorrhage was placed at the start of the algorithm because hemorrhage has been found to be the leading cause of preventable battlefield deaths.[6]

C Imminent or witnessed cardiac arrest?

ATLS/TCCC emphasizes the immediate treatment of life-threatening injuries identified in the primary survey. A patient in cardiopulmonary arrest or in extremis requires immediate and drastic therapeutic maneuvers if there is any hope of salvaging the patient's life. If the patient is not in arrest, the ATLS primary survey should be initiated. For patients in arrest, the utility of resuscitative thoracotomy or REBOA should be considered.

D CPR in progress >10 minutes (blunt trauma) or >15 minutes (penetrating trauma)?

The severely injured patient may present in extremis. Therapeutic maneuvers to treat severe hemorrhagic shock must be initiated immediately. For patients who are undergoing CPR and have no signs of life, the mechanism of injury (MOI) and the duration of CPR help determine when to declare further treatment futile. If CPR has been in progress for >10 minutes after a blunt MOI, or >15 minutes after a penetrating MOI, there is essentially no chance of survival, and the Western Trauma Association algorithm recommends that CPR should be stopped.[7]

E Injury above the diaphragm?

If the patient exhibits signs of life, is in profound refractory shock, or has been undergoing CPR for less than the time period specified, the use of resuscitative thoracotomy or REBOA may prove lifesaving. For injuries above the diaphragm, a resuscitative thoracotomy can allow definitive management of the thoracic injuries through the same incision used for aortic cross-clamping. The chest should be evaluated with chest x-ray, ultrasound, or bilateral chest tubes to determine whether the source of hemorrhage is within the chest or in the abdomen/pelvis. For injuries below the diaphragm in patients in profound hemorrhagic shock, REBOA is recommended in appropriate patients. As with resuscitative thoracotomy with aortic clamping, quality data showing that REBOA improves outcomes or survival is limited. Also, as with resuscitative thoracotomy with aortic clamping, if used inappropriately, REBOA can have complications such as mesenteric ischemia, paraplegia, and iatrogenic aortic, iliac, or femoral artery injury. At this time, REBOA is indicated for injuries below the diaphragm.[8] Before making the decision to employ REBOA or resuscitative thoracotomy, one must first determine the anatomic location of hemorrhage. Extended focused assessment with sonography in trauma (eFAST), chest x-ray, and pelvic x-ray can all be performed quickly in a critically injured patient to assess whether life-threatening bleeding is occurring in the chest, abdomen, or pelvis.[9,10]

F REBOA

The use of an endovascular balloon to occlude the aorta for the treatment of hemorrhagic shock was described during the Korean War but was not widely used until endovascular techniques became broadly adopted. Resuscitative thoracotomy with aortic cross-clamping for trauma gained acceptance and popularity in the 1960s and 1970s. With the revolution in endovascular approaches in the 1990s and early 2000s and the widespread use of balloon occlusion for the treatment of shock in patients with ruptured rAAA, there has been a renewed interest in REBOA for trauma patients.[10] Early techniques for REBOA for trauma were similar to the techniques described for balloon occlusion of the aorta in the treatment of ruptured AAA utilizing wires, long sheaths, and large complaint balloons. The newest generation of balloon-catheter devices specifically designed for REBOA in the emergent setting do not require wires (ie, no "over the wire" step), can be inserted through short 7F sheaths, and can be used with or without fluoroscopy.[9] REBOA can be broken down into six steps, each with its own considerations and potential complications:

a. Arterial access
b. Balloon positioning
c. Balloon inflation
d. Operative control of hemorrhage
e. Balloon deflation
f. Sheath removal

To facilitate appropriate placement of the aortic balloon to address different patterns of hemorrhage (ie, intraperitoneal vs. pelvic), it can be helpful to describe three zones of the descending aorta.

Zone 1 extends from the left SCA to the celiac artery.
Zone 2 extends from the celiac to the lowest renal artery.
Zone 3 extends from the lowest renal to the aortic bifurcation.

Inflation of the balloon in zone 1 is appropriate for intra-abdominal hemorrhage causing severe shock. Inflation in zone 3 is appropriate for pelvic hemorrhage or junctional hemorrhage from the groins. Balloons should not be inflated in zone 2 to avoid injury to visceral/renal branches.[11]

REBOA is contraindicated for injuries to the neck because it will not address hemorrhage from that location.[9] Although animal models seemed to indicate the safety of REBOA in the presence of traumatic brain injury (TBI), there are case reports of increased intracranial hemorrhage volumes after brief periods of REBOA.[12] Future studies may expand the known safe indications for REBOA.

A recent review evaluated the use of REBOA in multiple scenarios including trauma, postpartum hemorrhage, ruptured AAA, GI bleeding, and pelvic surgery.[13] Mortality in all patients was approximately 50%. Despite its empiric value, including rapid increase in SBP above, and slowed bleeding below the balloon, retrospective, registry studies to date have identified no clear mortality benefit with REBOA.[13] This is a rapidly evolving topic area and currently there are two prospective, multicenter trials under way, one in the United States and one in the United Kingdom, that are designed to provide better information about the use and effectiveness of REBOA for injury and shock.

G Resuscitative thoracotomy

Resuscitative thoracotomy is a salvage procedure associated with very high mortality and reserved for the most severely injured patients. Its use has decreased in recent decades as appreciation of its risk to providers and its relative futility in many scenarios has become clear. Recent efforts have sought to determine which patients are most likely to benefit from resuscitative thoracotomy and to focus its use on those patients. The Eastern Association for the Surgery of Trauma (EAST) has published guidelines in this regard. They divided patients by MOI (penetrating or blunt), presence or absence of signs of life (pupillary response, spontaneous ventilation, carotid pulse, measurable blood pressure, extremity movement, or cardiac electrical activity), and injury within or without the thorax. Of the six resulting categories, only the group with signs of life and a penetrating injury within the chest received a strong recommendation for resuscitative thoracotomy. A conditional recommendation against resuscitative thoracotomy was made for patients without signs of life and a blunt MOI. All other groups received a conditional recommendation for resuscitative thoracotomy.[14]

The goals of resuscitative thoracotomy are control of intrathoracic hemorrhage, release of cardiac tamponade, internal cardiac massage, and aortic occlusion to control bleeding below the diaphragm.[15] Resuscitative thoracotomy has six elemental steps:

a. Left anterolateral thoracotomy incision at the fourth or fifth rib space (which can be extended to a clam-shell incision if access to the right chest to repair injuries is needed)
b. Opening the pericardium
c. Control of cardiac injury
d. Temporary control of lung bleeding
e. Cross clamping of the aorta
f. Internal cardiac massage

After addressing cardiac injuries, intrathoracic sources of hemorrhage, and cross-clamping the aorta, the patient should be reassessed. If there has not been a return of vital signs, efforts at resuscitation should be discontinued.[15]

H Return of spontaneous circulation?

If the patient responds to resuscitative thoracotomy or REBOA, one must rapidly proceed or return to the primary survey/secondary survey of the ATLS algorithm so that all injuries can be rapidly diagnosed and treated. If vital signs cannot be restored, the patient should be declared dead.

I Massive hemorrhage?

Bleeding is the major cause of mortality in patients with trauma, second only to severe head injury, and major vascular injury is one of the leading causes of massive hemorrhage. The Hartford Consensus III meeting focused on addressing hemorrhage control especially in the civilian prehospital setting.[16] The U.S. Military's TCCC guidelines developed the acronym "MARCH" for the initial care of casualties after immediate threats have been suppressed. "M" indicates the need to first assess for massive hemorrhage. Although these guidelines are primarily directed toward prehospital treatment, the need to urgently address massive hemorrhage is equally relevant in the emergency room or trauma bay. In the most recent additions, ATLS has emphasized hemorrhage control in the assessment and treatment of circulation during, if not before, the ABCDEs of the primary survey. Monitoring of vital signs, physical examination, eFAST, chest x-ray, and diagnostic peritoneal lavage are adjuncts to the primary survey that assist a provider in diagnosing massive hemorrhage. Simultaneous control of hemorrhage and initiation of damage control resuscitation are essential in the survival of the severely injured patient.[17] Massive hemorrhage demands early, definitive management in the operating room (OR), with details dependent on the location of hemorrhage.

J Apply tourniquet, complete ATLS, and manage life-threatening injuries

If the source of hemorrhage is an extremity (almost always the result of injury to a large, named axial vessel), tourniquets provide rapid, effective, and safe hemorrhage control. In combat, the early application of tourniquets to control extremity hemorrhage before the onset of shock improved survival, and was not associated with limb loss from ischemia.[18] In civilian patients with a peripheral vascular injury, mortality was reduced 6-fold by the use of tourniquets.[19] The most effective tourniquet designs incorporate a windlass so that they can be tightened sufficiently to compress the arteries and the extremity. After the Boston Marathon bombing, 27 patients were treated with improvised tourniquets. However, many of these were found to be venous tourniquets only, which were not adequately controlling hemorrhage, emphasizing the importance of proper application.[20] Immediate use of a commercially available windlass tourniquet, such as the combat application tourniquet (CAT), will temporarily control hemorrhage and allow for completing a full assessment of the injured patient. Tourniquets can be left in place on extremities for up to 2 hours while other life-threatening injuries are managed. Nevertheless, operative exploration and management of extremity injuries should be pursued as soon as possible (see Chapter 63).

K Consider junctional tourniquet or REBOA

In contradistinction to compressible extremity hemorrhage, major vascular injuries in the groin, axilla, or torso are frequently noncompressible with traditional tourniquets or sometimes even by manual pressure. For injuries in the groin, pelvis, and abdomen, REBOA has been shown to be an effective method of hemorrhage control. Hemorrhage from the groin or axilla is potentially compressible but not by a traditional tourniquet. Major vascular injuries in these anatomic regions have been termed junctional vascular injuries (ie, junctional region between the torso and the extremities). Several devices have been designed to compress junctional vascular injuries including the Combat Ready Clamp (CRoC), SAM Junctional Tourniquet, and the Junctional Emergency Treatment Tool (JETT).[21] Successful use of the SAM Junctional Tourniquet in Afghanistan has been reported.[22] REBOA and junctional tourniquets are temporizing measures, and the patient's vascular injuries should be addressed urgently in the OR (see Chapter 62).

L Hard signs of vascular injury?

In the absence of massive hemorrhage, but suspicion of vascular injury, assessment for "hard signs" of vascular injury begins in the primary ATLS survey and continues in the secondary survey. The hard signs of vascular injury are massive or pulsatile bleeding, absence of pulse or continuous wave Doppler signal, bruit, thrill, and expanding hematoma. These signs indicate the presence of a major vascular injury, and additional diagnostic tests are unnecessary. The patient should be taken immediately to the OR for exploration and, if needed, on-table DSA to define the details of injury and allow potential endovascular treatment. Absent pulses should be reassessed with a handheld Doppler after the initiation of resuscitation and warming because the patient in severe shock, especially a young patient, may have significant peripheral vasoconstriction.[23] Once the vascular injury has been identified, management of the injury is dependent on the anatomic region in which the injury is located.

M Soft signs of vascular injury?

Significant vascular injuries are still possible without the obvious or hard signs. The soft signs of vascular injury are more subtle and include a reported history of major blood loss, penetrating wounds, or displaced fracture in close proximity to major vascular structures; nonexpanding hematoma; and evidence of injury to a peripheral nerve in close proximity to a major vessel.[24] The presence of soft signs of vascular injury warrant a thorough investigation with more advanced vascular imaging. Many vascular injuries are occult, and pose a significant diagnostic challenge. For example, secondary blast injuries from dozens of penetrating fragments caused a high rate of vascular injuries in Iraq and Afghanistan that were not detected on physical examination, and were only discovered with DSA.[25]

Ⓝ Calculate injured extremity index

The Injured Extremity Index (IEI) is useful refinement of the physical examination for detecting occult vascular injuries even when soft signs are not present. The IEI is the ratio of the SBP in the injured/uninjured extremity.

If the IEI is >0.9, major vascular injury in the injured extremity is ruled out.[26] This reduces the need for arteriography, conserving resources and time. However, caution should be exercised in interpreting the IEI in the setting of hypotension or hypothermia. It should be repeated after resuscitation and rewarming.[24] If any question remains of a vascular injury, close observation for 12 to 24 hours is needed.

Ⓞ Blunt trauma pattern suggests vascular injury?

Certain patterns of blunt trauma are associated with vascular injury even in the absence of hard and soft signs. Blunt thoracic aortic injury (BTAI), popliteal artery injuries associated with knee dislocation, and blunt cerebrovascular injuries (BCVIs) are examples of injuries that are often difficult to diagnose without advanced imaging. BTAI is usually caused by high-injury blunt or rapid deceleration mechanisms. Aircraft crashes, high-speed motor vehicle crashes (MVCs), and falls from significant height are mechanisms that should raise the suspicion for BTAI. Findings on chest x-ray obtained as an adjunct to the primary survey such as a widened mediastinum, sternal fractures, loss of the aortic knob, scapular fractures, upper rib fractures, and left apical pleural cap should raise suspicion for BTAI.[27] Knee dislocations, tibial plateau, and distal femur fractures have been associated with popliteal artery injuries. Popliteal artery injuries associated with a blunt MOI have a worse functional outcome and a higher rate of amputation than do penetrating injuries.[28] Therefore, the threshold should be low to perform advanced imaging to rule out arterial trauma with these injuries.

Although additional workup for BCVI is obvious in patients presenting with physical evidence like a seat belt sign to the neck, many BCVIs are very difficult to diagnose without focused advanced imaging. The consequences of a missed BCVI can be devastating, and there is often a window of opportunity to treat a BCVI before sequelae develop.[29] Determining which patients should be screened for BCVI is based on recognition of high-risk injury patterns. In the clinical guidelines of EAST, eight criteria that warranted further evaluation with advanced imaging were described. These were (1) neurologic abnormality unexplained by other injuries, (2) epistaxis from a suspected arterial source after blunt trauma, (3) Glasgow Coma Scale <8, (4) petrous bone fracture, (5) diffuse axonal injury, (6) cervical spine fracture of C1-C3 or involving the transverse foramen, (7) cervical spine fracture with subluxation or rotational mechanism, and (8) Lefort II or III fractures.[30] Surgeons at the University of Maryland have advocated for even broader screening for BCVIs after they found a significant number of BCVI on whole-body CT for patients

with blunt trauma who would not have received additional imaging based solely on the EAST guidelines.[29] Clinicians should be aware of certain vascular injuries that may only be apparent when a constellation of injuries is recognized.

Ⓟ Imaging confirms vascular injury?

In patients with soft signs, an abnormal IEI or a mechanism associated with vascular injury, advanced imaging to assess for blood vessel disruption is warranted. DSA has long been considered the standard for vascular imaging. It provides precise anatomic information and physiologic information such as flow rate and direction. In addition, DSA can easily be performed in the OR with plain films, a portable C-arm, or in a hybrid OR allowing one team of surgeons to address life-threatening injuries while a second team completes the diagnostic evaluation of the patient.

With the advent and increase in endovascular technologies, DSA also provides an opportunity to quickly treat injuries as they are identified.[31] Its downsides include need for contrast injection with concomitant risks for kidney injury or allergic reaction, the risk of access complications, and cost. CTA, especially multidetector CTA (MDCTA) has gradually replaced DSA for preoperative imaging for arterial injuries. CTA has been shown to be as accurate as DSA even in the presence of metallic fragments. It is also capable of imaging multiple anatomic regions at once.[32] CTA is quick, noninvasive, and offers diagnostic information about bones, lungs, solid organs, and soft tissues that DSA cannot provide. For patients who do not need immediate treatment in the OR, CTA has supplanted DSA as the first-line imaging modality of choice, although patterns of use vary among institutions and providers.

Although MRA and DUS have been shown to be accurate, they have significant limitations. MRA is time consuming, and contraindicated when metallic fragments are present, limiting its use in trauma. DUS is operator dependent, cannot simultaneously image multiple anatomic regions, and cannot image intrathoracic vascular structures.[33] Once a vascular injury has been identified, management of the injury is dependent on the anatomic region in which the injury is located.

Ⓠ Vascular injury location?

Specific treatment of vascular injuries of the neck, chest, abdomen, and extremities is discussed in Chapters 60, 61, 62, and 63, respectively.

Ⓡ Manage other injuries

If no vascular injury is found, other injuries are managed following ATLS/TCCC protocols (see B) and the patient is monitored for a potential occult vascular injury not initially detected.

Ⓢ Stop CPR

Resuscitation is stopped once members of the treating team agree that it is futile.

REFERENCES

1. Tai NRM, Rasmussen TE. Epidemiology of vascular injury. In: Rasmussen TE, Tai NRM, eds. *Rich's Vascular Trauma*. 3rd ed. Philadelphia, PA: Elsevier; 2016:13-20.
2. White JM, Stannard A, Burkhardt GE, Eastridge BJ, Blackbourne LH, Rasmussen TE. The epidemiology of vascular injury in the wars in Iraq and Afghanistan. *Ann Surg.* 2011;253(6):1184-1189.
3. Barmparas G, Inaba K, Talving P, et al. Pediatric vs adult vascular trauma: a National Trauma Databank review. *J Pediatr Surg.* 2010;45(7):1404-1412.
4. American College of Surgeons, Committee on Trauma. *Advanced Trauma Life Support Student (ATLS) Course Manual.* 9th ed. Chicago, IL: American College of Surgeons; 2012:ix.
5. Joint Trauma System, Committee on Tactical Combat Casualty Care. TCCC guidelines for medical personnel. http://jts.amedd.army.mil/index.cfm/committees/cotccc/guidelines. Accessed August 1, 2018.
6. Eastridge BJ, Mabry RL, Seguin P, et al. Death on the battlefield (2001–2011): implications for the future of combat casualty care. *J Trauma Acute Care Surg.* 2012;73(6 suppl 5):S431-S437.
7. Burlew CC, Moore EE, Moore FA, et al. Western Trauma Association critical decisions in trauma: resuscitative thoracotomy. *J Trauma Acute Care Surg.* 2012;73(6):1359-1363.
8. Brenner M, Bulger EM, Perina DG, et al. Joint Statement from the American college of Surgeons Committee on trauma (ACS COT) and the American College of Emergency Physicians regarding the clinical use of Resuscitative Balloon Occlusion of the Aorta (REBOA). *Trauma Surg Acute Care Open.* 2018;3:1-3.
9. Pasley J, Cannon J, Glaser J, et al. Joint trauma system clinical practice guideline: Resuscitative Endovascular Balloon Occlusion of the Aorta (REBOA) for Hemorrhagic Shock (JTS CPG 38). https://jts.amedd.army.mil/assets/docs/cpgs/JTS_Clinical_Practice_Guidelines_(CPGs)/REBOA_%20Hemorrhagic_Shock_31_Mar_2020_ID38.pdf. Accessed August 1, 2018.
10. Biffl WL, Fox CJ, Moore EE. The role of REBOA in the control of exsanguinating torso hemorrhage. *J Trauma Acute Care Surg.* 2015;78(5):1054-1058.
11. Johnson MA, Williams TK, Ferencz SE, et al. The effect of resuscitative endovascular balloon occlusion of the aorta, partial aortic occlusion and aggressive blood transfusion in traumatic brain injury and a swine multiple injuries model. *J Trauma Acute Care Surg.* 2017;83(1):61-70.
12. Stannard A, Eliason JL, Rasmussen TE. Resuscitative Endovascular Balloon Occlusion of the Aorta (REBOA) as an adjunct for hemorrhagic shock. *J Trauma.* 2011;71(6):1869-1872.
13. Morrison JJ, Galgon RE, Jansen JO, Cannon JW, Rasmussen TE, Eliason JL. A systematic Review of the use of resuscitative endovascular balloon occlusion of the aorta in

the management of hemorrhagic shock. *J Trauma Acute Care Surg*. 2016;80(2):324-334.

14. Seamon MJ, Haut ER, Van Arendonk K, et al. An evidence-based approach to patient selection for emergency department thoracotomy: a practice management guideline from the Eastern Association for the Surgery of Trauma. *J Acute Care Surg*. 2015;79(1):159-173.

15. Monchal T, Martin MJ, Streit S, et al. Joint trauma system clinical practice guideline: Emergent Resuscitative Thoracotomy (ERT) (JTS CPG 20). https://jts.amedd.army.mil/assets/docs/cpgs/JTS_Clinical_Practice_Guidelines_(CPGs)/Emergent_Resuscitative_Thoracotomy_ERT_18_Jul_2018_ID20.pdf. Accessed August 1, 2018.

16. Jacobs LM. The Hartford Consensus III: implementation of bleeding control. *Bull Am Coll Surg*. 2015;100(7):20-26.

17. American College of Surgeons, Committee on Trauma. *Advanced Trauma Life Support Student (ATLS) Course Manual*. 9th ed. Chicago, IL: American College of Surgeons; 2012:9-13.

18. Kragh JF, Walters TJ, Baer DG, et al. Survival with emergency tourniquet use to stop bleeding in major limb trauma. *Ann Surg*. 2009;249(1):1-7.

19. Teixeira PGR, Brown CVR, Emigh B, et al. Civilian prehospital tourniquet use is associated with improved survival in patients with peripheral vascular injury. *J Am Coll Surg*. 2018;226(5):769-776.

20. King DR, Larentzakis A, Ramly EP, Boston Trauma Collaborative. Tourniquet use at the Boston Marathon bombing: lost in translation. *J Trauma Acute Care Surg*. 2015;78(3):594-599.

21. Kragh JF, Lunati MP, Kharod CU, et al. Assessment of groin application of junctional tourniquets in a Manikin model. *Prehosp Disaster Med*. 2016;31(4):358-363.

22. Klotz JK, Leo M, Andersen BL, et al. First case report of SAM(r) Junctional tourniquet use in Afghanistan to control inguinal hemorrhage on the battlefield. *J Spec Oper Med*. 2014;14(2):1-5.

23. Rasmussen TE, Stockinger Z, Antevil J, et al. Joint trauma system clinical practice guideline: vascular injury (JTS CPG 45). https://jts.amedd.army.mil/assets/docs/cpgs/JTS_Clinical_Practice_Guidelines_(CPGs)/Vascular_Injury_12_Aug_2016_ID46.pdf. Accessed August 1, 2018.

24. Sise MJ. Diagnosis of vascular injury. In: Rasmussen TE, Tai NRM, eds. *Rich's Vascular Trauma*. 3rd ed. Philadelphia, PA: Elsevier; 2016:39-40.

25. Johnson ON 3rd, Fox CJ, White P, et al. Physical exam and occult post-traumatic vascular lesions: implications for the evaluation and management of arterial injuries in modern warfare in the endovascular era. *J Cardiovasc Surg (Torino)*. 2007;48(5):581-586.

26. Johansen K, Lynch K, Paun M, Copass M. Non-invasive vascular tests reliably exclude occult arterial trauma in injured extremities. *J Trauma*. 1991;31(4):515-519.

27. Demetriades D, Talving P, Inaba K. Blunt thoracic aortic injury. In: Rasmussen TE, Tai NRM, eds. *Rich's Vascular Trauma*. 3rd ed. Philadelphia, PA: Elsevier; 2016:39-40.

28. Mullenix PS, Steele SR, Andersen CA, Starnes BW, Salim A, Martin MJ. Limb salvage and outcomes among patients with traumatic popliteal vascular injury: an analysis of the National Trauma Data Bank. *J Vasc Surg*. 2006;44:94-100.

29. Bruns BR, Tesoriero R, Kufera J, et al. Blunt cerebrovascular injury screening guidelines: what are we willing to miss? *J Trauma Acute Care Surg*. 2014;76(3):691-695.

30. Bromberg WJ, Collier BC, Diebel LN, et al. Blunt cerebrovascular injury practice management guidelines: the Eastern Association for the Surgery of Trauma. *J Trauma*. 2010;68(2):471-477.

31. Dawson DL. Imaging for the evaluation and treatment of vascular trauma. In: Rasmussen TE, Tai NRM, eds. *Rich's Vascular Trauma*. 3rd ed. Philadelphia, PA: Elsevier; 2016:44-48.

32. White PW, Gillespie DL, Feurstein I, et al. Sixty-four slice multiple detector computed tomographic angiography in the evaluation of vascular trauma. *J Trauma*. 2010;68(1):96-102.

33. Patterson BO, Holt PJ, Cleanthis M, Tai N, Carrell T, Loosemore TM. Imaging vascular trauma. *Br J Surg*. 2012;99:494-505.

Micheal T. Ayad • David L. Gillespie

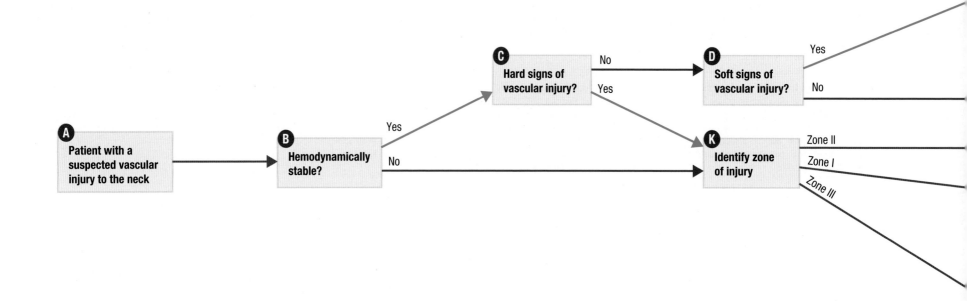

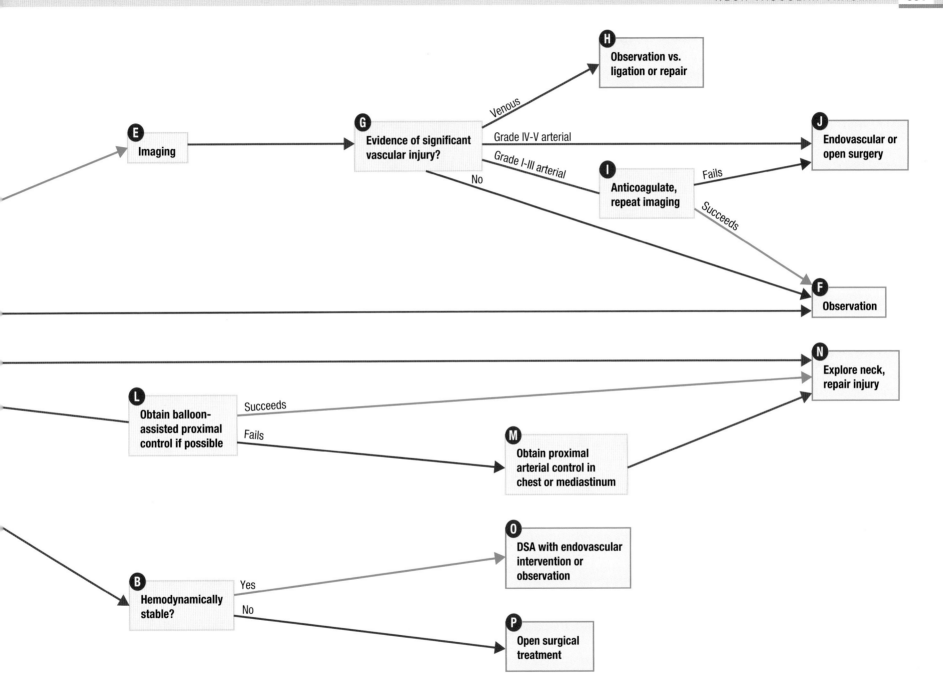

H Observation vs. ligation or repair

E Imaging

G Evidence of significant vascular injury?

Venous

Grade IV-V arterial

Grade I-III arterial

No

I Anticoagulate, repeat imaging

Fails

Succeeds

J Endovascular or open surgery

F Observation

N Explore neck, repair injury

L Obtain balloon-assisted proximal control if possible

Succeeds

Fails

M Obtain proximal arterial control in chest or mediastinum

O DSA with endovascular intervention or observation

B Hemodynamically stable?

Yes

No

P Open surgical treatment

(A) Patient with a suspected vascular injury to the neck

Vascular trauma is a leading cause of death and disability in younger patients and cervical vascular trauma accounts for 11% of such cases.[1,2] In patients with cervical trauma, the incidence of injury to major vascular structures is 25%.[3] Penetrating trauma is most common cause of cervical vascular trauma, with mortality rates ranging from 10% to 30%.[3] Cervical trauma presents a diagnostic and therapeutic challenge because many vital structures in the neck are juxtaposed in a small space. Anatomically, the neck spans the area from the base of the skull to the thoracic outlet. It contains the aerodigestive tract, brachial plexus, and other nerves as well as the carotid, subclavian, and vertebral vessels. Most cervical trauma results in multisystem injury and, therefore, prioritization of treatment complicates clinical decision making.

(B) Hemodynamically stable?

Hemodynamic stability is the first decision point in any trauma management protocol. A stable patient has a blood pressure that supports mentation, usually an SBP > 90 mm Hg, a heart rate between 60 and 100 beats/min, a favorable cardiac rhythm, and a secure airway. As long as there is hemodynamic stability, there is time to utilize appropriate diagnostic techniques and studies to evaluate the patient and ensure that no injuries were missed during the primary survey. Conversely, a hemodynamically unstable patient requires emergent intervention, which is dependent on the location of injury causing the instability.

In a patient with suspected vascular injury to the neck, once a primary trauma survey is performed, a search for vascular injury is undertaken. Significant vascular injury usually produces physical findings that can be detected by a trained examiner. Although a normal physical examination does not rule out a cervical vascular injury requiring treatment, it usually excludes clinically significant vascular injuries. Physical examination findings of vascular injury are classically divided into "hard signs" and "soft signs."

(C) Hard signs of vascular injury?

Hard signs of vascular injury include pulsatile bleeding, expanding hematoma, absent pulses distal to the injury, an audible bruit or a palpable thrill. Patients with hard signs should undergo operative exploration if the mechanism of injury is penetrating and the location of injury is apparent. When the site of injury is unclear (eg, shotgun blast with multiple entry injuries or blunt trauma), preoperative or intraoperative imaging is appropriate.

(D) Soft signs of vascular injury?

Soft signs of vascular injury include a history of prehospital blood loss, diminished pulse, moderate hematoma, and ipsilateral neurologic deficit. Patients with soft signs of vascular injury need to have a thorough evaluation and additional imaging to delineate any occult underlying vascular injury.

(E) Imaging

A normal physical examination does not completely rule out a vascular injury. Thus, patients with soft signs of cervical vascular injury need imaging to exclude an injury that may require treatment. DSA had historically been the gold standard for the diagnosis of vascular injury but has largely been replaced by CTA in the contemporary evaluation of patients with only soft signs of potential vascular injury. CTA has been shown to be accurate in detecting vascular injury in this setting. In a series of 20 patients with combat-related vascular injuries evaluated with 64-slice multidetector CTA, the study was deemed adequate in 94% of cases in yielding sufficiently high-resolution images. Presence of metallic fragments or orthopedic hardware did not interfere significantly with usefulness of imaging.[4-6]

DSA can also assist in the evaluation of potential cervical vascular trauma, particularly in the setting of blunt trauma with associated fractures, penetrating injury to the chest, zones I and III cervical injury, and with multiple pellet wounds. It also can be used intraoperatively if patients with soft signs of cervical vascular trauma were not evaluated with CTA before emergent surgery for other injuries.[7]

(F) Observation

In hemodynamically stable patients with no evidence of hard or soft signs of vascular injury or in hemodynamically stable patients with soft signs of vascular injury but negative imaging, close observation is the preferred approach. Observation obviates unnecessary initial interventions and allows the physician to detect any injury that has been missed on initial evaluation or develops in a delayed manner. Observation with repeat imaging, as needed, is also indicated for patients with mild (grade I-IV) arterial injuries being managed with anticoagulation.

(G) Evidence of significant vascular injury?

CTA evaluation findings direct the management of a patient with soft signs of trauma when no obvious source can be identified. Subsequent management depends on the severity (grade) of carotid or vertebral artery injuries:

Grade I injury: A luminal irregularity or dissection, with <25% narrowing of the lumen, is thought to result from stretching of the artery or a direct blow. Exposure of the thrombogenic subendothelial collagen puts patients at risk for thromboembolic stroke, which occurs in approximately 3% of such patients.[8]

Grade II injury: A dissection or intramural hematoma with ≥25% luminal narrowing, intramural thrombus, or raised intimal flap.

Grade III injury: A PSA that develops secondary to egress of blood into the subadventitial layer and can result from progression of grade II injuries. PSAs pose a risk of rupture, hemorrhage, and thromboembolism.

Grade IV injury is an occlusion, and *grade V injury* is a transection. Both are highly morbid injuries. Some authors feel that outcomes are generally independent of treatment efforts,[9,10] although others have suggested decreased stroke risk with heparin therapy for grade IV lesions.[11]

Bleeding or thrombosis of a major neck vein is not an unusual consequence of penetrating or blunt trauma, respectively. As such, potential venous injury should always be considered, whether it is isolated or associated with concomitant arterial injury.

(H) Observation vs. ligation or repair

Internal jugular vein (IJV) injury occurs in 20% of the victims of penetrating cervical trauma. Isolated injuries can manifest with hard or soft vascular injury signs; however, such patients are seldom unstable.[12] If isolated, venous bleeding will usually tamponade without significant compression of adjacent structures and can be managed conservatively.[12] If associated with other injuries that require neck exploration, ligation or repair can be performed. The IJV can be safely ligated if the injury is unilateral; however, such patients should be closely monitored for possible cerebral edema that is an uncommon but possible complication, especially with bilateral IJV ligation. Bilateral IJV ligation may also result in pseudotumor cerebri. As such, every effort to maintain at least one IJV patent should be made.[13] Venous lacerations involving <50% of the venous wall should be repaired primarily via lateral venography, whereas, lacerations with >50% loss usually need extensive repair using venous interposition or spiral panel grafts. Typically, such techniques do not have a role in acute management of penetrating neck trauma when time is critical.[14]

(I) Anticoagulate, repeat imaging

For grade I-III carotid or vertebral artery injury, anticoagulation is recommended to reduce stroke risk if not contraindicated by other injuries. Over time, 62% of nonocclusive dissections resolve with anticoagulation, supporting the Eastern Association for the Surgery of Trauma recommendations that these patients be treated with antiplatelet or anticoagulation therapy.[9] However, there is no prospective data supporting the type or duration of therapy, and hence treatment should be tailored to the patient, the lesion, and comorbid injuries.

In grade I injuries, exposure of the thrombogenic subendothelial collagen puts patients at increased risk for thromboembolic stroke.[8] Grade II injuries have a 70% risk of progression to grade III or IV despite full anticoagulation and only 10% of these injuries heal completely. Despite this progression rate to a higher grade lesion, anticoagulation seems to be protective against stroke and is recommended. It is recommended that these patients have repeat imaging 7 days postinjury to evaluate for progression.[8,9] Consensus opinion dictates that patients with grade III injuries (PSAs) should be initially anticoagulated or at least treated with antiplatelet agents to reduce stroke risk despite the inherent risk of injury progression. Reimaging should be performed at 7 days postinjury to determine whether aneurysmal growth or progression occurs, in which case endovascular treatment may be needed. For grade IV occlusions, some authors believe that outcomes are generally independent of treatment efforts,[10,11] although others have suggested decreased stroke risk with anticoagulation.[8] If neurologic symptoms suggesting embolization develop, or if repeat imaging shows PSA development, endovascular or open surgical treatment may be indicated.

J Endovascular or open surgery

In patients with grade I-IV carotid vascular injuries who failed medical therapy, surgical treatment is required. Endovascular therapy has gained more traction in recent years as the treatment of choice for surgically inaccessible lesions either as a primary treatment modality or as a temporizing method before more definitive repair, as the patient stabilizes.

In patients with grade I and II injuries, endovascular therapy with self-expanding stents avoids risk of excessive blood loss and possible cranial nerve injury that can occur with open surgery. Antiplatelet therapy must be instituted to assure long-term patency and sequential follow-up imaging is recommended. If accessible, open operative therapy remains the gold therapy with interposition grafting using GSV providing excellent results.[8,10]

Grade III injuries (PSAs) of the more accessible portions of the CCA and ICA are usually managed with open exposure and direct carotid repair.[15] For high cervical grade III injuries, stent-graft placement, with or without coil embolization, is acceptable. However, when concomitant injuries to the aerodigestive tract exist, open reconstruction with wide debridement and muscle coverage is more suitable.

Arterial transection (grade V) with resultant bleeding is treated by open surgical ligation or repair, depending on the extent of injury, neurologic status, and details of injury location. The ECA can be ligated without significant neurologic consequences. Every attempt at repairing the CCA and ICA should be made because outcomes are much worse in cases of ligation. Ligation should be reserved for severely unstable patients where repair and/or temporary shunting is not feasible and would delay management of other life-threatening injuries.

Management of the vertebral artery is also largely dependent on the patient's stability and the side of dominance of the vertebral artery. If the injury is to the nondominant vertebral artery, ligation is acceptable, particularly in an unstable patient. In general, the principle is to ligate the artery in unstable patients with multiple life-threatening injuries, and repair it in stable patients.[10]

K Identify zone of injury

In hemodynamically unstable patients or those with hard signs of vascular injury, emergent intervention is paramount to save life and/or function. In 1969, Monson et al. described three zones of cervical trauma with implications for technique of exposure and exploration.[13] Zone 1 encompasses the root of the neck and is defined by the area of the neck below the clavicles. Zone 2 spans between the clavicles and the angle of mandible. Zone 3 refers to the area of the neck superior to the angle of the mandible. More recently, a minor modification to the demarcation of the zones of the neck changed the anatomic delineations to zone 1 extending from the clavicles/sternum to the cricoid cartilage, zone 2 from the cricoid cartilage to the angle of the mandible, and zone 3 extending cephalad to the base of the skull.[16] In hemodynamically stable patients, if the zone of injury is not clear, preoperative CTA or intraoperative DSA may be required to more precisely plan treatment.

L Obtain balloon-assisted proximal control if possible

There are several damage control options available to mitigate vascular injuries in the neck. For injuries in zone I, balloon-assisted proximal control is valuable while expeditious preparation proceeds for definitive control. Using femoral or brachial access and fluoroscopic guidance, it may be possible to insert an over-the-wire occluding balloon for rapid proximal control of a bleeding innominate, CCA, or SCA. The balloon is sized to the estimated diameter of the proximal common carotid, subclavian, or innominate artery and inflated to nominal pressure when proximal control is needed for control of hemorrhage and during repair. Challenges to this approach occur in patients with aortoiliac occlusion, those with difficult aortic arch anatomy, and patients with shaggy atherosclerotic aortic arch disease. These technical challenges and their potential for complications should be weighed against the risk of hemorrhage associated with open proximal control. An additional advantage of intraluminal balloon occlusion is that a determination of the patient's tolerance to ligation can be determined; if the patient manifests focal neurologic deficit with occlusion, some form of repair with revascularization should be done, if at all possible.

M Obtain proximal arterial control in chest or mediastinum

In zone 1 injuries, if proximal balloon control is not possible, open surgical control must be obtained in the chest/mediastinum. For a penetrating injury above or below the left clavicle, the best approach for open control of the proximal left SCA is through an incision in the third interspace of the left chest. This high anterolateral thoracotomy allows adequate visualization of the root of the left SCA to gain vascular control. Once controlled, the surgeon can explore and repair the injured SCA through the standard supraclavicular incision.

The most common approach for open control of zone 1 vascular injuries is via a median sternotomy. This affords access to the ascending aorta, the brachiocephalic vein, and the pulmonary artery. The transverse aortic arch may be reached through this incision, although it may require a cervical extension. To fully control the innominate artery or the right subclavian artery or vein, the median sternotomy is extended to include a right cervical incision. Extension of the sternotomy into a left cervical incision will provide access to the left CCA. The mid- and distal left subclavian artery and vein are more challenging to access and require a left anterolateral thoracotomy in the third or fourth interspace, coupled with a left supraclavicular incision. Connecting these incisions with a vertical sternotomy is the "trapdoor" incision, which is much discussed but associated with significant morbidity and risk of causalgia.

N Explore neck, repair injury

Zone II major vascular injuries often require open exposure and repair. A cervical incision along the anterior border of the sternocleidomastoid muscle (extended CEA incision) is used. If bleeding is noted to be originating from a more proximal source, the cervical incision can be extended into a median sternotomy with an option to perform a trap door anterior thoracotomy, as needed. Alternatively, balloon occlusion of the arch vessel may be possible (see L). In some cases, rapid insertion of a balloon catheter (such as a Foley) into the penetrating wound tract, followed by inflation and outward traction may provide tamponade and temporize bleeding while preparations for definitive repair is made.

If bilateral cervical vascular injuries are present, either a transverse Kocher incision or bilateral cervical incisions will gain exposure to both carotid sheaths. If the arterial injury is known to involve only the left SCA, a supraclavicular incision can be utilized for exposure of the mid-to-distal left SCA. An infraclavicular incision can be utilized for exposure of the distal right and left subclavian arteries and the proximal axillary arteries.

Surgical options for repair include primary repair, bypass graft with autogenous vein or prosthetic graft, patch graft, or external carotid to internal carotid transposition for injuries near the carotid bulb. Liekweg et al. demonstrated improved outcomes for revascularization over ligation in noncomatose patients. However, in comatose patients, these authors recommend repair only if there is evidence of prograde flow.[17] Current practice is to revascularize all patients with penetrating injury regardless of neurologic deficits except for coma. Patients with Glasgow Coma Score <8 that is not related to hypovolemia, hypothermia, or intoxication are likely to have an adverse outcome regardless of management. If the presentation is delayed more than 3 to 4 hours postinjury, a head CT scan should be obtained. If an ischemic stroke is present, revascularization is contraindicated, because this may convert to a hemorrhagic infarct. In that setting, ligation is performed. If bypass grafting is performed for revascularization, ePTFE is appropriate for CCA injuries while autogenous vein should be used for ICA repairs given improved patency rates.[18] Prosthetic grafts should be avoided if possible in contaminated wounds.[19] If surgical repair is performed, a careful search for injury to other structures, especially the aerodigestive tract, is initiated. If such an injury is encountered, in addition to repair, the vascular suture line should be isolated by means of interposition of vascularized tissue. In this example, sternocleidomastoid muscle can be detached from its sternal head and rotated to cover the repair.

Vertebral artery injuries create varying degrees of difficulty for exposure based on the location of the injury. Most amenable to surgical repair are V1 segment injuries (origin to C6 transverse foramen). Exposure of the V1 segment is gained by retracting the sternocleidomastoid muscle laterally and the carotid sheath medially. The dissection is continued medial to the anterior scalene muscle until the vertebral vein is identified. If needed, the anterior scalene muscle can be divided to provide access to the SCA. Ligation and division of the vertebral vein allows excellent exposure of the V1 segment. Primary repair, transposition to the carotid artery, or GSV reconstruction provides options for open surgical repair. If the patient is deemed unstable, ligation should be considered. If the injury is more cephalad on the vertebral artery (V2 segment or higher), exposure is much more involved. Ligation of the V1 segment may be needed to control more distal hemorrhage. If direct exposure is required to the V2 segment, similar retraction of the sternocleidomastoid muscle and carotid sheath is performed. The cervical spine transverse processes are exposed after division of the anterior longitudinal ligament and paraspinous muscles. The anterior portion of the transverse processes is excised with a rongeur to provide access to the vertebral artery. Surgical repair in this tight space is difficult and hemorrhage control should be the main operative objective.

ⓞ DSA with endovascular intervention or observation

Owing to the difficulty in exposure and control of zone III injuries, endovascular treatment is the preferred option if the patient is hemodynamically stable. Selective DSA including intracranial anatomy is important to determine whether arterial occlusion will likely be tolerated because of adequate cerebral collateral circulation. The types of injuries that can be present with blunt and penetrating trauma are similar, although in the setting of blunt trauma, major arterial wall disruption is less likely. Endovascular therapy options include PTA to tack down intimal flaps and coil embolization and stents for PSAs. For intramural hematomas, intimal defects, or dissection with preserved distal flow, heparinization is appropriate for both grades I and II blunt injuries. Stenting may be needed to tack down the intima. If observation is selected as the treatment plan, repeat imaging is necessary in 1 to 2 weeks to ensure resolution of the lesion.

PSAs with contrast extravasation should be either observed (for small aneurysms) or stented with or without coil embolization. According to Feliciano, use of heparin is risky in this situation given the possibility of rupture.[18] Antiplatelet therapy should be used if a stent is placed. Nonetheless, results of more recent studies have been somewhat contradictory regarding antiplatelet versus anticoagulation therapy.[16] The consensus opinion from 2010 EAST guidelines suggest anticoagulation therapy while being alert toward the risk of bleeding associated with aggressive antithrombotic therapy.[9] For occlusions, anticoagulation is recommended to prevent distal thrombus propagation or embolization.

ⓟ Open surgical treatment

Zone III injuries in hemodynamically unstable patients require open surgical exposure and control. Nasal intubation and division of the posterior belly of the digastric muscle helps with distal exposure and subluxation of the mandible may be needed. In this zone, control of the distal ICA is particular difficult due to the anatomic constraints. Other methods to gain distal control are balloon occlusion devices with access through the CCA or site of injury. For resistant bleeding high in zone III, packing of the carotid canal with bone wax may allow tamponade for life-saving purposes.[18] After hemostasis is achieved with a damage control strategy, options include formal high cervical exploration for repair or ligation, arteriographic embolization or/and stenting, or 48-hour ICA balloon occlusion. In the 48-hour balloon occlusion technique, the Fogarty balloon is filled with contrast and the patient is monitored for signs of cerebral ischemia. If there is no sign of ischemia, the balloon remains in place until 48 to 72 hours postplacement, at which time it is deflated and removed. The patient should be imaged with a crossover arteriogram to rule out a PSA above the occlusion. If the patient manifests signs of ischemia, a bypass from the cervical ICA to the petrous ICA may be necessary and this requires the assistance of a neurosurgeon.[18] Surgical options for repair include ligation, primary repair, bypass graft with autogenous vein or prosthetic graft, patch graft, or external carotid to internal carotid transposition for injuries near the carotid bulb.[19] If bypass grafting is needed, autogenous vein should be used for ICA repairs given favorable size match and patency rates.[20]

Open surgical exposure and repair of zone III vertebral artery injuries pose a significant challenge to experienced vascular and trauma surgeons. Similar to zone II injuries, the vertebral artery in the zone III location is surrounded in the bony vertebral canal, making surgical visualization for repair difficult. Rather than proceeding with an arduous attempt at proper exposure, ligation of the V1 vertebral segment provides the most expeditious management. Follow-up endoluminal therapy with embolization is preferred if the patient demonstrates signs of continuous hemorrhage. If operative exposure

is deemed necessary, the sternocleidomastoid muscle should be divided from the skull base. Dissection in this region should expose the mastoid process. C1 and C2 lie just inferior to the mastoid process. Division of the muscle attachments to C1 and C2 allows for exposure of the V3 portion of the vertebral artery. Although V2 can be accessed by resection of the lateral process of the cervical process with a rongeur, this dissection is difficult.

REFERENCES

1. Daou B, Alkhalili K, Chalouhi N, et al. Epidemiology, pathophysiology, and treatment of traumatic cervical vascular injury. *Semin Spine Surg.* 2017;29(1):27-33.
2. Patel JA, White JM, White PW, Rich NM, Rasmussen TE. A contemporary, 7-year analysis of vascular injury from the war in Afghanistan. *J Vasc Surg.* 2018;68(6):1872-1879.
3. Kumar S, Weaver FA. Vascular injuries of the neck. In: *Emergency Vascular and Endovascular Surgical Practice.* 2nd ed. Boca Raton, FL: CRC Press; 2005:419.
4. White PW, Gillespie DL, Feurstein I, et al. Sixty-four slice multidetector computed tomographic angiography in the evaluation of vascular trauma. *J Trauma.* 2010;68(1): 96-102.
5. Schroeder JW, Ptak T, Corey AS, et al. ACR Appropriateness Criteria® penetrating neck injury. *J Am Coll Radiol.* 2017;14(11):S500-S505.
6. Greer LT, Kuehn RB, Gillespie DL, et al. Contemporary management of combat-related vertebral artery injuries. *J Trauma Acute Care Surg.* 2013;74(3):818-824.
7. Johnson ON, Fox CJ, O'Donnell S, et al. Arteriography in the delayed evaluation of wartime extremity injuries. *Vasc Endovascular Surg.* 2007;41(3):217-224.
8. Biffl WL, Moore EE, Offner PJ, Brega KE, Franciose RJ, Burch JM. Blunt carotid arterial injuries: implications of a new grading scale. *J Trauma.* 1999;47(5):845-853.
9. Bromberg WJ, Collier BC, Diebel LN, et al. Blunt cerebrovascular injury practice management guidelines: the Eastern Association for the Surgery of Trauma. *J Trauma.* 2010;68(2):471-477.
10. Karaolanis G, Maltezos K, Bakoyiannis C, Georgopoulos S. Contemporary strategies in the management of civilian neck zone II vascular trauma. *Front Surg.* 2017;4:56.
11. Wahl WL, Brandt MM, Thompson BG, Taheri PA, Greenfield LJ. Antiplatelet therapy: an alternative to heparin for blunt carotid injury. *J Trauma.* 2002;52(5):896-901.
12. Madsen AS, Bruce JL, Oosthuizen GV, Bekker W, Laing GL, Clarke DL. The selective non-operative management of penetrating cervical venous trauma is safe and effective. *World J Surg.* 2018;42(10):3202-3209.
13. Monson DO, Saletta JD, Freeark RJ. Carotid vertebral trauma. *J Trauma.* 1969;9(12):987-999.

14. Comerota AJ, Harwick RD, White JV. Jugular venous reconstruction: a technique to minimize morbidity of bilateral radical neck dissection. *J Vasc Surg*. 1986;3:322-329. doi:10.1016/0741-5214(86)90017-0.

15. Magge D, Farber A, Vladimir F, et al. Diagnosis and management of traumatic pseudoaneurysm of the carotid artery: case report and review of the literature. *Vascular*. 2008;16:350-355.

16. Sperry JL, Moore EE, Coimbra R, et al. Western Trauma Association critical decisions in trauma: penetrating neck trauma. *J Trauma Acute Care Surg*. 2013;75(6):936-940.

17. Liekweg WG Jr, Greenfield LJ. Management of penetrating carotid arterial injury. *Ann Surg*. 1978;188(5):587-592.

18. Feliciano DV. Management of penetrating injuries to carotid artery. *World J Surg*. 2001;25(8):1028-1035. Review. Erratum in: *World J Surg*. 2002;26(2):284.

19. Fox CJ, Gillespie DL, Weber MA, et al. Delayed evaluation of combat-related penetrating neck trauma. *J Vasc Surg*. 2006;44(1):86-93.

20. Rostomily RC, Newell DW, Grady MS, Wallace S, Nicholls S, Winn HR. Gunshot wounds of the internal carotid artery at the skull base: management with vein bypass grafts and a review of the literature. *J Trauma*. 1997;42(1):123-132.

Bruce Tjaden • Ali Azizzadeh

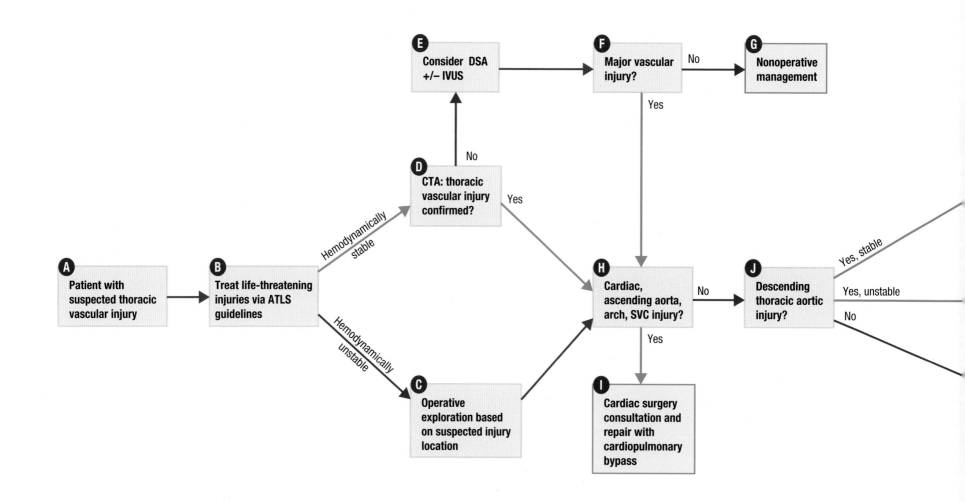

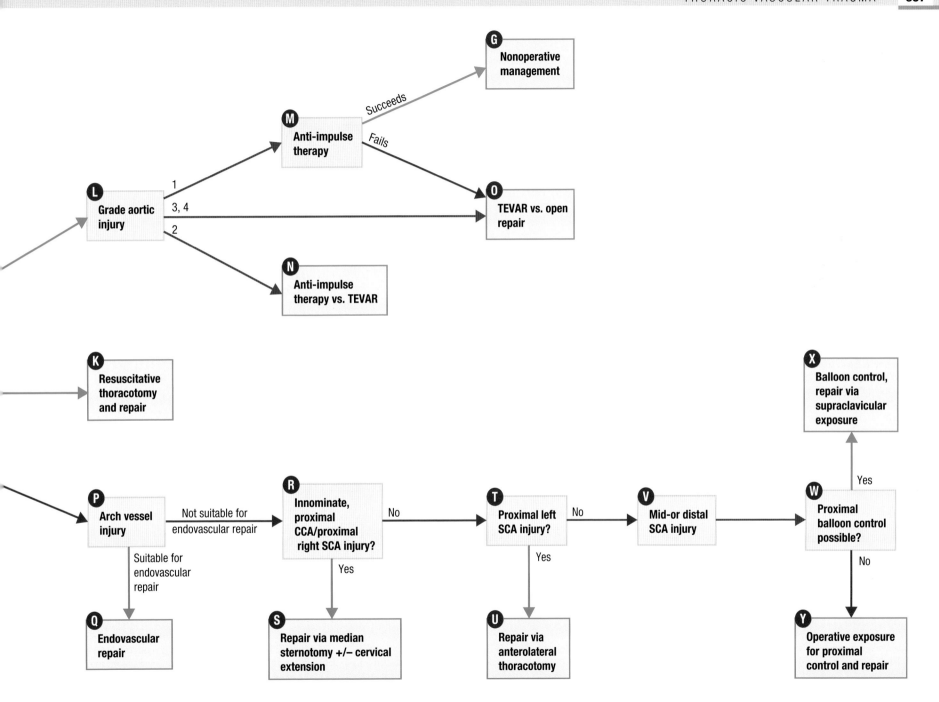

A Patient with suspected thoracic vascular injury

Both blunt and penetrating trauma have the potential to cause thoracic vascular injury (TVI). Blunt trauma is more common, and aortic injury is second only to head trauma in causes of death due to blunt force. The majority of blunt TVIs occur because of motor vehicle accidents.[1] Vascular injury may be suggested by hard signs (absent pulse, pulsatile hemorrhage, expanding hematoma, palpable thrill, audible bruit) or soft signs (mechanism/impact of injury, history of major hemorrhage, stable hematoma, diminished pulse, associated neurologic deficit, or proximity to a named vessel). Alternatively, hemodynamic instability due to internal bleeding may be the only manifestation of TVI.

B Treat life-threatening injuries via ATLS guidelines

Each patient with trauma should be treated according to ATLS guidelines. Specifically, these recommend the stepwise assessment and treatment of life-threatening injuries in a protocolized, orderly manner in every case depending on Airway, Breathing, Circulation, and Disability. The presence of a suspected TVI should not cause the treating physician to deviate from this pathway. Specifically, measures to secure a patent airway and air exchange should take precedence. After any necessary steps such as intubation to establish an airway have been performed, assessment of the patient's circulatory status can commence and TVI, if identified, may be treated. In some cases, placement of a chest tube during ATLS resuscitation may yield voluminous bleeding via the thoracostomy tube. In this case, the tube may need to be intermittently clamped (to prevent exsanguination) and released (to prevent tension hemothorax) as the patient is taken to the operating room. In this situation, we would usually proceed with a generous lateral thoracotomy to identify and repair the source of bleeding.

C Operative exploration based on suspected injury location

If the patient is hemodynamically unstable, immediate operative intervention should be undertaken with the surgeon's suspicion as to the likely site of injury dictating positioning, prepping, draping, and incision (see H and beyond). REBOA may be considered in selected patients with noncompressible torso hemorrhage below the diaphragm.

D CTA: thoracic vascular injury confirmed?

In patients who have TVI and are hemodynamically stable, imaging is obtained to guide intervention. Notably, this differs from the management of peripheral vascular trauma, in which the presence of hard signs would typically lead to exploration without imaging. Imaging for TVI is critical because of the widely different approaches that may be required to treat a TVI depending on the nature of the pathology (dissection vs. transection, active bleeding

vs. thrombosis and ischemia) and the specific relationship of the injury relative to the thoracic cage and major arterial branches. CTA provides excellent information about the type and location of injury that can guide the intervention and aid in device selection.[2] Furthermore, imaging findings such as active extravasation, perivascular fluid, and/or associated hematoma or hemothorax can provide useful information as to the severity of the injury and the need for emergent intervention.

E Consider DSA +/− IVUS

If CTA is nondiagnostic or cannot be obtained, consideration should be given to DSA with or without IVUS to identify and delineate the injury. IVUS is a useful adjunct to CTA, especially in cases where the CTA findings are equivocal or nondiagnostic. Examples include patients with a mediastinal hematoma without an identifiable aortic injury. In addition, some minor aortic injuries are more readily identifiable on IVUS when compared to CTA and DSA.[3] After a TVI has been localized, management can be planned.

F Major vascular injury?

Major TVI may be defined as injuries to medium or large vessels with active extravasation, impending rupture, or significant flow limitation. These injuries will likely require intervention, and, as such, mandate a careful consideration of risks and benefits of treatment strategies. On the other hand, minor TVI is defined as limited injuries to medium or large arteries, disruption of noncritical small arterial branches, and most venous injuries. Many of these minor TVIs can be managed without intervention.

G Nonoperative management

In patients with minor TVI, nonoperative management may be pursued unless there is need for surgical treatment of nonvascular injuries. If a patient is managed nonoperatively, close clinical follow-up is required, and repeat imaging (usually in the form of CTA) may be needed. For example, in a severely injured patient with a focal, nonflow limiting dissection in the SCA identified on initial trauma CT, we would obtain a brachial-brachial index, follow up the patient with serial neurovascular examinations, and repeat cross-sectional imaging in 24 to 72 hours.

H Cardiac, ascending aorta, arch, SVC injury?

Injury to the heart itself, the ascending aorta, the transverse arch, or the vena cava can be catastrophic. It has been suggested that only 3.5% to 5% of patients with blunt traumatic cardiac injuries will survive to hospitalization.[4] In one large autopsy series, cardiac injuries were present in 32% of blunt trauma fatalities, and the vast majority (78%) of the patients with cardiac injuries died on the scene.[5] Blunt injuries to the ascending aorta and/or aortic arch have been associated with an in-hospital mortality rate of 53%, and a 10-year survival of only 19%.[6] Penetrating injuries to the

heart or ascending aorta fare better than do blunt injuries, but are associated with high rates of prehospital and in-hospital mortality.[7] Data on SVC injury are sparse, but reports suggest that only 7% of patients with SVC injury will survive to be admitted.[8]

I Cardiac surgery consultation and repair with cardiopulmonary bypass

Repairs of these injuries are associated with a significant risk of mortality (57% in a contemporary large series) and should be undertaken by a cardiac surgeon.[9] A full discussion of the operative techniques for these injuries is outside the scope of this chapter.

J Descending thoracic aortic injury?

Injury to the descending thoracic aorta (DTA) most commonly occurs because of blunt trauma. Although blunt DTA injury is not extremely common (0.4% of trauma in our institutional registry),[10] it does carry a significant risk of mortality. More than 30% of blunt trauma fatalities in a large autopsy study were found to have a DTA injury.[11] The aorta is usually damaged near areas of anatomic fixation (eg, the ligamentum arteriosum, the bronchus, or the diaphragmatic hiatus). Penetrating trauma of the DTA is much less common, and usually presents as massive left-sided hemothorax or cardiac arrest due to hemorrhage. The mechanism of injury is less important than the patient's clinical status when determining management options.

K Resuscitative thoracotomy and repair

The management of cardiovascular collapse associated with DTA injury involves resuscitative emergency room thoracotomy. In this case, an expedient left anterolateral thoracotomy is performed. The left lung is retracted anteriorly and the aorta is identified. A clamp is placed distal to the origin of the left SCA artery. Care should be taken to avoid injury to the esophagus during clamp placement. The patient is rapidly transported to the operating room with the clamp in place for definitive repair.

L Grade aortic injury

DTA trauma is graded on the basis of the anatomy of the injury, because this determines management: grade 1 = intimal flap; grade 2 = intramural hematoma (IMH) or dissection; grade 3 = PSA; grade 4 = rupture.[12] Increasing injury grade is associated with increasing aortic-related mortality, and therefore higher grade injuries are treated more aggressively.[13] In a contemporary study, aortic-related mortality was significantly greater in grade 4 (37.5%) than in grade 3 (1.6%) and grades 1 and 2 (0%) injuries.[13] Most patients with a TVI involving the DTA who survive to reach the CT scanner or the operating room without a resuscitative thoracotomy will have had a blunt mechanism, and almost all of the following discussion arises from the blunt trauma literature. However, the same principles can be applied to penetrating mechanisms as well.

Ⓜ Anti-impulse therapy

Grade 1 injuries are intimal injuries, characterized by an intimal flap without external contour abnormality of the aortic wall. These are managed with anti-impulse therapy, consisting of pharmacologic treatment to achieve an SBP <120 and heart rate <60.[14,15] This is usually accomplished with labetalol and/or nicardipine infusions, because they are highly efficacious and easily titratable. These patients should undergo repeat CTA after 10 days to evaluate the injury for resolution, stability, or progression. If the lesion has not healed, repeat imaging after 4 to 6 weeks is recommended. Occasionally, the presence of a concomitant brain injury may preclude anti-impulse therapy (the requirement for an increased cerebral perfusion pressure may necessitate an SBP >120). In that case, or if appropriate SBP and heart rate parameters are simply not attainable, medical management will be impossible, and repair should be pursued.

Ⓝ Anti-impulse therapy vs. TEVAR

Grade 2 injuries involve the media of the aorta, and are characterized by an IMH with an external contour abnormality of the aorta, or a focal dissection. Until now, it has been recommended that these injuries be repaired, rather than medically managed.[15] However, this practice is evolving. In a recent survey conducted by the Aortic Trauma Foundation, respondents were equally divided between medical therapy and interventional therapy for grade 2 injuries.[16] We tend to approach these on a "case-by-case" basis, making an individualized decision depending on the size of the aortic injury, the severity of associated injuries, the overall condition of the patient, and the likelihood of patient compliance with medical therapy. For less severe grade 2 injuries, or in patients with other injuries that would make TEVAR very difficult, we have successfully employed medical management with very good outcomes, although with a slightly longer time to injury resolution when compared to grade 1 injuries.[17] For more significant grade 2 lesions, we typically intervene within 24 to 72 hours, after other associated injuries have been addressed (eg, laparotomy with control of intra-abdominal bleeding, fixation of unstable fractures). The safety of this delayed approach has been well demonstrated.[9,18-22]

TEVAR compares favorably to open surgery in the setting of blunt TVI involving the DTA,[9,23-25] and has been implemented in penetrating trauma as well.[26,27] The extent of aortic injury is usually fairly limited and well defined, although we often use IVUS to corroborate CT or angiographic findings and to ensure that the area of pathology is completely covered. In most cases, a short aortic stent graft (10 cm) will suffice. Oversizing is generally in accordance with the manufacturer's IFU, although we tend to err on the side of "less oversizing" in the setting of TEVAR for DTA TVI, as opposed to TEVAR for aneurysm. If coverage of the left SCA is required to obtain a proximal seal, we will do so in the absence of absolute contraindications (a previous CABG using a left internal mammary, a left vertebral artery terminating in a posterior inferior cerebellar artery [PICA], an occluded/absent right vertebral artery, or a patent left arm dialysis access). As suggested by the current Society for Vascular Surgery (SVS) guidelines, in the setting of trauma, coverage of the left SCA in the absence of absolute contraindications is associated with very low risk of complications.[15,28-30] If the left SCA is covered, we follow the patient postoperatively for signs of left upper extremity ischemia (arm pain with exertion, rest pain, vertebrobasilar insufficiency), and perform left SCA to carotid transposition or left carotid to SCA bypass with proximal SCA plugging/embolization if needed. Owing to the short extent of coverage and low risk of spinal cord ischemia, CSF drainage is not routinely used in TEVAR for TVI.[15] If bleeding from other traumatic injuries is a major concern, we will perform TEVAR with little or no systemic heparin.[15] We generally perform TEVAR for trauma via percutaneous access in one groin. The arterial puncture is "preclosed" using Proglide devices (Abbott, Abbott Park, IL), and the suture tail are tagged and left long for tightening at the completion of the operation. A floppy wire and marker pigtail catheter are used for initial DSA. The large sheath and thoracic endograft are delivered over a stiff wire (eg, Lunderquist wire; Cook Medical, Bloomington, IN). Additional angiography can be performed via the ipsilateral site using a "buddy wire" or the contralateral groin for sheath-less devices. After device deployment, completion DSA, and percutaneous hemostasis, the patients are generally transferred back to the ICU for neurovascular checks. Blood pressure and heart rate goals may be immediately liberalized after TEVAR. Midterm follow-up has demonstrated excellent results with low rates of complications after TEVAR for trauma, with technical success reported at >93%, and morality ranging between 4% and 9%.[10,31] CTA surveillance to identify and treat endograft-related complications is recommended (typically at 1 month, 6 months, 12 months, and yearly thereafter).

Ⓞ TEVAR vs. open repair

Grade 3 injuries are transmedial injuries, and are characterized by a PSA outpouching with an external contour abnormality of the aorta. Grade 4 injuries include frank ruptures and transections. Grade 3 injuries are treated urgently (<24 hours), whereas grade 4 injuries are treated emergently. There is a trend toward delayed repair (>24 hours) of stable grade 3 injuries,[16] with the exact time of intervention individualized depending on the presence of associated injuries and the overall condition of the patient. Coordination between other teams is necessary to ensure the most life-threatening injuries are addressed first. TEVAR is preferred to treat these injuries whenever possible. For grade 3 or 4 injuries, if TEVAR is not possible, open surgery is preferred over anti-impulse therapy. This is associated with significant risk of mortality (estimated at 13%-31% for open repair of DTA injury[10,32]) because medical management has not been validated in these high-grade aortic injuries. Open repair is performed with the patient positioned in the right lateral decubitus position with a dual-lumen endotracheal tube. A left lateral thoracotomy incision is made and the left lung is deflated. Left heart bypass with distal aortic perfusion is initiated after cannulating the left inferior pulmonary vein and either the left CFA or the distal DTA below the level of the injury. The aorta is clamped and opened, and the injured DTA is replaced with a large-diameter Dacron prosthesis, using a 4-0 polypropylene suture for the anastomoses.[12]

Ⓟ Arch vessel injury

Major injuries to the brachiocephalic vessels are uncommon, but are highly lethal—for example, blunt innominate injury is associated with a prehospital mortality rate of >90%.[33] Some of these injuries may be amenable to endovascular treatment, although open repair may be required in some cases, depending on the anatomy and severity of the injury. Specifically, consideration must be given to the proximity of any critical branches (a dominant vertebral artery, the origin of the right CCA, or a patent left internal mammary to coronary bypass graft), the size and length of the proximal/distal landing zones in the injured vessel (to ensure that appropriately sized devices are available), and the patient's access options (ideally, an accessible ipsilateral brachial or axillary artery and either femoral artery). When possible, endovascular repair is pursued.

Ⓠ Endovascular repair

Endovascular repair is an especially useful modality in SCA injuries, because the open exposure of this artery is associated with significant morbidity and mortality, and modern endovascular devices have demonstrated excellent results in this location.[34] In one series encompassing patients from two academic trauma centers, endovascular repair of axillo-SCA arterial injuries was associated with a statistically significant decrease in mortality (6% vs. 28%) and surgical site infections (0% vs. 26%) when compared to open repair.[34] In a review of published experience with axillo-SCA stent grafting for trauma, technical success was 97% with patency at 70 months of 84%.[35] In general, nitinol devices seem to perform significantly better than stainless steel devices in this location, and historical high failure rates reflect the use of earlier generation steel devices.[36] The proximal innominate or CCA injuries may also be treatable via endovascular means, although the risk of stroke should not be ignored. Data on the endovascular treatment of these vessels are sparse, and further research is needed in this area.

Ⓡ Innominate, proximal CCA/proximal right SCA injury?

The innominate artery, the proximal CCA, or the proximal right SCA artery are located centrally within the chest. Open repair of these injuries requires wide central exposure.

S Repair via median sternotomy +/− cervical extension

The procedure is initiated by incising the skin and subcutaneous tissue from the sternal notch to approximately the third intercostal space (for an upper sternotomy) or to the xiphoid process (for a full sternotomy).[37] The sternum is cleared of its anterior fascial attachments using electrocautery. The soft tissue behind the upper aspect of the sternum is cleared away using blunt finger dissection. A reciprocating saw is used to perform the sternotomy, and a Finochietto retractor is used to spread the two halves of the sternum laterally. The innominate vein may need to be retracted or divided to facilitate exposure of the great vessels. Proximal control can be achieved with clamp placement just distal to the arch. Distal control may require cervical extension of the incision onto the right or left neck—this is placed over the medial aspect of the sternocleidomastoid muscle, similar to the incision for a CEA. Vessel repair or interposition bypass is typically performed using a Dacron conduit.

T Proximal left SCA injury?

The proximal left SCA is located very posteriorly, and is not reliably reached through a median sternotomy.

U Repair via anterolateral thoracotomy

These injuries should be approached through a high left anterolateral thoracotomy. This is performed via a transverse incision over the third or fourth intercostal space, centered on the mid-clavicular line. After entering the pleural space above the rib, the left lung is retracted inferiorly and the proximal left SCA can be identified and clamped. Distal control can typically be achieved via a transverse supraclavicular incision. If further exposure of the intervening segment of the left SCA is needed, an upper median sternotomy can be performed, connecting the two previously exposed areas via a "trapdoor" approach.

V Mid- or distal SCA injury

Injuries to the mid- or distal SCA can be very challenging because of their location deep to the clavicle.

W Proximal balloon control possible?

If the proximal SCA is uninjured and major aortic/iliofemoral occlusive disease is absent, proximal balloon occlusion via femoral access should be considered, because this may obviate the need for a sternotomy or thoracotomy for proximal clamp placement.

X Balloon control, repair via supraclavicular exposure

Balloon occlusion may be achieved via a transfemoral approach. After establishing access in the usual manner, a long stiff wire can be placed into the ascending aorta, allowing for a sheath exchange for a 90-cm-long braided support sheath (7-9F, depending on the diameter of the required occlusion balloon). An angled catheter can be used to select the injured vessel with a soft wire, and an appropriately sized angioplasty balloon be positioned and inflated for proximal control. In the case of right-sided SCA injuries, heparinization should be strongly considered (other injuries permitting), because the wire and balloon catheter will need to traverse the arch. Distal control will require a periclavicular incision (usually supraclavicular) or rarely a mini-sternotomy.[38,39]

Y Operative exposure for proximal control and repair

If balloon occlusion is not possible, open exposure for both proximal and distal control should be obtained as described earlier.

Acknowledgment

The authors acknowledge Chris Akers, MA, for his assistance with the initial draft of the decision tree.

REFERENCES

1. Karmy-Jones R, Jurkovich GJ. Blunt chest trauma. *Curr Probl Surg.* 2004;41(3):211-380.
2. Mirvis SE, Shanmuganathan K, Miller BH, White CS, Turney SZ. Traumatic aortic injury: diagnosis with contrast-enhanced thoracic CT—five-year experience at a major trauma center. *Radiology.* 1996;200(2):413-422.
3. Azizzadeh A, Valdes J, Miller CC 3rd, et al. The utility of intravascular ultrasound compared to angiography in the diagnosis of blunt traumatic aortic injury. *J Vasc Surg.* 2011;53(3):608-614.
4. Fedakar R, Türkmen N, Durak D, Gündoğmuş UN. Fatal traumatic heart wounds: review of 160 autopsy cases. *Isr Med Assoc J.* 2005;7(8):498-501.
5. Teixeira P, Georgiou C, Inaba K, et al. Blunt cardiac trauma: lessons learned from the medical examiner. *J Trauma.* 2009;67(6):1259-1264.
6. Mosquera V, Marini M, Muñiz J, et al. Blunt traumatic aortic injuries of the ascending aorta and aortic arch: a clinical multicentre study. *Injury.* 2013;44(9):1191-1197.
7. Baillot R, Dontigny L, Verdant A, et al. Intrapericardial trauma: surgical experience. *J Trauma.* 1989;29(6):736-740.
8. Oschsner J, Crawford S, Debakey M. Injuries of the vena cava caused by external trauma. *Surgery.* 1961;49(3):397-405.
9. Estrera AL, Gochnour DC, Azizzadeh A, et al. Progress in the treatment of blunt thoracic aortic injury: 12-year single-institution experience. *Ann Thorac Surg.* 2010;90(1):64-71.
10. Estrera A, Miller C, Guajardo-Salinas G, et al. Update on blunt thoracic aortic injury: fifteen-year single-institution experience. *J Thorac Cardiovasc Surg.* 2013;145(3):S154-S158.
11. Teixeira P, Inaba K, Barmparas G, et al. Blunt thoracic aortic injuries: an autopsy study. *J Trauma.* 2011;70(1):197-202.
12. Azizzadeh A, Keyhani K, Miller CC 3rd, Coogan SM, Safi HJ, Estrera AL. Blunt traumatic aortic injury: initial experience with endovascular repair. *J Vasc Surg.* 2009;49(6):1403-1408.
13. Fortuna GRJ, Perlick A, DuBose JJ, et al. Injury grade is a predictor of aortic-related death among patients with blunt thoracic aortic injury. *J Vasc Surg.* 2016;63(5):1225-1231.
14. Fabian TC, Davis KA, Gavant ML, et al. Prospective study of blunt aortic injury: helical CT is diagnostic and antihypertensive therapy reduces rupture. *Ann Surg.* 1998;227(5):666-667.
15. Lee WA, Matsumura JS, Mitchell RS, et al. Endovascular repair of traumatic thoracic aortic injury: clinical practice guidelines of the Society for Vascular Surgery. *J Vasc Surg.* 2011;53(1):187-192. doi:10.1016/j.jvs.2010.08.027.
16. DeSoucy E, Loja M, DuBose J, Estrera A, Starnes B, Azizzadeh A. Contemporary management of blunt thoracic aortic injury: results of an EAST, AAST and SVS survey by the Aortic Trauma Foundation. *J Endovasc Resusc Trauma Manag.* 2017;1(1):4-8. https://www.jevtm.com/journal/index.php/jevtm/article/view/8/6.
17. Sandhu HK, Leonard SD, Perlick A, et al. Determinants and outcomes of nonoperative management for blunt traumatic aortic injuries. *J Vasc Surg.* 2018;67(2):389-398.
18. Demetriades D, Velmahos GC, Scalea TM, et al. Blunt traumatic thoracic aortic injuries: early or delayed repair—results of an American Association for the Surgery of Trauma prospective study. *J Trauma.* 2009;66(4):967-973.
19. Hemmila MR, Arbabi S, Rowe SA, et al. Delayed repair for blunt thoracic aortic injury: is it really equivalent to early repair? *J Trauma.* 2004;56(1):13-23.
20. Holmes JH 4th, Bloch RD, Hall RA, Carter YM, Karmy-Jones RC. Natural history of traumatic rupture of the thoracic aorta managed nonoperatively: a longitudinal analysis. *Ann Thorac Surg.* 2002;73(4):1149-1154.
21. Trust MD, Teixeira PGR. Blunt trauma of the aorta, current guidelines. *Cardiol Clin.* 2017;35(3):441-451.
22. Maggisano R, Nathens A, Alexandrova NA, et al. Traumatic rupture of the thoracic aorta: should one always operate immediately? *Ann Vasc Surg.* 1995;9(1):44-52.
23. Demetriades D, Velmahos GC, Scalea TM, et al. Operative repair or endovascular stent graft in blunt traumatic thoracic aortic injuries: results of an American Association for the Surgery of Trauma Multicenter Study. *J Trauma.* 2008;64(3):561.
24. Hoffer EK, Forauer AR, Silas AM, Gemery JM. Endovascular stent-graft or open surgical repair for blunt thoracic aortic trauma: systematic review. *J Vasc Interv Radiol.* 2008;19(8):1153-1164.
25. Dubose JJ, Azizzadeh A, Estrera AL, Safi HJ. Contemporary management of blunt aortic trauma. *J Cardiovasc Surg (Torino).* 2015;56(5):751-762.
26. Nasser R, Nakhla J, Sharif S, Kinon M, Yassari R. Penetrating thoracic spinal cord injury with ice pick extending into the aorta. A technical note and review of the literature. *Surg Neurol Int.* 2016;7(suppl 28):S763-S766.

27. Tamburrini A, Rehman SM, Votano D, et al. Penetrating trauma of the thoracic aorta caused by a knitting needle. *Ann Thorac Surg*. 2017;103(2):e193.

28. DuBose JJ, Leake SS, Brenner M, et al. Contemporary management and outcomes of blunt thoracic aortic injury: a multicenter retrospective study. *J Trauma Acute Care Surg*. 2015;78(2):360-369.

29. McBride CL, Dubose JJ, Miller CC 3rd, et al. Intentional left subclavian artery coverage during thoracic endovascular aortic repair for traumatic aortic injury. *J Vasc Surg*. 2015;61(1):73-79.

30. Matsumura JS, Lee WA, Mitchell RS, et al. The Society for Vascular Surgery Practice Guidelines: management of the left subclavian artery with thoracic endovascular aortic repair. *J Vasc Surg*. 2009;50(5):1155-1158.

31. Spiliotopoulos K, Kokotsakis J, Argiriou M, et al. Endovascular repair for blunt thoracic aortic injury: 11-year outcomes and postoperative surveillance experience. *J Thorac Cardiovasc Surg*. 2014;148(6):2956-2961.

32. Grigorian A, Spencer D, Donayre C, et al. National trends of thoracic endovascular aortic repair versus open repair in blunt thoracic aortic injury. *Ann Vasc Surg*. 2018;52: 72-78.

33. Cordova A, Bowen F, Price L, Dudrick S, Sumpio B. Traumatic innominate artery pseudoaneurysm in the setting of a Bovine Arch. *Ann Vasc Dis*. 2011;4(3):252-255.

34. Branco BC, Boutrous ML, DuBose JJ, et al. Outcome comparison between open and endovascular management of axillosubclavian arterial injuries. *J Vasc Surg*. 2016;63(3):702-709.

35. DuBose J, Rajani R, Gilani R, et al. Endovascular management of axillo-subclavian arterial injury: a review of published experience. *Injury*. 2012;43(11):1785-1792.

36. du Toit D, Lambrechts A, Stark H, Warren B. Long-term results of stent graft treatment of subclavian artery injuries: management of choice for stable patients? *J Vasc Surg*. 2008;47(4):739-743.

37. Starnes B, Arthurs Z. Vascular trauma: head and neck. In: Cronenwett K, Johnston K, eds. *Rutherford's Vascular Surgery*. 8th ed. Philadelphia, PA: Elsevier; 2015:2438-2450.e2.

38. Demetriades D, Chahwan S, Gomez H, et al. Penetrating injuries to the subclavian and axillary vessels. *J Am Coll Surg*. 1999;188(3):290-295.

39. Wind G, Valentine R. *Anatomic Exposures in Vascular Surgery*. 3rd ed. Philadelphia, PA: Wolters Kluwer Health; 2013.

Gregory A. Magee • Vincent L. Rowe

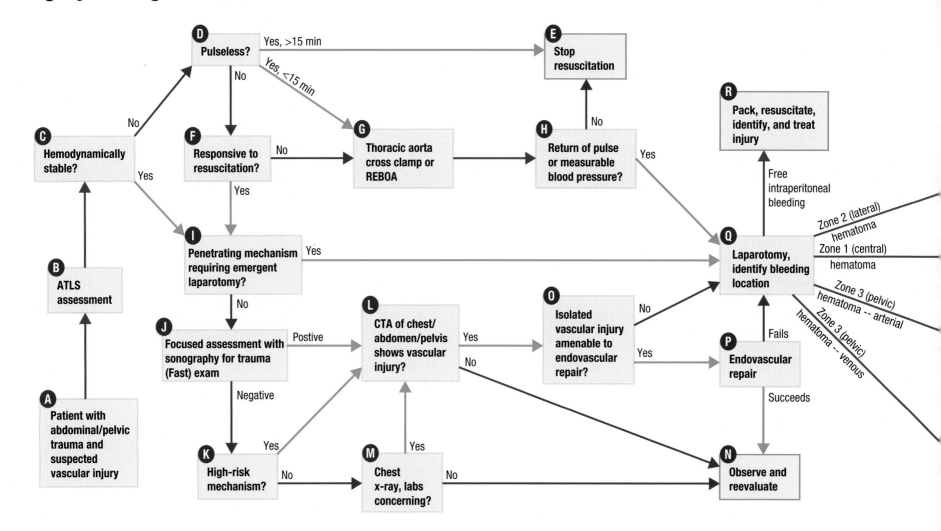

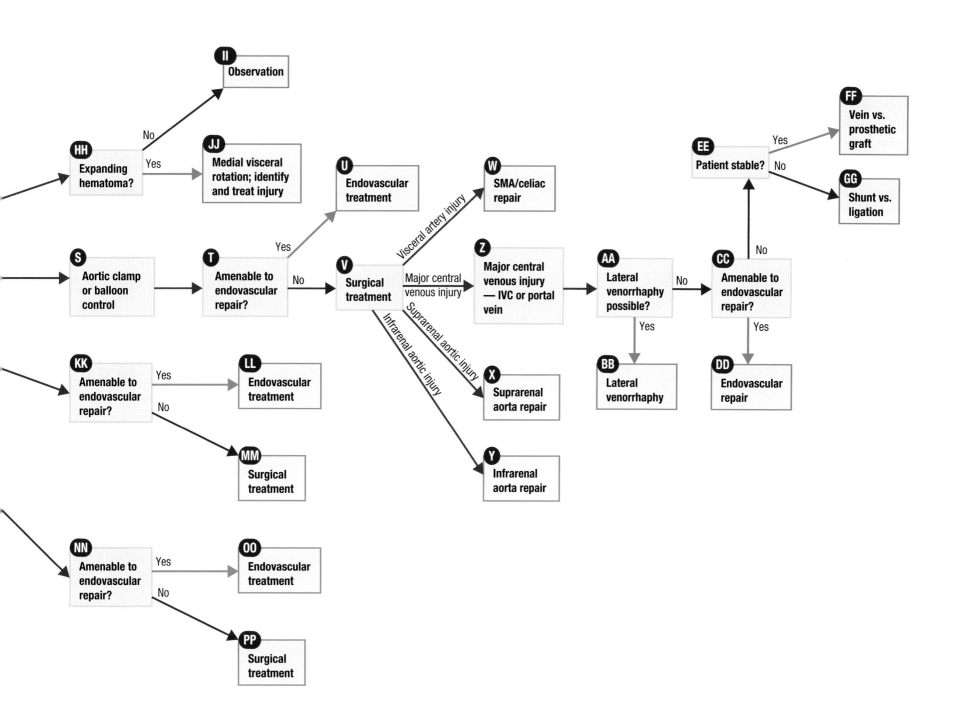

A Patient with abdominal/pelvic trauma and suspected vascular injury

All patients with penetrating abdominal, pelvic, or any high-force blunt trauma should be evaluated for possible vascular injury. Just over 2% of patients with trauma sustain a vascular injury and about 25% of vascular injuries occur in the abdomen with mortality rates that range from 25% to 50%.[1]

B ATLS assessment

Injured patients present with a broad array of problems requiring rapid diagnosis and treatment. ATLS was developed to provide a concise and methodical algorithm to assess and manage patients with trauma by addressing the most life-threatening issues first. This algorithm should be followed at initial evaluation and again if a patient's condition deteriorates.[2]

C Hemodynamically stable?

Hemodynamic instability requires rapid management. Any patient with abdominal/pelvic trauma who has an SBP < 90 mm Hg or a heart rate >120 beats/min should be considered hemodynamically unstable.

D Pulseless?

Femoral and carotid pulses should be checked as part of the primary ATLS survey. The trauma team should determine from the emergency medical service providers when the pulses were last palpable. The next step in management depends on whether the patient has been pulseless for >15 minutes. Guidelines recommend that patients who arrive pulseless for >15 minutes have essentially no chance of survival and, therefore, resuscitative efforts should be stopped.[3]

E Stop resuscitation

If the patient arrives to the hospital with >15 minutes of pulselessness, has no signs of life, or does not reestablish a pulse or measureable blood pressure after resuscitative thoracotomy, with thoracic aortic cross clamping, manual cardiac massage, and intracardiac epinephrine injection after adequate resuscitation, then resuscitative efforts should be stopped.

F Responsive to resuscitation?

Hemodynamically unstable patients with pulses are presumed to be hemorrhaging and should initially receive 1 L crystalloid bolus followed by PRBCs when available. If the SBP and heart rate return to normal after resuscitation, the patient is considered a "responder" and likely does not have substantial ongoing blood loss.

G Thoracic aorta cross clamp or REBOA

If the patient arrests in the hospital or <15 minutes before arrival with ongoing CPR, then a resuscitative thoracotomy should be considered.[3,4] Details of this procedure can be reviewed in Chapter 59. A contemporary, less invasive alternative to a thoracotomy with aortic cross clamping is REBOA. This is a temporizing maneuver to rapidly increase central blood pressure and decrease bleeding distal to the balloon, allowing time for restoration of blood volume (see Chapter 59).[5] REBOA is an ideal alternative to resuscitative thoracotomy so as to prevent cardiac arrest due to hypotension in a patient with abdominal or pelvic injury who is hypotensive despite resuscitation.

Patients who are not responsive to resuscitation likely have massive ongoing noncompressible torso hemorrhage that requires immediate action to prevent imminent cardiac arrest. This may be the most appropriate situation for the use of REBOA, especially for blunt trauma, with the balloon placed in the thoracic aorta if abdominal hemorrhage is suspected or infrarenal, if pelvic hemorrhage is suspected. Resuscitative thoracotomy in patients who do not respond to resuscitation is an alternative to REBOA and is preferred if an aortic injury is suspected or if there is significant hemorrhage in the left chest.

H Return of pulse or measurable blood pressure?

Following resuscitative thoracotomy or REBOA in a pulseless patient, the patient should be reassessed after all reasonable efforts at resuscitation have been performed. Resuscitative efforts should be stopped if there is no return of carotid or femoral pulses or measurable blood pressure. If pulses and measurable blood pressure are restored, the patient should proceed immediately to the operating room.

I Penetrating mechanism requiring emergent laparotomy?

Patients with a penetrating abdominal injury with peritonitis, evisceration, or hard signs of vascular injury (massive bleeding from wound, abdominal distention, refractory hypotension) should proceed expeditiously to the operating room for exploratory laparotomy for immediate control of hemorrhage. In the case of blunt trauma or a hemodynamically stable penetrating injury, further diagnostic imaging should be obtained.[6]

J Focused assessment with sonography for trauma (FAST) exam

A focused assessment with sonography for trauma (FAST) examination should be performed to evaluate for hemoperitoneum. A positive FAST examination finding in a hemodynamically unstable patient should prompt consideration for immediate exploratory laparotomy.[7] A positive FAST finding is defined as detection of fluid in the pericardium, the right upper quadrant of the abdomen, the left upper quadrant, or in the pelvis next to the bladder. The FAST examination has a reported sensitivity of 83% and specificity 99% to detect hemoperitoneum.[7]

K High-risk mechanism?

Patients with high-risk mechanisms, such as penetrating injury, high-speed motor vehicle accident, or fall from great height, should be further evaluated with a CTA (or plain CT if the patient cannot have contrast) to diagnose possible vascular injury.[8,9]

L CTA of chest/abdomen/pelvis shows vascular injury?

The positive and negative predictive value CTA has improved with modern multidetector scanners. A CTA scan can be helpful in patients without obvious need for immediate operation because a negative scan finding has been shown to effectively rule out intra-abdominal injury in asymptomatic patients with blunt trauma.[10] Overall, the sensitivity and specificity of CT to detect hollow viscous injury requiring operation is 85% and 96%, respectively.[11] Similarly, CTA scans are recommended when considering selective nonoperative management of penetrating abdominal trauma, with positive CTA findings prompting immediate operative repair.[12]

M Chest x-ray, labs concerning?

Dropping hemoglobin, elevated WBC count, and elevated lactate should raise concern for an intra-abdominal injury. Chest x-ray (CXR) findings with multiple rib fractures, hemothorax, and widened mediastinum should prompt a CTA. Because the sensitivity of a negative CXR and FAST examination finding is insufficient to rule out clinically significant injuries, a CTA should be performed unless there is low clinical suspicion.[13]

N Observe and reevaluate

Patients with a low-risk mechanism, negative FAST examination, normal CXR, and normal lab findings may be safely observed in the emergency department without further imaging and discharged if they remain clinically stable after a few hours.[8,9]

O Isolated vascular injury amenable to endovascular repair?

The use of endovascular repair of abdominal vascular trauma is still in its early stages because the frequency of associated injuries requiring open repair is very high. However, there are clear benefits of endovascular repair for some injuries. Endovascular covered stent placement for iliac artery injury can be performed faster and with less morbidity than for open repair in centers with experience and access to these techniques. In cases of isolated vascular injury that is amenable to endovascular repair, morbidity of a laparotomy can be avoided. Blunt abdominal aortic injuries occur in 0.03% of patients with blunt trauma and may be treated with EVAR if they are found to have a PSA or rupture.[14] It is important to recognize that endovascular repair of an arterial or venous injury does not preclude open repair of other injuries and may provide a useful adjunct. Examples include abdominal aortic injury with PSA or contained rupture, mesenteric or renal artery injury, iliac injuries, as well as pelvic bleeding. Similarly, endovascular techniques can be helpful for more accurate diagnosis and for hemorrhage control with localized intravascular balloon occlusion.

Ⓟ Endovascular repair

One common endovascular technique to treat isolated vascular trauma is deployment of a stent graft across the area of injury. This is more often used to treat arterial injury in a location where an appropriately sized stent graft can be successfully delivered and deployed. Another common technique is transcatheter embolization of bleeding vessels. Active extravasation in the setting of pelvic fractures can cause life-threatening hemorrhage. The source of bleeding is due to the disruption of the pelvic venous plexus in the majority of cases. Arteriographic embolization of bilateral internal iliac arteries with Gelfoam has a success rate of up to 90% in controlling hemorrhage without significant complications[15] (see OO for additional details of endovascular treatment of pelvic venous hemorrhage). Another common indication for embolization is for splenic injuries, which has decreased mortality and infection rates compared to splenectomy for grade IV and V splenic injuries.[16] If endovascular repair is not successful, open repair is undertaken.

Ⓠ Laparotomy, identify bleeding location

When possible, patients with suspected vascular trauma should be operated upon in a hybrid room equipped with DSA imaging equipment. An exploratory laparotomy should be performed when there are hard signs of vascular injury in the emergency department (massive bleeding from wound, abdominal distension, refractory hypotension). A midline laparotomy is performed and the abdomen is packed in all four quadrants to temporize bleeding, allow for resuscitation, and give the surgeon an opportunity to explore and locate the source(s) of hemorrhage. Distinct management is required for free intraperitoneal bleeding, a central (zone 1) hematoma, upper lateral (zone 2) hematoma, or a pelvic (zone 3) arterial or venous hematoma.

Ⓡ Pack, resuscitate, identify, and treat injury

Intraperitoneal bleeding can stem from a solid organ (liver or spleen), the mesentery, or a large vessel. Bleeding from solid organs should be controlled initially with packing. The surgeon should then evaluate for bleeding from the mesentery, controlling it with clamps, if necessary. Portal vein bleeding should be initially controlled with manual pressure around the foramen of Winslow (Pringle maneuver). Frequently, a segmental bowel resection may be required if its blood supply has been compromised in an effort to treat mesenteric hemorrhage. Questionably viable bowel should be left in place and a planned second-look laparotomy performed to ensure the remaining bowel is viable.

Ⓢ Aortic clamp or balloon control

A midline retroperitoneal hematoma may harbor an injury to the aorta, one of the visceral branches, or the IVC. Depending on the location of the central hematoma and bleeding site, aortic control is obtained at the supraceliac or infrarenal level. The most reliable

and expeditious method to expose the supramesocolic aorta and its visceral branches is with a left medial visceral rotation.[17] This is performed by mobilizing the left colon, left kidney, spleen, and tail of the pancreas toward the midline. The gastric fundus is also mobilized medially and the left diaphragmatic crus is divided at the aortic hiatus to expose and crossclamp the supraceliac aorta. Dissection inferiorly along the aorta leads to exposure of the celiac and SMA, which are usually within 1 to 2 cm of each other. With medial visceral rotation, the aorta is approached from its left lateral aspect; therefore, the trajectory of the celiac and SMA appear to be to the patient's right. If injury to either renal artery or vein is suspected, then the retroperitoneal exposure should be anterior to the left kidney because this provides better access to the juxtarenal aorta and bilateral renal arteries and veins. An alternative to aortic clamping is intraluminal balloon control. The balloon can be moved to the lowest location that allows for control of hemorrhage and adequate length of aorta for repair. An experienced provider can perform this technique quickly in a hybrid operating room. An inframesocolic midline hematoma should be approached similarly to open exposure of an aortic aneurysm with elevation of the transverse colon, right lateral retraction of the small bowel, and mobilization of the fourth portion of the duodenum by division of the ligament of Treitz.

Ⓣ Amenable to endovascular repair?

Once an aortic injury is controlled, the surgeon needs to decide how to repair it in the most expeditious manner. Supraceliac and infrarenal injuries that are not amenable to primary repair may be amenable to endovascular repair. However, in our experience, this is rarely feasible, because it requires correct sizing of the aorta, having appropriately sized endografts in stock, and access to immediately available fluoroscopy. If the patient is stable and the appropriate endograft inventory is available, there are some clear benefits of endovascular repair of aortic and iliac artery injuries. Open repair with a prosthetic graft has a high risk of infection if there is bowel contamination. Endografts are not without risk of infection in this scenario, but this risk may be lower because the graft is more protected from the contaminated field. Isolated injuries to one of the major aortic branches can be repaired with a stent graft. The role of endovascular repair may be most useful in the setting of intimal injuries with thrombosis as an alternative to surgical bypass because it may more quickly restore perfusion to the organ of interest. Especially in blunt trauma, CTA may demonstrate an intimal flap or thrombosed renal artery. Endovascular stenting (after suction or mechanical thrombolysis if needed) is appropriate in this situation if there is no prolonged warm renal ischemia time.[18] Although endovascular repair of aortic branches is usually achieved via femoral artery access, the proximal SMA can be quickly repaired with a stent graft via direct retrograde access at the root of the mesentery. The use of endovascular repair of traumatic injuries has increased over the past decade, and is currently most commonly performed for iliac arterial injury.

Ⓤ Endovascular treatment

If an injury to the aorta or visceral branches is amenable to endovascular repair, this should only be performed in a hybrid operating room without moving the patient off the table. Data regarding successful endovascular treatment of aortic and visceral branch vessels for trauma are limited to small case reports and series.

Ⓥ Surgical treatment

Open surgical treatment of zone 1 injuries depends on whether the injury is to the SMA/celiac, supra- or infrarenal aorta, or a major central vein.

Ⓦ SMA/celiac repair

A significant injury to the celiac artery can be treated with simple ligation because there is sufficient collateral circulation to the liver and stomach from the SMA in almost all cases. Similarly, the left gastric and splenic artery can be ligated. The common and proper hepatic should be repaired, usually with a vein graft, unless simple patch closure is possible. SMA injuries must be repaired, because ligation is almost universally fatal. If there is loss of flow in the SMA, a temporary shunt may be placed if repair and flow restoration will be delayed. Flow should be always confirmed in the shunt with a Doppler probe. In an unstable patient, such a shunt can be left in place and the patient returned to the operating room for definitive repair after hypothermia, acidosis, and coagulopathy have improved. Reconstruction of the SMA can be performed with reversed saphenous vein graft in an anatomic location, unless there is evidence of pancreatic injury and leak because this places the anastomoses at high risk of blowout. In the setting of a pancreatic leak, the proximal and distal ends of the SMA can be ligated in two layers and a bypass performed from the infrarenal aorta to the infracolic SMA away from the pancreatic leak. Heparinized saline can be injected locally, directed proximally and distally of the artery clamps if systemic heparinization is not possible because of bleeding risk. Relook laparotomy is generally recommended after SMA revascularization to evaluate the small bowel and ensure that no further bowel resection is necessary.

Ⓧ Suprarenal aorta repair

For injuries to the suprarenal aorta, the safest maneuver is to control the distal thoracic aorta in the chest before retroperitoneal abdominal exposure. Small aortic lacerations can occasionally be repaired primarily with 3-0 or 4-0 polypropylene sutures in a transverse orientation when possible to prevent stenosis; however, most injuries will require a complex reconstruction. Injuries to <50% of the aorta can usually be repaired with a patch using ePTFE, woven Dacron, or bovine pericardium. Often injuries are more destructive and require resection of a significant portion of the aorta. These cannot be repaired end to end because there is not sufficient mobility of the aorta, and as such interposition grafting using either ePTFE or woven Dacron is necessary. If there is bowel contamination, the area should be copiously irrigated before and after the graft is in position. Irrigation with saline-containing antibiotics may provide benefit and is recommended by some authors.[19,20] The retroperitoneum is tightly closed over the aorta if possible. Because this is frequently not achievable, the omentum should be mobilized and secured around the graft to protect against infection. Postoperative antibiotics should be administered for 1 to 3 days.[21]

Ⓨ Infrarenal aorta repair

An inframesocolic midline hematoma should be approached similarly to open exposure of an aortic aneurysm with elevation of the transverse colon, right lateral retraction of the small bowel, and mobilization of the fourth portion of the duodenum by division of the ligament of Treitz. This quickly exposes the infrarenal aorta and the crossing left renal vein, which can be divided if necessary. The aorta should be clamped below the renal arteries unless injured, in which case suprarenal aortic control should be obtained. Because suprarenal aortic exposure requires more time to expose a safe clamp location without damaging the renal or mesenteric branches, supraceliac clamping or balloon occlusion should be considered in this instance. After proximal control, the aorta is dissected distally to evaluate for injury. During this dissection, care must be taken to avoid injury to the IMA. The aorta should be repaired primarily or reconstructed, as described in X.

Ⓩ Major central venous injury—IVC or portal vein

If upon exploration of a zone 1 hematoma no aortic injury is found, then an IVC injury should be suspected. The IVC is most expeditiously exposed with a right medial visceral rotation. This is performed by elevating the right colon and performing a wide Kocher maneuver to mobilize the first and second portions of the duodenum medially. This allows for exposure of the infrahepatic IVC from the confluence of the common iliac veins to the liver.

A large, expanding hematoma behind the liver may represent injury to the retrohepatic IVC or hepatic veins. Manual compression of the liver should be applied immediately and the surgeon should alert the anesthesia team and blood bank to prepare for potentially rapid blood loss. If manual pressure does not control the hemorrhage, the right triangular and anterior coronary ligaments can be divided as an assistant continues to compress the liver with gentle inferior and medial traction. The right hepatic lobe is then elevated medially by the assistant to expose the retrohepatic IVC. If there is a small injury in the vein, the edges can be grasped with Judd Allis clamps to reduce blood loss and allow for lateral venorrhaphy with a running 4-0 polypropylene suture.

If elevating the right hepatic lobe produces exsanguinating hemorrhage, then a major venous injury that will require better vascular isolation with either an atriocaval shunt or total hepatic isolation is present. The assistant should resume manual compression while prompt control of the suprarenal IVC is obtained by placing an umbilical tape around the IVC and placing this through a 6-cm cut red rubber catheter as a Rummel tourniquet. The assistant should continue constant manual pressure and the surgeon should then perform a median sternotomy and open the pericardium longitudinally. The intrapericardial IVC is then controlled with a Rummel tourniquet. A right atrial to IVC caval shunt is then created using a modified 36F chest tube, after which both Rummels are tightened, effectively shunting the infrarenal IVC and renal vein blood directly to the right atrium, and reducing bleeding from the retrohepatic IVC. The retrohepatic IVC injury is then repaired with 4-0 polypropylene sutures if lateral venorrhaphy is possible. If there is a lengthy IVC injury, it can be reconstructed using an 18-mm externally supported ePTFE graft. An alternative to the atriocaval shunt is total hepatic vascular isolation, which is performed by clamping the suprahepatic IVC, suprarenal IVC, with a Pringle maneuver to clamp the portal triad, and a supraceliac aortic clamp, but this may not be hemodynamically tolerated.

For a portal vein or hepatic artery injury, manual compression with the thumb and index finger around the foramen of Winslow is used before placing a Debakey vascular clamp across the portal triad just to the right of the head of the pancreas (Pringle maneuver). This will provide vascular control and allow for assessment and repair of the injury.

ⒶⒶ Lateral venorrhaphy possible?

If there is a small venous injury or linear laceration, laterally venorrhaphy is usually possible, but destructive injuries with >50% of the circumference of the vessel will require a more complex reconstruction.

ⒷⒷ Lateral venorrhaphy

If lateral venorrhaphy is possible, Judd Allis clamps are placed across the edges of the vein or a Satinsky clamp is placed across the injury to allow closure with 4-0 polypropylene running sutures. Care must be taken to avoid excessive stenosis of the vein because this has a much higher likelihood to lead to thrombosis and pulmonary embolism.

ⒸⒸ Amenable to endovascular repair?

Retrohepatic IVC injuries are highly lethal because it is very challenging to achieve vascular isolation. Endovascular techniques such as balloon occlusion have been advocated in situations like these where hemorrhage is difficult to control.[22] Some have reported successful placement of aortic endografts in the IVC and/or iliac veins to repair venous injuries, and use of endovascular techniques for treatment of venous injuries will likely continue to increase and improve.[23]

Endovascular repair of the portal vein is not usually feasible because there is no direct access to the portal circulation from the systemic circulation, and there is usually little room to access the vein directly. However, this may be achievable through direct access of the superior mesenteric vein.

ⒹⒹ Endovascular repair

As with major arterial injuries, endovascular repair is only appropriate while the patient is still on the operating table in a hybrid operating room or with a mobile C-arm by an experienced provider. Surgical repair is performed if endovascular repair is not definitive.

ⒺⒺ Patient stable?

Once control of the major venous injury is obtained, the patient should be resuscitated via IV catheters placed in the upper extremities because lower extremity IV fluids will not be effective and will make venous repair more difficult. Continued hemodynamic instability may be due to insufficient venous return to the right atrium.

ⒻⒻ Vein vs. prosthetic graft

A large defect in the IVC or portal vein will require a patch repair with a bovine pericardial or woven Dacron patch. Larger injuries that involve >50% of the circumference will likely require an interposition graft. This takes time and can result in prolonged liver ischemia for portal vein and decreased cardiac return for IVC injuries. Therefore, a shunt can be helpful as a temporizing maneuver. A chest tube cut to 6 to 8 cm is usually a good fit and can be secured with proximal and distal Rummel tourniquets, as previously described. The proper hepatic artery can be ligated if necessary, but the portal vein needs to be spared.

An ePTFE prosthetic conduit can also be used and it has the benefit of being immediately available. Cryopreserved femoral veins are preferable to prosthetic grafts if there is bowel contamination because they are more resilient to infection, but are much more expensive. Autologous conduit reconstruction options include the femoral or internal jugular veins because they can be harvested with minimal morbidity and are of the appropriate size, but rarely practical at the index operation owing to hemodynamic stability.

Following major venous reconstruction, the patient should be put on systemic anticoagulation to prevent venous thrombosis and PE. If anticoagulation is not immediately possible, a temporary IVC filter can be placed. Long-term anticoagulation may be beneficial to reduce the likelihood of thrombosis.

ⒼⒼ Shunt vs. ligation

When the patient is not hemodynamically stable, major venous repair is not practical at the index operation. In these situations, an intravascular shunt can be used as an interim measure to decrease vascular congestion distal to the injury, and allow for delayed venous repair.[24] The IVC, iliac veins, and portal vein can be shunted using a large bore chest tube cut to appropriate length to allow several centimeters of the shunt into the vein on each side of the injury. The shunt should be secured in place with an umbilical tape Rummel tourniquet. Ligation of iliac veins or the IVC is occasionally necessary but leads to venous hypertension and can cause increased bleeding if there is major distal soft-tissue trauma. If the IVC or iliac veins are ligated, the legs should be wrapped and checked frequently for the development of compartment syndrome (see Chapter 51).

HH Expanding hematoma?

Zone 2 lateral retroperitoneal hematomas are typically caused by an injury to the renal artery, vein, or parenchyma. Penetrating injuries are more likely to have violation of the overlying fascia with ongoing bleeding, whereas blunt injuries rarely require surgical exploration.

II Observation

Zone 2 hematomas can be safely observed if they are not rapidly expanding. These may be examined by selective DSA either intra- or postoperatively to evaluate for small ongoing hemorrhage from vessels that can be percutaneously embolized as necessary.

JJ Medial visceral rotation; identify and treat injury

Lateral perirenal (zone 2) hematomas should be explored if they are large or expanding, because this likely is the manifestation of injury to the renal artery, vein, or a major injury to the renal parenchyma. The proximal renal artery and vein should be controlled either from a lateral approach with medial visceral rotation or with central exposure of the renal artery and vein by elevating the transverse mesocolon and exposing the infrarenal aorta (see Y). The lateral approach is performed by dividing the line of Toldt, opening the Gerota fascia, elevating the kidney, and controlling the renal hilum with a clamp or manual pressure. Immediate control of the right renal vein is usually not possible with the lateral approach. Once the proximal renal artery is controlled, the hematoma can be safely opened and repair of the renal artery or vein can ensue with primary repair or interposition bypass grafting with saphenous vein.

Renal arteries should be repaired especially if there is a solitary kidney. If there is a normal contralateral kidney and other injuries demand more urgent attention, a nephrectomy is acceptable. If revascularization of a renal artery is planned, the kidney can be packed with ice and cold saline can be injected into the distal end of the renal artery injury to reduce warm renal ischemia time and improve the likelihood of renal recovery. A destructive injury to the renal parenchyma usually requires nephrectomy.

KK Amenable to endovascular repair?

Endovascular treatment of pelvic hemorrhage is most commonly used when the source is the IIA because it can be readily embolized. CIA and EIA injuries can also be repaired endovascularly if the patient is hemodynamically stable or after proximal control is achieved.

LL Endovascular treatment

Hemorrhage from the IIA can be controlled by embolization with thrombin Gelfoam for small distal bleeding or with permanent coils or vascular plugs when there is a larger injury. As with renal artery injuries, endovascular repair of CIA and EIA injuries is most useful in the setting of intimal injury with placement of stent grafts. However, stent grafts can also be placed after open surgical control is obtained and may be useful in the setting of bowel contamination.

MM Surgical treatment

After penetrating trauma, a pelvic (zone 3) hematoma is evidence of an iliac artery or vein injury until proved otherwise. Proximal control should be obtained at or above the aortic bifurcation. The small bowel is retracted to the right and the peritoneum is opened longitudinally just above the pelvic brim. Distal control can then be obtained at the EIA by palpating it over the retroperitoneum as it rises out of the pelvis and exits under the inguinal ligament. Proximal CIA control can be obtained but careful dissection posteriorly is critical to avoid the adherent common iliac vein, because injury to this structure can be catastrophic.

Injuries from stab wounds can usually be repaired primarily, but gunshot injuries usually require reconstruction, because the energy of the projectile causes injury to the intima of the vessel proximal and distal to the area of vascular disruption. The saphenous vein is not of adequate size for bypass of the CIA or EIA; therefore, a prosthetic graft is usually required for in situ reconstruction. This is problematic if there is substantial contamination with bowel contents. In this situation, the surgeon should consider an extra-anatomic femoral-femoral crossover graft because this keeps the prosthetic graft out of the contaminated field and delayed in situ reconstruction can always be performed at a later date if needed, when the field is no longer contaminated. Alternatively, mobilization of the IIA can be performed with ligation of several branches. IIA can then be used as an excellent autologous conduit for CIA or EIA repair. Another option is a saphenous vein spiral or panel graft; however, this is a very time-consuming technique and not appropriate at the time of the initial operation. A temporary vascular shunt can be useful in these circumstances; a pediatric chest tube is usually an adequate size match for the iliac arteries. Cryopreserved artery or vein is another alternative conduit in a contaminated field if it is readily available, but such conduits are costly. Before placing a shunt or performing a bypass, the artery should be checked for adequate flow with a Doppler probe because frequently thrombus can form and propagate distally. An appropriately sized Fogarty thrombectomy catheter should be used to extract thrombus if present; completion DSA is performed to confirm complete thrombus extraction.

If the IIA is found to be injured during laparotomy, it can be surgically ligated. Ligation of bilateral IIAs should be avoided, because there is a risk of pelvic necrosis.

NN Amenable to endovascular repair?

Pelvic venous hemorrhage is most commonly associated with severe pelvic fractures, with bleeding originating from the sacral venous plexus. The first step in a hemodynamically unstable patient with venous hemorrhage from pelvic fractures is to reduce the pelvic space by placing a pelvic binder or sheet tight across the pelvis centered on the greater tuberosities of the femurs.[25] CTA should be performed to see if there is ongoing contrast extravasation. Methods for rapid intraoperative control of pelvic hemorrhage include preperitoneal pelvic packing,[26,27] temporary open control of bilateral IIAs at the time of laparotomy,[28] and angiographic embolization of bilateral IIAs,[29,30] with preferences depending on the experience of the center and surgeon.

OO Endovascular treatment

Gelfoam embolization of bilateral IIAs is used to decrease significant pelvic bleeding from fractures when the patient remains hemodynamically unstable after pelvic binding or external fixation. A blush on CTA is predictive of ongoing bleeding in these situations. Gelfoam provides temporary, but usually not permanent, occlusion to avoid potential complications of pelvic ischemia that would be associated with permanent coil occlusion of bilateral IIAs.

Placement of stent grafts in the iliac veins has been described, but it is rarely used in practice.[31] It would be most useful in the setting of an isolated iliac vein injury if the appropriate-sized covered stent was readily available and the patient was hemodynamically stable.

PP Surgical treatment

In blunt trauma, a zone 3 hematoma is presumed to be due to a pelvic fracture and should not be opened unless it is already partially opened, pulsatile, rapidly expanding, or the iliac pulse is absent.[32] In penetrating trauma or in the setting of a rapidly expanding pelvic hematoma, the common iliac vein can be circumferentially dissected out and controlled with a vessel loop; but if this is not possible without substantial blood loss, then a sponge stick can be used to compress the iliac veins and distal IVC to allow for better exposure. Once proximal and distal control of the iliac vessels is achieved, the hematoma can be opened in its entirety and the injury isolated. Repair of iliac vein injuries is recommended whenever possible because ligation is associated with a significant increase in mortality.[33]

As with the IVC and portal vein, the iliac veins should be repaired primarily if possible; and if not, then using patch repair or interposition graft. The options for autologous and prosthetic conduit are the same: femoral vein or internal jugular vein, ePTFE, or cryopreserved veins. If ePTFE is chosen, an externally reinforced graft is used. Autologous or cryopreserved grafts are preferable to prosthetic grafts if there is bowel contamination. Autologous vein harvest takes time and therefore should take place during a subsequent operation.

Following major venous reconstruction, the patient should be placed on systemic anticoagulation to prevent venous thrombosis and PE. If anticoagulation is not immediately possible, a temporary IVC filter can be placed. Long-term anticoagulation may be beneficial to reduce the likelihood of thrombosis.

REFERENCES

1. Branco BC, Musonza T, Long MA, et al. Survival trends after inferior vena cava and aortic injuries in the United States. *J Vasc Surg*. 2018;68(6):1880-1888.
2. ATLS Subcommittee; American College of Surgeons' Committee on Trauma; International ATLS working group. Advanced trauma life support (ATLS®): the ninth edition. *J Trauma Acute Care Surg*. 2013;74(5):1363-1366.
3. Burlew CC, Moore EE, Moore FA, et al. Western Trauma Association critical decisions in trauma: resuscitative thoracotomy. *J Trauma Acute Care Surg*. 2012;73(6):1359-1363.
4. Seamon MJ, Haut ER, Van Arendonk K, et al. An evidence-based approach to patient selection for emergency department thoracotomy: a practice management guideline from the Eastern Association for the Surgery of Trauma. *J Trauma Acute Care Surg*. 2015;79(1):159-173.
5. Biffl WL, Fox CJ, Moore EE. The role of REBOA in the control of exsanguinating torso hemorrhage. *J Trauma Acute Care Surg*. 2015;78(5):1054-1058.
6. Velmahos GC, Demetriades D, Toutouzas KG, et al. Selective nonoperative management in 1,856 patients with abdominal gunshot wounds: should routine laparotomy still be the standard of care? *Ann Surg*. 2001;234(3):395-402; discussion 402-393.
7. Rozycki GS, Ballard RB, Feliciano DV, Schmidt JA, Pennington SD. Surgeon-performed ultrasound for the assessment of truncal injuries: lessons learned from 1540 patients. *Ann Surg*. 1998;228(4):557-567.
8. Quinn AC, Sinert R. What is the utility of the Focused Assessment with Sonography in Trauma (FAST) exam in penetrating torso trauma? *Injury*. 2011;42(5):482-487.
9. Matsushima K, Khor D, Berona K, et al. Double Jeopardy in penetrating trauma: get FAST, get it right. *World J Surg*. 2018;42(1):99-106.
10. Benjamin E, Cho J, Recinos G, et al. Negative computed tomography can safely rule out clinically significant intra-abdominal injury in the asymptomatic patient after blunt trauma: Prospective evaluation of 1193 patients. *J Trauma Acute Care Surg*. 2018;84(1):128-132.
11. Abdel-Aziz H, Dunham CM. Effectiveness of computed tomography scanning to detect blunt bowel and mesenteric injuries requiring surgical intervention: a systematic literature review. *Am J Surg*. 2018;218(1):201-210.
12. Demetriades D, Hadjizacharia P, Constantinou C, et al. Selective nonoperative management of penetrating abdominal solid organ injuries. *Ann Surg*. 2006;244(4):620-628.
13. Schellenberg M, Inaba K, Bardes JM, et al. The combined utility of EFAST and CXR in blunt thoracic trauma. *J Trauma Acute Care Surg*. 2018. doi:10.1097/TA.0000000000001868.
14. Shalhub S, Starnes BW, Brenner ML, et al. Blunt abdominal aortic injury: a Western Trauma Association multicenter study. *J Trauma Acute Care Surg*. 2014;77(6):879-885; discussion 885.
15. Velmahos GC, Chahwan S, Hanks SE, et al. Angiographic embolization of bilateral internal iliac arteries to control life-threatening hemorrhage after blunt trauma to the pelvis. *Am Surg*. 2000;66(9):858-862.
16. Aiolfi A, Inaba K, Strumwasser A, et al. Splenic artery embolization versus splenectomy: analysis for early in-hospital infectious complications and outcomes. *J Trauma Acute Care Surg*. 2017;83(3):356-360.
17. Mattox KL, McCollum WB, Jordan GL, Beall AC, DeBakey ME. Management of upper abdominal vascular trauma. *Am J Surg*. 1974;128(6):823-828.
18. Lee JT, White RA. Endovascular management of blunt traumatic renal artery dissection. *J Endovasc Ther*. 2002;9(3):354-358.
19. Strider DV, Ratliff CR, Cherry KJ, Upchurch GR. Continuous betadine-bacitracin irrigation for vascular graft infections: a case series. *J Vasc Nurs*. 2018;36(1):40-44.
20. Umminger J, Krueger H, Beckmann E, et al. Management of early graft infections in the ascending aorta and aortic arch: a comparison between graft replacement and graft preservation techniques. *Eur J Cardiothorac Surg*. 2016;50(4):660-667.
21. Feliciano DV, Moore EE, Biffl WL. Western Trauma Association Critical Decisions in Trauma: Management of abdominal vascular trauma. *J Trauma Acute Care Surg*. 2015;79(6):1079-1088.
22. Reynolds CL, Celio AC, Bridges LC, et al. REBOA for the IVC? Resuscitative balloon occlusion of the inferior vena cava (REBOVC) to abate massive hemorrhage in retrohepatic vena cava injuries. *J Trauma Acute Care Surg*. 2017;83(6):1041-1046.
23. Chou EL, Colvard BD, Lee JT. Use of aortic endograft for repair of intraoperative iliocaval injury during anterior spine exposure. *Ann Vasc Surg*. 2016;31:207.e205-208.
24. Marinho de Oliveira Góes Junior A, de Campos Vieira Abib S, de Seixas Alves MT, Venerando da Silva Ferreira PS, Carvalho de Andrade M. To shunt or not to shunt? An experimental study comparing temporary vascular shunts and venous ligation as damage control techniques for vascular trauma. *Ann Vasc Surg*. 2014;28(3):710-724.
25. Routt ML, Falicov A, Woodhouse E, Schildhauer TA. Circumferential pelvic antishock sheeting: a temporary resuscitation aid. *J Orthop Trauma*. 2002;16(1):45-48.
26. Cothren CC, Osborn PM, Moore EE, Morgan SJ, Johnson JL, Smith WR. Preperitoneal pelvic packing for hemodynamically unstable pelvic fractures: a paradigm shift. *J Trauma*. 2007;62(4):834-839; discussion 839-842.
27. Burlew CC, Moore EE, Smith WR, et al. Preperitoneal pelvic packing/external fixation with secondary angioembolization: optimal care for life-threatening hemorrhage from unstable pelvic fractures. *J Am Coll Surg*. 2011;212(4):628-635; discussion 635-627.
28. DuBose J, Inaba K, Barmparas G, et al. Bilateral internal iliac artery ligation as a damage control approach in massive retroperitoneal bleeding after pelvic fracture. *J Trauma*. 2010;69(6):1507-1514.
29. Panetta T, Sclafani SJ, Goldstein AS, Phillips TF, Shaftan GW. Percutaneous transcatheter embolization for massive bleeding from pelvic fractures. *J Trauma*. 1985;25(11):1021-1029.
30. Velmahos GC, Toutouzas KG, Vassiliu P, et al. A prospective study on the safety and efficacy of angiographic embolization for pelvic and visceral injuries. *J Trauma*. 2002;53(2):303-308; discussion 308.
31. Mosquera Rey V, Fernández C, Zanabili A, Del Castro JA, Pandavenes MG, Alonso M. Endovascular repair of iliac vein laceration associated with complex pelvic fracture. *Ann Vasc Surg*. 2019;54:336.e9-336.e12.
32. Cestero RF, Plurad D, Green D, et al. Iliac artery injuries and pelvic fractures: a national trauma database analysis of associated injuries and outcomes. *J Trauma*. 2009;67(4):715-718.
33. Magee GA, Cho J, Matsushima K, et al. Isolated iliac vascular injuries and outcome of repair versus ligation of isolated iliac vein injury. *J Vasc Surg*. 2018;67(1):254-261.

David L. Dawson

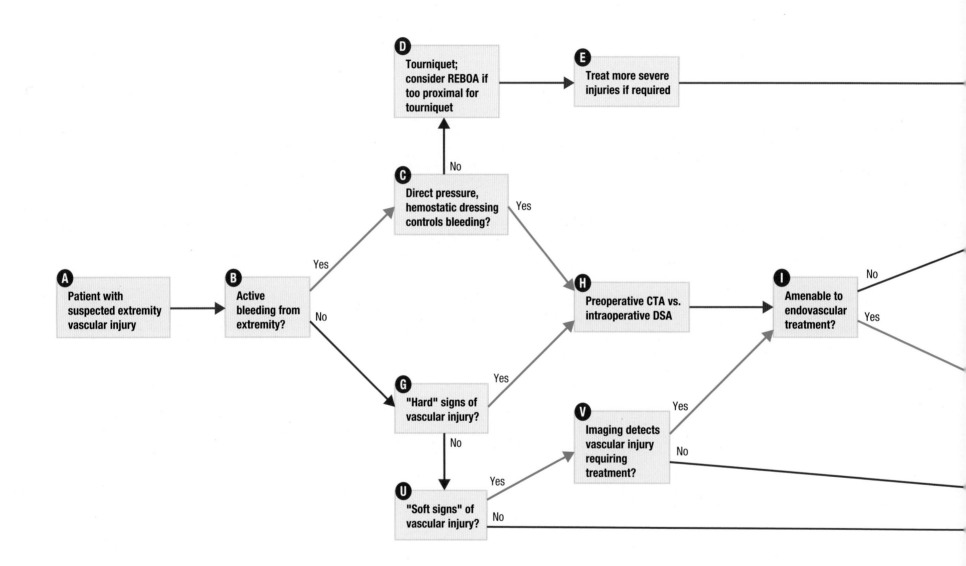

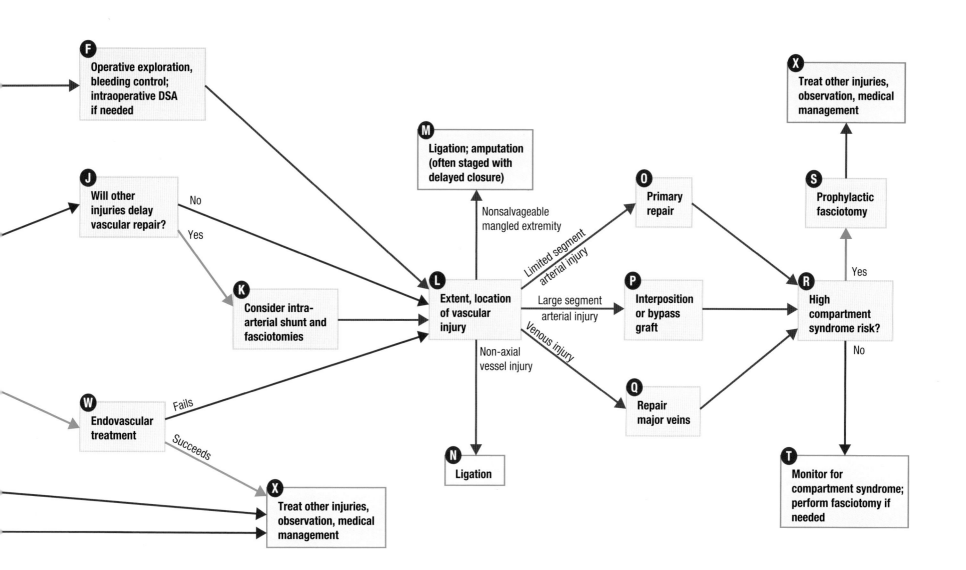

F Operative exploration, bleeding control; intraoperative DSA if needed

J Will other injuries delay vascular repair?

No

Yes

K Consider intra-arterial shunt and fasciotomies

W Endovascular treatment

Fails

Succeeds

M Ligation; amputation (often staged with delayed closure)

Nonsalvageable mangled extremity

L Extent, location of vascular injury

Limited segment arterial injury

Large segment arterial injury

Venous injury

Non-axial vessel injury

N Ligation

O Primary repair

P Interposition or bypass graft

Q Repair major veins

R High compartment syndrome risk?

Yes

No

S Prophylactic fasciotomy

X Treat other injuries, observation, medical management

T Monitor for compartment syndrome; perform fasciotomy if needed

X Treat other injuries, observation, medical management

A Patient with suspected extremity vascular injury

Extremity vascular injuries can be caused by either blunt or penetrating trauma.[1] In the setting of blunt trauma, extremity vascular injuries more likely result from high-energy injury mechanisms that lead to concomitant skeletal injuries (fractures, dislocations). Any penetrating trauma can directly injure vessels, but medium and high-energy gunshot wounds create cavitation that causes vascular injury beyond the ballistic track.

The American Association for the Surgery of Trauma (AAST), a multicenter registry, found that the majority of patients with extremity vascular injury were male (71%), often with severe injury patterns (32% with Injury Severity Score ≥15). Extremity arterial injuries were observed to be more common in the lower extremities. Extremity vascular injuries were associated with an 8% amputation and 13% hospital mortality rate.[2]

Analysis of the National Trauma Data Bank found that isolated lower extremity trauma with vascular injury was associated with approximately 10% risk of mortality or limb loss. Fatalities from lower extremity vascular trauma were often associated with a penetrating mechanism of injury and early onset of shock. Accordingly, hemorrhage control is a priority in ATLS (see Chapter 59).[3] In contrast, blunt vascular injuries, commonly involving the popliteal and tibial arteries, more often led to early limb loss.[4]

B Active bleeding from extremity?

During resuscitation of a patient with trauma, life-threatening injuries are identified and treated. Active blood loss from an extremity injury needs to be expeditiously controlled, because it can be fatal. Rapid cessation of ongoing blood loss is especially important when definitive care is delayed or if transfusion is not readily available.

C Direct pressure, hemostatic dressing controls bleeding?

Manual direct pressure is the first, and often best, treatment for extremity bleeding. Accurate application of digital or hand pressure to the bleeding source is key, and compression devices provide little or no advantage over manual pressure. Wrapping the bleeding site with bulky dressings is ineffective because it often does not apply pressure with needed accuracy.

When direct pressure with standard dressings is ineffective, a specialized dressing with a topical hemostatic agent may be packed into the wound and held with compression. Examples include chitosan (HemoCon), a factor concentrator, and kaolin-impregnated sponge (Quikclot), a mucoadhesive agent.[5] If direct pressure and hemostatic dressings cannot control bleeding, more aggressive measures are needed.

D Tourniquet; consider REBOA if too proximal for tourniquet

In the prehospital setting or before definitive operative treatment, a tourniquet should be used to control bleeding from extremity injuries that cannot be controlled by direct pressure. Commercially manufactured or improvised tourniquets can be used. The Combat Application Tourniquet (CAT Resources, LLC, Rock Hill, SC) is one commercial device used by the U.S. military that has become widely available in civilian practice. To be practical for self-aid, it was designed for one-handed application. The injured extremity is placed through the loop of the tourniquet band, 5 to 10 cm proximal to the injury, avoiding joints. The band is tightened and secured with a loop and pile (Velcro) strip. The tourniquet is tightened by turning a "windlass rod," which is secured with a clip. A second tourniquet can be placed proximal to the first if bleeding is not controlled.

The time of tourniquet application should be noted and written on the patient's skin with an indelible marker, to keep track of the ischemia time. The risk of nerve injury, rhabdomyolysis, and other complications increases with the duration of tourniquet application. Complications are low if the tourniquet time is <2 hours and high if it is >6 hours.

If the injury is too proximal for tourniquet use (ie, truncal or junctional), REBOA may be used as an alternative to proximal arterial clamping for patients in profound shock or with extensive proximal limb injuries (as may occur with traumatic amputations or blast injuries).[6-9] An aortic occlusion balloon is positioned in the distal abdominal aorta to control bleeding from pelvic, junctional, or proximal lower extremity.

Catheters that can be used for REBOA include compliant balloon catheters introduced over a 0.035″ guide wire (GORE Molding and Occlusion Balloon Catheter; Gore Medical, Flagstaff, AZ), through a 10F sheath; Coda Balloon Catheter (Cook Medical, Bloomington, IN) or Reliant Stent Graft Balloon Catheter (Medtronic, Minneapolis, MN) through a 12F sheath. The purpose-made ER-REBOA Catheter (Prytime Medical, Boerne, TX) is specifically designed for REBOA. It is introduced through a 7F femoral artery sheath without the need to track over a stiff guide wire.

Potential REBOA complications include access vessel injury and limb ischemia, balloon injury to the aorta or iliac arteries, spinal cord ischemia, or adverse sequelae from prolonged organ or lower body ischemia. As such, REBOA is only used when direct pressure or tourniquets cannot control hemorrhage. It is not an appropriate option for patients who cannot promptly receive definitive surgical care because potential complications must be recognized and treated immediately.

E Treat more severe injuries if required

Although the best limb-salvage outcomes are obtained with prompt revascularization,[10] damage control principles may dictate otherwise. Treatment of other life-threatening injuries may take precedence over definitive management of extremity vascular injuries ("life over limb"). This would include prioritizing hemorrhage control; correction of the "lethal triad" of coagulopathy, acidosis, and hypothermia; and management of chest, abdominal, and other injuries.

Although ischemia time >6 hours is associated with an increased risk of subsequent amputation, other factors, including the extent of associated soft-tissue or bone injuries, injury mechanism, anatomic site of injury, and the presence of compartment syndrome, are also important.[11]

F Operative exploration, bleeding control; intraoperative DSA if needed

The initial surgical treatment for major extremity vascular injury requires control of the bleeding vessel(s). Exploring a site of vascular injury without first controlling the vessel more proximally may be fraught with difficulty, blood loss, and risk of iatrogenic injury due to clumsy dissection or imprecise application of vascular clamps. The site of injury is often evident from the location of a penetrating injury or a displaced fracture. Intraoperative DSA can help localize injuries that are not evident at the time of surgical exploration. In most cases, proximal and distal exposure to allow direct visualization and clamping of the vessel is best. A hybrid endovascular technique with proximal balloon occlusion may be considered in select circumstances.[12] For more distal injuries, inflation of a padded pneumatic tourniquet provides a dry field with minimal ongoing bleeding.

G "Hard" signs of vascular injury?

"Hard signs" of vascular injury comprise a series of observations noted on the primary or secondary survey of a trauma patient that are indicative of significant vascular injury. They include pulsatile bleeding, an expanding hematoma, absent pulses distal to an extremity injury (if palpable elsewhere), an audible bruit, and a palpable thrill. When hard signs of vascular injury are present, definitive treatment is likely to be needed. If abnormal examination findings are attributed to a cause other than arterial injury (eg, pulse deficits caused by vasoconstriction owing to hypovolemic shock), serial evaluations are needed to confirm restoration of normal pulses after resuscitation.

H Preoperative CTA vs. intraoperative DSA

Vascular imaging helps localize and characterize vascular injury.[13] In a stable patient, preoperative CTA is often used.[14] DSA is needed in selected situations (eg, shotgun wound or when there is substantial CT artifact), or when endovascular therapy is planned. In an unstable patient or in one who requires immediate operative intervention, preoperative extremity CTA may not be feasible, and intraoperative DSA is performed in the operating room. In some cases of obviously localized arterial injury, imaging may not be required.

I Amenable to endovascular treatment?

Major vascular injuries identified with imaging are typically repaired surgically.[15] In selected cases, endovascular treatment is an option. Examples include use of therapeutic embolization to stop branch vessel bleeding, stenting to manage an intimal flap, or stent grafting to treat a PSA. An absolute contraindication to endovascular repair is inability to cross the injured segment with a guide wire. Hybrid approaches to vascular injury repair can include use of balloon occlusion for vascular control during a difficult surgical exposure (eg, subclavian artery). Endovascular treatment is less likely to have a role with high-energy trauma mechanisms, because there is often associated soft-tissue injury that requires surgical management.

J Will other injuries delay vascular repair?

Definitive vascular repair may be delayed if other injuries take precedence over vascular repair or transfer is needed. In such cases, a temporizing arterial shunt should be considered. Outcomes are poorer when limb warm ischemia time exceeds 6 hours, but ischemic injury to nerve and muscle starts earlier, and the ischemia-perfusion injury that contributes to the inflammatory shock state of trauma can be significant within 2 to 4 hours. Prolonged ischemia may lead to rhabdomyolysis and renal failure. More proximal interruption of blood flow, temperature, metabolic status, and other physiologic factors affect the threshold time for ischemic injury due to tourniquet use or delays in revascularization.

K Consider intra-arterial shunt and fasciotomies

If arterial repair is time consuming or the surgeon is not proficient in techniques for vascular reconstruction, then the use of a temporary shunt is a rapid, simple option that allows for distal blood flow when circumstances preclude prompt, definitive repair. Sundt, Argyle, and other shunts utilized for carotid surgery can be used. The injured segment is directly exposed. Proximal and distal control is obtained with vessel loops. The arterial injury is lengthened with scissors, and the shunt is introduced under direct vision and secured with a ligature (eg, O silk). Anticoagulation is not required to maintain shunt patency and its use may be associated with risk of bleeding from other injuries.

In a damage-control situation, temporary external fixation of skeletal injuries and shunt placement to temporarily restore blood flow may be sufficient surgical management for 24 hours or more. Also, shunt placement before orthopedic fixation of fractures appears to improve outcomes compared to delaying revascularization.[16] This may be the case during long operations with multiple surgical teams or in damage-control situations for which staged procedures are preferred to allow for correction of hemodynamic instability, coagulopathy, and hypothermia. If a patient leaves the operating room with a shunt in place, prophylactic fasciotomies should be considered. Fasciotomies are mandatory if the patient is transported to another facility with a shunt in place (see S).

L Extent, location of vascular injury

Operative strategies for management of extremity vascular injuries are based on the extent and location of the injury. Axial artery injuries are repaired or reconstructed depending on the extent of damage. Non-axial arteries can usually be ligated. Major vein injuries are repaired when possible, although ligation may be required. A mangled extremity requires evaluation of other injuries to determine if vascular repair versus amputation is the best course.

M Ligation; amputation (often staged with delayed closure)

Revascularization is not indicated if the extremity is not viable because of prolonged ischemia. Alternatively, it may be deemed not salvageable, because it is mangled and without sufficient soft tissue to cover an arterial repair, crushed with extensive tissue destruction, or with concomitant major nerve disruption or extensive nonreconstructable orthopedic injury. The Mangled Extremity Severity Score (MESS) was proposed as a means to predict extremity outcomes after trauma and to guide decisions for limb salvage versus primary amputation.[17] MESS considers age, duration, and severity of ischemia; severity of shock; and injury mechanism. Predictive scores to assess likelihood of amputation are based on clinical presentation; however, they have not been found to be reliable for all situations.[2,18] Therefore, a multidisciplinary approach with individualized assessment is crucial.[10] If extremity salvage is uncertain, but the patient is otherwise stable, repair of the vascular injury is recommended. If the patient is unstable or unlikely to recover from other injuries, arterial ligation and subsequent amputation may be required. If the multidisciplinary team concludes that the limb is not salvageable, arterial ligation and amputation is indicated, usually with an initial open amputation followed by secondary closure at a later time. In the setting of likely nonsurvivable concomitant injuries, extremity revascularization should not be attempted.

N Ligation

Ligation is appropriate for nonaxial (branch) arteries that do not require repair. Injuries to a single forearm or lower leg artery are also usually managed with ligation alone unless there is insufficient collateral circulation present.

O Primary repair

Short-segment or focal arterial injury can be managed with lateral suture repair or with debridement and primary anastomosis. If there is a noncircumferential defect in the vessel wall, debridement with vein patch angioplasty may also be an option. If a primary end-to-end repair is undertaken, care is ensured that minimal tension is present. In general, an arterial defect >2 cm cannot be reconstructed primarily without undue tension.

Technical factors contributing to successful repair include minimal tension, effective proximal and distal vascular control, use of loupe magnification, and fine interrupted monofilament sutures. Proximal and distal thrombectomy with a Fogarty balloon catheter should be considered before repair unless there is active proximal and backbleeding before clamping. Irrigation and direct intravascular administration of heparin is often sufficient because systemic anticoagulation is not needed for most surgical repairs of vascular injuries unless the procedure is prolonged and the injury is limited to the artery being repaired.[19]

Primary repair techniques avoid the use of prosthetic material, decreasing the risk of late infectious complications.

P Interposition or bypass grafts

When there is more extensive arterial injury (a >2-cm gap or segment that needs to be bridged), an interposition or bypass graft is required. The use of autologous vein conduit is preferred, for best patency and to reduce risk of graft infection. Preferential use of GSV from the uninjured extremity is a common surgical dictum, although superficial or deep vein from other locations may be considered. If there is extensive associated soft-tissue injury or loss of soft-tissue coverage, bypass grafts should have extra-anatomic routing through uninvolved tissue planes. In the setting of penetrating arterial injury, it is crucial for the artery proximal and distal to the area of injury to be securely ligated to avoid post bypass exsanguination through the site of original injury. In rare circumstances, when autologous vein is not available, cryopreserved vessels or ePFTE grafts can be used with reasonable initial success, although secondary reconstructions may be needed for subsequent graft thrombosis.[20]

Completion imaging, using DUS or DSA, should be routinely performed after complex vascular repair, because identification and correction of technical defects improves outcomes.[21]

Q Repair major veins

Major venous injuries should be preferentially repaired, rather than ligated.[22] Although ligation of major veins can be tolerated, compartment syndrome, early arterial graft failure, and need for amputation are more likely. Late complications due to venous HTN can be disabling. If venous injuries are repairable and the patient is stable, reconstruction of popliteal, femoral, common femoral, and iliac vein injuries are recommended because they will reduce acute venous HTN and late morbidity.

Techniques for venous injury repair include lateral venorrhaphy, end-to-end anastomosis, patch venoplasty, and interposition graft using autologous vein or prosthetic conduit. When both the artery and adjacent vein are injured, repair of both is advocated to reduce complications from venous HTN and improve flow through the arterial graft, although ligation of the injured vein is an acceptable option.[23]

Postoperative anticoagulation is indicated after repair of major venous injuries, because the risk of VTE is increased.[24] If there are other major injuries that contraindicate anticoagulation (eg, intracranial bleeding), use of mechanical sequential compression devices for VTE prophylaxis is a reasonable alternative.

R High compartment syndrome risk?

Prophylactic fasciotomy of muscular compartments distal to the vascular injury is indicated anytime compartment syndrome is diagnosed or expected,[25] or when interhospital transfer is planned. Risk factors for compartment syndrome include ischemia reperfusion, crush, extensive soft-tissue injury, hematoma, and long-bone fracture.

Compartment syndrome is more likely with long ischemia times (typically >6 hours; however, this depends on the extent of collateral circulation present), extensive soft-tissue injuries, and with concomitant arterial and venous injuries.[15] If the patient is unavailable for serial assessments or if a delayed fasciotomy is impractical, compartments should be opened prophylactically. When in doubt, fasciotomies of all compartments should be performed. The most common major errors with fasciotomies are delay and incomplete compartment release.

S Prophylactic fasciotomy

A complete fasciotomy involves releasing all compartments in the affected anatomic region over their full length, and widely opening the skin. When the diagnosis of acute compartment syndrome is correct, the muscles bulge outward through the incisions.

In the calf, the anterior, lateral, superficial posterior, and deep compartments should be released through two full-length incisions: one medial, one lateral. Incomplete fasciotomy can be the result of incorrect identification of the septum dividing the compartments. An initial transverse incision in the fascia overlying the septum between the anterior and lateral compartments, creating an "H" incision, helps avoid this error. The deep posterior compartment may not be adequately decompressed without release of the soleus muscle fibers from the tibia. The tibial neurovascular bundle should be exposed when the deep posterior compartment is fully decompressed. Another potential error is when fascial incisions are too short and less than the full extent of the fascial compartments.

Upper extremity fasciotomies are less commonly required.[26] Forearm compartment syndrome is more common than upper arm compartment syndrome. Volar and dorsal incisions are needed for decompression. Extension through the carpal tunnel into the palm may be needed.

Fasciotomy incisions can be managed with negative pressure wound therapy systems. In some cases, delayed closure of the skin is possible. In other situations, the open wounds require split thickness skin grafts for coverage.

T Monitor for compartment syndrome; perform fasciotomy if needed

Postoperative management after treatment of extremity vascular injuries should include appropriate fluid resuscitation, serial neurovascular checks, and avoidance of vasoconstrictor use.

Fasciotomy is indicated if symptoms and signs of compartment syndrome become manifest. These include pain out of proportion to the injury, pain with passive stretch, tense compartments, development of any new distal neurologic deficit, or high measured compartment pressures. Tissue edema peaks in the first 1 to 2 days after injury.

Measurement of compartment pressures may be considered if the clinical findings are equivocal. Normal compartment pressures (<10 mm Hg) can be reassuring. When compartment pressures rise to within 30 mm Hg of the diastolic blood pressure (delta pressure $\geq$30 mm Hg), capillary perfusion will be compromised and fasciotomy should be performed.[27] Early fasciotomy is associated with improved outcomes.[25]

U "Soft signs" of vascular injury?

"Soft signs" of vascular injury include a history of arterial bleeding in the field; penetrating injury or severe blunt trauma in proximity to major vessels; questionably reduced extremity pulses; small, nonpulsatile hematoma; or evidence of nerve injury. Because the clinical diagnosis of ischemia from arterial injury is not always straightforward, secondary or tertiary surveys should include measurement of limb blood pressures with a cuff and Doppler flow detector. An arterial pressure index (API) is calculated by dividing the pressure in the injured extremity by the pressure in an uninjured arm. The API should be measured anytime there is reason to suspect arterial injury, including penetrating trauma in proximity to major vessels, unstable fracture patterns, and posterior knee or elbow dislocations. This noninvasive vascular test can reliably exclude major occult arterial injury if the API is >0.9.[17] Presence of "soft signs" of vascular injury suggests that the need for intervention should be more thoroughly evaluated with arterial imaging.

V Imaging detects vascular injury requiring treatment?

When soft signs of vascular injury are present, but the index of suspicion is low, DUS may be sufficient to rule out a significant vascular injury.[28] This noninvasive modality should be considered when an accredited vascular laboratory is available. In cases when the index of suspicion is higher, or DUS not available, CTA is used, with DSA reserved for situations where CTA findings are unclear or CTA cannot be performed.

Minor vascular injuries identified with imaging (<50% stenosis, not associated with symptoms) are initially managed nonsurgically, with close observation to detect potential progression.[29] A focal, asymptomatic lesion associated with DUS peak systolic velocity ratio of <2.0 and not associated with a decreased API, is unlikely to progress.

W Endovascular treatment

There are several endovascular therapies potentially applicable to extremity vascular trauma.[30] Therapeutic embolization is the endovascular equivalent of arterial ligation. Options for embolization of traumatic injuries include metallic coils, cyanoacrylate, and gelatin sponge (Gelfoam). These modalities may be appropriate for branch vessels (eg, mid to distal profunda femoris artery) or when there are patent collateral pathways (eg, one injured tibioperoneal branch when others are patent). A self-expanding stent may be used to treat an intimal flap or dissection that creates a hemodynamically significant stenosis. Vessel wall disruption with bleeding or PSA is best treated with a stent graft. For extremity applications, self-expanding stents or stent grafts are most commonly used.

Postprocedure assessments should evaluate for vascular access site complications, including thrombosis and embolization, which may be more likely in the setting of shock or hypercoagulability. Routine postprocedural measurement of ABIs is recommended.

X Treat other injuries, observation, medical management

Often extremity vascular trauma is associated with other injuries that require treatment after vascular repair, not treated already. Antiplatelet therapy should be started, when possible, after arterial repair. Prophylaxis for VTE is appropriate for patients with trauma who remain hospitalized or immobilized using LMWH when not contraindicated by other injuries. Normal Doppler pressure measurements confirm the patency of arterial repairs. DUS in the first month after arterial reconstruction is useful to both assess the technical results and provide a baseline for future comparisons. When minor injuries are observed without surgical repair, follow-up DUS can evaluate for late complications (progression of stenosis, PSA, AVF).

REFERENCES

1. Slama R, Villaume F. Penetrating vascular injury: diagnosis and management updates. *Emerg Med Clin North Am.* 2017;35(4):789-801.
2. Scalea TM, DuBose J, Moore EE, et al. Western Trauma Association critical decisions in trauma: management of the mangled extremity. *J Trauma Acute Care Surg.* 2012;72(1):86-93.
3. American College of Surgeons Committee on Trauma. Advanced Trauma Life Support. 2018. https://www.facs.org/quality-programs/trauma/atls.
4. Kauvar DS, Sarfati MR, Kraiss LW. National trauma databank analysis of mortality and limb loss in isolated lower extremity vascular trauma. *J Vasc Surg.* 2011;53(6):1598-1603.
5. Granville-Chapman J, Jacobs N, Midwinter MJ. Pre-hospital haemostatic dressings: a systematic review. *Injury.* 2011;42(5):447-459.
6. Brenner M, Bulger EM, Perina DG, et al. Joint statement from the American College of Surgeons Committee on Trauma (ACS COT) and the American College of Emergency Physicians (ACEP) regarding the clinical use of Resuscitative

Endovascular Balloon Occlusion of the Aorta (REBOA). *Trauma Surg Acute Care Open.* 2018;3(1):e000154.

7. Brenner M, Teeter W, Hoehn M, et al. Use of resuscitative endovascular balloon occlusion of the aorta for proximal aortic control in patients with severe hemorrhage and arrest. *JAMA Surg.* 2018;153(2):130-135.

8. Davidson AJ, Russo RM, Reva VA, et al. The pitfalls of REBOA: risk factors and mitigation strategies. *J Trauma Acute Care Surg.* 2017. doi:10.1097/TA.0000000000001711.

9. DuBose JJ, Scalea TM, Brenner M, et al. The AAST prospective Aortic Occlusion for Resuscitation in Trauma and Acute Care Surgery (AORTA) registry: data on contemporary utilization and outcomes of aortic occlusion and resuscitative balloon occlusion of the aorta (REBOA). *J Trauma Acute Care Surg.* 2016;81(3):409-419.

10. Liang NL, Alarcon LH, Jeyabalan G, Avgerinos ED, Makaroun MS, Chaer RA. Contemporary outcomes of civilian lower extremity arterial trauma. *J Vasc Surg.* 2016;64(3):731-736.

11. Perkins ZB, Yet B, Glasgow S, et al. Meta-analysis of prognostic factors for amputation following surgical repair of lower extremity vascular trauma. *Br J Surg.* 2015;102(5):436-450.

12. D'Amours SK, Rastogi P, Ball CG. Utility of simultaneous interventional radiology and operative surgery in a dedicated suite for seriously injured patients. *Curr Opin Crit Care.* 2013;19(6):587-593.

13. Dawson DL. Imaging for the evaluation and treatment of vascular trauma. In: Rasmussen TE, Tai NRM, eds. *Rich's Vascular Trauma.* 3rd ed. Philadelphia, PA: Elsevier; 2015:44-56.

14. Fox N, Rajani RR, Bokhari F, et al. Evaluation and management of penetrating lower extremity arterial trauma: an Eastern Association for the Surgery of Trauma practice management guideline. *J Trauma Acute Care Surg.* 2012;73(5 suppl 4):S315-S320.

15. Faulconer ER, Branco BC, Loja MN, et al. Use of open and endovascular surgical techniques to manage vascular injuries in the trauma setting: a review of the Aast Proovit Registry. *J Trauma Acute Care Surg.* 2017. doi:10.1097/TA.0000000000001776.

16. Wlodarczyk JR, Thomas AS, Schroll R, et al. To shunt or not to shunt in combined orthopedic and vascular extremity trauma. *J Trauma Acute Care Surg.* 2018;85(6):1038-1042.

17. Johansen K, Lynch K, Paun M, Copass M. Non-invasive vascular tests reliably exclude occult arterial trauma in injured extremities. *J Trauma.* 1991;31(4):515-519; discussion 519-522.

18. Loja MN, Sammann A, DuBose J, et al. The mangled extremity score and amputation: time for a revision. *J Trauma Acute Care Surg.* 2017;82(3):518-523.

19. Loja MN, Galante JM, Humphries M, et al. Systemic anticoagulation in the setting of vascular extremity trauma. *Injury.* 2017;48(9):1911-1916.

20. Vertrees A, Fox CJ, Quan RW, Cox MW, Adams ED, Gillespie DL. The use of prosthetic grafts in complex military vascular trauma: a limb salvage strategy for patients with severely limited autologous conduit. *J Trauma.* 2009;66(4):980-983.

21. Feliciano DV. Pitfalls in the management of peripheral vascular injuries. *Trauma Surg Acute Care Open.* 2017;2(1):e000110.

22. Giannakopoulos TG, Avgerinos ED. Management of peripheral and truncal venous injuries. *Front Surg.* 2017;4:46.

23. Dua A, Desai SS, Ali F, Yang K, Lee C. Popliteal vein repair may not impact amputation rates in combined popliteal artery and vein injury. *Vascular.* 2016;24(2):166-170.

24. Frank B, Maher Z, Hazelton JP, et al. Venous thromboembolism after major venous injuries: competing priorities. *J Trauma Acute Care Surg.* 2017;83(6):1095-1101.

25. Farber A, Tan TW, Hamburg NM, et al. Early fasciotomy in patients with extremity vascular injury is associated with decreased risk of adverse limb outcomes: a review of the National Trauma Data Bank. *Injury.* 2012;43(9):1486-1491.

26. Branco BC, Inaba K, Barmparas G, et al. Incidence and predictors for the need for fasciotomy after extremity trauma: a 10-year review in a mature level I trauma centre. *Injury.* 2011;42(10):1157-1163.

27. McQueen MM, Court-Brown CM. Compartment monitoring in tibial fractures. The pressure threshold for decompression. *J Bone Joint Surg Br.* 1996;78(1):99-104.

28. deSouza IS, Benabbas R, McKee S, et al. Accuracy of physical examination, ankle-brachial index, and ultrasonography in the diagnosis of arterial injury in patients with penetrating extremity trauma: a systematic review and meta-analysis. *Acad Emerg Med.* 2017;24(8):994-1017.

29. Frykberg ER, Crump JM, Dennis JW, Vines FS, Alexander RH. Nonoperative observation of clinically occult arterial injuries: a prospective evaluation. *Surgery.* 1991;109(1):85-96.

30. Starnes BW, Arthurs ZM. Endovascular management of vascular trauma. *Perspect Vasc Surg Endovasc Ther.* 2006;18(2):114-129.

Karen Woo

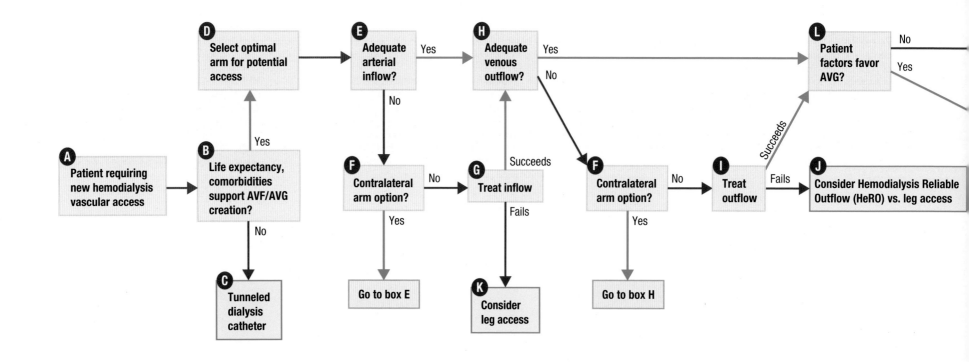

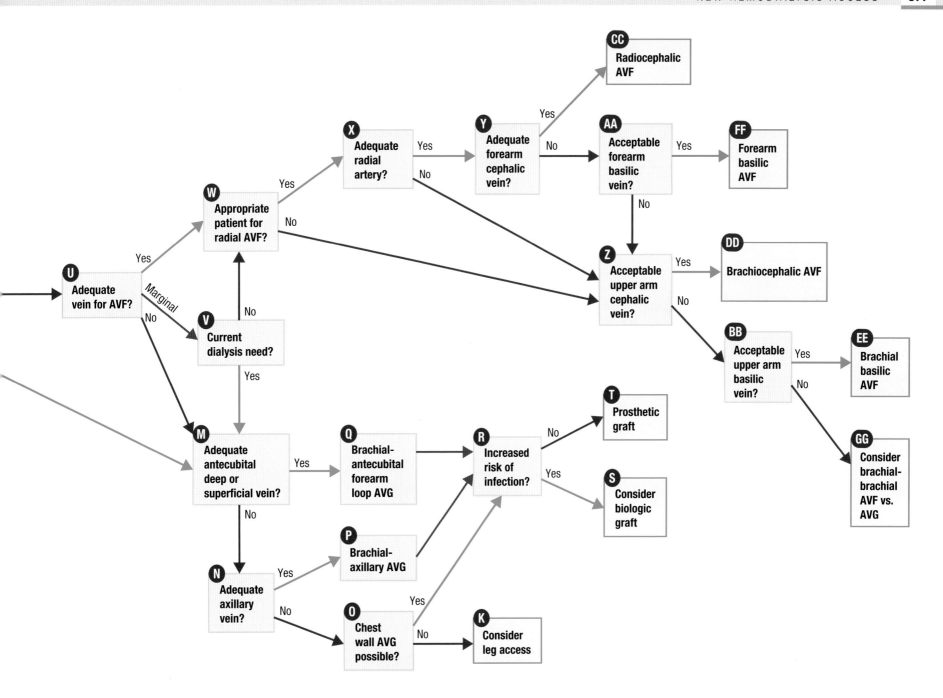

A Patient requiring new hemodialysis vascular access

In 2016, there were 451,000 hemodialysis-dependent patients in the United States.[1] Patients with stage IV CKD and ESRD should be educated on options for renal replacement and vascular access.[2] Patients who choose hemodialysis should be referred to a vascular access surgeon >6 months before they are anticipated to require hemodialysis. This allows for sufficient time for evaluation for an AVF or AVG. If a patient is determined to be a good candidate for an AVF, early referral allows adequate time for the AVF to mature or for a second AVF/AVG to be created if the initial AVF fails, so that the patient has a functional vascular access at the time of hemodialysis initiation. For predialysis patients who have been determined to be more appropriate for an AVG, the AVG should be created as close to the start of hemodialysis as possible. AVGs have a higher risk of infection and generally a lower patency than do AVFs.

B Life expectancy, comorbidities support AVF/AVG creation?

Patients with short life expectancy (<12 months) may not be good candidates for an AVF or AVG because the benefits may not outweigh the risks. Furthermore, patients with a short life expectancy may dialyze through a cuffed, tunneled dialysis catheter (TDC) without encountering the longer term complications of a TDC. Patients with chronic hypotension and/or poor cardiac output are also poor candidates for an AVF/AVG, which will more likely thrombose when blood pressure drops while on hemodialysis.[3,4] Ultimately, the choice between a permanent vascular access versus a TDC is one that should be made together with the patient, taking into account the patient's anatomy, comorbidities, functional status, and preferences. Overall, TDC is the best long-term vascular access option for only a small minority of hemodialysis patients (<10%).

C Tunneled dialysis catheter

TDC should be placed under DUS and fluoroscopic guidance. The right internal jugular is the preferred location given the direct path of the internal jugular vein into the SVC. Potential complications of insertion include pneumothorax, hemothorax, cardiac perforation, cardiac arrhythmia, thoracic duct laceration, wire embolism, and nerve injuries.[5] Catheter occlusion is one of the most common long-term complications of TDC, affecting 30% to 40% of patients at a rate of 0.5 to 3.42 episodes/1000 catheter-days. This generally occurs secondary to a fibrin sheath that develops around the catheter and can be treated with infusion of a fibrinolytic agent or mechanical removal of the sheath.[6,7] Catheter-related infection is another common long-term complication and is categorized into three types: exit-site infection, tunnel infection, and bacteremia.[8] Exit-site infections can often be treated with topical and systemic antibiotics without TDC removal. Tunnel infection and bacteremia require catheter removal and delayed replacement. The patient should have as long a "catheter holiday" as possible to allow the infection to be treated adequately. If necessary, a temporary noncuffed catheter can be placed for an individual hemodialysis session and removed thereafter. See Chapter 68 for further recommendations.

D Select optimal arm for potential access

The nondominant arm is optimal for AVF/AVG placement if it also has adequate anatomy, including large outflow veins, minimal or no previous vascular access operations, patent central veins, and normal arterial inflow. Creating the access in the patient's nondominant arm allows the patient to use the dominant arm during hemodialysis sessions. Furthermore, in the rare event of a disabling vascular access complication, the dominant arm would be spared. However, the dominant arm should be selected if the abovementioned anatomic requirements for durable access are not present in the nondominant arm.

E Adequate arterial Inflow?

A thorough physical examination should be performed on all patients before creation of an AVF/AVG. All upper extremity pulses should be examined and blood pressure should be measured in both arms. An upper extremity arterial DUS to assess waveforms of the brachial artery in the antecubital fossa, and the radial and ulnar arteries at the wrist is advisable to confirm normal arterial inflow. The waveform in the artery intended to serve as the inflow artery for the AVF/AVG should ideally be triphasic and the blood pressure should be equal in both arms. On DUS, the artery should have no more than a moderate degree of calcification. The brachial artery should have a minimum diameter of 3 mm and the radial and ulnar arteries should have a minimum diameter of 2 mm.

F Contralateral arm option?

If the patient does not have adequate arterial inflow or venous outflow in the nondominant arm, the contralateral arm should be evaluated for AVF/AVG creation before consideration of treating the inflow or outflow in the nondominant arm.

G Treat inflow

If neither arm has adequate arterial inflow at baseline, then the inflow of the nondominant arm should be treated, if possible, to establish an access site. Initial evaluation to localize the inflow stenosis is done with physical examination and DUS, followed by CTA or DSA as needed. Endovascular revascularization can usually be performed to correct arterial inflow in at least one arm. Rarely, open bypass may be needed (see Chapter 54).

H Adequate venous outflow?

A thorough history should include a detailed inventory of any central venous devices that the patient may have in place currently or in the past, including peripherally inserted central catheters, pacemakers, temporary central catheters, TDCs, and ports. Physical examination of the upper extremity and chest wall may reveal dilated collateral veins and/or arm swelling suggestive of central venous stenosis/obstruction. If there is any suspicion of compromised venous outflow, a CT venogram and/or catheter-based venogram should be performed. Ideally, there should be no evidence or suggestion of central venous stenosis on physical examination and/or imaging on the side where an AVF/AVG is being planned.

I Treat outflow

If neither arm has adequate venous outflow at baseline, the venous outflow of the optimal arm should be treated, if possible, to establish an access site. The preferred treatment for central venous stenosis is typically endovascular balloon venoplasty. A stent may be required if significant recoil occurs. Unfortunately, patency of bare-metal stents to improve venous outflow is poor, with 1-year primary patency of 30% to 40%.[9,10] Stents placed in the thoracic outlet region tend to fracture, resulting in occlusion and creating difficulty with recanalization. There is some evidence to suggest that the patency of stent grafts is superior.[10] In patients who have no other options for access and have a central occlusion on the ipsilateral side, open surgical options such as jugular venous turndown or bypass around the occlusion, if possible, may be considered.[11]

J Consider Hemodialysis Reliable Outflow (HeRO) vs. leg access

For patients with central venous stenosis/occlusion that cannot be successfully treated but can be crossed using endovascular techniques, the HeRO Graft (MeritMedical, South Jordan, UT) is an option for upper extremity access. The HeRO is a composite of a prosthetic graft and a catheter that is completely subcutaneous. The graft is anastomosed to arterial inflow in the arm, tunneled subcutaneously, and connected to the catheter portion in the shoulder area. The catheter portion extends into the jugular or subclavian vein and terminates in the right atrium. One-year primary patency rate is only 22%, but secondary patency is 60%.[12] On average, between 1.5 and 3 interventions per year are required to maintain HeRO patency and the device-related bacteremia rates are between 0.13 and 0.7 episodes per 1000 days, which equates to less than one episode of device-related bacteremia every 2.7 years.[12] One study of 36 HeRO grafts demonstrated that 7 grafts required excision because of infection over the study period.[13] A HeRO may be preferred to preserve lower extremity options for future access or in patients who do not have lower extremity access options.[14] In other cases, leg access is preferred (see K).

K Consider leg access

If no arm access is possible, thigh access can be considered. In evaluating a patient for a lower extremity vascular access, screening for significant PAD is imperative. Placement of a thigh vascular access in patients with significant PAD can result in ischemic steal, leading to limb-threatening ischemia, gangrene, and amputation. As such, patients with severe PAD should not undergo thigh vascular access without concomitant revascularization.

Thigh AVG, constructed from ePTFE, cryopreserved femoral vein, or bovine carotid artery can be placed in a loop or straight configuration. In the more commonly used loop AVG, inflow can be from the CFA, profunda, or SFA with outflow into the common femoral, femoral, or GSV vein. AVF in the thigh is preferentially constructed using the transposed femoral-popliteal vein. The femoral-popliteal vein is mobilized from the knee joint to the confluence of the deep femoral and femoral veins. It is then transposed through a superficial tunnel, tapered to avoid development of ischemic steal, and anastomosed to the SFA just proximal to the adductor hiatus. The femoral vein transposition AVF is a technically demanding operation involving a complex dissection and, as such, is reserved for good-risk patients.[15] Thigh AVF performed using the saphenous vein is less technically demanding; however, results are not satisfactory, because of the lack of dilation of the GSV over time.[16] To address this issue, some authors proposed using the GSV in a semipanel manner to increase the diameter.[17]

Prosthetic thigh AVGs are associated with a higher rate of infection than are arm AVGs. In one series of 125 thigh AVGs, 41% developed infection, requiring an intervention at 20 months of mean follow-up.[18] Femoral vein AVFs have been associated with 18% major complication rate; however, high maturation and patency rates—82% maturation rate and 56% 9-year secondary patency rate—were described in one large series.[19] In a recent meta-analysis, approximately 18% of thigh AVGs were abandoned because of infection compared with <2% of fistulas.[15] However, thigh AVGs had a lower incidence of ischemic complications compared to fistulas (21% vs. 7%).[15] In a comparison of thigh AVGs with long-term TDCs, despite a relatively high rate of thigh graft infection (21% at 1 year), thigh AVGs were associated with significantly higher infection-free survival rates.[20]

L Patient factors favor AVG?

There is increasing evidence that AVF may not have superior patency and function compared to AVG in all subgroups of ESRD patients. In particular, the elderly may be more appropriate for AVG over AVF creation.[21] Patients >65 years have inferior primary, primary assisted, and secondary patency and maturation of AVFs compared with patients <65 years old.[22] As such, elderly patients may not enjoy the benefits of AVF,

particularly if they have short life expectancy. Some authors have suggested that AVGs have equivalent patency and function as do AVFs for the first 18 months.[23] Thus, if a patient does not have a life expectancy longer than 18 months, the benefits of an AVF may not outweigh an AVG. In addition, a number of demographic characteristics and comorbidities may negatively affect AVF maturation and patency, including African-American race, female sex, CAD, and diabetes.[24] Ultimately, none of this evidence is conclusive and the decision between AVG versus AVF must be made on an individualized basis taking into account demographics, comorbidities, patient and family preferences, and lifetime access plan.

M Adequate antecubital deep or superficial vein?

A brachial or superficial vein that does not have wall thickening or thrombosis on DUS in the antecubital fossa and the upper arm is a potentially suitable candidate for venous outflow of a forearm AVG. A diameter of 3 mm or greater is ideal.[25] However, many hemodialysis patients have poor quality superficial veins due to repeated blood draws and IV catheter placements. Thus, if the only vein that is available has a diameter of <3 mm, it may be considered for AVF creation if it has an otherwise normal DUS appearance. No exact vein diameter criteria have been established. In the literature, vein diameters resulting in successful AVF vary widely, with diameters as low as 2 mm being reported. Measurement of vein diameter by DUS also varies depending on hydration status, room temperature, and use of a tourniquet. Each vascular access surgeon should be familiar with the techniques used by their vascular laboratory and should have DUS available in the operating room to reexamine the veins immediately before the operation.

N Adequate axillary vein?

An axillary vein in the upper arm of 3 mm or greater in diameter that is free of sclerosis and is patent throughout its course is a potentially suitable target for venous outflow for an upper arm AVG.

O Chest wall AVG possible?

A chest wall AVG requires normal axillary artery inflow and axillary vein outflow. The graft can be performed in a looped manner between the ipsilateral axillary artery and vein or in a "necklace" configuration between the axillary artery and the contralateral axillary vein. Both configurations are comparable with approximately 80% secondary patency at 12 months.[26] An ipsilateral axillary artery to axillary vein loop placed in the upper arm has also been described with similar patency outcomes.[27] For the ipsilateral axillary artery to axillary vein configuration, the grafts should be oriented such that the venous outflow can be easily accessed if angioplasty of the venous anastomosis is required in the future. In the right chest, the graft should be oriented clockwise and in the left chest, counterclockwise.

P Brachial-axillary AVG

A brachial-axillary AVG can be created in a gentle arc from the brachial artery in the antecubital fossa to the axillary vein, or in a looped manner from the mid/proximal brachial artery to the axillary vein. The median secondary patency of the upper arm AVG is approximately 20 months.[28] The most common reason for failure of AVGs is stenosis caused by intimal hyperplasia at the venous outflow anastomosis.[10] Use of a hybrid ePTFE graft reinforced with a self-expanding nitinol stent at the venous outflow end has been proposed to reduce the incidence of outflow stenosis by creating a more favorable transition from the graft to the vein.[29] However, evidence is lacking to support this theory.[30]

Q Brachial-antecubital forearm loop AVG

The forearm loop AVG is created using the antecubital brachial artery as inflow and the antecubital brachial vein and cephalic or basilic vein as outflow. The secondary patency of the forearm loop AVG is approximately 80% at 12 months.[31]

R Increased risk of infection?

Patients who are immunocompromised secondary to medications and/or comorbidities, those with a chronic infection, or those who have had vascular access infections in the past are at an increased risk of AVG infection. The infection rate of upper extremity AVG has been reported to be anywhere from 3.5% to 19.7%.[32] In a study of 1023 upper extremity AVG, the infection rate was 9% with a median of 168 days at time of infection.[33] If this is the case, biologic rather than prosthetic conduit for AVGs should be considered.

S Consider biologic graft

A number of biologic grafts are available and have been used for vascular access including bovine carotid artery, bovine ureter, bovine mesenteric vein, cryopreserved human vein, and cryopreserved human artery. Of the bovine conduits, the bovine carotid artery is the most commonly used. In a randomized trial of bovine carotid artery and ePTFE AVGs, the bovine carotid artery had higher primary (60.5% vs. 10.1% at 12 months, $P = 0.0062$) and primary-assisted patency (60.5% vs. 20.8% at 12 months, $P = 0.012$), with fewer interventions required to maintain patency (1.3 vs. 2.5 per patient-year, $P = 0.014$).[34] The same trial also demonstrated that upper arm ePTFE AVGs had 0.3 episodes of infection per patient-year compared to 0 episodes for bovine carotid artery AVGs ($P = 0.008$).[34] Cryopreserved femoral and saphenous vein, as well as cryopreserved femoral artery, have also been used to create AVGs.[35] Cryopreserved vein is associated with higher patency than is cryopreserved artery with a secondary patency rate at 5 years of 58% versus 42%, respectively.[35]

ⓣ Prosthetic graft

A number of types of prosthetic grafts are available and can be used for AVG construction. However, none have been shown to have superior patency or lower complication rates. The most commonly used is the ePTFE graft. Other available materials are heparin-bonded ePTFE and multilayer early-access grafts. ePTFE grafts are available as a conventional single-diameter tube and tapered versions, that include a 4- to 7-mm taper and a 6- to 8-mm taper. Randomized comparisons of tapered grafts compared to conventional grafts have not demonstrated differences in access-related hand ischemia or patency.[36-38] Heparin-bonded ePTFE has not been shown to improve patency over conventional ePTFE grafts.[39,40]

Grafts that are not intended for early access typically require 2 to 3 weeks of tissue ingrowth after AVG creation before the graft can be accessed for hemodialysis without access site extravasation. Early-cannulation grafts, however, can be accessed as soon as 24 hours after AVG creation. There are four commercially available early-access grafts in the United States. One is a three-layer ePTFE graft. The outer layer has larger pores intended to promote tissue ingrowth. The middle layer is for reinforcement to promote durability. The inner layer has smaller pores to reduce permeability.[41] The second is composed of a self-sealing, nonwoven, synthetic nanofiber.[42] The third is a three-layer graft composed of polyetheruethaneurea and a siloxane-containing surface-modifying additive.[43] The fourth is also a three-layer graft with the inner and outer layer being ePTFE and a low-bleed elastomeric middle layer.[44] The 12-month primary patency of all the early cannulation grafts ranges from 43% to 63% and the 12-month secondary patency ranges from 70% to 86%.[45] Early cannulation does not appear to adversely affect graft patency.[45]

ⓤ Adequate vein for AVF?

In general, a basilic or cephalic vein that is 2.5 mm or greater in diameter that is free of sclerotic areas on DUS is a good candidate for AVF creation. Vein diameters between 2 and 2.5 mm may have marginal success with AVF creation.

ⓥ Current dialysis need?

Patients who are already hemodialysis dependent have a more urgent need for a functional long-term vascular access. AVG has been shown to be associated with early catheter removal and fewer catheter days than is AVF, which requires months to mature before use.[46] Patients who are hemodialysis dependent or imminently dialysis dependent may be more appropriate for an AVG than for an AVF. A number of factors should be taken into account when making this decision. Marginal vein quality, limited life expectancy, and obese body habitus are factors that may sway the decision toward AVG.

ⓦ Appropriate patient for radial AVF?

Radiocephalic access has been shown to have lower patency and maturation when compared with upper arm access in patients >65 years, women, and patients with diabetes.[22,47] Elderly age combined with diabetes markedly increase the risk of radiocephalic access failure to mature.[47] Although the evidence regarding any one of these characteristics is not conclusive, patients with increasing numbers of these adverse characteristics are not good candidates for radial AVF, and as such, should have a more proximal site selected.

ⓧ Adequate radial artery?

A radial artery of 2 mm in diameter at the wrist by DUS without significant proximal stenosis is typically adequate for AVF construction. Radial arteries <2 mm in diameter are associated with increased rates of AVF nonmaturation.[47] No more than a moderate degree of calcification in the area of the anastomosis is advisable to limit technical difficulties. Furthermore, calcified radial arteries may not dilate sufficiently after creation of the AVF to permit adequate access flow and effective dialysis. There is limited evidence to suggest that patients with diabetes and extensive radial artery calcification have worse patency rates than those with normal radial arteries, suggesting that patients with extensive radial artery calcifications should not undergo radial-cephalic AVF.[48] Ultimately, the surgeon must judge whether the artery is healthy enough to be clamped and sewn. If there is doubt based on preoperative imaging, the artery can be explored to make this determination.

ⓨ Adequate forearm cephalic vein?

A forearm cephalic vein of 2.0 mm in diameter or greater throughout with minimal sclerosis on DUS is generally considered adequate for construction of a radial-cephalic fistula.[47]

ⓩ Acceptable upper arm cephalic vein?

An upper arm cephalic vein of 2.5 mm or greater in diameter throughout with minimal sclerosis on DUS is generally considered adequate for construction of an upper arm brachial-cephalic fistula.[25]

ⒶⒶ Acceptable forearm basilic vein?

A forearm basilic vein diameter ≥2 to 2.5 mm throughout, with minimal sclerosis on DUS, is generally considered adequate for construction of a radial-basilic AVF.[25]

ⒷⒷ Acceptable upper arm basilic vein?

An upper arm basilic vein of 2.5 mm or greater in diameter throughout with minimal sclerosis on DUS is generally considered adequate for construction of a brachial-basilic fistula.[25]

ⒸⒸ Radiocephalic AVF

The classic Brescia-Cimino fistula was described in 1966 as a side-to-side anastomosis of the radial artery to the largest available neighboring vein through a 3-cm incision over the area of the radial pulse.[49] One of the most common causes of primary radiocephalic AVF failure is a juxta-anastomotic stenosis that occurs where the cephalic vein turns toward the radial artery. The piggyback straight-line onlay technique (pSLOT) has been shown to decrease the incidence of primary failure due to juxta-anastomotic stenosis.[50] In the pSLOT technique, the posterior aspect (underside) of the cephalic vein is anastomosed to the anterior aspect of the radial artery in a side-to-side manner. Care is taken to dissect the outflow vein further in the subcutaneous tissue to ensure that the vein has a straighter lie without an abrupt turn. An alternative technique is the radial artery deviation and reimplantation (RADAR) technique that is intended to minimize manipulation of the vein and reduce the risk of juxta-anastomotic stenosis in the swing segment. In RADAR, the radial artery is ligated at the wrist.[51] The distal end of the artery, proximal to the ligation, is turned toward the cephalic vein. An anastomosis is then created from the end of the artery to the side of the vein. The radiocephalic AVF can also be constructed distally in the snuffbox where the vessels lie parallel and in close proximity.[52] The end of the vein is anastomosed to the side of the artery. Despite the smaller diameter of the vessels in the snuffbox location, studies have shown no significant difference in primary and secondary patency up to 18 months.[53]

ⒹⒹ Brachiocephalic AVF

Brachiocephalic AVFs are typically performed through a transverse incision in the antecubital fossa.[54] The cephalic vein is transected and an anastomosis is created from the end of the cephalic vein to the side of the brachial artery. When ultrasound is available in the operating room, it is recommended that the brachial artery and cephalic vein be imaged before making the incision. If the surgeon thinks that the distance between the cephalic vein and brachial artery is too large for the operation to be performed through a single transverse incision, two parallel incisions may be used, one over the cephalic vein and one over the brachial artery. This allows for more extensive dissection of the cephalic vein if necessary and mobilization of the vein with branch ligation. The distal end of the vein is then tunneled under the skin bridge for the anastomosis. Use of a 6- to 7-mm arteriotomy in the brachial artery and liberal use of a venous footplate has been associated with increased primary functional patency at 12 months.[55] A footplate is created by transecting the cephalic vein near a branch point. The branch vein is also transected 2 to 3 mm from the cephalic vein. The bridge between the cephalic vein and the branch are divided, creating a footplate that is then used to create the end-to-side anastomosis. Similar to the radiocephalic fistula, the juxta-anastomotic area is at risk for stenosis if there is a sharp turn in the vein.[56] Care should be taken to perform extended dissection in this area to ensure a straight lie of the cephalic vein.

EE Brachial basilic AVF

Brachial basilic AVF can be created in a single-stage or two-stage manner. Although the basilic vein is a "superficial vein," in the upper arm, it is not anatomically located in an immediate subcutaneous position needed for access. Thus, the basilic vein must be transposed to a more superficial and anterolateral position to allow for cannulation. In the single-stage procedure, the entire basilic vein is dissected out, transposed to a superficial position, and anastomosed to the brachial artery in the antecubital fossa. In the two-stage procedure, the basilic vein is anastomosed to the brachial artery in the antecubital fossa in the first operation, and at the second operation, the fistula is superficialized. Typically, 4 to 6 weeks elapse between the first and second stages to allow for maturation of the fistula. Using either approach, the basilic vein can be superficialized by passing it through a superficial tunnel or placing the vein in a superficial pocket by creating a skin flap that is no more than 5 mm thick. If tunneling is used in a two-stage approach, the fistula is divided distal to the anastomosis, passed through the tunnel, and reanastomosed to itself. Using a superficial pocket in the two-stage approach obviates the need for a new anastomosis.

There is some evidence to suggest that the two-stage approach may be more durable and cost-effective than the one stage procedure.[57] One meta-analysis demonstrated no difference in 1-year primary and secondary patency rates between the one-stage and two-stage approach, despite the veins in the two-stage group being smaller in diameter.[58] Three of the eight studies included in the meta-analysis preferentially reserved two-stage transpositions for patients with smaller veins. Primary patency at 12 months for the one-stage transpositions was 26% to 70% and 13% to 87% for the two-stage transpositions (P = 0.33). Secondary patency at 12 months for the one-stage transpositions was 77% to 86% and 62% to 95% for the two-stage transpositions (P = 0.98). Similarly, there was no difference in primary failure with a rate of 15% to 45% in patients with one-stage transpositions and 10% to 42% in patients with two-stage transpositions (P = 0.46). This suggests that for smaller basilic veins, the two-stage approach may be preferred. Another meta-analysis also demonstrated no difference in 1-year primary and secondary patency and 2-year secondary patency.[59] However, the two-stage procedure had significantly improved 2-year primary patency rates despite no difference in complications. The 2-year secondary patency for one-stage transpositions ranged from 41% to 80% and 61% to 86% for the two-stage transpositions (P < 0.001).

FF Forearm basilic AVF

The forearm basilic AVF can be created using either the radial artery or the ulnar artery as inflow.[60] The course of the basilic vein in the forearm can vary somewhat; and depending on the individual patient's anatomy, the distal segment of the basilic vein may need to be mobilized and transposed in order for it to be anastomosed to the radial or ulnar artery. The reported outcomes of forearm basilic AVF are relatively poor, with approximately 50% primary and 70% secondary patency at 1 year.[60-62] Maturation rates, when reported, are as low as 60%.[60] However, the complication rates of vascular-access-related hand ischemia and infection are very low. The forearm basilic AVF allows for preservation of upper arm vascular access sites and is a particularly attractive option in younger patients with long life expectancies who may need numerous permanent vascular access sites over their lifespan.

GG Consider brachial-brachial AVF vs. AVG

The brachial-brachial AVF is a technically challenging operation, with high rates of maturation failure in up to 50% and primary patency at 12 months ranging between 24% and 77%.[63,64] The brachial vein is a thin-walled, deep vein with numerous small tributaries that must all be carefully dissected and ligated. The brachial-brachial AVF can be created in one stage or in two stages, in the same manner as the brachial-basilic AVF. The limited evidence that is available supports better outcomes with the two-stage approach.[63,64] Although brachial-brachial AVF maturation and patency rates are inferior to brachiocephalic and brachiobasilic AVF, the brachiobrachial AVF offers an autogenous alternative for patients who do not have adequate upper extremity superficial veins.

REFERENCES

1. U.S. Renal Data System. 2017 USRDS annual data report: epidemiology of kidney disease in the United States. Bethesda, MD: National Institutes of Health, National Institute of Diabetes and Digestive and Kidney Diseases; 2017.
2. Vascular Access Work Group. Clinical practice guidelines for vascular access. *Am J Kidney Dis.* 2006;48(suppl 1):S248-S273.
3. Puskar D, Pasini J, Savic I, Bedalov G, Sonicki Z. Survival of primary arteriovenous fistula in 463 patients on chronic hemodialysis. *Croat Med J.* 2002;43(3):306-311.
4. Chang TI, Paik J, Greene T, et al. Intradialytic hypotension and vascular access thrombosis. *J Am Soc Nephrol.* 2011;22(8):1526-1533.
5. Bream PR Jr. Update on insertion and complications of central venous catheters for hemodialysis. *Semin Intervent Radiol.* 2016;33(1):31-38.
6. Ponce D, Mendes M, Silva T, Oliveira R. Occluded tunneled venous catheter in hemodialysis patients: risk factors and efficacy of alteplase. *Artif Organs.* 2015;39(9):741-747.
7. Brady PS, Spence LD, Levitin A, Mickolich CT, Dolmatch BL. Efficacy of percutaneous fibrin sheath stripping in restoring patency of tunneled hemodialysis catheters. *AJR Am J Roentgenol.* 1999;173(4):1023-1027.
8. Miller LM, Clark E, Dipchand C, et al. Hemodialysis tunneled catheter-related infections. *Can J Kidney Health Dis.* 2016;3:2054358116669129.
9. Kundu S. Review of central venous disease in hemodialysis patients. *J Vasc Interv Radiol.* 2010;21(7):963-968.
10. Ginsburg M, Lorenz JM, Zivin SP, Zangan S, Martinez D. A practical review of the use of stents for the maintenance of hemodialysis access. *Semin Intervent Radiol.* 2015;32(2):217-224.
11. Wooster M, Fernandez B, Summers KL, Illig KA. Surgical and endovascular central venous reconstruction combined with thoracic outlet decompression in highly symptomatic patients. *J Vasc Surg Venous Lymphat Disord.* 2019;7(1):106-112.e3.
12. Al Shakarchi J, Houston JG, Jones RG, Inston N. A review on the Hemodialysis Reliable Outflow (HeRO) graft for haemodialysis vascular access. *Eur J Vasc Endovasc Surg.* 2015;50(1):108-113.
13. Katzman HE, McLafferty RB, Ross JR, Glickman MH, Peden EK, Lawson JH. Initial experience and outcome of a new hemodialysis access device for catheter-dependent patients. *J Vasc Surg.* 2009;50(3):600-607, 607.e1.
14. Steerman SN, Wagner J, Higgins JA, et al. Outcomes comparison of HeRO and lower extremity arteriovenous grafts in patients with long-standing renal failure. *J Vasc Surg.* 2013;57(3):776-783; discussion 782-773.
15. Antoniou GA, Lazarides MK, Georgiadis GS, Sfyroeras GS, Nikolopoulos ES, Giannoukas AD. Lower-extremity arteriovenous access for haemodialysis: a systematic review. *Eur J Vasc Endovasc Surg.* 2009;38(3):365-372.
16. Pierre-Paul D, Williams S, Lee T, Gahtan V. Saphenous vein loop to femoral artery arteriovenous fistula: a practical alternative. *Ann Vasc Surg.* 2004;18(2):223-227.
17. Alomran F, Boura B, Mallios A, De Blic R, Costanzo A, Combes M. Tagliatelle technique for arteriovenous fistula creation using a great saphenous vein semipanel graft. *J Vasc Surg.* 2013;58(6):1705-1708.
18. Cull JD, Cull DL, Taylor SM, et al. Prosthetic thigh arteriovenous access: outcome with SVS/AAVS reporting standards. *J Vasc Surg.* 2004;39(2):381-386.
19. Bourquelot P, Rawa M, Van Laere O, Franco G. Long-term results of femoral vein transposition for autogenous arteriovenous hemodialysis access. *J Vasc Surg.* 2012;56(2):440-445.
20. Ong S, Barker-Finkel J, Allon M. Long-term outcomes of arteriovenous thigh grafts in hemodialysis patients: a comparison with tunneled dialysis catheters. *Clin J Am Soc Nephrol.* 2013;8(5):804-809.
21. Woo K, Ulloa J, Allon M, et al. Establishing patient-specific criteria for selecting the optimal upper extremity vascular access procedure. *J Vasc Surg.* 2017;65(4):1089-1103.e1081.
22. Misskey J, Faulds J, Sidhu R, Baxter K, Gagnon J, Hsiang Y. An age-based comparison of fistula location, patency, and

maturation for elderly renal failure patients. *J Vasc Surg.* 2018;67(5):1491-1500.

23. Lee T, Qian J, Thamer M, Allon M. Tradeoffs in vascular access selection in elderly patients initiating hemodialysis with a catheter. *Am J Kidney Dis.* 2018;72(4):509-518.

24. Lok CE, Allon M, Moist L, Oliver MJ, Shah H, Zimmerman D. Risk equation determining unsuccessful cannulation events and failure to maturation in arteriovenous fistulas (REDUCE FTM I). *J Am Soc Nephrol.* 2006;17(11):3204-3212.

25. Wilmink T, Corte-Real Houlihan M. Diameter criteria have limited value for prediction of functional dialysis use of arteriovenous fistulas. *Eur J Vasc Endovasc Surg.* 2018;56(4):572-581.

26. Gale-Grant O, Chemla ES. Single-center results of a series of prosthetic axillary-axillary arteriovenous access grafts for hemodialysis. *J Vasc Surg.* 2016;64(6):1741-1746.

27. Hunter JP, Nicholson ML. Midterm experience of ipsilateral axillary-axillary arteriovenous loop graft as tertiary access for haemodialysis. *J Transplant.* 2014;2014:908738.

28. Lok CE, Sontrop JM, Tomlinson G, et al. Cumulative patency of contemporary fistulas versus grafts (2000-2010). *Clin J Am Soc Nephrol.* 2013;8(5):810-818.

29. Habibollahi P, Mantel MP, Rosenberry T, Leeser DB, Clark TWI. Outcomes of a polytetrafluoroethylene hybrid vascular graft with preloaded nitinol stent at the venous outflow for dialysis vascular access. *Ann Vasc Surg.* 2019;55:210-215.

30. Benedetto F, Spinelli D, Pipito N, et al. Initial clinical experience with a polytetrafluoroethylene vascular dialysis graft reinforced with nitinol at the venous end. *J Vasc Surg.* 2017;65(1):142-150.

31. Keuter XH, De Smet AA, Kessels AG, van der Sande FM, Welten RJ, Tordoir JH. A randomized multicenter study of the outcome of brachial-basilic arteriovenous fistula and prosthetic brachial-antecubital forearm loop as vascular access for hemodialysis. *J Vasc Surg.* 2008;47(2):395-401.

32. Akoh JA. Prosthetic arteriovenous grafts for hemodialysis. *J Vasc Access.* 2009;10(3):137-147.

33. Harish A, Allon M. Arteriovenous graft infection: a comparison of thigh and upper extremity grafts. *Clin J Am Soc Nephrol.* 2011;6(7):1739-1743.

34. Kennealey PT, Elias N, Hertl M, et al. A prospective, randomized comparison of bovine carotid artery and expanded polytetrafluoroethylene for permanent hemodialysis vascular access. *J Vasc Surg.* 2011;53(6):1640-1648.

35. Harlander-Locke MP, Lawrence PF, Ali A, et al. Cryopreserved venous allograft is an acceptable conduit in patients with current or prior angioaccess graft infection. *J Vasc Surg.* 2017;66(4):1157-1162.

36. Dammers R, Planken RN, Pouls KP, et al. Evaluation of 4-mm to 7-mm versus 6-mm prosthetic brachial-antecubital

37. Polo JR, Ligero JM, Diaz-Cartelle J, Garcia-Pajares R, Cervera T, Reparaz L. Randomized comparison of 6-mm straight grafts versus 6- to 8-mm tapered grafts for brachial-axillary dialysis access. *J Vasc Surg.* 2004;40(2):319-324.

38. Han S, Seo PW, Ryu JW. Surgical outcomes of forearm loop arteriovenous fistula formation using tapered versus non-tapered polytetrafluoroethylene grafts. *Korean J Thorac Cardiovasc Surg.* 2017;50(1):30-35.

39. Allemang MT, Schmotzer B, Wong VL, et al. Heparin bonding does not improve patency of polytetrafluoroethylene arteriovenous grafts. *Ann Vasc Surg.* 2014;28(1):28-34.

40. Zea N, Menard G, Le L, et al. Heparin-bonded polytetrafluoroethylene does not improve hemodialysis arteriovenous graft function. *Ann Vasc Surg.* 2016;30:28-33.

41. Hinojosa CA, Soto-Solis S, Olivares-Cruz S, Laparra-Escareno H, Gomez-Arcive Z, Anaya-Ayala JE. Early cannulation graft Flixene for conventional and complex hemodialysis access creation. *J Vasc Access.* 2017;18(2):109-113.

42. Yilmaz S. Early experience with a novel self-sealing nanofabric vascular graft for early hemodialysis access. *Vascular.* 2016;24(4):421-424.

43. Kakkos SK, Topalidis D, Haddad R, Haddad GK, Shepard AD. Long-term complication and patency rates of Vectra and IMPRA Carboflo vascular access grafts with aggressive monitoring, surveillance and endovascular management. *Vascular.* 2011;19(1):21-28.

44. Glickman M. Early cannulation graft: acuseal. *J Vasc Access.* 2016;17(suppl 1):S72-S74.

45. Al Shakarchi J, Inston N. Early cannulation grafts for haemodialysis: an updated systematic review. *J Vasc Access.* 2019;20(2):123-127.

46. Leake AE, Yuo TH, Wu T, et al. Arteriovenous grafts are associated with earlier catheter removal and fewer catheter days in the United States Renal Data System population. *J Vasc Surg.* 2015;62(1):123-127.

47. Mousa AY, Dearing DD, Aburahma AF. Radiocephalic fistula: review and update. *Ann Vasc Surg.* 2013;27(3):370-378.

48. Georgiadis GS, Georgakarakos EI, Antoniou GA, et al. Correlation of pre-existing radial artery macrocalcifications with late patency of primary radiocephalic fistulas in diabetic hemodialysis patients. *J Vasc Surg.* 2014;60(2):462-470.

49. Brescia MJ, Cimino JE, Appel K, Hurwich BJ. Chronic hemodialysis using venipuncture and a surgically created arteriovenous fistula. *N Engl J Med.* 1966;275(20):1089-1092.

50. Bharat A, Jaenicke M, Shenoy S. A novel technique of vascular anastomosis to prevent juxta-anastomotic stenosis following arteriovenous fistula creation. *J Vasc Surg.* 2012;55(1):274-280.

51. Sadaghianloo N, Declemy S, Jean-Baptiste E, et al. Radial artery deviation and reimplantation inhibits venous

juxta-anastomotic stenosis and increases primary patency of radial-cephalic fistulas for hemodialysis. *J Vasc Surg.* 2016;64(3):698-706.e1.

52. Letachowicz K, Golebiowski T, Kusztal M, Letachowicz W, Weyde W, Klinger M. The snuffbox fistula should be preferred over the wrist arteriovenous fistula. *J Vasc Surg.* 2016;63(2):436-440.

53. Siracuse JJ, Arinze A, Levin SR, et al. Snuffbox arteriovenous fistulas have similar outcomes and patency as wrist arteriovenous fistulas. *J Vasc Surg.* 2019. doi:10.1016/j.jvs.2018.11.030.

54. Bender MH, Bruyninckx CM, Gerlag PG. The brachiocephalic elbow fistula: a useful alternative angioaccess for permanent hemodialysis. *J Vasc Surg.* 1994;20(5):808-813.

55. Kim JJ, Gifford E, Nguyen V, et al. Increased use of brachiocephalic arteriovenous fistulas improves functional primary patency. *J Vasc Surg.* 2015;62(2):442-447.

56. Brahmbhatt A, Remuzzi A, Franzoni M, Misra S. The molecular mechanisms of hemodialysis vascular access failure. *Kidney Int.* 2016;89(2):303-316.

57. Ghaffarian AA, Griffin CL, Kraiss LW, Sarfati MR, Brooke BS. Comparative effectiveness of one-stage versus two-stage basilic vein transposition arteriovenous fistulas. *J Vasc Surg.* 2018;67(2):529-535.e1.

58. Cooper J, Power AH, DeRose G, Forbes TL, Dubois L. Similar failure and patency rates when comparing one- and two-stage basilic vein transposition. *J Vasc Surg.* 2015;61(3):809-816.

59. Jun Yan Wee I, Mohamed IH, Patel A, Choong A. A systematic review and meta-analysis of one-stage versus two-stage brachiobasilic arteriovenous fistula creation. *J Vasc Surg.* 2018;68(1):285-297.

60. Schwein A, Georg Y, Lejay A, et al. Promising results of the forearm basilic fistula reveal a worthwhile option between radial cephalic and brachial fistula. *Ann Vasc Surg.* 2016;32:5-8.

61. Al Shakarchi J, Khawaja A, Cassidy D, Houston JG, Inston N. Efficacy of the ulnar-basilic arteriovenous fistula for hemodialysis: a systematic review. *Ann Vasc Surg.* 2016;32:1-4.

62. Glowinski J, Glowinska I, Malyszko J, Gacko M. Basilic vein transposition in the forearm for secondary arteriovenous fistula. *Angiology.* 2014;65(4):330-332.

63. Kotsis T, Moulakakis KG, Mylonas SN, Kalogeropoulos P, Dellis A, Vasdekis S. Brachial artery-brachial vein fistula for hemodialysis: one- or two-stage procedure—a review. *Int J Angiol.* 2016;25(1):14-19.

64. Jennings WC, Sideman MJ, Taubman KE, Broughan TA. Brachial vein transposition arteriovenous fistulas for hemodialysis access. *J Vasc Surg.* 2009;50(5):1121-1125; discussion 1125-1126.

Dirk M. Hentschel • C. Keith Ozaki

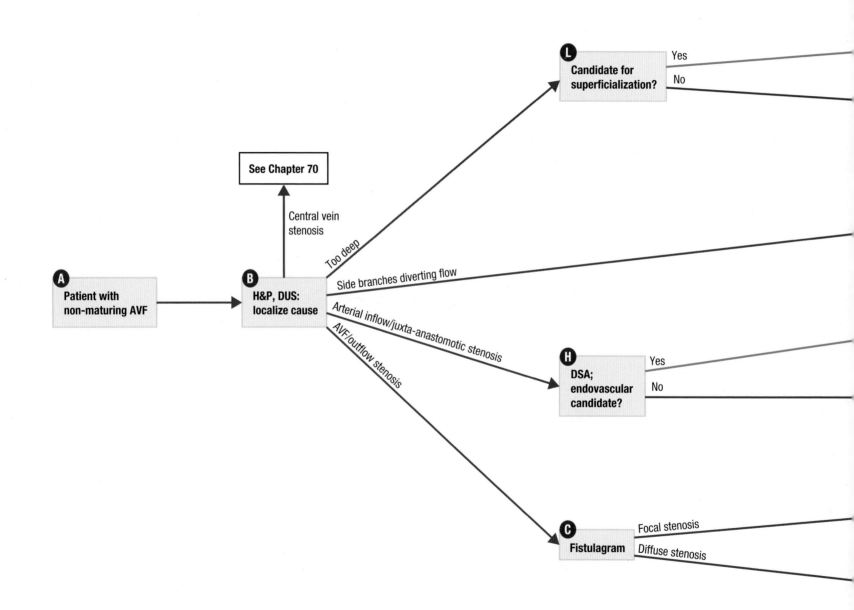

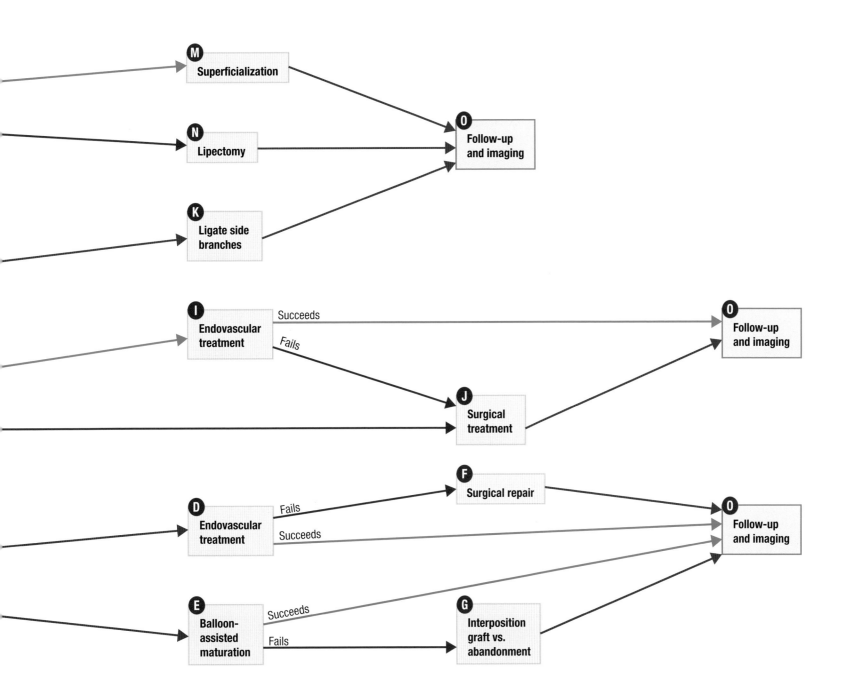

A Patient with non-maturing AVF

Large clinical trials and series have documented strikingly high rates (>50%) of non-maturation of AVFs.[1] The pathophysiology of non-maturation is not completely understood, but likely includes intimal hyperplasia and failure of flow- and pressure-induced outward vascular remodeling.[2] Risk factors for non-maturation include more distal arm location (eg, distal radial-cephalic AVF), advanced age, systemic vascular disease, female gender, small initial vein diameter, local adipose phenotype, and surgical experience.[3-5]

Various criteria exist for a "mature" AVF. Under our practical guidelines, a mature fistula meets the following criteria: vein ≥6 mm in diameter, ≤6 mm deep from the skin, has a flow rate of ≥600 mL/min, has ≥15 cm of length suitable for cannulation, and has a sufficiently thick wall for cannulation. Our clinical observation is that it usually takes at least 6 weeks for the vein wall to thicken sufficiently to withstand repeated needle cannulation. If the physical examination is abnormal at 6 to 8 weeks, the chances of maturation without intervention are low,[1,6] and, therefore, we actively pursue interventions to facilitate maturation.

In describing AVFs, it is important to use uniform terminology.[7,8] The artery and vein are connected at the *arterial anastomosis*. The *juxta-anastomotic* segment extends 2 cm on either side of the anastomosis. In the antegrade direction (ie, toward the venous outflow), the *inflow segment* is located between the juxta-anastomotic segment and the *body of the access*, the segment that is used for the actual cannulation. The body of the access then drains into the forearm/upper arm cephalic/basilic/brachial *outflow veins*. In a transposed upper arm access, the segment mobilized toward the axilla is called the *swing point segment*. The *cephalic arch* is the most central portion of the cephalic vein that lies in the delta-pectoral groove, immediately proximal to its confluence with the axillary vein. For upper extremity access, the *central veins* include subclavian and brachiocephalic veins as well as the SVC.

B H&P, DUS: localize cause

Most causes of AVF non-maturation can be diagnosed using physical examination, and supplemented with DUS, as necessary. DUS is a useful adjunct that can be used to measure the fistula dimensions and depth relative to the skin, and to identify areas of stenosis, tortuosity, the presence of large side branches; arterial inflow and venous outflow can also be evaluated. DUS can also be used to calculate access flow rates (best measured where there is laminar flow such as in the inflow artery 2 cm retrograde from the anastomosis)[9]; such flow measurement may miss the contribution of retrograde inflow from the distal artery, which is particularly common in forearm access.

Stenosis within the inflow segment or body of the access is the most frequent cause of AVF failure to mature. Most stenoses

are focal, but they can be more diffuse and require different treatments. The area of stenosis can often be identified by inspection or physical examination because the stenosis leads to a change in the character of the access with a transition in pulsatility (increased or decreased) and an associated thrill antegrade to the change in pulsatility. The area of stenosis may be confirmed by DUS.

Poor arterial inflow or a juxta-anastomotic stenosis is identified by a diminished pulse at the anastomosis that does not improve with compression of the AVF inflow segment (ie, segment of AVF between juxta-anastomosis and body). Presence of a prominent pulse in the AVF typically denotes a significant downstream stenosis. It is important to remember that, on occasion, more than one fistula stenosis may occur (eg, both juxta-anastomotic and outflow stenoses).

Failure of an AVF to mature can occur if large side branches in the inflow segment or body of the AVF divert significant blood flow away from the main AVF outflow vein. These can be often identified by visual inspection, or in deeper lying AVF, confirmed with DUS. If they are significant, compression of these side branches should augment the flow in the AVF, as detected by increased pulsatility on physical examination or DUS.

In some cases, the body of the AVF may be too deep (ie, >6 mm from the skin surface) to allow accurate cannulation even though the diameter of the vein is adequate. This is apparent by inspection and palpation of the access, but can be confirmed by DUS.

Rarely, failure of an AVF to mature can result if central venous stenosis impedes venous return such that AVF flow is limited. In such cases, arm swelling is usually present, and AVF flow may be elevated.

C Fistulagram

A fistulagram provides additional diagnostic imaging for the underlying mechanisms of access dysfunction and, more importantly, provides an opportunity for endovascular intervention. In the context of immature AVFs, the access site for the fistulagram should be guided by the physical examination. Within the first 6 weeks of AVF creation, puncture can cause profound spasm in the access that can lead to inadvertent puncture of the AVF back wall with the development of a hematoma, and even access occlusion. In the case of these early cannulations for diagnostic imaging, we prefer retrograde puncture of the brachial artery at the elbow using only the internal 3-Fr dilator of a micropuncture sheath. This allows imaging of both forearm and upper arm AVFs with antegrade flow of contrast, which identifies angiographic flow pattern as well as sites of stenoses. Angiographic images can be shared among providers and is less operator dependent than is DUS. In an access that has had more time to mature, we directly access the inflow segment of the AVF in an antegrade direction, first using only the internal dilator of a micropuncture set. This can be

exchanged for a 5-Fr vascular sheath if endovascular treatment is required. DUS is a helpful adjunct for small-diameter AVFs or AVFs that are otherwise difficult to cannulate. Subsequent treatment selection depends on whether there is focal or diffuse stenosis in the AVF.

In patients not yet on dialysis, the quantity of iodinated contrast for a fistulagram can usually be limited to <5 mL to reduce the likelihood of renal injury. Carbon dioxide can be used as a contrast agent to avoid or limit the use of iodinated contrast and is safe when reflux into the arterial circulation is avoided.

D Endovascular treatment

In current practice, focal stenoses of the AVF inflow segment, body, and venous outflow are treated initially with PTA. If more than one stenosis exists, the more central one is treated first to avoid exposing the peripheral angioplasty site to elevated intra-access pressures from the more distal central stenosis, which can potentially lead to access disruption and contrast extravasation.[10] A retrograde sheath may cause such severe spasm that the flow within the access stops. For this reason, we use an antegrade sheath or arterial puncture to image the outflow first, before the expected intervention. We routinely give 2000 to 4000 units of IV heparin at the onset of the procedure to prevent access thrombosis.

For initial interventions, we use a 5-Fr vascular sheath and limit balloon diameters to 3 to 5 mm, particularly in the inflow segment. Gradual increase of flow over time facilitates shear stress-pressure relationships that favor outward venous remodeling and maturation.[11-13] Stenoses in the venous outflow that are detected early are often associated with valve mechanisms and, thus, undersizing the balloon diameter relative to the vein diameter avoids injury to the vein itself. However, this can disrupt the ring of the venous valve. With this approach, "less" intervention is often "more," and repeat PTA can be performed within 1 to 2 weeks, as needed. This staged approach is usually more successful in maturing a vein than in attempting to achieve a perfect angiographic result at the time of the first balloon dilation at the cost of a higher incidence of PTA-related vein injury.[10]

Some brachial-cephalic AVFs require early intervention of the cephalic arch. In our opinion, the cephalic arch has to be approximately 8 mm in diameter to accommodate adequate flow volumes without increased intra-access pressure. We use stent grafts to treat cephalic arch stenoses, based on reports that suggest a benefit over PTA or bare-metal stents alone.[14,15] We place 8 × 50 or 8 × 100 self-expanding stent grafts that may not be fully expanded at the time of deployment to avoid stretch injury of immature cephalic veins, but can be fully dilated at a later point when the cephalic vein diameter has increased.

Focal stenoses or occlusions that can be navigated successfully with a guidewire should be treated with PTA alone. Longer length outflow stenoses (ie, >2 cm or segmental disease) and specific locations (eg, cephalic arch) may favor the use of a stent graft because most stenoses are prone to recurrence. Stents and stent grafts should be specifically avoided in the cannulation zone.

After sheath removal, access sites have to be compressed manually, because the skin overlying an immature AVF is not particularly adherent, and, thus, prone to development of a hematoma. After removal of a retrograde sheath (more so than for antegrade sheath), the access vein may go into complete spasm and flow will stop. Unless carefully managed, this will lead to pulsatile bleeding from the sheath insertion site. We typically occlude the inflow and the sheath insertion site, and then only gradually restore flow through the access.

E Balloon-assisted maturation

AVFs with diffusely small diameter outflow veins can be remediated by an endovascular approach referred to as "BAM"—balloon-assisted maturation.[10] This process entails repeated segmental disruptive dilation of the body of the access using long balloons, starting with balloon diameters of 4 to 5 mm and lengths of 8 to 12 cm. The balloon diameters are increased in 1- to 2-mm steps, with the timing of the repeat interventions spaced between 1 and 3 weeks, as dictated by patient age and comorbidities, until a target diameter is reached. Care needs to be exercised to occlude the inflow during balloon deflation and the outflow stenoses need to be treated first. Both strategies tend to limit the intraluminal pressure and minimize the extent of the hematoma associated with vein disruption.

F Surgical treatment

A focal stenosis in the outflow fistula vein that recurs shortly after initial endovascular therapy is best treated using surgical patch angioplasty. We prefer to use autogenous vein for patching, usually harvested from a large side branch. Occasionally, transposition of the vein (ie, transposition of an upper arm cephalic vein over to the basilic/axillary veins) or a jump graft beyond a focal stenosis or occlusion is necessary.

G Interposition graft vs. abandonment

Diffuse stenoses that are refractory to PTA can be treated with an interposition graft provided there is a sufficient segment of the AVF that is mature or uninvolved to merit salvage. This approach can lead to more rapid access use when compared with abandonment and creation of a new access. However, abandonment may be appropriate if the entire access is stenotic.

H DSA; endovascular candidate?

DSA is used to define details of arterial inflow or juxta-anastomotic stenoses, to help determine whether endovascular or open surgical revision is optimal. In most cases, PTA and intraluminal

stenting are favored for proximal SCA lesion. Although the less invasive endovascular approach is also appealing for stenoses in the axillary or brachial arteries, these are relatively easy to expose and, given superior long-term outcomes, are usually best treated with an open surgery using vein patch angioplasty. Patient risk for open surgery and likelihood of successful endovascular treatment are key factors that determine the optimal approach. Juxta-anastomotic stenoses are nearly always approached with surgical revision.

I Endovascular treatment

Endovascular treatment in the SCA usually is done with bare-metal stenting. PTA alone may be used if axillary or brachial stenoses are not treated surgically. Arterial inflow lesions in small, calcified radial arteries can sometimes also be successfully treated with PTA.[16] Although juxta-anastomotic stenoses are best treated with open surgical repair using patch angioplasty, there are some anastomotic configurations that lend themselves to stent-graft placement across the anastomosis (eg, brachial-cephalic AVF anastomosis after DRIL procedure). After successful stent placement, patients are typically maintained on clopidogrel or full-dose anticoagulation for the initial 6 months after endovascular treatment with continued treatment depending on the success of the access in terms of maturation, successful cannulation, and the number of remedial procedures.

J Surgical treatment

Standard surgical techniques such as endarterectomy, patch angioplasty, and bypass can be used to treat arterial inflow or juxta-anastomotic stenoses, with the choice contingent on individual patient circumstances. When using autogenous vein for reconstructions, it is important to preserve future access sites within the context of a lifetime access plan. Biologic and ePTFE grafts can be used as an alternative conduit to salvage the access, with the configuration dictated by the distribution of the arterial inflow or venous outflow stenoses. For example, a juxta-anastomotic stenosis in a brachial-cephalic AVF can be remediated with an interposition ePTFE graft based off the brachial artery proximal to the stenotic anastomosis. Similarly, a stenotic lesion in a radial artery inflow for a distal radial-cephalic AVF can be remediated by resiting the inflow source of the AVF to a more proximal artery, preferably the proximal radial rather than the brachial artery at the antecubital fossa using autogenous or prosthetic conduit (ie, "proximalization"). The new anastomosis between the conduit and outflow vein should be configured in an end/end manner (either anatomically or functionally) in this setting to optimize the distal perfusion to the hand and avoid the potential for hand ischemia that could occur from having dual AVFs. A sterile tourniquet positioned above the elbow (inflated to about 50 mm Hg above SBP) and an Esmark bandage to exsanguinate the arm can help control arterial inflow and venous

backbleeding in this setting, simplifying dissection of the reoperative field.[17]

K Ligate side branches

Location of significant side branches should be marked using DUS before the start of the procedure. Significant side branches are identified by observing an increased flow on DUS when the main AVF outflow vein is compressed. The procedure itself is performed by making a series of small longitudinal incisions approximately 5 mm from the main outflow vein of the access, dissecting out the side branches, and ligating them with 4-0 monofilament permanent suture. We avoid braided suture material in this setting because we have observed an inflammatory reaction that can lead to stenosis in the adjacent access segment. After ligation of all previously identified side branches, a continuous-wave Doppler is placed just distal to the AVF anastomosis and the main outflow vein is occluded (distal to the sites of the ligated side branches). Complete cessation of flow in the AVF confirms that all of the side branches have been ligated. If flow is still detected in the AVF depending on the Doppler signal, the probe is moved along the course of the outflow vein until there is a transition from "flow present" to "none," indicating the location of an occult side branch that requires ligation. Although endovascular coil embolization can be used to occlude side branches with equal long-term efficacy,[18] we prefer simple surgical ligation, which is possible in most patients under local anesthesia.

L Candidate for superficialization?

If the AVF cannot be cannulated because it is too deep, it may be possible to elevate the vein to a more superficial position, similar to a second stage of a brachial-basilic fistula. This process requires that the vein is sufficiently tortuous or redundant such that there is an additional length of vein to span the requisite distance from the deep to superficial tissue. If the vein is not sufficiently redundant, this process of superficialization can create an unacceptable amount of tension on the outflow vein, leading to stenosis and/or retraction back into the deeper tissue. If patients are not candidates for superficialization, lipectomy is an acceptable alternative.

M Superficialization

After the location of the fistula is marked with the help of DUS, an incision is made over the fistula and the fistula is dissected out completely. It is then elevated by suturing the fascia deep to the fistula. The arm is closed in one layer keeping the fistula immediately below the skin. Stenotic lesions within the body of the access can be addressed at the time of the superficialization with either a patch angioplasty or diseased segment excision with primary reanastomosis. Unfortunately, the latter approach sacrifices a segment of the vein and may, if the vein itself is not sufficiently redundant, further complicate superficialization.

Ⓝ Lipectomy

Lipectomy offers an alternative method to reduce the depth of an access relative to the surface of the skin without having to perform an anastomosis.[19,20] DUS is used preoperatively to mark deep portions of the access and any significant side branch locations that merit ligation. Transverse incisions are made (about 2 in. apart over the deep portions of the access), and thin skin flaps are raised. The outflow vein is then completely exposed by dividing the overlying fascia and adipose tissue while any significant side branches are ligated with 4-0 monofilament sutures. Finally, the subcutaneous fat pads are removed with sharp dissection, essentially leaving the access vein immediately below the undersurface of the skin. The skin is reapproximated at the site of the transverse incisions, but no attempt is made to close the deeper tissue. The extremity is wrapped gently with an ace bandage (left intact for 48-72 hours) and the patients are instructed to elevate their arm as much as possible to prevent the development of a hematoma in the dead space between the access and the skin.

Ⓞ Follow-up and imaging

Careful follow-up is necessary after all interventions to facilitate maturation because additional procedures may be required. The appropriate follow-up interval varies with the individual access, but usually patients are seen and reevaluated with physical examination and DUS within 2 to 3 weeks of their initial treatment, and then monthly thereafter until maturation. We instruct patients on how to examine their access and educate them in terms of the signs associated with a failing access (eg, loss of thrill/bruit, increased pulsatility). Furthermore, patients are also encouraged to perform hand exercises to facilitate maturation.[21]

REFERENCES

1. Dember LM, Beck GJ, Allon M, et al. Effect of clopidogrel on early failure of arteriovenous fistulas for hemodialysis: a randomized controlled trial. *JAMA*. 2008;299:2164-2171.
2. Franzoni M, Walsh MT. Towards the identification of hemodynamic parameters involved in arteriovenous fistula maturation and failure: a review. *Cardiovasc Eng Technol*. 2017;8:342-356.
3. Lilly MP, Lynch JR, Wish JB, et al. Prevalence of arteriovenous fistulas in incident hemodialysis patients: correlation with patient factors that may be associated with maturation failure. *Am J Kidney Dis*. 2012;59:541-549.
4. Lok CE, Allon M, Moist L, Oliver MJ, Shah H, Zimmerman D. Risk equation determining unsuccessful cannulation events and failure to maturation in arteriovenous fistulas (REDUCE FTM I). *J Am Soc Nephrol*. 2006;17:3204-3212.
5. Goodkin DA, Pisoni RL, Locatelli F, Port FK, Saran R. Hemodialysis vascular access training and practices are key to improved access outcomes. *Am J Kidney Dis*. 2010;56:1032-1042.
6. Beathard GA, Arnold P, Jackson J, Litchfield T, Physician Operators Forum of RMSL. Aggressive treatment of early fistula failure. *Kidney Int*. 2003;64:1487-1494.
7. Swinnen J. Duplex ultrasound scanning of the autogenous arterio venous hemodialysis fistula: a vascular surgeon's perspective. *Australas J Ultrasound Med*. 2011;14:17-23.
8. Vascular Access Work G. Clinical practice guidelines for vascular access. *Am J Kidney Dis*. 2006;48(suppl 1):S176-S247.
9. Ko SH, Bandyk DF, Hodgkiss-Harlow KD, Barleben A, Lane J 3rd. Estimation of brachial artery volume flow by duplex ultrasound imaging predicts dialysis access maturation. *J Vasc Surg*. 2015;61:1521-1527.
10. Miller GA, Goel N, Khariton A, et al. Aggressive approach to salvage non-maturing arteriovenous fistulae: a retrospective study with follow-up. *J Vasc Access*. 2009;10:183-191.
11. Wong V, Ward R, Taylor J, Selvakumar S, How TV, Bakran A. Factors associated with early failure of arteriovenous fistulae for haemodialysis access. *Eur J Vasc Endovasc Surg*. 1996;12:207-213.
12. Fry DL. Certain histological and chemical responses of the vascular interface to acutely induced mechanical stress in the aorta of the dog. *Circ Res*. 1969;24:93-108.
13. Tohda K, Masuda H, Kawamura K, Shozawa T. Difference in dilatation between endothelium-preserved and -desquamated segments in the flow-loaded rat common carotid artery. *Arterioscler Thromb*. 1992;12:519-528.
14. Rajan DK, Falk A. A randomized prospective study comparing outcomes of angioplasty versus VIABAHN stent-graft placement for cephalic arch stenosis in dysfunctional hemodialysis accesses. *J Vasc Interv Radiol*. 2015;26:1355-1361.
15. Dukkipati R, Lee L, Atray N, Kajani R, Nassar G, Kalantar-Zadeh K. Outcomes of cephalic arch stenosis with and without stent placement after percutaneous balloon angioplasty in hemodialysis patients. *Semin Dial*. 2015;28:E7-E10.
16. Turmel-Rodrigues L, Boutin JM, Camiade C, Brillet G, Fodil-Cherif M, Mouton A. Percutaneous dilation of the radial artery in nonmaturing autogenous radial-cephalic fistulas for haemodialysis. *Nephrol Dial Transplant*. 2009;24:3782-3788.
17. Sadaghianloo N, Dardik A, Jean-Baptiste E, et al. Salvage of early-failing radiocephalic fistulae with techniques that minimize venous dissection. *Ann Vasc Surg*. 2015;29:1475-1479.
18. Davies MG. Management of arteriovenous fistula side branches: ligation or coil embolization. *J Vasc Surg*. 2019;70:e34.
19. Barnard KJ, Taubman KE, Jennings WC. Accessible autogenous vascular access for hemodialysis in obese individuals using lipectomy. *Am J Surg*. 2010;200:798-802; discussion 802.
20. Bourquelot P, Tawakol JB, Gaudric J, et al. Lipectomy as a new approach to secondary procedure superficialization of direct autogenous forearm radial-cephalic arteriovenous accesses for hemodialysis. *J Vasc Surg*. 2009;50:369-374.e1.
21. Salimi F, Majd Nassiri G, Moradi M, et al. Assessment of effects of upper extremity exercise with arm tourniquet on maturity of arteriovenous fistula in hemodialysis patients. *J Vasc Access*. 2013;14:239-244.

Sarah E. Gray • Scott A. Berceli

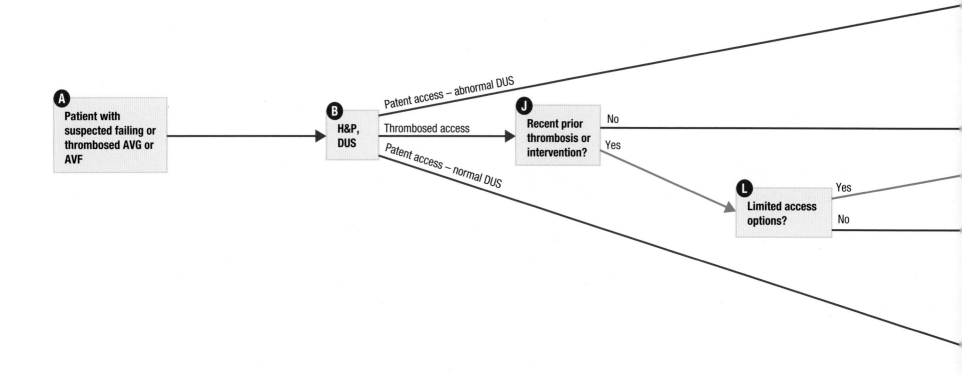

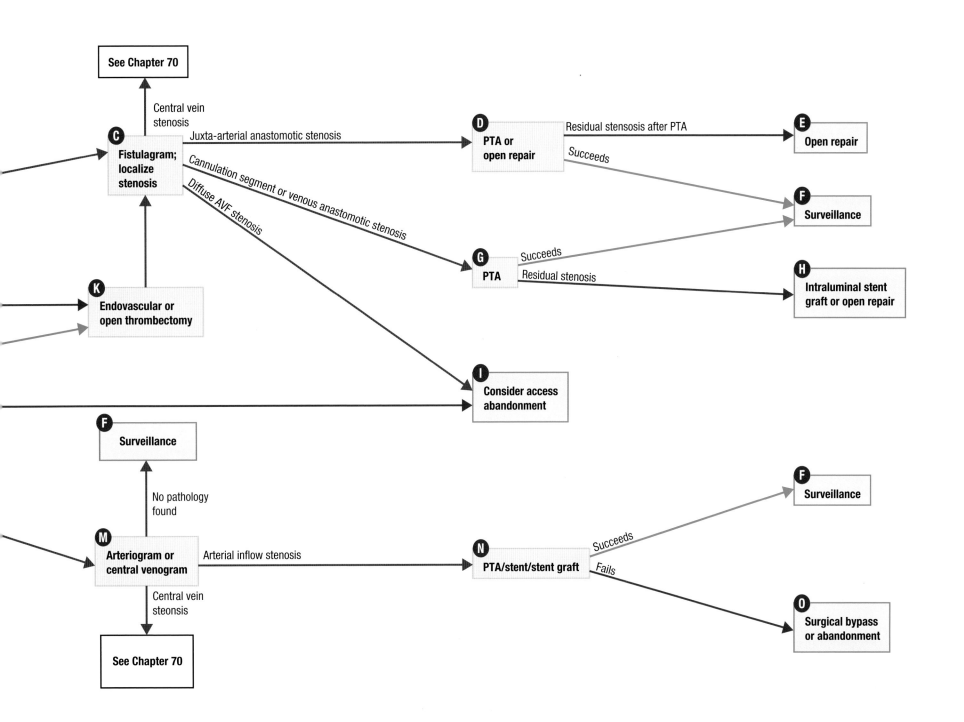

See Chapter 70

Central vein stenosis

C Fistulagram; localize stenosis

Juxta-arterial anastomotic stenosis

D PTA or open repair

Residual stensosis after PTA

E Open repair

Succeeds

F Surveillance

Cannulation segment or venous anastomotic stenosis

Diffuse AVF stenosis

K Endovascular or open thrombectomy

G PTA

Succeeds

Residual stenosis

H Intraluminal stent graft or open repair

I Consider access abandonment

F Surveillance

No pathology found

M Arteriogram or central venogram

Arterial inflow stenosis

N PTA/stent/stent graft

Succeeds

F Surveillance

Fails

O Surgical bypass or abandonment

Central vein steonsis

See Chapter 70

A Patient with suspected failing or thrombosed AVG or AVF

Patients with dysfunctional or thrombosed AVGs and AVFs may present with a variety of clinical signs and symptoms, and are often referred for evaluation directly from the dialysis center. These include increased venous collateralization across the arm or chest, swelling or pain in the access limb, increased pulsatility or loss of thrill within the access, difficulty cannulating the access, or prolonged bleeding following decannulation. Access surveillance parameters may also reveal dysfunction, such as high venous pressures during dialysis, a decrease in flow rate, an abnormal recirculation, or a stenosis in the venous outflow.

B H&P, DUS

If a patient has a suspected dysfunctional or thrombosed access, the next step is a directed physical examination in combination with DUS. Physical examination should include inspection, palpation, and auscultation, with each element providing an important clue to the underlying pathology. A normal AVF should be easily compressible with a palpable thrill at the anastomosis and along the first few centimeters of the vein, and an audible bruit throughout. Examination of an AVG is similar to that of an AVF, although a thrill may only be present in the outflow vein immediately adjacent to the graft. A strong or water-hammer pulse in the graft suggests venous outflow obstruction.[1] Prospective observational studies have shown a high correlation between physical examination findings and angiographic abnormalities.[2-4] Therefore, if the diagnosis is readily apparent following examination of the access, DUS may be omitted. However, if the diagnosis is unclear, DUS may confirm the suspected pathology and facilitate a more directed angiographic approach. DUS can serve as a nice adjunct to the physical examination because it is noninvasive, reproducible, inexpensive, readily available, and does not require the use of iodinated contrast. Unfortunately, DUS is not definitive for the evaluation of the central veins within the thorax.

C Fistulagram; localize stenosis

A fistulagram should be performed to help define the anatomic cause responsible for access dysfunction and should include detailed imaging of the central venous outflow. The dialysis access should be viewed as a circuit from the heart through the arterial inflow and then the venous outflow back to the heart. Accordingly, it may be necessary to image the entire circuit on the basis of the clinical suspicion of the underlying problem. A diagnostic fistulagram is typically performed through a small-caliber sheath placed near the arterial anastomosis and oriented toward the venous outflow. It can reveal the location and extent of stenosis(es), as well as visualize other abnormalities (eg, aneurysms). It is important to note that not all stenoses require intervention. According to the 2019 NKF-KDOQI guidelines, intervention is only warranted in accesses with a "functionally significant" stenosis, defined as a

>50% reduction in lumen diameter in combination with clinical symptoms or hemodynamic abnormalities.[5] Clinical manifestations of stenosis may include swelling of the extremity, increased venous collaterals, change in character of the thrill, or prolonged bleeding after decannulation. Hemodynamic abnormalities include a reduction in urea clearance (>0.2 units) or a reduction in access flow rate (<400-500 mL/min in AVFs; <600 mL/min in AVGs).[5] The location of the stenosis will determine the best course of action (see also Chapter 70).

D PTA or open repair

Juxta-arterial stenoses, defined nominally as lesions within 2 cm of the anastomosis, may be treated with PTA or open repair. PTA is performed through a sheath oriented toward the anastomosis placed through the fistula or arterial inflow vessel and care is taken not to injure the inflow artery during the procedure. Open surgical options include patch angioplasty, resiting the anastomosis to a more proximal arterial location, or revision using an interposition segment of vein or prosthetic graft. In comparison to endovascular approaches, open surgical revision of juxta-anastomotic lesions yields superior primary patency at 12 months.[6-8] Although less durable, PTA confers several advantages including uninterrupted use of the access and the opportunity for treatment outside of the hospital environment. Given these benefits, it is reasonable to consider PTA as the initial treatment approach for these lesions. Stents and stent grafts are not recommended for treatment of angioplasty failure, although stent grafts can be placed in the setting of post-angioplasty access rupture.

E Open repair

Recalcitrant or early recurrent stenoses after PTA are associated with poor graft survival.[9] Although secondary endovascular intervention of these lesions can achieve an acceptable technical success, continued patency is compromised.[10] Therefore, open surgical revision of residual or recurrent juxta-arterial anastomotic lesions is recommended. Surgical revision includes patch angioplasty using either vein or bovine pericardium, resiting the anastomosis to a more proximal arterial location, or revision using an interposition segment of vein or prosthetic graft.

F Surveillance

Data regarding routine surveillance of AVFs and AVGs are somewhat controversial. The 2019 NKF-KDOQI guidelines find no supporting evidence for routine AVF surveillance and recommend against routine AVG surveillance.[5] Although routine surveillance of AVFs using either flow measurements or DUS may reduce the risk of thrombosis, secondary patency of the access is not improved.[11] In contrast, routine monitoring of AVGs does not appear to impact either thrombosis or secondary patency rates. Lacking data to support a robust surveillance program, attentive clinical monitoring is the prudent strategy to maximize access

functionality and should be part of the routine during each dialysis session.

G PTA

The venous anastomosis is the most common site of clinically significant stenoses in AVGs, accounting for approximately 60% of such lesions.[12] In AVFs, lesions within the cannulation segment of the vein are less common but still account for 29% of the culprit lesions.[13] Supported by an excellent technical success rate (>90%), PTA is the procedure of choice for these *de novo* venous lesions.[14] Although the use of cutting over conventional balloons for treatment of distal vein AVG stenoses improves 1-year patency, mid-vein AVF lesions do not demonstrate a similar improvement with the use of cutting balloons.[15] Although conceptually attractive, the role of antiproliferative pharmacologic therapies delivered by drug-eluting balloons remains in evolution.[16,17]

H Intraluminal stent graft or open repair

Supported by two randomized trials, the use of stent grafts for the endovascular treatment of distal vein AVG lesions improves primary patency, compared to the use of balloon PTA alone.[18-20] This survival advantage for stent grafts is balanced by the risk of stent migration, shortening of the available cannulation segment, and, most importantly, loss of vein length for future access revisions. On the basis of these concerns, an open surgical approach for recurrent or residual lesions of the vein distal to an AVG may be preferable. Although data regarding the use of stent grafts in the cannulation segment of AVFs are limited, retrospective reviews have raised concerns about increased risk of infection, strut protrusion, and hemorrhage.[21] As such, open surgical revision via patch angioplasty or interposition grafting for these lesions is recommended.

I Consider access abandonment

In one prospective study of dysfunctional access, 33% of AVFs and 12.5% of AVGs were found to have at least two stenotic sites. In cases where these stenotic sites are discrete, targeted endovascular or open surgical treatment is viable. However, in cases of diffuse or multiple tandem stenoses, the potential for a durable repair is unlikely. In these cases, access abandonment should be considered. It may be possible to replace the involved segment of AVF with a prosthetic graft while saving the original arterial inflow and venous outflow. This essentially converts an AVF to an AVG, but can preserve another access option, remembering the fact that patients with ESRD need a lifetime plan for their renal replacement therapy.

It is important to balance the need for reliable dialysis access with the finite number of possible access options. Tolerance of repeated interventions on a single access will vary by patient and will be influenced by a variety of factors such as patient age, life expectancy, and number of other access options. In a patient with other options for upper extremity access, it is reasonable to consider abandoning an AVF or AVG after the second thrombotic event.[10]

J Recent prior thrombosis or intervention?

Although intervention of the thrombosed access yields acceptable secondary patency rates, intermediate and long-term success is reduced in comparison to interventions performed for stenosis. The inflammation and endothelial trauma associated with thrombus formation, coupled with the frequent occurrence of chronic adherent thrombi, likely account for this outcome difference. Reocclusion within 1 month of intervention is a poor prognostic marker for long-term success, and an assessment of alternative access options is warranted.[22]

K Endovascular or open thrombectomy

Both open surgical and endovascular thrombectomy are options for treatment of an occluded access. Although these approaches have similar technical success in reestablishing flow, 1-year patency appears to be slightly improved in individuals undergoing surgical intervention.[23] Primary post-intervention patency rates for surgical approaches range between 51% and 84% at 1 year, whereas endovascular primary post-intervention patency rates range from 18% to 70% at 1 year. However, with endovascular repair benefiting from the ability to perform repeat interventions, the secondary patency for these approaches is nearly equivalent with rates of 69% to 95% and 44% to 89% for the surgical and endovascular interventions, respectively.[23] Given the less invasive and often more efficient delivery of care associated with an endovascular approach, it is reasonable to defer open versus endovascular repair decision to surgeon judgment and local expertise, in the majority of cases. Exceptions include patients with pulmonary HTN, right to left shunt, or access infection, in whom percutaneous clot dissolution is contraindicated.

Both AVG and AVG thromboses should be treated within 48 hours to avoid placement of a catheter, although AVGs can be salvaged up to a month after thrombosis. Improved post-intervention patency has been suggested to provide a more durable revision if AVF salvage is untaken within 24 hours of thrombosis. A similar benefit in early AVG intervention has not been observed.[24]

Numerous devices are available for percutaneous thrombectomy, including those that incorporate rotational, hydrodynamic, or pharmacomechanical mechanisms. Although there are limited data directly comparing these techniques, several studies suggest that rotational thrombectomy is associated with a higher technical success rate, shorter procedural time, and better secondary patency at 1 year.[25,26]

Although hypercoagulability, hypotension, or external compression can predispose to access occlusion, a reduction in flow secondary to laminated thrombus or a hyperplastic stenosis is the mechanism for failure in the majority of cases. Accordingly, a fistulagram should be routinely performed and repair of anatomic abnormalities initiated to maximize post-intervention outcomes.[27]

L Limited access options?

Central venous obstruction or multiple access failures may result in limited access options for a given patient. In these individuals, failure to maintain a functional access can be life-threatening and the tolerance for multiple access salvage procedures is increased.

M Arteriogram or central venogram

Some patients may present with a normal DUS but persistent access dysfunction. In these patients, central vein stenosis or proximal arterial stenosis may be the culprit. Patients with inflow stenosis may have a weak pulse in the AVF or AVG when it is compressed or the access may collapse with elevation. Central vein abnormalities will be associated with significant swelling of the extremity and prominent collateralization of the superficial veins along the shoulder. Any of these signs should prompt an evaluation with either arteriography or central venography, as appropriate, remembering that the dialysis access is a circuit. If no pathology is found on imaging, careful follow-up is required.

N PTA/stent/stent graft

If a functionally significant arterial inflow stenosis is discovered, PTA is typically the first line of treatment because of the ease of procedure and good technical success. Nevertheless, the optimal treatment should be dictated by the anatomic location and natural history of the lesion. Stenting may be considered for lesions that are resistant to PTA alone. The common culprit lesion at the origin of the SCA responds well to the combination of PTA and intraluminal stenting. Stent grafts can be used in lieu of stents and are particularly useful in calcified lesions at high risk for rupture.

O Surgical bypass or abandonment

If PTA and stenting/stent grafting fail to ameliorate the inflow lesion, open surgical revision should be considered via interposition graft or patch angioplasty. The various surgical approaches are within the skill set of most vascular surgeons that treat arterial insufficiency. However, the decision algorithm should factor in the magnitude of the surgical procedure and the anticipated access patency. Access abandonment may be a better alternative in certain cases.

REFERENCES

1. Beathard GA. Physical examination of the dialysis vascular access. *Semin Dial*. 2007;11:231-236.
2. Asif A, Leon C, Orozco-Vargas LC, et al. Accuracy of physical examination in the detection of arteriovenous fistula stenosis. *Clin J Am Soc Nephrol*. 2007;2:1191-1194.
3. Tessitore N, Bedogna V, Melilli E, et al. In search of an optimal bedside screening program for arteriovenous fistula stenosis. *Clin J Am Soc Nephrol*. 2011;6:819-826.
4. Leon C, Asif A. Physical examination of arteriovenous fistulae by a renal fellow: does it compare favorably to an experienced interventionalist? *Semin Dial*. 2008;21:557-560.
5. Lok CE, Huber TS, Lee T, et al; KDOQI Vascular Access Guideline Work Group. KDOQI clinical practice guideline for vascular access: 2019 update. *Am J Kidney Dis*. 2020;75(4)(suppl 2):S1-S164.
6. Napoli M, Prudenzano R, Russo F, Antonaci AL, Aprile M, Buongiorno E. Juxta-anastomotic stenosis of native arteriovenous fistulas: surgical treatment versus percutaneous transluminal angioplasty. *J Vasc Access*. 2010;11:346-351.
7. Argyriou C, Schoretsanitis N, Georgakarakos EI, Georgiadis GS, Lazarides MK. Preemptive open surgical vs. endovascular repair for juxta-anastomotic stenoses of autogenous AV fistulae: a meta-analysis. *J Vasc Access*. 2015;16:454-458.
8. Tessitore N, Mansueto G, Lipari G, et al. Endovascular versus surgical preemptive repair of forearm arteriovenous fistula juxta-anastomotic stenosis: analysis of data collected prospectively from 1999 to 2004. *Clin J Am Soc Nephrol*. 2006;1:448-454.
9. Lilly RZ, Carlton D, Barker J, et al. Predictors of arteriovenous graft patency after radiologic intervention in hemodialysis patients. *Am J Kidney Dis*. 2001;37:945-953.
10. Malka KT, Flahive J, Csizinscky A, et al. Results of repeated percutaneous interventions on failing arteriovenous fistulas and grafts and factors affecting outcomes. *J Vasc Surg*. 2016;63:772-777.
11. Tonelli M, James M, Wiebe N, Jindal K, Hemmelgarn B. Ultrasound monitoring to detect access stenosis in hemodialysis patients: a systematic review. *Am J Kid Dis*. 2008;51:630-640.
12. Maya ID, Oser R, Saddekni S, Barker J, Allon M. Vascular access stenosis: comparison of arteriovenous grafts and fistulas. *Am J Kidney Dis*. 2004;44:859-865.
13. Turmel-Rodrigues L, Mouton A, Birmelé B, et al. Salvage of immature forearm fistulas for haemodialysis by interventional radiology. *Nephrol Dial Transplant*. 2001;16:2365-2371.
14. Beathard GA, Litchfield T. Effectiveness and safety of dialysis vascular access procedures performed by interventional nephrologists. *Kidney Int*. 2004;66:1622-1632.
15. Saleh HM, Gabr AK, Tawfik MM, Abouellail H. Prospective, randomized study of cutting balloon angioplasty versus conventional balloon angioplasty for the treatment of hemodialysis access stenoses. *J Vasc Surg*. 2014;60:735-740.
16. Katsanos K, Karnabatidis D, Kitrou P, Spiliopoulos S, Christeas N, Siablis D. Paclitaxel-coated balloon angioplasty vs. plain balloon dilation for the treatment of failing dialysis access: 6-month interim results from a prospective randomized controlled trial. *J Endovasc Ther*. 2012;19:263-272.

17. Kitrou PM, Katsanos K, Spiliopoulos S, Karnabatidis D, Siablis D. Drug-eluting versus plain balloon angioplasty for the treatment of failing dialysis access: final results and cost-effectiveness analysis from a prospective randomized controlled trial (NCT01174472). *Eur J Radiol.* 2015;84: 418-423.

18. Vesely T, DaVanzo W, Behrend T, Dwyer A, Aruny J. Balloon angioplasty versus Viabahn stent graft for treatment of failing or thrombosed prosthetic hemodialysis grafts. *J Vasc Surg.* 2016;64:1400-1410.e1.

19. Haskal ZJ, Saad TF, Hoggard JG, et al. Prospective, randomized, concurrently-controlled study of a stent graft versus balloon angioplasty for treatment of arteriovenous access graft stenosis: 2-year results of the RENOVA Study. *J Vasc Interv Radiol.* 2016;27:1105-1114.e3.

20. Falk A, Maya ID, Yevzlin AS. A prospective, randomized study of an expanded polytetrafluoroethylene stent graft versus balloon angioplasty for in-stent restenosis in arteriovenous grafts and fistulae: two-year results of the RESCUE Study. *J Vasc Interv Radiol.* 2016;27:1465-1476.

21. Zink JN, Netzley R, Erzurum V, Wright D. Complications of endovascular grafts in the treatment of pseudoaneurysms and stenoses in arteriovenous access. *J Vasc Surg.* 2013;57:144-148.

22. Crikis S, Lee D, Brooks M, Power DA, Ierino FL, Levidiotis V. Predictors of early dialysis vascular-access failure after thrombolysis. *Am J Nephrol.* 2008;28:181-189.

23. Tordoir JH, Bode AS, Peppelenbosch N, van der Sande FM, de Haan MW. Surgical or endovascular repair of thrombosed dialysis vascular access: is there any evidence? *J Vasc Surg.* 2009;50:953-956.

24. Hsieh MY, Lin L, Chen TY, et al. Timely thrombectomy can improve patency of hemodialysis arteriovenous fistulas. *J Vasc Surg.* 2018;67:1217-1226.

25. Yang CC, Yang CW, Wen SC, Wu CC. Comparisons of clinical outcomes for thrombectomy devices with different mechanisms in hemodialysis arteriovenous fistulas. *Catheter Cardiovasc Interv.* 2012;80:1035-1041.

26. Gregory LB, Grandas OH, Tayidi IT, et al. Contemporary clinical and financial analysis of open versus percutaneous mechanical thrombectomy for occluded hemodialysis access. *J Vasc Surg.* 2018;67:e5-e6.

27. Chang TI, Paik J, Greene T, et al. Intradialytic hypotension and vascular access thrombosis. *J Am Soc Nephrol.* 2011;22:1526-1533.

Raphael Blochle • Linda M. Harris

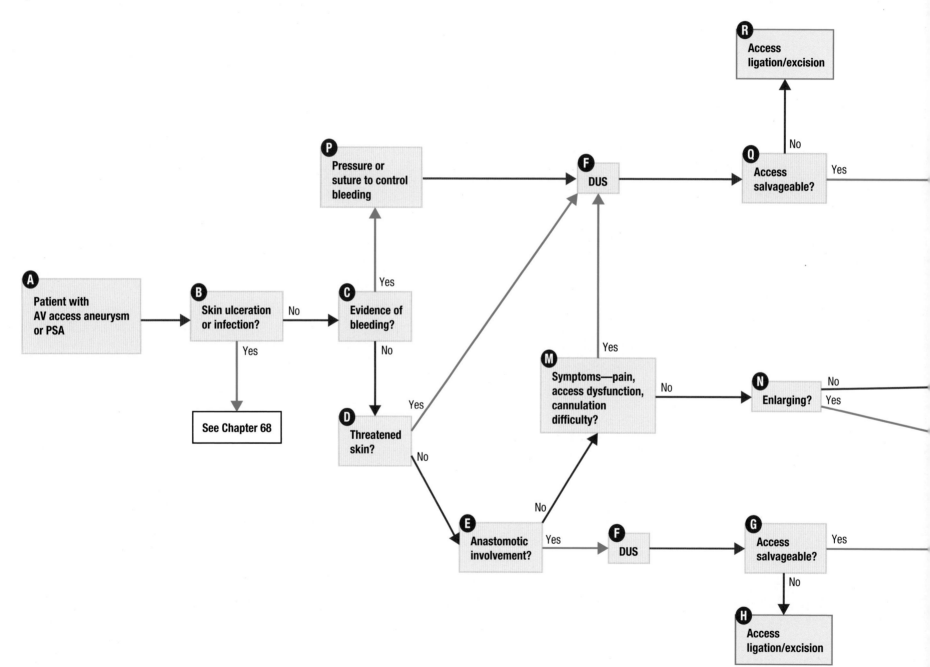

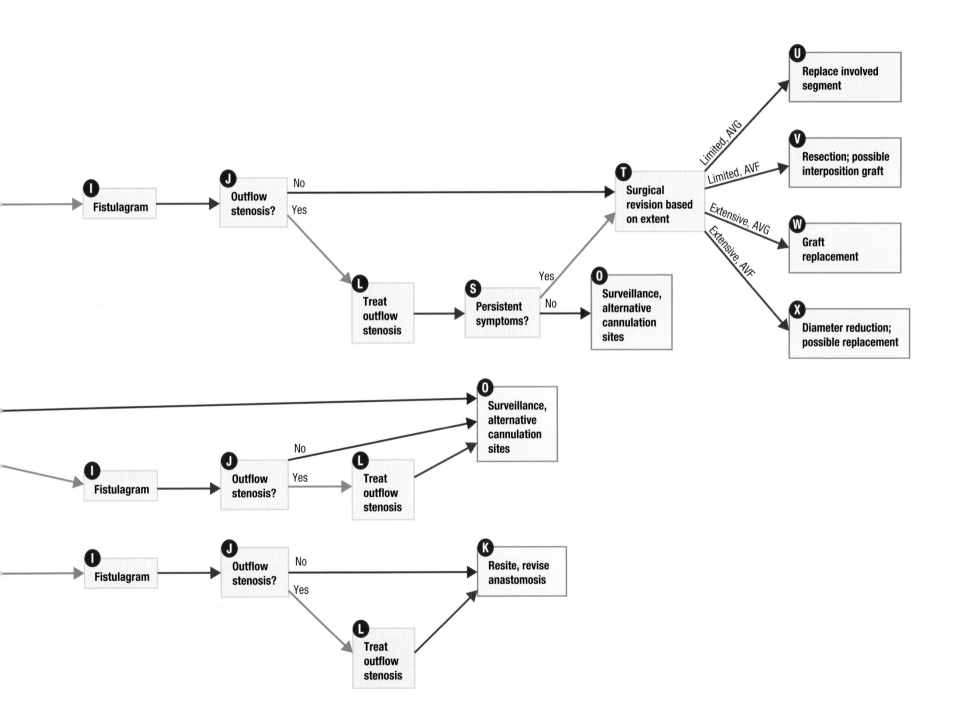

A Patient with AV access aneurysm or PSA

An aneurysm is defined as a circumscribed dilation of all three layers of a vessel wall, whereas a PSA is a defect in the vessel or prosthetic material that is walled off by the surrounding external fibrous tissue. Accordingly, true AV access aneurysms can only develop in AVFs, whereas PSAs can develop in both AVFs and AVGs. True aneurysms can form adjacent to stenoses in AVFs, next to vein valves or junctions, or diffusely along the access outflow vein. PSAs are related to the trauma from repetitive punctures at the same site. The reported prevalence of access aneurysms and PSAs is quite broad, with a range of 5% to 60%.[1,2] The hemodynamic changes that result from the construction of an AVF lead to the dilation of the outflow vein and, thus, the development of diffuse aneurysmal change is an expected outcome. However, access aneurysms and PSAs can become problematic and lead to difficulty with cannulation, access thrombosis, high-output CHF, and are associated with an increased bleeding and infection risk. They may also cause pain, and are cosmetically unappealing to patients. Additional factors that contribute to their development include poor cannulation technique, older access age, and outflow obstruction. Treatment goals for patients with access aneurysms and PSAs are to preserve the access, avoid the use of tunneled dialysis catheters, and prevent associated complications. Dialysis center personnel should be educated on the appropriate cannulation technique to reduce their incidence.

B Skin ulceration or infection?

AV access should be examined during each dialysis session for evidence of infection and/or ulceration. Ulcerations typically result from thinning of the skin from repetitive punctures at the same site and increase in the risk of bleeding complications. The incidence of infections is estimated to be 11% to 35% over the lifetime of an AVG,[3] but quite low for AVF. The presence of aneurysmal degeneration at an anastomosis may be related to infection with a low virulent organism or an adjacent outflow stenosis.[4] Accesses with associated skin ulceration should be presumed infected and treated accordingly. The management of access-related infections is detailed in Chapter 68.

C Evidence of bleeding?

Bleeding from an AV access, which is not easily controlled with gentle digital pressure, requires both a temporary and longer term solution. It is worth emphasizing that access-related bleeding can be a true life-threatening, surgical emergency that requires early recognition and definitive treatment. Bleeding is frequently related to increased venous pressures from an outflow stenosis, infection, or aneurysmal degeneration with thinning of the overlying skin and ulceration. It can occur in a normal access after decannulation from puncture sites in patients on anticoagulation or antiplatelet agents, particularly when anticoagulation is supratherapeutic. Before assuming that the etiology of bleeding is due to anticoagulants or antiplatelet agents, patients should be assessed for the presence of thin/threatened skin ± an aneurysm, infection, and outflow stenosis. The management of venous outflow stenoses and access-related infections are addressed in Chapters 70 and 68, respectively.

D Threatened skin?

Patients with threatened skin over an AV access require intervention to prevent bleeding or infection. Skin threat can be due to underlying aneurysms, PSAs or trauma from repeated punctures. Concerning or threatened skin appears thin, shiny, and usually with loss of pigmentation. The threatened skin is often firm and adherent to the underlying access in contrast to being supple and easily movable. The overlying skin with these characteristics is at increased risk of breakdown, ulceration, and exposure of the underlying access with consequent bleeding.

E Anastomotic involvement?

Dilation of the access in the region of the anastomosis from either an aneurysm or a PSA merits further imaging to determine whether the anastomosis itself is involved. Involvement of the anastomosis with degeneration is more serious than is mid-access aneurysmal degeneration, and routinely requires intervention.[2,5,6] Involvement of the anastomosis can be associated with infection of the AVG or AVF.

F DUS

DUS is a very useful adjunct to physical examination for the assessment of AV access. It is noninvasive, reproducible, inexpensive, readily available, and does not require the use of iodinated contrast. It can be used to screen for the presence of infection, as suggested by perigraft fluid or inflammation around the access. Furthermore, it can help identify potential intraluminal stenoses distal to the aneurysm or PSA. Unfortunately, DUS is not definitive for the evaluation of the central veins within the thorax. To fully evaluate the aneurysm or PSA, the DUS should assess the maximal size of the dilation, the location, and size of the neck (for PSAs), presence of thrombus within the aneurysm sac, and relationship to branches or the anastomosis. If the anastomosis is actively involved with aneurysmal degeneration, an assessment needs to be made as to whether the access is salvageable.[6]

G Access salvageable?

Some accesses with aneurysmal or pseudoaneurysmal involvement of the anastomoses may be salvageable. However, it is important to determine the etiology of the aneurysmal degeneration to prevent recurrence. All infected AVGs with anastomotic involvement require excision and should be deemed nonsalvageable. A small subset of infected AVFs with aneurysmal involvement may be salvageable provided that the infectious process is limited (ie, peri-access fluid), the organisms are nonvirulent, and the remaining segment of the access is uninvolved.

H Access ligation/excision

Accesses with aneurysms or PSAs involving the anastomoses that are deemed nonsalvageable can be ligated or excised. Ligation is the simpler approach, but it may not adequately address the anastomotic aneurysm or PSA. Excision or partial excision is preferable in most cases and can be performed concomitant with repair of the donor artery. All of the prosthetic material should be removed for anastomotic aneurysms/PSAs in the presence of infection. Occasionally, a small segment of prosthetic material can be left at the arterial anastomosis when graft infection is far removed and the para-anastomotic graft material is well incorporated. However, this small remnant of prosthetic material may become infected and, thus, longer term follow-up is mandatory.[7] AVFs deemed nonsalvageable owing to an infected anastomotic aneurysm/PSA should be excised because the organism that led to the degeneration of the vessel increases the likelihood of future bleeding. Arterial reconstruction should be performed with autogenous tissue as either a vein patch or an interposition graft with the choice dictated by the quality of the tissue and the extent of the infection. Ligation of the inflow/artery has been demonstrated to be safe in select cases and may be an option for patients with such extensive infection that arterial reconstruction is prohibitive.[8]

I Fistulagram

A fistulagram should be performed and the full extent of the outflow tract, including the central veins, should be imaged to exclude other venous outflow stenosis.

J Outflow stenosis?

Stenoses in the outflow tract of an access can lead to venous HTN, which can contribute to the development of aneurysms/PSAs. These stenotic lesions typically occur just distal to the aneurysmal segment and/or in the central outflow veins. Notably, Rajput et al.[9] reported that up to 80% of patients with access aneurysm/PSA had a concomitant central lesion. The presence of a central vein stenosis is suggested by arm edema, tense aneurysms, prolonged access bleeding, high venous pressures, and accesses that are not completely decompressed with arm elevation.[10]

K Resite, revise anastomosis

Anastomotic arterial aneurysms or PSAs can be repaired by revising or resiting the anastomosis with the choice dictated by the anatomy and the quality of the tissue. The anastomotic aneurysm can sometimes be revised by mobilizing a redundant proximal portion of the AVF or AVG and redoing the anastomosis. Alternatively, a segment of autogenous or prosthetic material can be used as an interposition graft between the access and the original anastomosis after excising the aneurysmal portion.

Similarly, the anastomosis can be resited more proximal on the arterial tree by mobilizing the access or using an interposition graft. In this scenario, the original anastomosis can be patched using a segment of the original AVF or AVG if a suitable segment of vein is not available. The involved aneurysm sac itself does not need to be debrided, unless the overlying skin is ulcerated. Aneurysmal degeneration at the venous anastomosis will usually resolve after treating the outflow stenosis distal to the degenerated segment. If the aneurysmal degeneration is extensive, the anastomosis can be resited more centrally on the outflow vein and the original anastomosis patched or simply ligated. Alternatively, the aneurysmal outflow vein can be reduced in size, as outlined later (see X).

Ⓛ Treat outflow stenosis

Details of treating venous outflow stenoses are discussed in Chapter 70.

Ⓜ Symptoms—pain, access dysfunction, cannulation difficulty?

The mere presence of an access aneurysm or a PSA is not an indication for intervention and there are no specific size criteria for intervention in the absence of symptoms. The presence of pain, access dysfunction, high-output CHF, and difficulty with cannulation may necessitate treatment in the addition to the presence of infection and the risk of bleeding addressed earlier.[1] The presence of an aneurysm or a PSA can also contribute to access thrombosis. Management of access thrombosis is addressed in Chapter 66.

Ⓝ Enlarging?

The natural history of most access aneurysms/PSAs is to increase in size, although their rate of growth is poorly defined. There are no absolute size thresholds for intervention and, thus, a slowly enlarging aneurysm/PSA is probably not worrisome in the absence of other symptoms. Aneurysms/PSAs that enlarge acutely are more concerning and it is important to evaluate other contributing factors (eg, infection) or complications (eg, spontaneous bleeding) that may merit intervention.

Ⓞ Surveillance, alternative cannulation sites

Simple surveillance is appropriate in the setting of a stable or slowly growing access aneurysm/PSA, provided that there are no other associated symptoms. Assessment of the access should be part of the routine physical examination with each dialysis session and the various access-care providers should be trained to recognize access-related complications. Dialysis centers should be advised to cannulate alternative sites, remote from the aneurysm/PSA, to prevent further access degeneration.[11] In the rare scenario where there are no alternative sites, dialysis nurses should be encouraged to cannulate the lateral or medial aspect of the aneurysm/pseudoaneurysm, away from the area of thinning skin.

Ⓟ Pressure or suture to control bleeding

Initial control of any access bleeding can usually be obtained by direct digital pressure, which should be applied directly over the puncture site with sufficient pressure to stop the bleeding, but not occlude the access. Compression of the access outflow (ie, distal to the bleeding site) should be avoided because it increases the luminal pressure and potentially increases the bleeding. Tourniquets should also be avoided because they increase the likelihood of access thrombosis and the risk of arm/hand ischemia if left in place for a prolonged period of time. Prolonged bleeding not responsive to pressure may be controllable with a figure-8 or U-stitch at the bleeding site. Such a suture is placed while an assistant controls inflow and outflow with the goal of controlling the bleeding while avoiding access ligation. Those requiring suture control of access bleeding should be further evaluated to determine whether there is an underlying cause for the bleeding that may require intervention (ie, infection, outflow stenosis, skin erosion). The suture is not a definitive therapy for the bleeding, and intervention should be relatively urgent to prevent recurrent hemorrhage. If skin erosion is present, the patient will need definitive surgical repair.

Ⓠ Access salvageable?

A determination of whether the access is salvageable can be made depending on the history, physical examination, and DUS findings. The generic criteria for functional access include an adequate flow rate, a suitable access diameter, and an acceptable depth relative to the surface of the skin. The concerns are somewhat different in the case of access aneurysms/PSAs because patients are typically using their access when concerns arise. Fortunately, access salvage is possible for the majority of the patients with uninfected, symptomatic aneurysms/PSAs that do not involve the anastomosis. The potential exceptions include patients with diffuse degeneration of the access and those with refractory central vein stenoses or occlusions.

Ⓡ Access ligation/excision

Accesses that are deemed nonsalvageable can be either ligated or excised. Ligation is certainly simpler, although it can lead to thrombosis of the aneurysm or PSA. This can result in the development of an inflammatory response in the aneurysm/PSA similar to that seen with IV catheter-associated thrombophlebitis. Furthermore, the large, thrombosed aneurysms/PSAs do not usually resolve and can be unsightly to patients from a cosmetic standpoint. Excision may be a better option, although the trade-offs are the larger operation and the extent of the incision. The donor artery can by patched with a segment of the vein that comprised the access in the case of AVF or the very proximal segment of the access (either AVF or AVG) can be simply oversewn, exercising caution not to narrow the lumen of the artery. For accesses deemed nonsalvageable, it may be beneficial to delay ligation or

excision until a new, alternative access has matured. The index access can be safely maintained for 2 to 3 months in the absence of infection by treating any associated stenoses in the interim and by cannulating sites remote from the aneurysm/PSA.

Ⓢ Persistent symptoms?

Patients with persistent symptoms after correction of a venous outflow stenosis will require additional treatment. Indeed, the majority of symptomatic aneurysms and PSAs will require further intervention.

Ⓣ Surgical revision based on extent

Patients with persistent symptoms and/or threatened skin after correction of any outflow stenosis require further revision. The optimal treatment is dependent on the extent of the degenerative process and the type of access.[12,13] Both open surgical and endovascular options are available, with the latter generally reserved for emergent indications. Fortunately, access salvage is feasible in the majority of cases, with patency rates after revision ranging from 52% to 100% at 1 year.[1,2,4] The intervention(s) should be orchestrated in such a manner that the access can be used continuously, obviating the need for a tunneled dialysis catheter.

Ⓤ Replace involved segment

Patients with PSAs involving a limited segment of their AVG can be treated with replacement of the involved segment. Similar to the treatment of patients with localized graft infection, proximal and distal control of the index graft can be obtained away from the involved segment and then a new graft can be tunneled through a separate plane. The requisite incision for the exposure can then be closed before excising and/or debriding the degenerated area. The uninvolved segment of the original graft can be used continuously for dialysis. It can be helpful to mark the area of ideal cannulation on the skin for the benefit of both the patient and dialysis nurses.[14,15] Cannulation in the new graft segment should be delayed 3 to 6 weeks to allow incorporation. Limited AVG PSAs can also be excluded with the use of a stent graft.[16-18] Although relatively simple, the potential downside of stent-graft repair includes loss of cannulation zone, failure of incorporation into surrounding tissue, and the introduction of foreign tissue into a potentially infected field. Furthermore, the use of stent grafts for this indication is not approved by the Food and Drug Administration. As such, they are generally reserved for emergent indications and for patients who are at prohibitive operative risk.

Ⓥ Resection; possible interposition graft

Similar to the scenario with AVGs, it is usually possible to revise an AVF in patients with limited aneurysms or PSAs while preserving sufficient cannulation zones to sustain uninterrupted dialysis. Notably, the outflow vein of an AVF often elongates and becomes tortuous, concomitant with the increase in diameter that leads to the development of the aneurysm. Accordingly, it may be possible to mobilize the nonaneurysmal sections and construct an end-to-end anastomosis after resection of the aneurysm. More extensive aneurysms can be treated with plication or some other form of diameter reduction treatment as outlined later (see X). An interposition graft can also be used to replace the aneurysmal segment using either autogenous or prosthetic conduit. Alternatively, a stent graft could also be placed across the aneurysm/PSA, although there is the potential for a size mismatch between the afferent and efferent vein segments in addition to the limitations noted earlier (see U).

W Graft replacement

The degenerative process in the AVG may occur throughout the graft to such an extent that local treatment is not feasible. This is usually seen in old grafts that have been cannulated throughout their length and essentially have a series of PSAs caused by the disruption of graft fabric. Provided that the venous outflow is adequate, these grafts can usually be salvaged because the arterial anastomosis and proximal segment of the graft are typically not involved. Graft salvage or replacement can be accomplished in either a single- or two-stage process.[19] In the two-stage approach, the upstream portion of the graft is replaced first. The proximal anastomosis is performed to the uninvolved segment of the original graft near the anastomosis and the downstream anastomosis performed to a segment of the degenerated graft, preserving a sufficient length of the old graft that can be used for continuous dialysis, precluding the need for a tunneled dialysis catheter. The remaining segment of the old graft is replaced during the second stage after the new proximal segment of the graft is incorporated (and suitable for cannulation). The original venous anastomosis, similar to the arterial anastomosis, can usually be preserved. Ideally, the new graft segments should be tunneled through an uninvolved tissue plane, as outlined earlier for the "limited involvement" scenario (see U). The single-stage approach essentially combines the two procedures and involves tunneling a new AVG through a new tissue plane while preserving the original arterial and venous anastomoses.

X Diameter reduction; possible replacement

Symptomatic AVFs with diffuse aneurysmal degeneration can usually be salvaged by reducing their diameter or replacing the involved segment, as outlined for AVGs with extensive involvement (see W). It is imperative to first correct any venous outflow stenoses, as outlined in the decision algorithm. A variety of creative "diameter-reducing" strategies have been described, but all entail excising a segment of the aneurysmal access wall along with the redundant overlying skin.[20-23] An incision is made over the aneurysmal segment of the AVF and vascular control is obtained both proximally and distally. A longitudinal incision is then made in the aneurysmal vein, preferentially on the medial or lateral wall to avoid

having the subsequent suture line underlie future cannulation sites. A longitudinal segment of excess vein in the aneurysmal segment is then excised and a more appropriate-sized AVF (eg, 8-mm lumen) is then created with a long, continuous suture using a temporary mandrill, typically a red rubber catheter, a Foley catheter, or a small chest tube. The redundant overlying skin is then excised and the remaining skin reapproximated over the new, smaller AVF. The diameter-reducing procedures can be performed as a single- or two-stage procedure (proximal followed by distal after incorporation), with the goal of the latter approach being to maintain continuous dialysis through the AVF and avoid the use of a tunneled catheter. Ideally, the skin incision over the aneurysmal access should be positioned on the lateral aspect of the aneurysm and the dissection of skin overlying the future cannulation zone limited to allow earlier cannulation after the revision. All thrombus within the lumen of the aneurysmal access should be removed as part of the procedure. Unfortunately, the vessel wall of aneurysmal AVFs can degenerate, typically from diffuse calcification within the wall, to the point that they are not pliable enough to salvage with the diameter-reducing approach. In that scenario, the involved segments can be replaced with either a prosthetic or autogenous graft (see W) performed as a single- or two-stage procedure with the new conduit tunneled through an uninvolved tissue plane.

REFERENCES

1. Balaz P, Bjorck M. True aneurysm in autologous hemodialysis fistulae: definitions, classification and indications for treatment. *J Vasc Access.* 2015;16(6):446-453.
2. Inston N, Mistry H, Gilbert J, et al. Aneurysms in vascular access: state of the art and future developments. *J Vasc Access.* 2017;18:464-472.
3. Kim CY, Guevara CJ, Engstrom BI, et al. Analysis of infection risk following covered stent exclusion of pseudoaneurysms in prosthetic arteriovenous hemodialysis access grafts. *J Vasc Interv Radiol.* 2012;23:69-74.
4. Lazarides MK, Georgiadis GS, Argyriou C. Aneurysm formation and infection in AV prosthesis. *J Vasc Access.* 2014;15(suppl 7):S120-S124.
5. Siedlecki A, Barker J, Allon M. Aneurysm formation in arteriovenous grafts: associations and clinical significance. *Semin Dial.* 2007;20:73-77.
6. Watson KR, Gallagher M, Ross R, et al. The aneurysmal arteriovenous fistula—morphological study and assessment of clinical implications. A pilot study. *Vascular.* 2015;23:498-503.
7. Ryan SV, Calligaro KD, Scharff J, Dougherty MJ. Management of infected prosthetic dialysis arteriovenous grafts. *J Vasc Surg.* 2004;39:73-78.
8. Schanzer A, Ciaranello AL, Schanzer H. Brachial artery ligation with total graft excision is a safe and effective approach to prosthetic arteriovenous graft infections. *J Vasc Surg.* 2008;48:655-658.

9. Rajput A, Rajan DK, Simons ME, et al. Venous aneurysms in autogenous hemodialysis fistulas: is there an association with venous outflow stenosis. *J Vasc Access.* 2013;14:126-130.
10. Salman L, Beathard G. Interventional nephrology: physical examination as a tool for surveillance for the hemodialysis arteriovenous access. *Clin J Am Soc Nephrol.* 2013;8:1220-1227.
11. Marticorena RM, Hunter J, Macleod S, et al. The salvage of aneurysmal fistulae utilizing a modified buttonhole cannulation technique and multiple cannulators. *Hemodial Int.* 2006;10:193-200.
12. Pasklinsky G, Meisner RJ, Labropoulos N, et al. Management of true aneurysms of hemodialysis access fistulas. *J Vasc Surg.* 2011;53:1291-1297.
13. Al-Thani H, El-Menyar A, Al-Thani N, et al. Characteristics, management, and outcomes of surgically treated arteriovenous fistula aneurysm in patients on regular hemodialysis. *Ann Vasc Surg.* 2017;41:46-55.
14. Sigala F, Kontis E, Sassen R, Mickley V. Autologous surgical reconstruction for true venous hemodialysis access aneurysms—techniques and results. *J Vasc Access.* 2014;15:370-375.
15. Belli S, Parlakgumus A, Colakoglu T, et al. Surgical treatment modalities for complicated aneurysms and pseudoaneurysms of arteriovenous fistulas. *J Vasc Access.* 2012;13:438-445.
16. Hedin U, Engstrom J, Roy J. Endovascular treatment of true and false aneurysms in hemodialysis access. *J Cardiovasc Surg.* 2015;56:599-605.
17. Fotiadis N, Shawyer A, Namagondlu G, Iyer A, Matson M, Yaqoob MM. Endovascular repair of symptomatic hemodialysis access graft pseudoaneurysms. *J Vasc Access.* 2014;15:5-11.
18. Zink JN, Netzley R, Erzurum V, Wright D. Complications of endovascular grafts in the treatment of pseudoaneurysms and stenoses in arteriovenous access. *J Vasc Surg.* 2013;57:144-148.
19. Georgiadis GS, Lazarides MK, Panagoutsos SA, et al. Surgical revision of complicated false and true vascular access-related aneurysms. *J Vasc Surg.* 2008;47:1284-1291.
20. Woo K, Cook PR, Garg J, Hye RJ, Canty TG. Midterm results of a novel technique to salvage autogenous dialysis access in aneurysmal arteriovenous fistulas. *J Vasc Surg.* 2010;51:921-925, 925.e1.
21. Hossny A. Partial aneurysmectomy for salvage of autogenous arteriovenous fistula with complicated venous aneurysms. *J Vasc Surg.* 2014;59:1073-1077.
22. Hakim NS, Romagnoli J, Contis JC, Akoh J, Papalois VE. Refashioning of an aneurysmatic arterio-venous fistula by using the multifire GIA 60 surgical stapler. *Int Surg.* 1997;82:376-377.
23. Vo T, Tumbaga G, Aka P, Behseresht J, Hsu J, Tayarrah M. Staple aneurysmorrhaphy to salvage autogenous arteriovenous fistulas with aneurysm-related complications. *J Vasc Surg.* 2015;61(2):457-462.

Joseph-Vincent V. Blas • David L. Cull

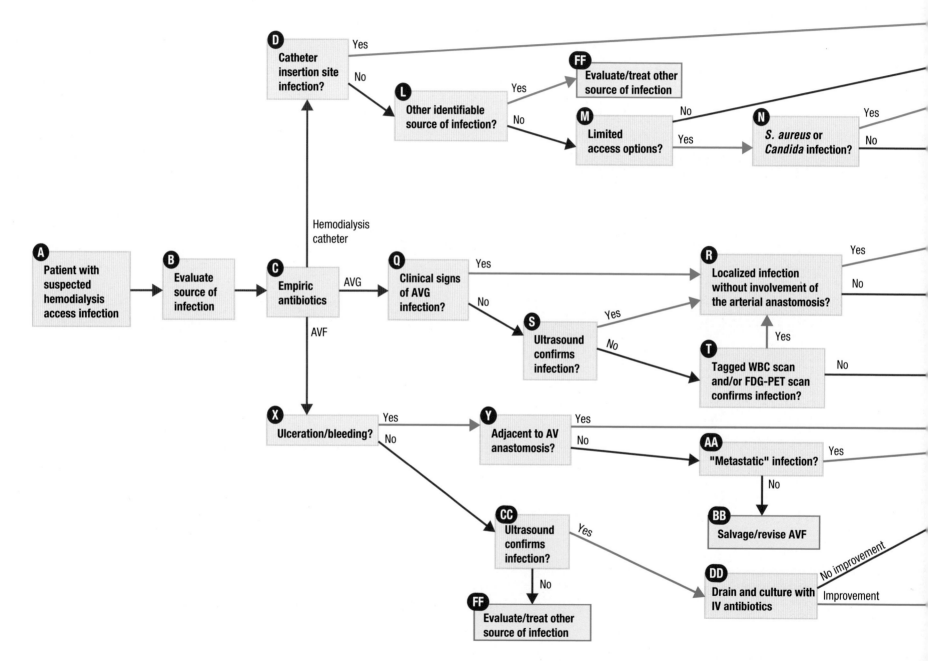

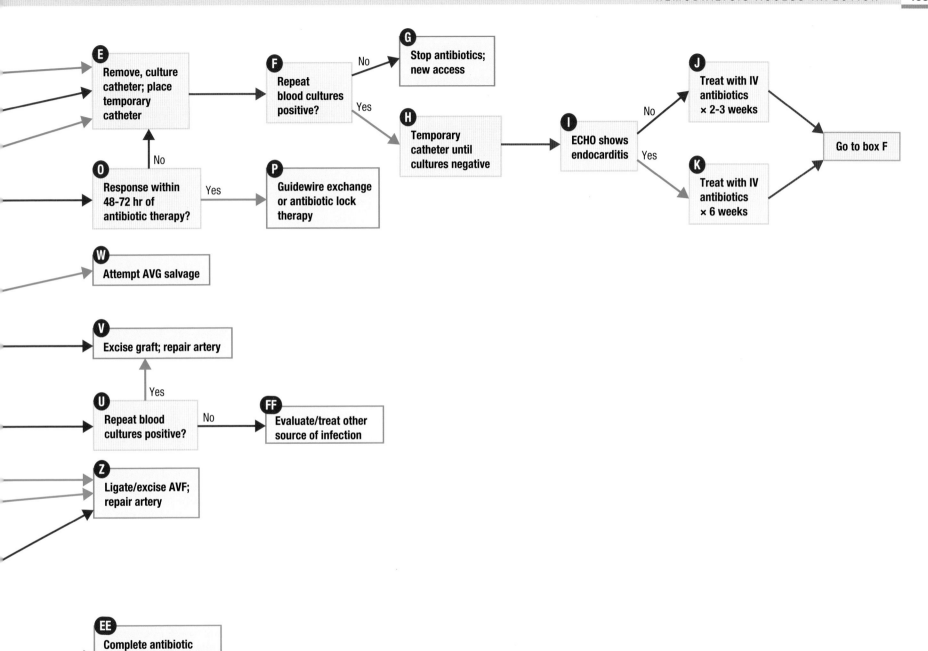

A Patient with suspected hemodialysis access infection

Suspected hemodialysis (HD) access infection is based on clinical findings of systemic infection (eg, fever, warmth, pain, redness, ulceration, or induration) in any patient with an AV access. By far, cuffed tunneled HD catheter infections are the most common. The incidence of bacteremia in patients with HD catheters is approximately 50% at 6 months. The most sensitive findings in patients with catheter-related infections include fever and/or chills. The rate of AVG infection is between 4% and 20% per year. AVF infections occur infrequently (<5% per year).[1-4] Cellulitis, abscess, PSA, or hematoma are the typical findings of AVF infections that usually occur secondary to puncture site complications (eg, hematoma and/or PSA). The risk of infection is increased in AVFs accessed using the "buttonhole" cannulation technique.[5] *Staphylococcus aureus* and *Staphylococcus epidermidis* are the most common pathogens associated with any HD access infection.[2,3,6]

B Evaluation source of infection

The initial evaluation for a suspected HD access infection includes laboratory tests (eg, complete blood count) and blood cultures. If possible, blood cultures should be obtained before the initiation of antibiotics. Paired blood cultures should be obtained (one from the central catheter and one from a peripheral vein) in patients with a suspected catheter infection. Alternatively, one can obtain two central blood cultures from different catheter lumen separated by 10 to 15 minutes.[7]

C Empiric antibiotics

Empiric broad-spectrum antibiotics that cover both gram-positive and gram-negative organisms should be started to treat suspected infection. Vancomycin is administered for gram-positive coverage and either gentamicin or ceftazidime for gram-negative organisms. IV vancomycin (20 mg/kg) is administered as a loading dose followed by 500 mg in the last 30 to 60 minutes of each dialysis session. In patients allergic or intolerant to vancomycin, daptomycin (7-9 mg/kg) can be substituted. Gentamicin (1-2 mg/kg) is administered after each HD session. Ceftazidime (2 g) can be substituted for patients intolerant to gentamicin. Empiric coverage for multidrug-resistant (MDR) gram-negative bacilli, such as *Pseudomonas aeruginosa*, is indicated for patients with neutropenia and severe sepsis, or patients with documented colonization by such organisms. Modification of antibiotic therapy is dictated by the culture results.[7] Subsequent treatment depends on the type of access infected: HD catheter, AVG, or AVF.

D Catheter insertion site infection?

Clinical findings suggestive of catheter insertion site infection are local erythema and exit-site purulence and/or drainage. Fever is the most sensitive finding for catheter-related infection. The majority of catheter-associated bacteremia occurs in the absence of local signs of infection. Gross exit-site purulence is found in only 5% to 10% of patients with catheter-associated bacteremia. Positive blood culture results occur in approximately 60% to 80% of patients with a central catheter and fever or chills.[8,9]

E Remove, culture catheter; place temporary catheter

If the catheter insertion site appears infected, the exudate should be collected and sent for culture and gram stain analysis. Antibiotic therapy should be tailored to the culture results. If exit-site or incisional-site purulence is present, the cuffed (tunneled) catheter should be promptly removed and the tip of the catheter sent for culture and gram stain analysis. A temporary "holiday" without central catheter access is advisable until the subsequent HD session. A temporary catheter is placed at a separate, uninfected site.[7]

F Repeat blood cultures positive?

After catheter removal, antibiotic therapy should be tailored to the infecting organism. Additional blood cultures are obtained 48 to 96 hours after initiation of antibiotics to determine whether to continue antibiotics.[7]

G Stop antibiotics; new access

Antibiotics are stopped after removal of the catheter if blood culture results are negative, after which the patient is evaluated for new HD access placement (see Chapter 64).[7]

H Temporary catheter until cultures negative

Temporary (noncuffed) catheter, placed after removal of infected tunneled catheter (see E), should continue to be used for dialysis until repeat blood culture results are negative.

I ECHO shows endocarditis

Persistent positive blood culture results, despite antibiotic therapy, mandates ECHO to assess for bacterial endocarditis. If detected, this must be treated with a prolonged course of antibiotics before placing a new access.

J Treat with IV antibiotics × 2-3 weeks

Patients without bacterial endocarditis are treated with a limited course of IV antibiotics (2-3 weeks) before repeating blood cultures to determine whether antibiotics can be stopped and new HD access planned.

K Treat with IV antibiotics × 6 weeks

Patients with evidence of bacterial endocarditis are treated with prolonged IV antibiotics (4-6 weeks).[10] Blood cultures are repeated after treatment for endocarditis. Future placement of cuffed catheter access is dictated by those results.

L Other identifiable source of infection?

In the absence of catheter insertion-site or incisional-site infection and with negative blood culture results, evaluation for an alternative source of infection should be done. Common infections in HD-dependent patients include upper or lower respiratory tract infections (eg, pneumonia), urinary tract infections, GI tract infections, diabetic foot ulcer infections, other skin/soft-tissue infections (eg, cellulitis), osteomyelitis, and tuberculosis. If found, such infections should be treated. If no other source of infection is found, the catheter is presumed to be infected.

M Limited access options?

If there remains high suspicion for catheter infection (eg, severe sepsis, hemodynamic instability, or "metastatic" infection) but without local signs of infection, the tunneled catheter should be removed except in rare cases when no other access is possible.[7,11] A "metastatic" infection is defined as hematogenous seeding at remote sites (eg, spine, distal extremity) due to bacteremia.[11] More aggressive efforts than usual should be undertaken to salvage the tunneled catheter if limited alternative access options are available.[8-10,12]

N *S. aureus* or *Candida* infection?

Candida or *Staphylococcus aureus* bacteremia on initial blood cultures should prompt removal of the tunneled catheter because of the increased risk of persistent fever and bacteremia if catheter salvage is attempted.[8,13]

O Response within 48-72 hr of antibiotic therapy?

The patient is monitored for 48 to 72 hours for clinical improvement (decreasing WBC, defervescence of fever, or resolution of sepsis).[9,14] Persistent fevers, sepsis, or failure to clinically improve on IV antibiotics should prompt removal of the tunneled, cuffed catheter.

P Guidewire exchange or antibiotic lock therapy

With clinical improvement, salvage of the tunneled catheter insertion site may be attempted with either exchange of the catheter over a wire or antibiotic lock therapy. Because no direct comparison between antibiotic lock therapy and guidewire catheter exchange has been reported to identify superiority of one strategy over the other, the choice is based on institutional experience and preference.

Guidewire catheter exchange is effective in highly selected patient populations.[9,15] Exchange of the cuffed catheter over a guidewire after 48 to 72 hours of systemic antibiotics, with resolution of fever, and absent local signs of infection is a reasonable alternative to catheter removal in patients with limited access and without *S. aureus* or *Candida* infections. Repeat blood cultures ("surveillance" cultures) are obtained after exchange of the catheter. Positive blood culture results after catheter exchange mandates removal of the catheter because of the low likelihood of resolving the bacteremia. In patients who undergo catheter exchange, systemic IV antibiotics are continued for 3 weeks.

"Cure" of bacteremia occurs in 67% to 75% of patients, and depends on the microbial species causing the infection. More failures are observed in patients with gram-positive bacteria or *Candida* species infections. The incidence of "metastatic" infections (eg, endocarditis, septic arthritis, or osteomyelitis) is observed in approximately 20% of patients.[14-19]

Antibiotic lock therapy is also a reasonable alternative in patients with limited access. Culture-specific concentrated antibiotics (eg, vancomycin or cefazolin) and heparin is combined into a solution for instillation into each catheter lumen after each dialysis session for 3 weeks. Systemic antibiotics are concurrently administered. Catheter salvage (ie, resolution of fever and clearance of "surveillance" blood cultures) is reported in 40% to 70% of patients and is highly dependent on the specific bacterial species isolated. Failure of therapy (ie, recurrent or persistent fever or bacteremia) occurs in about one-third to two-fifths of patients. Recurrent or persistent bacteremia is highest in patients with *Staphylococcus aureus or Candida* species.[8,9,13,20,21]

Q Clinical signs of AVG infection?

Clinical signs of AVG infection include warmth, erythema, tenderness, pain, ulceration, and/or drainage at the access site. Abandoned AVGs (eg, thrombosed AVGs) can be a source of infection and should also be evaluated for local signs of infection.[22-25]

R Localized infection without involvement of the arterial anastomosis?

An AVG infection is localized if it is limited to a discrete segment of the graft and does not involve the arterial anastomosis. Different treatment is required if the anastomoses are infected. An ultrasound of the graft should be obtained if one is unable to determine the extent of graft infection and/or to differentiate localized graft infection from widespread graft infection.[26,27]

S Ultrasound confirms infection?

In patients with systemic signs of infection, but without local signs of AVG infection, an ultrasound should be obtained. Complex fluid along the graft ("perigraft fluid"), within the tunnel or at the anastomoses on ultrasound is concerning for infection.[26,27] Positive ultrasound findings for nonlocalized graft infection should prompt complete graft excision and arterial repair.

T Tagged WBC scan and/or FDG-PET scan confirms infection?

Patients with persistent bacteremia, no identifiable alternate source of infection, and a normal graft ultrasound should have additional diagnostic imaging, such as indium-tagged WBC scans or fluorodeoxyglucose positron emission tomography (FDG-PET) scans. The intensity and extent of activity seen on the indium-tagged WBC scan can quantify the severity of infection.

Abandoned grafts have been shown to have positive scan findings with subclinical infection (ie, asymptomatic) because a significant number of thrombosed grafts can be colonized by bacteria. Indium-tagged WBC scan sensitivity nears 100% and specificity for graft infection is greater than 85%. FDG-PET scans, which are easier to perform than are tagged WBC scans, show increased uptake in the AVG with infection.[22,24,25,28-30]

U Repeat blood cultures positive?

If repeat blood culture results remain positive, the AVG should be excised; otherwise, another source of infection should be sought (see L).

V Excise graft; repair artery

Infections involving the entire graft and/or the arterial anastomosis should be treated by resecting the entire graft and repairing the artery.[31-35] In some situations, a widespread graft infection spares the arterial anastomosis. Dense scarring around the arterial anastomosis can complicate the arterial repair. For brachial artery–based AVGs distal to the profunda brachial branch, resection of the prosthetic material and ligation of the brachial artery is an alternative to brachial artery repair. Perfusion of the hand is usually sustained by the profunda brachial artery. No hand ischemic symptoms were reported in a single-center review of 21 patients treated in this way.[36] Alternatively, a short, well-incorporated "cuff" of graft can be left on the artery with an acceptable low risk of persistent/recurrent graft infection (~15%). Close clinical and, possibly, ultrasound surveillance is necessary to identify patients with persistent or recurrent infection when a prosthetic cuff is left. Evidence of persistent/recurrent infection, for example, nonhealing incisions or persistent bacteremia, warrants resection of the remaining prosthetic cuff with repair of the artery, reconstruction/revascularization, or ligation. Revascularization can be done in an extra-anatomic or "in situ" manner. Autogenous conduit (eg, saphenous or femoral vein) or, alternatively, cryopreserved conduit is recommended.[1,33,37-39]

W Attempt AVG salvage

Localized infections without involvement of the arterial anastomosis may be treated with partial graft excision (eg, excision of the infected segment with "bypass" in a clean field around the site of infection). Although reinfection does occur (~15%-40%), secondary graft patency can be significantly extended with this technique.[31-35,37]

X Ulceration/bleeding?

Ulceration and/or bleeding along an AVF mandates urgent evaluation and intervention. A clinical assessment of the extent and location of ulceration and the site of bleeding is necessary to determine treatment options.

Y Adjacent to AV anastomosis?

Ulceration or bleeding near the AV anastomosis renders the fistula unsalveageable in most cases. The primary objective of intervention is to prevent hemorrhage and sepsis. This generally requires sacrifice of the fistula.

Z Ligate/excise AVF; repair artery

If the ulceration is adjacent to the AV anastomosis, or if nonanastomotic infection does not resolve with incision, drainage, and antibiotics, ligation of the fistula, and excision and debridement of the infected tissue is performed. The artery is repaired with autogenous vein patch angioplasty. If the segment of artery is unsuitable for repair or requires resection, revascularization or ligation can be performed. Revascularization can be done with an "in situ" or extra-anatomic bypass. For extra-anatomic bypass, the artery is resected and oversewn, and a bypass performed through a sterile field. "In situ" revascularization is done with an autogenous conduit or a cryopreserved conduit. Ligation of the brachial artery in HD accesses that arise from the brachial artery distal to the profunda brachii has been shown to be well tolerated because the profunda brachial artery perfuses the hand adequately in most cases. Broad-spectrum antibiotic (typically, vancomycin plus an aminoglycoside) treatment is given for a total of 6 weeks. Conversion to pathogen-specific antibiotics is performed after return of blood culture results.[36,39-41]

AA "Metastatic" infection?

"Metastatic" infections secondary to AVF include endocarditis, septic thromboemboli to the distal extremity, osteomyelitis, or spinal epidural abscess. Any "metastatic" infection warrants prompt AVF ligation, excision, and repair of the artery.[11,41]

BB Salvage/revise AVF

Revision options for nonanastomotic AVF infections include simple excision of the ulcer or site of bleeding, resection of a short portion of the AVF with anastomosis, or ligation plus excision and bypass around the area with autogenous vein. If an autogenous vein is not available, then bypass using cryopreserved or prosthetic conduit can be utilized. Two weeks of broad-spectrum antibiotics is indicated in patients whose blood culture results were negative. In patients with positive blood culture results (bacteremia), 6 total weeks of culture-specific antibiotics is indicated.[1,41,42]

CC Ultrasound confirms infection?

Ultrasound should be obtained if one is unable to identify an AVF infection based on clinical examination alone. Ultrasound can identify the presence of complicated fluid collections such as hematomas, seromas, lymphatic fluid collections, or phlegmon that indicate local infection. If the ultrasound finding is normal, other sources of infection need to be evaluated.

DD Drain and culture with intravenous antibiotics

Fluid collections identified by ultrasound around the AVF not adjacent to the anastomosis should undergo incision and drainage. Wound cultures should be sent for analysis and IV antibiotic therapy initiated. Improvement with drainage and systemic antibiotics permits an attempt at fistula salvage. If improvement does not occur, excision and arterial repair is indicated.

EE Complete antibiotic therapy and utilize AVF

Two weeks of broad-spectrum antibiotics is indicated in patients whose blood culture results are negative after AVF fluid collection incision and drainage. In patients with positive blood culture results (bacteremia), 6 total weeks of culture-specific antibiotics is indicated. If the patient's fever has resolved and the WBC count has returned to normal, the fistula can be used for HD. Because most AV fistula infections occur at cannulation sites, these areas should be avoided for future access.[40-42]

FF Evaluate/treat other source of infection

If initially suspected hemodialysis access infection is not confirmed, other potential sources for systemic infection should be evaluated and treated as appropriate. Common infections in hemodialysis-dependent patients include upper or lower respiratory tract infections (eg, pneumonia), urinary tract infections, gastrointestinal tract infections, diabetic foot ulcer infections, other skin/soft tissue infections (eg, cellulitis), osteomyelitis, and tuberculosis.

REFERENCES

1. Padberg FT Jr., Calligaro KD, Sidawy AN. Complications of arteriovenous hemodialysis access: recognition and management. *J Vasc Surg*. 2008;48:55S-80S.
2. Stevenson KB, Hannah EL, Lowder CA, et al. Epidemiology of hemodialysis vascular access infections from longitudinal infection surveillance data: predicting the impact of NKF-DOQI clinical practice guidelines for vascular access. *Am J Kidney Dis*. 2002;39:549-555.
3. D'Amato-Palumbo S, Kaplan AA, Feinn RS, Lalla RV. Retrospective study of microorganisms associated with vascular access infections in hemodialysis patients. *Oral Surg Oral Med Oral Pathol Oral Radiol*. 2013;115:56-61.
4. Almasri J, Alsawas M, Mainou M, et al. Outcomes of vascular access for hemodialysis: a systematic review and meta-analysis. *J Vasc Surg*. 2016;64:236-243.
5. Al-Jaishi AA, Liu AR, Lok CE, Zhang JC, Moist LM. Complications of the arteriovenous fistula: a systematic review. *J Am Soc Nephrol*. 2017;28:1839-1850.
6. Fysaraki M, Samonis G, Valachis A, et al. Incidence, clinical, microbiological features and outcome of bloodstream infections in patients undergoing hemodialysis. *Int J Med Sci*. 2013;10:1632-1638.
7. Mermel LA, Allon M, Bouza E, et al. Clinical practice guidelines for the diagnosis and management of intravascular catheter-related infection: 2009 Update by the Infectious Diseases Society of America. *Clin Infect Dis*. 2009;49:1-45.
8. Krishnasami Z, Carlton D, Bimbo L, et al. Management of hemodialysis catheter-related bacteremia with an adjunctive antibiotic lock solution. *Kidney Int*. 2002;61:1136-1142.
9. Poole CV, Carlton D, Bimbo L, Allon M. Treatment of catheter-related bacteraemia with an antibiotic lock protocol: effect of bacterial pathogen. *Nephrol Dial Transplant*. 2004;19:1237-1244.
10. Allon M, Daugirdas J, Depner TA, Greene T, Ornt D, Schwab SJ. Effect of change in vascular access on patient mortality in hemodialysis patients. *Am J Kidney Dis*. 2006;47:469-477.
11. Kovalik EC, Raymond JR, Albers FJ, et al. A clustering of epidural abscesses in chronic hemodialysis patients: risks of salvaging access catheters in cases of infection. *J Am Soc Nephrol*. 1996;7:2264-2267.
12. Sychev D, Maya ID, Allon M. Clinical management of dialysis catheter-related bacteremia with concurrent exit-site infection. *Semin Dial*. 2011;24:239-241.
13. Maya ID, Carlton D, Estrada E, Allon M. Treatment of dialysis catheter-related Staphylococcus aureus bacteremia with an antibiotic lock: a quality improvement report. *Am J Kidney Dis*. 2007;50:289-295.
14. Tanriover B, Carlton D, Saddekni S, et al. Bacteremia associated with tunneled dialysis catheters: comparison of two treatment strategies. *Kidney Int*. 2000;57:2151-2155.
15. Robinson D, Suhocki P, Schwab SJ. Treatment of infected tunneled venous access hemodialysis catheters with guidewire exchange. *Kidney Int*. 1998;53:1792-1794.
16. Marr KA, Sexton DJ, Conlon PJ, Corey GR, Schwab SJ, Kirkland KB. Catheter-related bacteremia and outcome of attempted catheter salvage in patients undergoing hemodialysis. *Ann Intern Med*. 1997;127:275-280.
17. Shaffer D. Catheter-related sepsis complicating long-term, tunnelled central venous dialysis catheters: management by guidewire exchange. *Am J Kidney Dis*. 1995;25:593-596.
18. Ashby DR, Power A, Singh S, et al. Bacteremia associated with tunneled hemodialysis catheters: outcome after attempted salvage. *Clin J Am Soc Nephrol*. 2009;4:1601-1605.
19. Mokrzycki MH, Zhang M, Cohen H, Golestaneh L, Laut JM, Rosenberg SO. Tunnelled haemodialysis catheter bacteraemia: risk factors for bacteraemia recurrence, infectious complications and mortality. *Nephrol Dial Transplant*. 2006;21:1024-1031.
20. Capdevila JA, Segarra A, Planes AM, et al. Successful treatment of haemodialysis catheter-related sepsis without catheter removal. *Nephrol Dial Transplant*. 1993;8:231-234.
21. Peterson WJ, Maya ID, Carlton D, Estrada E, Allon M. Treatment of dialysis catheter-related Enterococcus bacteremia with an antibiotic lock: a quality improvement report. *Am J Kidney Dis*. 2009;53:107-111.
22. Ayus JC, Sheikh-Hamad D. Silent infection in clotted hemodialysis access grafts. *J Am Soc Nephrol*. 1998;9:1314-1317.
23. Beathard GA. Bacterial colonization of thrombosed dialysis arteriovenous grafts. *Semin Dial*. 2015;28:446-449.
24. Bachleda P, Kalinova L, Vachalova M, Koranda P. Unused arteriovenous grafts as a source of chronic infection in haemodialysed patients with relevance to diagnosis of Fluorodeoxyglucose PET/CT examination. *Ann Acad Med Singapore*. 2012;41:335-338.
25. Carlos MG, Juliana R, Matilde N, et al. Hidden clotted vascular access infection diagnosed by fluorodeoxyglucose positron emission tomography. *Nephrology (Carlton)*. 2008;13:264-265.
26. Scheible W, Skram C, Leopold GR. High resolution real-time sonography of hemodialysis vascular access complications. *AJR Am J Roentgenol*. 1980;134:1173-1176.
27. Finlay DE, Longley DG, Foshager MC, Letourneau JG. Duplex and color Doppler sonography of hemodialysis arteriovenous fistulas and grafts. *Radiographics*. 1993;13:983-989.
28. Brunner MC, Mitchell RS, Baldwin JC, et al. Prosthetic graft infection: limitations of indium white blood cell scanning. *J Vasc Surg*. 1986;3:42-48.
29. Williamson MR, Boyd CM, Read RC, et al. 111 In-labeled leukocytes in the detection of prosthetic vascular graft infections. *AJR Am J Roentgenol*. 1986;147:173-176.
30. Palestro CJ, Vega A, Kim CK, Vallabhajosula S, Goldsmith SJ. Indium-111-labeled leukocyte scintigraphy in hemodialysis access-site infection. *J Nucl Med*. 1990;31:319-324.
31. Walz P, Ladowski JS. Partial excision of infected fistula results in increased patency at the cost of increased risk of recurrent infection. *Ann Vasc Surg*. 2005;19:84-89.
32. Schwab DP, Taylor SM, Cull DL, et al. Isolated arteriovenous dialysis access graft segment infection: the results of segmental bypass and partial graft excision. *Ann Vasc Surg*. 2000;14:63-66.
33. Ryan SV, Calligaro KD, Scharff J, Dougherty MJ. Management of infected prosthetic dialysis arteriovenous grafts. *J Vasc Surg*. 2004;39:73-78.
34. Schutte WP, Helmer SD, Salazar L, Smith JL. Surgical treatment of infected prosthetic dialysis arteriovenous grafts:

total versus partial graft excision. *Am J Surg*. 2007;193:385-8; discussion 388.

35. Sgroi MD, Kirkpatrick VE, Resnick KA, Williams RA, Wilson SE, Gordon IL. Less than total excision of infected prosthetic PTFE graft does not increase the risk of reinfection. *Vasc Endovascular Surg*. 2015;49:12-15.

36. Schanzer A, Ciaranello AL, Schanzer H. Brachial artery ligation with total graft excision is a safe and effective approach to prosthetic arteriovenous graft infections. *J Vasc Surg*. 2008;48:655-658.

37. Padberg FT Jr., Smith SM, Eng RH. Accuracy of disincorporation for identification of vascular graft infection. *Arch Surg*. 1995;130:183-187.

38. Calligaro KD, Veith FJ, Valladares JA, McKay J, Schindler N, Dougherty MJ. Prosthetic patch remnants to treat infected arterial grafts. *J Vasc Surg*. 2000;31:245-252.

39. Lok CE, Huber TS, Lee T, et al; KDOQI Vascular Access Guideline Work Group. KDOQI clinical practice guideline for vascular access: 2019 update. *Am J Kidney Dis*. 2020;75(4) (suppl 2):S1-S164.

40. Stevenson KB. Management of hemodialysis vascular access infection. In: Gray RJ, Sands JJ, eds. *Dialysis Access: A Multidisciplinary Approach*. 1st ed. Philadelphia, PA: Lippincott Williams & Wilkins; 2002.

41. Gilmore J. KDOQI clinical practice guidelines and clinical practice recommendations—2006 updates. *Nephrol Nurs J*. 2006;33:487-488.

42. Taylor B, Sigley RD, May KJ. Fate of infected and eroded hemodialysis grafts and autogenous fistulas. *Am J Surg*. 1993;165:632-636.

Salvatore T. Scali • Thomas S. Huber

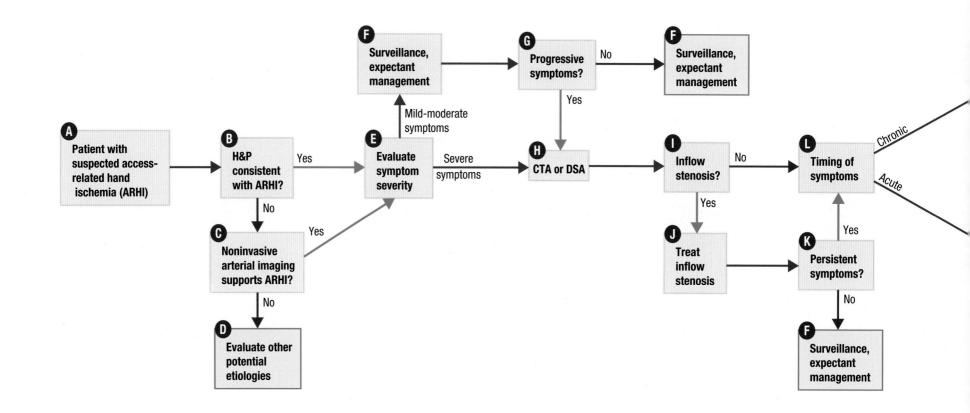

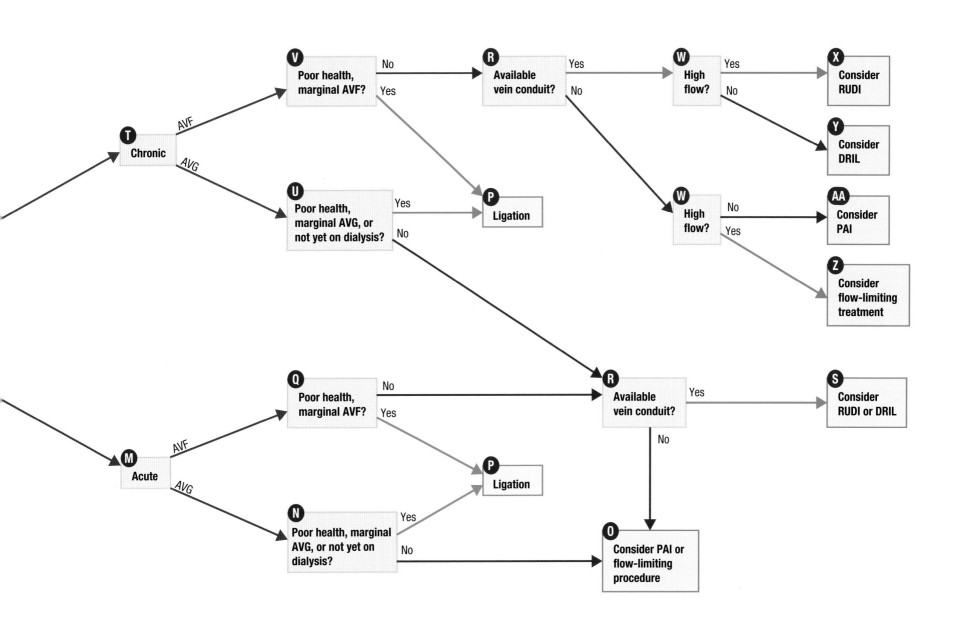

Ⓐ Patient with suspected access-related hand ischemia

The construction of an AV hemodialysis access creates a low-resistance, high-flow circuit through which blood is preferentially directed depending on pressure gradients.[1] The compensatory responses to the creation of the access include an increase in the cardiac output, vasodilation of the inflow and outflow arteries (ie, relative to the anastomosis), and the development of collateral vessels. The net effect of these hemodynamic changes is such that the perfusion pressure of the tissue distal to the AV anastomosis is usually reduced, with the common scenario being a decrease in the perfusion to the hand after a brachial artery–based AV access.[2] The decrease in distal perfusion or "physiological steal" is usually well tolerated, but patients may become symptomatic if the quantity of blood flow resulting from the compensatory mechanisms is inadequate for the metabolic needs of the tissue, resulting in the classic symptoms of acute and/or chronic ischemia. This phenomenon is commonly referred to as the "steal syndrome," although this is likely a misnomer because the blood flow simply follows pressure gradients and the contribution of any retrograde blood from the artery immediately distal to the anastomosis is fairly minimal.[3] A variety of other more appropriate terms have been used to describe this phenomenon including access-related hand ischemia (ARHI) and hemodialysis access–induced distal ischemia, although they have not been as widely adopted. Accordingly, the terminology ARHI and AV-access steal are used interchangeably throughout the decision tree and text.

Some type of steal-related symptoms occur in up to 20% of AV accesses based off the brachial artery near the antecubital fossa,[2,4-6] but only up to 2% of those originate from the distal radial artery.[7] The underlying hemodynamic mechanisms responsible for the brachial artery– and radial artery–based steal syndrome are similar, although the contribution of retrograde flow from the artery distal to the anastomosis (ie, retrograde flow through the distal radial artery from the palmar arch) is a more significant contributor for the radial artery–based procedures. Some type of remedial treatment to reverse the steal-related symptoms is required in up to 10% of brachial artery–based accesses.[2,4-6,8-10] Huber at al.[11] reported from the Hemodialysis Fistula Maturation (HFM) Study, a prospective study to identify predictors of AVF maturation, that 7% of the patients developed some type of steal-related symptoms, whereas 4% required a remedial, corrective procedure. These findings were corroborated by a systemic review of the complications associated with AVF by Al-Jaishi et al.[12] that reported a rate of 0.05 events/1000 patient-days for AV-access steal among >2500 patients.

Several predictors for the development of AV-access steal have been identified, and can be considered factors that put patients at "high risk." These include advanced age, female sex, diabetes mellitus, PAD, large access outflow conduits (eg, translocated femoral vein), multiple prior access procedures, distal brachial artery–based procedures (ie, brachial artery at antecubital fossa), and prior episodes of ARHI.[6,9,13-16] The HFM Study identified diabetes (OR 13.6), female sex (OR 3.2), outflow vein capacitance (OR 2.8), CAD (OR 2.6), and vein diameter (OR 1.6) as clinical predictors for remedial treatment.[11]

Ⓑ H&P consistent with ARHI?

The diagnosis of ARHI is largely a clinical one depending on the presence of signs and symptoms consistent with acute or chronic ischemia. The traditional symptoms of acute ischemia include the six P's—pain, paresthesia, paralysis, pulselessness, pallor, and poikilothermia, whereas those for chronic ischemia include exertional pain (ie, claudication), rest pain, or tissue loss. Among the acute symptoms, the presence of motor compromise (ie, paralysis) is the most worrisome and mandates immediate attention and remediation. The pulse examination can be somewhat misleading in that patients can have symptoms consistent with the steal syndrome despite the presence of a palpable pulse distal to the AV anastomosis (ie, radial pulse with brachial artery–based access) and vice versa in that patients may be completely asymptomatic despite the absence of a distal pulse. Similarly, noninvasive testing with arterial pressure and Doppler waveforms of the brachial, radial, ulnar, and digital vessels may also be misleading because patients may have symptoms consistent with ischemia despite only a moderate decrease in the various measurements (eg, brachial/radial pressures, WBI [wrist/brachial/index]). It is important to emphasize that the differential diagnosis of hand pain or numbness after an AV access is very limited and underscores the fact that all hand discomfort must be assumed to be ischemic in origin (ie, steal) until proved otherwise.[17] The dialysis history may provide some insight and aid in the diagnosis of AV-access steal because any hypotension or hypovolemia associated with the dialysis run may exacerbate the hemodynamic perturbation from the AVF and may precipitate symptoms in patients who are otherwise asymptomatic.

Ⓒ Noninvasive arterial imaging supports ARHI?

Noninvasive imaging may provide some additional support to corroborate the diagnosis of AV-access steal in equivocal cases. However, it is worth reemphasizing that the diagnosis of AV-access steal is largely a clinical one and that the differential diagnosis of hand pain after the creation of an access is very limited and has to be presumed to be related to the steal phenomenon until proved otherwise. The noninvasive arterial imaging should include pressure measurements and the corresponding velocity waveforms for the brachial, radial, ulnar, and digital vessels. These should be obtained with the access patent and compressed in an attempt to quantify its hemodynamic contribution. Unfortunately, there are no threshold pressure measurements that correspond to ARHI and the range of wrist and/or finger pressures can be somewhat broad, similar to the lower extremity pressures and indices in patients with claudication and ischemic rest pain. Several studies have attempted to identify an *intraoperative* digital pressure threshold that corresponds to *postoperative* ischemic symptoms, although findings have been somewhat equivocal.[16,18]

Ⓓ Evaluate other potential etiologies

Patients with atypical symptoms and those with normal noninvasive testing can be monitored closely and other diagnoses excluded. However, it is worth reemphasizing that the differential diagnosis of hand pain or numbness after an access is very limited.[17] Fortunately, patients with ESRD undergoing hemodialysis access are typically seen by their health care team thrice weekly. Assessment for access patency and any related complications, including ARHI, should be part of the routine assessment before cannulation.

Ⓔ Evaluate symptom severity

The natural history of the ARHI remains poorly defined. Patients with mild symptoms may improve, whereas those with severe ischemic rest pain associated with tissue loss do not improve and require some type of remedial treatment. Some of the patients with intermediate or more moderate symptoms may improve without intervention, although they likely require close follow-up. The Society for Vascular Surgery had developed a grading system (grade 0—no symptoms; grade 1—mild, cool extremity, few symptoms; grade 2—moderate, intermittent symptoms during dialysis, claudication; grade 3—severe, ischemic rest pain, tissue loss), although the system does not provide much guidance for the moderate group and has not been prospectively validated.[19] Although not necessary for diagnosis, it may be helpful to obtain noninvasive arterial studies as a baseline for any future intervention.

All patients with severe or grade 3 symptoms (rest pain, tissue loss) merit treatment to prevent long-term disability. In addition, a subset of patients with moderate or grade 2 symptoms (intermittent symptoms, claudication) also likely merit treatment, although the thresholds for intervention are somewhat less clear; some form of mild hand numbness may be tolerable but any motor compromise certainly merits intervention. It is important to remember that the overwhelming majority of hand dysfunction after access creation is related to the access itself, although more recent data would suggest that the responsible mechanism may be more than the hemodynamic changes alone.[20]

The treatment goals for patients with ARHI are to reverse the symptoms and salvage the access, if at all possible, although the prevention of further disability is the paramount concern. From a hemodynamic standpoint, this entails improving or augmenting the distal perfusion pressure. There are a variety of remedial treatment strategies and they should be viewed as complementary rather than as competitive, with the optimal choice dictated by the clinical scenario. The determinants include the acuity of symptoms, the patient's underlying comorbidities, timing of dialysis needs (ie, CKD vs. ESRD), type of access (ie, AVG vs. AVG), quality of access (ie, likelihood of maturation, anticipated long-term patency), contributing mechanisms (eg, presence of inflow stenosis, high flow vs. low flow), future access options, the availability of autogenous conduit, surgeon expertise, and patient preference. The remedial treatments for access salvage are all quite good in terms of reversing the ischemic symptoms (both acute and chronic) and salvaging the access itself. Given the fact that the remedial procedures reverse the adverse hemodynamic changes associated with the access, the acute symptoms should improve immediately, whereas any associated tissue loss should heal within a relatively short period of time, typically a month.

AV-access steal may occur after radial artery–based accesses, although the incidence is much less than that reported for the brachial-based procedures.[7,21] The responsible hemodynamic changes resulting from the access are comparable, although somewhat different given the dual blood supply to the hand through the radial and ulnar arteries. The available remedial treatment options are dictated by the underlying contributing causes of the hemodynamic changes but include correction of any inflow lesions, flow reduction, ligation (or embolization) of the distal radial artery to prevent retrograde perfusion, and access ligation.[7,21]

The creation of an AV access can result in severe sensorimotor dysfunction distal to the access in the setting of only mild to moderate ischemia, termed ischemic monomelic neuropathy.[22,23] Although this is likely within the spectrum of AV-access steal, it may be a distinct entity that has been attributed to the development of severe ischemic neuropathy despite adequate skin and muscle perfusion. The published experience is somewhat limited, although the condition appears to be increased among patients with diabetes, PAD, and preexisting peripheral neuropathy. Optimal treatment includes immediate recognition and remedial treatment, typically with access ligation, although the sensorimotor symptoms may not be reversible.[24]

F Surveillance, expectant management

Given the potential adverse sequelae, all patients with mild to moderate symptoms of ARHI merit close follow-up, ideally with an access surgeon familiar with the full range of remedial treatment strategies. Assessment for access patency and any related complications, including ARHI, should be part of the routine assessment before cannulation in the dialysis center and all associated health care providers should be familiar with the symptoms of ARHI and the importance of timely referral to an access surgeon. Patients should also be educated about the potential symptoms and provided with instructions to contact the appropriate health care provider.

G Progressive symptoms?

Progression of symptoms from grade 1 (mild, cool extremity) or grade 2 (intermittent symptoms, claudication) to grade 3

(ischemic rest pain, tissue) merits timely referral to an access surgeon for definitive treatment. Notably, the symptoms can range anywhere along the spectrum of acute and chronic ischemia, similar to the more common situation of lower extremity arterial occlusive disease. The presence of any motor compromise, including fine motor control (eg, inability to button a shirt) is particularly worrisome and likely merits referral and intervention.

H CTA or DSA

Patients requiring remedial treatment for their AV-access steal should undergo additional imaging (ie, CTA or DSA) to exclude any potential inflow lesion. The presence of significant arterial occlusive disease in the inflow (eg, subclavian artery stenosis) or outflow (eg, diffuse occlusive disease of the radial and ulnar artery in the forearm) vessels may further exacerbate the hemodynamic changes and symptoms associated with the AV access.

I Inflow stenosis?

Inflow lesions that are not hemodynamically significant at baseline may become hemodynamically significant after the construction of an AV access because of increased blood flow across the stenosis, similar to the effect of exercise or intra-arterial vasodilators in patients with aortoiliac occlusive disease. Notably, Kokkosis et al.[25] reported that one-third of the patients in their series with severe steal symptoms had a contributory arterial inflow lesion (ie, subclavian or brachial). Noninvasive arterial imaging before the index access procedure (ie, preoperatively) may help exclude an arterial inflow lesion and should be mandatory in patients deemed high risk for ARHI.

J Treat inflow stenosis

All hemodynamically significant inflow lesions in patients with ARHI should be treated. There are a variety of endovascular and open surgical approaches to treat the various inflow lesions with the choice dictated by the anatomic location and extent of the lesion. The common lesion at the origin of the left SCA usually responds well to endovascular treatment with an intraluminal stent.

K Persistent symptoms?

The presence of moderate to severe symptoms after correction of any inflow lesions merits further evaluation and definitive treatment.

L Timing of symptoms

Treatment of AHRI depends on whether symptoms are acute or chronic. Acute symptoms typically develop immediately after the access construction. Notably, the onset of acute, severe symptoms tends to be worse with AVGs versus AVFs, as might be predicted by the hemodynamic changes associated with the construction of an AV communication with a large outflow conduit, typically 6 mm.[5]

The distribution of remedial interventions was roughly trimodal in one of the largest series for the DRIL procedure, with a third of the patients requiring treatment within 0 to 7 days, 8 to 30 days and >30 days.[26] Patients with chronic ischemia often present with digital tissue loss months after their index access procedure, typically in the setting of long-standing diabetes and severe arterial occlusive disease in the forearm and hand. Although the underlying hemodynamic changes and the options for remedial treatment are basically the same for acute and chronic ischemia, the timing of the symptoms is relevant for the specific treatment choice.

M Acute

The choice of the optimal remedial treatment for both acute and chronic symptoms is a relatively complex clinical decision that is impacted by a variety of factors, as detailed earlier (see E). The major clinical decision is whether to pursue further attempts at salvage or simply ligate the access. In the acute setting, this decision is largely driven by the type and quality of the access and the patient's underlying comorbidities.

N Poor health, marginal AVG, or not yet on dialysis?

The optimal treatment for patients with advanced comorbidities with acute, persistent ARHI after placement of an AVG is likely ligation. Admittedly, this is somewhat of a judgment call in terms of the severity of the underlying medical conditions. Furthermore, this may commit these patients to dialysis with tunneled catheter because their alternative permanent access options may be limited. Patients with CKD and no imminent need for dialysis may also be better served with access ligation. It is not advisable to perform a series of remedial procedures on patients who are not actively on dialysis given the limited life expectancy of AVGs.[27] It is difficult to predict exactly when a patient will progress from CKD to ESRD with the requirement for renal replacement therapy, and, thus, most providers elect to defer placement of an AVG until dialysis is imminent.

O Consider PAI or flow-limiting procedure

The potential remedial treatments for AVG salvage in the acute setting include PAI or some variant of a flow-limiting (banding) procedure. Both are effective and have their proponents. The DRIL and RUDI are not recommended because of the limited longer term patency of most AVGs and the requirement for autogenous conduit. The PAI converts an access based off the brachial artery at the antecubital fossa to one based off the more proximal brachial artery using a small-caliber prosthetic conduit and may represent a variation of a flow-limiting strategy.[28,29] A variety of flow-limiting strategies have been described (eg, narrowing of the anastomosis, diameter reduction of the outflow graft), with the ultimate goal of augmenting the distal perfusion pressure while maintaining sufficient flow through the access for effective dialysis.[30,31] Achieving this hemodynamic result may be difficult, but it can be augmented with the aid of intraoperative noninvasive monitoring of digital perfusion.[31]

A small percentage of patients will have persistent symptoms of numbness or paresthesia after all of the remedial interventions despite hemodynamic improvement. This is likely related to an ischemic nerve injury and may not be reversible.[22] The diagnostic conundrum in this scenario is whether the ongoing symptoms are related to ongoing ischemia or residual ischemic neuropathy from the initial event. Noninvasive imaging with upper extremity arterial pressures and waveforms may be helpful in this setting. Access ligation remains an option.

P Ligation

Access ligation should reverse the hemodynamic changes associated with the access, and, hopefully, reverse symptoms. This is generally performed through a small incision over the access immediately downstream to the arterial anastomosis, where the access is dissected out locally and ligated with a large-diameter ligature. It is worth reemphasizing that ESRD requires a lifetime plan with committed providers and that an episode of ARHI is a strong predictor of future events with subsequent accesses, and, thus, it is not always feasible to simply resite the access on the contralateral extremity. Accordingly, *preoperative* strategies should be developed to reduce the incidence of ARHI during subsequent access creations including assessment (and correction) of any arterial inflow stenoses, avoiding siting the access at the brachial artery near the antecubital fossa, and the avoidance of using large conduits (eg, femoral vein) when feasible. It may also be worthwhile to explore transplantation and/or peritoneal dialysis in this cohort of patients.

Q Poor health, marginal AVF?

The optimal treatment for patients with advanced comorbidities and acute, persistent ARHI after placement of an AVF is likely ligation. Admittedly, this is somewhat of a judgment call in terms of the severity of the underlying medical conditions and the likelihood of the AVF maturation. The clinical judgment of the surgeon in terms of the likelihood of maturation has proved to be quite accurate, with the determinants being the quality of the artery (eg, diameter, calcification) and vein (eg, diameter, presence of intimal hyperplasia).[32] Interestingly, larger outflow veins are associated with an increased incidence of both ARHI and maturation.[11,33] It can be helpful to generate a remedial plan for ARHI at the time of the index access procedure and we frequently challenge the trainees during the procedure to develop a plan of action to address the hypothetical call from the recovery room nurse stating that the patient cannot move the hand and is experiencing severe pain. The dialysis status (ie, CKD vs. ESRD) tends to be less of a concern for AVFs (vs. AVGs) because they are often constructed well in

advance of the anticipated start date for dialysis to account for the obligatory period of maturation.

R Available vein conduit?

The definitive remedial options for access salvage include the DRIL, RUDI, PAI, and some variation of a flow-limiting procedure. As noted earlier, the various approaches are complementary and all can reverse the adverse hemodynamic changes associated with the access. Both the DRIL and the RUDI require a suitable segment of autogenous conduit. The exact criteria remain undefined, but a segment of saphenous vein ≥3 mm is preferable given the experience with its use as a conduit for lower extremity revascularization.[26] Upper extremity veins should generally be avoided and reserved for future access options.

S Consider RUDI or DRIL

The RUDI effectively converts an access based off the brachial artery at the antecubital fossa to one based off a more distal inflow site, typically the proximal radial artery.[34] It may also have a role for steal symptoms related to "high-flow" fistulas and has been reported to have a role for AVFs causing high-output CHF and/or symptomatic venous HTN, independent of any symptoms related to ARHI.[34] Notably, Misskey et al.[35] compared their outcomes with the RUDI and DRIL and reported that the procedures were associated with comparable outcomes in terms of patency, relief of symptoms, and survival.

The DRIL procedure is essentially a brachial artery bypass with the proximal anastomosis sited proximal to the fistula anastomosis and the distal anastomosis sited distal to the fistula anastomosis. Concomitant with the bypass, the brachial artery immediately distal to the fistula anastomosis is ligated to prevent any retrograde flow. This approach has been reported to effectively salvage the access and reverse the ARHI in >80% of the cases.[36] Illig et al.[37] measured intra-arterial pressures before and after the DRIL procedure and demonstrated that it effectively reverses the hemodynamic change.

T Chronic

The choice of optimal remedial treatment for both acute and chronic symptoms is complicated (see E). The major clinical decision is whether to pursue further attempts at salvage or simply ligate the access. In the case of chronic ischemic symptoms, the access has presumably been functional or at least patent for some time, so salvage is more often pursued.

U Poor health, marginal AVG, or not yet on dialysis?

Patients with advanced comorbidities and/or marginally functional AVG with chronic symptoms of ARHI, particularly those with CKD but not yet on dialysis, should undergo ligation. Good-risk patients with a functional AVG and chronic

symptoms of ARHI should likely undergo access salvage and all of the remedial procedures are potential options. The potential exceptions include AVGs that have required multiple remedial procedures to maintain functional patency and the rare patient with CKD and a long-standing AVG that has not progressed to needing dialysis. The major treatment determinant is really the expected patency rate of the AVG. Given the fairly limited long-term patency rates of an AVG, it does not make too much sense to harvest a segment of autogenous conduit for the RUDI or DRIL, although there are select clinical scenarios (ie, AVG patent long term) where this may be worthwhile. Similar to the acute setting, both the PAI and flow-limiting therapies are viable options and do not require autogenous vein.

V Poor health, marginal AVF?

Remedial treatment to salvage the AVF is appropriate for majority of patients with chronic symptoms of ARHI. The potential exceptions include marginal AVFs that have required multiple remedial procedures to maintain functional patency and/or patients with advanced comorbidities and such poor overall health in terms of life expectancy and functional status that they cannot or should not undergo an access salvage procedure. This is similar to the scenario with AVGs. The threshold for access salvage should be somewhat lower for AVFs (relative to AVGs) given their patency advantage. All of the remedial procedures are potential options for access salvage, with the optimal choice dictated by the availability of autogenous conduit and the underlying hemodynamic changes in terms of the flow rate.

W High flow?

The optimal access salvage procedure for patients with AVFs and chronic symptoms may be partially contingent on the flow rate through the fistula. Although the threshold for "high-flow" fistulas is not universal, a flow rate of >1200 mL/min is generally considered "high flow."[29,38] These higher flow rates result from the chronic changes associated with the creation of an AV access (ie, outflow vein dilation, inflow artery vein dilation, increased cardiac output) and are more commonly seen with AVFs given the relative flow restriction through the nondistensible prosthetic accesses (typically 6-mm ePTFE). Remedial access salvage therapies that limit the flow through the access (ie, flow limiting, RUDI) may be optimal for these "high-flow" AVFs, and, conversely, the PAI and DRIL may be better suited for lower flow AVFs (ie, <1200 L/min). Notably, the flow-limiting therapies may not be effective for patients with extensive tissue loss.[39] Admittedly, the PAI converts an autogenous access to a composite prosthetic/autogenous access in this setting.

X Consider RUDI

The RUDI converts an access based off the brachial artery at the antecubital fossa to one based off a more distal inflow site, typically the proximal radial artery (see S).[34] It may have a role for steal symptoms related to "high-flow" fistulas and has been reported to have a role for AVFs causing high-output CHF and symptomatic venous HTN, independent of any symptoms related to hand ischemia.[34]

Ⓨ Consider DRIL

The DRIL is essentially a brachial artery bypass with the proximal anastomosis sited proximal to the fistula anastomosis and the distal anastomosis sited distal to the fistula anastomosis (see S). Concomitant with the bypass, the brachial artery immediately distal to the fistula anastomosis is ligated to prevent any retrograde flow. This approach has been reported to effectively salvage the access and reverse the ARHI in more than 80% of the cases.[36,40]

Ⓩ Consider flow-limiting treatment

A variety of flow-limiting strategies have been described (eg, narrowing of the anastomosis, diameter reduction of the outflow graft) with the ultimate goal of augmenting the distal perfusion pressure while maintaining sufficient flow through the access for effective dialysis (see O).[30,31,41,42] Achieving this hemodynamic result may be difficult, but can be augmented with the aid of intraoperative noninvasive monitoring of the digital perfusion.[31]

ⒶⒶ Consider PAI

The PAI converts an access based off the brachial artery at the antecubital fossa to one based off the more proximal brachial artery using a small caliber prosthetic conduit (see O).[28,29]

Acknowledgment

The author acknowledges and appreciates the assistance of Salvatore T. Scali, MD, who provided significant contributions and editorial oversight in the development of this chapter.

REFERENCES

1. Wixon CL, Hughes JD, Mills JL. Understanding strategies for the treatment of ischemic steal syndrome after hemodialysis access. *J Am Coll Surg.* 2000;191:301-310.
2. Papasavas PK, Reifsnyder T, Birdas TJ, Caushaj PF, Leers S. Prediction of arteriovenous access steal syndrome utilizing digital pressure measurements. *Vasc Endovascular Surg.* 2003;37:179-184.
3. Vaes RH, Tordoir JH, Scheltinga MR. Blood flow dynamics in patients with hemodialysis access-induced hand ischemia. *J Vasc Surg.* 2013;58:446-451.
4. Keuter XH, Kessels AG, de Haan MH, Van Der Sande FM, Tordoir JH. Prospective evaluation of ischemia in brachial-basilic and forearm prosthetic arteriovenous fistulas for hemodialysis. *Eur J Vasc Endovasc Surg.* 2008;35:619-624.
5. Lazarides MK, Staramos DN, Kopadis G, Maltezos C, Tzilalis VD, Georgiadis GS. Onset of arterial "steal" following

6. Morsy AH, Kulbaski M, Chen C, Isiklar H, Lumsden AB. Incidence and characteristics of patients with hand ischemia after a hemodialysis access procedure. *J Surg Res.* 1998;74:8-10.
7. Chemla E, Raynaud A, Carreres T, et al. Preoperative assessment of the efficacy of distal radial artery ligation in treatment of steal syndrome complicating access for hemodialysis. *Ann Vasc Surg.* 1999;13:618-621.
8. Schanzer H, Eisenberg D. Management of steal syndrome resulting from dialysis access. *Semin Vasc Surg.* 2004;17:45-49.
9. Suding PN, Wilson SE. Strategies for management of ischemic steal syndrome. *Semin Vasc Surg.* 2007;20:184-188.
10. Tordoir JH, Dammers R, Van Der Sande FM. Upper extremity ischemia and hemodialysis vascular access. *Eur J Vasc Endovasc Surg.* 2004;27:1-5.
11. Huber TS, Larive B, Imrey PB, et al. Access-related hand ischemia and the Hemodialysis Fistula Maturation Study. *J Vasc Surg.* 2016;64:1050-1058.
12. Al-Jaishi AA, Liu AR, Lok CE, Zhang JC, Moist LM. Complications of the arteriovenous fistula: a systematic review. *J Am Soc Nephrol.* 2017;28:1839-1850.
13. Davidson D, Louridas G, Guzman R, et al. Steal syndrome complicating upper extremity hemoaccess procedures: incidence and risk factors. *Can J Surg.* 2003;46:408-412.
14. Huber TS, Hirneise CM, Lee WA, Flynn TC, Seeger JM. Outcome after autogenous brachial-axillary translocated superficial femoropopliteal vein hemodialysis access. *J Vasc Surg.* 2004;40:311-318.
15. Kusztal M, Weyde W, Letachowicz W, et al. Influence of autologous arteriovenous fistula on the blood supply to the hand in very elderly hemodialyzed patients. *J Vasc Access.* 2005;6:83-87.
16. Valentine RJ, Bouch CW, Scott DJ, et al. Do preoperative finger pressures predict early arterial steal in hemodialysis access patients? A prospective analysis. *J Vasc Surg.* 2002;36:351-356.
17. Namazi H, Majd Z. Carpal tunnel syndrome in patients who are receiving long-term renal hemodialysis. *Arch Orthop Trauma Surg.* 2007;127:725-728.
18. Goff CD, Sato DT, Bloch PH, et al. Steal syndrome complicating hemodialysis access procedures: can it be predicted? *Ann Vasc Surg.* 2000;14:138-144.
19. Sidawy AN, Gray R, Besarab A, et al. Recommended standards for reports dealing with arteriovenous hemodialysis accesses. *J Vasc Surg.* 2002;35:603-610.
20. Rehfuss JP, Berceli SA, Barbey SM, et al. The spectrum of hand dysfunction after hemodialysis fistula placement. *Kidney Int Rep.* 2017;2:332-341.
21. Miller GA, Khariton K, Kardos SV, Koh E, Goel N, Khariton A. Flow interruption of the distal radial artery: treatment for

proximal angioaccess: immediate and delayed types. *Nephrol Dial Transplant.* 2003;18:2387-2390.

finger ischemia in a matured radiocephalic AVF. *J Vasc Access.* 2008;9:58-63.
22. Hye RJ, Wolf YG. Ischemic monomelic neuropathy: an under-recognized complication of hemodialysis access. *Ann Vasc Surg.* 1994;8:578-582.
23. Thermann F, Kornhuber M. Ischemic monomelic neuropathy: a rare but important complication after hemodialysis access placement—a review. *J Vasc Access.* 2011;12:113-119.
24. Coscione AI, Gale-Grant O, Maytham GD. Early access ligation resolves presumed ischaemic monomelic neuropathy in a patient with recurrence of central venous occlusion. *J Vasc Access.* 2015;16:344-346.
25. Kokkosis AA, Abramowitz SD, Schwitzer J, Nowakowski S, Teodorescu VJ, Schanzer H. Inflow stenosis as a contributing factor in the etiology of AV access-induced ischemic steal. *J Vasc Access.* 2014;15:286-290.
26. Huber TS, Brown MP, Seeger JM, Lee WA. Midterm outcome after the distal revascularization and interval ligation (DRIL) procedure. *J Vasc Surg.* 2008;48:926-932.
27. Huber TS, Carter JW, Carter RL, Seeger JM. Patency of autogenous and PTFE upper extremity arteriovenous hemodialysis accesses: a systematic review. *J Vasc Surg.* 2003;38(5):1005-1011.
28. Thermann F, Wollert U. Proximalization of the arterial inflow: new treatment of choice in patients with advanced dialysis shunt-associated steal syndrome? *Ann Vasc Surg.* 2009;23(4):485-490.
29. Zanow J, Kruger U, Scholz H. Proximalization of the arterial inflow: a new technique to treat access-related ischemia. *J Vasc Surg.* 2006;43:1216-1221.
30. Miller GA, Goel N, Friedman A, et al. The MILLER banding procedure is an effective method for treating dialysis-associated steal syndrome. *Kidney Int.* 2010;77:359-366.
31. Thermann F, Ukkat J, Wollert U, Dralle H, Brauckhoff M. Dialysis shunt-associated steal syndrome (DASS) following brachial accesses: the value of fistula banding under blood flow control. *Langenbecks Arch Surg.* 2007;392:731-737.
32. Farber A, Imrey PB, Huber TS, et al. Multiple preoperative and intraoperative factors predict early fistula thrombosis in the Hemodialysis Fistula Maturation Study. *J Vasc Surg.* 2016;63:163-70.e6.
33. Dageforde LA, Harms KA, Feurer ID, Shaffer D. Increased minimum vein diameter on preoperative mapping with duplex ultrasound is associated with arteriovenous fistula maturation and secondary patency. *J Vasc Surg.* 2015;61(1):170-176.
34. Loh TM, Bennett ME, Peden EK. Revision using distal inflow is a safe and effective treatment for ischemic steal syndrome and pathologic high flow after access creation. *J Vasc Surg.* 2016;63(2):441-444.
35. Misskey J, Yang C, MacDonald S, Baxter K, Hsiang Y. A comparison of revision using distal inflow and distal

revascularization-interval ligation for the management of severe access-related hand ischemia. *J Vasc Surg*. 2016;63:1574-1581.

36. Scali ST, Huber TS. Treatment strategies for access-related hand ischemia. *Semin Vasc Surg*. 2011:128-136.

37. Illig KA, Surowiec S, Shortell CK, Davies MG, Rhodes JM, Green RM. Hemodynamics of distal revascularization-interval ligation. *Ann Vasc Surg*. 2005;19:199-207.

38. Scheltinga MR, van HF, Bruyninckx CM. Surgical banding for refractory hemodialysis access-induced distal ischemia (HAIDI). *J Vasc Access*. 2009;10:43-49.

39. Thermann F. Intervention for access-induced ischemia: which option is the best? *J Vasc Access*. 2015;16(suppl 9):S102-S107.

40. Katz S, Kohl RD. The treatment of hand ischemia by arterial ligation and upper extremity bypass after angioaccess surgery. *J Am Coll Surg*. 1996;183:239-242.

41. Zanow J, Petzold K, Petzold M, Krueger U, Scholz H. Flow reduction in high-flow arteriovenous access using intraoperative flow monitoring. *J Vasc Surg*. 2006;44:1273-1278.

42. Vaes RH, Wouda R, Teijink JA, Scheltinga MR. Venous side branch ligation as a first step treatment for haemodialysis access induced hand ischaemia: effects on access flow volume and digital perfusion. *Eur J Vasc Endovasc Surg*. 2015;50(6):810-814.

Karl A. Illig

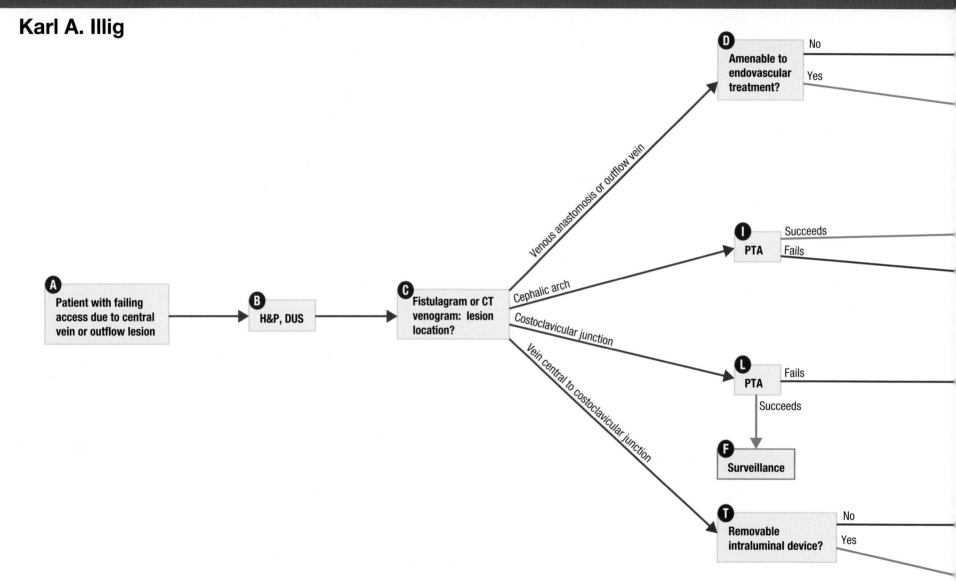

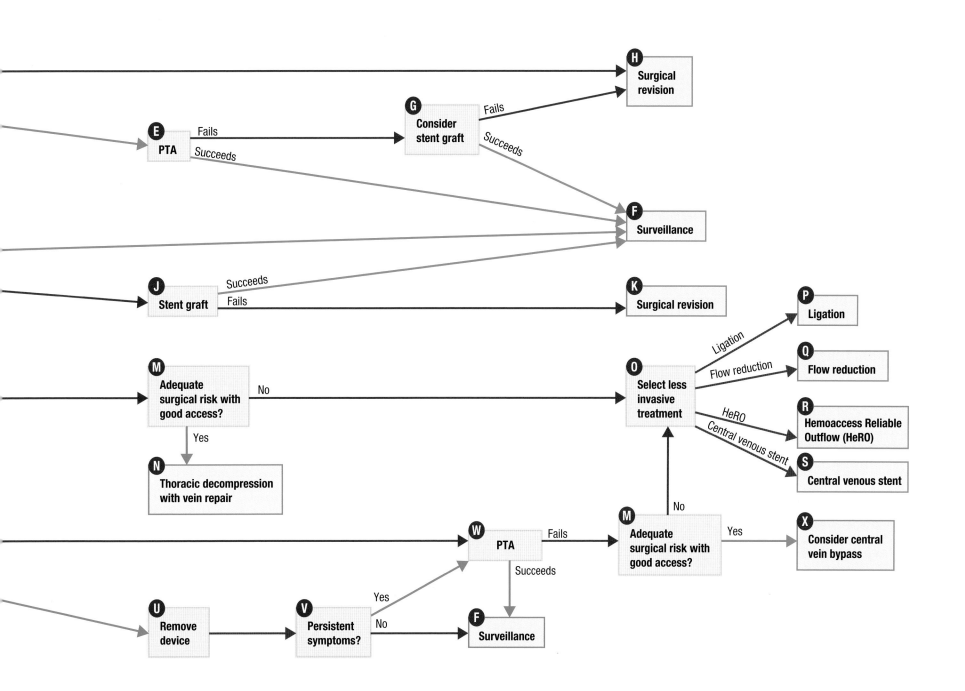

Ⓐ Patient with failing access due to central vein or outflow lesion

Venous outflow stenoses or occlusions are a common mode of access failure for both AVFs and AVGs. Indeed, venous outflow stenoses, typically at the venous anastomosis, represent the most common etiology for AVG access dysfunction and thrombosis.[1] The decision analysis and the accompanying text discuss the treatment of a patient with a failing access due to outflow stenoses. In this context, the venous outflow is considered anything central to the cannulation zone, encompassing all of the venous return from the functional portion of the access to the heart. Treatment algorithms for these lesions are fairly well established and defined by clinical practice guidelines.[2-4]

Ⓑ H&P, DUS

Dialysis patients with central vein or outflow stenoses, by definition, display some evidence of increased pressure in the access circuit. Clinically, this is manifested as a swollen arm, although the chest, breast, neck, and/or face can also swell depending on the anatomy of venous return and the presence of other venous obstructions. In the most extreme case, this can lead to the development of SVC syndrome. Other clues suggesting outflow stenoses include marked superficial varicosities, access thrombosis, elevated circuit pressures during dialysis, inefficient dialysis, high recirculation rates, and chest or shoulder pain during dialysis. Patients are typically referred to a surgeon or interventionalist by their nephrologist or dialysis center for these complaints. Physical examination in combination with DUS of the access and the venous outflow are the initial diagnostic steps. Pulsatile access suggests a venous outflow stenosis and it is often possible to identify the site of the stenosis depending on the transition of the pulse to a thrill. An edematous extremity suggests a central stenosis or occlusion. The physical findings can be corroborated by DUS, which, in many ways, is an extension of the physical examination. Unfortunately, DUS is not particularly helpful for directly imaging the central veins given the limitations of the bony thorax.

Ⓒ Fistulagram or CT venogram: lesion location?

A catheter-based fistulagram or CT venogram should be obtained to further define the anatomy in patients with access dysfunction and presumed venous outflow stenoses. Most clinicians proceed directly to fistulagram, particularly because the majority of patients will require concomitant endovascular treatment. It is convenient to divide the venous outflow problems into five general categories, based on the type of access and the anatomic location of the lesion. These include venous anastomotic stenosis, venous outflow stenosis, cephalic arch stenosis, costoclavicular junction (CCJ) stenosis, and stenosis of vein central to CCJ. The AVG venous anastomotic stenosis and venous outflow are addressed together because their treatment algorithm is essentially the same.

Ⓓ Amenable to endovascular treatment?

A stenosis at the venous anastomosis of an AVG or the venous outflow of either an AVF or AVG is a common finding and a leading cause of access failure. Indeed, venous anastomotic stenoses are the leading cause of AVG dysfunction. However, it is important to differentiate the presence of an *asymptomatic* venous anastomotic stenosis from a hemodynamically significant stenosis associated with access dysfunction or clinical symptoms. There is likely no indication for treatment of asymptomatic venous outflow stenoses and the clinical practice of surveillance with prophylactic PTA of these lesions has been demonstrated to be ineffective (and potentially harmful) in a number of randomized trials.[5]

The majority of venous anastomotic and outflow stenoses are amenable to endovascular treatment and the endovascular approach is typically the first line of therapy, as emphasized by the NKF-KDOQI guidelines.[2] The clinical determinants include the ability to pass a suitable wire across the stenosis, the character of the venous outflow beyond the area of stenosis (eg, diameter of outflow vein, absence of central vein stenoses), and patient history in terms of prior interventions at the same site. Long-segment, diffuse outflow lesions and those that recur early after PTA alone likely merit more aggressive, definitive treatment with a stent graft or open surgery.

Ⓔ PTA

PTA is the preferred first line of treatment for *de novo* AVG venous anastomotic and outflow stenoses. However, some consideration should be given to the placement of a stent graft, given the evolving body of literature supporting that approach (see G). PTA should be performed with relatively large balloons; we typically use 8-mm balloons for the venous anastomosis and 10-mm balloons for outflow lesions despite the fact that most of the prosthetic accesses are 6 mm in diameter. Oversizing the balloon relative to the graft has proved to be safe and is associated with good outcomes, although caution should be exercised with biologic grafts that may be more prone to disruption. Lesions refractory to standard PTA balloons can be treated with either high pressure or cutting balloons and the latter may be associated with improved outcomes.[2-4] Alternatively, a small wire (eg, 0.018) can be placed across the lesion and used in combination with a standard angioplasty balloon to "score" the hyperplastic lesion, similar to a cutting balloon. It is important for the outflow lesion to be completely effaced (ie, no residual stenosis) after PTA because residual stenoses predict early recurrence. Of note, anastomotic lesions result from intimal hyperplasia rather than from atherosclerosis and, as such, are prone to recoil.

Ⓕ Surveillance

Patients undergoing endovascular treatment for outflow and central venous lesions are typically seen within a month of their procedure with a DUS. Any hemodynamically significant stenosis associated with clinical symptoms is addressed as outlined throughout the algorithm. The recurrence rate after the various endovascular treatments is significant, particularly for PTA alone. We usually defer further surveillance (ie, beyond the early postprocedure visit) to the dialysis center because most centers have some type of monitoring or surveillance protocol. Surveillance with prophylactic intervention for *asymptomatic* venous lesions has not shown to be beneficial.[5]

Ⓖ Consider stent graft

The presence of a residual stenosis after PTA merits additional treatment with either a stent graft or surgical revision. Similar to the preceding steps in the algorithm, the endovascular approach is usually preferred. However, it is important to consider the patient's overall lifetime access plan and not compromise future access options by placing a stent across an outflow vein that could support a future access (eg, cephalic arch stent with compromise of axillary vein outflow). Several prospective, randomized trials have demonstrated the superiority of stent grafts for the treatment of AVG venous anastomotic stenoses, although the supporting evidence for the treatment of venous outflow stenoses is not as compelling.[6-9] Stent grafts may provide a theoretic advantage over open cell stents in terms of decreased ingrowth of hyperplastic tissue. Placement of a stent graft can be considered as an alternative to PTA for *de novo* lesions, although cost considerations likely favor the use of PTA alone.

Ⓗ Surgical revision

Open surgical revision is an excellent treatment option for venous anastomotic and outflow lesions not amenable to endovascular treatment and those lesions that recur early.[2-4] Outcomes are typically more durable than those for endovascular therapy, although this advantage is offset by the more invasive nature of the procedure. Surgical options include patch angioplasty or the use of an interposition graft. The choice is usually dictated by the extent of the intimal hyperplasia, although we favor the use of an interposition graft for venous anastomotic lesions and typically use an 8-mm PTFE graft in an attempt to increase the size of the anastomosis. The size discrepancy between the new interposition graft (8 mm) and the old graft (typically 6 mm) can be overcome by spatulating the graft–graft anastomosis. The choice of patch or graft material (ie, prosthetic vs. autogenous) is usually dictated by the type of access (ie, AVG vs. AVF) and the availability of a suitable segment of vein; for an AVF, attempts should be made to preserve an all-autogenous conduit. Stenoses or occlusion of the axillary vein can be treated with an axillary-jugular bypass if the ipsilateral jugular vein is patent and its central runoff is unobstructed. Another operation that has been used in this setting is jugular venous turndown, where a patent internal jugular vein, in the setting of a normal ipsilateral innominate vein outflow, is anastomosed to the ipsilateral axillary vein to bypass the subclavian vein occlusion.[10]

① PTA

Stenoses at the cephalic arch (ie, the terminal portion of the cephalic vein at its confluence with the axillary vein) represent a distinct group of venous outflow stenoses. Indeed, there has been a greater appreciation of these lesions and their unique biologic response to treatment in the past several years.[11] The management of basilic vein "swing" segment stenoses (ie, terminal portion of the basilic vein at the axillary vein junction) for the brachial-basilic AVF is similar and most of the treatment principles apply.

Standard balloon PTA is the initial treatment option for the *de novo* cephalic arch lesions. These stenoses can span the length of the arch, but are usually not so diffuse that PTA is precluded. These lesions can rupture with oversizing of the balloon and, thus, we favor balloon diameters of 6 to 8 mm in the majority of patients. Notably, the cephalic arch can be somewhat difficult to image during a routine fistulagram and full-strength iodinated contrast (vs. diluted or half-strength contrast) is often necessary, particularly in the case of residual stenosis.

① Stent graft

The presence of a residual stenosis merits additional treatment with either a stent graft or surgical revision. Both are effective treatment options for residual cephalic arch lesions, with the choice dictated by the quality of the access, the patient's operative risk, and future access options. The determinants of surgical risk in this setting include comorbidities, life expectancy, and dependency (ie, home vs. facility, ambulatory vs. nonambulatory). These concerns are relevant for all of the endovascular versus open surgical decisions detailed throughout the algorithm, but perhaps most relevant in this setting given the equipoise between the treatment options.[12]

Stent grafts are a better treatment option than are open-cell stents, as suggested by several recent studies.[11,13-15] Precise placement of the stent graft in this setting is crucial to avoid compromising the deep venous outflow and future access options. Stent grafts should not be placed across the CCJ because the anatomic forces in the thoracic outlet can lead to stent fracture with central vein thrombosis. Anecdotally, this has led to the development of life-threatening SVC syndrome in two patients referred to our practice.

① Surgical revision

Surgical revision of residual or recurrent cephalic arch stenoses is likely optimal for adequate risk patients. The cephalic arch is somewhat difficult to expose because the cephalic vein dives deep from its superficial course at the deltopectoral groove as it drains into the axillary vein. Accordingly, direct repair is somewhat problematic and requires division of the muscle. A better alternative is to transpose the distal aspect of the cephalic vein onto the axillary vein in the axilla. This can be accomplished by making a longitudinal incision over the distal cephalic and a second incision more proximal in the axilla. The distal cephalic vein can be dissected free, transected, and then tunneled through a subcutaneous tissue to facilitate the anastomosis.[16] Fortunately, the cephalic vein tends to elongate and become more tortuous after AVF creation, and this redundancy helps facilitate both vein mobilization and a tension-free anastomosis.

① PTA

Stenosis or occlusion at the CCJ represents a separate category among the venous outflow problems given the associated anatomic constraints. Unlike the other regions of the access venous outflow (eg, upper arm brachial and axillary vein), the central veins at the CCJ are surrounded and potentially compressed by the structures that comprise the thoracic outlet, specifically the clavicle, first rib, and anterior scalene muscle. This area can be identified by looking carefully at the shadow of the bones during a fistulagram after digital subtraction, but it is just central to the jugular/subclavian confluence and is typically surrounded by fairly short, localized collaterals in affected patients. There has been an increased awareness of the significance of the CCJ compression to access dysfunction over the past decade and an appreciation that the associated lesions cannot be effectively treated without bony decompression (ie, claviculectomy or first rib resection), similar to the treatment of venous thoracic outlet.[17-20]

Similar to the other venous outflow lesions, PTA is likely the recommended initial treatment. Although PTA alone is unlikely to be a definitive, long-term solution, it appears to be effective in the short term and there are no data to suggest that it is ineffective or compromises future options. High-pressure balloons are frequently required given the refractory nature of the hyperplastic lesions contributing to the stenosis. A balloon diameter of 8 to 10 mm is usually sufficient and oftentimes the practical limit given the extrinsic compression from the thoracic outlet.

① Adequate surgical risk with good access?

Residual and/or recurrent stenoses are common after balloon PTA of CCJ lesions because of extrinsic compression. Generically, the early technical success rates for PTA alone exceed 90%, but the primary patency is only 50% at 6 months and 25% at 12 months, respectively.[21-24] Thus, the management of recurrent or residual stenosis is a chronic, ongoing problem. Given these high rates of residual stenosis and/or recurrence, the relevant question is not whether there is a persistent stenosis or occlusion, but rather whether the lesion is associated with significant symptoms in terms of arm swelling or access dysfunction. The index balloon PTA can often serve as a temporizing solution to allow the development of additional venous collaterals. Indeed, it is not uncommon to see patients with patent, functional accesses without upper extremity swelling despite a central vein occlusion.[25] Regardless, patients with persistent symptoms likely merit further treatment.

More definitive treatment of the recurrent CCJ or more central lesions is contingent on the quality of the access in terms of its anticipated long-term patency and the patient's overall general health and operative risk. An aggressive approach at access salvage seems reasonable for a mature AVF that has functioned for a while without problems, but may not be indicated for an AVG that has been associated with multiple thromboses. Treatment of these CCJ and more central lesions also needs to be viewed within the patient's lifetime access plan because failure to address the central lesion likely precludes further access attempts in the ipsilateral extremity. The determinants of surgical risk include comorbidities, life expectancy, and dependency (ie, home vs. facility, ambulatory vs. nonambulatory). Remedial open, surgical treatments for failing dialysis accesses span a relatively broad range in terms of their magnitude (eg, minor [vein patch angioplasty] vs. more major [thoracic decompression with venous reconstruction]) and potential patient disability. Appropriate surgical judgment entails weighing the risks of the procedure against the benefits. Accordingly, thoracic decompression and central vein bypass should be reserved for good-risk patients with good access.

① Thoracic decompression with vein repair

The optimal treatment for stenoses or occlusions at the CCJ in good-risk patients with a good access entails thoracic decompression to eliminate the extrinsic compression along with treatment of the intraluminal lesion.[18-20] This can be accomplished by means of an anterior scalene and first rib resection through an infraclavicular or a paraclavicular approach, both of which allow for a first interspace sternotomy if more extensive venous reconstruction is required.[26] Alternatively, the decompression can be performed with a claviculectomy, which is tolerated remarkably well from a functional standpoint.[27] The patency of the vein should be reassessed after decompression with a fistulagram. Although most advocate conservative treatment for residual stenoses in the setting of the *venous* thoracic outlet,[17] it has been our impression that this scenario is different in the setting of a high-flow dialysis access. First, the venous HTN and the associated sequelae (ie, swelling) are exacerbated. Second, the high flow predisposes patients with stenosis to turbulence that creates a positive feedback loop for further intimal hyperplasia and stenosis. Accordingly, it is our belief that these lesions should be treated aggressively with PTA ± intraluminal stenting or venous reconstruction. The long-term patency rates for the reconstructions performed in the setting of venous thoracic outlet (93% at 1 year) are excellent and even better (100% at 1 year) among the small cohort of patients undergoing reconstruction for dialysis-related stenoses.[28]

O Select less invasive treatment

There are several less invasive treatment options for patients who are not candidates for thoracic decompression or central venous bypass. These include ligation, the Hemoaccess Reliable Outflow (HeRO) Vascular Access Device (Hemosphere, Inc., Minneapolis, MN), flow reduction, and central venous stenting. Each of these has advantages and disadvantages that must be evaluated for each patient in the context of the clinician's experience.

P Ligation

Access ligation will reduce venous HTN and its associated sequelae. It will essentially "cure" the presenting symptoms of pain and swelling, even in the presence of a central vein occlusion. The obvious downside to ligation is the fact that the access is sacrificed. Furthermore, failure to treat the underlying cause of the problem effectively precludes the ipsilateral extremity from further permanent access attempts. The short- and long-term consequences of access ligation should be thoroughly discussed with the patient.

Q Flow reduction

The quantity of blood flow through the access can be reduced in an attempt to reduce the venous HTN and associated sequelae as an alternative to correcting the outflow lesion. This option is particularly relevant for "high-flow" access with flow rates exceeding 1.2 mL/min. There are a variety of "flow-reducing therapies" including "banding" or the RUDI.[29-31] The various "banding" procedures should likely be performed using some type of physiologic assessment such as real-time flow measurements to assure the desired outcome because they require striking the tenuous balance between sufficient access flow to sustain effective dialysis, yet low enough to avoid complications. The RUDI essentially converts a brachial artery–based access to a radial artery–based access. Not surprisingly, symptomatic central vein lesions are more common after brachial artery–based than are radial artery–based procedures.[32,33] These approaches are used more commonly for the treatment of access-related hand ischemia (see Chapter 69).

R Hemoaccess Reliable Outflow (HeRO)

The HeRO Vascular Access Device is a hybrid graft-catheter system that can be used for patients with refractory central vein occlusive disease.[34,35] The catheter component is inserted across the stenoses or occlusion with the tip or outflow positioned at the SVC–atrial junction, similar to a tunneled dialysis catheter. The catheter component is then coupled to the upper extremity access using the 6-mm ePTFE graft component of the system. Notably, the HeRO system can also be used to create a *de novo* access if the anticipated life expectancy of the index access is limited. This approach does not actually address the central venous

lesion, but creates a reasonable outflow (catheter—5-mm ID) into the atrium. Unfortunately, the catheter delivery system is quite large (19 F) and can be difficult to insert across a tight lesion. Longer term patency rates and infectious complications are both reasonable.[36,37]

S Central venous stent

The placement of a central venous stent should be considered as a last resort in patients with CCJ stenoses or occlusions. There is a significant amount of data demonstrating that these stents perform poorly in the nondecompressed thoracic outlet for patients with venous thoracic outlet stenosis and the results are likely applicable to dialysis patients with CCJ lesions.[17] Unfortunately, stents are prone to kinking and fracture from the extrinsic compression. Their use should generally be reserved for only the oldest/sickest patient with a limited life expectancy and no other reasonable access options (eg, contralateral extremity) or other viable solutions for the CCJ lesion.

Caution should also be exercised when placing an intraluminal stent across and retained endoluminal device (eg, pacer wire) because the stent can essentially "trap" the device and complicate future attempts at removal although the natural history of the devices in this setting is poorly described.

T Removable intraluminal device?

Clinically significant stenoses can develop within the most distal segment of the venous outflow track between the CCJ and the atrium. Unlike the region of the thoracic outlet, the central veins in this anatomic region (ie, innominate vein, SVC) are surrounded by soft tissue and, thus, are more amenable to endovascular treatment.[2-4]

Intraluminal devices (eg, tunneled dialysis catheter, pacer leads) can narrow the lumen of the central venous outflow and contribute to the access-related venous HTN and clinical sequelae. Pacemaker wires can be particularly problematic and it has been our anecdotal impression that they can stimulate in intense hyperplastic response that is refractory to traditional balloon PTA. A common scenario is to have a tunneled dialysis catheter contralateral to the AVF or AVG that is obstructing the central venous outflow. Notably, the concerns about intraluminal devices are also relevant for the more proximal regions of the central venous outflow addressed earlier.

U Remove device

All intraluminal devices that are obstructing the lumen of the venous outflow should be removed if at all possible. Admittedly, they may need to be reinserted, but it is optimal to resite in a location such that they do not obstruct the venous outflow (eg, common femoral vein). Subcutaneous defibrillators and leadless pacers are a reasonable alternative, as indicated, and should likely be used preferentially in patients with CKD and ESRD.[38,39]

V Persistent symptoms?

Removal of any intraluminal device should, ideally, result in the resolution of the clinical symptoms that precipitated the investigation. However, this series of events is relatively uncommon and further, definitive treatment is usually necessary.

W PTA

Balloon PTA should be the first line of therapy after the removal of any intraluminal device for patients with persistent symptoms. The brachiocephalic veins can usually be dilated with fairly large balloons, typically 10 to 14 mm. Similarly, the SVC can also be dilated with large balloons. It has been our anecdotal experience that the junction of the superior vena cava and the right atrium is prone to rupture. Accordingly, balloon dilation in this region should be approached with caution and it has been our practice to have a 13-mm stent graft immediately available and perform the index PTA through an appropriate size sheath such that it would accommodate the covered stent should the need arise. The potential sequelae of disrupting the central veins can be further minimized by occluding or thrombosing the AVF or AVG, thereby reducing the associated elevated venous pressures. The access can be temporarily occluded with a PTA balloon and/or intentionally thrombosed with a planned thrombectomy after the central vein disruption is treated or heals.

A residual stenosis or the development of a recurrent stenosis after central vein PTA is commonplace. Remedial treatment should be dictated by the presence of recurrent symptoms. Fortunately, these lesions tend to develop somewhat slowly, oftentimes allowing for the development of collateral pathways, and, thus, the presence of recurrent stenosis does not always translate into recurrent symptoms.

X Consider central vein bypass

There may be a small subset of patients who may benefit from a central venous bypass to treat persistent symptoms and salvage-associated access. Limited published experience has been favorable; however, it is important to emphasize that this approach requires a median sternotomy.[26,40] It has been our impression that the venous collaterals tend to be deep (ie, azygous), and, thus, the surgical dissection is not too different from that in patients without a central vein lesion.

REFERENCES

1. Maya ID, Oser R, Saddekni S, Barker J, Allon M. Vascular access stenosis: comparison of arteriovenous grafts and fistulas. *Am J Kidney Dis*. 2004;44:859-865.
2. Vascular Access Work Group. Clinical practice guidelines for vascular access. *Am J Kidney Dis*. 2006;48(suppl 1):S248-S273.
3. Sidawy AN, Spergel LM, Besarab A, et al. The Society for Vascular Surgery: clinical practice guidelines for the surgical placement and maintenance of arteriovenous hemodialysis access. *J Vasc Surg*. 2008;48:2S-25S.

4. Thomas M, Nesbitt C, Ghouri M, Hansrani M. Maintenance of hemodialysis vascular access and prevention of access dysfunction: a review. *Ann Vasc Surg*. 2017;43:318-327.

5. Ravani P, Quinn RR, Oliver MJ, et al. Pre-emptive correction for haemodialysis arteriovenous access stenosis. *Cochrane Database Syst Rev*. 2016;(1):CD010709.

6. Haskal ZJ, Trerotola S, Dolmatch B, et al. Stent graft versus balloon angioplasty for failing dialysis-access grafts. *N Engl J Med*. 2010;362:494-503.

7. Haskal ZJ, Saad TF, Hoggard JG, et al. Prospective, randomized, concurrently-controlled study of a stent graft versus balloon angioplasty for treatment of arteriovenous access graft stenosis: 2-year results of the RENOVA Study. *J Vasc Interv Radiol*. 2016;27:1105-1114.e3.

8. Vesely T, DaVanzo W, Behrend T, Dwyer A, Aruny J. Balloon angioplasty versus Viabahn stent graft for treatment of failing or thrombosed prosthetic hemodialysis grafts. *J Vasc Surg*. 2016;64:1400-1410.e1.

9. Yang HT, Yu SY, Su TW, Kao TC, Hsieh HC, Ko PJ. A prospective randomized study of stent graft placement after balloon angioplasty versus balloon angioplasty alone for the treatment of hemodialysis patients with prosthetic graft outflow stenosis. *J Vasc Surg*. 2018;68:546-553.

10. Puskas JD, Gertler JP. Internal jugular to axillary vein bypass for subclavian vein thrombosis in the setting of brachial arteriovenous fistula. *J Vasc Surg*. 1994;19(5):939-942.

11. Kim SM, Yoon KW, Woo SY, et al. Treatment strategies for cephalic arch stenosis in patients with brachiocephalic arteriovenous fistula. *Ann Vasc Surg*. 2019;54:248-253.

12. Vasanthamohan L, Gopee-Ramanan P, Athreya S. The management of cephalic arch stenosis in arteriovenous fistulas for hemodialysis: a systematic review. *Cardiovasc Intervent Radiol*. 2015;38(5):1179-1185.

13. Rajan DK, Falk A. A Randomized Prospective Study comparing outcomes of angioplasty versus VIABAHN stent-graft placement for cephalic arch stenosis in dysfunctional hemodialysis accesses. *J Vasc Interv Radiol*. 2015;26(9):1355-1361.

14. Jones RG, Willis AP, Tullett K, Riley PL. Results of stent graft placement to treat cephalic arch stenosis in hemodialysis patients with dysfunctional brachiocephalic arteriovenous fistulas. *J Vasc Interv Radiol*. 2017;28:1417-1421.

15. Miller GA, Preddie DC, Savransky Y, Spergel LM. Use of the Viabahn stent graft for the treatment of recurrent cephalic arch stenosis in hemodialysis accesses. *J Vasc Surg*. 2018;67:522-528.

16. Sigala F, Sassen R, Kontis E, Kiefhaber LD, Forster R, Mickley V. Surgical treatment of cephalic arch stenosis by central transposition of the cephalic vein. *J Vasc Access*. 2014;15:272-277.

17. Illig KA, Doyle AJ. A comprehensive review of Paget-Schroetter syndrome. *J Vasc Surg*. 2010;51:1538-1547.

18. Glass C, Dugan M, Gillespie D, Doyle A, Illig K. Costoclavicular venous decompression in patients with threatened arteriovenous hemodialysis access. *Ann Vasc Surg*. 2011;25:640-645.

19. Illig KA, Gabbard W, Calero A, et al. Aggressive costoclavicular junction decompression in patients with threatened AV access. *Ann Vasc Surg*. 2015;29:698-703.

20. Illig KA. Management of central vein stenoses and occlusions: the critical importance of the costoclavicular junction. *Semin Vasc Surg*. 2011;24:113-118.

21. Agarwal AK. Central vein stenosis. *Am J Kidney Dis*. 2013;61:1001-1015.

22. Massara M, De Caridi G, Alberti A, Volpe P, Spinelli F. Symptomatic superior vena cava syndrome in hemodialysis patients: mid-term results of primary stenting. *Semin Vasc Surg*. 2016;29:186-191.

23. Horikawa M, Quencer KB. Central venous interventions. *Tech Vasc Interv Radiol*. 2017;20:48-57.

24. Krishna VN, Eason JB, Allon M. Central venous occlusion in the hemodialysis patient. *Am J Kidney Dis*. 2016;68:803-807.

25. Shi Y, Zhu M, Cheng J, Zhang J, Ni Z. Venous stenosis in chronic dialysis patients with a well-functioning arteriovenous fistula. *Vascular*. 2016;24:25-30.

26. Molina JE. A new surgical approach to the innominate and subclavian vein. *J Vasc Surg*. 1998;27:576-581.

27. Green RM, Waldman D, Ouriel K, Riggs P, Deweese JA. Claviculectomy for subclavian venous repair: long-term functional results. *J Vasc Surg*. 2000;32:315-321.

28. Edwards JB, Brooks JD, Wooster MD, Fernandez B, Summers K, Illig KA. Outcomes of venous bypass combined with thoracic outlet decompression for treatment of upper extremity central venous occlusion. *J Vasc Surg Venous Lymphat Disord*. 2019;7(5):660-664.

29. Loh TM, Bennett ME, Peden EK. Revision using distal inflow is a safe and effective treatment for ischemic steal syndrome and pathologic high flow after access creation. *J Vasc Surg*. 2016;63(2):441-444.

30. Miller GA, Goel N, Friedman A, et al. The MILLER banding procedure is an effective method for treating dialysis-associated steal syndrome. *Kidney Int*. 2010;77:359-366.

31. Thermann F, Ukkat J, Wollert U, Dralle H, Brauckhoff M. Dialysis shunt-associated steal syndrome (DASS) following brachial accesses: the value of fistula banding under blood flow control. *Langenbecks Arch Surg*. 2007;392:731-737.

32. Trerotola SO, Kothari S, Sammarco TE, Chittams JL. Central venous stenosis is more often symptomatic in hemodialysis patients with grafts compared with fistulas. *J Vasc Interv Radiol*. 2015;26(2):240-246.

33. Arnaoutakis DJ, Deroo EP, McGlynn P, et al. Improved outcomes with proximal radial-cephalic arteriovenous fistulas compared with brachial-cephalic arteriovenous fistulas. *J Vasc Surg*. 2017;66:1497-1503.

34. Allan BJ, Prescott AT, Tabbara M, Bornak A, Goldstein LJ. Modified use of the Hemodialysis Reliable Outflow (HeRO) graft for salvage of threatened dialysis access. *J Vasc Surg*. 2012;56:1127-1129.

35. Davis KL, Gurley JC, Davenport DL, Xenos ES. The use of HeRo catheter in catheter-dependent dialysis patients with superior vena cava occlusion. *J Vasc Access*. 2016;17(2):138-142.

36. Al SJ, Houston JG, Jones RG, Inston N. A Review on the Hemodialysis Reliable Outflow (HeRO) graft for haemodialysis vascular access. *Eur J Vasc Endovasc Surg*. 2015;50(1):108-113.

37. Katzman HE, McLafferty RB, Ross JR, Glickman MH, Peden EK, Lawson JH. Initial experience and outcome of a new hemodialysis access device for catheter-dependent patients. *J Vasc Surg*. 2009;50:600-607.e1.

38. Dhamija RK, Tan H, Philbin E, et al. Subcutaneous implantable cardioverter defibrillator for dialysis patients: a strategy to reduce central vein stenoses and infections. *Am J Kidney Dis*. 2015;66:154-158.

39. Da Costa A, Axiotis A, Romeyer-Bouchard C, et al. Transcatheter leadless cardiac pacing: the new alternative solution. *Int J Cardiol*. 2017;227:122-126.

40. Wooster M, Fernandez B, Summers KL, Illig KA. Surgical and endovascular central venous reconstruction combined with thoracic outlet decompression in highly symptomatic patients. *J Vasc Surg Venous Lymphat Disord*. 2019;7:106-112.e3.

Thom Rooke

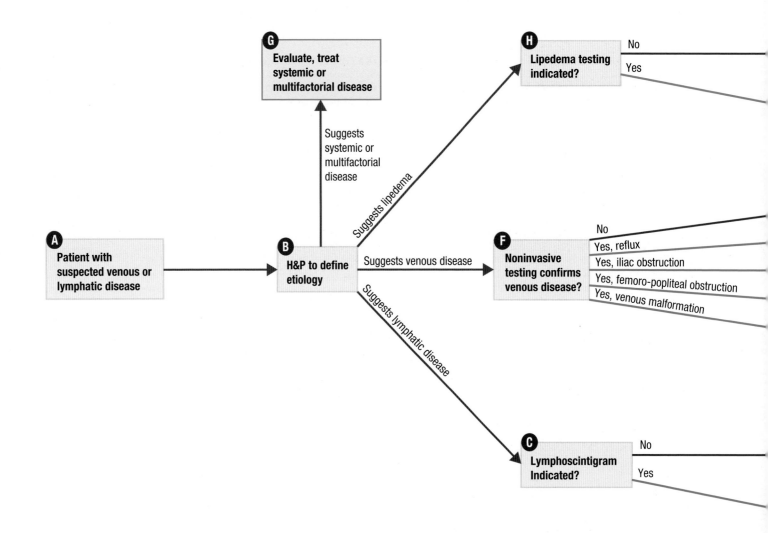

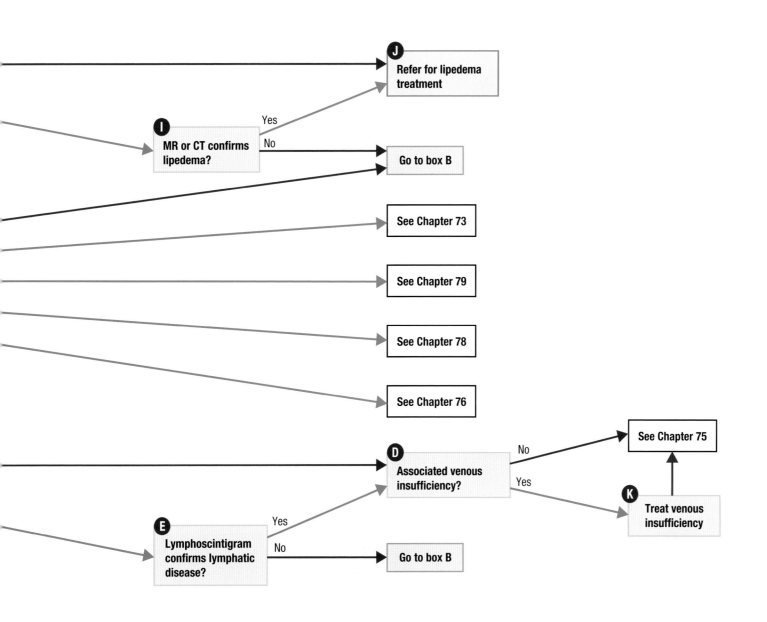

Ⓐ Patient with suspected venous or lymphatic disease

Chronic venous disease, lymphedema, and lipedema are all extremely common conditions. Chronic venous disease (including chronic venous obstruction, venous incompetence, varicose veins, and other forms) affects 50% or more of the population, especially in those >50 to 60 years of age.[1] Lymphedema (swelling caused by obstruction or reflux in lymphatic vessels) is one of the most common conditions afflicting humans. There are millions of cases in the United States (many of which have occurred following cancer, radiation therapy, trauma, infection, or other causes). It is estimated that there are >100 million people worldwide with lymphedema.[2] Lipedema (a congenital condition involving the abnormal deposition of fatty tissue over the low lower trunk and legs) may affect up to 10% of the female population, although there is considerable uncertainty regarding this figure.[3]

Ⓑ H&P to define etiology

A thorough H&P should be performed to try to differentiate between venous disease, lymphedema, and lipedema. *Venous disease* is suggested by a history of varicose veins, superficial phlebitis, previous DVT, limb swelling, pain/ache, pruritis, or superficial lower extremity ulceration(s).[4] *Lymphedema* is suggested by limb swelling that occurs spontaneously in infancy or during puberty; it can also develop after trauma, surgery, or infection. *Lipedema* typically includes a familial pattern and lack of improvement with compression therapy and/or weight loss.

PE findings suggestive of *venous disease* include limb swelling associated with pain/tenderness, skin discoloration due to hemosiderin deposition, red, weeping skin ulceration(s) with prominent granulation tissue that are typically located near the medial malleolus.[5] *Lymphedema* is characterized by limb, ankle, and foot swelling associated with induration and sclerotic-appearing skin. The pathognomonic Stemmer sign is often used to assess this; it is the inability to pinch the skin at the base of the second toe, and it suggests that the skin has developed "orange peel" rigidity.[6] Lymphedema typically involves the foot and toes (which are often "square" or sausage shaped). "Firm" (nonpitting) edema, Bier spots,[7] and/or ski-jump nails[8] are also common findings. With *lipedema*, the swelling always stops at the ankles and spares the feet. Localized pain, swelling, or inflammation may be clues to musculoskeletal or other nonvascular systemic problems described in Box G.

Next steps in management depend on whether the H&P suggests lymphedema, venous disease, lipedema, or another systemic disease.

Ⓒ Lymphoscintigram indicated?

Lymphedema is usually diagnosed on the basis of H&P, but a lymphoscintigram can be valuable when the diagnosis is uncertain.[9] A radioactive colloid tracer is injected into the affected region of the limb, and its subsequent movement (or lack of

movement) through the lymphatic vessels is assessed. Abnormal transport is indicative of lymphedema. Because lymphedema is often incurable, lymphoscintigraphy helps confirm the diagnosis, and hence prognosis, for the patient (and providers). However, it seldom leads to definitive treatment, and, as such, is not usually performed when the clinical diagnosis is clear.

Ⓓ Associated venous insufficiency?

Lymphedema is difficult to treat and usually impossible to cure; so even when the H&P and testing (lymphoscintigraphy) suggest that the patient has lymphedema, it is important to confirm that a potentially treatable condition such as venous disease is not a cofactor in the production of limb swelling. If there is concern that venous insufficiency might be present along with lymphedema, further evaluation including venous testing is indicated (see F). If detected, treatment of both venous and lymphatic disease is indicated.

Ⓔ Lymphoscintigram confirms lymphatic disease?

If lymphoscintigraphy fails to confirm lymphedema, alternative conditions should be sought. If the lymphoscintigram is positive, then lymphedema is likely to be present.[10] In some cases, it is desirable to investigate a patient with lymphedema to determine whether there is a secondary cause such as invasive tumor or lymph node involvement,[11] or whether the lymphedema might be treatable (with lymphatic bypass or some other surgical procedure). These evaluations typically require some type of imaging (CT/MRI/DUS) or even lymphangiography.

Ⓕ Noninvasive testing confirms venous disease?

Although in many vascular laboratories DUS is the primary means of noninvasively testing for venous disease, physiologic tests (including air or strain gauge plethysmography) may be useful in many clinical settings. Venous DUS evaluation should include both a supine examination to evaluate for acute or chronic obstruction as well as an upright examination to evaluate for abnormal venous reflux. The next steps depend on the laboratory findings/diagnosis: reflux from valvular incompetence (see Chapter 73), leg venous obstruction (see Chapter 78), iliac venous obstruction (see Chapter 79), and venous malformation (see Chapter 76). If vascular testing fails to confirm venous disease, then alternative explanations should be evaluated.

In certain patients with a diagnosis of venous disease, the question of proximal venous obstruction (May–Thurner syndrome, or vena cava obstruction) may arise. In many patients, this cannot be adequately assessed by ultrasound because of body habitus or other issues. CT/MRI or IVUS are often used to clarify this situation.[12]

Ⓖ Evaluate, treat systemic or multifactorial disease

Bilateral leg edema raises the possibility of systemic problems including those related to the heart, kidneys, or liver dysfunction or failure. Hypoproteinemia, poor nutritional status, thyroid disease

with myxedema, and drug effects can also mimic venous disease or lymphedema.

In many cases, the cause of limb edema is multifactorial.[13] When a problem (venous disease, lymphedema, systemic disease, medication effect, etc.) is identified but does not account for the entire clinical picture, the possibility that multiple causes are present should be entertained. It is often necessary to go back to the original step of H&P to detect additional possibilities.

Ⓗ Lipedema testing indicated?

Lipedema is primarily a clinical diagnosis, but when there is uncertainty, an MR or CT can be helpful to distinguish between subcutaneous adipose tissue and edema fluid. In some cases, venous testing and/or lymphoscintigraphy is performed to rule out venous or lymphatic disease.[14] If lipedema appears to be the obvious clinical diagnosis, the patient can be referred for treatment without additional testing.

Ⓘ MR or CT confirms lipedema?

If leg imaging confirms lipedema by demonstrating the presence of subcutaneous fat, the patient can be referred for treatment. If testing fails to confirm lipedema, then alternative explanations should be evaluated.

Ⓙ Refer for lipedema treatment

Physical therapy (wrapping, massage, pneumatic pumps) and overall weight loss may be helpful for patients with lipedema and is the initial recommended treatment. It should be emphasized that dieting alone will not "cure" lipedema. The only definitive treatment involves liposuction; when lipedema is severe, referral to a plastic surgeon or other liposuction practitioners may be appropriate. Weight loss does not treat lipedema and should not be recommended.

Ⓚ Treat venous insufficiency

If venous insufficiency coexists with lymphedema, it should be evaluated for treatment, which may be more definitive than specific treatment of lymphedema. See Chapters 73, 78, and 79 for a discussion of treatment for valvular incompetence, leg venous obstruction, and iliac venous obstruction, respectively.

REFERENCES

1. Beebe-Dimmer JL, Pfeifer JR, Engle JS, Schottenfeld D. The epidemiology of chronic venous insufficiency and varicose veins. *Ann Epidemiol*. 2005;15(3):175-184.
2. Rockson SG, Rivera KK. Estimating the population burden of lymphedema. *Ann N Y Acad Sci*. 2008;1131:147-154. doi:10.1196/annals.1413.014.
3. Fife CE, Maus EA, Carter MJ. Lipedema: a frequently misdiagnosed and misunderstood fatty deposition syndrome. *Adv Skin Wound Care*. 2010;23(2):81-92; quiz 93-94.

4. Kistner RL. Diagnosis of chronic venous insufficiency. *J Vasc Surg*. 1986;3(1):185-188.

5. Onida S, Lane T, Davies A. Clinical presentation and assessment of patients with venous disease. In: Gloviczki P, ed. *Handbook of Venous and Lymphatic Disorders*. Boca Raton, FL: CRC Press; 2017:chap 29.

6. Laredo J, Lee BB. Lymphedema. In: Mowatt-Larssen E, Desai S, Dua A, Shortell C, eds. *Phlebology, Vein Surgery and Ultrasonography*. Cham, Switzerland: Springer International Publishing; 2014:chap 23.

7. Dean SM, Zirwas M. Bier spots are an under-recognized cutaneous manifestation of lower extremity lymphedema: a case series and brief review of the literature. *Ann Vasc Surg*. 2014;28:1935.e13-e16.

8. Dean SM. "Ski-jump" toenails—A phenotypic manifestation of primary lymphedema. *Vasc Med*. 2015;20(3):268-268.

9. Kalawat TC, Chittoria RK, Reddy PK, Suneetha B, Narayan R, Ravi P. Role of lymphoscintigraphy in diagnosis and management of patients with leg swelling of unclear etiology. *Indian J Nucl Med*. 2012;27(4):226-230. doi:10.4103/0972-3919.115392.

10. Rooke TW, Felty CL. Lymphedema: pathophysiology, classification, and evaluation. In: Gloviczki P, Forum AV, eds. *Handbook of Venous and Lymphatic Disorders: Guidelines of the American Venous Forum*. 4th ed. Boca Raton, FL: CRC Press; 2017:chap 61.

11. Paskett ED, Dean JA, Oliveri JM, Harrop JP. Cancer-related lymphedema risk factors, diagnosis, treatment, and impact: a review. *J Clin Oncol*. 2012;30(30):3726-3733.

12. McLafferty RB. The role of intravascular ultrasound in venous thromboembolism. *Semin Intervent Radiol*. 2012;29(1):10-15. doi:10.1055/s-0032-1302446.

13. Thaler HW, Pienaar S, Wirnsberger G, Roller-Wirnsberger RE. Bilateral leg edema in an older woman. *Z Gerontol Geriatr*. 2015;48(1):49-51.

14. Warren Peled A, Kappo EA. Lipedema: diagnostic and management challenges. *Int J Women's Health*. 2016;8:389-395. doi:10.2147/IJWH.S106227.

Steven Elias

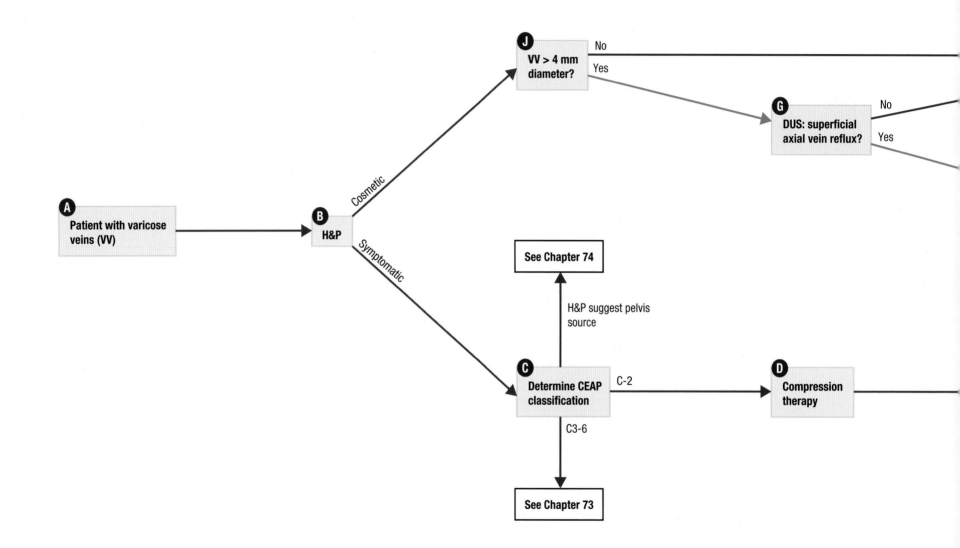

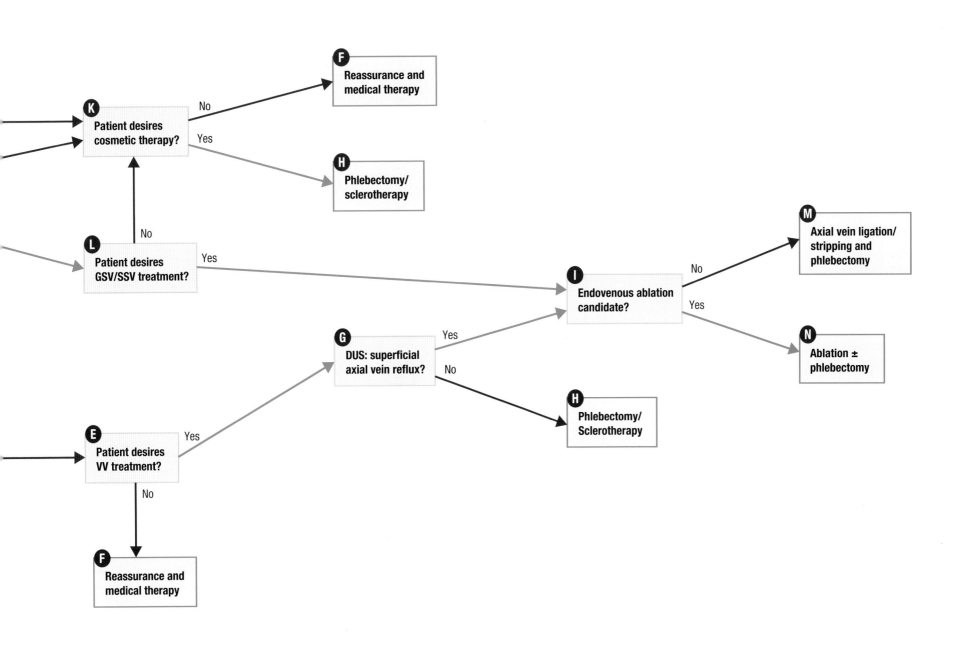

A Patient with varicose veins (VV)

VVs represent a common condition that is present in >40% of women and 25% of men >50 years of age.[1] Patients present with concerns about symptoms, cosmesis, complications, or future risks associated with VVs. Because VVs are not limb- or life-threatening, measurement of treatment success is improvement in quality of life. As such, it is important to gain an understanding of the patient's personal goals for treatment of their VVs. Some patients are only concerned about controlling symptoms such as pain or edema, whereas others are concerned about the appearance of the limb. The use of treatment decision algorithms must consider the patient's objectives to achieve the best possible results in each individual situation. Because VVs represent a chronic, often recurrent problem, it is important to incorporate education and health awareness into the treatment plan to encourage patients to make lifestyle changes that will limit their risk of recurrence.

B H&P

A detailed venous H&P is critical to identify whether patients have significant symptoms and whether these are likely due to venous disease. Patients may present with symptoms of diffuse leg ache, pain, or edema and may inaccurately ascribe these to their coexisting visible VVs. Differentiating symptoms caused by venous insufficiency from musculoskeletal conditions, neuropathy, arterial disease, and other potential sources is critical to successfully treating patients with VVs. Lower extremity symptoms typically caused by venous disease may be described by the acronym HASTI—heaviness, aching, swelling, throbbing, and itching, as well as tiredness or warmth. Most symptoms worsen as the day progresses and the leg is more dependent. They are exacerbated by prolonged standing and improved by walking, because the calf muscle pump ejects blood from the leg reducing venous HTN, unless the patient has deep venous outflow obstruction resulting in venous claudication.[2] Symptoms that occur with movement or when the patient is lying supine typically are unrelated to venous disease. Common nonvenous causes of symptoms in patients with visible VVs include sciatica, hip/knee joint degeneration, arthritis, plantar fasciitis, obesity, and lymphedema.

On physical examination, it is important to identify the size, location, and type of venous abnormality (VV, reticular vein, or spider vein). The leg should be examined for edema and skin changes, including the presence of hyperpigmentation, lipodermatosclerosis, atrophie blanche, and healed or open leg ulcers. Physical examination should also include the arterial system, because compression therapy for VVs can negatively impact patients with severe PAD.

In summary, the goal of the H&P is to determine the severity and distribution of the patient's symptoms and signs and to determine whether these are due to VVs. Identifying nonvenous conditions that may be responsible for the patient's symptoms is equally important. Finally, if patients primarily have cosmetic goals for treatment, determining these goals and whether they are realistic is necessary to achieve patient satisfaction after treatment.

C Determine CEAP classification

To standardize the reporting of venous disorders, the CEAP classification was developed to allow for uniform patient or populations comparisons. CEAP is divided into patient clinical presentation (C), etiology (E), anatomic distribution (A), and underlying pathophysiology (P). Using the clinical or C component of the CEAP classification is a useful way of categorizing the severity of vein disease and determining the best management pathway.[3] C1 patients have only spider veins and/or telangiectasias, which are typically only of cosmetic concern and may be treated with sclerotherapy. C2 patients, by definition, have VVs that can be either Cs (symptomatic) or Ca (asymptomatic). Patients with C3-C6 disease may have VVs; however, they lack venous drainage from the limb, which results in edema and skin changes, differentiating them from C2 patients. The treatment for patients with C3-C6 venous disease is considered medically necessary to prevent further tissue damage or progression to ulceration, whereas the treatment for C2 patients may be medically warranted if the patient has significant symptoms, typically pain or itching. This chapter focuses on the management of patients with C2 venous disease (VVs) only. C3-C6 venous disease treatment is discussed in Chapter 73. Pelvic congestion syndrome, a condition also associated with VVs, is discussed in Chapter 74.

D Compression therapy

Compression therapy, with medical grade graduated compression stockings, is recommended for most patients with VVs.[4] Compression stockings are effective in decreasing symptom severity in patients who have aching or heaviness in the legs and they are useful for controlling edema in patients with C3 venous disease. In C2 patients who do not have leg edema, patients may individualize therapy and use compression if their symptoms improve with the compression stockings. There is little clinical evidence to support the misconception that compression stockings prevent progression of disease.

Typically, these low-compression (20-30 mm Hg) stockings are well tolerated. Many insurance providers require that patients undergo treatment with compression stockings for a period of 3 to 6 months with venous disease and will only provide coverage for those whose symptoms do not improve.

E Patient desires VV treatment?

Patients should be educated about the natural history of VV regardless of whether treatment is provided. They should understand that VVs are a chronic hereditary condition that cannot be cured; VVs will tend to recur if intervention is performed, but that recurrence usually takes many years to occur. Patients are often concerned about the risk of DVT or other major complications and these issues should be discussed. Patients' goals for treatment should be determined and the clinician must ensure that these expectations are realistic for each individual depending on their disease severity, leg condition, and comorbidities. Given the same level of symptoms, some patients may prefer conservative medical management, whereas others will desire further evaluation leading to potential VV treatment.

F Reassurance and medical therapy

If patients do not desire interventional treatment for VV, they should be reassured that, in general, no major sequelae are likely to occur, and that intervention can be performed in the future if symptoms worsen. The condition will often gradually progress with the development of additional VV, and if symptoms start to affect their quality of life, patients are encouraged to return to consider interventional treatment. Compression therapy can improve symptoms but is unlikely to halt development of new VVs. As such, patients are encouraged to use them only for symptom relief.

G DUS: superficial axial vein reflux?

Key anatomic information concerning the source of venous insufficiency and VV etiology is provided by DUS examination of the limb.[3] A systematic search for venous reflux and obstruction is performed to identify the specific pathway of disease bringing high venous pressure to the offending VVs. Venous HTN can be caused by abnormal venous reflux or venous obstruction and both should be identified on venous DUS examination. The deep, superficial, and perforator systems should be examined to develop a map of all sources of venous insufficiency. Approximately 85% to 90% of patients with VVs are found to have disease in an underlying superficial axial source (typically the GSV, small saphenous vein [SSV]), or anterior accessory saphenous vein). In 10% to 15% of cases, however, VVs are found with no underlying axial vein reflux or obstruction. This is an important differentiation, because the presence of axial vein reflux contributing to VVs requires axial vein ablation, whereas isolated VVs are treated with local sclerotherapy or excision.

Key elements of the DUS examination needed for appropriate procedure planning and insurance authorization include the following:

1. Supine and upright position imaging
2. Evaluation of the deep and superficial venous systems
3. Size of superficial axial veins and VVs
4. Highest origin of reflux and lowest point of reflux in the axial veins
5. Source of reflux into visible VVs (which superficial axial vein?)

H Phlebectomy/sclerotherapy

In patients with visible VVs (symptomatic or asymptomatic), but no superficial, deep, or perforator vein incompetence, treatment can be performed using either phlebectomy or sclerotherapy. In general, smaller veins (4-5 mm) respond better to sclerotherapy than do larger veins (>5 mm); however, good results have been reported with phlebectomy for small veins and sclerotherapy for large veins by practitioners with expertize.[5] Sclerotherapy tends to have higher risk for skin pigmentation and/or matting, and requires multiple treatments, whereas phlebectomy involves incisions, some form of anesthesia, and a higher risk of nerve injury. Both options are viable and the decision is often made on the basis of physician and patient preference. Many vein specialists now place sclerosant in the veins before phlebectomy. This helps treat any missed veins and causes spasm in the veins after injection, thereby decreasing bleeding with subsequent phlebectomy.

ⓘ Endovenous ablation candidate?

The treatment of choice for incompetence of the GSV or SSV is currently endovenous ablation using a thermal or nonthermal approach.[6,7] In a randomized trial of 500 patients, Rasmussen et al. compared endovenous ablation and ultrasound-guided foam sclerotherapy (UGFS) with surgical stripping for patients with GSV reflux and symptomatic VVs. At 3 years, both endovenous ablation and surgical stripping had >90% rates of saphenous closure compared to 74% for UGFS (P < 0.01). Interestingly, the rate of recurrent VVs and quality-of-life scores were similar in all groups during follow-up. This trial found that all treatment modalities were efficacious in improving quality of life, but more GSV recanalization and more reoperations were seen after UGFS. Current reasons to perform open stripping and ligation would be for insurance noncoverage of endovenous ablation, multiple failed attempts at endovenous ablation with recanalization, or venous aneurysms, particularly at the saphenofemoral or saphenopopliteal junction. Thermal ablation methods are able to effectively close saphenous veins with diameters as large as 20 mm, so it is rare that the size of the saphenous vein alone limits the use of an endovenous approach. Hyperpigmentation of the skin may occur in patients with little subcutaneous tissue where the saphenous vein is close to the skin. For the best cosmetic result, particularly in fair skinned patients, stripping may be preferred over endovenous ablation in such cases.

ⓙ VV > 4 mm diameter?

When patients present with asymptomatic VVs of cosmetic concern, the size of the veins may determine whether a DUS examination is needed. Smaller (<5 mm) veins have a lower chance of superficial axial incompetence as a source; the incompetence of the superficial axial vein may, in fact, be secondary to the VVs that are draining into it and may cause it to become incompetent. In general, these patients do well with phlebectomy or sclerotherapy alone.[8] For patients with VVs > 4 mm diameter, DUS evaluation for axial reflux should be performed, because axial vein ablation may be needed for effective cosmetic treatment to reduce the risk of recurrence.

ⓚ Patient desires cosmetic therapy?

Patients seeking cosmetic treatment for asymptomatic VVs should be educated on what to realistically expect from the therapy in terms of what can and cannot be accomplished. They also need to understand that sclerotherapy will yield improvement but not perfection in most patients and that the full benefit takes at least 6 weeks and maybe as long as 6 months to achieve. The patient should also understand that multiple sessions are usually required to achieve successful results from sclerotherapy, depending on the number of VVs requiring treatment. Not every patient desiring cosmetic treatment will be appropriate for treatment for a multitude of reasons: elevated expectations, body habitus, skin type, advanced age, failed cosmetic treatment in the past, and inability to self-pay.

ⓛ Patient desires GSV/SSV treatment?

In the asymptomatic patient with cosmetic concerns about their VVs, the presence of significant superficial axial incompetence (ie, large volume of reflux, large axial vein diameter, and prolonged reflux) indicate that axial vein ablation may be beneficial. If the visible VVs are filled from a superficial axial incompetent vein that has significant reflux, the vein specialist can consider treating this axial vein primarily, with good cosmetic results. This is a very specific set of criteria and, in general, endovenous ablation is not performed for purely cosmetic VVs. When conducted in select, appropriate patients, however, it can minimize incisions, bleeding, pigmentation, and/or multiple sclerotherapy treatments. The decision about whether to pursue incompetent axial vein ablation in patients with asymptomatic VVs will depend on the severity of reflux and the patient's perspective of the magnitude of adding axial ablation to local VV treatment.

ⓜ Axial vein ligation/stripping and phlebectomy

If saphenous ligation and stripping is performed, it should be performed using an inversion pin technique with tumescent anesthesia. Inversion pin stripping invaginates the vein and leaves a tract only as large as the vein after removal, leading to less bleeding and less pain. The use of tumescent anesthesia allows for hydrodissection of the vein for ease of stripping and acts to tamponade the vein channel, thus decreasing bleeding and pain. Applying lessons learned from endovenous ablation, the branches at the junction need not be dissected. The vein only needs to be ligated and divided. Ideally, during this procedure, phlebectomy of large VVs should also be performed.

ⓝ Ablation ± phlebectomy

There are many choices currently available for endovenous ablation of the saphenous veins.[7,9] These can be divided into two categories: thermal tumescent (TT) and nonthermal nontumescent (NTNT). It is beyond the scope of this chapter to discuss when to use which

technique, but the references given have a full discussion regarding this.[10] TT methods include radiofrequency and laser-based saphenous ablation and require tumescent anesthesia. NTNT methods include mechanic-chemical ablation and ablation using cyanoacrylate glue and do not require tumescent anesthesia leading to a shorter procedure with potentially less patient discomfort. Harlock et al. performed a meta-analysis of NTNT versus TT therapies for patients with GSV insufficiency and VVs.[11] Their review indicated that these methods achieved similar rates of saphenous closure and improvement in quality of life, but intraprocedural pain scores were significantly lower for NTNT therapies.

Another decision required is whether phlebectomy of associated large varicosities should be performed at the time of endovenous ablation or be staged, typically 3 to 6 months after the ablation procedure. This is dependent on physician and patient preference. Long-term results are essentially equal in terms of quality-of-life improvement at 6 to 12 months. Simultaneous phlebectomy removes most of the visible VVs immediately, decreases future adjuvant procedures, prolongs recovery, but may require more extensive dissection than does the staged approach. Staged phlebectomy may not be needed in 50% patients after endovenous ablation, because the VVs decrease in size after eliminating the source of venous HTN. Monahan reported that in a series of patients with symptomatic VVs and GSV insufficiency treated with radiofrequency ablation alone, complete resolution occurred in 42% of above-knee VVs and 26% of below-knee VVs.[12] The majority of those that did not completely resolve decreased in size by an average of 35% after ablation. In many of these patients, only sclerotherapy was needed to subsequently eliminate the remaining bothersome VVs.

REFERENCES
1. Rabe E, Pannier F. Epidemiology of chronic venous disorders. In: Gloviczki P, ed. *Handbook of Venous and Lymphatic Disorders*. 4th ed. Boca Raton, FL: CRC Press; 2017.
2. National Institute for Health and Care Excellence. Varicose veins: diagnosis and management. NICE guidelines. Manchester, England: National Institute for Health and Care Excellence; 2013:25.
3. Gloviczki P, Comerota AJ, Dalsing MC, et al. The care of patients with varicose veins and associated chronic venous disease: clinical practice guidelines of the Society for Vascular Surgery and the American Venous Forum. *J Vasc Surg*. 2011;53:2S-48S.
4. Rabe E, Partsch H, Hafner J, et al. Indications for medical compression stockings in venous and lymphatic disorders: an evidence based consensus statement. *Phlebology*. 2018;33:163-184.
5. Einarsson E, Eklof B, Neglen P. Sclerotherapy or surgery as treatment for varicose veins: a prospective randomized study. *Phlebology*. 1993;8:22-26.

6. Rasmussen L, Lawaetz M, Serup J, et al. Randomized clinical trial comparing endovenous laser ablation, radiofrequency ablation, foam sclerotherapy and surgical stripping for great saphenous varicose veins with three-year follow-up. *J Vasc Surg Venous Lymphat Disord*. 2013;1:349-356.

7. Elias S. Evaluating options to treat superficial vein disease in 2018. *Endovasc Today*. 2018;17:36-40.

8. Pittaluga P, Chastenet S, Rea B, Barbe R. Midterm results of the surgical treatment of varices by phlebectomy with the conservation of a refluxing saphenous vein. *J Vasc Surg*. 2009;50:107-118.

9. Kheirelseid EAH, Crowe G, Sehgal R, et al. Systematic review and meta-analysis of randomized controlled trials evaluating long-term outcomes of endovenous management of lower extremity varicose veins. *J Vasc Surg Venous Lymphat Disord*. 2018;6:256-270.

10. Kugler N, Brown KR. An update on the currently available nonthermal ablative options in the management of superficial venous disease. *J Vasc Surg Venous Lymphat Disord*. 2017;5:422-429.

11. Harlock JA, Elias F, Qadura M, Dubois L. Meta-analysis of non-tumescent based versus tumescent-based endovenous therapies for patients with great saphenous insufficiency and varicose veins. *J Vasc Surg Venous Lymphat Disord*. 2018;6:779-788.

12. Monahan DL. Can phlebectomy be deferred in the treatment of varicose veins? *J Vasc Surg*. 2005;42:1145-1149.

Katharine L. McGinigle • William A. Marston

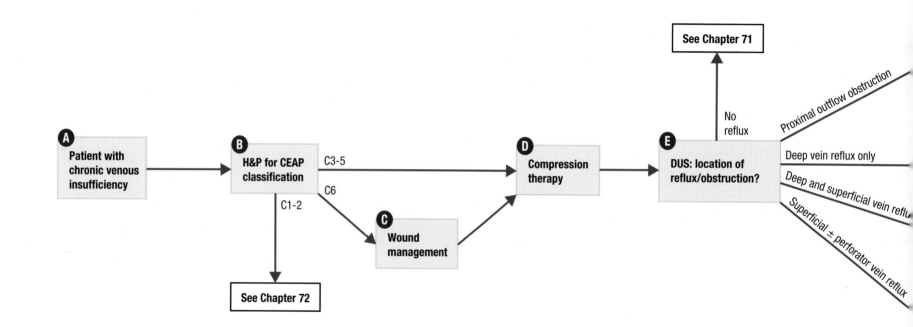

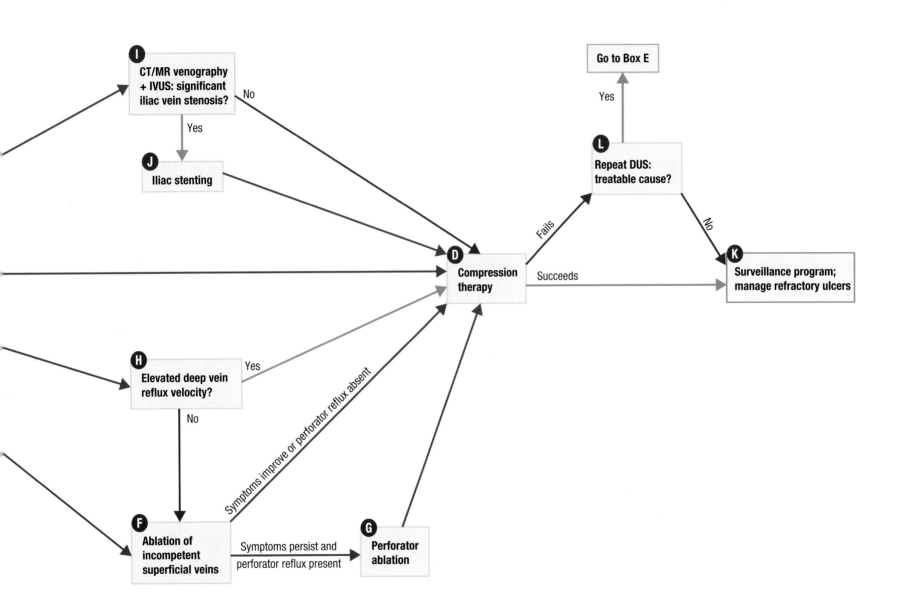

A Patient with chronic venous insufficiency

The prevalence and economic impact of chronic venous insufficiency (CVI) continue to increase in the United States. Prevalence of chronic venous disease varies widely by geographic location and severity of disease. Varicose veins are more prevalent in Western countries and are more common in patients who are female, obese, or have an occupation that requires prolonged standing.[1] CVI tends to be more equally distributed between males and females, with up to 8% of adults having trophic changes and 1% of adults having a venous ulcer.[1,2] Treatment of CVI can consume a significant amount of resources and it is important to have an established best practice algorithm that can maximize the efficiency of care to reduce resource utilization and the cost of care.

B H&P for CEAP classification

A thorough H&P is critical in determining risk factors and treatment of CVI. The patient's medical history should be investigated for prior history of arterial or venous thromboembolism, prior interventional therapies for venous disease, and any history of hypercoagulability. A family history for these events may suggest an increased possibility of hypercoagulability in the patient.

CVI is described by the CEAP classification, which provides guidance for further evaluation and treatment. CEAP stands for clinical, etiologic (congenital, primary, secondary), anatomy (superficial, deep, perforator), and pathophysiology (reflux, obstruction).[3] Physical examination is important to assign the correct CEAP clinical classification (see subsequent table) for the patient. In addition, the patient's symptoms can be scored using a system like the Venous Clinical Severity Score (VCSS). This score correlates with the severity of symptoms and should be calculated both pre- and posttreatment to determine treatment outcome.[2]

The physical examination should also evaluate for venous abnormalities, such as truncal varicose veins suggestive of iliocaval venous obstruction. Specific characteristics of the affected limb should be assessed, including the presence and severity of edema, any skin changes such as hyperpigmentation or lipodermatosclerosis, or ulceration. Venous ulcers usually present initially on the medial malleolar portion of the lower leg, but may become more extensive. They are associated with hyperpigmentation. It is also important to examine the lower extremity arterial system as well, given the coexistence of arterial insufficiency in 10% to 20% of patients with venous disease. If strong pedal pulses are not confirmed, noninvasive vascular laboratory studies should be performed to assess potential coexistent arterial disease.

This chapter discusses management of patients with C3-6 disease. C2 disease is discussed in Chapter 72. C1 (cosmetic) disease is not considered in this book.

CEAP Clinical Score and Associated Physical Examination Findings	
CEAP Clinical Score	**Physical Examination Findings**
C0	No visible or palpable varicose veins
C1	Telangiectasias
C2A	Asymptomatic varicose veins
C2B	Symptomatic varicose veins
C3	Lower extremity edema due to varicose veins
C4	Lipodermatosclerosis
C5	Healed venous ulcer
C6	Active venous ulcer

C Wound management

The most severe clinical classification, C6 disease, describes patients with active venous ulcers. As with all patients having suspected CVI, compression therapy is a critical fundamental component of ulcer therapy,[2-4] and has received a grade 1A recommendation to increase the healing rate of venous ulcers in the Society for Vascular Surgery/American Venous Forum venous ulcer guideline document.[4,5] (For details of compression therapy, see D.) In addition to compression therapy, patients with active venous ulcers require aggressive, multidisciplinary workup to identify all potential factors limiting the normal healing of the wound, including venous HTN, bacterial overgrowth, inflammatory mediator upregulation, and tissue necrosis. This assessment allows generation of a treatment plan to addresses modifiable risk factors, extent of vascular (venous and arterial) involvement, and wound management.[6-8] The quality of the wound bed is critical to the success of any wound healing plan; debridement, control of exudate, and control of bacterial colonization are recommended.[9] Topical dressings such as alginates and foams will maintain a moist environment while managing exudate. Although compression therapy is required for closure of venous ulcers, the ESCHAR trial demonstrated that the addition of an appropriate venous intervention to treat CVI to compression therapy can reduce the risk of ulcer recurrence to 12% from 28% at 1 year.[10] If neither venous nor arterial disease is suspected in a patient with a lower extremity wound, then atypical etiologies including malignancy, infection, vasculitis, and others must be considered. Punch biopsies in the wound bed and at the wound margin can help differentiate these diagnoses but are not needed for typical venous ulcers.[11]

D Compression therapy

C3-C5 disease with lower extremity edema, skin hyperpigmentation, lipodermatosclerosis, or healed venous ulcers is treated with medical grade graduated compression therapy with custom fit stockings of at least 20 to 30 mm Hg.[12] The rationale for compression is to assist the calf muscle pump in returning venous blood to the heart in the face of lower extremity venous HTN. For this reason, knee-high stockings are usually sufficient; however, patients with significant swelling and varicosities behind the knee or in the thigh may be more comfortable wearing thigh-high stockings. Compression alone can successfully ameliorate symptoms and prevent the progression of venous disease. The most commonly used compression is a graded pressure elastic stocking, which a patient can don and doff daily. Inelastic compression wraps or Velcro-based compression systems (Circaids) may also be used and in theory provide higher support for the calf muscle pump when ambulating, but a lower resting pressure, which may increase the safety of this method of compression. Single or multilayer bandaging systems can also be utilized and are favored when patients have active severe edema that prevents sizing for an appropriate compression stocking. These bandages can achieve rapid reduction in severe swelling so that patients can be fit for a standard elastic compression stocking for long-term treatment. In some cases, patients experience relief of symptoms from consistent use of compression stockings and this is a reasonable treatment method if the patient is engaged and willing to apply the compression daily. For those who do not experience relief with compression or who cannot or will not apply compression daily, additional evaluation and potential intervention is indicated.

Compression therapy is the mainstay of treatment for patients with venous insufficiency, regardless of source.[12] In addition, compression therapy mitigates postoperative symptoms for patients undergoing ablative or stenting procedures.

E DUS: location of reflux/obstruction?

Patients with C3-C6 CVI not responsive to compression therapy need appropriate venous evaluation to determine whether the pathophysiology of their leg symptoms results from venous obstruction or reflux. The recommended test is a venous DUS. This study is relatively inexpensive, noninvasive, and allows for determination of the anatomic location of venous reflux or obstruction. A complete DUS evaluation for venous obstruction includes compression B-mode ultrasound and color Doppler insonation from the common femoral vein to the posterior tibial and peroneal veins at the ankle as well as the great and small saphenous veins.[13] Compression maneuvers and examination of flow patterns with augmentation identify the presence of either acute or chronic venous obstruction. Venous reflux is due to venous valvular incompetence that allows for reversal of flow and resultant venous HTN in the lower extremity. Importantly, venous reflux can occur in the presence or absence of venous obstruction. For an accurate reflux assessment, the patient must be upright with the leg externally rotated and minimally weight-bearing.[13] Presence of bidirectional flow with retrograde flow present for

>0.5 seconds on DUS indicates clinically significant venous reflux. The same criteria are used to assess the competence of perforator veins connecting the deep and superficial venous systems.[13] If no reflux or obstruction is detected, other causes of leg swelling should be evaluated (see Chapter 71).

F Ablation of incompetent superficial veins

If DUS reveals superficial (with or without perforator) venous reflux without deep venous insufficiency in patients with C3-C6 CVI not responsive to compression therapy, intervention to ablate the refluxing superficial vein is indicated. Interventional treatment options for superficial vein reflux include injection of foam sclerosant agents, radiofrequency ablation, endovenous laser ablation, and venous ligation and stripping.

Vemulapalli et al. published a systematic review of 57 studies representing over 100,000 patients comparing compression alone to endovascular procedures, endovascular versus open therapies, and different endovascular procedures.[14] Owing to heterogeneity and high risk of bias, meta-analysis was only possible for studies comparing stripping with radiofrequency and laser ablation and revealed that all techniques have similar short-term bleeding risk, long-term symptom scores, and 1- to 2-year reflux recurrence rates.[14] Endovenous ablation is thus considered first-line therapy because it is less invasive and causes less initial pain.[15] Historically, foam sclerotherapy has had higher recanalization rates,[14,16,17] but this area is evolving to include other sclerosing agents and pharmacomechanical techniques including cyanoacrylate glue,[18,19] which may have more comparable results. Additional details regarding the choice of ablation therapy type can be found in Chapter 72.

Patients with superficial reflux may also have perforator vein reflux. According to Mendes et al., patients with superficial and perforator vein incompetence and a normal deep venous system experience significant improvement in hemodynamic parameters and clinical symptom score after superficial ablation alone.[20] In fact, 71% of previously incompetent perforator veins were either absent or competent on postoperative venous DUS. For this reason, many venous specialists prefer to treat superficial disease first in patients with combined superficial and perforator incompetence and only treat the incompetent perforator later if the patient has ongoing symptoms and a persistent incompetent perforator. But some venous specialists prefer to treat both superficial and perforator incompetence at the same time to eliminate all sources of venous HTN, particularly if the incompetent perforator is particularly large.

G Perforator ablation

After ablation of incompetent superficial veins, if symptoms persist or recur, patients should be restudied with venous DUS to evaluate for reflux in the perforating veins. A perforator vein is judged incompetent if it is larger than 3 mm in diameter and demonstrates reverse or bidirectional DUS flow for >0.5 seconds with compression and release.[13,21] Perforating veins can be surgically treated in a way similar to that for the superficial veins, that is, with radiofrequency or endovenous laser ablative techniques or with foam sclerotherapy.[12] Surgical ligation may be performed, but these techniques have generally been abandoned because of the high risk of wound-healing complications associated with the poor condition of the skin in the area of the incompetent perforator.

H Elevated deep vein reflux velocity?

Patients presenting with CVI are frequently found to have concomitant deep and superficial venous valvular insufficiency.[22] In these patients, it may be difficult to determine how much the superficial system contributes to the patient's symptoms and whether they will experience improvement if superficial ablation is performed. Measuring the maximal reflux velocity in common femoral, femoral, and popliteal veins (from the reflux tracings obtained using DUS) provides predictive data for treatment. If the maximal deep vein reflux velocities are lower than approximately 10 cm/s, one can proceed with ablation of the superficial veins and expect clinical improvement in symptoms in most patients.[22] Patients with deep vein reflux velocities >10 cm/s are more likely to have persistent symptoms even after ablation of the superficial system. Although some improvement may occur, these patients typically require long-term compression therapy for their deep reflux anyway, and should be informed that they may experience continued symptoms despite successful superficial ablation.

I CT/MR venography + IVUS: significant iliac vein stenosis?

Patients with findings of proximal venous outflow obstruction on DUS (lack of phasicity and respiratory variation in the common femoral vein) should undergo further imaging to evaluate the iliac veins.[13,23] Obstruction of the iliofemoral venous system can be primary from external compression (May–Thurner syndrome or mass effect from pelvic pathology) or secondary due to postthrombotic changes. Common femoral vein findings suggestive of iliac vein obstruction on DUS are highly specific for outflow obstruction, but not very sensitive. If there remains a high suspicion for iliac vein outflow obstruction despite a normal common femoral waveform, direct DUS of the iliac veins can sometimes provide good visualization, or CT or MR venography can be done. All of these methods can provide specific information to determine whether there is obstruction of the iliac veins or IVC (for discussion of IVC obstruction, see Chapter 80). If there are positive findings on these, or if the diagnosis is still uncertain, IVUS is recommended.[24] IVUS is considered to be the gold standard for obstruction of the iliac veins and IVC because it is the most accurate for defining the extent and severity of venous involvement.[25,26] Venography is typically performed at the time of IVUS but is less accurate for diagnosing venous stenosis.

J Iliac stenting

For patients with CVI and associated iliac venous stenosis, iliac vein stent placement is recommended. The stents restore luminal cross-sectional area, improve venous return, and relieve venous HTN in the affected limb.[12] Technical success and long-term patency are more likely with single or multiple short-segment stenoses rather than long-segment occlusions.[25] There are no specifically designed stents for the venous system, but large (12-24 mm) diameter Wallstents are commonly used. IVUS should be used to determine the length of abnormal vein requiring stenting. Stent diameter should be determined using the IVUS to measure the area of the normal vein proximal and distal to the obstruction.[26] For appropriate stent selection, a simple calculation of the area of each stent should be performed and then matched to the area of the normal vein.

K Surveillance program; manage refractory ulcers

After successful treatment of CVI, either using conservative or endovascular/surgical management, a surveillance program is needed to determine the need and duration of compression therapy. This determination is made depending on symptoms, clinical findings, and progression of disease. The VCSS can be helpful in monitoring these factors over time.[12]

If venous ulcerations persist (4-6 weeks with local wound care/compression therapy) despite successful treatment of the superficial system, and in the absence of proximal outflow obstruction or DVT, more advanced strategies for wound healing are required. Punch biopsies should be performed to investigate for squamous cell carcinoma of the skin, referred to as a Marjolin ulcer. This entails multiple 3- to 6-mm punch biopsies taken at the base and margin of the wound. For patients with active ulcers and signs and symptoms of infection, microbiologic cultures should be obtained to direct appropriate antibiotic therapy.[9]

Modifiable risk factors are important to evaluate and address when treating patients with venous ulcers, recognizing that location, size, and duration of the ulcer are the most important predictors of healing.[27] Many biologic dressings that may improve wound closure rates are available. The American Venous Forum and Society for Vascular Surgery clinical practice guidelines suggest using a cultured allogeneic bilayer skin replacement (with both epidermal and dermal layers) in addition to compression therapy for venous ulcers that have not improved with 4 to 6 weeks of standard wound management.[9] Autogenous split-thickness skin grafting is another option to promote more rapid wound closure, but the evidence on short- and long-term outcomes is sparse, and, as such, this is only recommended for wounds with >25 cm^2 surface area.[9,28]

🅛 Repeat DUS: treatable cause?

If symptoms persist after endovascular/surgical treatment for CVI, a repeat venous DUS should be performed to search for an anatomic cause for persistent or recurrent symptoms. The differential diagnosis includes missed symptomatic perforator reflux, endovenous heat-induced thrombosis and resulting DVT, post-thrombotic syndrome causing deep vein reflux, and/or recurrent proximal outflow obstruction. In addition, GSV recanalization post ablation, reported in 12% of patients at 1 year, may be the contributing cause of recurrent symptoms.[17] If residual reflux or obstruction is detected, additional evaluation and potential treatment is required (see E).

If no further pathology is identified and no ulcers are present, symptom management with leg elevation, compression therapy, and horse chestnut seed extract are recommended. On the basis of a Cochrane Review of 17 studies, horse chestnut seed extract taken as capsules twice daily, reduces leg pain, edema, and pruritis.[29]

Acknowledgment

We thank and acknowledge Duke Pfitzinger, DO for his assistance in drafting this chapter.

REFERENCES

1. Beebe-Dimmer JL, Pfeifer JR, Engle JS, Schottenfeld D. The epidemiology of chronic venous insufficiency and varicose veins. *Ann Epidemiol*. 2005;15(3):175-184.
2. Criqui MH, Jamosmos M, Fronek A, et al. Chronic venous disease in an ethnically diverse population: the San Diego Population Study. *Am J Epidemiol*. 2003;158(5):448-456.
3. Eklof B, Rutherford RB, Bergan JJ, et al. Revision of the CEAP classification for chronic venous disorders: consensus statement. *J Vasc Surg*. 2004;40(6):1248-1252.
4. Korn P, Patel ST, Heller JA, et al. Why insurers should reimburse for compression stockings in patients with chronic venous stasis. *J Vasc Surg*. 2002;35(5):950-957.
5. Mayberry JC, Moneta GL, Taylor LM Jr, Porter JM. Fifteen-year results of ambulatory compression therapy for chronic venous ulcers. *Surgery*. 1991;109(5):575-581.
6. O'Donnell TF Jr, Passman MA, Marston WA, et al. Management of venous leg ulcers: clinical practice guidelines of the Society for Vascular Surgery (R) and the American Venous Forum. *J Vasc Surg*. 2014;60(2 suppl):3S-59S.
7. Wittens CH. Manuscripts from the European Venous Course 2016. *Phlebology*. 2016;31(1 suppl):3-4.
8. Alavi A, Sibbald RG, Phillips TJ, et al. What's new: management of venous leg ulcers: treating venous leg ulcers. *J Am Acad Dermatol*. 2016;74(4):643-664; quiz 665-666.
9. O'Donnell TF Jr, Passman MA. Clinical practice guidelines of the Society for Vascular Surgery (SVS) and the American Venous Forum (AVF)—Management of venous leg ulcers. Introduction. *J Vasc Surg*. 2014;60(2 suppl):1S-2S.
10. Barwell JR, Davies CE, Deacon J, et al. Comparison of surgery and compression with compression alone in chronic venous ulceration (ESCHAR study): randomised controlled trial. *Lancet*. 2004;363(9424):1854-1859.
11. Alavi A, Sibbald RG, Phillips TJ, et al. What's new: Management of venous leg ulcers: approach to venous leg ulcers. *J Am Acad Dermatol*. 2016;74(4):627-640; quiz 641-642.
12. Gloviczki P, Dalsing MC. *Handbook of Venous Disorders: Guidelines of the American Venous Forum*. 3rd ed. London, England: Hodder Arnold; 2009.
13. Neumyer MM. Ultrasound diagnosis of venous disease. In: Pellerito JS, Polak JF, eds. *Introduction to Vascular Ultrasonogrphy*. 7th ed. Philadelphia, PA: Elsevier; 2019.
14. Vemulapalli S, Parikh K, Coeytaux R, et al. Systematic review and meta-analysis of endovascular and surgical revascularization for patients with chronic lower extremity venous insufficiency and varicose veins. *Am Heart J*. 2018;196:131-143.
15. Gloviczki P, Comerota AJ, Dalsing MC, et al. The care of patients with varicose veins and associated chronic venous diseases: clinical practice guidelines of the Society for Vascular Surgery and the American Venous Forum. *J Vasc Surg*. 2011;53(5 suppl):2S-48S.
16. O'Hare JL, Earnshaw JJ. Randomised clinical trial of foam sclerotherapy for patients with a venous leg ulcer. *Eur J Vasc Endovasc Surg*. 2010;39(4):495-499.
17. Biemans AA, Kockaert M, Akkersdijk GP, et al. Comparing endovenous laser ablation, foam sclerotherapy, and conventional surgery for great saphenous varicose veins. *J Vasc Surg*. 2013;58(3):727-734.e1.
18. Yang GK, Parapini M, Gagnon J, Chen JC. Comparison of cyanoacrylate embolization and radiofrequency ablation for the treatment of varicose veins. *Phlebology*. 2019;34(4):278-283.
19. Radak D, Djukic N, Neskovic M. Cyanoacrylate embolisation: a novelty in the field of varicose veins surgery. *Ann Vasc Surg*. 2019;55:285-291.
20. Mendes RR, Marston WA, Farber MA, Keagy BA. Treatment of superficial and perforator venous incompetence without deep venous insufficiency: is routine perforator ligation necessary? *J Vasc Surg*. 2003;38(5):891-895.
21. Sandri JL, Barros FS, Pontes S, Jacques C, Salles-Cunha SX. Diameter-reflux relationship in perforating veins of patients with varicose veins. *J Vasc Surg*. 1999;30(5):867-874.
22. Marston WA, Brabham VW, Mendes R, Berndt D, Weiner M, Keagy B. The importance of deep venous reflux velocity as a determinant of outcome in patients with combined superficial and deep venous reflux treated with endovenous saphenous ablation. *J Vasc Surg*. 2008;48(2):400-405; discussion 405-406.
23. Needleman L, Cronan JJ, Lilly MP, et al. Ultrasound for lower extremity deep venous thrombosis: multidisciplinary recommendations from the society of radiologists in ultrasound consensus conference. *Circulation*. 2018;137(14):1505-1515.
24. Neglen P, Raju S. Intravascular ultrasound scan evaluation of the obstructed vein. *J Vasc Surg*. 2002;35(4):694-700.
25. Crowner J, Marston W, Almeida J, McLafferty R, Passman M. Classification of anatomic involvement of the iliocaval venous outflow tract and its relationship to outcomes after iliocaval venous stenting. *J Vasc Surg Venous Lymphat Disord*. 2014;2(3):241-245.
26. Gagne PJ, Tahara RW, Fastabend CP, et al. Venography versus intravascular ultrasound for diagnosing and treating iliofemoral vein obstruction. *J Vasc Surg Venous Lymphat Disord*. 2017;5(5):678-687.
27. Marston WA, Ennis WJ, Lantis JC 2nd, et al. Baseline factors affecting closure of venous leg ulcers. *J Vasc Surg Venous Lymphat Disord*. 2017;5(6):829-835.e1.
28. Jones JE, Nelson EA, Al-Hity A. Skin grafting for venous leg ulcers. *Cochrane Database Syst Rev*. 2013;(1):CD001737.
29. Pittler MH, Ernst E. Horse chestnut seed extract for chronic venous insufficiency. *Cochrane Database Syst Rev*. 2006;(1):CD003230.

Erica E. Nelson • Robert B. McLafferty

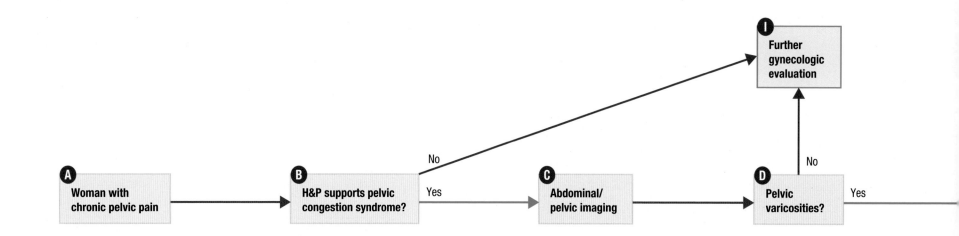

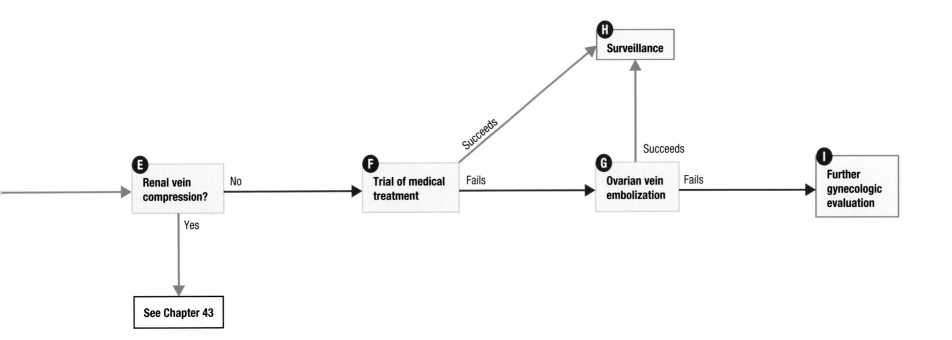

A Woman with chronic pelvic pain

Chronic pelvic pain (CPP) afflicts approximately 15% of women between the ages of 18 and 50.[1-3] Etiology as well as the derived symptoms can vary widely. Pelvic congestion syndrome (PCS) can cause CPP from pelvic varicosities, most often emanating from large incompetent left and/or right ovarian veins. Symptoms from PCS typically are gravity dependent and consist of left and/or right lower quadrant aching, throbbing, and/or stinging from prolonged standing or sitting. Dyspareunia, postcoital pelvic pain, dysmenorrhea, and abnormal uterine bleeding can also occur with PCS. Unlike other causes of CPP, symptoms are typically relieved when supine.

B H&P supports pelvic congestion syndrome?

A gynecologic history and physical examination that includes an awareness of PCS remains paramount to making the diagnosis. In women with no identifiable cause of CPP and complete evaluation, more than 80% will be diagnosed with PCS.[4] Risk for PCS rises with increasing number of pregnancies, and early signs can include pelvic pain during pregnancy and/or the early postpartum period. Dyspareunia and especially postcoital pelvic pain can occur with PCS. Retrograde venous flow and congestion of the perimetrial and myometrial veins can cause edema of the uterine wall, leading to dysmenorrhea and/or abnormal uterine bleeding. Although these symptoms may indicate other gynecologic diagnoses, the sine qua non of PCS is left and/or right lower quadrant aching, throbbing, and/or stinging from prolonged standing or sitting that is relieved, all or in part, by being supine. Other symptoms indicative of PCS may include worsening of this pain before menstruation as well as left flank or leg pain/swelling with prolonged standing. Flank pain could indicate an associated diagnosis of left renal vein compression syndrome (see Chapter 43), whereas leg pain/swelling, an associated diagnosis of symptomatic varicose veins. The absence of these symptoms does not preclude the presence of pelvic varicosities, particularly if the symptoms are confounded by other diagnoses or the patient is asymptomatic. Symptoms more specific to other causes of CPP are beyond the scope of this chapter and require further gynecologic evaluation.

Most often in PCS, routine gynecologic physical examination is normal. However, nondescript, mild ovarian tenderness may be noted on bimanual examination. More important findings that lead to a high suspicion of PCS include the presence of varicosities on the vulva, perineum, inguinal region, and gluteal folds. Specific findings such as a pelvic mass or significant focal tenderness require further gynecologic evaluation.

C Abdominal/pelvic imaging

In most women, transvaginal ultrasound is performed for the assessment of CPP.[5] Pelvic varicosities can be observed in patients with PCS as multiple dilated vascular/tubular structures around the uterus and ovaries. Color-flow imaging should be performed for detection of arterial and/or venous flow. The presence of dilated tortuous periovarian vessels >4 mm; sluggish flow of <3 cm/s and a dilated arcuate vein in the myometrium are highly suggestive of the presence of pelvic varicosities. Other maneuvers that may be necessary in visualizing pelvic varicosities include insonation while in the upright position during a Valsalva maneuver. The absence of the abovementioned finding does not rule out the presence of pelvic varicosities and PCS. Associated symptoms in other parts of the abdomen may warrant further imaging such as abdominal ultrasound or CT.

Depending on the presentation of CPP and the results from transvaginal ultrasound, multiplanar imaging may be indicated. MRI provides excellent contrast and resolution of the pelvic anatomy and vasculature. The ovarian veins and pelvic varices can appear as abnormally dilated vascular structures. The dilated veins, typically varying from 4 to 10 mm in diameter, will appear hypointense on T1-weighted images and hyperintense on T2. With contrast enhancement, timing should focus on the venous phase. The MRI should also evaluate for left renal vein compression/obstruction between the aorta and the SMA (see Chapter 43). Compression of this vein can lead to higher venous pressures in the left ovarian vein that could result in pelvic varicosities. In addition, MRI may reveal other causes of CPP diagnoses stemming from adnexal, uterine, urologic, GI, or musculoskeletal etiologies. CT is generally a poor imaging test for the pelvic organs, but if ordered, requires a prior pregnancy test in women of childbearing years.

D Pelvic varicosities?

If no pelvic varicosities are noted on imaging, then further gynecologic evaluation such as diagnostic laparoscopy is warranted to evaluate for any missed, subtle, or equivocal findings that could cause CPP. Depending on the evaluation algorithm used for CPP by the gynecologist, pelvic varicosities can be initially discovered by diagnostic laparoscopy.

Most commonly, PCS stems from pelvic varicosities that involve tributaries to the left ovarian vein. The left ovarian vein becomes dilated and can range from 4 to 10 mm in diameter. The pampiniform venous plexus that drains into the ovarian vein is equally enlarged and can predominate in varying degrees around the uterus. The myometrium and perimetrium of the uterus have venous lakes that drain into the pampiniform plexus as well as into the uterine veins. Left and right uterine veins drain into tributary veins, leading to each corresponding internal iliac vein. The right ovarian vein usually drains directly into the IVC, inferior to the right renal vein. Understanding the anatomy and the probable source of venous incompetence remains pivotal to a targeted appropriate treatment.[6]

E Renal vein compression?

If pelvic varicosities are confirmed, imaging should also evaluate potential left renal vein compression/obstruction between the aorta and the SMA. If left renal vein compression is identified, then renal vein compression syndrome should be evaluated and potentially treated (see Chapter 43).

F Trial of medical treatment

There are several important principles to be adhered to when considering medical treatment of PCS. Unfortunately, medical treatments of PCS have had mixed results and long-term studies are lacking. Ovarian suppression using combination hormonal contraception or progestin therapy alone has been the mainstay medical treatment.[7,8] Trials with gonadotrophin-releasing hormone (GrNH) agonists can be diagnostic as well as therapeutic. Side effects of estrogen hormonal therapy include headache, nausea, mood changes, decreased libido, and potentially harmful elevated blood pressure and VTE. Progestin therapy can cause weight gain and GrNH agonists cause menopausal symptoms. Other treatments used with little to no objective study have included biofeedback, intravenous dihydroergotamine, and horse chestnut seed extract.[9-11]

Given the myriad of treatment options and potential side effects, it is important for gynecologists to both prescribe and monitor treatment. In patients with few comorbidities and a firm diagnosis of PCS, medical treatment does not have to be trialed before offering endovascular treatment. That said, if such patients are not interested in a procedural solution, they still should be offered a trial of medical treatment. In patients with moderate to high comorbidities, and/or another confounding gynecologic diagnosis, medical treatment is usually warranted before recommending a procedural solution. Lastly, in those patients with equivocal symptoms and minimal to no imaging evidence of PCS, a period of observation or medical treatment may be both therapeutic and diagnostic. Partnership between the gynecologist and vascular specialist provides the best treatment options for such patients.

G Ovarian vein embolization

An incompetent left ovarian vein is the primary cause in the large majority of women with PCS. Although there has been no standardization of the endovascular treatment for ablating ovarian veins, virtually all procedures have involved the use of varying lengths and diameters of coils.[12] Other adjuvant embolization techniques include sclerotsants, gel foam, and glue.[12-14] To provide a better fulcrum for more stable catheter access, percutaneous access should be obtained through the right common femoral vein. After selective venography and catheterization of the left renal vein followed by the left ovarian vein, stable wire access well into the distal ovarian vein is desired to pass a longer hydrophilic sheath or guiding catheter to the midportion of the ovarian vein. This working catheter will allow passage of smaller straight or slightly curved catheters over a wire to the distal portion of the ovarian vein.

The patient should then be placed in approximately 20° to 30° reverse Trendelenburg to maximize blood pooling in the pelvic varicosities. Power injection of contrast should be avoided because the injection pressures and jets from the catheters can rupture pelvic varicosities. In addition to a well-controlled hand injection of diluted contrast for initial pelvic venography, close attention should be paid to the amount of contrast injected and where it travels. When considering the use of sclerotherapy for large pelvic varicosities leading into the ovarian vein, pooling of contrast should be observed over a period of 3 to 5 minutes. Often, it lingers longer. If washout of contrast is relatively quick, sclerotherapy may be contraindicated because of perceived risk of drainage into the portal circulation. Sodium tetradecyl sulfate at a 3% concentration can be mixed 50:50 with contrast and injection into the varicosities should not be more than what provided adequate visualization of them on initial venography—typically 5 to 10 mL. Following this, coils with attached synthetic fibers should be tightly deployed in the ovarian vein starting at the pelvic brim to 2 to 3 cm inferior to the left renal vein. Rarely, the right ovarian vein may need to be embolized and not uncommonly, right internal jugular vein access is necessary because of the acute inferior angle off the inferior vena cava. In cases where symptomatology of PCS is in combination with symptomatic varicose veins of the vulva, inguinal areas and/or gluteal folds, attention should be brought to venography and potential embolization of abnormal tributaries of the right and/or left internal iliac veins using similar techniques. The success rate of ovarian vein embolization in patients with PCS who undergo this treatment has been outstanding. A review of 866 women undergoing embolization demonstrated a 99.8% initial technical success (vein occlusion).[15] Numerous other studies have shown complete or significant improvement in PCS symptoms over the short in >90% of women.[16-18] Although more long-term studies are needed, one has estimated the recurrence rate of reflux to be 13% at 5 years.[15]

❶ Surveillance

In the first 24 hours following successful sclerotherapy of pelvic varicosities and embolization of the ovarian vein, the patient may experience a wide range of pain. Most women will have mild to moderate discomfort from the inflammatory response of sclerotherapy and thrombosis of the varicosities. Most often, these symptoms are well controlled with anti-inflammatory medication or, rarely, with short-term narcotics. Within 1 to 2 weeks, acute symptoms should resolve, and most patients will have significant to complete resolution of symptoms.[16] The vascular specialist should follow up with the patient in 4 to 6 weeks. Assuming improvement, no further imaging is necessary and subsequent follow-up can be with the gynecologist, as would be the case for women managed with medical treatment,

❶ Further gynecologic evaluation

If during the H&P, the diagnosis points to another etiology, the gynecologist will pursue a different course of recommendations regarding observation, further imaging, consultation, and/or treatment. In the setting of PCS, ovarian vein embolization rarely fails, either from a technical inability or recurrence. The infrequent failure requires further evaluation by the gynecologist in conversation with the patient and the vascular specialist. Options include open ligation of the ovarian vein via a retroperitoneal approach or hysterectomy ± bilateral salpingo-oophorectomy. Historically, ovarian vein ligation has been described from just a few centers[19] and with the current endovascular tools, techniques, and outcomes, this procedure is virtually extinct. Outcomes from hysterectomy ± removal of the adnexa for PCS may be more mixed. Published results are limited and one small study reported only 67% of woman pain free after the procedure.[20] PCS typically affects women in the childbearing years, and hysterectomy, especially with oophorectomy, should be avoided unless for other gynecologic indications, or if symptoms continue to be severe when all other treatments have failed.

REFERENCES

1. Twiddy H, Bradshaw A, Chawla R, Johnson S, Lane N. Female chronic pelvic pain: the journey to diagnosis and beyond. *Pain Manag.* 2017;7(3):155-159.
2. Carey ET, Till SR, As-Sanie S. Pharmacologic management of chronic pelvic pain in women. *Drugs.* 2017;77(3):285-301.
3. Engeler DS, Baranowski AP, Dinis-Oliverira P, et al. The 2013 EAU guidelines on chronic pelvic pain: is management of chronic pelvic pain a habit, a philosophy, or a science? 10 years of development. *Eur Urol.* 2013;64(3):431-439.
4. White JV, Schwartz LB, Ryjewski C. Management of pelvic congestion syndrome and perineal varicosities. In: Gloviczki P, ed. *Handbook of Venous and Lymphatic Disorders: Guidelines of the American Venous Forum.* 4th ed. Boca Raton, FL: CRC Press; 2017:685-696.
5. Whitely MS, Dos Santos SJ, Harrison CC, Holdstock JM, Lopez AJ. Transvaginal duplex ultrasonography appears to be the gold standard investigation for the haemodynamic evaluation of pelvic venous reflux in the ovarian and internal iliac veins in woman. *Phlebology.* 2015;30(10):706-713.
6. Beckett D, Dos Santos SJ, Dabb EB, Shiangoli I, Price BA, Whiteley MS. Anatomical abnormalities of the pelvic venous system and their implications for endovascular management of pelvic venous reflux. *Phlebology.* 2018;33(8):567-574.
7. Gavrilov SG, Turischeva OO. Conservative treatment of pelvic congestion syndrome: indications and opportunities. *Curr Med Res Opin.* 2017;33(6):1099-1103.
8. Tu FF, Hahn D, Steege JF. Pelvic congestion syndrome—associated pelvic pain: a systematic review of diagnosis and management. *Obstet Gynecol Surv.* 2010;65(5):332-340.
9. Newman DK. Pelvic disorders in women: chronic pelvic pain and vulvodynia. *Ostomy Wound Manage.* 2000;46(12):48-54.
10. Reginald PW, Beard RW, Kooner JS, et al. Intravenous dihydroergotamine to relieve pelvic congestion with pain in young women. *Lancet.* 1987;2(8555):351-353.
11. Suter A, Bommer S, Rechner J. Treatment of patients with venous insufficiency with fresh plant horse chestnut seed extract: a review of 5 clinical studies. *Adv Ther.* 2006;23(1):179-190.
12. Daniels JP, Champaneria R, Shah L, Gupta JK, Birch J, Moss JG. Effectiveness of embolization or sclerotherapy of pelvic veins for reducing chronic pelvic pain: a systematic review. *J Vasc Interv Radiol.* 2016;27(10):1478-1486.
13. Cordts PR, Eclavea A, Buckley PJ, DeMaioribus CA, Cockerill ML, Yeager TD. Pelvic congestion syndrome: early clinical results after transcatheter ovarian vein embolization. *J Vasc Surg.* 1998;28(5):862-868.
14. Marcelin C, Izaaryene J, Castelli M, et al. Embolization of the ovarian vein for pelvic congestion syndrome with ethylene vinyl alcohol copolymer (Onyx®). *Diagn Interv Imaging.* 2017;98(12):843-848.
15. Hansari V, Abbas A, Bhandari S, Caress AL, Seif M, McCollum CN. Trans-venous occlusion of incompetent pelvic veins for chronic pelvic pain in women: a systematic review. *Eur J Obstet Gynecol Reprod Biol.* 2015;185:156-163.
16. Kim HS, Malhotra AD, Rowe PC, Lee JM, Venbrux AC, et al. Embolotherapy for pelvic venous congestion syndrome: long-term results. *J Vasc Interv Radiol.* 2006;17(2, pt 1):289-297.
17. Hocguelet A, Le Bras Y, Balian E, et al. Evaluation of the efficiency of endovascular treatment of pelvic congestion syndrome. *Diagn Interv Imaging.* 2014;95(3):301-306.
18. Nasser F, Cavalcante RN, Affonso BB, Messina ML, Carnevale FC, de Gregorio MA. Safety, efficacy, and prognostic factors in endovascular treatment of pelvic congestion syndrome. *In J Gynaecol Obstet.* 2014;125(1):65-68.
19. Richardson GD. Management of pelvic venous congestion and perineal varicosities. In: Gloviczki P, ed. *Handbook of Venous Disorders: Guidelines of the American Venous Forum.* 3rd ed. London, England: Edward Arnold Ltd; 2009:617-626.
20. Beard RW, Kennedy RG, Ganger KF, et al. Bilateral oophorectomy and hysterectomy in the treatment of intractable pelvic pain associated with pelvic congestion syndrome. *Br J Obstet Gynaecol.* 1991;98:988-992.

Audra A. Duncan

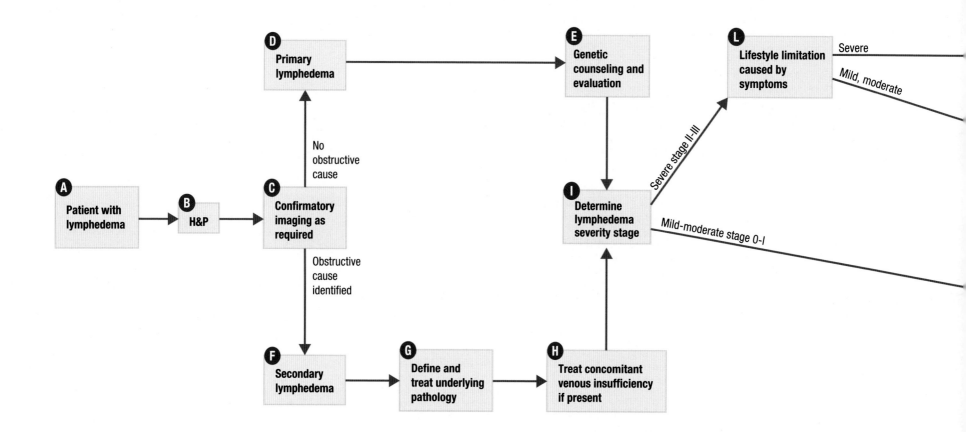

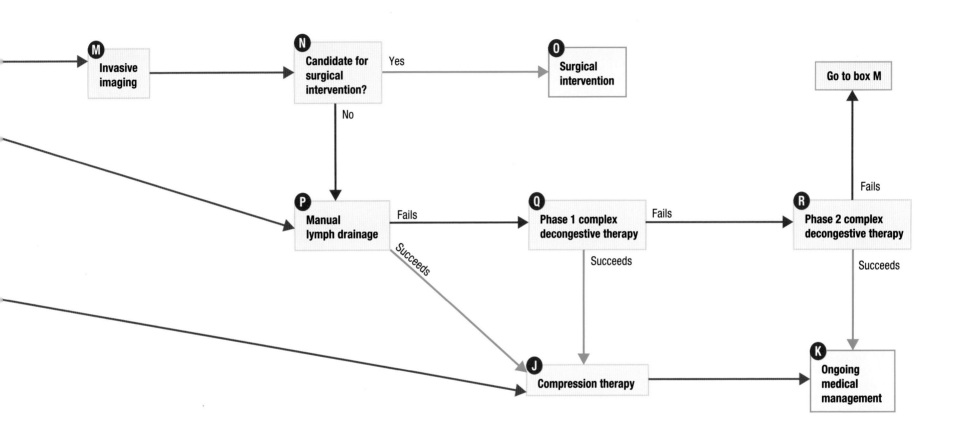

A   Patient with lymphedema

Frequently, patients with unilateral or bilateral edema can be considered to have lymphedema based solely on H&P. Confirmatory imaging or laboratory studies may support the diagnosis, but in many cases are not required. Primary lymphedema is a hereditary disease that results in agenesis, hypoplasia, or obstruction of distal lymphatic vessels, or obstruction of proximal lymphatics or lymph nodes. It is rare, with an incidence of 1.2 cases per 100,000 persons <20 years of age, with a 3.5:1 female preponderance and a 3:1 likelihood of unilateral (vs. bilateral) involvement.[1] Secondary, or acquired, lymphedema can occur much more frequently depending on the cause. For example, upper extremity lymphedema after breast cancer treated with axillary dissection occurs in up to 40% of patients.[2] Primary lymphedema occurs most frequently in the lower extremities, whereas secondary lymphedema can result from destruction of lymphatics and lymph nodes in the upper or lower extremity, depending on the cause.

B   H&P

Age of onset of primary lower extremity lymphedema can often aid in the diagnosis. Congenital lymphedema is diagnosed at birth or within the first year, whereas lymphedema praecox (~90% of primary lymphedema) typically occurs at puberty through 30 years of age. Lymphedema tarda (~10% primary lymphedema) is usually diagnosed at age 35 years and older. Family history may help elucidate familial causes, such as Milroy disease (see E), and syndromes, many of which are autosomal dominant.[3] Alternatively, a history suggestive of acquired lymphedema, which may involve the upper extremity, would include exposure to parasites, history of cancer, previous surgery, trauma or burns, pregnancy, bacterial and fungal infections, dermatitis, and rheumatoid arthritis.[4]

Physical findings include pitting edema in early stages progressing to liposclerosis in later stages. Edema tends to be cylindrical and includes the toes and fingers, with a "buffalo hump" over the forefoot or dorsum of the hand. Ulceration, brown pigmentation, or lipodermatosclerosis is rare, differentiating lymphedema from venous disease. The Stemmer sign is pathognomonic for lymphedema and occurs when the skin of the interdigital webs cannot be tented because of loss of elasticity.

C   Confirmatory imaging as required

Imaging may be used when H&P does not provide a definitive diagnosis. Frequently, imaging is needed solely to exclude venous disease.

CT or MRI can differentiate between lymphedema, which typically has a honeycomb edema appearance, compared to other causes of edema. The location of the edema will differ as well, with lymphedema occurring in the epifascial layer, venous edema in the epifascial and subfascial, and lipedema demonstrating fat without edema fluid.

Lymphoscintigraphy can be performed to confirm the diagnosis in cases where H&P alone is not adequate, or in cases when overlapping symptoms occur such as with combined venous incompetence. Lymphoscintigraphy requires injection of a radiolabeled tracer into the interdigital space of the affected foot or hand for observation of the activity pattern. Normal limbs will demonstrate lymph channels and transport of tracer to the inguinal nodes by 60 minutes. In patients with primary lymphedema, such channels may be absent or incompetent. In lymphangiectasia, the tracer will fill abnormal, dilated lymph channels without delay of transport.[5] In secondary lymphedema, where the lymph nodes have been destroyed by infection or blocked by other causes such as tumor, the lymphatic channels, but not the lymph nodes, may fill. Further management depends on whether an obstructive cause (secondary lymphedema) is identified versus nonobstructive primary lymphedema is present.

D   Primary lymphedema

Primary lymphedema is usually unilateral and more common in women. Primary lymphedema is commonly categorized by age of presentation (see B). It can also be categorized by the underlying morphology (ie, obliteration of lymphatics vs. hyperplasia of lymphatics), or by anatomy (distal vs. proximal lymphatic obstruction).

E   Genetic counseling and evaluation

Most patients with primary lymphedema develop the condition spontaneously with no preexisting family or personal history. Milroy disease[6] (also known as hereditary lymphedema or Nonne–Milroy–Meige syndrome) has been mapped to an abnormality of the *FLT4* gene, which codes for VEGFR-3 in the development of the lymphatic system. The defect results in lymphatic hypoplasia. Lymphedema distichiasis is associated with an abnormality of the *FOXC2* gene, and hypotrichosis-lymphedema-telangiectasis linked to the *SOX18* gene. Genetic mapping allows early identification of patients with possible hereditary lymphedema who can then be counseled and guided in risk factor modification.[7-9] Even patients with nonhereditary primary lymphedema should be counseled about risk factor control including the use of compression stockings or garments, good skin hygiene, and limb elevation, to decrease the possibility of lymphedema developing in the contralateral limb.

F   Secondary lymphedema

The most common worldwide cause of secondary lymphedema is infection. It is typically caused by parasites *Wuchereria bancrofti*, *Brugia malayi*, and *B. timori*, which are spread by mosquito vectors and lead to filiriasis. The larvae transmitted by the mosquito migrate to the lymph vessels and nodes, develop into microfilariae-producing adults, and destroy the lymphatic system in the process. These adult nematodes can live in the host for years.

In developed countries, secondary lymphedema is most commonly caused by cancers, surgical interruption of lymphatics or resection of lymph nodes, radiation, and, less frequently, recurrent skin infections such as cellulitis.[10,11]

G   Define and treat underlying pathology

Depending on the underlying etiology of secondary lymphedema, treatment of the pathology does not necessarily change the course of lymphedema and its associated complications. For example, although it is important to manage bancroftian filariasis with antifilarial medication, once the lymph nodes are destroyed by the adult worms, the process cannot be reversed. It is important to recognize infection as a cause to institute the correct treatment. Other secondary etiologies such as postsurgical causes, can be defined by clinical history, and are best treated with prevention. For example, improvements in axillary sentinel node detection have markedly decreased the need for extensive axillary node dissection with resultant reduction in upper extremity lymphedema.

H   Treat concomitant venous insufficiency if present

In many cases of secondary lymphedema, concomitant venous insufficiency (or phlebolymphedema) may be present, exacerbating symptoms. The edema noted in pure venous disease is low-protein, whereas primary or secondary lymphedema occurs with accumulation of interstitial, protein-rich fluid. When venous insufficiency occurs, however, venous HTN may overload the capacity of the lymphatics to drain from the limb, and mixed lymphedema and venous edema result. Diagnosis requires venous imaging (ie, DUS of deep and superficial veins for competency and patency), CT venography, or contrast venography, and lymphoscintigraphy if necessary. Although treatment of venous insufficiency (see Chapter 73) may subsequently improve lymphatic drainage, it is often necessary to institute nonsurgical treatment of lymphedema concomitantly.[12]

I   Determine lymphedema severity stage

Latent stage (stage 0) is defined by the absence of clinical edema, but with fluid and fibrosis around the lymphatics. Stage I lymphedema is defined by pitting edema that resolves with elevation, and no fibrosis is present. Stage II is defined as nonpitting edema that does not resolve with elevation and is accompanied by moderate to severe subcutaneous fibrosis. Stage III lymphedema has irreversible edema due to repeated episodes of fibrosis, inflammation, and infection (referred to as elephantiasis because of its appearance).[13]

J   Compression therapy

The mainstay of treatment for primary lymphedema is compression stockings and garments of graduated pressure ranging from 30 to 40 mm Hg proximally, 40 to 50 mm Hg in the midportion, and 50 to 60 mm Hg in the distal portion of the limb. These garments are typically measured and custom-fitted. It may be difficult or impossible for patients with diabetes, neuropathy, or arthritis of the lower limbs or hands to use higher pressure stockings, and lower pressure 20 to 30 mm Hg or 30 to 40 mm Hg may be more practical for this subset of patients to facilitate daily use.

Compression stockings for the leg and garments for the arm may be constructed of spandex, nylon, latex, cotton, and/or silk, and the resulting material may alter the patients' preference of garment type. Patients are therefore advised to try on several stocking/garment types before committing to a specific one; ideally, the stocking/garment should be comfortable enough for daily use. Insurance may or may not cover these products, making treatment compliance difficult, especially because the stockings/garments need to be worn daily and replaced several times each year. Most surgical supply stores offer a range of sizes to allow good fit without the expense of custom-fittings. In addition to the stockings, patients may need to purchase supplies to facilitate donning the stocking such as a metal frame and/or rubber gloves. Initial use of the stockings/garments should be witnessed by the therapist to assure the patient is capable of donning and doffing, and that the fit is adequate for the condition. Often, patients with severe edema will also need manual lymph drainage (MLD; see Q) or phase 1 and 2 complex decongestive therapy (CDT; see R) before being able to wear standard compression.

Ⓚ Ongoing medical management

Patients at risk for primary and secondary lymphedema can institute daily measures to minimize symptoms. These include the following:

1. For lower limbs, exercise to improve calf muscle pump function to increase lymphatic limb flow
2. Range-of-motion and stretching exercises
3. Elevation of the limb above the level of the heart both during the day and by elevating the limb at night in bed
4. Maintaining a healthy weight with a balanced diet with adequate fluid and low sodium
5. Avoiding pressure to the affected limb (such as blood pressure cuffs, tight clothing, and heavy shoulder bags).

One of the most critical aspects of risk factor modification is skin hygiene. However, maintaining daily skin hygiene can be difficult in patients with morbid obesity, poor social support, or other comorbidities that limit the ability to wash regularly.[14] The affected limb should be washed at least daily with soap and water and treated immediately with a hypoallergenic, fragrance-free emollient cream to prevent skin cracks. Loose-fitting cotton or wicking clothing should be worn, and the skin protected from trauma such as direct injury or sunburn. Any cuts, scrapes, or puncture wounds should be promptly cleaned. Patients with chronic lymphedema may develop intertriginous fungal infections that can primarily be treated or prevented with topical clotrimazole cream (1%) or miconazole nitrate lotion or cream (2%). In rare cases, oral antifungal agents may be needed to treat recalcitrant infections.

The use of pharmacologic therapy is generally ineffective for treating lymphedema. Diuretics are often tried early in the development of lymphedema, but do not provide durable relief. There is some evidence that benzopyrones (flavonoids) may stimulate tissue macrophages and proteolysis, reduce intercellular protein concentration, and promote tissue softening and remodeling, but clinical efficacy is not yet established.[15] Intralymphatic steroid injections and autologous lymphocyte injections have been described, but their efficacy remains unproved.[16,17]

Ⓛ Lifestyle limitation caused by symptoms

Depending on the stage of disease, limitations can range from minimal (ie, well managed with compression) to devastating (home bound with immobility). Unfortunately, many cases of severe lymphedema result in loss of work and poor social and financial status, which limits the ability to obtain health care resources such as manual lymphatic drainage (MLD), compression garments, or aid with hygiene, thereby exacerbating the lymphedema and associated skin infections.

Ⓜ Invasive imaging

Contrast lymphangiography is primarily used for surgical planning of lymphatic reconstruction, such as a lymphovenous anastomosis. Lipid-soluble, iodine-based contrast is injected into lymphatics before imaging.[18] Because the study can be painful for the patient, and potentially exacerbate symptoms, it is rarely performed. Therefore, few interventionalists are experienced in performing the technique. As such, this imaging is typically only performed at high-volume tertiary centers. If a main channel lymphatic is identified, this may potentially be used as the conduit of a lymphovenous anastomosis, whereas if diffuse small lymphatics are identified, lymphatic grafting may be required.

Ⓝ Candidate for surgical intervention?

Excisional or physiologic procedures to increase lymphatic transit from the limb have been used to treat lymphedema. Although they have been reported to be used in up to 5% to 15% of patients with lymphedema, more recent literature shows a much lower utilization of these procedures. In general, indications for intervention include (1) gross enlargement of a limb that is not responsive to conservative therapy and that interferes with activities of daily living or (2) recurrent skin infections. Before consideration of resection or lymphatic bypass, decongestive therapy needs to be prescribed so as to optimize/stabilize limb edema.

Ⓞ Surgical intervention

Options for surgical treatment include either subcutaneous tissue resection or reconstruction (autologous lymphatic grafting or lymphovenous anastomosis).[19,20] Surgery should only be considered if thorough medical therapy has been followed for >6 months and has failed. Waiting too long to intervene, however, can result in fibrosis of tissues, and irreversibility of symptoms despite surgery. Lymphatic grafting is performed by harvesting one to four lymph vessels from the thigh and performing lympholymphatic anastomoses.[19] Lymphatic grafts can be harvested from the patient's thigh as a transposition and one end remains attached to the inguinal lymph nodes. Using an operating microscope, one to four lymph vessels are anastomosed to the affected leg lymph vessels using 10-0 absorbable suture. Lymphovenous anastomoses are performed by suturing groin lymphatics to the great saphenous vein, also using fine suture under the operating microscope.[20] Subcutaneous resection techniques that eliminate the space where lymphedema accumulates have previously been performed via large open incisions, although more recently the use of liposuction has been described. Abnormal skin is resected concomitantly and may require skin grafting.

Ⓟ Manual lymph drainage

The technique of MLD is designed to redirect lymph and interstitial proteins to functioning lymphatic territories. Proximal congestion in the trunk, groin, buttock, or axilla is treated first, and then distal to proximal massage is performed to provide gentle skin distraction to stimulate the contractility of lymph-collecting vessels. MLD is unique compared to other types of massage in that it targets the skin with gentle, superficial pressure to stimulate the lymph vessels to contract and improve lymph flow. A trained MLD therapist performs this massage in sequential steps by dividing the body into treatment territories. Typically, the trunk is divided into six areas and the territory adjacent to the affected limb is treated first to prepare it to accept incoming lymph. Next, MLD is used to gradually treat the limb from the most distal aspect first. The treatment is repeated, working from proximal to distal but applying massage from distal to proximal to encourage lymph flow from abnormal beds into functional sites.[21] Although MLD is typically used for extremities, other body sites such as face or breast can be treated similarly if affected.

Ⓠ Phase 1 complex decongestive therapy

CDT phase 1 includes elevation, MLD, an exercise regimen, skin care, and multilayered low-stretch wrapping.[22] Elevation of the limb to 30° to 45° is typically recommended, although routine compliance is more important than is the absolute elevation. Elevation alone is often the first line of treatment for early stage I lymphedema that may still be reversible but is also a critical component of CDT. If reduction in limb size is achieved through elevation, the reduction must be maintained with a compression system, because elevation alone does not provide long-term benefit in patients with severe lymphedema. MLD is then performed to redirect lymph and interstitial proteins to functioning lymphatic territories. For compression during phase 1 CDT, low-stretch elastic wrapping techniques that are comfortable for the patient at rest are used. In addition to the low-stretch elastic, foam padding may be added under the wrap for comfort. In phase 1 CDT, the wraps are worn 24 hours each day except during MLD and bathing.

Ⓡ Phase 2 complex decongestive therapy

Phase 2 is home-based maintenance therapy with daytime pressure garments, night wrapping, self-administered MLD, and continued exercise and skin care.[22] Home-based phase 2 CDT is planned once maximal gain from phase 1 is achieved, typically after 2 to 6 weeks. Education is the prime goal before phase 2 can begin. A referral to a local therapist is given, if available, along with options for long-term management. Return appointments are typically at 3, 6, and 12 months, every 6 months for 3 years, and then annually thereafter if the patient is stable.

The patient converts from using low-stretch wraps day and night to applying pressure stockings/garments only during the day in phase 2. Because compliance in wearing these stockings/garments is critical to maintain the improvement achieved in phase 1 CDT, the patient must be comfortable donning the stockings/garments and wearing it all day.

As an alternative to CDT, some have recommended the use of intermittent pneumatic compression. In several early publications, long-term maintenance of edema reduction was maintained in 90% of 49 patients using pneumatic compression and absolute reduction in ankle girths of 4.6 cm was achieved.[23] However, a poor response was noted in 80% of patients who had chronic lymphedema for >10 years. Bergan et al. in 1998 randomized 35 patients to three groups: (1) unicompartment pneumatic compression pump (50 mm Hg), (2) three-compartment pump (50 mm Hg in each cell), and (3) multicompartment gradient pressure pump (10 cells ranging in pressure from 80 mm Hg distally to 30 mm Hg proximally).[24] Group 3 achieved a markedly improved reduction in limb volume, indicating that if pneumatic compression is used, a multicompartmental device is superior. The risks of pneumatic compression compared to CDT include genital or truncal edema, as well as the potential formation of fibrosis adjacent to the proximal aspect of the pump.[25] Although most authors agree that pneumatic compression alone is not superior to CDT, there is no consensus on the role of intermittent pneumatic compression as an adjunct to CDT phase 1 or 2.

REFERENCES

1. Rockson SG. Diagnosis and management of lymphatic vascular disease. *J Am Coll Cardiol*. 2008;52:799-806.
2. Ribeiro Pereira ACP, Koifman RJ, Bergmann A. Incidence and risk factors of lymphedema after breast cancer treatment: 10 years of follow-up. *Breast*. 2017;36:67-73.
3. Kinmoth JB, Taylor GW, Tracy GD, Marsh JD. Primary lymphedema: clinical and lymphangiographic studies of a series of 107 patients in which the lower limbs were affected. *Br J Surg*. 1957;45(189):1-9.
4. Rockson SG. Lymphedema. *Am J Med*. 2001;110:288-295.
5. Gloviczki P, Calcano D, Schirger A, et al. Noninvasive evaluation of the swollen extremity: experience with 190 lymphoscintigraphic examinations. *J Vasc Surg*. 1989;9:683-689.
6. Milroy WF. An undescribed variety of hereditary edema. *N Y Med J*. 1892;56:505-508.
7. Spiegel R, Ghalamkarpour A, Daniel-Spiegel E, Vikkula M, Shalev SA. Wide clinical spectrum in a family with hereditary lymphedema type I due to a novel missense mutation in VEGFR3. *J Human Gene*. 2006;51(10):846-850.
8. Sutkowska E, Gil J, Stembalska A, Hill-Bator A, Szuba A. Novel mutation in the FOXC2 gene in three generations of a family with lymphoedema-distichiasis syndrome. *Gene*. 2012;498(1):96-99.
9. Kartopawiro J, Bower NI, Karnezis T, et al. Arap3 is dysregulated in a mouse model of hypotrichosis-lymphedema-telangiectasia and regulates lymphatic vascular development. *Hum Mol Genet*. 2014;23(5):1286-1297.
10. Hoerauf A. Control of filarial infections: not the beginning of the end, but more research is needed. *Curr Opin Infect Dis*. 2003;16:403-410.
11. Bockarie MJ. Mass treatment to eliminate filariasis in Papua New Guinea. *N Engl J Med*. 2002;347:1841-1848.
12. Raju S, Owen S Jr, Neglen P. Reversal of abnormal lymphoscintigraphy after placement of venous stents for correction of associated venous obstruction. *J Vasc Surg*. 2001;34:779-784.
13. Casley-Smith JR, Foldi M, Ryan TJ, et al. Lymphedema: summary of the 10th International Congress of Lymphology Working Group discussions and recommendations, Adelaide, Australia, August 10-17, 1985. *Lymphology*. 1985;18:175.
14. Scheinfeld NS. Obesity and dermatology. *Clin Dermatol*. 2004;22:303-309.
15. Casley-Smith JR. The pathophysiology of lymphedema and the action of benzo-pyrones in reducing it. *Lymphology*. 1988;21:190-194.
16. Fyfe NC. Intralymphatic steroid therapy for lymphoedema: preliminary studies. *Lymphology*. 1982;15:23-28.
17. Katoh I. Intraarterial lymphocytes injection for treatment of lymphedema. *Jpn J Surg*. 1984;14:331-334.
18. Kinmoth JB. *The Lymphatics; Diseases, Lymphography and Surgery*. London, England: Edward Arnold; 1972.
19. Baumeister RGH, Fink U, Tatsch K, Frick A. Microsurgical lymphatic grafting: first demonstration of patent grafts by indirect lymphography and long term follow-up studies. *Lymphology*. 1994;27(suppl):787.
20. Gloviczki P, Fisher J, Hollier LH, Pairolero PC, Schirger A, Wahner HW. Microsurgical lymphovenous anastomosis for treatment of lymphedema: a critical review. *J Vasc Surg*. 1988;7:647-652.
21. Williams AF. A randomized controlled crossover study of manual lymphatic drainage therapy in women with breast cancer-related lymphoedema. *Eur J Cancer Care (Engl)*. 2002;11:254-261.
22. Lymphology Association of North America. Applications for the LANA Exam and Recertication. http://www.clt-lana.org/
23. Pappas CJ. Long-term results of compression treatment for lymphedema. *J Vasc Surg*. 1992;16:555-562.
24. Bergan JJ. Lymphedema: a comparison of compression pumps in the treatment of lymphedema. *Vasc Surg*. 1998;32:455-462.
25. Mayrovitz HN. Interface pressures produced by two different types of lymphedema therapy devices. *Phys Ther*. 2007;87:1379-1388.

Daniel F. Geersen • Cynthia Shortell

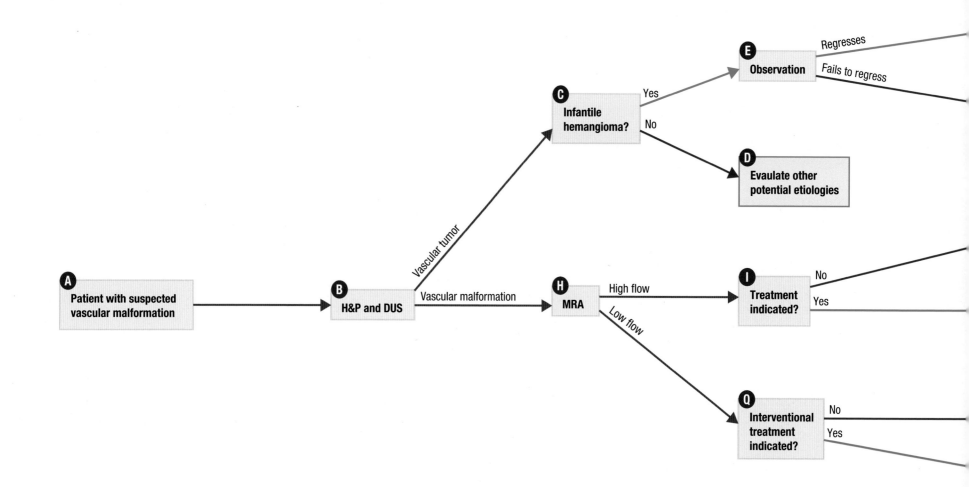

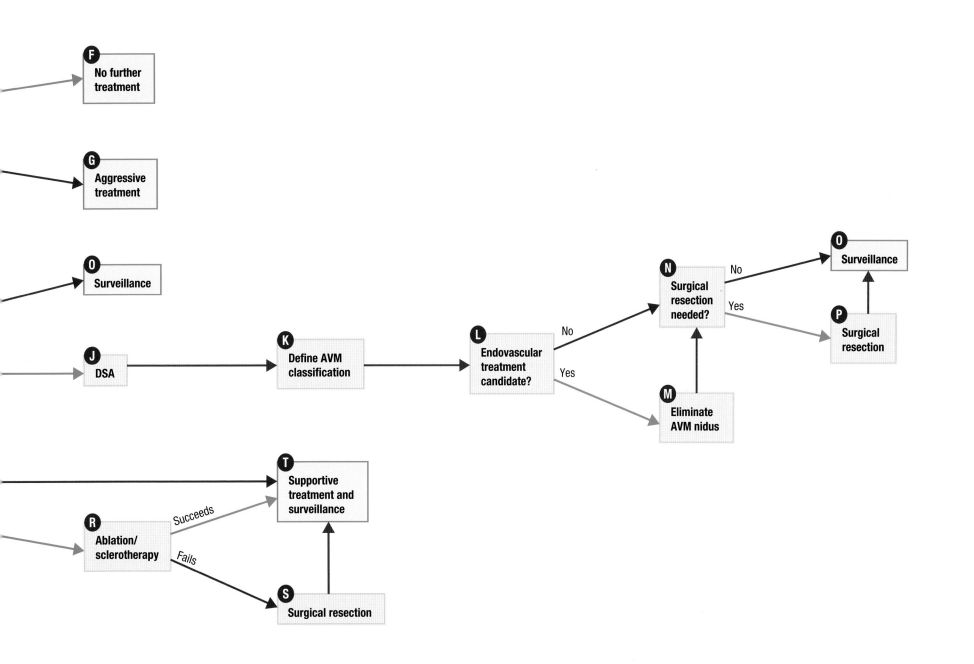

A Patient with suspected vascular malformation

Vascular anomalies remain both diagnostic and treatment challenges to treating physicians because they are uncommon, often not well understood, and create great concern and anxiety for patients and their families. The terminology used to describe and classify vascular anomalies is essential for proper diagnosis and treatment. The 2018 classification system established by the International Society for the Study of Vascular Anomalies (ISSVA) is now a widely accepted system used to categorize vascular anomalies into two types: (1) vascular malformations (VMs) and (2) vasoproliferative or vascular tumors such as hemangioma.[1]

VMs are categorized into four categories: (1) simple, (2) combined, (3) of major named vessels, and (4) associated with other anomalies.

- Simple VMs include slow flow (capillary malformations [CMs], lymphatic malformations [LMs], and venous malformations) and fast flow (arteriovenous malformations and arteriovenous fistula).
- Combined VMs encompass capillary-venous, capillary-lymphatic, capillary-arteriovenous, lymphatic-venous, capillary-lymphatic-venous, capillary-lymphatic-arteriovenous, capillary-venous-arteriovenous, and capillary-lymphatic-venous-arteriovenous malformations.
- VMs of major named vessels include "channel type" or "truncal" and affect lymphatics, veins, and arteries. They include anomalies of vessel origin, course, number, length, diameter (aplasia, hypoplasia, stenosis, ectasia/aneurysm), valves, communication (AVF), or persistence of an embryonal vessel. Finally,
- VM associated with other anomalies include Klippel-Trenaunay syndrome (KTS), Parkes Weber syndrome (PWS), Servelle-Martorell syndrome, Sturge-Weber syndrome, Limb CM with congenital nonprogressive limb overgrowth, Maffucci syndrome, macrocephaly without CM, microcephaly without CM, CLOVES syndrome (congenital lipomatous overgrowth, VMs, epidermal nevi, and scoliosis/skeletal/spinal anomalies), Proteus syndrome, Bannayan-Riley-Ruvalcaba syndrome, and CLAPO syndrome (CM of the lower lip, LM of the face and neck, asymmetry, and partial/generalized overgrowth).[1,2]

The distinction between vascular tumors and VM is based on histopathologic assessment of increased cell turnover. Unlike vascular tumors, VMs comprise abnormally formed channels lined by endothelial cells and do not have abnormal cellular proliferation. They are congenital, often go unnoticed at birth, grow proportionally with the individual, and never regress. Vascular tumors, formerly classified as hemangiomas, are true neoplasms with pathologic and abnormal cell proliferation.[3,4]

B H&P and DUS

Vascular tumors can often be differentiated from VM of childhood based on time of presentation, physical appearance, and rate of growth and/or involution. VMs are differentiated among themselves based on arterial/venous flow (low vs. high) and complexity (simple vs. combined vs. associated other anomalies). VMs commonly encountered by vascular surgeons are described below.

Vascular Tumors

Infantile hemangioma (IH), a benign tumor of the endothelium, is the most common neoplasm of infancy. Between 30% and 50% are visible at birth as a pale spot, ecchymotic area, or telangiectatic stain, although the median age at appearance is 2 weeks after birth. IH affects 5% of white infants, is rare in dark-skinned individuals, is more frequent in premature infants, and is two to three times more common among females than males.[5] Most IHs are single (80%) and involve the head and neck (60%), trunk (25%), or extremity (15%). IHs have a unique but classic growth pattern. During the first 9 months of the child's life, IH rapidly proliferates (proliferating phase), with 80% of tumor growth achieved in the first 3 months.[6] The tumor appears red if it involves only the superficial dermis and bluish-purplish in color when it occupies the deep dermis. After 9 months of age, the tumor enters the involuting phase with characteristic shrinkage of size and fading of the bright color of the tumor. The tumor becomes less tense and the skin pales at the center of the lesion. Involution is complete in most children by 3.5 years of age.[6] On physical examination, the lesions range from bright red to dark purple, typically located on the face, neck, or trunk, and are spongy and blanch with pressure. They typically are not painful unless they are the rare tumor that presses against other vital structures such as the orbit, airway, or visceral organs.

The diagnosis of IH can generally be made based on their classic growth pattern. Less than 10% require imaging for definitive diagnosis. DUS is the first-line confirmatory study and will demonstrate a well-circumscribed hypervascular mass. Low-resistance waveforms are seen with associated significant venous drainage. MRI should be obtained if these findings are not seen on DUS.

Vascular Malformations

VMs are primarily classified based on their flow rate, because this is the major determinant of treatment: slow flow (CMs, LMs, or venous malformations) and fast flow (arteriovenous malformation and arteriovenous fistula). These lesions can also have combined components, such as a mixed lymphaticovenous malformation, or be associated with other anomalies, such as in KTS and PWS.[1,2] As such, the clinical presentation of VM is extremely variable and ranges from an asymptomatic birthmark to a life-threatening condition. Diagnosis and treatment planning present a major challenge to physicians because they are rare, occurring in fewer than 1 in 100,000 people in the United States. To start, the clinical examination including DUS should differentiate a high-flow lesion from a low-flow one.

Low-Flow VM: Simple

Low-flow VMs are slow to progress and usually do not have a bruit or thrill. The patient may present with skin warmth, a mass, port wine stain, or limb length discrepancy. A large "bird's nest" deformity of veins is common, and frequently adults have been treated for venous reflux disease only later to be found to have a low-flow VM.

Capillary malformations (CMs), found in 0.5% of the population, were initially and erroneously referred to as "port wine stain."[7] CMs affect the capillaries in the papillary dermis and commonly appear as a macular, pink, or purple stain that is present at birth and persists throughout life.[7] The majority of CMs appear on the face and within the trigeminal nerve distribution, especially ophthalmic (V1) and maxillary (V2) divisions.[8] CMs in the V1 or midline distribution warrant MRI as these findings are predictive of central nervous system (leptomeningeal) involvement and subsequent seizure disorders (ie, Sturge-Weber syndrome). With adulthood, the facial stains tend to darken and thicken into a "cobblestone" appearance and can distort facial features, including the underlying bony structures. Cerebral angiography can detect abnormal cortical veins and parenchymal contrast stasis associated with CNS involvement.[8]

Lymphatic malformations (LMs), incorrectly referred to as "lymphangioma" in the past, are single endothelial cell–lined vascular channels, pouches, or vesicles filled with lymphatic fluid. The majority of LMs (75%) occurring in the cervicofacial region are categorized by the size of the lymphatic chamber: macrocystic (>2 cm), microcystic (<2 cm), or mixed.[7] These lesions are often present at birth and appear as small, crimson dome-shaped nodules caused by intralesional bleeding. LMs do not regress but expand and contract based on the amount of inflammation, lymphatic fluid present, and the presence of bleeding. Macrocystic LMs can enlarge significantly, causing soft tissue and bony facial distortion. This tissue distortion can lead to frequent episodes of bleeding and cellulitis.[7]

Venous malformations are the most common type of VM, affecting 1% to 4% of individuals. They are present at birth and are composed of masses of veins and venules of different dimensions.[9] Clinically, they appear as bluish, soft, compressible lesions found on the face, limbs, or trunk. They tend to grow proportionally with the child and increase in size with puberty, hormonal changes, or infection. Venous malformations show a predisposition to thrombosis and phlebolith formation. DUS will identify the intralesional calcifications, formed as a result of venous stasis and inflammation that are pathognomonic of VM.[10] Venous malformations may incorporate lymphatic tissue and are often seen in many of the combined VM like KTS.

Low-Flow VM: Combined

Combined low-flow VMs include KTS and *CLOVES syndrome*, and manifest within a wide-ranging spectrum.

KTS is a rare congenital disorder characterized by combined capillary and venous malformations, ± associated lymphatic anomalies, and limb overgrowth. Cutaneous vascular stains (port wine stains) and limb hypertrophy are often present at birth, with the port wine stain involving the affected limb. The cutaneous CMs are classified as geographic (dark red-purple in color and sharply demarcated) or blotchy/segmental (irregularly shaped resembling that of a country or continent). Venous malformations characteristic of KTS result from persistence of avalvular embryonal veins (lateral thigh and sciatic vein) and present as dilated tortuous varicosities typically located over the anterolateral thigh and leg. Limb hypertrophy is secondary to soft tissue and bony overgrowth, although the presence of venous malformations and lymphedema may be contributing factors.

Patients with KTS are at risk for complications including localized intravascular coagulopathy and thromboembolism with increased risk for superficial thrombophlebitis, and less commonly DVT and PE, chronic venous insufficiency/lymphedema, bleeding, pain, cellulitis, and limb length discrepancy.

Initial screening should employ venous DUS to identify anomalies of the superficial and deep systems and confirm low flow, compressible vascular channels, valvular incompetence, and venous abnormalities including atresia or aneurysms. MRI or MRA is the diagnostic imaging of choice to define the nature and extent of the mixed vascular anomalies. MRI will accurately define the venous and lymphatic abnormalities, as well as soft tissue and bony overgrowth. MRV should be considered for patients with perineal involvement, as these patients may have large pelvic varicosities, increasing their risk for PE.

High-Flow VM

High-flow arterial VMs (AVMs) often present as a macular stain, with excess warmth of the skin, pulsatility, thrill, bruit, edema that continues despite elevation, hypertrophy, limb length discrepancy, pain, bleeding, infections, and ulcers. Long-standing untreated lesions may have the appearance of a dialysis fistula with tight scarred or thinning skin. High-flow lesions typically progress and can result in limb loss, life-threatening hemorrhage, or heart failure. Patients presenting with high-flow AVM should have an echocardiogram to evaluate potential heart strain (PWS).[11]

AVMs develop from an identifiable source vessel called the "nidus," which is central to an abnormal connection of arterial and venous vessels. They comprise 10% to 20% of VMs and arise from birth defects of both the arterial and venous vessels that result in high-flow fistulous connections, which make treatment of these lesions complex.[12] AVMs are usually present at birth, but do not become apparent until the first or second decade of life. Although these lesions are most commonly found intracranially, they can appear in soft tissues or bone of the limbs and trunk, and in viscera. AVMs have a reliable natural history consisting of four

distinct stages: quiescent, growing, symptomatic, and decompensating and are thought to expand in response to certain stimuli such as trauma or puberty.[13] If visible on PE, they are seen as telangiectasias or macular stains that can be mistaken for CM or IHs. They are slightly compressible and pulsatile with a palpable thrill, typically not accompanied by pain, and associated with frequent episodes of bleeding.[14]

The Hamburg, ISSVA, Schobinger, and angiographic classifications have been used to better differentiate AVM based on their developmental biology, with lesions described as truncular versus extratruncular. Truncular forms involve the main vessel trunks, often directly communicating with an artery and vein, described as an A-V fistula. These develop in the latter half of embryologic development and therefore are less likely to recur after treatment. The much more common extratruncular forms develop early when the vascular system is in its reticular stage and are mesodermal tissue remnants with angioblasts in the extremities. This nidus of angioblasts allows for recurrence after treatment. Extratruncular AVMs always have a nidus of angioblasts, whereas it is possible for a truncular AVM to have a direct fistulous connection without a nidus.[12,15,16]

Imaging plays an important role in the diagnosis and operative planning of AVM. As with other VMs, DUS and MRI can identify high-flow patterns as well as determine the extent of the lesion. DUS will confirm the multispacial and hypervascular AVM lesion, whereas MRI helps to define the extent of AVM and its relationship to surrounding structures or organs. Unlike other VMs, CTA can be valuable, especially for evaluating bony AVMs. DSA can also be utilized for defining an AVM nidus, its feeding and draining vessels, and is essential prior to sclerotherapy, endovascular treatment, or surgical intervention.[17]

High-Flow VM: Combined

Similar to KTS, PWS is a combined VM, but with capillary-arteriovenous and/or LMs with high-flow characteristics. PWS is characterized by large CMs of an extremity, soft tissue and bone hypertrophy of the affected limb, and multiple microscopic fast-flow AVM. Presentation can be similar to that of KTS with port wine stain and limb hypertrophy; however, because of the high-flow arteriovenous shunting, these patients may display limb venous ulcerations and high-output cardiac failure, especially in the neonatal period.

⒞ Infantile hemangioma?

H&P will help to differentiate a vascular tumor from a VM, as described in Box B. IHs occur most often in premature infants, females, and Caucasians and are the most common vascular tumors in children. Growth can be observed in the first 2 years of life, with most resolving spontaneously without any need for therapy. For lesions that do not respond in this manner, that is, characteristic proliferation and involution, or those that present of a darker

purple color, on an extremity, with bruits or rapid growth, other diagnosis must be evaluated for other causality including tufted angioma, kaposiform hemangioendothelioma, fibrosarcoma, or angiosarcoma.[18]

⒟ Evaulate other potential etiologies

Tufted angioma and kaposiform hemangioendothelioma are rare vascular tumors that typically present during infancy or early childhood. They may be associated with Kasabach-Merritt phenomenon, a life-threatening complication characterized by severe thrombocytopenia and coagulopathy. These suspected masses should be evaluated with DUS and biopsy to rule out consumptive platelet trapping (Kasabach-Merritt phenomenon).[18]

⒠ Observation

IH should be observed as most regress within the first 2 years of life, if not within the first decade. If they regress, no further treatment is indicated. Although most are small cutaneous lesions, hemangiomas can also be large, disfiguring lesions with serious complications. "Watchful waiting" is appropriate for most lesions, with approximately 10% resulting in complications requiring intervention or management by a multidisciplinary team of specialists.

⒡ No further treatment

Most cutaneous IHs are uncomplicated and require no intervention. IHs that recede require no further treatment or surveillance.

⒢ Aggressive treatment

Cutaneous IH may ulcerate, leading to pain, bleeding, scarring, and/or infection. Other lesions may cause functional impairment and/or disfigurement after a proliferative phase. Ulceration is the most common complication of IH, occurring in 16% of patients.[5] It is particularly frequent when IHs are rapidly proliferating and located in trauma- or pressure-susceptible regions. Airway compromise may occur in patients with airway hemangiomas. These hemangiomas can develop in children who do not have cutaneous hemangiomas. Risk is higher for IH located in a cervicofacial, mandibular, or "beard" distribution. Airway IH must be considered in any child with cutaneous hemangioma in a cervicofacial mandibular distribution and progressive hoarseness and stridor. Periorbital hemangiomas may compromise normal visual development. The majority of IHs that lead to visual complications involve the upper medial eyelid, but any lesion in the periorbital location can pose a threat to vision. Early and regular examination by an ophthalmologist familiar with periorbital hemangioma and their complications is mandatory. Hemangiomas of the ear may obstruct the auditory canal. IH of the tongue, oral cavity, and aerodigestive tract may interfere with feeding, swallowing, and speech.

Systemic steroid therapy should be considered for problematic IHs that are too large to be treated with local injection. Systemic pharmacotherapy includes prednisolone and propranolol. For symptomatic IH that impair vision, breathing, and swallowing, treatment is warranted. Intralesional administration of corticosteroids is indicated for small, well-localized IH that obstruct vision or the nasal airway. Treatment is also recommended for lesions located in aesthetically important areas (eyelid, nose, lip).[19] Injectable or systemic corticosteroids can be used to reduce the overall mass effect and inflammation. Long-term risks of these medications are well known and include growth retardation. Prednisolone (3 mg/kg) is administered in the morning for 30 days. The dose should then be tapered every 2 to 4 weeks until discontinued between 10 and 12 months of age. Treatment is successful in nearly all patients, with 88% of lesions regressing. For patients experiencing side effects such as cushingoid appearance (20%) and decrease in height gain (12%), the therapy should be tapered quicker than anticipated.[19] Systemic pharmacotherapy treatment should also include beta blockade using oral propranolol, recognizing that in infants, propranolol can cause bronchospasm, bradycardia, hypotension, hypoglycemia, seizures, and hyperkalemia.[19] Propranolol, a nonselective beta-blocker, causes regression of IH and has recently been found to be efficacious in treating problematic hemangiomas. The mechanism of action is unclear. Propranolol (2 mg/kg/d) divided into two or three daily doses is then tapered until it is discontinued around 1 year of age. Abrupt cessation can result in rebound growth and is not recommended. Treatment is successful in approximately 90% of tumors. If this treatment modality is unsuccessful, then second-line drugs for the treatment of IH include interferon and vincristine. These agents are rarely used as most tumors respond well to propranolol and corticosteroids.

More aggressive nonsurgical or surgical resection is reserved for those patients unresponsive to medical management. Laser therapy can be utilized to treat bleeding lesions, residual hemosiderin deposition, and painful ulcerated lesions. Pulsed laser treatment of proliferating IH has been advocated by some, but almost all IH lesions are beyond the reach of the laser.

Operative excision of IH lesions is used primarily for cosmesis; approximately 50% of patients have residual skin changes after IH involution, including hypo- or hyperpigmentation, excess skin, or fibrofatty tissue. Operative treatment should be avoided during the proliferative phase as these lesions typically respond well to pharmacotherapy. Operative intervention should only be employed during the involuted phase (after 3 years of age) when IHs are smaller and less vascular (than during the proliferative phase). Circular lesions should be excised with a circular incision closed with a purse string–like closure. The resultant circular scar can subsequently be excised

and closed linearly. This technique reduces the overall length of the incision by one-third if the original tumor had been excised with an elliptical excision.[19]

Ⓗ MRA

MRA is the primary imaging type after initial DUS used to confirm high- versus low-flow VM and plan potential treatment. The T2-weighted images show low-flow lesions as bright signals, with the dilated veins noted. The high-flow lesions are identified by shunting, and MRA captures the true extent of such lesions, including fistulous connections, soft tissue, and musculoskeletal involvement. Further, with software advancements capturing the maximal intensity projections, the lesion is isolated and dynamic flow acquisitioned.[20] Although CTA can at times better evaluate the osseous structures, for example, orbit of the eye, MRA provides the most critical data, especially differentiating whether a lesion can be treated surgically.[21,22]

If additional information is required to characterize the degree of shunting by an AVM, scintigraphy can aid in detecting micro-AV shunting in the soft tissues. Additional, unrecognized lesions can be identified by whole-body blood pool scintigraphy utilizing radioisotope tagged erythrocytes.[23,24]

Ⓘ Treatment indicated?

Indications for endovascular and surgical intervention of high-flow VM include pain, recurrent ulcerations/bleeding, or perturbed cardiac function.[13] Treatment decisions must always consider overall patient risk and benefit.

Ⓙ DSA

If the VM is characterized as a high-flow lesion that requires treatment, then DSA should be performed to define the AVM nidus, delineate feeding versus draining vessels, and provide a road map to plan therapy. DSA is essential prior to sclerotherapy, endovascular treatment, or surgical intervention.

Ⓚ Define AVM classification

Identifying high-flow AVM architecture (Type I–IIIb) is critical for treatment planning and treatment success. This includes defining the AVM nidus as well as the inflowing (arterial) and outflowing (venous) vessels (see Figure 76-1).

Ⓛ Endovascular treatment candidate?

Management of an AVM can involve embolization alone or in combination with surgical excision. Based on MRA and DSA, it must be determined whether access to the AVM can be achieved to allow embolization without eliminating future access to the nidus, because the nidus can recruit new vessels after treatment. This can be a complex decision depending on the characteristics of the AVM and is based substantially on operator experience.

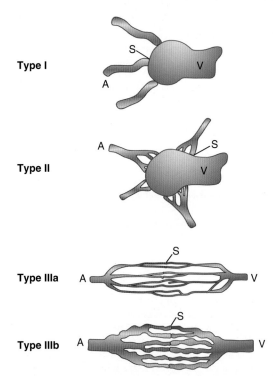

Figure 76-1. Arteriovenous Fistula Anatomic Classification.[20] Type I (arteriovenous fistula): at most three separate arteries shunted to a single draining vein. Type II (arteriolovenous fistula): multiple arterioles shunted into a single draining vein. Type III (arteriolovenulous fistula): multiple shunts between the arterioles and venules.[2]

Ⓜ Eliminate AVM nidus

The goal of AVM treatment is to eliminate the nidus, which can be approached from both the arterial and venous side. Arterial embolization must be carefully planned. Proximal arterial occlusion that prohibits future access to the nidus can result in more unwanted growth of the AVM. Proximal arterial occlusion can also create ischemia, especially in extratruncular lesions of the extremities. As such, coil embolization or proximal arterial ligation is being abandoned, and interventionalists now recommend approaching from the venous side, even in high-flow AVMs, with obliteration of the nidus by back-filling, while preserving arterial supply to peripheral tissues. This approach also reduces the risk of distal embolization of sclerosants or coils. One can then further embolize the nidus from the arterial side if needed, with greater success and precise delivery. Poorly executed interventions that fail to obliterate the nidus can stimulate the AVM to transition from a "dormant to proliferative" state. This in turn can cause massive growth and unmanageable complications.[25,26]

The tools utilized for AVM endovascular intervention are considerable. However, the risk of embolo-sclerotherapy is real, so that careful planning for next steps based on extensive experience is essential. A combination approach is often recommended to treat AVMs including transvenous, transarterial, and direct puncture. In addition, combinations of embolic agents can be employed including liquid sclerosants, polymerizing agents like onyx, N-butyl cyanoacrylate (nBCA), venous coils, and occlusion balloons.

Because the goal of therapy is to alter flow dynamics, coils can be used quite effectively in low-flow lesions. However, high-flow lesions often are not completely occluded by coils alone, because thrombosis is also required for effective management.[25-27] Therefore, using coils in combination with agents like onyx, with the coils acting as "rebar" and the onyx as cement, provides an effective option. Additionally, single venous outflow AVM can typically be occluded with treatment even if there are multiple arterial components. The number and location of coils placed in the extremities should be considered because atrophy of the lesion can lead to coil erosion through the surrounding tissues or skin and cause pressure and sensitivity to the patient. Balloons can be helpful during treatment, positioned to direct nidal injection, or obstruct outflow to allow filling of the nidus and increase the local concentration of various sclerosant agents.

Onyx is an excellent choice in treating high-flow lesions, because unlike coils, it can reach the nidus. As a polymerizing agent, it is similar to nBCA but onyx has a delayed polymerization when injected into the vessel, in addition to less adhesive action, which provides the operator with greater control of the product and projection of the material into the nidus. nBCA will polymerize on contact with any ionic solution and therefore has less risk of drift within the nidus. Like onyx, it also induces an acute inflammatory reaction with the exothermic reaction. Unfortunately, nBCA is considered palliative as long-term imaging has shown reabsorption of the product.[26-28] Both products can embolize, so careful imaging of vessels distal to the nidus must be performed to avoid cases where distal embolization is likely to occur.

Ethanol is an extremely powerful sclerosant that can be used to treat some AVM. It denudes endothelial cells and the vessel wall is effectively fractured to the level of the elastic lamina, resulting in platelet aggregation and thrombosis. Because the endothelium is denuded, angiogenesis is eliminated, and the lesion is effectively prohibited from regeneration.[29,30] Ethanol should be reserved for larger AVMs requiring treatments that are more destructive and should be avoided when treating complex and dynamic lesions involving not only the vascular system but also any system (eg, skin or nerves) that could inadvertently be injured by the treatment. The risks of ethanol include pulmonary hypertension from either arterial spasm or micro-thromboemboli and can result in cardiac

arrest.[29,32] Close monitoring with general anesthesia and use of a pulmonary artery catheter are recommended. Dose should be limited to 1 mL/kg.[29-34] When treating superficial malformations, ethanol can be used but has a high risk of skin necrosis and nerve damage. The inflammation from ethanol use can also be treated with hydrocortisone and NSAIDs.

Other liquid sclerosing agents include sodium tetradecyl sulfate (STS), polidocanol, doxycycline, and bleomycin. STS is a fatty acid salt with detergent properties similar to polidocanol. These agents being detergents act on the lipid structures of the endothelial cells, causing lysis and thrombosis. Both can cause distal thrombosis and embolization and are not as effective for large high-flow AVMs. The lower flow venous malformations are effectively treated with these agents, especially in the foam mixtures.[34]

Doxycycline and bleomycin are mild sclerosants effective for the low lymphatic components of venous malformations. The amounts of agent used should be considered as bleomycin can cause hair loss, pulmonary fibrosis, and pigmentation.[33,34]

Ⓝ Surgical resection needed?

With the advent of endovascular therapy (sclerotherapy and embolization), surgical excision, once considered the "gold standard," is less often required for AVM treatment. The goal of endovascular therapy is to eliminate the AVM nidus completely or to decrease the AVM to a "manageable" size for surgical excision. Integration of endovascular therapy into the treatment paradigm has markedly improved surgical outcomes by reducing bleeding, better localizing the lesion, and reducing the size of lesion to be excised.[35]

A multidisciplinary team must make the decision for surgical excision, because multiple specialties are often required for successful treatment of the AVM. The need for tissue expanders, skin grafts, and potential risk for nerve injury with en bloc resection must be addressed. If endovascular treatment options are exhausted or other less invasive interventions are felt to be suboptimal, surgical resection should be considered.

Ⓞ Surveillance

Regular monitoring should be considered in every patient who has been diagnosed with a VM. Future growth as well as recurrence after initial treatment is likely.[15,26] Early signs of recurrence include erythema, superficial telangiectasia, swelling, pulsations, palpable thrill, bleeding, and a recurrent ballotable mass. DUS may be necessary to monitor and confirm for recurrent growth. As most malformations are chronic, the patient's subjective complaints are used as a benchmark for reintervention. This also applies to patients with VM that do not initially require treatment.

Ⓟ Surgical resection

The goal of surgical resection is complete excision to normal margins, with removal of both the AVM nidus and involved tissue and

skin. Ligation of the feeding vessels into the nidus alone should never be performed as this leads to rapid recruitment of collaterals and heightened vascularity and prevents an arterial endovascular approach. When considering resection of an AVM, it is paramount to realize that these lesions are rarely curable, so operative treatment should focus on disease control. Diffuse lesions have higher recurrence rates and are more challenging to treat. Operative planning involving a multidisciplinary team is essential because resection of these lesions can create large defects that may require flap coverage or formal reconstruction and should only be performed if the benefit of AVM removal greatly outweighs the risks of the surgical excision. Large excisions that do not allow for primary closure can be managed with temporary wound-assisted closure devices or rotational/free flaps. For limb AVM, especially those with associated loss of function, excision may require amputation.

Ⓠ Interventional treatment indicated?

Conservative management can be a long- or short-term treatment plan for low-flow VM depending on the patient's current symptoms, risks to the limb or organ system involved, and functional imitations. If risk of intervention outweighs benefits or current interventions have provided maximal effectiveness, conservative measures may be engaged. These include, but are not limited to, compression, medicinal management, physical therapy, and surveillance.

Leg length discrepancy differentiates KTS and PWS from other low-flow VM. All patients with leg length discrepancy should be followed closely with regular documentation of the distance between the anterior superior iliac spine and medial malleolus, especially during rapid growth periods. Generally, less than 2 cm leg length discrepancy is considered inconsequential and can be managed with shoe lifts. Leg length discrepancies greater than 2 cm often require treatment to halt the continued excessive limb growth. These patients should be referred to an orthopedic specialist familiar with KTS treatment. Patients with limb hypertrophy have an increased risk for embryonal tumors such as Wilms tumor and hepatoblastoma.[36] Tumor screening is essential and includes serial renal DUS and serum alpha-fetoprotein measurements for all these patients until age 8.[36]

Asymptomatic LMs can be observed. LMs are unique among VM in that they not only serve as a source of infection, causing cellulitis and bacteremia, but are also affected by illness occurring elsewhere in the body, increasing the response to infection. Indications for treatment include deformity, dysfunction, leakage into body cavities or from the skin, and recurrent infections.

Ⓡ Ablation/sclerotherapy

Interventional treatment options for VMs depend on both the extent of the lesion and the location. Typically, functional or aesthetic limitations will drive the initiation of therapy. Primary treatment involves staged sclerotherapy and embolization prior to surgical excision. Sclerotherapy with absolute ethanol is effective for treatment of large, extensive VM, but should be used with caution as it can damage nerves, cause skin necrosis, and induce systemic toxicity.[37,38] Other common sclerosants used include 3% STS and bleomycin. Surgery is rarely first-line therapy but may be considered in an effort (1) to ligate efferent veins to improve the results with sclerotherapy, (2) to remove residual VM after sclerotherapy, (3) to remove lesion resistant to sclerotherapy, or (4) in localized lesions amenable to complete excision.[39]

For patients with KTS, ablative CO_2 laser therapy is recommended for complicated (bleeding, leaking, ulcerated) superficial vascular stains and lymphatic blebs, whereas pulsed dye laser therapy is effective in lightening CMs. Endovenous laser/radiofrequency ablation or sclerotherapy can be employed for treatment of symptomatic venous and lymphatic disease with good result. Early ablation of embryonal veins in young children has been proposed for severely symptomatic venous disease with venous treatment extending into adulthood.[3] Treatment of the venous malformation does not prevent limb overgrowth.

Resection is not usually necessary for isolated CMs. Laser ablative therapy, such as the pulsed dye laser (580-595 nm), significantly improves the color of the stain when laser treatment is begun in infancy and when applied to CM of the lateral face.[40] Noticeable lightening is typically seen in greater than 75% of patients, with better results achieved when therapy is initiated early. Therefore, it is recommended that laser treatment commence before 6 months of age. Surgery is reserved for lesions that are refractory to ablative treatment or are causing significant disfigurement.[41]

Sclerosants are first-line therapy for microcytic LMs that do not respond to conservative management. Sclerosant options include absolute ethanol, doxycycline, STS, or picibanil (OK-432).[8] These agents cause irreversible damage to the endothelium, inducing local inflammation and ultimately fibrosis with the goal of obliterating the lesion. Unfortunately, sclerotherapy does not work well for macrocytic lesions; the only potentially curative modality is surgical resection.

S Surgical resection

Resection is not usually necessary for isolated CM as most lesions respond well to laser therapy. Surgery is reserved for CM lesions that are refractory to ablative treatment or are causing significant disfigurement.[41]

Unfortunately, sclerotherapy does not work well for macrocytic LMs; the only potentially curative modality is surgical resection. For LM, the goals of surgical resection focus on gross debulking of defined anatomic field, limiting blood loss, and minimizing damage to surrounding structures. Extensive radical resection can be morbid and is typically performed at the expense of surrounding normal structures.[42] Because the operations can be lengthy, surgical resection should be delayed until the patient is 6 months old. Surgical resection requires a team approach as these lesions can be surgically challenging because of the considerable tissue expansion by the LM, risk for postoperative leaks, infection, and need for creative skin incisions. Every effort should be made to try to remove the whole LM lesion, as reoperations can be more difficult.

For VM, surgery is rarely first-line therapy. Surgery may be considered in an effort to (1) ligate efferent veins to improve the results with sclerotherapy, (2) remove residual VM after sclerotherapy, (3) remove lesions resistant to sclerotherapy, or (4) remove localized lesions amenable to complete excision.[39] It is important to recognize that resection can be arduous and technically demanding; thus, it should not be undertaken without a goal in mind and after thorough consideration of all operative risks.

In patients with KTS, surgical resection is reserved for local superficial disease and indicated for managing bleeding, lymph leakage, and ulceration. Surgical debulking of the VM is not recommended and certainly not feasible for malformations extending deep into muscle and bone. Debulking of overgrown soft lymphatic tissue and amputation can be considered in patients disabled by severe progressive overgrowth and a heavy large limb. These procedures should only be undertaken in centers with established resources and expertise.

T Supportive treatment and surveillance

Conservative management of low-flow VM involves compression garments, lymphatic massage, physical therapy, and physical activity, depending on the specific location and type of VM. When the leg is involved, compression stockings should extend from the foot to above the affected area; typically, these stockings need to be custom made. Reducing edema and venous hypertension decreases the risk of recurrent cellulitis and skin breakdown. Treatment for LMs should begin with expectant management of symptomatic lesions, such as pain control and compression for intralesional bleeding and antibiotics for infection, which can often be life threatening.

As with all VM, the management of patients with KTS requires a multidisciplinary approach. Treatment should be individualized and based upon the extent of disease and complications. Patients with KTS are at risk for chronic venous insufficiency and lymphedema, and the sequela of these chronic conditions. Medical management of KTS involves pain management, treatment and prevention of limb infection, and treatment of coagulation disorders. Pain is a significant source of morbidity for KTS patients, and treatment should focus on targeting the source of pain—infection, superficial or deep venous thrombosis, neuropathic pain, and contractures.[43] Reducing the burden of VM including intraosseous/articular disease should be the goal of therapy. Patients with KTS can be plagued with recurrent cellulitis and lymphangitis, especially those with associated lymphatic anomalies. Antibiotic therapy should be empiric and target beta-hemolytic streptococci and methicillin-sensitive *Staphylococcus aureus*. Coverage should include MRSA for limb infection resistant to first-line antibiotic therapy. For patients suffering from superficial thrombophlebitis, the presence of phleboliths, and chronic coagulopathy, as evidenced by elevated D-dimer and low fibrinogen, low-dose aspirin should be initiated.[44] Low-dose aspirin appears to be beneficial in patients with venous malformations, with improvement in leg pain and swelling.[44] Sirolimus has emerged as a potential therapeutic option for patients with complex venous-lymphatic VM, with studies showing dramatic size reduction of the vascular anomalies and marked improvement in pain, quality of life, functional impairment, bleeding, and coagulation parameters.[42] Consultation with hematology is recommended for treatment protocols and therapy.[42]

REFERENCES

1. ISSVA classification for vascular anomalies© (Approved at the 20th ISSVA Workshop, Melbourne, April 2014, last revision May 2018). http://www.issva.org/UserFiles/file/ISSVA-Classification-2018.pdf
2. Mulliken JB, Glowacki J. Classification of pediatric vascular lesions. *Plast Reconstr Surg*. 1982;70(1):120-121.
3. Mulliken JB, Glowacki J. Hemangiomas and vascular malformations in infants and children: a classification based on endothelial characteristics. *Plast Reconstr Surg*. 1982;69(3):412-422.
4. Van Aalst JA, Bhuller A, Sadove AM. Pediatric vascular lesions. *J Craniofac Surg*. 2003;14(4):566-583.
5. Haggstrom AN, Drolet BA, Baselga E, et al; Hemangioma Investigator Group. Prospective study of infantile hemangiomas: demographic, prenatal, and perinatal characteristics. *J Pediatr*. 2007;150(3):291-294.
6. Berenguer B, Mulliken JB, Enjolras O, et al. Rapidly involuting congenital hemangioma: clinical and histopathologic features. *Pediatr Dev Pathol*. 2003;6(6):495-510.
7. Colletti G, Valassina D, Bertossi D, Melchiorre F, Vercellio G, Brusati R. Contemporary management of vascular malformations. *J Oral Maxillofac Surg*. 2014;72(3):510-528.
8. Burrows PE, Mulliken JB, Fellows KE, Strand RD. Childhood hemangiomas and vascular malformations: angiographic differentiation. *AJR Am J Roentgenol*. 1983;141(3):483-488.
9. Pappas DC Jr, Persky MS, Berenstein A. Evaluation and treatment of head and neck venous vascular malformations. *Ear Nose Throat J*. 1998;77(11):914-916, 918-922.
10. Hochman M, Adams DM, Reeves TD. Current knowledge and management of vascular anomalies, II: malformations. *Arch Facial Plast Surg*. 2011;13(6):425-433.
11. Rienhoff WF. Congenital arteriovenous fistula. *Bull Johns Hopkins Hosp*. 1924;35:271-284.

12. Lee BB, Baumgartner I, Berlien HP, et al. Consensus Document of the International Union of Angiology (IUA)-2013 Current concepts of the management of arteriovenous malformations. *Int Angiol*. 2013;32(1):9-36.

13. Greene AK, Orbach DB. Management of arteriovenous malformations. *Clin Plast Surg*. 2011;38(1):95-106.

14. Christison-Lagay ER, Fishman SJ. Vascular anomalies. *Surg Clin North Am*. 2006;86(2):393-425, x.

15. Lee BB, Do YS, Yakes W, Kim DI, Mattassi R, Hyun WS. Management of arterial-venous shunting malformations (AVM) by surgery and embolosclerotherapy. A multidisciplinary approach. *J Vasc Surg*. 2004;39:590-600.

16. St-Amant M, Gaillar Tasnadi G. Epidemiology and etiology of congenital vascular malformations. *Semin Vasc Surg*. 1993; 6:200-203.

17. Lowe LH, Marchant TC, Rivard DC, Scherbel AJ. Vascular malformations: classification and terminology the radiologist needs to know. *Semin Roentgenol*. 2012;47(2): 106-117.

18. Mulliken JB, Enjolras O. Congenital hemangiomas and infantile hemangioma: missing links. *J Am Acad Dermatol*. 2004;50(6):875-882.

19. Enjolras O, Mulliken JB, Boon LM, Wassef M, Kozakewich HP, Burrows PE. Noninvoluting congenital hemangioma: a rare cutaneous vascular anomaly. *Plast Reconstr Surg*. 2001;107(7):1647-1654.

20. Léauté-Labrèze C, Harper JI, Hoeger PH. Infantile haemangioma. *Lancet*. 2017;390:85.

21. Revencu N, Boon LM, Mulliken JB, Enjolras O, Cordisco MR, Burrows PE. Parkes Weber syndrome, vein of Galen aneurysmal malformation, and other fast-flow vascular anomalies are caused by RASA 1 mutations. *Human Mut*. 2009; 29:959-965.

22. Wassef M, Blei F, Adams D, et al. Vascular anomalies classification: recommendations from the international society for the study of vascular anomalies. *Pediatrics*. 2015;136:e203-e214.

23. Lee BB, Mattassi R, Choe YH, Vaghi M, Ahn J M, Kim DI. Critical role of duplex ultrasonography for the advanced management of venous malformation (VM). *Phlebology*. 2005;20:28-37.

24. Lidsky ME, Spritzer CE, Shortell CK. The role of dynamic contrast-enhanced magnetic resonance imaging in the diagnosis and management of patients with vascular malformations. *J Vasc Surg*. 2012;56(3):757-764.

25. Dubois J, Alison M. Vascular anomalies: what a radiologist needs to know. *Pediatr Radiol*. 2010;40:895-905.

26. Lee BB, Mattassi R, Kim BT, Kim DI, Ahn JM, Choi JY. Contemporary diagnosis and management of venous and AV shunting malformation by whole body blood pool scintigraphy (WBBPS). *Int Angiol*. 2004;23:355-367.

27. Lee BB, Mattassi R, Kim BT, Park JM. Advanced management of arteriovenous shunting malformation with Transarterial Lung Perfusion Scintigraphy (TLPS) for follow up assessment. *Int Angiol*. 2005;24:173-184.

28. Charité—University Medicine Berlin. Minimally Invasive Tumor Therapy (MITT). http://www.radiology-berlin.de/mitt-en/gefaessfehlbildungen.html. Accessed May 13, 2018.

29. Grady RM, Sharkey AM, Bridges ND. Transcatheter coil embolization of a pulmonary arteriovenous malformation in a neonate. *Br Heart J*. 1994;71:370-371.

30. Velat GJ, Reavey-Cantwell JF, Sistrom C, Smullen D, Fautheree GL, Whiting J. Comparison of N-butyl cyanoacrylate and onyx for the embolization of intracranial arteriovenous malformation: analysis of fluoroscopy and procedure times. *Neurosurgery*. 2008;63(1 suppl 1):ONS73-8; discussion ONS78-80.

31. Natarajan SK, Born D, Ghodke B, Britz GW, Sekhar LN. Histopathological changes in brain arteriovenous malformations after embolization using Onyx or N-butyl cyanoacrylate. Laboratory investigation. *J Neurosurg*. 2009;111:105-113.

32. Yakes WF, Pevsner P, Reed M, Donohue HJ, Ghaed N. Serial embolizations of an extremity AVM with alcohol via direct puncture. *AJR Am J Roentgenol*. 1986;146:1038-1044.

33. Shin BS, Do YS, Cho HS, Hahm TS, Kim CS. Effects of repeat bolus ethanol injections on cardiopulmonary hemodynamic changes during embolectomy of arteriovenous malformations of the extremities. *J Vasc Interv Radiol*. 2010;21:81-89.

34. Shin BS, Do YS, Lee BB, Kim DI, Chung IS, Cho HS. Multistage ethanol sclerotherapy of soft-tissue arteriovenous malformations: effect on pulmonary arterial pressure. *Radiology*. 2005;235:1072-1077.

35. Upton J, Taghinia A. Special considerations in vascular anomalies: operative management of upper extremity lesions. *Clin Plast Surg*. 2011;38:143-151.

36. Clericuzio CL, Martin RA. Diagnostic criteria and tumor screening for individuals with isolated hemihyperplasia. *Genet Med*. 2009;11(3):220-222.

37. Berenguer B, Burrows PE, Zurakowski D, Mulliken JB. Sclerotherapy of craniofacial venous malformations: complications and results. *Plast Reconstr Surg*. 1999;104:1-11, discussion 12-15.

38. Cabrera J, Cabrera J Jr, Garcia-Olmedo MA. Sclerosants in microfoam. A new approach in angiology. *Int Angiol*. 2001;20(4):322-329.

39. Eifert S, Villavicencio JL, Kao TC, Taute BM, Rich NM. Prevalence of deep venous anomalies in congenital vascular malformations of venous predominance. *J Vasc Surg*. 2000;31(3):462-471.

40. Yuan KH, Gao JH, Huang Z. Adverse effects associated with photodynamic therapy (PDT) of port-wine stain (PWS) birthmarks. *Photodiagn Photodyn Ther*. 2012;9(4):332-336.

41. Buckmiller LM, Richter GT, Suen JY. Diagnosis and management of hemangiomas and vascular malformations of the head and neck. *Oral Dis*. 2010;16(5):405-418.

42. Adams DM, Trenor CC III, Hammill AM, et al. Efficacy and safety of sirolimus in the treatment of complicated vascular anomalies. *Pediatrics*. 2016;137(2):e20153257.

43. Lee A, Driscoll D, Gloviczki P, Clay R, Shaughnessy W, Stans A. Evaluation and management of pain in patients with Klippel-Trenaunay syndrome: a review. *Pediatrics*. 2005;115(3):744-749.

44. Nguyen JT, Koerper MA, Hess CP, et al. Aspirin therapy in venous malformation: a retrospective cohort study of benefits, side effects, and patient experiences. *Pediatr Dermatol*. 2014;31(5):556-560.

Margaret E. Smith • Thomas W. Wakefield

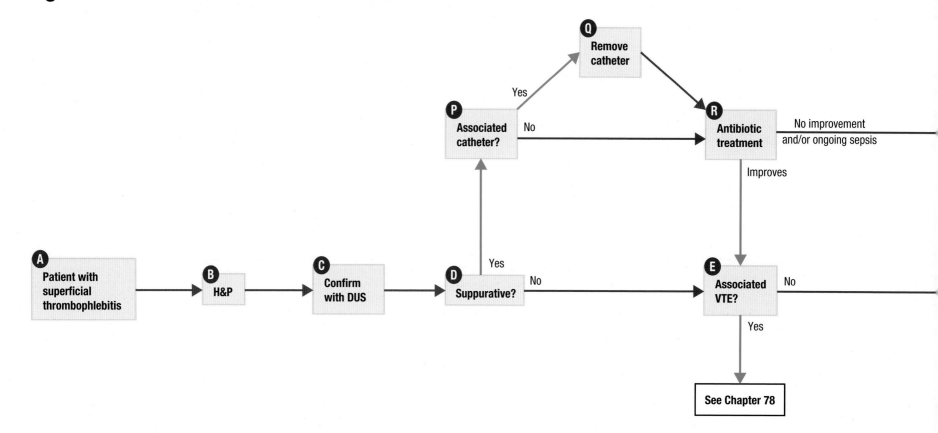

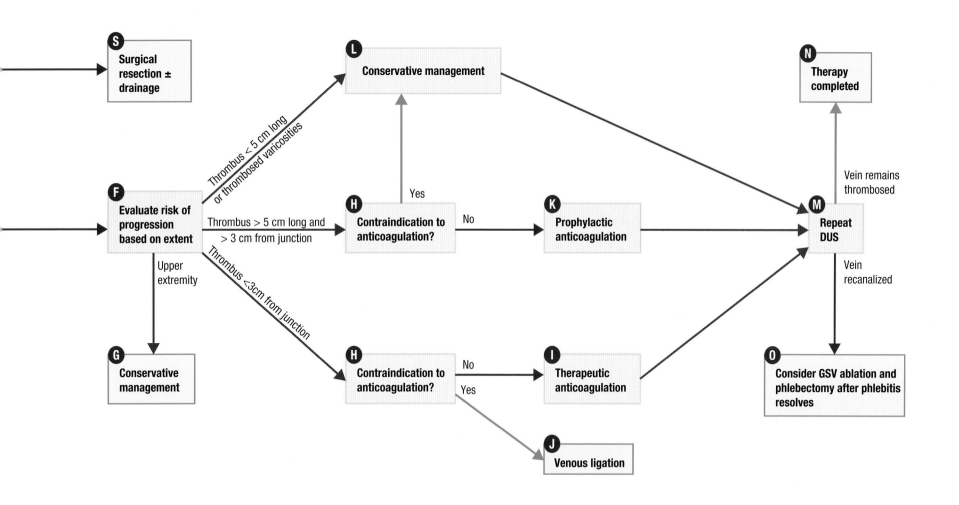

A Patient with superficial thrombophlebitis

Superficial venous thrombophlebitis (SVT) affects nearly 125,000 patients in the United States annually.[1] However, this is likely underestimated because many cases are subclinical and not reported. The average age of diagnosis is 55 to 64 years, with females more often affected than are males. Varicose veins, present in two-thirds of patients, are the most commonly reported risk factors and up to 70% of patients with SVT may have associated superficial venous insufficiency.[1] Additional factors increasing the prevalence of SVT include obesity, tobacco use, history of DVT, pregnancy, oral contraceptive and hormone replacement therapy, immobilization and/or recent surgery, IV catheterization, active malignancy, autoimmune disease, and inherited thrombophilia.[2,3]

B H&P

Initial evaluation of a patient with SVT should include a careful history to evaluate for the presence of risk factors or a hypercoagulable disorder. Patients with SVT most commonly present with erythema and tenderness overlying the distribution of a superficial vein, along with a palpable "cord" (thrombus within the vein) and edema of the surrounding soft tissue. Malaise and a low-grade fever may be present. The most common location of SVT is the GSV and its tributaries; however, any superficial veins of the upper or lower extremities may be affected.[4]

C Confirm with DUS

DUS is used to confirm the presence of SVT, because this is an accurate, noninvasive method to determine the extent of involvement in the superficial and deep venous systems. DUS findings characteristic of SVT include a dilated vein with a lack of compressibility and a lack of echoes from within the lumen. Venogram, CT-venogram, and MR-venogram are not recommended as first-line imaging.

D Suppurative?

Suppurative superficial venous thrombophlebitis (SSVT), or septic SVT is suspected in a patient with fever, leukocytosis, severe local pain, a tender palpable cord, and purulent drainage at the site of the involved vessel.[5] Prompt identification and management is necessary because SSVT may be lethal owing to its association with septicemia. Factors that increase the prevalence of SSVT include steroid use, injection drug use, and associated burns.[6]

E Associated VTE?

Concomitant DVT is present in 5% to 40% of patients with SVT.[1] Thrombus in the GSV is most likely to propagate into the deep system; however, up to 16% of patients with small saphenous vein (SSV) thrombus may develop DVT or PE.[7] Approximately 25% of identified DVTs are noncontiguous with the site of SVT, occasionally occurring in the contralateral extremity.[8] Consequently,

DUS of bilateral extremities should be performed routinely in all patients with SVT.[9] If a patient with SVT has associated VTE, more aggressive treatment is required (see Chapter 78).

F Evaluate risk of progression based on extent

SVT carries a significant risk of progression to DVT and subsequent PE. In patients diagnosed with SVT, 6% to 44% suffered from a DVT, 20% to 30% had an asymptomatic PE, and 2% to 13% developed a symptomatic PE.[3] In addition, in a population-based study of nearly 11,000 patients, the incidence of VTE in the first 3 months following an SVT diagnosis was 70 times greater than that in the general population.[10] Proximity of the SVT to saphenofemoral junction (SFJ) is associated with greater risk of progression to DVT.[11] Therefore, the distance from the SFJ to the thrombus within the GSV (<3 cm or greater) must be assessed by DUS. This, and the length of the thrombus, determines the aggressiveness of management of GSV SVT. The same logic is applied to SVT in the SSV, measuring from the saphenopopliteal junction (SPJ). Upper extremity SVT is much less likely to progress and, as such, is managed conservatively.

In addition to location and extent of SVT burden impacting risk of progression, patients with SVT have an increased likelihood of an underlying hypercoagulable state or malignancy. No current recommendations exist to define which patients merit workup for hypercoagulable states; however, as many as 35% of patients with SVT may have an associated disorder.[12] Evaluation of hypercoagulable states and malignancy should be considered in all patients, especially when the episode of SVT is recurrent or unprovoked, that is, not associated with instrumentation, varicosities, or known high-risk clinical states (eg, immobilization, pregnancy, history of DVT). In patients with a hypercoagulable state or malignancy, the risk of progression to DVT is higher and anticoagulation may be recommended regardless of SVT location or length.

G Conservative management

Upper extremity SVT is most often associated with trauma secondary to an IV cannula or infusion, resulting in caustic endothelial damage. Extension of an upper extremity SVT to the deep system with subsequent VTE is rare when compared to SVT of the lower extremity.[13] Treatment of nonsuppurative upper extremity SVT consists of prompt removal of an IV catheter, if present, and applying warm compresses. Although upper extremity SVT is poorly studied, guidelines suggest treatment with oral anti-inflammatory drugs, topical diclofenac gel, or topical heparin gel until resolution of symptoms or for up to 2 weeks.[9,14] Systemic anticoagulation is not indicated.

H Contraindication to anticoagulation?

Patients should be evaluated for contraindication to anticoagulation therapy before initiating treatment. Common contraindications include significant thrombocytopenia, acute clinically

significant bleeding, severe bleeding diathesis, previous history of intracranial hemorrhage, recent GI hemorrhage, and recurrent iatrogenic falls in patients at higher bleeding risk. Individual risk versus benefit analysis for therapeutic and prophylactic anticoagulation must be incorporated into treatment decision making for patients with relative contraindications to anticoagulation.

I Therapeutic anticoagulation

Treatment of SVT has primarily been evaluated for GSV thrombus >3 cm distal to the SFJ, with minimal evidence available to guide treatment of SVT ≤3 cm from the SJF. Prophylactic anticoagulation is the recommended treatment regimen for SVT >5 cm long and >3 cm from the SFJ, and has been suggested as treatment for SVT <3 cm from the SFJ, regardless of length.[9] However, given the close proximity to the SFJ and risk of extension into the deep venous system and VTE, we suggest a more aggressive approach. Thus, for patients with SVT <3 cm from the SFJ, we use therapeutic anticoagulation, in accordance with treatment guidelines for lower extremity DVT. Although a few studies have included patients with SVT of the SSV, we also recommend therapeutic anticoagulation for SVT <3 cm from the SPJ because of similar risk of extension into the deep venous system.

J Venous ligation

Venous disconnection and ligation is appropriate in patients with contraindications to anticoagulation and SVT <3 cm from the SFJ or SPJ to prevent extension into the deep system. Compared to anticoagulation, venous ligation has superior symptom relief and reduction of thrombus extension; however, anticoagulation minimizes complications and is superior in prevention of VTE.[15] Therefore, anticoagulation is the first-line therapy for thrombus <3 cm from the SFJ or SPJ, with venous ligation reserved for those unable to be anticoagulated.

K Prophylactic anticoagulation

Treatment for SVT ≥5 cm in length and at least 3 cm away from to the SFJ or SPJ includes prophylactic dose anticoagulation to prevent extension and reduce the risk of VTE. The CALISTO trial in 2010, a randomized double-blind trial of 45 days of prophylactic fondaparinux versus placebo for patients with lower extremity SVT at least 5 cm long, found that fondaparinux significantly reduced the rate of DVT or PE by 85%.[16] The fondaparinux treatment group also had lower rates of extension and recurrence without an increased incidence of major bleeding. A 2018 Cochrane review, including 33 randomized controlled trials and 7120 patients, summarized that LMWH and nonsteroidal anti-inflammatory drugs (NSAIDs) reduced SVT extension and recurrence but had no effect on the development of symptomatic VTE.[3] In 2017, a trial comparing 6 weeks of prophylactic fondaparinux to 6 weeks of daily rivaroxaban found rivaroxaban was noninferior to fondaparinux in the prevention of DVT, PE, and progression or recurrence of SVT.[17] These data suggest that rivaroxaban, a less expensive and more patient-friendly treatment option, may be appropriate for patients with SVT. However, further research on direct oral anticoagulants is necessary before these are considered as first-line treatment for SVT. On the basis of current evidence and the American College of Chest Physicians (ACCP) guidelines, patients with lower extremity SVT at least 5 cm in length and >3 cm from the SFJ or SPJ should be treated with prophylactic fondaparinux (2.5 mg subcutaneously) for 45 days (grade 2B) over prophylactic LMWH (grade 2C).[9]

L Conservative management

For SVT <5 cm in length or thrombophlebitis of thrombosed varicosities, anticoagulation is not recommended (grade 2B).[9] In these cases of mild disease, treatment includes ambulation, warm compresses, elastic compression, intermittent elevation, and NSAIDs.[18,19] NSAIDs have been shown in multiple studies to effectively control and alleviate local symptoms and significantly reduce the risk of SVT extension and/or recurrence compared to placebo.[3] However, NSAIDs do not significantly affect the development of VTE and therefore are the primary treatment modality only for mild SVT (<5 cm in length), for patients with SVT >5 cm long and ≥3 cm distal to the SFJ or SPJ who cannot receive prophylactic anticoagulation, and for those patients with thrombosed varicosities.

M Repeat DUS

DUS should be performed after cessation of anticoagulation or resolution of phlebitis to document anatomic resolution of the thrombus and to evaluate the patency of the affected vein(s), because this determines subsequent management.[20]

N Therapy completed

If the vein with SVT remains thrombosed after treatment is completed and symptoms have resolved, no further treatment is needed, and the patient is counseled to return if recurrence occurs.

O Consider (interval) GSV ablation and phlebectomy after phlebitis resolves

Phlebectomy, in most cases, is not beneficial in the acute phase of SVT. However, given a 10% to 20% risk of recurrent SVT, venous ablation of veins that recanalize and demonstrate axial reflux after SVT should be considered, with appropriate patient counseling. Similarly, if SVT has involved varicosities that recanalize, phlebectomy of the involved varicosities is considered optimal treatment after the resolution of phlebitis, typically after 3 to 6 months.[7,15]

P Associated catheter?

SSVT is most commonly associated with the use of an IV catheter and occurs in up to 2% of peripheral catheter vein insertions.[14] The risk of SSVT increases when peripheral IV catheters remain inserted for >3 days.[7]

Q Remove catheter

Treatment of SSVT requires prompt removal of inciting IV catheter.

R Antibiotic treatment

Patients with SSVT are at risk of developing bacteremia and require prompt administration of IV antibiotics. For patients with peripheral vein SSVT, broad-spectrum antibiotics with activity against Staphylococci and Enterobacteriaceae should be initiated. SSVT of the jugular vein is often associated with normal oropharyngeal flora, and antibiotics should include a beta-lactamase resistant beta-lactam antibiotic.[6] Antibiotics should be tailored to qualitative blood cultures and susceptibility results when available.

S Surgical resection ± drainage

Patients with SSVT that do not respond appropriately to antimicrobial therapy and have persistent sepsis require surgical management for infection source control. Operative interventions include local exploration, abscess drainage, and full venous resection to the extent that brisk back bleeding is encountered and is anatomically feasible. Incision and drainage alone is often inadequate because the septic focus is not removed and source control is not achieved.[6,19]

REFERENCES

1. Meissner MH, Wakefield TW, Ascher E, et al. Acute venous disease: venous thrombosis and venous trauma. *J Vasc Surg.* 2007;46(suppl S):25s-53s.
2. Decousus H, Quere I, Presles E, et al. Superficial venous thrombosis and venous thromboembolism: a large, prospective epidemiologic study. *Ann Intern Med.* 2010;152(4):218-224.
3. Di Nisio M, Wichers IM, Middeldorp S. Treatment for superficial thrombophlebitis of the leg. *Cochrane Database Syst Rev.* 2018;2:CD004982.
4. Leon L, Giannoukas AD, Dodd D, Chan P, Labropoulos N. Clinical significance of superficial vein thrombosis. *Eur J Vasc Endovasc Surg.* 2005;29(1):10-17.
5. Hammond JS, Varas R, Ward CG. Suppurative thrombophlebitis: a new look at a continuing problem. *South Med J.* 1988;81(8):969-971.
6. Spelman D. Suppurative (septic) thrombophlebitis. *UpToDate.* 2018. https://www.uptodate.com/contents/suppurative-septic-thrombophlebitis. Accessed May 2, 2018.
7. Coleman D. Superficial thrombophlebitis. In: Lanzer P, ed. *PanVascular Medicine.* 2nd ed. Berlin, Heidelberg: Springer-Verlag; 2015:4483-4487.
8. De Weese MS. Nonoperative treatment of acute superficial thrombophlebitis and deep femoral venous thrombosis. In: Ernst CB, Stanley JC, eds. *Current Therapy in Vascular Surgery.* Philadelphia, PA: BC Decker.
9. Kearon C, Akl EA, Comerota AJ, et al. Antithrombotic therapy for VTE disease: antithrombotic therapy and prevention of thrombosis, 9th ed: American College of chest physicians evidence-based clinical practice guidelines. *Chest.* 2012;141(2):e419S-e496S.
10. Cannegieter SC, Horvath-Puho E, Schmidt M, et al. Risk of venous and arterial thrombotic events in patients diagnosed with superficial vein thrombosis: a nationwide cohort study. *Blood.* 2015;125(2):229-235.
11. Dalsing MC. The case against anticoagulation for superficial venous thrombosis. *Dis Mon.* 2010;56(10):582-589.
12. Hanson JN, Ascher E, DePippo P, et al. Saphenous vein thrombophlebitis (SVT): a deceptively benign disease. *J Vasc Surg.* 1998;27(4):677-680.
13. Sassu GP, Chisholm CD, Howell JM, Huang E. A rare etiology for pulmonary embolism: basilic vein thrombosis. *J Emerg Med.* 1990;8(1):45-49.
14. Di Nisio M, Peinemann F, Porreca E, Rutjes AW. Treatment for superficial infusion thrombophlebitis of the upper extremity. *Cochrane Database Syst Rev.* 2015;(11):Cd011015.
15. Sullivan V, Denk PM, Sonnad SS, Eagleton MJ, Wakefield TW. Ligation versus anticoagulation: treatment of above-knee superficial thrombophlebitis not involving the deep venous system. *J Am Coll Surg.* 2001;193(5):556-562.
16. Decousus H, Prandoni P, Mismetti P, et al. Fondaparinux for the treatment of superficial-vein thrombosis in the legs. *N Engl J Med.* 2010;363(13):1222-1232.
17. Beyer-Westendorf J, Schellong SM, Gerlach H, et al. Prevention of thromboembolic complications in patients with superficial-vein thrombosis given rivaroxaban or fondaparinux: the open-label, randomised, non-inferiority SURPRISE phase 3b trial. *Lancet Haematol.* 2017;4(3):e105-e113.
18. Lee JT, Kalani MA. Treating superficial venous thrombophlebitis. *J Natl Compr Canc Netw.* 2008;6(8):760-765.
19. Gloviczki PE, Dalsing MC, Eklof B, Lurie F, Wakefield TW, Gloviczki ML; American Venous Forum. *Handbook of Venous and Lymphatic Disorders.* Boca Raton: CRC Press; 2017.
20. Scovell SD, Ergul EA, Conrad MF. Medical management of acute superficial vein thrombosis of the saphenous vein. *J Vasc Surg Venous Lymphat Disord.* 2018;6(1):109-117.

Peter Henke

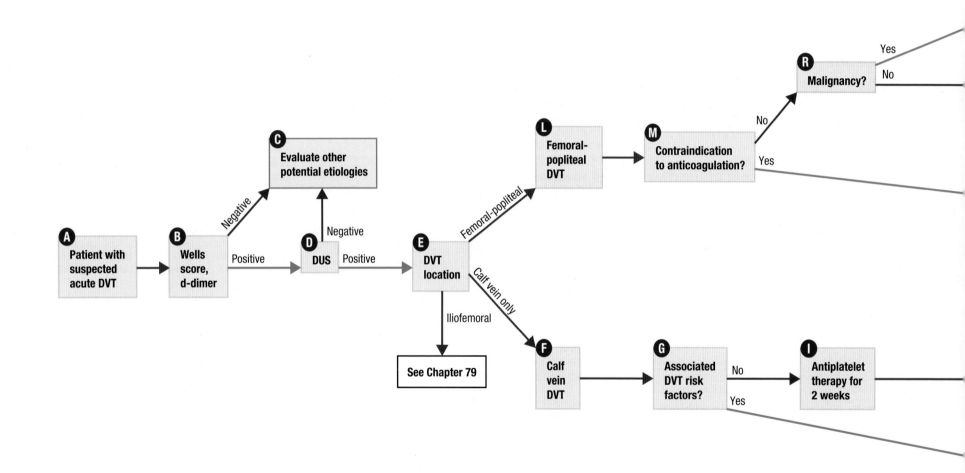

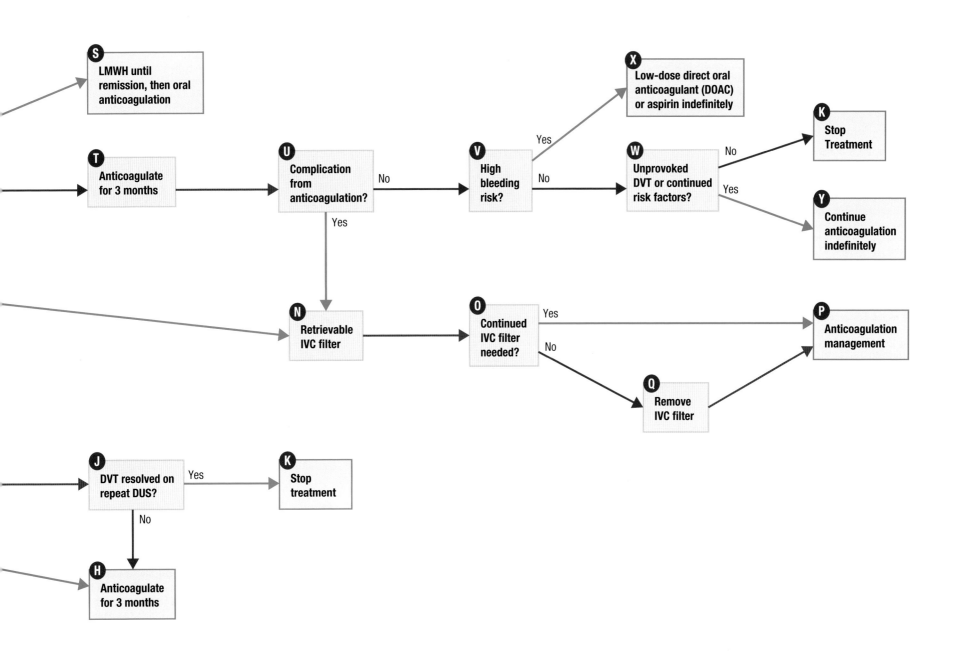

A Patient with suspected acute DVT

Patients with suspected acute DVT often present with acute onset of swelling, pain, and rubor in the affected limb. PE can present concomitantly with shortness of breath, tachycardia, hypoxia, and, occasionally, hemoptysis. Initial laboratory studies specific to DVT/PE on presentation include a complete blood count and D-dimer level. If pulmonary symptoms predominate, then a chest x-ray, pulse oxygenation, and, possibly, a CT of the chest with IV contrast are ordered.

B Wells score, D-dimer

In a patient with suspected DVT, the Wells score is calculated to increase certainty of diagnosis.[1] It is obtained by the summation of several factors, each of which is assigned 1 point. Additive sums of 2 or higher indicates that the probability of DVT is likely; a score <2 indicates a low probability of DVT. In patients with bilateral symptoms, the more symptomatic leg is used.

Scored factors include active cancer (patient receiving treatment for cancer within the previous 6 months or currently receiving palliative treatment); paralysis, paresis, or recent plaster immobilization of the lower extremities; recently bedridden for 3 days or more, or major surgery within the previous 12 weeks requiring regional or general anesthesia; localized tenderness along the distribution of the deep venous system; entire leg swollen; calf swelling at least 3 cm larger than that on the asymptomatic side (measured 10 cm below tibial tuberosity); pitting edema confined to the symptomatic leg; collateral superficial veins (nonvaricose); and previously documented DVT. Alternative diagnoses at least as likely as DVT trigger a subtraction of 2 points.[5]

Table 78-1. **Wells Score Table for DVT**	
Present	**Score**
Lower limb trauma or surgery or immobilization in a plaster cast	+1
Bedridden for more than 3 days or surgery within the last 4 wk	+1
Tenderness along the line of femoral or popliteal veins (NOT only calf tenderness)	+1
Entire limb swollen	+1
Calf more than 3 cm bigger circumference, 10 cm below tibial tuberosity	+1
Pitting edema	+1
Dilated collateral superficial veins (non-varicose)	+1
Past history of confirmed DVT	+1
Malignancy (including treatment up to 6 mo previously)	+1
Intravenous drug use	+3
Alternative diagnosis as more likely than DVT	−2

D-Dimer is a product of fibrin cleavage by plasmin and serves as a clinically useful marker of fibrinolysis. A low D-dimer (<0.5 mg/L) is used to exclude DVT in low-risk patients. Conversely, a high D-dimer (>0.5 mg/L) in combination with positive risk factors is associated with DVT in 70% of cases.[1] Therefore, D-dimer assessment has a high sensitivity but a low specificity for diagnosing DVT. Other proposed biomarkers for DVT such as factor VIII have been studied. However, their use is limited because, as acute phase reactants, their levels are often elevated in inflammatory states without the presence of DVT.[2]

C Evaluate other potential etiologies

Several alternative disease processes mimic the symptoms of DVT and should be considered in the differential diagnosis of acute DVT. These include cellulitis, osteoarthritis, lymphedema, chronic venous insufficiency, PAD, trauma, neuropathy, superficial thrombophlebitis, muscle tears, Baker cyst, varicose veins, May-Thurner syndrome, and systemic diseases leading to lower extremity swelling such as nephrotic syndrome, glomerulonephritis, or cirrhosis.[3]

D DUS

DUS should be obtained for any patient presenting with a suspected acute DVT. It is highly sensitive, specific (>95% for both), and reproducible, making it the ideal diagnostic test.[4] An acute DVT will demonstrate an echogenic mass in the lumen of the vein that is noncompressible by the DUS probe. In addition, the walls of the vein involved in acute DVT are not as echogenic because they commonly are in a chronic post-thrombotic state. Venous blood flow is often impeded with a lack of augmentation (ie, flow reversal with respiration is not present in the acute state).[5]

E DVT location

Therapy and intervention should be tailored to the affected anatomic location. Iliofemoral DVT, calf vein DVT, and femoral/popliteal DVTs are all treated differently, although leg elevation and anticoagulation are common to each. Iliofemoral DVT is considered in detail in Chapter 79.

F Calf vein DVT

Patients with calf vein (tibial, gastrocnemius, or soleal) DVT often present with mild swelling and/or tenderness of the calf. DUS is used to identify the amount of clot burden and its proximity to the popliteal vein, which help determine the type and course of treatment. In addition to considering anticoagulation, compression and leg elevation are important for this patient population.

G Associated DVT risk factors?

Patients presenting with calf vein DVT should be assessed for risk factors that would more likely lead to propagation of thrombus into the popliteal vein, such as malignancy, obesity, use of oral contraceptives (OCPs), trauma, immobility, and history of DVT

or PE. Patients with such risk factors are considered for anticoagulation treatment.

H Anticoagulate for 3 months

For patients with calf vein DVT who have significant risk factors for femoral-popliteal thrombus extension or PE, the recommended treatment is anticoagulation with LMWH or fondaparinux, followed by a vitamin K antagonist (VKA), or a DOAC for at least 3 months with reevaluation for continuation or cessation of anticoagulation (grade 1B evidence). Femoral-popliteal thrombus propagation may complicate isolated calf vein thrombosis in up to 23% of untreated patients.[6] Therefore, guidelines from the American College of Chest Physicians (ACCP) include treatment of idiopathic calf vein with either 3 months of anticoagulation[7,8] when risk factors for VTE are present (grade IIb evidence). For patients with calf vein DVT but without risk factors, anticoagulation can be considered if conservative measures including aspirin do not result in thrombus or symptom resolution.

I Antiplatelet therapy for 2 weeks

If the patient is at low risk of calf vein thrombus extension, antiplatelet therapy with aspirin (81-160 mg daily) for 2 weeks with DUS follow-up is recommended.[8]

J DVT resolved on repeat DUS?

If the calf vein DVT has resolved on repeat DUS after antiplatelet treatment, no further treatment is needed. If residual calf vein DVT persists, initiation of anticoagulation is recommended to decrease risk of recurrence; however, this decision should be balanced by bleeding risk because direct supporting evidence is lacking.

K Stop treatment

If DUS shows that the calf vein DVT has resolved, antiplatelet or anticoagulation treatment should be stopped and the patient counseled to return if new symptoms develop. Similarly, after 3 months of anticoagulation in a patient with a provoked DVT and low-risk factors for recurrent DVT, anticoagulation is stopped.

L Femoral-popliteal DVT

Thrombotic disease involving this segment comprises the bulk of DVT incidence, carries higher morbidity than does calf DVT, and has a higher risk of clot extension and PE.[9] Patients present with rubor, swelling, pain, and, if associated with a PE, shortness of breath, and hypoxia. The differential diagnosis should include cellulitis, superficial thrombophlebitis, and necrotizing fasciitis. DUS is very accurate in diagnosing DVT in this location.[1,4,5] Risk factor assessment is critical in these patients because it will dictate the type and course of treatment. All patients should receive parenteral anticoagulation following the diagnosis—most frequently with LMWH or fondaparinux and followed by a VKA or, more recently, a DOAC (grade IA evidence).[8]

Ⓜ Contraindication to anticoagulation?

Certain contraindications in patients with DVTs prohibit the use of systemic anticoagulation. These include recent or active bleeding, severe renal or liver disease, severe thrombocytopenia (ie, <70,000/mm³), recent surgical procedure (<2 weeks), and history of intracranial bleeding (traumatic, surgical or idiopathic).[10]

Ⓝ Retrievable IVC filter

Patients with DVT and contraindications to anticoagulation should be considered for PE protection in the form of an IVC filter. IVC filters can either be permanent or retrievable, inserted under fluoroscopy or ultrasound.[10] If patients have irreversible risk for continued VTE, permanent IVC filters are recommended in part because they have fewer complications compared to retrievable filters that are not removed. This is the case in patients with chronic thromboembolic pulmonary hypertension (CTPH) undergoing pulmonary thromboembolectomy, where the ACCP recommends permanent filter placement before or at the time of the procedure (grade 2C evidence). However, in most patients with acute DVT who cannot be anticoagulated, a retrievable IVC filter is recommended because it can be removed to reduce the risk of late complications when the VTE risk decreases. With >95% protection from PE, the kind of IVC filter used should be tailored to each patient. Less established indications for IVC filter usage include the presence of free-floating thrombus tails in the iliofemoral system.[11-13]

Commonly, filter placement technique involves deployment of the filter, under fluoroscopic guidance, into an infrarenal position to minimize the risk of filtered occlusive thrombus occluding the renal vein outflow. This is generally performed from the femoral or internal jugular vein access. When performing the procedure, the choice of imaging modality for deployment, location of deployment, route of access, and anatomic variations must be considered.[14] Filter placement carries low morbidity and mortality and provides adequate protection against PE, although filters can be associated with progression/recurrence of DVT, as well as IVC thrombosis. Commonly used retrievable filters include OPTEASE filter (3-week retrieval recommendation), the Gunther-Tulip filter (2-week removal recommendation), the G2 Express filter, and the Celect filter. Despite these complications, there has been a recent increase in retrievable filters for prophylaxis of PE in patients with time-limited contraindications to anticoagulation.

Ⓞ Continued IVC filter needed?

The American Heart Association guidelines recommend that patients who receive retrievable IVC filters be periodically evaluated for filter removal within the specific filter's retrieval window (grade 1C evidence).[10] The Food and Drug Administration (FDA) issued a safety alert in 2014 recommending IVC filter removal as soon as is clinically appropriate and shared the responsibility of filter removal equally between the implanting physician and the clinician responsible for the ongoing care of patients in whom a retrievable IVC filter has been placed. In many instances, the filters are not removed during the index hospitalization once the bleeding risk for prophylactic anticoagulation is passed. Improved surveillance and follow-up of these patients is important to allow for prompt removal of the filter to decrease complications such as caval wall penetration, filter fracture or migration, caval thrombosis, and DVT.[15]

Ⓟ Anticoagulation management

If the IVC filter needs to remain in place, then anticoagulation should be started as soon as clinically feasible once anticoagulation or active bleeding complications have resolved to prevent DVT propagation[10,13] (grade 1B evidence). Nevertheless, the need for the filter should continue to be assessed periodically. Once the filter is removed, anticoagulation use should be reevaluated and appropriately managed according to the patient's DVT burden and recurrence risks. One suggestion is for periodic DUS every 6 months to monitor for DVT recurrence to guide anticoagulation maintenance.

Ⓠ Remove IVC filter

The standard technique for IVC filter removal usually involves the use of a snare and sheath combination to engage, collapse, and retrieve the filter. Depending on the manufacturer, access is usually through the right jugular vein for introduction of the sheath and snare combination. The reported success rates are 80% to 90%, with success rates often correlating inversely with dwell time.[15] There are other methods for removing IVC filters (depending on the manufacturer and the filter position), although a thorough discussion of these techniques is outside the scope of this chapter.

Ⓡ Malignancy?

Patients with a history of malignancy are at higher risk of DVT. Approximately 20% of all new DVT diagnoses are associated with occult malignancy.[16] As such, all patients with primary unprovoked DVT need full evaluation for an underlying, malignant process.[17] The mechanisms contributing to the hypercoagulable state in malignancy are multifactorial.[18] About 28% of the surgical procedures for malignancy are complicated by DVT.[19] Although all forms of malignancy are suspect, mucin-producing tumors such as adenocarcinoma, small cell lung tumors, GI cancers, and ovarian cancers are most often associated with DVT.[20]

Ⓢ LMWH until remission, then oral anticoagulation

For patients with DVT and active malignancy, aggressive anticoagulation is recommended. LMWH is superior to a VKA,[21] and a VKA is not advised in this scenario. However, recent data suggest DOACs, particularly rivaroxaban, may be as efficacious as is LMWH in cancer patients.[22] If the cancer is in remission, VKA or DOACs are prescribed until the risk of DVT recurrence is judged to be low (often based on periodic surveillance of cancer). For cancers that cannot be effectively treated, anticoagulation is continued indefinitely.

Ⓣ Anticoagulate for 3 months

In patients with a DVT not due to malignancy, standard treatment dictates the use of LMWH or fondaparinux with eventual transition to VKA or DOAC (grade IA evidence). DOACs are now first-line therapy, because of their improved safety profile (compared with VKA or LMWH), decreased risk of intracranial bleeding, and availability of reversal agents.[8] For patients with a provoked DVT (caused by a known and temporary factor), 3 months of anticoagulation is recommended. For patients with an unprovoked DVT, or a persistent provoking factor(s) such that recurrent risk is high, lifelong anticoagulation is recommended if bleeding risk is low.[8] Genetic and other tests can be performed to attempt to detect an etiology (ie, factor V Leiden, antiphospholipid antibody tests, etc.) to aid in making informed family decisions, but knowledge of these genetic diseases frequently does not alter the course of treatment.[23]

Ⓤ Complication from anticoagulation?

Most complications from anticoagulation include bleeding (GI, intracranial, etc.) which can be fatal. In one meta-analysis involving 12 RCTs,[24] DOACs were shown to significantly reduce the risk of overall major bleeding, fatal bleeding, intracranial bleeding, clinically relevant nonmajor bleeding, and total bleeding. There was no significant difference in major GI bleeding between DOACs and VKAs, making DOACs a favorable consideration for long-term anticoagulation. When complications of anticoagulation occur, treatment must be modified depending on the bleeding risk and underlying DVT etiology.

Ⓥ High bleeding risk?

Patients with high bleeding risk include those with a recent history of ischemic stroke (risk of hemorrhagic conversion), intracranial hemorrhage, or recent surgery. In this patient population, IVC filters can be placed to decrease the risk of PE.

Ⓦ Unprovoked DVT or continued risk factors?

In patients with an unprovoked DVT or those with continued risk factors for recurrent DVT, lifelong anticoagulation is recommended if the bleeding risk is low (see T). In patients with a *provoked* DVT follow-up at 3 months and checking the D-dimer levels while on anticoagulation is recommended. If this result is positive (>0.5 mg/dL), then these patients should continue treatment. If the result is negative (<0.5 mg/dL), treatment may stop when considering other factors, including patient preference.[25]

Ⓧ Low-dose direct oral anticoagulant (DOAC) or aspirin indefinitely

For some patients, indefinite aspirin or a prophylactic dose of DOAC (eg, 2.5 mg daily of rivaroxaban) is recommended if the risk of bleeding is moderate. This has been shown to reduce the rate of major vascular events with improved clinical benefits, although the rates of recurrent VTE reduction were not statistically significant.[26,27] Thus, therapeutic aspirin or prophylactic dose DOAC is beneficial for patients with unprovoked DVT if they are at high risk for recurrence but too high a bleeding risk for full-dose DOAC.

ⓨ Continue anticoagulation indefinitely

For patients with an unprovoked DVT, recurrent VTE or ongoing high-risk, prolonged anticoagulation is recommended if the bleeding risk is low so that benefits outweigh the harms.[8] Further, use of the DOAC rivaroxaban is associated with a significant decrease in recurrent VTE without a significant increase in bleeding incidence.[28]

REFERENCES

1. Hull RD, Stein PD, Ghali WA, Cornuz J. Diagnostic algorithms for deep vein thrombosis: work in progress. *Am J Med.* 2002;113(8):687-688.
2. Rosendaal FR. High levels of factor VIII and venous thrombosis. *Thromb Haemost.* 2000;83(1):1-2.
3. Kahn SR. The clinical diagnosis of deep venous thrombosis: integrating incidence, risk factors, and symptoms and signs. *Arch Intern Med.* 1998;158(21):2315-2323.
4. Zierler BK. Screening for acute DVT: optimal utilization of the vascular diagnostic laboratory. *Semin Vasc Surg.* 2001;14(3):206-214.
5. Comerota AJ, Katz ML, Hashemi HA. Venous duplex imaging for the diagnosis of acute deep venous thrombosis. *Haemostasis.* 1993;23(suppl 1):61-71.
6. Philbrick JT, Becker DM. Calf deep venous thrombosis. A wolf in sheep's clothing? *Arch Intern Med.* 1988;148(10):2131-2138.
7. Kearon C, Akl EA, Comerota AJ, et al. Antithrombotic therapy for VTE disease: antithrombotic therapy and prevention of thrombosis, 9th ed: American College of Chest Physicians Evidence-Based Clinical Practice Guidelines. *Chest.* 2012;141(2 suppl):e419S-e96S.
8. Kearon C, Akl EA, Ornelas J, et al. Antithrombotic therapy for VTE disease: CHEST guideline and expert panel report. *Chest.* 2016;149(2):315-352.
9. Cornuz J, Ghali WA, Hayoz D, Stoianov R, Depairon M, Yersin B. Clinical prediction of deep venous thrombosis using two risk assessment methods in combination with rapid quantitative D-dimer testing. *Am J Med.* 2002;112(3):198-203.
10. DeYoung E, Minocha J. Inferior vena cava filters: guidelines, best practice, and expanding indications. *Semin Intervent Radiol.* 2016;33(2):65-70.
11. Baadh AS, Zikria JF, Rivoli S, Graham RE, Javit D, Ansell JE. Indications for inferior vena cava filter placement: do physicians comply with guidelines? *J Vasc Interv Radiol.* 2012;23(8):989-995.
12. PREPIC Study Group. Eight-year follow-up of patients with permanent vena cava filters in the prevention of pulmonary embolism the PREPIC (Prévention du Risque d'Embolie Pulmonaire par Interruption Cave) randomized study. *Circulation.* 2005;112(3):416-422.
13. Sing RF, Fischer PE. Inferior vena cava filters: indications and management. *Curr Opin Cardiol.* 2013;28(6):625-631.
14. Doe C, Ryu RK. Anatomic and technical considerations: inferior vena cava filter placement. *Semin Intervent Radiol.* 2016;33(2):88-92.
15. Kuyumcu G, Walker TG. Inferior vena cava filter retrievals, standard and novel techniques. *Cardiovasc Diagn Ther.* 2016;6(6):642-650.
16. Bergqvist D, Caprini JA, Dotsenko O, Kakkar AK, Mishra RG, Wakefield TW. Venous thromboembolism and cancer. *Curr Probl Surg.* 2007;44(3):157-216.
17. Oger E, Leroyer C, Le Moigne E, et al. The value of a risk factor analysis in clinically suspected deep venous thrombosis. *Respiration.* 1997;64(5):326-330.
18. Rickles FR, Falanga A. Molecular basis for the relationship between thrombosis and cancer. *Thromb Res.* 2001;102(6):V215-V224.
19. Clagett GP, Reisch JS. Prevention of venous thromboembolism in general surgical patients. Results of meta-analysis. *Ann Surg.* 1988;208(2):227-240.
20. Levitan N, Dowlati A, Remick SC, et al. Rates of initial and recurrent thromboembolic disease among patients with malignancy versus those without malignancy. Risk analysis using Medicare claims data. *Medicine (Baltimore).* 1999;78(5):285-291.
21. Lee AY, Levine MN, Baker RI, et al. Low-molecular-weight heparin versus a coumarin for the prevention of recurrent venous thromboembolism in patients with cancer. *N Engl J Med.* 2003;349(2):146-153.
22. Smith M, Wakam G, Wakefield T, Obi A. New trends in anticoagulation therapy. *Surg Clin North Am.* 2018;98(2):219-238.
23. Connors JM. Thrombophilia testing and venous thrombosis. *N Engl J Med.* 2017;377(12):1177-1187.
24. Chai-Adisaksopha C, Crowther M, Isayama T, Lim W. The impact of bleeding complications in patients receiving target-specific oral anticoagulants: a systematic review and meta-analysis. *Blood.* 2014;124(15):2450-2458.
25. Palareti G, Cosmi B, Legnani C, et al. D-dimer testing to determine the duration of anticoagulation therapy. *N Engl J Med.* 2006;355(17):1780-1789.
26. Brighton TA, Eikelboom JW, Mann K, et al. Low-dose aspirin for preventing recurrent venous thromboembolism. *N Engl J Med.* 2012;367(21):1979-1987.
27. Becattini C, Agnelli G, Schenone A, et al. Aspirin for preventing the recurrence of venous thromboembolism. *N Engl J Med.* 2012;366(21):1959-1967.
28. Weitz JI, Lensing AWA, Prins MH, et al. Rivaroxaban or aspirin for extended treatment of venous thromboembolism. *N Engl J Med.* 2017;376(13):1211-1222.

Marc A. Passman

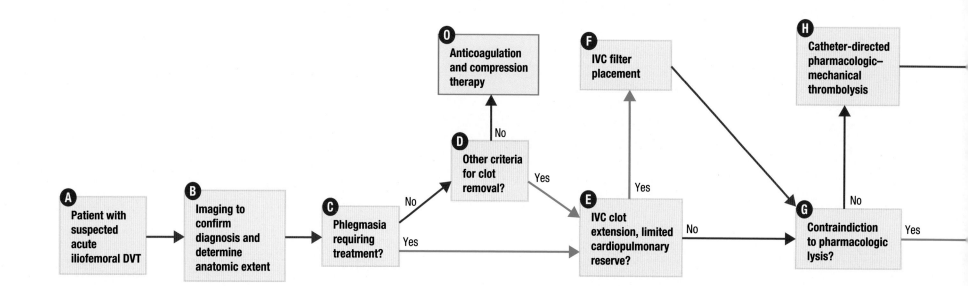

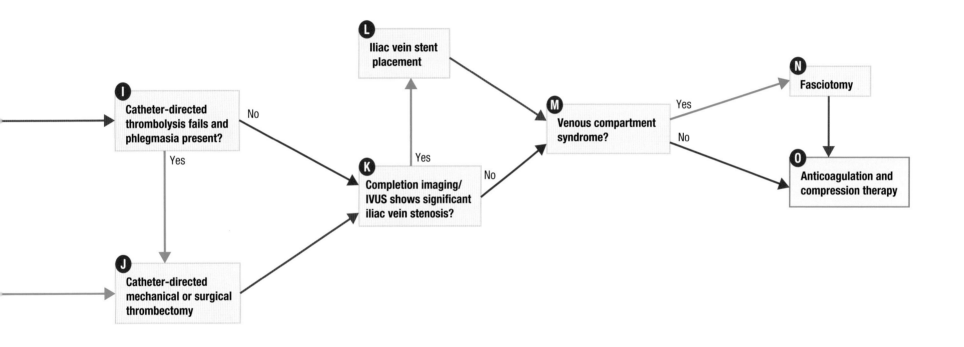

(A) Patient with suspected acute iliofemoral DVT

Iliofemoral DVT involves complete or partial thrombosis of the iliac vein and/or the common femoral vein, ± extension into the IVC and is often associated with femoropopliteal DVT.[1] Iliofemoral DVT accounts for one quarter of all cases of DVT.[2,3] It usually presents with sudden onset of unilateral lower extremity pain and swelling, which is more severe than femoropopliteal DVT alone on initial presentation, with bilateral symptoms suggesting possible involvement of the IVC.[4] Progression to massive edema and cyanosis (phlegmasia cerulea dolens) is more likely with iliofemoral than femoropopliteal DVT and, as such, iliofemoral DVT is associated with a higher risk of adverse outcomes, including recurrent VTE and post-thrombotic syndrome.[5] In selected patients with iliofemoral DVT, therapeutic strategies to reduce or remove thrombus have resulted in improved long-term vessel patency and reduced post-thrombotic syndrome relative to anticoagulation alone.[6] Evidence-based guidelines support catheter-based therapy for selected patients with iliofemoral DVT, although benefit is equivocal for those with femoral–popliteal DVT.[7-9] Patients with femoral–popliteal DVT should be treated with standard anticoagulation recommendations (see Chapter 78).

(B) Imaging to confirm diagnosis and determine anatomic extent

Diagnostic evaluation should begin with a lower extremity venous DUS to confirm presence and anatomic location of DVT (see Chapter 78). Whereas DUS has a mean sensitivity and specificity of 97% and 94%, with a mean positive and negative predictive value of 97% and 98%, for symptomatic proximal DVT, direct imaging of the iliac veins and IVC can be limited by excess bowel gas, large body habitus, postsurgical abdomen, and prior IVC filter.[10] Indirect findings in the common femoral vein that suggest iliac venous outflow issues can include continuous venous flow, absent respiratory variation, and inability to augment with Valsalva. These findings cannot differentiate nonocclusive thrombus from extrinsic compression. CT or MR venography should be performed when there is a high clinical suspicion of iliofemoral DVT to confirm diagnosis and to help guide further decisions for possible clot removal options.[11-13]

(C) Phlegmasia requiring treatment?

For patients with severe iliofemoral DVT causing critical venous outflow obstruction, clinical findings consistent with severe venous congestion will be present. Phlegmasia alba dolens ("painful white edema" or "milk leg"), classically seen during pregnancy and postpartum, may indicate iliofemoral compression resulting in associated lymphedema, but is not necessarily associated with iliofemoral DVT if limb ischemia is absent. Phlegmasia cerulea dolens ("painful blue edema") is characterized by sudden severe pain, swelling, cyanosis, and edema of the affected leg resulting from acute massive venous thrombosis compromising venous

outflow and, eventually, arterial inflow. Progression to venous ischemic gangrene and potential risk of limb loss can occur when high compartment pressure from venous outflow obstruction compromises arterial tissue perfusion. In addition to venous assessment, arterial segmental Doppler testing and ABIs are needed to assess arterial perfusion. Neurologic function of the leg should be documented and assessment for potential compartment syndrome should be performed (see Chapter 51).

(D) Other criteria for clot removal?

Current evidence-based guidelines support consideration for possible venous clot removal options in select patients with first-time acute iliofemoral DVT (<14 days), who are ambulatory with good functional status, low risk of bleeding, life expectancy >1 year, and have severe symptoms of venous congestion or ischemia.[5,7,8,9,14,15] Although these criteria should be considered independently, they are not mutually inclusive or exclusive. Each decision point is most critically driven by clinical severity of symptoms and limb risk, which may still justify proceeding with venous intervention based on risk–benefit profile independent of these criteria.[16] There may also be additional considerations for venous clot removal options for patients with recurrent iliofemoral DVT or those presenting with thrombosis of a previously placed venous stent, based on acuity and severity of venous congestion, although there are no current evidence-based guidelines addressing these scenarios.[17] Ultimately, the decision of whether to proceed with venous clot removal options for these clinical scenarios is based on balancing the potential margin of symptomatic improvement, potential to prevent post-thrombotic syndrome, and improved quality of life versus the overall risk of therapy, including bleeding, PE, and recurrent DVT.

(E) IVC clot extension, limited cardiopulmonary reserve?

Although catheter-directed clot removal may be associated with asymptomatic radiographic evidence of PE, symptomatic PE is relatively a rare complication.[18] Placement of IVC filters in conjunction with catheter-directed thrombolysis or operative thrombectomy of iliofemoral DVT is not routinely recommended.[5] IVC filters should be selectively considered in patients with DVT extending into the IVC or those with markedly limited cardiopulmonary reserve, especially if there has been previous PE (see Chapter 82).[19] IVC filter placement might also be considered in patients undergoing catheter-directed thrombolysis in which excessive manipulation of thrombus is anticipated based on thrombus burden and planned catheter approach, although there is no specific guidelines to determine this potential. IVC filters should not be used when operative thrombectomy is required, given the risk of dislodgement with passage of operative thrombectomy catheters.

(F) IVC filter placement

If an IVC filter is placed, a retrievable filter should be used, unless there is an independent indication for permanent filter placement

(see Chapter 78). There should be a plan for filter retrieval shortly after catheter-directed therapy is completed.

(G) Contraindication to pharmacologic lysis?

CDT for iliofemoral DVT that includes use of lytic agents is associated with increased risk of bleeding. Absolute contraindications to lytic therapy include active bleeding, recent head trauma (within 3 months), intracranial hemorrhage, stroke (within 3 months), intracranial AVM, neoplasm, or intracranial aneurysm; and neurosurgery (within 3 months), major surgery (within 3 weeks), known bleeding diathesis, and pregnancy. Relative contraindications that increase bleeding risk but in which lysis may be considered under special circumstances include age >75 years, minor head trauma, prior GI or urinary tract bleeding, seizures, recent arterial puncture at a noncompressible site, thrombocytopenia (platelet <100,000), recent lumbar puncture or epidural catheter, oral anticoagulation medication, poorly controlled HTN, and postpartum (<1 week) and recent prolonged cardiopulmonary resuscitation. In each scenario, the relative benefit of catheter-directed thrombolysis needs to be weighed against the potential risk of bleeding.[7-9,20]

(H) Catheter-directed pharmacologic–mechanical thrombolysis

Percutaneous CDT (pharmacologic or pharmaco-mechanical) is recommended as a first-line treatment strategy for thrombus removal in patients with iliofemoral DVT because of the greater risk of complications with surgical thrombectomy.[5] Thrombolytic dosing depends on the pharmacologic agent, method of delivery, and anticipated duration of therapy, and practitioners should be familiar with pharmacologic profiles of the lytic agent used. A strategy of pharmaco-mechanical thrombolysis that combines lytics with mechanical catheter thrombectomy options, including aspiration, rheolytic, rotational, or ultrasonic-assisted devices, should be considered over catheter-directed pharmacologic thrombolysis alone because this improves the efficiency of thrombolysis (>50% lysis in 83%-100% of patients undergoing pharmaco-mechanical), reduces lytic doses and procedure times (76 ± 34 minutes for pharmaco-mechanical vs. 18 ± 8 hours for catheter-directed thrombolysis alone), and lessens bleeding complications (<1% major bleeding with 4.2%-14% patients with minor bleeding requiring a transfusion for pharmaco-mechanical lysis).[21,22]

(I) Catheter-directed thrombolysis fails and phlegmasia present?

If CDT is unsuccessful or technically not possible, there are contraindication(s) to thrombolytic agent, or the patient has ongoing limb-threatening phlegmasia, then surgical iliofemoral thrombectomy should be considered in patients who are appropriate surgical candidates to avoid amputation.

J Catheter-directed mechanical or surgical thrombectomy

Open surgical venous thrombectomy is recommended in selected patients who are candidates for anticoagulation but in whom thrombolytic therapy is contraindicated or unsuccessful.[5,23] Alternatively, mechanical thrombectomy catheter alone (without use of lytic agents) may be considered in patients who can still be anticoagulated but are at higher risk for operative approaches. Occasionally, a hybrid strategy that combines open surgical approaches with use of mechanical thrombectomy catheters can be an option to facilitate clot removal. Important technical considerations include preoperative imaging to demonstrate the proximal extent of thrombus, intraoperative use of positive end-expiratory pressure to reduce the risk of PE, intraoperative completion venography to ensure patency of the iliac vein, stenting of any identified iliac vein lesions, use of a temporary AVF to reduce early rethrombosis, and need for postoperative anticoagulation.[24] Operative technique is usually performed from a femoral approach using balloon thrombectomy catheters for the more proximal iliac vein segments and Esmarch compression from distal ankle/calf to proximal thigh for the distal thrombus based on valve directional flow. For extension of clot into the IVC, transabdominal approach may also be required for direct thrombectomy of the IVC. Although thrombectomy does appear to be associated with improved long-term outcomes after iliofemoral DVT, the overall quality of the data supporting its use as a primary therapy is low, and there is little evidence allowing a reliable risk versus benefit analysis.[25]

K Completion imaging/IVUS shows significant iliac vein stenosis?

Underlying compressive or obstructive iliac vein lesions can cause or contribute to iliofemoral DVT.[14] After patency of iliofemoral vein segments is restored, additional imaging should be performed to evaluate for a potential residual iliac vein lesion >50% diameter reduction, which may be present in two-thirds of patients.[26] Single-plane venography is relatively insensitive in detecting iliocaval compression. Multiplanar venography can improve sensitivity, especially in the presence of venous collateral drainage. IVUS has been shown to be more sensitive for assessing treatable iliofemoral vein stenosis compared with multiplanar venography and can detect residual thrombus that may be missed by venography. IVUS more frequently leads to revised treatment plans and the potential for improved clinical outcome.[27]

L Iliac vein stent placement

If a significant iliac vein stenosis is identified, a stent should be placed to prevent recurrent thrombosis. Flexible, large-diameter, self-expanding stents, extending into the IVC and common femoral vein, if indicated, are preferred for use in the iliac veins.[5] Adequate inflow and outflow through the stent is required and should be free of residual thrombus. If adequate inflow or outflow cannot

be established, additional operative thrombectomy/endophlebectomy to remove any residual thrombus, intimal defects, and scar tissue may be required in conjunction with stent placement.

M Venous compartment syndrome?

With prolonged severe leg swelling, patients with iliofemoral DVT are at risk for venous compartment syndrome. Compartment syndrome should be suspected if there is ongoing severe pain, diminished pulses, decreased motor function, numbness, or a pale color of the affected limb despite restoration of venous patency. If diagnosis is in question, intracompartmental pressures can be measured with a needle transducer connected to a catheter inserted into the compartment (see Chapter 51). A pressure >30 mm Hg is associated with compartment syndrome and fasciotomy is indicated.

N Fasciotomy

If compartment syndrome is present, fasciotomy should be performed (see Chapter 51).

O Anticoagulation and compression therapy

For patients who do not require iliofemoral thrombus removal or after such treatment, standard therapeutic anticoagulation and compression therapy is recommended based on current evidence-based guidelines[5,6] (see Chapter 78). For patients who underwent iliofemoral thrombus removal, once patency has been achieved, standard therapeutic anticoagulation should be continued. If a stent is needed, additional extended therapeutic anticoagulation beyond 6 months may be required to maintain stent patency.[28] Although iliofemoral patency has been restored, there may still be leg swelling, especially if there is associated femoropopliteal DVT. Graduated compression stockings (at least 30-40 mm Hg) are also an essential component after DVT to reduce symptomatic swelling, although impact on post-thrombotic syndrome may be equivocal (20% incidence of mild-to-moderate and 11% severe post-thrombotic syndrome).[6,29]

REFERENCES

1. Vedantham S, Millward SF, Cardella JF, et al. Society of interventional radiology position statement: treatment of acute iliofemoral deep vein thrombosis with use of adjunctive catheter-directed intrathrombus thrombolysis. *J Vasc Interv Radiol.* 2006;17(4):613-616.
2. Liu D, Peterson E, Dooner J, et al. Diagnosis and management of iliofemoral deep vein thrombosis: clinical practice guideline. *CMAJ.* 2015;187(17):1288-1296.
3. Vedantham S, Thorpe PE, Cardella JF, et al.; CIRSE and SIR Standards of Practice Committees. Quality improvement guidelines for the treatment of lower extremity deep vein thrombosis with use of endovascular thrombus removal. *J Vasc Interv Radiol.* 2009;20(7 suppl):S227-S239.
4. Hill SL, Martin D, McDannald ER Jr, Donato AT. Early diagnosis of iliofemoral venous thrombosis by Doppler examination. *Am J Surg.* 1988;156:11-15.
5. Watson LI, Armon MP. Thrombolysis for acute deep vein thrombosis. *Cochrane Database Syst Rev.* 2004;(4):CD002783.
6. Enden T, Haig Y, Kløw NE, et al.; CaVenT Study Group. Long-term outcome after additional catheter-directed thrombolysis versus standard treatment for acute iliofemoral deep vein thrombosis (the CaVenT study): a randomised controlled trial. *Lancet.* 2012;379:31-38.
7. Meisner MD, Gloviczki P, Comerota AJ, et al. Early thrombus removal strategies for acute deep vein thrombosis: clinical practice guidelines of the society for vascular surgery and the American venous forum. *J Vasc Surg.* 2012;55:1449-1462.
8. Kearon C, Akl EA, Ornelas J, et al. Antithrombotic therapy for VTE disease CHEST guideline and expert panel report. *Chest.* 2016;149(2):315-352.
9. Vendantham S, Goldhaber SZ, Julian JA, et al. Pharmacomechanical catheter-directed thrombolysis for deep-vein thrombosis. *N Engl J Med.* 2017;377:2240-2252.
10. Kearon C, Julian JA, Math M, Newman TE, Ginsberg JS. Noninvasive diagnosis of deep venous thrombosis. McMaster diagnostic imaging practice guidelines initiative. *Ann Intern Med.* 1998;128:663-677.
11. Orbell JH, Smith A, Burnand KG, Waltham M. Imaging of deep vein thrombosis. *Br J Surg.* 2008;95:137-146.
12. Thomas SM, Goodacre SW, Sampson FC, van Beek EJ. Diagnostic value of CT for deep vein thrombosis: results of a systematic review and meta-analysis. *Clin Radiol.* 2008;63:299-304.
13. Bates SM, Jaeschke R, Stevens SM, et al. Diagnosis of DVT: antithrombotic therapy and prevention of thrombosis, 9th ed: American College of Chest Physicians evidence-based clinical practice guidelines. *Chest.* 2012;141(2 suppl):e351S-e418S.
14. Vedantham S, Thorpe PE, Cardella JF, et al. Quality improvement guidelines for the treatment of lower extremity deep vein thrombosis with use of endovascular thrombus removal. *J Vasc Interv Radiol.* 2006;17:435-447.
15. Watson L, Broderick C, Armon MP. Thrombolysis for acute deep vein thrombosis. *Cochrane Database Syst Rev.* 2016;(11):CD002783.
16. Mewissen MW, Seabrook GR, Meissner MH, Cynamon J, Labropoulos N, Haughton SH. Catheter-directed thrombolysis for lower extremity deep venous thrombosis: report of a national multicenter registry. *Radiology.* 1999;211:39-49.
17. Neglén P, Hollis KC, Olivier J, Raju S. Stenting of the venous outflow in chronic venous disease: long-term stent related outcome, clinical, and hemodynamic result. *J Vasc Surg.* 2007;46:979-990.
18. Kölbel T, Alhadad A, Acosta S, Lindh M, Ivancev K, Gottsäter A. Thrombus embolization into IVC filters during

catheter-directed thrombolysis for proximal deep venous thrombosis. *J Endovasc Ther.* 2008;15:605-613.

19. Arko FR, Davis CM III, Murphy EH, et al. Aggressive percutaneous mechanical thrombectomy of deep venous thrombosis: early clinical results. *Arch Surg.* 2007;142:513-518.

20. Vedantham S, Piazza G, Sista AK, Goldenberg NA. Guidance for the use of thrombolytic therapy for the treatment of venous thromboembolism. *J Thromb Thrombolysis.* 2016;41:68-80.

21. Karthikesalingam A, Young EL, Hinchliffe RJ, Loftus IM, Thompson MM, Holt PJ. A systematic review of percutaneous mechanical thrombectomy in the treatment of deep venous thrombosis. *Eur J Vasc Endovasc Surg.* 2011;41:554-565.

22. Dasari TW, Pappy RM, Hennebry TA. Pharmacomechanical thrombolysis of acute and chronic symptomatic deep vein thrombosis: a systematic review of literature. *Angiology.* 2012;63:138-145.

23. Plate G, Einarsson E, Ohlin P, Jensen R, Qvarfordt P, Eklöf B. Thrombectomy with temporary arteriovenous fistula: the treatment of choice in acute iliofemoral venous thrombosis. *J Vasc Surg.* 1984;1:867-876.

24. Eklof B, Arfvidsson B, Kistner RL, Masuda EM. Indications for surgical treatment of iliofemoral vein thrombosis. *Hematol/Oncol Clin North Am.* 2000;14:471-482.

25. Casey ET, Munrad MH, Zumeta Garcia M, et al. Treatment of acute iliofemoral deep vein thrombosis: a systematic review and meta-analysis. *J Vasc Surg.* 2012;55(5):1463-1473.

26. Lin PH, Zhou W, Dardik A, et al. Catheter-direct thrombolysis versus pharmacomechanical thrombectomy for treatment of symptomatic lower extremity deep venous thrombosis. *Am J Surg.* 2006;192:782-788.

27. Gagne PJ, Tahara RW, Fastabend CP, et al. Venography versus intravascular ultrasound for diagnosing and treating iliofemoral vein obstruction. *J Vasc Surg Venous Lymphati Disord.* 2017;5(5):678-681.

28. Protack CD, Bakken AM, Patel N, Saad WE, Waldman DL, Davies MG. Long-term outcomes of catheter directed thrombolysis for lower extremity deep venous thrombosis without prophylactic inferior vena cava filter placement. *J Vasc Surg.* 2007;45:992-997.

29. Prandoni P, Lensing AW, Prins MH, et al. Below-knee elastic compression stockings to prevent the post-thrombotic syndrome: a randomized, controlled trial. *Ann Intern Med.* 2004;141:249-256.

Aleem K. Mirza • Manju Kalra

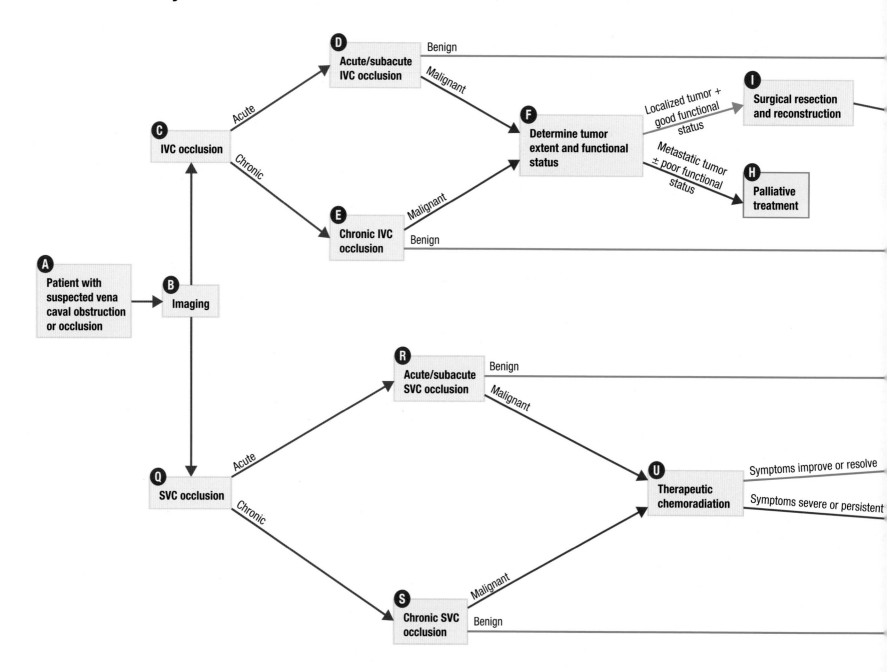

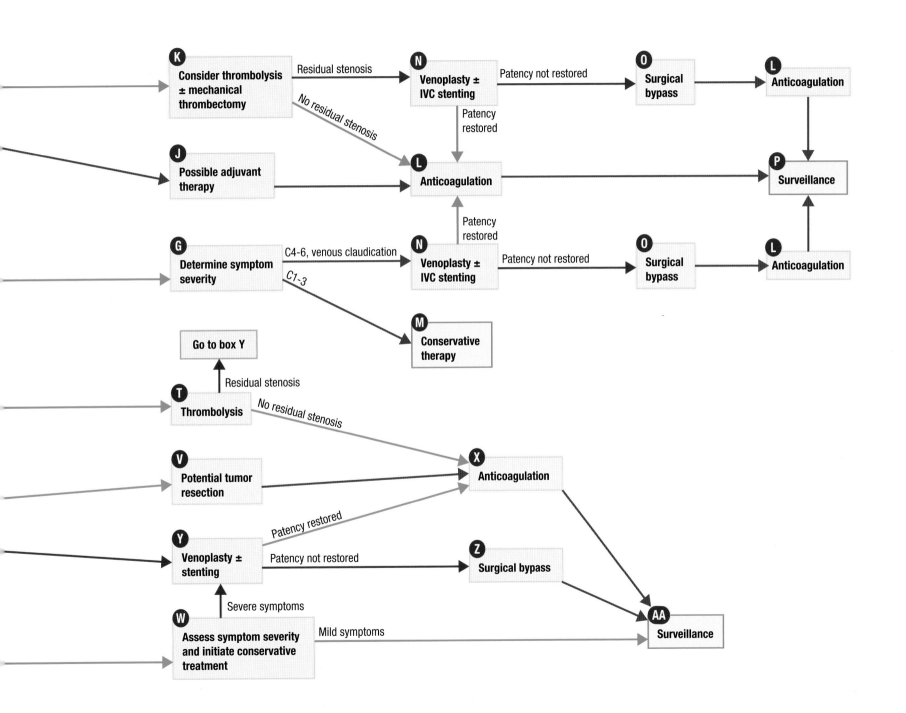

A Patient with suspected vena caval obstruction or occlusion

IVC occlusion can be caused by central propagation of iliofemoral venous thrombosis, thrombosis around an IVC filter, or compression or invasion by tumor. It is often underdiagnosed because lower extremity signs and symptoms predominate without specific signs of IVC occlusion. Unfortunately, extension of acute iliofemoral thrombosis to the IVC portends worse patient outcomes, including doubling of mortality.

SVC or innominate vein occlusions most often occur secondary to metastatic lung cancer with compression by mediastinal lymphadenopathy or primary mediastinal malignancy in 60% of cases.[1-3] However, the escalating use of central venous catheters and cardiac pacemakers is contributing to a rapid increase in nonmalignant etiologies of SVC occlusion and have overtaken the more traditional nonmalignant etiologies of mediastinal fibrosis, granulomatous fungal disease, previous radiation to the mediastinum, retrosternal goiter, and aortic dissection.

Signs and symptoms of venous congestion of the lower extremities and head, neck, and upper extremities resulting from IVC and SVC occlusion, respectively, are determined by the duration, progression, and extent of the venous occlusive disease and by the amount of collateral venous circulation that develops. The degree of symptoms may not accurately reflect the extent of vena caval stenosis/occlusion, so imaging is necessary to confirm the diagnosis and plan treatment.

B Imaging

The initial imaging modality for patients with suspected IVC obstruction is DUS. However, DUS may be limited because of patient obesity or overlying bowel gas. Indirect evidence from loss of femoral venous phasicity and waveform blunting may suggest IVC obstruction. Once suspected CT or MR venography is necessary for definitive diagnosis and treatment planning, the latter being the superior imaging modality, especially in patients with an associated tumor. Anatomic extent of thrombosis is classified according to whether the IVC involvement is infrarenal, suprarenal, or both, ± additional uni-/bilateral iliac vein involvement.[4]

SVC occlusion is classified into four venographic (DSA, CT venography, or MR venography) patterns originally described by Stanford and Doty,[5] each having a different venous collateral network depending on the site and extent of SVC obstruction. Type I is partial SVC occlusion, whereas type II is complete or near-complete SVC obstruction, with flow in the azygos vein remaining antegrade. Type III is 90% to 100% SVC obstruction with reversed azygos blood flow, whereas type IV is extensive mediastinal central venous occlusion with venous return occurring through the IVC.

Although the SVC itself cannot be directly visualized, SVC obstruction can be suggested by DUS of the central veins (internal jugular, subclavian, and innominate). Plain film radiographs may detect an underlying lung malignancy or mediastinal mass often associated with SVC obstruction. However, either CT or MR venography is essential for confirming SVS obstruction and evaluating the extent of the occlusion.

C IVC occlusion

The annual number of IVC thromboses in the United States is estimated at 5000 with an incidence of 1.7 and 1.8/100,000 in men and women, respectively.[6] Thrombosis associated with IVC filters is increasingly common as more filters are placed and often not removed.[6] In the long-term, IVC filters are associated with total and partial IVC thrombosis in 7.3% and 5.2% of patients, respectively.[7] Significant sequelae of untreated IVC thrombosis include post-thrombotic syndrome occurring in up to 90% of patients, venous claudication in 45%, PE in 30%, and rarely phlegmasia and renal failure from extension across renal veins.[8,9] Management of IVC occlusion depends on whether it is acute or chronic. Acute IVC occlusion is defined if symptoms have been present <14 days, subacute if between 15 and 28 days, and chronic if >28 days.

D Acute/subacute IVC occlusion

Signs and symptoms of acute/subacute IVC thrombosis are similar to those of iliofemoral DVT, but lower extremity symptoms (heaviness, pain, swelling, discoloration, and cramping) may be preceded by nonspecific back, abdominal, or pelvic pain and genital swelling. Risk factors for acute thrombosis of the IVC are the same as those for iliofemoral DVT (see Chapter 78). Additional risk factors unique to IVC thrombosis include the presence of congenital IVC anomalies and unretrieved IVC filters. Congenital anomalies, including absence of the infrarenal or suprarenal/hepatic IVC with azygos continuation, have a prevalence of 0.5% to 1.0% in the general population and 2% to 3% in patients with congenital cardiac defects. Congenital anomalies are associated with eventual IVC thrombosis in 60% to 80% of patients who have them. Symptoms are precipitated by thrombosis of the robust collaterals that initially keep these patients asymptomatic into adulthood, when additional factors enhance thrombosis risk. Tumors arising from or compressing/invading the IVC and IVC filters can also cause luminal obstruction and thrombosis of the IVC; however, this process is usually insidious and associated with concomitant development of adequate collaterals, thereby making an acute presentation extremely rare.

Anticoagulation is the principal treatment of acute/subacute IVC thrombosis and should be initiated at the time of diagnosis. Additional adjunctive treatment modalities are instituted selectively depending on the severity of the presentation and the potentially rare cases associated with malignancy.

E Chronic IVC occlusion

Fibrotic transformation of IVC thrombus commences after 2 weeks and progresses thereafter with the resultant effect of stenosis or occlusion. Signs and symptoms of chronic IVC occlusion range from none to those of advanced chronic venous insufficiency with lower extremity venous claudication, swelling, lipodermatosclerosis, and venous ulceration depending on the extent of iliofemoral venous occlusion. Isolated caval occlusion may be asymptomatic, especially if slow to develop, because of concomitant collateralization of flow around the occluded segment.

The presence of nonretrieved IVC filters is the most common predisposing factor for chronic IVC thrombosis. Other predisposing risk factors include recurrent thrombosis in the setting of hypercoagulable states, IVC compression or invasion by tumor, and congenital anomalies/atresia. Therapeutic anticoagulation is the initial treatment in this chronic setting, with additional treatment dependent on whether the chronic occlusion is associated with a malignant tumor versus a benign thrombotic problem.

F Determine tumor extent and functional status

Tumors can cause IVC thrombosis that can present acutely, but more often chronically, as collateral circulation develops with gradual tumor compression or invasion of the IVC. The most common primary IVC tumor is leiomyosarcoma, preferentially affecting women aged 50 to 60 years. It is usually intracaval, invades surrounding structures, and metastasizes early. Other tumors invade the IVC from outside, the most common being retroperitoneal sarcoma, which usually affects the infrarenal IVC, although invasion can occur at any level.[10] Tumor thrombus within the IVC is most frequently seen with renal cell carcinoma, with extension into the suprarenal IVC occurring in 40% of cases and right atrial extension in 10%.[11] As occlusion of the IVC from intraluminal tumor growth or extrinsic compression occurs gradually, lower extremity swelling is an infrequent symptom, seen in <30% of patients at presentation. Patients typically present with abdominal/back pain, fatigue, or nonspecific symptoms related to the malignancy.

Treatment of IVC occlusion by a tumor depends on whether the tumor is resectable and considers the functional and surgical risk status of the patient. Imaging with CT, MR, and/or PET scanning is used to define the exact location and tumor extent and whether metastases exist. If the tumor is locally resectable and without metastatic involvement, preoperative evaluation should be performed to determine if the patient's functional status and surgical risk justify tumor and IVC resection with reconstruction.

G Determine symptom severity

In patients with chronic, benign IVC occlusion, the clinical spectrum is very wide, with severity of symptoms dependent largely on the degree of collateralization. Symptoms range from lower extremity swelling alone in well-compensated patients to venous stasis, ulceration, and/or chronic back and pelvic pain. It is important to grade the severity of venous insufficiency and reserve intervention (endovascular or surgical) for patients with CEAP clinical class 4 to 6 or young patients with lifestyle-limiting venous claudication. Conservative management is appropriate for patients with CEAP clinical class 1 to 3 (see Chapter 73).

Ⓗ Palliative treatment

Patients with aggressive tumor types, distant metastases, and/or poor functional status or excessive surgical risk should be offered palliative treatment. Palliative treatment for the IVC occlusion includes anticoagulation, graduated compression stockings, and palliative oncologic treatment for those patients with tumors.

Ⓘ Surgical resection and reconstruction

For patients with tumors involving <60% of the IVC diameter over a short (<7 cm) segment, bovine pericardium patch venoplasty can be used after tumor resection. For patients with >60% diameter involvement, or >7 cm length involvement, with poor collateral flow around the obstruction, IVC replacement is necessary. This should be performed with externally supported ePTFE (resists compression in the abdomen), utilizing grafts ranging from 12 to 20 mm in diameter.[12] Unlike arterial anastomoses, we recommend that the ePTFE rings be persevered on the graft immediately adjacent to the venous anastomosis to prevent anastomotic stenosis. Five-year patency rates are reported as high as 90% to 92%.[12] Operative challenges unique to IVC replacement include control of the iliocaval confluence and anomalous lumbar vein anatomy. Replacement across the pararenal IVC can be completed without renal vein reconstruction depending on drainage of the kidney through collateral veins, but renal vein reimplantation is preferred to prevent renal failure. Retrohepatic and suprahepatic tumor/IVC resection and replacement can require several additional technical adjuncts, including total hepatic vascular isolation and selective use of cardiopulmonary bypass and hypothermia.[13] For patients with chronic occlusion of the IVC and adequate collateralization, tumor plus infrarenal IVC resection without graft replacement is recommended.

Ⓙ Possible adjuvant therapy

Traditionally, surgical resection has been considered the only therapeutic modality for tumors involving the IVC, especially primary leiomyosarcomas. In recent years, pre-/intra- and postoperative radiation therapy as well as newer chemotherapeutic drugs are being used in conjunction with surgical resection. Other retroperitoneal tumors invading the IVC may also be suitable for adjuvant treatment depending on the histological type. A multidisciplinary team approach with involvement of an oncologist is best suited for management of these complex patients.

Ⓚ Consider thrombolysis ± mechanical thrombectomy

CDT and/or pharmaco-mechanical catheter-directed thrombolysis (PMCT) should be considered in all severely symptomatic, functionally sound patients with an acute/subacute IVC thrombosis and low bleeding risk. The advantages in terms of invasiveness and safety of catheter-directed treatment over surgical thrombectomy and systemic thrombolysis are proven, making it the procedure of choice for early thrombus removal.[14] The completeness of thrombus resolution decreases with increasing duration between onset of thrombosis and initiation of therapy. The long-term benefit of decreasing the incidence of post-thrombotic syndrome has also been demonstrated in observational studies. However, prospective evaluation including the recently published ATTRACT trial have not been able to conclusively prove this fact, leading to conflicting guidelines by the American College of Chest Physicians (ACCP) and the American Heart Association. Regardless, the results of the ATTRACT trial should not prevent use of PMCT in the appropriate patient with acute IVC and/or iliofemoral thrombosis in clinical practice. The technical details of CDT and PMCT are discussed in Chapter 79.

Ⓛ Anticoagulation

The ACCP recommends management of acute lower extremity proximal DVT with IV anticoagulation followed by 3 months of oral anticoagulation in instances of provoked DVT. In instances of unprovoked DVT, anticoagulation should be extended for at least 12 months with consideration of indefinite therapy, especially in patients with cancer.[15] There are no separate guidelines for management of IVC thrombosis; however, the larger thrombus burden of IVC occlusion, with greater propensity for immediate and long-term morbidity, mandates early and effective anticoagulation, evaluation for predisposing factors, and aggressive correction of modifiable risks. In our practice, IV unfractionated heparin is initiated once the diagnosis is made, with subsequent conversion to oral anticoagulation to complete the course of treatment, sometimes lifelong, if risk factors for recurrent thrombosis remain present.

Following balloon venoplasty ± stenting for IVC occlusion/stenosis, periprocedural anticoagulation with unfractionated heparin to maintain an activated clotting time of 250 to 300 seconds is usually followed by a single dose of therapeutic LMWH, with immediate initiation of long-term oral anticoagulation. The duration of therapy is based on various risk factors, such as underlying hypercoagulability, technical outcome of the intervention, and quality of venous inflow.[16] Although there are no specific guidelines regarding the use of antiplatelet therapy, it may have a role following IVC recanalization and stenting for chronic occlusion, especially following reintervention. The pathology of restenosis within venous stents is felt to be different from that of intimal hyperplasia in the arterial tree. Interestingly, one provider group reports use of lifelong antiplatelet therapy in conjunction with variable length of oral anticoagulation (see section F), whereas another does not use it at all. Both report similar early and late results in terms of patency of IVC stents.[16,17]

After open reconstruction with ilio-/femorocaval bypass with ringed ePTFE, therapeutic anticoagulation is continued lifelong.[18] After resection and reconstruction of the IVC with large-diameter ePTFE for malignant IVC tumors, therapeutic anticoagulation for at least 1 year with an oral agent is standard practice.[12]

Ⓜ Conservative therapy

For patients with chronic IVC occlusion but with mild symptoms (C1-3), conservative management with a combination of compression stockings, lifestyle modification, lower extremity elevation, and anticoagulation is appropriate.

Ⓝ Venoplasty ± IVC stenting

Following treatment for acute/subacute IVC thrombosis with CDT/PMCT, untreated residual luminal stenosis has been shown to be associated with a 73% incidence of rethrombosis compared with only 13% in patients undergoing additional treatment with venoplasty ± stenting.[19] As many as 60% of patients require adjunctive venoplasty ± stenting in contemporary practice.[6] The IVC is typically stented using the single-barrel technique, often with a Wallstent (Boston Scientific) in combination with the large-diameter (20 mm) Gianturco stents (Cook Medical, Bloomington, IN) to add more radial force and reinforce the weaker distal ends of the Wallstent.

In the setting of chronic benign occlusion of the IVC, venoplasty ± stenting should be considered in severely symptomatic patients (C4-6 or lifestyle-limiting venous claudication), because successful intervention is associated with significant relief of symptoms, including healing of venous ulcers. Although it can be technically challenging, recanalization with balloon venoplasty and self-expandable stents has been shown to be safe and effective with patency rates >85% at 36 months.[16] The technique is not different from that described for iliac vein stenting for May–Thurner syndrome (see Chapter 79). The addition of concurrent right internal jugular vein access is often helpful, providing through-and-through femoral-jugular access to facilitate wire crossing of highly fibrotic iliocaval segments. Self-expandable stents such as Wallstents and Gianturco stents should be used in the setting of endofibrosis commonly seen in chronic occlusion. IVUS is an invaluable adjunct to identify fibrotic webs and ensure that no disease segment is left uncovered. Although many configurations have been described for recreating the iliocaval confluence (double barrel, side butting, side piercing), it is best recreated by extending stents into the common iliac veins with proximal extension significantly into the IVC in a parallel stent fashion.[16] Initial technical success at recanalization of the IVC is reported as 85% to 90% in the two series with significant experience.[16,17] Although primary patency is only 78% and 52% at 3 and 5 years, respectively, secondary patency is excellent at 91% to 93% inspite of the lengthy, complex endovenous reconstruction.

If endovenous recanalization is not possible or successful, surgical bypass can be considered.

O Surgical bypass

Open surgical reconstruction for IVC occlusion with femorocaval or iliocaval bypass is extremely challenging, and patency is adversely affected by low venous pressure, poor inflow secondary to infrainguinal chronic post-thrombotic venous changes, and frequent thrombophilia in these patients. In addition, ringed ePTFE is the only conduit available in large enough caliber and long enough length to bypass these long, occlusive lesions. Successful bypass around an IVC occlusion provides excellent relief of venous stasis symptoms and promotes ulcer healing. However, unlike short iliofemoral or iliocaval bypasses to the distal IVC performed for iliac vein occlusions, secondary patency of femorocaval bypasses at 1 and 5 years is only 76% and 67%, respectively.[18] These invasive procedures should therefore only be considered for patients with severe disability from the condition and after unsuccessful or failed endovenous reconstruction.

P Surveillance

Following intervention and before hospital discharge, patients should undergo imaging to confirm early patency. Imaging usually includes DUS after balloon venoplasty and stenting and CT or MR venography following open surgical reconstruction. Surveillance imaging with the same modalities is indicated at 3, 6, and 12 months, and annually thereafter. Graduated compression stockings must be prescribed for all patients. If recurrent thrombosis or stenosis occurs, it can potentially be retreated with endovenous techniques.

Q SVC occlusion

The frequency of symptomatic SVC occlusion in the United States is about 15,000 patients per year.[20] Although malignancy, specifically lung cancer and lymphomas, remains the most common causes (60%),[21] the etiology of benign SVC occlusion has changed significantly from mediastinal fibrosis to predominantly indwelling central venous catheters, given their escalating use and association with thrombosis. Signs and symptoms of venous congestion of the head, neck, and upper extremities are determined by the duration and extent of the venous occlusive disease and by the amount of collateral venous circulation that develops. Although not specifically defined in the setting of SVC occlusion, the definitions of acute, subacute, and chronic timelines are similar to those described for other large vein occlusions/thrombosis; acute <14 days, subacute 14 to 28 days, and chronic >28 days utilized for the purpose of guiding choice of therapy.

R Acute/subacute SVC occlusion

Patients with acute/subacute catheter-related thrombosis or compression by a rapidly enlarging mediastinal tumor (usually a lymphoma) present with facial swelling, headache, and shortness of breath, especially with exertion. The most frequent cause of acute SVC occlusion is thrombosis associated with long-term indwelling intravenous catheters or pacemaker wires. In patients with ESRD, asymptomatic SVC occlusion may be unmasked upon creation of AV access with rapid development of arm swelling and neck engorgement. Although SVC occlusion from tumor compression may cause acute symptoms, it usually results in a more chronic presentation. Management of acute SVC occlusion depends on whether the etiology is benign (catheter related thrombosis) or associated with a malignant tumor.

S Chronic SVC occlusion

Chronically symptomatic SVC occlusion leads to insidious development of venous HTN of the head and upper extremities that may cause a feeling of fullness in the head and neck, dyspnea on exertion, orthopnea, headache, dizziness, or syncope or visual symptoms. Patients may complain of confusion, or cough. Physical examination reveals dilated neck veins; swelling of the face, neck, or eyelids; prominent chest wall collaterals; ecchymosis; and cyanosis of the face. Symptoms may also involve the upper extremity, with swelling and exertional fatigue. Symptoms of malignant SVC obstruction, whether acute or chronic, may include hemoptysis, hoarseness, dysphagia, weight loss, lethargy, or palpable cervical tumor or lymph nodes, in addition to symptoms of head and neck venous congestion. Patients with lymphoma may also present with fever and night sweats. Chronic benign SVC occlusion can be caused by mediastinal fibrosis or granulomatous fungal disease, such as histoplasmosis.[21-23] Previous radiotherapy to the mediastinum, retrosternal goiter, and aortic dissection can also cause chronic SVC occlusion. The risk of venous thrombosis is increased in patients with thrombophilia such as factor V Leiden mutation and deficiencies in circulating natural anticoagulants, such as anti-thrombin III, protein S, and protein C. Management of chronic SVC occlusion depends on whether the etiology is thrombosis from benign pathology or associated with a malignant tumor.

T Thrombolysis

CDT should be considered in most patients with benign acute/subacute SVC obstruction and symptoms severe enough to warrant intervention. These are usually young, functional patients with indwelling catheters or treatable mediastinal fibrosis who do not have contraindications to thrombolysis. This is followed by IV unfractionated heparin or LMWH, followed by warfarin, to prevent recurrence and protect the venous collateral circulation. Mechanical thrombectomy is not usually performed in the SVC due to concern for precipitating cardiac bradycardia. If a provoking intravascular catheter is present, it is ideally removed, but may be retained if no other access is possible. Success with thrombolysis is greater in patients with acute versus subacute presentation. More frequently than not however, thrombolysis alone is not sufficient treatment for acute SVC thrombosis and is usually followed by more definitive therapy in the form of balloon venoplasty and stenting to treat the underlying stenotic lesion unmasked by successful thrombolysis.

U Therapeutic chemoradiation

Primary mediastinal malignant tumors leading to SVC occlusion include mediastinal lymphoma, medullary or follicular carcinoma of the thyroid, thymoma, teratoma, angiosarcoma, and synovial cell carcinoma.[1,20] Primary thoracic malignant tumors leading to SVC occlusion, include non-small cell lung cancer is the cause in 50%, followed by small cell lung cancer (22%), lymphoma (12%), metastatic cancer (9%), germ cell cancer (3%), and thymoma (2%).[20]

Symptoms of SVC syndrome caused by mediastinal malignancy frequently improve after irradiation, chemotherapy, or combination chemo-radiation based on tumor histology. Resolution of symptoms occurs in 80% of patients within 4 weeks, especially in those with tumor histology that is chemosensitive and this should be first-line therapy in these patients with very likely no direct intervention required for the SVC.[24] In patients being relegated to definitive or preoperative radiation therapy if symptoms of SVC occlusion are sufficiently severe, balloon venoplasty and stenting may be required before radiation can be started because the symptoms are likely to worsen secondary to radiation-induced inflammation and swelling at the site of SVC compression by the tumor. If symptoms are severe and persist after chemoradiation, venoplasty and stenting can be performed. Usually, symptomatic relief is immediate in 95% of patients, adequate, and long-lasting enough such that reintervention is rarely necessary.[24]

V Potential tumor resection

Surgical reconstruction of the SVC should be considered with tumor resection and reconstruction of the SVC through a medium sternotomy in patients with a life expectancy >1 year, usually those with lymphoma, thymoma, or metastatic medullary carcinoma of the thyroid gland.[25] This is usually accomplished with a large caliber ringed ePTFE interposition graft. It is important to determine the feasibility of complete tumor resection based on preoperative imaging with MR or CT venography. Extra-anatomic subcutaneous bypass between the jugular vein and the femoral vein using a composite saphenous vein graft is an alternative in the setting of incapacitating symptoms of head and neck venous congestion, failed/unsuccessful endovenous intervention, and a surgically unresectable mediastinal tumor.[26]

W Assess symptom severity and initiate conservative treatment

Conservative medical measures should be instituted in every patient with SVC occlusion to relieve symptoms of venous congestion regardless of the severity and extent of disease and may suffice as sole treatment in patients with mild symptoms. These measures include elevation of the head during the night on pillows, modifications of daily activities by avoiding bending over, and avoidance of wearing constricting garments or a tight collar. Diuretic therapy is an adjunct to help decrease, at least temporarily, excessive edema of the neck and head while definitive therapy is planned. For patients with more severe or persistent symptoms, venoplasty and stenting is then indicated.

ⓧ Anticoagulation

In the absence of evidence-based guidelines, use of anticoagulation and/or antiplatelet therapy is routine in the short-term for SVC occlusion, but variable in type and duration at the discretion of the interventionist. The majority of patients, especially those with malignancy and catheter-related thrombosis, usually receive oral anticoagulation for 3 to 6 months (or life for ongoing cancer) and those with mediastinal fibrosis often antiplatelet therapy alone.[27,28] Following open reconstruction with SVC bypass, anticoagulation with heparin is commenced within 24 hours with conversion to oral anticoagulation before discharge. Patients with spiral saphenous vein or femoral vein grafts who have no underlying coagulation abnormality are maintained on warfarin for 3 months only. Those with underlying coagulation disorders and most patients with long ePTFE grafts are kept on lifelong anticoagulation.

ⓨ Venoplasty ± stenting SVC

Endovascular therapy with stenting of the SVC/innominate veins has been the first line of therapy for symptomatic SVC obstruction of malignant etiology for over 2 decades, given the excellent symptom relief combined with only the need for short- to mid-term patency related to the shorter life expectancy of these patients. Endovascular treatment has now also become accepted as first-line therapy for benign causes of SVC occlusion.[29] Most studies have emphasized the need for customizing treatment with a combination of thrombolysis, balloon angioplasty, and stenting depending on the etiology and acuity of the obstruction in order to achieve an initial technical success rates of 90% to 100%.[30] PTA alone is rarely performed in the primary setting, except occasionally when avoiding stents across the confluence of the innominate veins but has a role in the treatment of in-stent restenosis. In the absence of availability of dedicated venous stents, large caliber (10-16 mm), self-expanding stents like Wallstents (Boston Scientific Corp., Natick, MA), Smart stents (Cordis Endovascular, Warren, NJ), Protégé stents (ev3, Plymouth, MN), E*Luminexx (Bard GmbH/Angiomed, Karlsruhe, Germany), Sinus-XL (OptiMed Medizinische Instrumente GmbH, Ettlingen, Germany), and Zilver Vena (Cook Medical Inc., Bloomington, IN) stents have been used most frequently because of flexibility and availability in multiple sizes and lengths.[22,23] Stentgrafts have been used in recent years in an attempt to improve patency in malignant SVC obstruction.[21]

Symptomatic relief is immediate and comparable to that following open surgical reconstruction. Inspite of excellent early success with balloon venoplasty and stenting, primary patency at 1 and 3 years is reported at 70% and 44%, with ongoing need for secondary interventions to maintain patency. Our early experience with stentgrafts for initial treatment of benign SVC stenosis has been encouraging in the short term with reduced symptom recurrence (29% vs. 60%, $P < 0.05$) and need for reintervention (15% vs. 39% at 12 months) for covered when compared with uncovered stents, respectively.

ⓩ Surgical bypass

Open surgical bypass should be considered in patients with benign SVC obstruction if a long occlusion (Doty IV lesion) could not be crossed, or after stent thrombosis with no further endovenous options. Given the longevity of patients with benign SVC occlusion, it is not surprising that some opt for surgical treatment if repeated endovenous interventions have been required. Careful evaluation of the patient's symptom severity, effect on quality of life, and medical fitness is important for patient selection. Preoperative imaging should be performed to confirm and identify a source of inflow for the bypass procedure. DUS of the lower extremities is also recommended to identify a suitable venous conduit (GSV to fashion a spiral vein conduit or femoral vein). Collateralization across the midline is usually adequate to decompress both sides with a single graft from the internal jugular or innominate vein to the central SVC or right atrial appendage.[31-33] Open surgical treatment for SVC occlusion has excellent long-term results with good relief from symptoms, depending on etiology, conduit, and the length of venous reconstruction. In a single-center series, primary and secondary patency rates of all the grafts at 5 years were 45% and 75%, respectively. Of the different graft types, spiral SVGs performed best, with an 86% secondary patency rate at 5 years.[32,34]

⒜⒜ Surveillance

Surveillance is mandatory as many patients with treated SVC occlusion will experience recurrence of symptoms from stenosis developing within a stent or bypass graft. Unfortunately, DUS provides only indirect evidence of patency of the intrathoracic SVC, stent, or bypass graft. CT or conventional contrast venography is therefore recommended postendovenous therapy at 3 to 6 months and 1 year, and annually thereafter, with baseline imaging obtained before discharge following open bypass. MR venography can also be used after surgery and is recommended before discharge and once at 3 to 6 months, at 1 year, and annually thereafter. Primary patency of bypass grafts is not significantly superior to current results of endovenous intervention; however, in our comparative experience, stenoses requiring intervention occurred mostly in the first 1 to 2 years, following which there was maintained, durable long-term graft patency, unlike with SVC stenting when the need for reintervention persisted.[29] Bypass graft patency can be inferred from freedom

from symptoms, and imaging after the first year needs to be only performed in symptomatic patients or in asymptomatic patients with known nonsignificant stenosis.

Mechanisms of stenosis within SVC stents and bypasses for benign disease include intimal hyperplasia, fibrosis and extrinsic compression from mediastinitis, and tumor ingrowth in malignant disease. Patients with malignant SVC occlusion have a shortened life expectancy with an overall survival at 12 months as low as 30%. These patients therefore rarely require reintervention, so surveillance can be relaxed.[22] There is a greater incidence of restenosis in patients with benign SVC obstruction due to mediastinitis compared with central line-related thrombosis.

All significant restenoses are symptomatic and merit venography and reintervention, which can usually be accomplished by endovenous means sometimes complimented by thrombolysis for acute occlusion in both SVC stents and bypass/interposition grafts.[29,31] Endovenous intervention remains an invaluable adjunctive measure to improve long-term graft patency. Approximately half of all patients treated with venoplasty ± stenting will require at least one reintervention within the first 2 years, and some patients with stents will require reinterventions every few months. The latter are associated with a higher risk of perforation and acutely life-threatening pericardial effusion caused by high pressure balloon angioplasty to treat resistant restenoses. This acute life-threatening complication requires immediate pericardiocentesis in conjunction with treatment of the rupture with a stentgraft.

REFERENCES

1. Rice TW, Rodriguez RM, Light RW. The superior vena cava syndrome: clinical characteristics and evolving etiology. *Medicine (Baltimore)*. 2006;85(1):37-42.
2. Parish JM, Marschke RF Jr, Dines DE, Lee RE. Etiologic considerations in superior vena cava syndrome. *Mayo Clin Proc*. 1981;56(7):407-413.
3. Chen JC, Bongard F, Klein SR. A contemporary perspective on superior vena cava syndrome. *Am J Surg*. 1990;160(2):207-211.
4. Crowner J, Marston W, Almeida J, McLafferty R, Passman M. Classification of anatomic involvement of the iliocaval venous outflow tract and its relationship to outcomes after iliocaval venous stenting. *J Vasc Surg Venous Lymphat Disord*. 2014;2(3):241-245.
5. Stanford W, Doty DB. The role of venography and surgery in the management of patients with superior vena cava obstruction. *Ann Thorac Surg*. 1986;41(2):158-163.
6. Alkhouli M, Bashir R. Inferior vena cava filters in the United States: less is more. *Int J Cardiol*. 2014;177(3):742-743.
7. Wang SL, Siddiqui A, Rosenthal E. Long-term complications of inferior vena cava filters. *J Vasc Surg Venous Lymphat Disord*. 2017;5(1):33-41.

8. White RH. The epidemiology of venous thromboembolism. *Circulation*. 2003;107(23 suppl 1):I4-I8.

9. Kahn SR. The post-thrombotic syndrome: the forgotten morbidity of deep venous thrombosis. *J Thromb Thrombolysis*. 2006;21(1):41-48.

10. Bower TC, Mendes BC, Toomey BJ, et al. Outcomes of 102 patients treated with segmental inferior vena cava resection and graft replacement for malignant disease. *J Vasc Surg*. 2014;59:36S-36S.

11. Pouliot F, Shuch B, LaRochelle JC, Pantuck A, Belldegrun AS. Contemporary management of renal tumors with venous tumor thrombus. *J Urol*. 2010;184(3):833-841.

12. Bower TC, Nagorney DM, Cherry KJ Jr, et al. Replacement of the inferior vena cava for malignancy: an update. *J Vasc Surg*. 2000;31(2):270-281.

13. Sarmiento JM, Bower TC, Cherry KJ, Farnell MB, Nagorney DM. Is combined partial hepatectomy with segmental resection of inferior vena cava justified for malignancy? *Arch Surg*. 2003;138(6):624-630; discussion 30-31.

14. Casey ET, Murad MH, Zumaeta-Garcia M, et al. Treatment of acute iliofemoral deep vein thrombosis. *J Vasc Surg*. 2012;55(5):1463-1473.

15. Kearon C, Akl EA, Ornelas J, et al. Antithrombotic therapy for VTE disease CHEST guideline and expert panel report. *Chest*. 2016;149(2):315-352.

16. Erben Y, Bjarnason H, Oladottir GL, McBane RD, Gloviczki P. Endovascular recanalization for nonmalignant obstruction of the inferior vena cava. *J Vasc Surg Venous Lymphat Disord*. 2018;6(2):173-182.

17. Murphy EH, Johns B, Varney E, Raju S. Endovascular management of chronic total occlusions of the inferior vena cava and iliac veins. *J Vasc Surg Venous Lymphat Disord*. 2017;5(1):47-59.

18. Garg N, Gloviczki P, Karimi KM, et al. Factors affecting outcome of open and hybrid reconstructions for nonmalignant obstruction of iliofemoral veins and inferior vena cava. *J Vasc Surg*. 2011;53(2):383-393.

19. Hartung O, Benmiloud F, Barthelemy P, Dubuc M, Boufi M, Alimi YS. Late results of surgical venous thrombectomy with iliocaval stenting. *J Vasc Surg*. 2008;47(2):381-387.

20. Wilson LD, Detterbeck FC, Yahalom J. Superior vena cava syndrome with malignant causes. *N Engl J Med*. 2007;356(18):1862-1869.

21. Gwon DI, Ko GY, Kim JH, Shin JH, Yoon HK, Sung KB. Malignant superior vena cava syndrome: a comparative cohort study of treatment with covered stents versus uncovered stents. *Radiology*. 2013;266(3):979-987.

22. Maleux G, Gillardin P, Fieuws S, Heye S, Vaninbroukx J, Nackaerts K. Large-bore nitinol stents for malignant superior vena cava syndrome: factors influencing outcome. *AJR Am J Roentgenol*. 2013;201(3):667-674.

23. Fagedet D, Thony F, Timsit JF, et al. Endovascular treatment of malignant superior vena cava syndrome: results and predictive factors of clinical efficacy. *Cardiovasc Intervent Radiol*. 2013;36(1):140-149.

24. Rowell NP, Gleeson FV. Steroids, radiotherapy, chemotherapy and stents for superior vena caval obstruction in carcinoma of the bronchus. *Cochrane Database Syst Rev*. 2001;(4):CD001316.

25. Dartevelle PG, Chapelier AR, Pastorino U, et al. Long-term follow-up after prosthetic replacement of the superior vena cava combined with resection of mediastinal-pulmonary malignant tumors. *J Thorac Cardiovasc Surg*. 1991;102(2):259-265.

26. Graham A, Anikin V, Curry R, McGuigan J. Subcutaneous jugulofemoral bypass: A simple surgical option for palliation of superior vena cava obstruction. *J Cardiovasc Surg*. 1995;36:615-617.

27. Rosch J, Bedell JE, Putnam J, Antonovic R, Uchida B. Gianturco expandable wire stents in the treatment of superior vena cava syndrome recurring after maximum-tolerance radiation. *Cancer*. 1987;60(6):1243-1246.

28. Irving JD, Dondelinger RF, Reidy JF, et al. Gianturco self-expanding stents: clinical experience in the vena cava and large veins. *Cardiovasc Intervent Radiol*. 1992;15(5):328-333.

29. Rizvi AZ, Kalra M, Bjarnason H, Bower TC, Schleck C, Gloviczki P. Benign superior vena cava syndrome: stenting is now the first line of treatment. *J Vasc Surg*. 2008;47(2):372-380.

30. Barshes NR, Annambhotla S, El Sayed HF, et al. Percutaneous stenting of superior vena cava syndrome: treatment outcome in patients with benign and malignant etiology. *Vascular*. 2007;15(5):314-321.

31. Kalra M, Gloviczki P, Andrews JC, et al. Open surgical and endovascular treatment of superior vena cava syndrome caused by nonmalignant disease. *J Vasc Surg*. 2003;38(2):215-223.

32. Doty DB, Doty JR, Jones KW. Bypass of superior vena cava. Fifteen years' experience with spiral vein graft for obstruction of superior vena cava caused by benign disease. *J Thorac Cardiovasc Surg*. 1990;99(5):889-895; discussion 95-96.

33. Moore W, Hollier, LH. Reconstruction of the superior vena cava and central veins. In: Bergan J, Yao JST, eds. *Venous Disorders*. Philadelphia, PA: WB Saunders; 1991:517-527.

34. Doty JR, Flores JH, Doty DB. Superior vena cava obstruction: bypass using spiral vein graft. *Ann Thorac Surg*. 1999;67(4):1111-1116.

Afsha Aurshina • Anil Hingorani

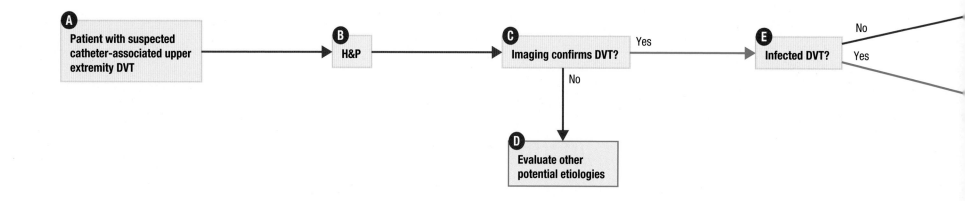

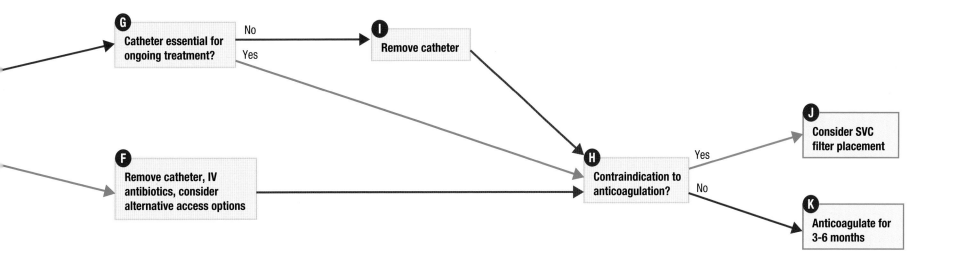

A Patient with suspected catheter-associated upper extremity DVT

Upper extremity DVT constitutes 4.4% of all DVTs, almost half of which are catheter-related (45%).[1,2] Upper extremity DVT can be either primary or secondary. Primary upper extremity DVT is either idiopathic or related to effort thrombosis (Paget–Schroetter syndrome, see Chapter 57). Secondary upper extremity DVT develops in patients with cancer or in association with central venous catheters. Catheter-associated upper extremity DVT can be defined as intraluminal thrombus of the brachial, axillary, or subclavian vein(s) secondary to an indwelling catheter with the causality presumed to result from infective, mechanical, chemical irritation, venous stasis, or thrombogenic reaction to the catheter coating.[3,4]

B H&P

Patients with catheter-related upper extremity DVT have been described as asymptomatic in 5% to 62% of cases.[1,5] When symptomatic, patients present with pain, swelling, or erythema, located in the neck, chest, or arm.[5-10] As severity of venous congestion progresses, engorgement of collateral veins along the chest wall or extremity can also be observed; phlegmasia cerulea dolens is very rare in the upper extremities.[11] PE occurs in 5 to 20% of patients with upper extremity DVT.[12] Another important chronic complication of upper extremity DVT is development of painful and swollen upper extremity caused by post-thrombotic syndrome (4%-35%).[13]

C Imaging confirms DVT?

DUS is the mainstay for diagnosis of upper extremity DVT,[4] which can be confirmed when there is direct visualization of thrombus, absence of color flow within the vein, lack of compressibility of the affected venous segment, loss of phasicity, or minimal change in flow with augmentation maneuvers. These findings may not be apparent when the thrombus is located in the proximal subclavian or brachiocephalic vein or if the veins are not well visualized due to the overlying bony structures.[14] It is essential to consider upper extremity DVT as a source for patients presenting with PE and no evidence of lower extremity DVT. When the clinical suspicion for upper extremity DVT is high and DUS fails to reveal thrombosis, additional testing using computed tomography venography (CTV) or magnetic resonance venography (MRV) is recommended. The D-dimer test can also be conducted to exclude the diagnosis of DVT and search for alternate causes. Catheter-directed venography remains the gold standard to diagnose central thrombosis; however, it is seldom used.

D Evaluate other potential etiologies

If imaging does not reveal DVT as a cause for upper extremity swelling, other diagnoses, such as lymphedema, need to be evaluated.

E Infected DVT?

If DUS is positive for DVT, it is important to determine if the thrombus is infected because this can result in systemic sepsis and embolization of infected thrombus. Fever, leukocytosis, positive blood cultures, or cutaneous signs of infection at the catheter insertion site suggest an infected DVT. If a DVT is infected, definitive treatment beyond anticoagulation is required.

F Remove catheter, IV antibiotics, consider alternative access options

Patients with suspected or proven infected DVT in association with a catheter require prompt removal of the catheter and initiation of IV antibiotic therapy targeted to blood cultures, if positive. The removed catheter tip should also be cultured. Patients with concomitant septic PE will require removal of the source, that is, thrombectomy and/or venectomy of the affected vein, provided the patient will tolerate such a procedure. Should the patient require continued central venous catheter access, an alternative site for a temporary (nontunneled) catheter should be sought. More permanent central venous access should not be placed until the patient is blood culture–free for >48 hours or based on infectious disease specialists' recommendations.

G Catheter essential for ongoing treatment?

For patients with a noninfected catheter-associated DVT who require continued central venous access, the recommendation is to leave the catheter in place and treat around it with anticoagulation. Jones et al. described complete resolution of thrombus in 46% of patients on follow-up with up to 75% thrombus resolution noted in patients in whom catheter was removed <48 hours after diagnosis of catheter-related upper extremity DVT.[15] This study also revealed that catheter (associated with DVT) removal and placement of a new catheter at another site often resulted in recurrent catheter-associated DVT at the new catheter placement site. If the catheter associated with the DVT is not essential, it should be removed.

H Contraindication to anticoagulation?

Absolute contraindications to anticoagulation include intracranial bleeding, severe active bleeding, and recent brain, eye, or spinal cord surgery. Relative contraindications include uncontrolled HTN, thrombocytopenia, prior GI bleeding, history of falls, and severe anemia. If anticoagulation is contraindicated, consideration may be given to SVC filter placement.

I Remove catheter

In order to prevent further catheter-induced venous thrombosis, the catheter should be removed if it is not essential for ongoing treatment.

J Consider SVC filter placement

Compared with lower extremity DVT, upper extremity DVT has a lower risk of PE. The use of SVC filters should be considered in rare cases of patients with PE and contraindications for anticoagulation.[16,17] Given the substantially lower risk of clinically significant PE, the potential benefit must outweigh the risks of filter placement, including filter dislocation and development of the SVC syndrome due to thrombotic occlusion of the filter. Thus, this is considered only in patients in whom even a small PE might be fatal, namely those with severe underlying cardiopulmonary disease and a high risk for progressive thrombosis when not anticoagulated.

K Anticoagulate for 3-6 months

The current recommendation based on the American College of Chest Physicians' (ACCP) guidelines for treatment of upper extremity DVT is anticoagulation for 3 to 6 months.[15,18,19] This consists of initial treatment with IV unfractionated heparin, subcutaneous LMWH or fondaparinux with transition to warfarin, or alternate direct oral anticoagulants.

REFERENCES

1. Munoz FJ, Mismetti P, Poggio R, et al. Clinical outcome of patients with upper-extremity deep vein thrombosis: results from the RIETE registry. *Chest.* 2008;133(1):143-148.
2. Liem TK, Yanit KE, Moseley SE, et al. Peripherally inserted central catheter usage patterns and associated symptomatic upper extremity venous thrombosis. *J Vasc Surg.* 2012;55(3):761-767.
3. Lee AY, Levine MN, Butler G, et al. Incidence, risk factors, and outcomes of catheter-related thrombosis in adult patients with cancer. *J Clin Oncol.* 2006;24(9):1404-1408.
4. Crawford JD, Liem TK, Moneta GL. Management of catheter-associated upper extremity deep venous thrombosis. *J Vasc Surg Venous Lymphat Disord.* 2016;4(3):375-379.
5. Kuter DJ. Thrombotic complications of central venous catheters in cancer patients. *Oncologist.* 2004;9(2):207-216.
6. Ge X, Cavallazzi R, Li C, Pan SM, Wang YW, Wang FL. Central venous access sites for the prevention of venous thrombosis, stenosis and infection. *Cochrane Database Syst Rev.* 2012;(3):CD004084.
7. Murray J, Precious E, Alikhan R. Catheter-related thrombosis in cancer patients. *Br J Haematol.* 2013;162(6):748-757.
8. Baskin JL, Pui CH, Reiss U, et al. Management of occlusion and thrombosis associated with long-term indwelling central venous catheters. *Lancet (London, England).* 2009;374(9684):159-169.
9. Tilney ML, Griffiths HJ, Edwards EA. Natural history of major venous thrombosis of the upper extremity. *Arch Surg.* 1970;101(6):792-796.
10. Joffe HV, Kucher N, Tapson VF, Goldhaber SZ. Upper-extremity deep vein thrombosis: a prospective registry of 592 patients. *Circulation.* 2004;110(12):1605-1611.

11. Gloviczki P, Kazmier FJ, Hollier LH. Axillary-subclavian venous occlusion: the morbidity of a nonlethal disease. *J Vasc Surg*. 1986;4(4):333-337.

12. Hingorani A, Ascher E, Marks N, et al. Morbidity and mortality associated with brachial vein thrombosis. *Ann Vasc Surg*. 2006;20(3):297-300.

13. Elman EE, Kahn SR. The post-thrombotic syndrome after upper extremity deep venous thrombosis in adults: a systematic review. *Thromb Res*. 2006;117(6):609-614.

14. Hingorani A, Ascher E, Lorenson E, et al. Upper extremity deep venous thrombosis and its impact on morbidity and mortality rates in a hospital-based population. *J Vasc Surg*. 1997;26(5):853-860.

15. Jones MA, Lee DY, Segall JA, et al. Characterizing resolution of catheter-associated upper extremity deep venous thrombosis. *J Vasc Surg*. 2010;51(1):108-113.

16. Ascher E, Hingorani A, Tsemekhin B, Yorkovich W, Gunduz Y. Lessons learned from a 6-year clinical experience with superior vena cava Greenfield filters. *J Vasc Surg*. 2000;32(5):881-887.

17. Usoh F, Hingorani A, Ascher E, et al. Long-term follow-up for superior vena cava filter placement. *Ann Vasc Surg*. 2009;23(3):350-354.

18. Debourdeau P, Kassab Chahmi D, Le Gal G, et al. 2008 SOR guidelines for the prevention and treatment of thrombosis associated with central venous catheters in patients with cancer: report from the working group. *Ann Oncol*. 2009;20(9):1459-1471.

19. Kearon C, Akl EA, Ornelas J, et al. Antithrombotic therapy for VTE disease: CHEST guideline and expert panel report. *Chest*. 2016;149(2):315-352.

Zein M. Saadeddin • Rabih A. Chaer

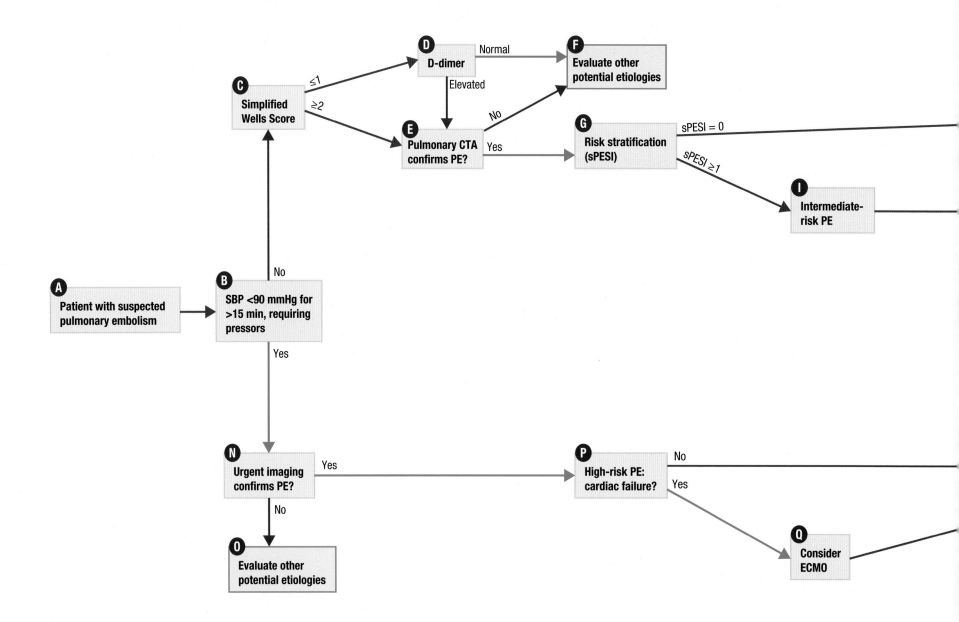

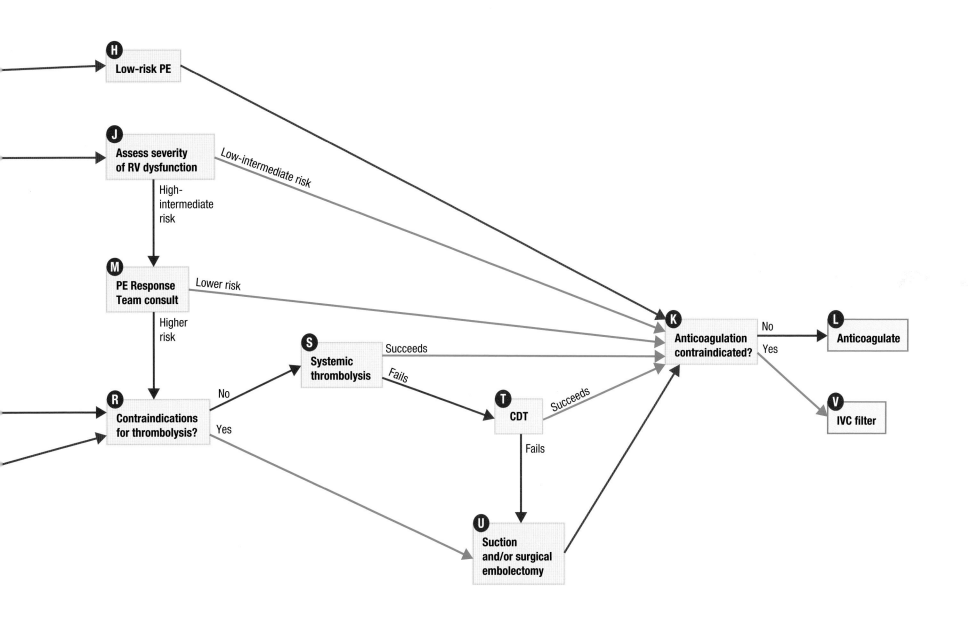

A Patient with suspected pulmonary embolism

Acute PE is the third leading cause of cardiovascular mortality and the most common cause of preventable in-hospital death.[1] Clinical presentation of PE varies from completely asymptomatic to acutely fatal. In 25% of patients, sudden death occurs as the very first manifestation of PE.[2] Given its nonspecific presentation, it is crucial that a high level of suspicion is maintained as treatment is usually highly successful. Suspicion for PE is increased in patients presenting with dyspnea, chest pain, or syncope with or without hemoptysis. Although dyspnea and chest pain, often pleuritic, are the most common symptoms,[3] <1% of patients presenting with syncope have PE.[4] Despite its infrequency, the presence of syncope may indicate a state of reduced hemodynamic reserve. Common clinical signs include tachypnea, tachycardia, signs of DVT, rales and/or decreased breath sounds, and rarely fever, mimicking pneumonia. Hypotension and shock are rare (~5%) yet critical clinical signs.[3]

B SBP<90 mm Hg for >15 min, requiring pressors

The initial step for patients with suspected PE is to assess hemodynamic stability. If the SBP is <90 mm Hg for >15 minutes, or if the patient is requiring blood pressure support, urgent evaluation and treatment of the PE is required. For hemodynamically stable patients with suspected PE, pretest probability is calculated to determine the extent of diagnostic evaluation needed.

C Simplified Wells score

The Wells score has been simplified and validated for improved clinical pretest probability calculation in patients with potential PE (see Table 82-1).[5]

Table 82-1. Simplified Wells Score

Risk Factors[5]	Simplified Score[5]
Previous PE or DVT	1
Heart rate ≥100 beats/min	1
Surgery or immobilization within the past 4 weeks	1
Hemoptysis	1
Active cancer	1
Clinical signs of DVT	1
Alternative diagnosis less likely than PE	1

This scoring system assigns points for various risk factors and provides a cumulative score when added together. Patients with Wells score of ≥2 require imaging to rule out PE. Data on the validity of its clinical prediction rules in pregnancy are still lacking.[5]

D D-dimer

Routine laboratory testing in patients with PE is nonspecific; elevated inflammatory markers, including WBC, LDH, ESR, and CRP, can be observed. Plasma D-dimer, a marker of fibrin formation, increases during an acute venous thrombosis because of the simultaneous activation of coagulation and fibrinolysis pathways. It is a sensitive test with a high negative predictive value (NPV) that is useful in patients with low probability of PE. Normal D-dimer levels (<500 µg/L) rule out acute PE, eliminating the need for unnecessary imaging. D-dimer test, however, has a very low specificity because fibrin is increased in a wide range of conditions including malignancy, trauma, surgery, inflammation, and bleeding. An elevated level is not sufficient to diagnose PE. The specificity of D-dimer test decreases even further among the elderly, increasing false-positive rates. Compared with the standard nonadjusted threshold (500 µg/L), age-adjusted D-dimer threshold (age × 10 µg/L) increases the rates of PE exclusion in patients ≥50 years of age.[6]

E Pulmonary CTA confirms PE?

Combined with clinical probability, pulmonary CTA is the imaging test of choice in patients with high suspicion for PE as it allows for adequate visualization of the pulmonary vasculature to at least the segmental level.[7] Based on the PIOPED II trial, multidetector pulmonary CTA has a sensitivity of 83% and a specificity of 96% and a high predictive value particularly with a concordant clinical assessment.[7,8] In patients with a strong suspicion for PE despite a negative pulmonary CTA, further testing such as ventilation/perfusion (V/Q) scans may be considered.[9] Pulmonary CTA should also be performed in those with low Wells or modified Geneva pretest probability scores who have elevated D-dimer (≥500 µg/L) levels. It is also done urgently to diagnose PE in hemodynamically unstable patients.

F Evaluate other potential etiologies

Patients with a normal D-dimer and low pretest probability for PE do not require further evaluation or treatment for PE. If clinical symptoms are present, other etiologies should be evaluated.

G Risk stratification (sPESI)

Once confirmed in hemodynamically stable patients, PE risk should be stratified using a risk stratification scoring system. The most commonly used is the pulmonary embolism severity index (PESI), which has been simplified to sPESI with prognostic accuracy similar to the original PESI.[10] Patients with at least one of the following risk factors (age > 80, cancer, CHF, COPD, heart rate >100, SBP <100 mm Hg, oxygen saturation <90%) are considered to have *intermediate-risk* PE, whereas those with none have a *low-risk* PE.

Patients classified as low-risk PE (sPESI = 0) have PE-associated mortality up to 1.0%, whereas those with sPESI ≥1

have PE-related mortality up to 11%.[5] Although not currently part of the sPESI, the presence of concomitant DVT has been found to be significantly associated with increased risk of death within 30 days of PE diagnosis and might possibly offer enhanced risk stratification for intermediate-risk PE patients.[11]

H Low-risk PE

PE risk is classified as low, intermediate, or high based on the anticipated 30-day mortality risk, which depends on several factors. Normotensive patients with confirmed PE identified as *low risk* (or nonmassive) using clinical prognostic scores (sPESI = 0) have excellent short-term prognosis. Further cardiac biomarker testing and imaging have poor predictive values for adverse outcomes and are not necessary in these patients.[5,12] Patients with low-risk PE can usually be safely discharged early on anticoagulation for outpatient care depending on their compliance history and social background.[12] Mortality risk is typically <1%.

I Intermediate-risk PE

Hemodynamically stable patients with sPESI score ≥1 constitute the *intermediate-risk* group (or submassive). Within this category, further risk assessment should be established based on right ventricular (RV) functional status using ECHO or pulmonary CTA, along with cardiac biomarkers.[5,13,14] In a large randomized controlled trial, death or hemodynamic decompensation occurred in 5.6% of patients with intermediate-risk PE treated with anticoagulation alone.[15]

J Assess severity of RV dysfunction

Elevated biomarkers, particularly cardiac troponins, have been shown to add important prognostic value. Hemodynamically stable patients with confirmed PE and elevated troponin levels had 5-fold increased risk of death. Serum B-type natriuretic peptide (BNP) and N-terminal [NT] proBNP (NT-proBNP) levels can increase with RV dilation and are also associated with increased mortality in normotensive PE patients.[13] The optimal prognostic cutoff for NT-proBNP is a plasma concentration >600 pg/mL.

Although ECHO is not recommended in the routine diagnostic workup of hemodynamically stable patients with suspected PE,[5] it is useful for prognostic stratification. The presence of RV dysfunction seems to increase short-term mortality by more than 2-fold.[16] On ECHO, RV dysfunction is defined as a right-to-left ventricular (RV/LV) end-diastolic diameter ratio of >1. On pulmonary CTA, RV enlargement is defined as an RV/LV end-diastolic dimensional ratio ≥0.9, which is also associated with a 2-fold increased risk of 30-day mortality.[14]

Based on these factors, the intermediate-risk group is further subdivided into: *intermediate-high* risk (with both RV dysfunction on cardiac imaging *and* an abnormal cardiac biomarker [troponins, BNP, or NT-proBNP]) and *intermediate-low* risk (with only one of these two findings present). See Table 82-2.

Table 82-2. Types of Acute PE

Early Mortality Risk		Risk Parameters and Scores				
		Shock/Hypotension	sPESI ≥1	RV Dysfunction on Imaging	Cardiac Laboratory Biomarkers[a]	
High		+	(+)[b]	+	(+)[b]	
Intermediate	Intermediate-high	−	+	Both positive		
	Intermediate-low	−	+	Either one (or none) positive		
Low		−	−	Assessment optional: If assessed, both negative[c]		

[a]Biomarkers of myocardial injury (eg, elevated cardiac troponin levels) or RV dysfunction (eg, elevated B-type natriuretic peptide [BNP] or N-terminal proBNP levels).
[b]sPESI risk stratification or cardiac testing is not required in patients with hypotension or shock.
[c]Patients with sPESI = 0 with signs of RV dysfunction on imaging or elevated biomarkers are considered as intermediate-low risk.
PE, pulmonary embolism; RV, right ventricle; sPESI, simplified pulmonary embolism severity index.

🅚 Anticoagulation contraindicated?

Anticoagulation is the principal treatment for PE, but in some cases may be contraindicated because of active bleeding or high bleeding risk. The risk-benefit of anticoagulation must always be evaluated, especially in cases of relative contraindications to anticoagulation, such as recent major surgery, stroke, or severe thrombocytopenia. Absolute contraindications, such as intracranial hemorrhage, severe active bleeding, and recent eye or spinal surgery, preclude anticoagulation and are an indication for IVC filter placement.

🅛 Anticoagulate

Unless contraindicated, all patients presenting with acute PE should receive anticoagulation to prevent early death and recurrent events regardless of whether advanced therapies are also indicated. Anticoagulation is the mainstay of therapy and should be initiated early during the diagnostic workup. The standard duration of anticoagulation should cover a period of at least 3 months.[5,12] In the acute PE phase, parenteral anticoagulants (eg, unfractionated heparin [UFH], LMWH, or fondaparinux) should be first initiated followed by a vitamin K antagonist (warfarin) with UFH "bridging" for at least 5 days or until the INR reaches the target therapeutic level (2.0-3.0). Although LMWH or fondaparinux is favored because of its lower risk of major bleeding or heparin-induced thrombocytopenia (HIT), UFH is preferred in high-risk PE patients with hypotension and in patients with renal insufficiency (creatinine clearance <30 mL/min) or severe obesity (BMI > 40 kg/m²).[5,17]

Although warfarin continues to be an important oral anticoagulant, its use may be challenging because of numerous drug-drug, drug-food interactions, and genetic polymorphisms with the need for routine INR monitoring. Novel oral anticoagulants, including factor Xa inhibitors (rivaroxaban, apixaban, edoxaban) and direct thrombin inhibitors (dabigatran) are alternative options that do not require monitoring, dose adjustments, or prolonged UFH

bridging time. They were shown to be noninferior to vitamin K antagonists with a significantly lower risk of bleeding complications in patients with acute VTE.[5,18]

🅜 PE Response Team consult

Intermediate-high risk PE is best managed by a multidisciplinary team because of the lack of evidence favoring one of several possible management options. In 2012, the Massachusetts General Hospital introduced the first PE Response Team (PERT).[19] The concept of PERT involves mobilizing select experts with competency in treating PE from cardiovascular medicine, vascular and cardiac surgery, interventional radiology and cardiology, hematology, emergency medicine, and pulmonary/critical care all to provide a timely assessment and management plan that would deliver the best care for intermediate- and high-risk PE patients.[19] Those judged to be at higher risk are considered for more aggressive treatment, whereas those at lower risk or not candidates for more aggressive treatment are managed with anticoagulation.

🅝 Urgent imaging confirms PE?

In patients with suspected PE who are hypotensive or unstable, urgent imaging to diagnose potential PE is needed. Pulmonary CTA is the preferred imaging technique if it is immediately available and the patient sufficiently stable (see Section E). Bedside transthoracic echocardiography (TTE) is most helpful in hemodynamically unstable patients with suspected PE when pulmonary CTA is not immediately available or hypotension is uncontrolled. The absence of TTE signs of RV overload or dysfunction practically excludes PE as the cause while instantaneously examining other possible causes of shock, including pericardial tamponade, valvular dysfunction, or ventricular dysfunction.[5] It can also identify intracardiac clot in transit.

🅞 Evaluate other potential etiologies

In addition to massive PE, other possible causes of hypotension and shock can include tension pneumothorax, pericardial

tamponade, cardiogenic shock from MI, life-threatening arrhythmia, valvular dysfunction, acute aortic dissection, and septic shock. Life support should be prioritized before evaluating these different etiologies.

🅟 High-risk PE: cardiac failure?

Hemodynamically unstable patients with PE who have sustained hypotension and cardiogenic shock, or cardiac arrest are classified as *high-risk* (or massive)[5,20] and have a high risk of short-term mortality, exceeding 60% in those requiring cardiopulmonary resuscitation.[20] Hemodynamic and respiratory support should be immediately initiated along with empiric anticoagulation, preferably intravenous UFH, in preparation for systemic thrombolysis.[5]

🅠 Consider ECMO

Transportable ECMO assistance systems can be helpful in critical situations, ensuring circulation and oxygenation until definitive diagnosis or management is established. It is generally indicated in any cardiorespiratory failure that is potentially reversible or has failed therapies; contraindications are relative (for an otherwise critically ill patient) and mainly include poor baseline functional status, futile diagnosis, and advanced age.[21] For those with massive PE and cardiac failure, ECMO can unload the acutely failing right heart to provide hemodynamic and respiratory support until thrombus is auto-lysed or another treatment is planned (eg, surgical or aspiration thrombectomy). Although it is reasonable to offer ECMO to unstable high-risk PE patients as a last resort, the decision should be individualized while taking into consideration comorbidities and available expertise to avoid providing futile care.

🅡 Contraindications for thrombolysis?

Risk factors for bleeding and contraindications to thrombolysis have not been exclusively studied in PE but have been extrapolated from experience and guidelines for patients with MI.[12,20] It is unclear to what extent these contraindications apply for CDT in unstable patients, but it seems reasonable to avoid using thrombolysis in patients who need aggressive treatment but have major contraindications, particularly when alternative treatments are available (eg, aspiration thrombectomy).[22]

🅢 Systemic thrombolysis

Compared to anticoagulation, systemic thrombolysis can rapidly restore pulmonary perfusion by promptly reducing thrombus burden, leading to lower pulmonary artery pressure and improved RV function, arterial oxygenation, and hemodynamic status. The net mortality benefit from thrombolysis depends on the patient's presentation and is often offset by the risk of bleeding. Current guidelines clearly endorse IV thrombolysis in hemodynamically unstable patients with PE and no contraindications.[5,12,20] The most widely used regimen is 100 mg of alteplase (recombinant tissue plasminogen activator [rtPA]) over 2 hours; reteplase and desmoteplase have similar outcomes.[5] Heparin infusion is typically held during thrombolysis.

Although indicated in high-risk PE, use of systemic thrombolysis remains controversial for intermediate-risk PE. The Pulmonary Embolism Thrombolysis trial, which assessed the outcomes of fibrinolytic (tenecteplase) therapy in patients with intermediate-risk PE as compared to heparin alone, found that those in the fibrinolysis group were 56% less likely to die or have hemodynamic collapse. However, this net benefit was at the expense of a significantly increased risk of major bleeding.[15] It is reasonable to consider systemic thrombolysis for selected patients with *intermediate-high* risk PE if bleeding risk is low.[5,12]

Concern over bleeding prompted the investigation of the role of half-dose systemic thrombolysis. One trial of 121 patients with "moderate" PE showed that a lower-dose regimen of rtPA resulted in immediate reduction of pulmonary HTN maintained at 28 months as compared to heparin only with no bleeding events in either groups.[23] Although appealing, evidence in favor of half-dose fibrinolytics is preliminary.[19] Current practice is more in favor of catheter-based techniques or surgical embolectomy in those with advancing hemodynamic decompensation and contraindications to systemic thrombolysis, with choice dependent on available expertise. Following successful systemic thrombolysis, anticoagulation is initiated. If systemic thrombolysis is not effective, CDT or suction/surgical embolectomy can be considered.

T CDT

The limitations and complications of systemic thrombolysis are shifting current practice toward CDT that can be done with much lower rtPA doses.[24,25] Standard CDT directly delivers rtPA into the pulmonary artery thrombus through a multiside-hole catheter[5,12,24]; ultrasound-assisted thrombolysis (USAT) involves the additional use of ultrasound to facilitate thrombolytic permeation and is widely used, with studies supporting its efficacy and safety.[24-26] No prospective comparative study has shown USAT superiority over standard catheters, and an ongoing randomized clinical trial is currently comparing the outcomes of these techniques.[27] For patients at high bleeding risk with major contraindications for rtPA, interventional options without lytics, such as suction thrombectomy, are generally preferable (see Section U). Following successful CDT, anticoagulation is continued. If unsuccessful, patients are considered for mechanical embolectomy.

The ULTIMA trial, the first trial to study CDT for intermediate-risk PE, showed that USAT with anticoagulation significantly improved RV function at 24 hours as compared to anticoagulation alone, with no major bleeding in either groups.[26] However, in the real world, CDT is not entirely risk-free and can

be associated with bleeding events and rarely with device-related adverse events like cardiac valve injuries.[28] A recent meta-analysis of 20 studies (2009-2017) with 1168 patients treated with CDT showed that the pooled estimate for major bleeding was 1.4% for intermediate-risk PE and 6.7% for high-risk PE.[29]

U Suction and/or surgical embolectomy

For patients at high risk for bleeding from thrombolysis, suction embolectomy is a good treatment option. Interventional options can include thrombus fragmentation or aspiration without lytic agents, although their safety and efficacy remain controversial. For thrombus fragmentation, rotating pigtail catheters have been widely used in the past. Because of the risk of distal embolization, adjunctive aspiration thrombectomy may be needed, so fragmentation is reserved for high-risk PE. Thrombus aspiration may be performed alone or as adjunct to catheter thrombolysis. The simplest aspiration technique uses any 5F to 9F end-hole catheter or 10F to 14 F dedicated steerable aspiration catheters. Novel large-bore suction systems, such as the Flowtriever (Inari Medical, Irvine, CA) and the Indigo System CAT 8 Aspiration Catheter (Penumbra Inc., Alameda, CA), are currently evaluated in ongoing studies and appear promising.[24]

Surgical embolectomy is reserved for patients with massive central PE in whom thrombolysis is contraindicated or has failed or those who are not eligible for catheter-based interventions. It is performed through a median sternotomy using a normothermic cardiopulmonary bypass where the main pulmonary artery is opened, the thrombotic material is removed, the right chambers of the heart are explored for possible thrombus, and patent foramen ovale, if present, is closed. It rapidly reduces RV afterload and has good results.[30] Outcomes have improved in the past two decades, with mortality declining from 30% to well below 10% with appropriate expertise.[31] Anticoagulation is initiated after surgery.

V IVC filter

IVC filters are generally recommended in patients with acute PE with contraindications to anticoagulation or recurrent PE despite adequate anticoagulation.[32] A recent randomized trial (PREPIC 2) evaluated the safety and efficacy of retrievable IVC filters plus anticoagulation as compared to anticoagulation alone in preventing PE recurrence. By 3 months, recurrent PE occurred in six patients (3.0%; all fatal) in the filter group and in three patients (1.5%; two fatal) in the control group (relative risk [RR] with filter, 2.00; P = 0.50); results were similar at 6 months. Based on these findings, the trial does not support the liberal use of IVC filters beyond the indications mentioned.[33] However, because it is uncertain if there is benefit to IVC filter placement in anticoagulated patients with high-risk PE (eg, with hypotension; see Section P), recommendations against their insertion may not apply to this select subgroup of patients.[12]

Acknowledgment

I would like to express my sincere gratitude to my partner and colleague Dr. Efthimios Avgerinos, MD, for providing his invaluable guidance, comments, suggestions, and expertise that were invaluable for the completion of this work.

REFERENCES

1. Kahn S, Houweling A, Granton J, et al. Long-term outcomes after pulmonary embolism. *Blood Coagul Fibrinolysis.* 2014;25(5):407-415. doi:10.1097/mbc.0000000000000070.
2. Centers for Disease Control and Prevention. *Venous Thromboembolism (Blood Clots).* Atlanta, GA: CDC; 2015. www.cdc.gov/ncbddd/dvt/data.html. Accessed April 2, 2018.
3. Stein P, Beemath A, Matta F, et al. Clinical characteristics of patients with acute pulmonary embolism: data from PIOPED II. *Am J Med.* 2007;120(10):871-879. doi:10.1016/j.amjmed.2007.03.024.
4. Oqab Z, Ganshorn H, Sheldon R. Prevalence of pulmonary embolism in patients presenting with syncope. A systematic review and meta-analysis. *Am J Emerg Med.* 2018;36(4):551-555. doi:10.1016/j.ajem.2017.09.015.
5. Konstantinides SV, Torbicki A, Agnelli G, et al. 2014 ESC guidelines on the diagnosis and management of acute pulmonary embolism: the task force for the diagnosis and management of acute pulmonary embolism. *Eur Heart J.* 2014;35:3033-3069, 3069a-3069k.
6. Righini M, Van Es J, Den Exter P. Age-adjusted d-dimer cutoff levels to rule out pulmonary embolism: the ADJUST-PE Study. *J Vasc Surg.* 2014;59(5):1469. doi:10.1016/j.jvs.2014.03.260.
7. Stein P, Hull R. Multidetector computed tomography for the diagnosis of acute pulmonary embolism. *Curr Opin Pulm Med.* 2007;13(5):384-388. doi:10.1097/mcp.0b013e32821acdbe.
8. Mos I, Klok F, Kroft L, et al. Safety of ruling out acute pulmonary embolism by normal computed tomography pulmonary angiography in patients with an indication for computed tomography: systematic review and meta-analysis. *J Thromb Haemost.* 2009;7(9):1491-1498. doi:10.1111/j.1538-7836.2009.03518.x.
9. Moores L, Kline J, Portillo A, et al. Multidetector computed tomographic pulmonary angiography in patients with a high clinical probability of pulmonary embolism. *J Thromb Haemost.* 2015;14(1):114-120. doi:10.1111/jth.13188.
10. Jiménez D, Aujesky D, Moores L, et al. Simplification of the pulmonary embolism severity index for prognostication in patients with acute symptomatic pulmonary embolism. *Arch Intern Med.* 2010;170(15):1383. doi:10.1001/archinternmed.2010.199.
11. Becattini C, Cohen A, Agnelli G, et al. Risk stratification of patients with acute symptomatic pulmonary embolism based on presence or absence of lower extremity DVT. *Chest.* 2016;149(1):192-200. doi:10.1378/chest.15-0808.

12. Kearon C, Akl E, Ornelas J, et al. Antithrombotic therapy for VTE disease. *Chest.* 2016;149(2):315-352. doi:10.1016/j .chest.2015.11.026.

13. Bajaj A, Rathor P, Sehgal V, et al. Prognostic value of biomarkers in acute non-massive pulmonary embolism: a systematic review and meta-analysis. *Lung.* 2015;193(5):639-651. doi:10.1007/s00408-015-9752-4.

14. Becattini C, Agnelli G, Germini F, Vedovati MC. Computed tomography to assess risk of death in acute pulmonary embolism: a meta-analysis. *Eur Respir J.* 2014;43(6):1678-1690. doi:10.1183/09031936.00147813.

15. Meyer G, Vicaut E, Danays T, et al. Fibrinolysis for patients with intermediate-risk pulmonary embolism. *N Engl J Med.* 2014;370(15):1402-1411. doi:10.1056/nejmoa1302097.

16. Carrier M, Righini M, Wells P, et al. Subsegmental pulmonary embolism diagnosed by computed tomography: incidence and clinical implications. A systematic review and meta-analysis of the management outcome studies. *J Thromb Haemost.* 2010;8(8):1716-1722. doi:10.1111/j.1538-7836.2010.03938.x.

17. Leentjens J, Peters M, Esselink AC, Smulders Y, Kramers C. Initial anticoagulation in patients with pulmonary embolism: thrombolysis, unfractionated heparin, LMWH, fondaparinux, or DOACs? *Br J Clin Pharmacol.* 2017;83(11):2356-2366. doi:10.1111/bcp.13340.

18. van der Hulle T, Kooiman J, den Exter PL, Dekkers OM, Klok FA, Huisman MV. Effectiveness and safety of novel oral anticoagulants as compared with vitamin K antagonists in the treatment of acute symptomatic venous thromboembolism: a systematic review and meta-analysis. *J Thromb Haemost.* 2014;12(3):320-328. doi:10.1111/jth.12485.

19. Dudzinski D, Horowitz J. Start-up, organization and performance of a multidisciplinary pulmonary embolism response team for the diagnosis and treatment of acute pulmonary embolism. *Rev Esp Cardiol.* 2017;70(1):9-13. doi:10.1016/j.rec.2016.05.025.

20. Jaff M, McMurtry M, Archer S, et al. Management of massive and submassive pulmonary embolism, iliofemoral deep vein thrombosis, and chronic thromboembolic pulmonary hypertension: a scientific statement from the American Heart Association. *Circulation.* 2011;123(16):1788-1830. doi:10.1161/cir.0b013e318214914f.

21. Extracorporeal Life Support Organization–ECMO and ECLS. *Elsoorg.* http://www.elso.org/. Accessed April 9, 2018.

22. Avgerinos E, Abou Ali A, Liang N, et al. Predictors of failure and complications of catheter-directed interventions for pulmonary embolism. *J Vasc Surg Venous Lymphat Disord.* 2017;5(3):303-310. doi:10.1016/j.jvsv.2016.12.013.

23. Sharifi M, Bay C, Skrocki L, Rahimi F, Mehdipour M; "MOPETT" Investigators. Moderate pulmonary embolism treated with thrombolysis (from the "MOPETT" trial). *Am J Cardiol.* 2013;111(2):273-277. doi:10.1016/j.amjcard.2012 .09.027.

24. Avgerinos E, Chaer R. Catheter-directed interventions for acute pulmonary embolism. *J Vasc Surg.* 2015;61(2):559-565. doi:10.1016/j.jvs.2014.10.036.

25. Tapson V, Sterling K, Jones N. A randomized trial of the optimum duration of acoustic pulse thrombolysis procedure in acute intermediate-risk pulmonary embolism. *JACC Cardiovasc Interv.* 2018;11(14):1401-1410. doi:10.1016/j. jcin.2018.04.00.

26. Kucher N, Boekstegers P, Müller OJ, et al. Randomized, controlled trial of ultrasound-assisted catheter-directed thrombolysis for acute intermediate-risk pulmonary embolism. *Circulation.* 2014;129:479-486.

27. Avgerinos ED, Mohapatra A, Rivera-Lebron B, et al. Design and rationale of a randomized trial comparing standard vs. ultrasound-assisted thrombolysis for submassive pulmonary embolism (SUNSET sPE). *J Vasc Surg Venous Lymphat Disord.* 2018;6(1):126-132.

28. Avgerinos E, Liang N, El-Shazly O, et al. Improved early right ventricular function recovery but increased complications with catheter-directed interventions compared with anticoagulation alone for submassive pulmonary embolism. *J Vasc Surg Venous Lymphat Disord.* 2016;4(3):268-275. doi:10.1016/j.jvsv.2015.11.003.

29. Avgerinos E, Saadeddin Z, Abou Ali A, et al. A meta-analysis of outcomes of catheter-directed thrombolysis for high- and intermediate-risk pulmonary embolism. *J Vasc Surg Venous Lymphat Disord.* 2018;6(4):530-540. doi:10.1016/j .jvsv.2018.03.010.

30. Aymard T, Kadner A, Widmer A, et al. Massive pulmonary embolism: surgical embolectomy versus thrombolytic therapy—should surgical indications be revisited? *Eur J Cardiothorac Surg.* 2012;43(1):90-94. doi:10.1093/ejcts/ ezs123.

31. Neely R, Byrne J, Gosev I, et al. Surgical embolectomy for acute massive and submassive pulmonary embolism in a series of 115 patients. *Ann Thorac Surg.* 2015;100(4):1245-1252. doi:10.1016/j.athoracsur.2015.03.111.

32. Konstantinides S, Barco S, Lankeit M, Meyer G. Management of pulmonary embolism. *J Am Coll Cardiol.* 2016;67(8):976-990. doi:10.1016/j.jacc.2015.11.061.

33. Mismetti P, Laporte S, Pellerin O, et al. Effect of a retrievable inferior vena cava filter plus anticoagulation vs anticoagulation alone on risk of recurrent pulmonary embolism. *JAMA.* 2015;313(16):1627. doi:10.1001/jama.2015.3780.

Brajesh K. Lal

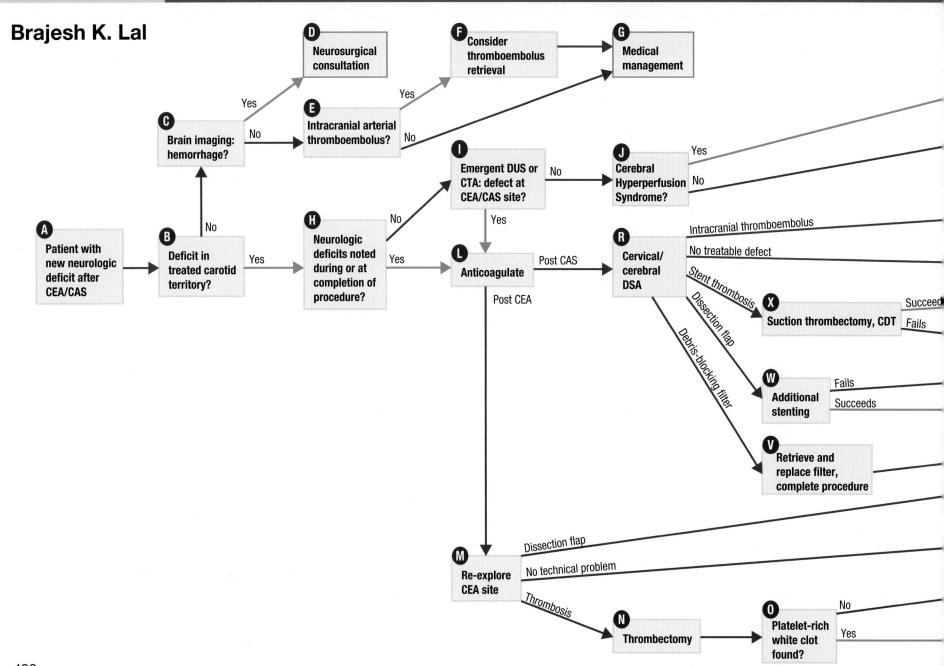

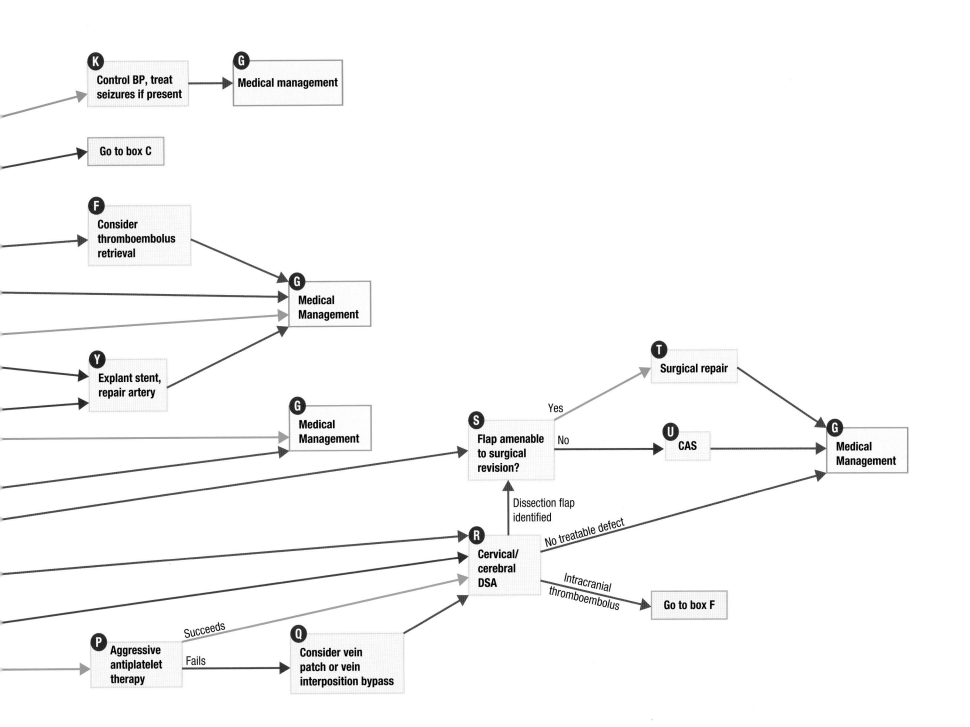

A Patient with new neurologic deficit after CEA/CAS

Neurologic deficits after carotid revascularization (CEA or CAS) procedures are relatively infrequent. Currently existing Society for Vascular Surgery and American Heart Association guidelines recommend target neurologic deficit rates of no more than 3% for asymptomatic patients and 6% for symptomatic patients undergoing CEA or CAS.[1,2] More recent experience from clinical trials and national databases suggest even lower acceptable thresholds for this complication.[3,4] Over 90% of neurologic deficits after CEA or CAS are a result of atheroembolization from the carotid bifurcation plaque with subsequent ischemic brain injury; a small proportion are from hyperperfusion and intracerebral hemorrhage.[5] CREST showed that most strokes after CEA or CAS were minor (81%), ischemic (90%), in the anterior circulation (94%), and on the ipsilateral side (88%).[6] Strokes are more frequent within 24 hours of CAS (60%) and CEA (43%), with fewer occurring post-treatment days 1 to 7 (21% CAS, 33% CEA) or days 8 to 30 (19% CAS, 24% CEA).[6] This chapter focuses on the management of neurologic deficits that occur within the first week of CEA or CAS.

B Deficit in treated carotid territory?

The great majority of periprocedural neurologic complications occur on the ipsilateral side of the CEA or CAS. Ipsilateral symptoms are a strong indicator of a periprocedural atheroembolic event, although, if they are immediate, they can be associated with prolonged clamp time during CEA. After transfemoral CAS, the contralateral carotid territory can be affected by atheroemboli from aortic arch catheter manipulation. When a postprocedure neurologic deficit does not occur within the treated carotid territory, additional nonembolic causes must be considered and potential hemorrhage excluded.

C Brain imaging: hemorrhage?

The first step in the evaluation of a patient with a new neurologic deficit on the side contralateral to the revascularization procedure, once the patient's airway and hemodynamic status have been secured, is rapid brain imaging to rule out hemorrhage or potentially retrievable large vessel embolization. Hemorrhage can be assessed with emergent brain CT. To detect a potentially treatable intracranial embolus, CTA, MRA, or rarely DSA is required.

D Neurosurgical consultation

The presence of intracranial hemorrhage with or without accompanying cerebral edema should prompt aggressive management of HTN, upright positioning of the patient, and neurosurgical consultation for consideration of cranial decompression and evacuation of the hematoma.

E Intracranial arterial thromboembolus?

The presence of intracranial arterial occlusion on contrast imaging, in combination with a perfusion deficit in the distal cerebral cortex on MR imaging, likely indicates atheroembolic occlusion.

F Consider thromboembolus retrieval

Acute occlusive intracranial arterial thrombus/embolus in the ICA or middle cerebral artery (MCA) should prompt immediate neuroradiologic and stroke team consultation. The patient should be evaluated for potential intracranial intra-arterial thrombus retrieval with or without locally delivered lytic therapy. For centers not having this treatment modality readily available, expeditious transfer of the patient to the closest facility that can offer such treatment should be considered. Several recent trials have confirmed the potential to reverse brain ischemia and its consequent deficits, especially when treatment is initiated within the first 4 to 6 hours of the event.[7] (For details of this treatment, see Chapter 9.)

G Medical management

Medical management of neurologic deficits after CEA or CAS is focused on the underlying cause. Because most result from atheroemboli, antiplatelet and statin therapy are important, just as they are after CEA or CAS without complications. If the cause of a post-CEA/CAS neurologic deficit has not been identified, a potential cardiac or arch source of embolism should be investigated. Echocardiography should be performed to rule out a cardiac source of emboli, with chest CTA recommended for aortic arch evaluation if not done previously. Many of the cryptogenic strokes after CAS or CEA result from unrecognized atrial fibrillation and are best managed with anticoagulation.

H Neurologic deficits noted during or at completion of procedure?

If a new neurologic deficit is observed during or immediately after the procedure, there should be high suspicion for a potentially reversible technical problem. It could result from distal dissection or intimal flap elevation, platelet-rich thromboembolization, or thrombosis. When a new early deficit is observed, anticoagulation is initiated and CEA reexploration or CAS arteriography is performed emergently. Events occurring at later timepoints are evaluated with other imaging.

I Emergent DUS or CTA: defect at CEA/CAS site?

When neurologic deficits are not present at the completion of CEA or CAS, but arise within hours or days, emergent imaging may disclose an underlying correctable problem. The imaging modality most rapidly available for making this determination may vary between hospitals. The choice between DUS or a CTA is based primarily on expediency, but if available, CTA provides much more information, including intracranial assessment.

J Cerebral Hyperperfusion Syndrome?

Cerebral hyperperfusion syndrome is an uncommon cause of neurologic deficits after carotid revascularization (<1%).[8] Its pathophysiology is related to dysregulation of cerebrovascular autoregulation that results in markedly increased cerebral blood flow with resulting cerebral edema. It usually occurs after treatment of a severe ICA stenosis in a patient who has severe contralateral carotid disease and can occur after CEA or CAS. Symptoms occur typically within 30 days of the procedure and most often within the first 5 days.[8] It is usually accompanied by HTN, headaches, nausea, and, in more severe cases, seizures and cerebral edema on brain imaging. Headache in a patient who has had a recent carotid revascularization is often the first sign of cerebral hyperperfusion and needs to be treated seriously. Transcranial Doppler (TCD) assessment that demonstrates high flow velocities in the MCA on the revascularized side can assist in the diagnosis. Severely reduced MCA blood flow velocity on the side of the carotid stenosis at baseline may indicate a higher risk of postoperative reperfusion injury. In addition, a 1.5-fold increase in MCA velocity after revascularization may predict the occurrence of hyperperfusion injury. In most cases of delayed ipsilateral neurologic deficit after CEA or CAS, the cause will be embolization, which should be evaluated when hyperperfusion syndrome is ruled out.

K Control BP, treat seizures if present

Management of cerebral hyperperfusion syndrome is focused on aggressive blood pressure control to reduce intracranial pressure, as well as monitoring for intracranial bleeding. If the condition progresses to intracranial bleeding, the prognosis is not favorable and up to 30% of patients will remain partially disabled, while mortality rates may be as high as 50%. SBP is lowered to <100 mm Hg if otherwise tolerated, which usually results in improvement of headache and reduction in TCD MCA flow velocity. Seizures and cerebral edema require neurologic consultation and treatment with antiseizure medication and steroids. Any patient with intracranial bleeding needs prompt neurosurgical consultation for consideration of potential cerebral decompression.

L Anticoagulate

If neurologic deficits are observed during or immediately after CEA or CAS, or if emergent cervical imaging demonstrates filling defects within the carotid artery at the repair site/within the stent, intravenous anticoagulation must be started immediately with an aim to achieve target activated clotting time between 250 and 300 seconds. Subsequent management depends on whether the event occurred after CEA or CAS.

M Re-explore CEA site

Early neurologic deficit after CEA should prompt immediate re-exploration of the operative site to evaluate and potentially treat a surgical site problem.[9] Expeditious return to the operating room is needed to restore flow in an occluded artery, tack down a dissection flap, or remove endarterectomy site thrombus and offers the only chance to prevent further brain injury. An exception to this general principle is if a normal completion DUS or DSA was done at the conclusion of the CEA, but the patient develops a very early neurologic deficit. In such a case, emergent DUS to confirm CEA patency followed by urgent CTA may be more prudent than reexploration.

Reoperation must be performed recognizing that further thrombus could embolize during the operative procedure itself and, as such, meticulous, gentle handling of the arteries is critical with early distal ICA control. After controlling the CCA and ECA, the endarterectomy site should be opened and inspected for thrombus, a dissection flap, or other technical problem as well as the presence of back-bleeding from the ICA. Treatment depends on whether thrombus or a distal flap/technical problem is found. If neither is present, cerebral DSA is performed to identify potential large vessel occlusion amenable to clot retrieval. If ICA back-bleeding is not observed, the arteriotomy should be extended if possible to ensure that a dissection has not occurred beyond the distal endpoint of the endarterectomy.

Ⓝ Thrombectomy

If thrombus is encountered, it is gently grasped and extracted with forceps. If this thrombus has been occlusive, it may have propagated a variable distance into the ICA. If ICA back-bleeding is not observed after extraction of visible thrombus, gentle and limited ICA thromboembolectomy should be performed. A No. 2 Fogarty balloon catheter should be used for sequential ICA thrombectomy by advancing the catheter in 2 cm increments to a maximum distance of approximately 10 cm. More distal balloon expansion is avoided as it could result in carotid cavernous sinus fistula. If back-bleeding results, low-pressure contrast DSA may be performed to ensure complete thrombus removal and extended to exclude intracranial large vessel thrombus. Any technical issues found after thrombus removal need correction before reclosing the endarterectomy site.

Ⓞ Platelet-rich white clot found?

In rare circumstances, a patient can develop a platelet-rich white clot "carpeting" of the endarterectomized surface that can embolize and result in neurologic deficits immediately after CEA. On reexploration, typical thrombosis is not encountered. Instead, platelet-rich fibrin aggregates (white clot) can be found lining the endarterectomized surface and/or patch. These appear in a typical "moth-eaten" pattern on imaging.

Ⓟ Aggressive antiplatelet therapy

If platelet-rich fibrin thrombus is identified at the CEA site, it is removed, and an antiplatelet infusion must be immediately initiated to prevent immediate recurrence during surgical repair. Options include starting an infusion of GPIIb/IIIa inhibitors, abciximab (IV bolus of 0.25 mg/kg, followed by 0.125 μg/kg/min

[max 10 μg/min]) or tirofiban (IV bolus of 25 μg/kg for 30 minutes followed by maintenance dose of 0.1 μg/kg/min).[10]

Ⓠ Consider vein patch or vein interposition bypass

After clearing the operative site of the platelet-rich fibrin aggregates and initiating an antiplatelet infusion, the next step in the procedure is to eliminate the inciting cause of the white clot. If aggregation recurs in the operating room and a synthetic patch was used at the initial procedure, then a vein patch should be used for arterial closure. Most recommend using proximal GSV or jugular vein. If the endarterectomized arterial surface is aggressively laden with white clot, then arterial replacement with a vein interposition graft needs to be considered.

Ⓡ Cervical/cerebral DSA

After successful ICA thrombectomy or treatment of platelet-rich aggregates at the surgical site, or if no technical defect is found at the endarterectomy site, on-table cervical/cerebral DSA should be performed to ensure adequate treatment of all arterial defects and to exclude large vessel intracranial emboli that might be amenable to retrieval. A careful angiographic assessment for dissection flaps must be made within the operative field.

Ⓢ Flap amenable to surgical revision?

A dissection flap can occur at the distal endpoint of the endarterectomized ICA if the plaque is inadequately feathered or not tacked down. Similarly, incomplete clearance of proximal plaque in the CCA can create a dissection flap if the endarterectomized plane is not uniform. If a dissection flap is identified at reexploration, it is repaired, usually by extending the endarterectomy and achieving a better endpoint. If the dissection flap is very distal, it may not be accessible for surgical revision, in which case CAS may need to be considered to treat the dissection flap.

Ⓣ Surgical repair

Usually the ICA arteriotomy needs to be extended to appropriately identify and correct a dissection flap at the distal endpoint. Extending the endarterectomy may achieve a good endpoint and treat a local dissection. If not, the flap must be tacked down, in a step-wise fashion, with interrupted 7-0 monofilament sutures (knot on the outside). Dissection flaps located along the endarterectomized surface should be removed and endpoints (or rough spots in the endarterectomized surface) secured with interrupted 7-0 sutures.

Ⓤ CAS

Dissection flaps that extend too far proximal or distal for adequate surgical repair can be treated with CAS.[11] If the flap is identified in the operating room with the endarterectomy site open, then a stent can be positioned and deployed expeditiously, with back-bleeding from the ICA providing embolic protection. If the

flap is identified later, a stent can be deployed through a transfemoral route, though adequate embolic protection must be instituted during the procedure.[12]

Ⓥ Retrieve and replace filter, complete procedure

If a neurologic defect occurs during CAS, the patient's anticoagulation must be maintained to an ACT between 250 and 300 seconds and a DSA performed. If a distal embolic protection filter is being utilized, large volume periprocedural microembolization may block the filter and result in a no-reflow phenomenon that causes contrast hold-up at the filter.[13] The proximal artery must be carefully aspirated with a catheter and the filter must be retrieved, taking care to capture and close the filter within its retrieval sheath to prevent distal embolization.[14] This should result in restoration of prograde cerebral flow on subsequent DSA, with reversal of neurologic deficits. If stenting has not been completed, a new filter (or flow reversal device) must be placed prior to completing the stenting and angioplasty procedure.

Ⓦ Additional stenting

Aggressive post-stenting angioplasty with balloon sizes in excess of 5 mm, balloons positioned outside of the stent during angioplasty, oversized stents, aggressive wire manipulation, prograde movement of the sheath, or shifting of the distal protection filter may all result in arterial injury and dissection flaps located in the proximal CCA or distal ICA arterial territories. These must be searched for carefully on multiplane DSA because they may not be readily visible. If identified, additional stenting is used to treat the dissection flap.

Ⓧ Suction thrombectomy, CDT

Inadequate periprocedural antithrombotic and antiplatelet therapy, undersizing of the stent, distal or proximal dissections, and stent collapse from excessive calcification can result in primary stent thrombosis. Several suction aspiration catheter devices are now available to address this infrequent complication and must be used immediately if stent thrombosis occurs. This may be followed by thrombolysis via a selectively placed catheter. If necessary, neuroradiologic consultation may be required intraoperatively to accomplish this.

Ⓨ Explant stent, repair artery

Dissections and stent thrombosis can generally be addressed with endovascular means. In the eventuality that resources are not available or reintervention has failed, and the patient presents with progressive symptoms, stent explantation and surgical repair of the carotid artery should be considered.[15] In patients with a stable neurologic deficit and stent thrombosis not amenable to endovascular treatment, anticoagulation to prevent distal thrombus propagation, rather than stent removal, is recommended. CEA in the setting of a freshly implanted stent may offer technical challenges, particularly if the stent was placed because of anatomic considerations (high or low lesions, radiation field, tracheostomy stoma). Arterial replacement with prosthetic or autogenous conduit may be necessary.

REFERENCES

1. Ricotta JJ, Aburahma A, Ascher E, Eskandari M, Faries P, Lal BK. Updated society for vascular surgery guidelines for management of extracranial carotid disease. *J Vasc Surg.* 2011;54(3):e1-e31. doi:10.1016/j.jvs.2011.07.004.
2. Brott TG, Halperin JL, Abbara S, et al. 2011 ASA/ACCF/AHA/AANN/AANS/ACR/ASNR/CNS/SAIP/SCAI/SIR/SNIS/SVM/SVS Guideline on the management of patients with extracranial carotid and vertebral artery disease a report of the American College of Cardiology Foundation/American Heart Association task force on practice guidelines, and the American Stroke Association, American Association of Neuroscience Nurses, American Association of Neurological Surgeons, American College of Radiology, American Society of Neuroradiology, Congress of Neurological Surgeons, Society of Atherosclerosis Imaging and Prevention, Society for Cardiovascular Angiography and Interventions, Society of Interventional Radiology, Society of NeuroInterventional Surgery, Society for Vascular Medicine, and Society for Vascular Surgery. *J Am Coll Cardiol.* 2011;57(8):e16-e94. doi:10.1016/j.jacc.2010.11.006.
3. Brott TG, Hobson RW, Howard G, et al. Stenting versus endarterectomy for treatment of carotid-artery stenosis. *N Engl J Med.* 2010;363:11-23. doi:10.1056/NEJMoa0912321.
4. Lichtman JH, Jones MR, Leifheit EC, et al. Carotid endarterectomy and carotid artery stenting in the US Medicare population, 1999-2014. *JAMA.* 2017;318(11):1035-1046. doi:10.1001/jama.2017.12882.
5. Ascher E, Markevich N, Schutzer RW, Kallakuri S, Jacob T, Hingorani AP. Cerebral hyperperfusion syndrome after carotid endarterectomy: predictive factors and hemodynamic changes. *J Vasc Surg.* 2003;37(4):769-777. doi:10.1067/mva.2003.231.
6. Hill MD, Brooks W, Mackey A, et al. Stroke after carotid stenting and endarterectomy in the Carotid Revascularization Endarterectomy versus Stenting Trial (CREST). *Circulation.* 2012;126(25):3054-3061. doi:10.1161/CIRCULATIONAHA.112.120030.
7. Goyal M, Menon BK, van Zwam WH, et al. Endovascular thrombectomy after large-vessel ischaemic stroke: a meta-analysis of individual patient data from five randomised trials. *Lancet (London, England).* 2016;387(10029):1723-1731. doi:10.1016/S0140-6736(16)00163-X.
8. Moulakakis KG, Mylonas SN, Sfyroeras GS, Andrikopoulos V. Hyperperfusion syndrome after carotid revascularization. *J Vasc Surg.* 2009;49(4):1060-1068. doi:10.1016/j.jvs.2008.11.026.
9. Rockman CB, Jacobowitz GR, Lamparello PJ, et al. Immediate reexploration for the perioperative neurologic event after carotid endarterectomy: is it worthwhile? *J Vasc Surg.* 2000;32(6):1062-1070. doi:10.1067/mva.2000.111284.
10. King S, Short M, Harmon C. Glycoprotein IIb/IIIa inhibitors: the resurgence of tirofiban. *Vascul Pharmacol.* 2016;78:10-16. doi:10.1016/j.vph.2015.07.008.
11. Anzuini A, Briguori C, Roubin GS, et al. Emergency stenting to treat neurological complications occurring after carotid endarterectomy. *J Am Coll Cardiol.* 2001;37(8):2074-2079. doi:10.1016/S0735-1097(01)01284-0.
12. Marone EM, Coppi G, Tshomba Y, Chiesa R. Eight-year experience with carotid artery stenting for correction of symptomatic and asymptomatic post-endarterectomy defects. *J Vasc Surg.* 2010;52(6):1511-1517. doi:10.1016/j.jvs.2010.06.167.
13. Roffi M, Baumgartner RW, Eberli FR. Images in cardiology. No reflow during carotid stenting. *Heart.* 2006;92(4):538. doi:10.1136/hrt.2005.070896.
14. Casserly IP, Abou-Chebl A, Fathi RB, et al. Slow-flow phenomenon during carotid artery intervention with embolic protection devices: predictors and clinical outcome. *J Am Coll Cardiol.* 2005;46(8):1466-1472. doi:10.1016/j.jacc.2005.05.082.
15. Moulakakis KG, Lazaris AM. Emergent carotid stent removal after carotid stent thrombosis. *Ann Vasc Surg.* 2018;46:401-406. doi:10.1016/j.avsg.2017.08.014.

Evan Lipsitz

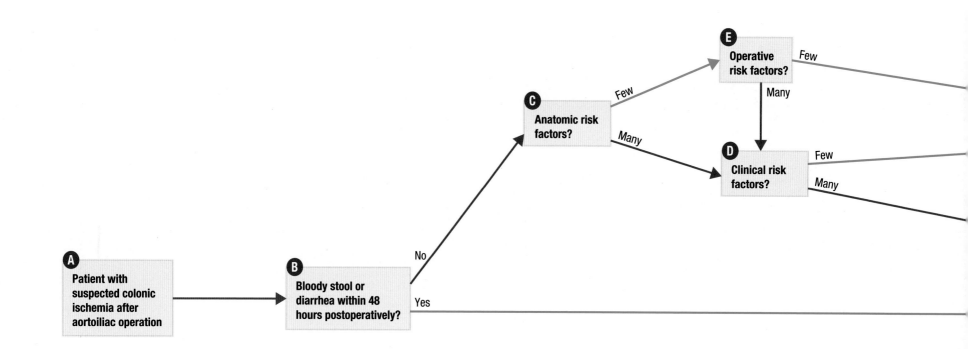

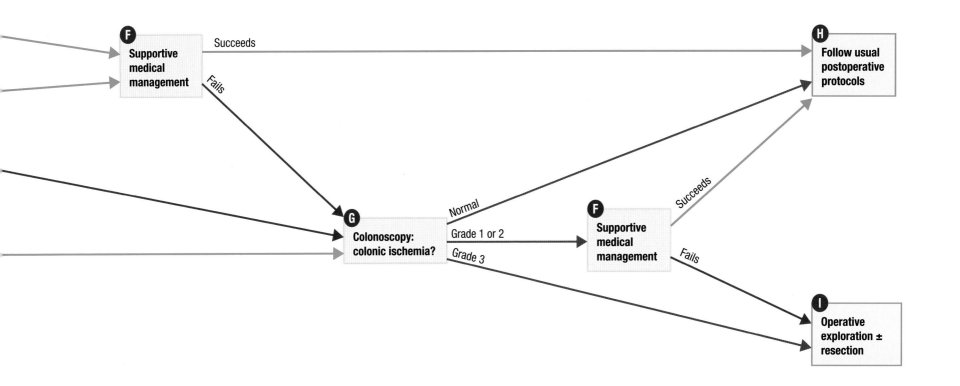

A Patient with suspected colonic ischemia after aortoiliac operation

Patients undergoing aortoiliac surgery are at risk for a number of complications including colonic ischemia. When this complication occurs, the consequences can be devastating. Anywhere from 1% to 3% of patients undergoing aortoiliac surgery for nonruptured AAA develop colon ischemia: 3% to 6% of those having open repair and 0.5% to 2% having endovascular repair.[1,2] In the setting of repair for a ruptured AAA, these percentages can increase 5- to 15-fold. A high index of suspicion and attention to perioperative risk factors are important for timely diagnosis and therapy. The most significant risk factor is an operation performed in the setting of ruptured aneurysm with coexisting hypotension.[1-3]

B Bloody stool or diarrhea within 48 hours postoperatively?

The presence of any of these findings is suggestive of ischemic colitis and should prompt immediate, and careful, colonoscopy.[4] Because most cases of colonic ischemia after aortic operation involve only the rectosigmoid colon, some authors recommend sigmoidoscopy in lieu of colonoscopy as it is often more readily available, and the diagnosis can be confirmed with this study alone.[5] Other concerning signs and symptoms for colonic ischemia postaortic surgery include persistent tachycardia, increased intravenous fluid requirements, and increasing leukocytosis and/or lactic acidosis. If colonic ischemia is suspected in the absence of these findings, the patient's preprocedural risk factors and anatomy should be reviewed for factors that may make ischemia more likely.

C Anatomic risk factors?

There are several preprocedural anatomic features that increase the risk of postoperative colonic ischemia. Unilateral or bilateral IIA occlusion is one such risk factor.[2,6,7] In some cases, a unilateral or bilateral IIA embolization is required to facilitate endovascular repair. Some authors have advocated staging the occlusion from the time of repair and performing staged embolization when bilateral coverage is required.[8] This clinical scenario is becoming less frequent with the advent of branched iliac endografts. When the IIA has been occluded, it is important to assess whether the occlusion was performed at the level of the main trunk or the primary IIA branches. In the latter setting, collaterals may be negatively impacted. Because many cases of colonic ischemia are caused by microembolization, it may also arise in the presence of patent IIAs.[8,9]

The preoperative status and intraoperative handling of the IMA have not been found to be a major predictive factor of colonic ischemia by the majority of authors.[2,10] It is important to note whether the IMA was occluded preoperatively and, if not, whether it was ligated/covered or reimplanted. If it was ligated or covered, an assessment of its size and flow should be reviewed if possible. The status of the SMA and the celiac artery as well as the presence of mesenteric collaterals should also be assessed.[11] If a large meandering mesenteric artery is seen on a preprocedural imaging and the IMA ligated or covered, suspicion for colonic ischemia should be high.

Other important independent risk factors for colonic ischemia include female gender, the presence of a "shaggy" aorta, smoking, CHF, HTN, CKD, and a history of pelvic radiation that may compromise the internal iliac and pelvic collaterals.[1,12-14] The risk of colon ischemia increases with the number of factors present.

D Clinical risk factors?

In addition to the presence of bloody stools or diarrhea, clinical factors that may indicate colonic ischemia include unexplained sepsis, decreased urine output, hemodynamic instability, peritonitis and/or abdominal pain, hypothermia, or evidence of diffuse microembolization. Suggestive laboratory abnormalities include leukocytosis, elevated lactate, and/or acidosis.[15] The risk of colon ischemia increases with the number of factors present.

E Operative risk factors?

The most significant operative risk factor for postaortic surgery colonic ischemia is aortic repair performed for rupture in the setting of concomitant hemorrhagic shock. Other significant operative risk factors include excessive blood loss and transfusion requirement, prolonged operative time, prolonged cross-clamp time, supraceliac location of the proximal clamp, preoperative renal insufficiency, and the need for an aortobifemoral reconstruction.[12,16] Operative iatrogenic vascular injury and the performance of an open versus endovascular repair have also been cited as risk factors. The risk of colon ischemia increases with the number of factors present.

F Supportive medical management

In the absence of suggestive clinical factors and operative risk factors, supportive medical management should be provided. This includes fluid resuscitation, broad-spectrum antibiotics, and bowel rest. Parenteral nutrition is used when indicated.

G Colonoscopy: colonic ischemia?

If colonoscopy/sigmoidoscopy does not show ischemic changes, the usual postoperative protocols may be followed. If suggestive clinical features persist, supportive medical management and a further search for the underlying cause are indicated. When colonic ischemia is present, therapy depends upon the grade seen on colonoscopy or sigmoidoscopy.[16] Grade 1 ischemia is defined as mucosal involvement alone and is usually transient. Grade 2 ischemia involves the mucosa and the muscularis, and while the injury may heal, there is the potential for future fibrosis and stricture formation. Grade 3 ischemia is defined by transmural necrosis and results in gangrene and perforation. Grades 1 and 2 ischemia are treated with supportive medical management and close observation. If clinical deterioration is evident, operative exploration is indicated. Grade 3 ischemia requires operative exploration and resection as needed. Supportive medical management is indicated throughout this second periprocedural period.[17]

H Follow usual post operative protocols

General principles of fluid management, awaiting return of bowel function, and progressive resumption of activity should be followed. The time course of events will clearly be different for patients undergoing open versus endovascular repair.

I Operative exploration ± resection

In the setting of Grade 3 ischemia, operative exploration will almost certainly include partial colonic resection and is best accomplished via laparotomy. In the setting of clinical deterioration with Grade 1 or 2 ischemia, laparotomy or laparoscopy may be performed, with the latter done only when a thorough and complete inspection is possible. Fifty percent of patients who develop colonic ischemia will require intervention, with substantial morbidity and mortality of 40% to 50%.[1,2]

REFERENCES

1. Moghadamyeghaneh Z, Sgroi MD, Chen SL, Kabutey NK, Stamos MJ, Fujitani RM. Risk factors and outcomes of postoperative ischemic colitis in contemporary open and endovascular abdominal aortic aneurysm repair. *J Vasc Surg*. 2016;63(4):866-872.
2. Ultee KH, Zettervall SL, Soden PA, et al; Vascular Study Group of New England. Incidence of and risk factors for bowel ischemia after abdominal aortic aneurysm repair. *J Vasc Surg*. 2016;64(5):1384-1391.
3. Becquemin JP, Majewski M, Fermani N, et al. Colon ischemia following abdominal aortic aneurysm repair in the era of endovascular abdominal aortic repair. *J Vasc Surg*. 2008;47:258-263.
4. Megalopoulos A, Vasiliadis K, Tsalis K, et al. Reliability of selective surveillance colonoscopy in the early diagnosis of colonic ischemia after successful ruptured abdominal aortic aneurysm repair. *Vasc Endovascular Surg*. 2007;41(6):509-515.
5. Assadian A, Senekowitsch C, Assadian O, Hartleb H, Hagmüller GW. Diagnostic accuracy of sigmoidoscopy compared with histology for ischemic colitis after aortic aneurysm repair. *Vascular*. 2008;16(5):243-247.
6. Farivar BS, Kalsi R, Drucker CB, Goldstein CB, Sarkar R, Toursavadkohi S. Implications of concomitant hypogastric artery embolization with endovascular repair of infrarenal abdominal aortic aneurysms. *J Vasc Surg*. 2017;66(1):95-101.
7. Lin PH, Chen AY, Vij A. Hypogastric artery preservation during endovascular aortic aneurysm repair: is it important?

Semin Vasc Surg. 2009;22(3):193-200. doi:10.1053/j.semvascsurg.2009.07.012.

8. Miller A, Marotta M, Scordi-Bello I, Tammaro Y, Marin M, Divino C. Ischemic colitis after endovascular aortoiliac aneurysm repair: a 10-year retrospective study. *Arch Surg.* 2009;144(10):900-903.

9. Dadian N, Ohki T, Veith FJ, et al. Overt colon ischemia after endovascular aneurysm repair: the importance of micro-embolization as an etiology. *J Vasc Surg.* 2001;34(6):986-996.

10. Senekowitsch C, Assadian A, Assadian O, Hartleb H, Ptakovsky H, Hagmüller GW. Replanting the inferior mesentery artery during infrarenal aortic aneurysm repair: influence on postoperative colon ischemia. *J Vasc Surg.* 2006;43(4):689-694.

11. Zhang WW, Kulaylat MN, Anain PM, et al. Embolization as cause of bowel ischemia after endovascular abdominal aortic aneurysm repair. *J Vasc Surg.* 2004;40(5):867-872.

12. Bjorck M, Troëng T, Bergqvist D. Risk factors for intestinal ischaemia after aortoiliac surgery: a combined cohort and case-control study of 2824 operations. *Eur J Vasc Endovasc Surg.* 1997;13:531-539.

13. Dardik H. Regarding "Incidence of and risk factors for bowel ischemia after abdominal aortic aneurysm repair." *J Vasc Surg.* 2017;65(4):1244-1245.

14. Toya N, Baba T, Kanaoka Y, Ohki T. Embolic complications after endovascular repair of abdominal aortic aneurysms. *Surg Today.* 2014;44(10):1893-1899.

15. Levison JA, Halpern VJ, Kline RG, Faust GR, Cohen JR. Perioperative predictors of colonic ischemia after ruptured abdominal aortic aneurysm. *J Vasc Surg.* 1999;29(1):40-45; discussion 45-47.

16. Champagne BJ, Darling RC III, Daneshmand M, et al. Outcome of aggressive surveillance colonoscopy in ruptured abdominal aortic aneurysm. *J Vasc Surg.* 2004;39(4):792-796.

17. Geraghty PJ, Sanchez LA, Rubin BG, et al. Overt ischemic colitis after endovascular repair of aortoiliac aneurysms. *J Vasc Surg.* 2004;40(3):413-418.

Michael C. Bounds • Eric D. Endean

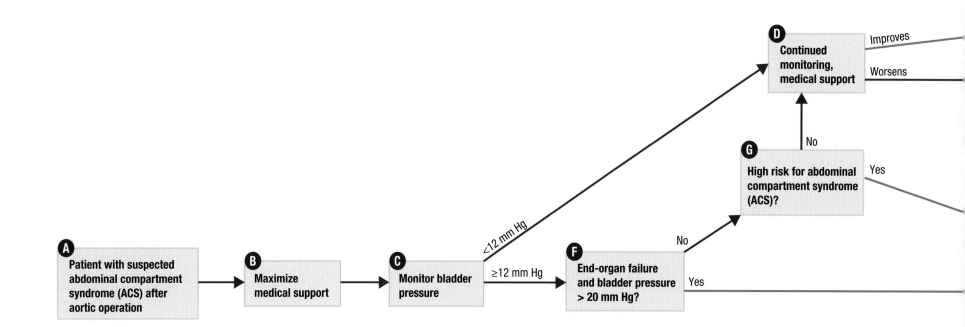

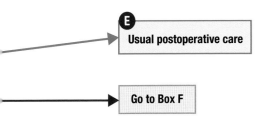

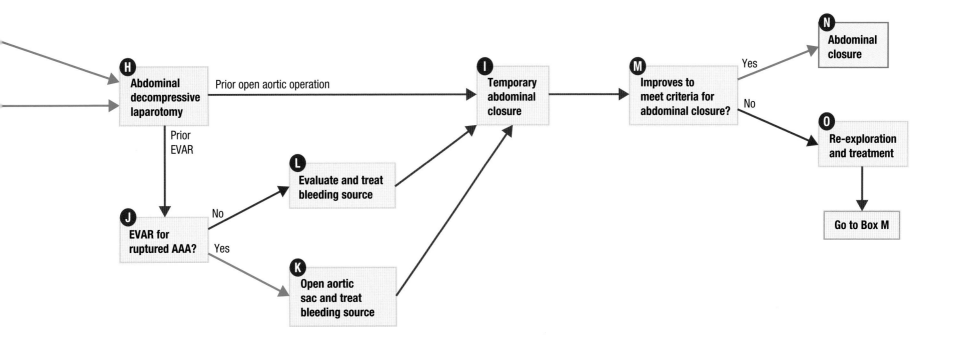

A **Patient with suspected abdominal compartment syndrome after aortic operation**

Abdominal compartment syndrome (ACS) is a condition in which intra-abdominal pressure (IAP) is elevated and, if untreated, can result in multisystem organ failure. Although the dangers of IAP have been recognized since the 1860s, the first use of the term ACS was in 1984, when Kron et al. described the development of the condition after aortic aneurysm repair.[1] Elevated IAP can occur after aortic surgery with a rise in intra-abdominal volume, either secondary to ongoing hemorrhage or with fluid sequestration within the abdominal cavity. This third spacing is exacerbated by massive resuscitation, ischemia-reperfusion injury, and stimulation of proinflammatory mediators to induce the release of oxygen free radicals and promote capillary leak. IAP is further increased with the use of positive-pressure ventilation and with decreased abdominal wall compliance.[2] Elevated IAP can decrease venous return, increase cardiac afterload, decrease lung compliance, and directly compress the heart. The condition is associated with a mortality of >50%.[2] ACS can develop after aortic surgery, with risk factors as outlined later.

EVAR, particularly in the setting of ruptured AAA (rAAA) may reduce the patient's inflammatory response and subsequent development of ACS.[3] However, ACS can still develop after EVAR, and when it does occur, it is associated with a mortality as high as 60% to 83%.[4,5] The incidence of ACS development after EVAR for rAAA is about 7.5%, as measured in a recent NSQIP study.[5]

In the setting of rAAA, the pathophysiologic mechanisms that lead to ACS development are likely different with EVAR compared to open repair. ACS that occurs after open repair is associated with over-resuscitation with crystalloid, whereas its development after EVAR is associated with increased requirement for blood transfusion, suggesting that ongoing bleeding is a primary mechanism of increased IAP.[4,5]

Patients undergoing either open or endovascular aortic surgery may develop ACS, which in turn greatly increases morbidity and mortality.[6] ACS is associated with a number of risk factors, including the following:

- Preoperative need for intubation and ventilatory support
- Large-volume resuscitation
- Perioperative shock
- Coagulopathy
- Massive transfusion
- Aortic rupture pathology[5,7,8]

Increased number and severity of these risk factors correlate with a higher likelihood of the development of ACS. When any of these are present, close monitoring for the potential development of ACS is needed.

B **Maximize medical support**

Clinical suspicion for development of ACS should lead to prompt escalation of care with close monitoring and maximization of medical management. A number of adjunctive measures should be pursued when a patient is at high risk for development of ACS, but does not exhibit clear indications for decompressive laparotomy. Medical support may prevent the development of ACS by reducing IAP and correcting fluid balance.[9]

Preventive interventions include the following:

- Enteral decompression with nasogastric and/or rectal tubes
- Reverse Trendelenburg positioning
- Neuromuscular blockade
- Adequate sedation and pain control
- Optimized ventilator settings
- Minimizing fluid resuscitation and use diuretics as tolerated to achieve negative fluid balance[10]
- Correction of coagulopathy

C **Monitor bladder pressure**

For patients at risk for ACS, bladder pressure measurements (which reflect IAP) can provide an objective means for clinical decision making. The World Society of the Abdominal Compartment Syndrome has defined IAP >12 mm Hg as intra-abdominal hypertension, whereas IAP >20 mm Hg with end-organ failure constitutes ACS. Abdominal perfusion pressure is defined as MAP – IAP. Abdominal perfusion pressure of 60 mm Hg can also be used as a threshold for diagnosing ACS.[10] IAP < 12 mm Hg is an indication of continued pressure monitoring and medical support, whereas IAP ≥ 12 mm Hg may require abdominal decompression, depending on the presence of end-organ failure and the risk factors for ACS that are present.

D **Continued monitoring, medical support**

In patients with suspected ACS but IAP < 12 mm Hg, or in patients with higher IAP but no end-organ failure who are not high risk for ACS, continued clinical and bladder pressure monitoring is indicated, with continued medical support to reduce the likelihood of ACS (see B). If the clinical scenario and IAP improve, usual postoperative care in continued. However, if IAP increases to ≥12 mm Hg or the clinical scenario worsens, the need for decompressive laparotomy must be reevaluated.

E **Usual postoperative care**

Without predisposing risk factors associated with ACS, standard postoperative management is indicated.

F **End-organ failure and bladder pressure >20 mm Hg?**

In the setting of elevated bladder pressure (>12 mm Hg) without signs of clinical deterioration or end-organ failure, ongoing monitoring with continued medical support is indicated.

End-organ failure combined with bladder pressure >20 mm Hg is the hallmark of ACS and requires emergent decompressive laparotomy. End-organ failure is manifested by renal failure with oliguria, pulmonary failure with respiratory decline and increased peak airway pressures, and/or cardiac failure with decreased cardiac output and increased pulmonary capillary wedge pressure. The high morbidity and mortality associated with ACS is secondary to the consequences of end-organ failure, and it is therefore of utmost importance that the clinician has a high level of suspicion for ACS development when multiple risk factors are present. Clinical experience may prove more valuable than strict bladder pressure criteria in preventing the disastrous consequences of ACS development.[11] It should be noted that much of the data regarding monitoring for ACS and its subsequent development are limited by the lack of prospective randomized trials.

G **High risk for abdominal compartment syndrome (ACS)?**

In patients with IAP ≥ 12 mm Hg, but without end-organ failure, the presence of multiple risk factors for ACS (see A) is a potential indication for preemptive decompressive laparotomy. Data supporting this treatment in patients without associated end-organ failure are insufficient to make firm recommendations,[10,11] but this approach obviates the difficulties in monitoring for and detecting ACS, and may mitigate the associated high morbidity and mortality that comes with the condition. Although data are limited, primary abdominal decompressive laparotomy appears to be associated with decreased intestinal ischemia, lower rates of dialysis, shorter duration of open abdomen, lower in-hospital mortality, and higher primary fascial closure rates.[12] Clinical judgment considering all risk factors in the context of the patient's overall condition is required to make this decision, but a liberal application of decompressive laparotomy is generally recommended.

H **Abdominal decompressive laparotomy**

For patients with ACS, the most reliable and expeditious treatment modality is decompressive laparotomy. This procedure also allows for exploration of the abdomen and surgical correction of any contributing factors such as on-going hemorrhage or infarcted bowel.

Although there have been attempts at less invasive methods of ACS management, the gold standard remains decompressive laparotomy. Interventions with percutaneous intraperitoneal drain placement or placement of lytic catheters in areas of known hematoma have shown some promise, but large trials are lacking to support their routine use and application. Use of both intraperitoneal drains and lytic catheter methods are also limited by length of time to onset of action, inability to assess intra-abdominal contents, and potential worsening of hemorrhage.[9]

It should be noted that ACS associated with EVAR treatment of ruptured AAA may present a special case. When ACS develops at the initial operation and requires concurrent laparotomy, there is a nearly sixfold increase in 30-day mortality[5] which may be secondary to ongoing bleeding. Thus, management of ACS after EVAR requires special considerations (see J).

Ⓘ Temporary abdominal closure

There are numerous methods for temporary abdominal closure, including use of Bogota bags, and other "homemade" vacuum dressings, bridging meshes, and the Abthera open abdomen negative pressure (vacuum) system (Acelity and KCI, San Antonio, TX).[2,8,12,13] Although it is beyond the scope of this chapter to debate the merits of these various methods, the critical characteristics of temporary closure include management of increased IAP, maintenance of sterility, and the ability to perform multiple relook operations. With vacuum dressings, the rate of closure has been reported to be >90%.[12]

Ⓙ EVAR for ruptured AAA?

In the setting of EVAR for rAAA, consideration must be given to ongoing bleeding/endoleak as the etiology for development of ACS. Unlike in open aortic surgery, where bleeding from lumbar vessels and the IMA is controlled with suture ligature, in EVAR performed for rupture, a type II endoleak can result in ongoing hemorrhage, enlarging retroperitoneal hematoma, and resultant clinical decline.[4,5,7]

Ⓚ Open aortic sac and treat bleeding source

For patients who develop ACS following EVAR for ruptured AAA, consideration should be given to opening the aneurysm sac for ligation of lumbar vessels, the IMA, or additional points of bleeding within the sac if no other cause for ongoing hemorrhage (type 1 or 3 endoleak) has been determined.[4] If there is any concern regarding ongoing hemorrhage secondary to type 1 or 3 endoleak, the sac should not be opened and the patient should be immediately treated with endovascular evaluation and repair of the technical problem or conversion to open repair.

Ⓛ Evaluate and treat bleeding source

Intra-abdominal hemorrhage, especially after open AAA repair, should be considered as a cause for the development of ACS and treated operatively when present. In addition to bowel edema from resuscitation, a large retroperitoneal hematoma can occupy space and contribute to the formation of ACS. Careful evacuation of such a hematoma is recommended.

Ⓜ Improves to meet criteria for abdominal closure?

Before attempting abdominal closure after decompressive laparotomy, the patient must be clinically stable with normal IAP, resolution of ACS pathology, and maximal treatment of risk factors. Quantitative parameters include improvement in pulmonary function with decreasing oxygen requirements and peak airway pressures, restoration of renal function, and improvement in cardiac function with hemodynamic stabilization. In addition, the abdominal wall must have sufficient laxity to allow fascial approximation without an increase in IAP. There are no strict criteria for determining when it is safe to proceed to abdominal closure, but the patient should demonstrate improvement in the physiologic parameters that led to the diagnosis of ACS.

Ⓝ Abdominal closure

At the time of abdominal closure, attention to supportive care must be maintained with reestablishment of abdominal domain. With prolonged open abdomen, direct fascial closure may not be possible, and adjuncts such as bridging meshes or component separation may be required.[8] Appropriate abdominal wall laxity for primary closure can be verified intraoperatively by monitoring bladder pressures while performing partial or complete closure.[8]

Ⓞ Re-exploration and treatment

With ongoing clinical instability or deterioration, relook laparotomy may be indicated. At that exploration, other etiologies must be considered, including the presence of infarcted bowel that would require resection.

REFERENCES

1. Kron IL, Harman PK, Nolan SP. The measurement of intra-abdominal pressure as a criterion for abdominal re-exploration. *Ann Surg.* 1984;196:28-30.
2. Loftus IM, Thompson MM. The abdominal compartment syndrome following aortic surgery. *Eur J Vasc Endovasc Surg.* 2003;25:97-109.
3. Makar RR, Badger SA, O'Donnell ME, Loan W, Lau LL, Soong CV. The effects of abdominal compartment hypertension after open and endovascular repair of a ruptured abdominal aortic aneurysm. *J Vasc Surg.* 2009;49:866-872.
4. Rubenstein C, Bietz G, Davenport DL, Winkler M, Endean ED. Abdominal compartment syndrome associated with endovascular and open repair of ruptured abdominal aortic aneurysms. *J Vasc Surg.* 2015;61:648-654.
5. Adkar SS, Turley RS, Benrashid E, Cox MW, Mureebe L, Shortell CK. Laparotomy during endovascular repair of ruptured abdominal aortic aneurysms increases mortality. *J Vasc Surg.* 2017;65:356-361.
6. Ersryd S, Djavani-Gidlund K, Wanhainen A, Björck M. Editor's choice—Abdominal compartment syndrome after surgery for abdominal aortic aneurysm: a nationwide population based study. *Eur J Vasc Endovasc Surg.* 2016;52:158-165.
7. Mehta M, Darling RC, Roddy SP, et al. Factors associated with abdominal compartment syndrome complicating endovascular repair of ruptured abdominal aortic aneurysms. *J Vasc Surg.* 2005;42:1047-1051.
8. Mayer D, Rancic Z, Meier C, Pfammatter T, Veith F, Lachat M. Open abdomen treatment following endovascular repair of ruptured abdominal aortic aneurysms. *J Vasc Surg.* 2009;50:1-7.
9. Karkos CD, Menexes GC, Patelis N, Kalogirou TE, Giagtzidis IT, Harkin DW. A systematic review and meta-analysis of abdominal compartment syndrome after endovascular repair of ruptured abdominal aortic aneurysms. *J Vasc Surg.* 2014;59:829-842.
10. Kirkpatrick AW, Roberts DJ, Waele JD, et al. Intra-abdominal hypertension and the abdominal compartment syndrome: updated consensus definitions and clinical practice guidelines from the World Society of the Abdominal Compartment Syndrome. *Intensive Care Med.* 2013;39:1190-1206.
11. Björck M, Wanhainen A. Management of abdominal compartment syndrome and the open abdomen. *Eur J Vasc Endovasc Surg.* 2014;47:279-287.
12. Acosta S, Seternes A, Venermo M, et al. Open abdomen therapy with vacuum and mesh mediated fascial traction after aortic repair: an international multicentre study. *Eur J Vasc Endovasc Surg.* 2017;54:697-705.
13. Acosta S, Wanhainen A, Björck M. Temporary abdominal closure after abdominal aortic aneurysm repair: a systematic review of contemporary observational studies. *Eur J Vasc Endovasc Surg.* 2016;51:371-378.

Jahan Mohebali • Matthew J. Eagleton

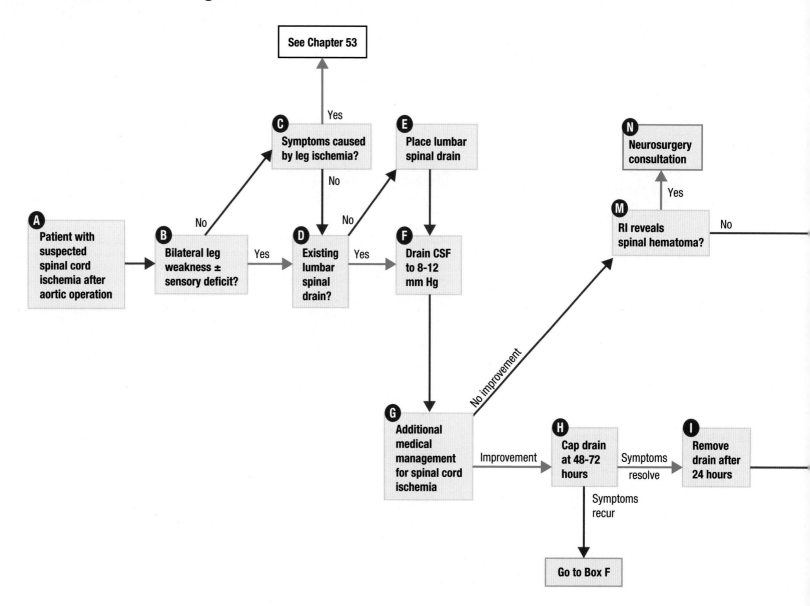

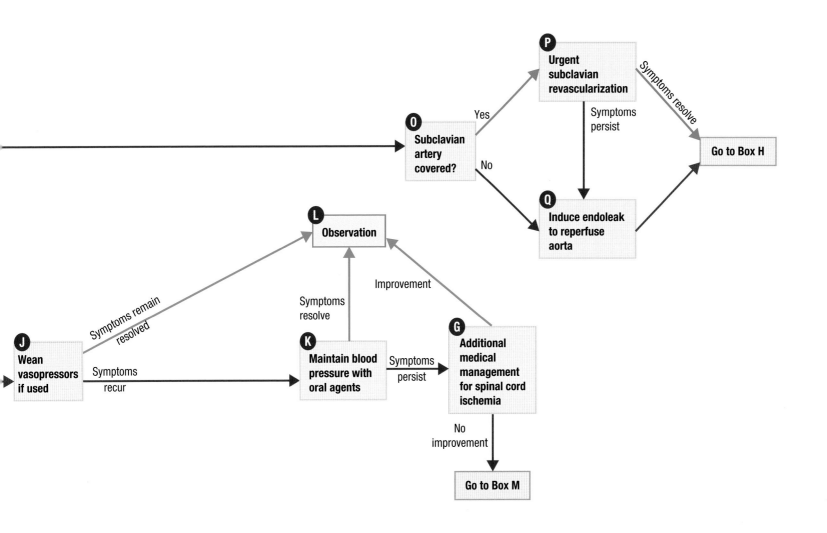

A Patient with suspected spinal cord ischemia after aortic operation

Spinal cord ischemia (SCI) is a devastating potential complication of aortic surgery. Its incidence is most directly affected by the extent of aortic repair, with longer segments of aortic exclusion or replacement placing patients at higher risk.[1,2] Rates of SCI after open and endovascular repair of AAA are very low (<0.2%).[3,4] Patients are at increased risk after AAA repair if there are prolonged procedural times, extensive intra-aortic graft manipulation resulting in embolization, coil embolization of a hypogastric artery, or treatment of aortic rupture.[3,5] The development of SCI following TEVAR is more frequent, ranging from 2% to 10%, with the majority of symptoms presenting in a delayed manner (see Chapter 20).[6-10] SCI associated with TAAA repair also varies ranging from 2% to 21% depending on the extent of repair.[4,11-13] In addition to the extent of coverage, independent risk factors for the development of SCI after TEVAR are renal insufficiency, prolonged fluoroscopy time, sustained hypotension, and occlusion of a collateral network artery (such as the subclavian or hypogastric artery).[14]

B Bilateral leg weakness ± sensory deficit?

Lower extremity weakness following aortic surgery can occur because of a variety of etiologies, and SCI accounts for approximately 40% of these reasons. Other etiologies include acute lower extremity ischemia, cerebrovascular accidents, exacerbation of chronic neurologic comorbidities, peripheral neuropathy, and metabolic encephalopathy.[4] Workup of acute postoperative lower extremity weakness must include the patient's history, clinical presentation, and risk factors for SCI.

SCI symptoms following aortic surgery can vary from mild paraparesis to flaccid paralysis, and these may be associated with sensory deficits. Although symptoms are often bilateral, they can be asymmetric in both presentation and severity. Temporal presentation can also vary. Symptoms can develop immediately upon arousal from anesthesia, or in a more delayed manner, up to days to weeks following the primary operation. Patients who present immediately with flaccid paralysis are less likely to recover and more likely have irreversible spinal cord damage. Prompt evaluation and treatment are essential for all causes of lower extremity weakness following aortic surgery to provide the best chance of recovery. Even with aggressive treatment, many patients having SCI do not return to baseline functional levels. In addition, occurrence of SCI symptoms is associated with a dramatically reduced long-term survival.[4,15]

C Symptoms caused by leg ischemia?

The second most common cause of lower extremity weakness with or without sensory loss following aortic surgery is lower extremity ischemia. Unlike SCI, this is less likely to occur bilaterally.

Diagnosis is facilitated by physical examination findings of a cool, pale, pulseless lower extremity in association with a possible motor or sensory deficit. For management of ALI, see Chapter 53.

D Existing lumbar spinal drain?

The use of prophylactic spinal drainage for all aortic operations is controversial. Two randomized studies have demonstrated reduced incidence of SCI by placing spinal drains before open aortic surgery.[16,17] Coselli et al. reported an incidence of paraplegia and paraparesis in 13% of patients without the use of spinal drains, whereas those with spinal drains had a 2.6% rate of paraparesis and no paraplegia. Svensson et al. demonstrated a nearly 75% risk reduction (43%-12%) of paraparesis/paraplegia in those undergoing repairs of types I and II TAAA with the use of a spinal drain and intrathecal papaverine.

Although these protocols have gained credibility for their application to open aortic surgery, there has been no randomized trial of lumbar spinal drain use to prevent SCI associated with endovascular aortic surgery. Given the relative rarity of SCI with EVAR, its routine use is not indicated. Similarly, given the high risk associated with extensive TAAA treatment (types II and III TAAA), most surgeons would use perioperative lumbar spinal drainage in patients undergoing endovascular treatment of such thoracic aortic anatomy.

Controversy exists in the use of prophylactic lumbar spinal drainage in the setting of TEVAR for TAA. The following three strategies are employed: (1) mandatory drainage for all patients; (2) selective drainage for patients considered at high risk for SCI; (3) selective drainage for patients who develop symptoms of SCI. When choosing mandatory drainage, surgeons must weigh the risk and benefit of routine spinal drainage and its associated potential complications (see Box M). Those considered at high risk for SCI are discussed in Box A.

E Place lumbar spinal drain

If a routine lumbar spinal drain has not been placed, most would advocate drain placement and use of CSF drainage in the setting of acute SCI following aortic surgery. The Alabama protocol[18] calls for neurologic assessment of patients following TEVAR every 2 hours for the initial 8 hours, and then every 4 hours if there is no change in neurologic status. If patients develop motor deficits worse than 4/5, or significant sensory loss, then immediate lumbar spinal drain placement is mandated.[18] This is augmented with pharmacologic increase in MAP, as discussed later. If there are neurologic deficits but maintained >4/5 motor function, an MRI of the thoracic and lumbar spine is obtained, if feasible. If MRI findings exclude an alternate etiology and there is evidence of reversible ischemia, a spinal drain is placed. One of the keys to the success of a selective lumbar spinal drain protocol is the institutional capability of timely placement. In hospitals where this is not possible, protocols for routine preoperative drain placement should be adopted, at least in high-risk patients.

F Drain CSF to 8-12 mm Hg

Most lumbar spinal drain protocols call for drainage of CSF to maintain CSF pressure from 8 to 12 mm Hg, or approximately 10 to 16 cm H_2O. A serious risk of lumbar spinal drainage is the development of a subdural hematoma potentially caused by stretching and tearing of subdural veins during CSF drainage.[19] As such, most experts advocate judicious use of CSF drainage, with hourly limits on the total volume drained (20-30 mL/h). In addition, patients are frequently kept in a supine position (<30° head of bed elevation) to avoid potential fluctuations in CSF and cerebral perfusion pressure.

G Additional medical management for spinal cord ischemia

In addition to lumbar spinal drains, the mainstay of therapy for patients who experience symptoms attributable to SCI is augmentation of blood pressure. Hypotension and fluctuations in SBP have been shown to be associated with the development of delayed SCI.[20] In fact, 90% of patients who experience delayed-onset SCI either had episodes of SBP < 130 mm Hg or 15 mm Hg fluctuations in SBP. Therefore, pharmacologic strategies to maintain SBP > 140 mm Hg and cardiac index >2.5 L/min/m² should be adopted.[20,21] Some experts have suggested more aggressive blood pressure augmentation, driving the MAP > 110 mm Hg.[22] In addition, transfusion to maintain a hemoglobin >10 g/dL has been recommended.

A number of other pharmacologic adjuncts, including corticosteroids, naloxone, barbiturates, and mannitol, have been investigated for preventing the development of SCI following open aortic surgery. None have been evaluated for use in the endovascular patient population, and none have been demonstrated to have effects on outcomes for patients who have developed SCI symptoms in the postoperative period.[21,23]

H Cap drain at 48-72 hours

The exact time for maintenance of lumbar spinal drainage of CSF is unknown. Most would advocate continuation of drainage for no less than 24 hours or until neurologic symptoms have plateaued.[18] Others advocate for a longer drainage period ranging from 3 to 7 days depending on the severity of symptoms.[21,22] On the basis of animal studies, it appears that there is a change in the anatomic morphology of the paraspinous arteries and arterioles providing a substrate for improved cord perfusion.[24] In this canine model, paraspinous vascular remodeling had occurred by 5 days after intercostal/lumbar artery occlusion. This may serve as a framework to drive clinical decision making regarding patients with persistent SCI symptoms and an intact spinal drain, such that its value after 5 days may be of limited use.

I Remove drain after 24 hours

Following resolution of SCI symptoms, a process should be initiated to remove the lumbar spinal drain and limit intravenous vasopressor use. Initially, the spinal drain is not removed but simply capped. This allows for easy reinitiation of drainage if symptoms recur within the first few hours. If the patient remains symptom-free, or with stable, permanent symptoms after the drain has been capped for 24 hours, it is removed.

(J) Wean pressors if used

In addition to removing the lumbar spinal drain, removal of pharmacologic blood pressure augmentation should commence after SCI symptoms resolve or plateau. This should be done gradually to prevent rapid fluctuations in blood pressure, which may cause recurrence of SCI symptoms.

(K) Maintain blood pressure with oral agents

Once IV vasopressors are eliminated, strict caution should be taken when reinitiating any preoperative medications with hypotensive effects. In some situations, patients are intolerant of cessation of the IV vasopressors without the administration of oral hypertensive agents such as midodrine or pseudoephedrine. There are limited data reporting outcomes of the use of oral hypertensive agents in patients with resistant or persistent SCI.

(L) Observation

Patients recovering from SCI following aortic surgery require close attention and monitoring following their recovery. Special care should be taken to avoid hypotensive episodes, especially in patients who are on renal replacement therapy because dialysis episodes can reinitiate their symptoms. Long-term survival for patients who develop SCI symptoms is worse than in those who do not.[4,15] DeSart et al. demonstrated that estimated mean survival in those with and without SCI was 37 versus 72 months, respectively.[15] In patients with SCI and functional improvement, mean estimated survival was 54 months, whereas in those with permanent, nonrelenting deficits, mean survival was only 9 months.

(M) MRI reveals spinal hematoma?

If spinal drainage and medical management of acute SCI do not result in resolution of symptoms, the possibility of spinal hematoma must be considered. Hemorrhagic complications following lumbar spinal drain placement for open or endovascular aortic repair range from 3% to 4%.[25,26] These must be differentiated into neuraxial complications including epidural or intraspinal hematoma, and those occurring intracranially, either of which may or may not result in bloody CSF drainage and/or neurologic deficit. Despite guidelines from the American Society of Regional Anesthesia and Pain Medicine regarding timing of antiplatelet cessation,[27] Mazzeffi et al. did not find any association with preoperative aspirin or clopidogrel use and actual bleeding complications.[26] In fact, in their study, the only patient who developed an epidural hematoma was not taking any antiplatelet medications. Moreover, bloody spinal drain output was not necessarily predictive of

neuraxial hematoma, even in cases where it was associated with paraplegia. Similarly, Wynn et al. noted bloody drainage in 5% of their cases, yet none of these patients had neuraxial hematoma.[25] It should be noted, however, that 70% of these patients had some form of intracranial hemorrhage that was associated with high mortality and further supported the authors' protocol to obtain both spinal *and* head CT in any patient with bloody drainage and abnormal neurologic findings.

Because epidural hematomas are outside the CSF space, they are often not associated with bloody drainage.[28] Given the inability to predict these complications, deficits refractory to the measures mentioned in Boxes A-D should be evaluated with MRI, which has the benefit of identifying both neuraxial blood and/or cord ischemia. In cases with concomitant bloody drain output where no neuraxial hematoma is identified, strong consideration should be given to intracranial imaging. Lastly, patients who are unable to undergo MRI secondary to instability, stent-graft composition, or other factors, should obtain spinal CT.

(N) Neurosurgery consultation

If a spinal hematoma is identified, emergent neurosurgical consultation is obtained to ensure timely decompression, as needed, with the aim at preservation of cord function.

(O) Subclavian artery covered?

Although the development of SCI during or after extensive aortic surgery was thought to primarily result from interruption of blood flow to the Artery of Adamkiewicz,[29] Griepp et al. challenged this view by demonstrating that patients with less extensive aneurysms and fewer than 10 interrupted segmental arteries failed to develop paraplegia.[30] Furthermore, these authors showed that postoperative SCI was reversible in some instances. Jacobs and Backes later postulated that multiple vessels were responsible for spinal cord perfusion,[31,32] a notion that was ultimately formalized by Griepp as the "collateral network concept."[33] This concept postulates that a series of inflow vessels consisting of segmental (intercostal, lumbar), internal iliac, and subclavian arteries perfuse a richly anastomotic vascular bed that ultimately supplies the spinal cord. Thus, elimination of one of these inflow sources should not consistently result in cord ischemia, assuming compensatory flow is provided via other inflow sources. The Cleveland group confirmed this by demonstrating that in any case of aortic endografting (segmental artery coverage) where an additional inflow vessel was occluded (hypogastric or subclavian), immediate SCI rates increased from 24% to 73%.[4] Thus, it should be emphasized that in cases where subclavian or internal iliac coverage is anticipated, preemptive revascularization should be employed, if possible when there is a high risk for development of SCI.[4,34-36]

(P) Urgent subclavian revascularization

The Society for Vascular Surgery has developed guidelines recommending routine subclavian revascularization in all elective

aortic endografting procedures where subclavian artery origin coverage is anticipated.[36] Although these guidelines are based on data that show only a trend toward increased odds of paraplegia (OR, 2.69, 95% CI, 0.75-9.68), they are meant to prevent additional adverse outcomes of arm and vertebrobasilar ischemia that demonstrated statistically significant association with subclavian coverage.[37] Although no specific data exist regarding urgent subclavian revascularization, in cases where SCI persists after aortic surgery despite implementation of treatment outlined in Boxes A to H, timely augmentation/restoration of subclavian blood flow by means of angioplasty/stent or carotid-subclavian bypass may prove beneficial.

(Q) Induce endoleak to reperfuse aorta

An alternate approach to reverse acute SCI is to induce an aortic sac endoleak to reperfuse potential branches to the spinal cord that arise from the excluded aorta.[38] This can be accomplished by gaining access between the distal stent graft and aortic or iliac wall. Once in this location, a type Ib endoleak may be induced by the placement of a balloon expandable stent—thus disrupting the distal seal. Once the patient has recovered, the endoleak can be reversed with occlusion of this secondary stent. Neither the effectiveness of this technique nor the timing of reversal of the endoleak is known. It may be considered in patients with recurrent symptoms or in those who develop symptoms on emergence from anesthesia in the operating room despite use of other adjuncts.

REFERENCES

1. Greenberg R, Eagleton M, Mastracci T. Branched endografts for thoracoabdominal aneurysms. *J Thorac Cardiovasc Surg*. 2010;140(6 suppl):S171-S178.
2. Feezor RJ, Martin TD, Hess PJ Jr, et al. Extent of aortic coverage and incidence of spinal cord ischemia after thoracic endovascular aneurysm repair. *Ann Thorac Surg*. 2008;86(6):1809-1814; discussion 14.
3. Berg P, Kaufmann D, van Marrewijk CJ, Buth J. Spinal cord ischemia after set-graft treatment for infra-renal abdominal aortic aneurysms. Analysis of the Eurostar database. *Eur J Vasc Endovasc Surg*. 2001;22:342-347.
4. Eagleton MJ, Shah S, Petkosevek D, Mastracci TM, Greenberg RK. Hypogastric and subclavian artery patency affects onsent and recovery of spinal cord ischemia associated with aortic endografting. *J Vasc Surg*. 2014;59:89-94.
5. Peppelenbosch N, Cuypers PW, Vahl AC, Vermassen F, Buth J. Emergency endovascular treatment for ruptured abdominal aortic aneurysm and the risk of spinal cord ischemia. *J Vasc Surg*. 2005;42(4):608-614.
6. Ullery BW, Cheung AT, Fairman RM, et al. Risk factors, outcomes, and clinical manifestations of spinal cord ischemia following thoracic endovascular aortic repair. *J Vasc Surg*. 2011;54(3):677-684.

7. Lee WA, Daniels MJ, Beaver TM, Klodell CT, Raghinaru DE, Hess PJ Jr. Late outcomes of a single-center experience of 400 consecutive thoracic endovascular aortic repairs. *Circulation*. 2011;123(25):2938-2945.

8. Fairman RM, Criado F, Farber M, et al. Pivotal results of the medtronic vascular talent thoracic stent graft system: the VALOR trial. *J Vasc Surg*. 2008;48(3):546-554.

9. Matsumura JS, Cambria RP, Dake MD, et al. International controlled clinical trial of thoracic endovascular aneurysm repair with the Zenith TX2 endovascular graft: 1-year results. *J Vasc Surg*. 2008;47(2):247-257; discussion 57.

10. Buth J, Harris PL, Hobo R, et al. Neurologic complications associated with endovascular repair of thoracic aortic pathology: incidence and risk factors. a study from the European Collaborators on Stent/Graft Techniques for Aortic Aneurysm Repair (EUROSTAR) registry. *J Vasc Surg*. 2007;46(6):1103-1110; discussion 10-11.

11. Chiesa R, Melissano G, Marrocco-Trischitta MM, Civilini E, Setacci F. Spinal cord ischemia after elective stent-graft repair of the thoracic aorta. *J Vasc Surg*. 2005;42(1):11-17.

12. Black JH III, Cambria RP. Contemporary results of open surgical repair of descending thoracic aortic aneurysms. *Semin Vasc Surg*. 2006;19(1):11-17.

13. Greenberg RK, Lu Q, Roselli EE, et al. Contemporary analysis of descending thoracic and thoracoabdominal aneurysm repair: a comparison of endovascular and open techniques. *Circulation*. 2008;118(8):808-817.

14. Sobel JD, Vartanian SM, Gasper WJ, Hiramoto JS, Chuter TA, Reilly LM. Lower extremity weakness after endovascular repair with multibranched thoracoabdominal stent grafts. *J Vasc Surg*. 2014:1-7.

15. DeSart K, Scali ST, Feezor RJ, et al. Fate of patients with spinal cord ischemia complicating thoracic endovascular aortic repair. *J Vasc Surg*. 2013;58:635-642.

16. Coselli JS, LeMaire SA, Koksoy C, Schmittling ZC, Curling PE. Cerebrospinal fluid drainage reduces paraplegia after thoracoabdominal aortic aneurysm repair: results of a randomized clinical trial. *J Vasc Surg*. 2002;35(4):631-639.

17. Svensson LG, Hess KR, D'Agostino RS, et al. Reduction of neurologic injury after high-risk thoracoabdominal aortic operation. *Ann Thorac Surg*. 1998;66:132-138.

18. Keith CJ Jr, Passman MA, Carignan MJ, et al. Protocol implementation of selective postoperative lumbar spinal drainage after thoracic aortic endograft. *J Vasc Surg*. 2012;55(1):1-8; discussion 8.

19. Dardik A, Perler BA, Roseborough GS, Williams GM. Subdural hematoma after thoracoabdominal aortic aneurysm repair: an underreported copmlication of spinal fluid drainge? *J Vasc Surg*. 2002;36:47-50.

20. Sandhu HK, Evans JD, Tanaka A, et al. Flucturations in spinal cord perfusion pressure: a harbinger of delayed paraplegia after thoracoabdominal aortic repair. *Sem Thorac Cardioavasc Surg*. 2017;29:451-459.

21. Tanaka A, Safi HJ, Estrera AE. Current strategies of spinal cord protection during thoracoabdominal aortic surgery. *Gen Thorac Cardiovasc Surg*. 2018;66:307-314.

22. Hanna JM, Andersen ND, Aziz H, Shah AA, McCann RL, Hughes GC. Results with selective preoperative lumbar drain placement for thoracic endovascular aortic repair. *Ann Thorac Surg*. 2013;95(6):1968-1974; discussion 74-75.

23. Wynn MM, Acher CW. A modern theory of spinal cord ischemia/injury in thoracoabdominal aortic surgery and its implications for prevention of paralysis. *J Cardiothorac Vasc Anesth*. 2014;28:1088.

24. Etz CD, Kari FA, Mueller CS, Brenner RM, Lin HM, Griepp RB. The collateral network concept: remodeling of the arterial collateral network after experimental segmental artery sacrifice. *J Thorac Cardiovasc Surg*. 2011;141:1029-1036.

25. Wynn MM, Mell MW, Tefera G, Acher CW. Complications of spinal fluid drainage in thoracoabdominal aortic aneurysm repair: a report of 486 patients treated from 1987 to 2008. *J Vasc Surg*. 2009;49:29-34.

26. Mazzeffi M, Abuelkasem E, Drucker CB, et al. Contemporary single-center experience with prophylactic cerbrovascular fluid drainage for thoracic endovascular aortic repair in patients at high risk for ischemic spinal cord injury. *J Cardiothorac Vasc Anesth*. 2108;32:883-889.

27. Narouze S, Benzon HT, Provenzano DA, et al. Interventional spine and pain procedures in patients on antiplatelet and anticoagulant medications (second edition): guidelines from the American Society of Regional Anesthesia and Pain medicine, the European Society of Regional Anaesthesia and Pain Therapy, the American Academy of Pain Medicine, the international Neuromodulation Society, the North American neuromodulation Society, and the World Institute of Pain. *Reg Anesth Pain Med*. 2018;43:225-262.

28. Weaver KD, Wiseman DB, Farber M, Ewend MG, Marston W, Keagy BA. Complications of lumbar drainage after thoracoabdominal aneurysm repair. *J Vasc Surg*. 2001;34:224-262.

29. Kieffer E, Richard T, Chiras J, Godet G, Cormier E. Preoperative spinal cord arteriography in aneurysmal disease of the descending thoracic and thoracoabdominal aorta; preliminary results in 45 patients. *Ann Vasc Surg*. 1989;3:34-46.

30. Griepp RB, Ergin MA, Galla JD, et al. Looking for the artery of Adamkiewicz: a quest to minimize paraplegia after operations for aneurysms of the descending thoracic and thoracoabdominal aorta. *J Thorac Cardiovasc Surg*. 1996;112(5):1202-1213; discussion 13-15.

31. Jacobs MJ, de Mol BA, Elenbaas T, et al. Spinal cord blood supply in patients with thoracoabdominal aortic aneurysms. *J Vasc Surg*. 2002;35(1):30-37.

32. Backes WH, Nijenhuis RJ, Mess WH, Wilmink FA, Schurink GW, Jacobs MJ. Magnetic resonance angiography of collateral blood supply to the spinal cord in thoraic and thoracoabdoimnal aortic aneurysm patients. *J Vasc Surg*. 2008;48:362-372.

33. Griepp EB, Griepp RB. The collateral network concept: minimizing paraplegia secondary to thoracoabdominal aortic aneurysm resection. *Tex Heart Inst J*. 2010;37(6):672-674.

34. Sobel JD, Vartanian SM, Gasper WJ, Hiramoto JS, Chuter TA, Reilly LM. Lower extremity weakness after endovascular aneurysm repair with multibranched thoracoabdominal stent grafts. *J Vasc Surg*. 2015;61:623-629.

35. Melissano G, Bertoglio L, Mascia D, et al. Spinal cord ischemia is multifactorial: what is the best protocol. *J Cardiovasc Surg (Torino)*. 2016;57:191-201.

36. Matsumura JS, Lee WA, Mitchell RS, et al. The Society for Vascular Surgery Practice Guidelines: managment of the left subclavian artery with thoracic endovascular aortic repair. *J Vasc Surg*. 2009;50:1155-1158.

37. Rizvi AZ, Murad MH, Fairman RM, Erwin PJ, Montori VM. The effect of left subclavian artery coverage on morbidity and mortality in patients undergoing endovascular thoracic aortic interventions: a systematic review and meta-analysis. *J Vasc Surg*. 2009;50(5):1159-1169.

38. Reilly LM, Chuter TA. Reversal of fortune: induced endoleak to resolve neurological deficit after endovascular repair of thoracoabdominal aortic aneurysm. *J Endovasc Ther*. 2010;17(1):21-29.

Thomas L. Forbes

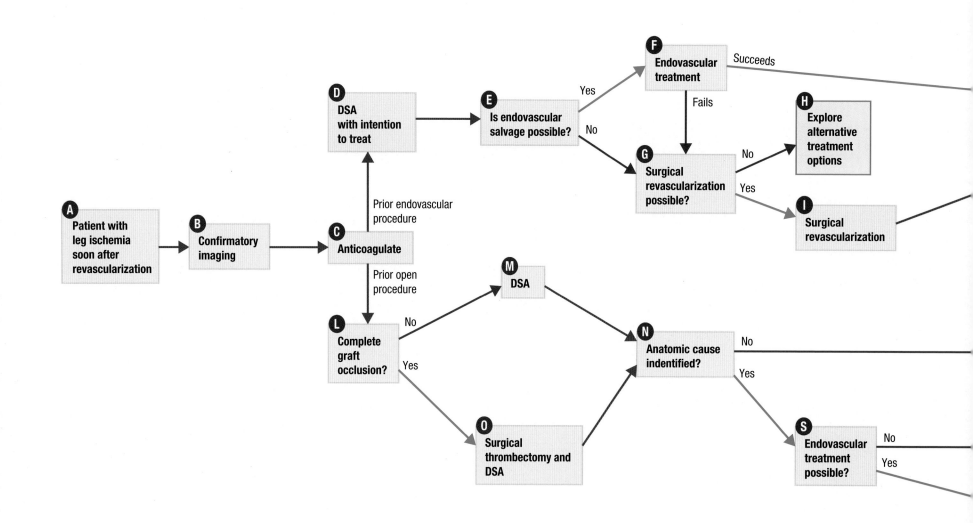

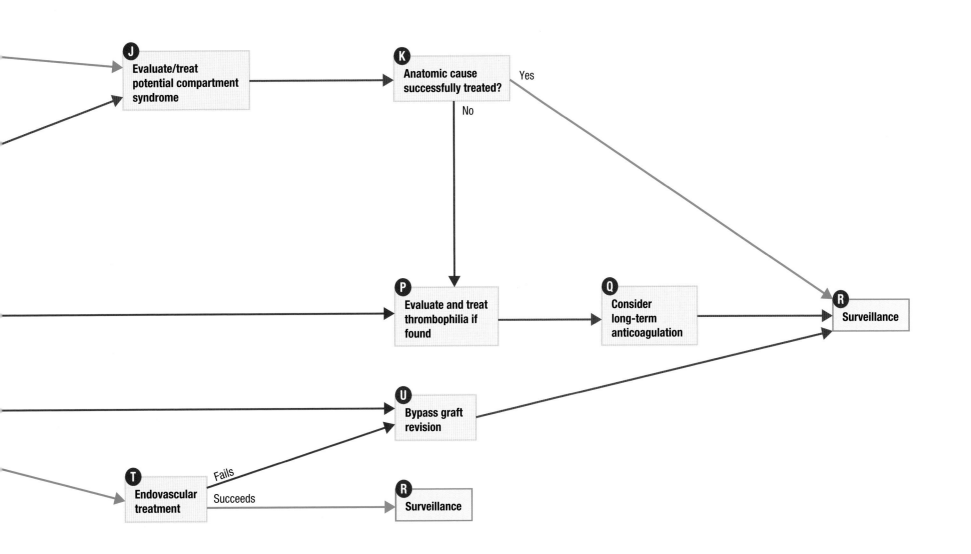

A   Patient with leg ischemia soon after revascularization

This chapter focuses on early failure of open surgical or percutaneous lower extremity revascularization. By definition, an early failure occurs within the initial 30 days post the procedure, but most occur in the immediate postprocedure period. Attempts have been made to utilize patient and disease characteristics to predict the risk of postprocedure arterial, stent, or graft thrombosis,[1] but most of these events are multifactorial in nature and precipitating causes include technical issues, anatomic constraints, iatrogenic injuries, and previously unrecognized hypercoagulable states. Whether revascularization was performed for claudication or CLI, early revascularization failure often results in the patient experiencing new-onset ischemic rest pain, although symptom severity depends on the status of collateral vessels in the limb. Immediately post the procedure, pulses and Doppler signals should be regularly monitored in both the index foot and bypass graft (if applicable). Any change in pulse or Doppler signal status, or new or worsening ischemic symptoms, should prompt a high index of suspicion for a failing revascularization that should be confirmed with imaging. In rare cases, if pretreatment symptoms were minimal (mild claudication alone), then reintervention may not be advisable if recurrent symptoms and ABI are unchanged from pretreatment and salvage of the revascularization is unlikely. Patients' comorbidities and postoperative condition should be considered when the options of reintervention are being considered.

B   Confirmatory imaging

If reintervention is necessary, depending on the clinical status of the patient, then confirmatory imaging of a failing, or failed, revascularization should be performed promptly to plan rapid treatment. DUS is usually the most expeditious method for confirming graft or artery occlusion after intervention. In some instances, CTA may be useful to disclose a potential cause for failure, such as unrecognized inflow disease.

C   Anticoagulate

If arterial or graft thrombosis is confirmed, an IV bolus of heparin should be administered promptly (75-100 units/kg), followed by continuous IV heparin infusion until corrective management can be instituted. Subsequent management depends on whether the revascularization was endovascular or open surgery.

D   DSA with intention to treat

Although percutaneous revascularization procedures for CLI have a high (96%) technical success rate, the 5-year amputation-free survival rate can be as low as 41% in some series.[2] Patients with diabetes demonstrate reduced primary patency rates after percutaneous treatment of lower extremity atherosclerotic disease, possibly due to a more advanced stage of distal artery disease.[3] Despite a higher reintervention rate, patients with diabetes, and others with risk factors predictive of reduced primary patency, can attain equivalent short-term secondary patency and limb-salvage rates.

Complications of percutaneous revascularization resulting in early ischemic symptoms include initial failure to cross the lesion (4%), arterial dissection, residual stenosis (4%), and distal embolization (2.3%), resulting in a 30-day amputation rate of 2%.[4,5] Despite these relatively poor long-term results, an aggressive approach to restoration of patency after early failure of a percutaneous revascularization procedure is warranted, unless it was performed with marginal expectation for success. Patients experiencing post-endovascular revascularization leg ischemia should be returned urgently to the endovascular suite and a diagnostic arteriogram performed. Access should generally be performed from the contralateral common femoral artery, with intention to treat the thrombosis and any culprit lesions, unless prior CTA imaging or clinical circumstances have ruled out potential salvage.

E   Is endovascular salvage possible?

The diagnostic arteriogram (in conjunction with CTA if performed) will determine whether an endovascular salvage procedure is possible. Generally, shorter lesions, especially if thrombotic, are more amenable to a redo percutaneous revascularization procedure. The etiology of these lesions could include iatrogenic occlusions or stenoses, incompletely treated atherosclerotic lesions, thrombosis, or distal embolization. Special attention should be paid to the inflow and outflow arteries beyond the initial procedure to uncover any previously unidentified and untreated lesions.

F   Endovascular treatment

In the longer term, a surgical bypass after failed endovascular interventions can offer improved amputation-free survival (45% vs. 27%) compared to repeat endovascular interventions, as reported in several series.[6] However, early failure of an endovascular revascularization procedure can be salvaged with a purely percutaneous procedure if the thrombus burden is not too extensive. Depending on the clinical status of the limb, different endovascular strategies should be considered. CDT can be considered for lesser degrees of ischemia where the time necessary for this treatment does not add additional risk for limb loss. In appropriately selected individuals, CDT following failed endovascular procedures can result in similar chances of clinical success, 30-day mortality rates (4% vs. 8%, $P = 0.4$), but longer hospitalizations compared to percutaneous thrombectomy.[7] CDT is not appropriate in the immediate limb-threatened situation if the expected time needed to restore circulation is longer than that with open surgery. Endovascular thrombus removal can be done with several techniques. After crossing the thrombosed region with a wire, suction thrombectomy can be attempted for focal thrombosis or mechanical thrombolysis for a more extensive clot. In a series of 94 patients with CLI, 31 who had initially been treated with endovascular strategies, percutaneous mechanical thrombectomy had a 68% technical success rate with the absence of end-stage renal failure being a strong predictor of success (hazard ratio of 3.3).[7] If patency can be established, arteriography may reveal a residual stenosis that can be treated with balloon angioplasty and/or stenting. Many operators employ a distal embolic protection device, especially when treating infrainguinal thrombosis.[8] Distal embolization of atherosclerotic debris can be salvaged with percutaneous suction embolectomy. A previously unidentified inflow stenosis should be treated if detected. If thrombectomy is not successful or underlying lesions cannot be treated with an endovascular approach, then options for surgical treatment should be evaluated, assuming the symptoms are severe enough to warrant intervention that is more aggressive.

G   Surgical revascularization possible?

If a percutaneous endovascular procedure is not possible, then a timely surgical revascularization procedure is often necessary for limb salvage. Arteriography or CTA should evaluate whether there is an acceptable origin and target artery for bypass. If the thrombosed region is infrainguinal, it is important for the arteriogram to be timed and performed in such a way to reveal tibial target vessels and flow into the foot. If the thrombosis is suprainguinal, evaluation of an acceptable artery for bypass origin must be evaluated, in the context of the patient's overall surgical risk. Depending on the type of bypass required, assessment for adequate venous conduit may be required. Timing of the bypass procedure is dictated by the severity of limb ischemia (see Chapter 53) and the medical condition and comorbidities of the patient. For cases of thrombosis of an endovascular procedure, a hybrid approach involving surgical balloon catheter thrombectomy combined with redo endovascular treatment may be possible if the thrombus cannot be extracted via an endovascular approach. Clinicians and patients should be aware that secondary bypasses after failed percutaneous approaches often have worse results compared to primary bypass procedures in patients with infrainguinal arterial disease. As reported by the Bypass versus Angioplasty for Severe Ischemia of the Limb (BASIL) trialists, patients undergoing primary bypass procedures had better amputation-free survival and limb salvage (85% vs. 73%) compared to patients who received secondary bypasses following a failed percutaneous approach with a median follow-up of 7 years.[9,10]

H   Explore alternative treatment options

If neither endovascular nor surgical revascularization is possible, IV anticoagulation should be continued to allow time for the ischemic symptoms to potentially improve if collateral circulation improves. However, depending on the severity of resulting ischemia, the risks of limb loss are high. Blind exploration of a distal tibial vessel in search of an outflow vessel for bypass can be performed with intraoperative arteriography, recognizing that the chance of success is low. Alternative treatment options such as intermittent compression or negative pressure devices are discussed in Chapter 45 in the event that acute ischemia does not mandate prompt amputation (see Chapter 53).

I Surgical revascularization

If a percutaneous salvage procedure is not possible or fails to restore adequate circulation, open surgical revascularization is often possible. Whether an endovascular-first strategy "burns bridges" for subsequent bypass options is somewhat controversial.[11] Regardless, BASIL investigators have reported poorer outcomes following secondary bypass procedures compared to primary procedures in patients with CLI (85% vs. 73%).[12] Decision making and details for supra- and infrainguinal surgical revascularization are discussed in Chapters 46 and 47.

J Evaluate/treat potential compartment syndrome

Depending on the severity of acute ischemia after early revascularization thrombosis, and the rapidity with which circulation is restored, calf compartment syndrome may develop. Diagnosis and treatment of compartment syndrome with four-compartment fasciotomy are discussed in detail in Chapter 51.

K Anatomic cause successfully treated?

If an anatomic cause for endovascular treatment failure is successfully treated, such that repeat failure is unlikely, the patient is followed with standard surveillance. However, if no underlying anatomic cause for endovascular treatment failure is found, or if the persisting anatomic situation is such that repeat failure is more likely, evaluation for thrombophilia and potential anticoagulation is appropriate.

L Complete graft occlusion?

Early graft failure following supra- or infrainguinal arterial bypass occurs in up to 5% of cases.[13] Along with confirming complete graft thrombosis/occlusion, prior DUS or CTA imaging should also evaluate the inflow and outflow arteries of the bypass to identify any previously unidentified culprit lesions that may have precipitated the graft thrombosis. If graft occlusion is complete, arteriography is delayed until after surgical graft thrombectomy, but if incomplete or with only focal thrombosis, arteriography may reveal potential endovascular treatment options.

M DSA

If imaging demonstrates low flow and not total graft occlusion, arteriography is performed to help identify an anatomic cause for graft thrombosis. In some cases, endovascular treatment of the underlying lesion may be possible during this procedure.

N Anatomic cause identified?

Graft occlusion can be precipitated by inflow and outflow artery or anastomotic stenoses, inadequate outflow, and in the case of vein grafts, by twisting the graft, missed valve leaflets, or patent tributaries (if in situ bypass), and even compression by surrounding structures or hematoma.[14] If a culprit anatomic lesion is detected by arteriogram, it is evaluated for endovascular or surgical treatment. If no anatomic lesion is found, a hypercoagulable evaluation is undertaken.

O Surgical thrombectomy and DSA

In the instances of early perioperative complete graft thrombosis, the patient should be returned to the operating room for open balloon catheter thrombectomy of the bypass graft. Some operators have suggested the use of intraoperative rheolytic thrombectomy to reduce trauma to vein grafts, but a benefit compared to balloon thrombectomy has not been proved. If there is a high suspicion that one anastomosis has caused the thrombosis (more often the distal), this anastomosis is taken down first to allow thrombectomy and correction of any anastomotic defect found. Oftentimes, both anastomoses need to be taken down to adequately thrombectomize the graft, especially if thrombectomy is made difficult by thrombosed vein graft valve leaflets. In cases of prosthetic grafts, thrombectomy via a graftotomy at the hood of the graft anastomosis may allow adequate thrombectomy of the full length of the graft without taking down the other anastomosis. The contralateral lower extremity should always be prepped into the operative field in case an additional vein conduit is required. After thrombectomy, completion arteriography should be performed to confirm adequate thrombectomy and detect any underlying cause for graft thrombosis. Subsequent management depends on whether an anatomic cause for graft thrombosis is identified.

P Evaluate and treat thrombophilia if found

If no culprit lesion is identified, then a hypercoagulable state (thrombophilia) should be considered as a possible reason for early graft failure. The common hypercoagulable states associated with increased risk of arterial thrombosis include antithrombin III deficiency, antiphospholipid syndrome, protein C and S deficiency, activated protein C resistance, and prothrombin mutations.[15] Diagnosis and treatment of thrombophilia are discussed in detail in Chapter 92. Graft or artery thrombosis can also be due to heparin-induced thrombocytopenia (HITT), a relatively common prothrombotic drug reaction that features platelet-activating IgG antibodies.[16] The immunologic response is transitory and is confirmed by the presence of thrombocytopenia and a positive HITT immunologic assay. Alternatives to heparin include Argatroban in these instances.[17] Diagnosis and treatment of HITT are discussed in detail in Chapter 91. Hematology consultation is recommended for evaluation and subsequent follow-up.

Q Consider long-term anticoagulation

Long-term anticoagulation (6-12 months) is often recommended for patients who experience graft or interventional treatment site thrombosis without any underlying cause found or treated. Although this is not strongly supported by literature, it is commonly practiced as the last possible step to prevent rethrombosis. Antiplatelet therapy is continued in such patients as part of a generalized atherosclerotic risk reduction strategy. For patients with proven thrombophilia, chronic oral anticoagulation therapy is usually indicated to prevent rethrombosis, depending on the specific state identified (see Chapter 92).

R Surveillance

After surgical or endovascular treatment of early graft or interventional site thrombosis, increased vigilance is required during surveillance, because the likelihood of rethrombosis may be increased after the first episode due to the reintervention itself, intimal injury associated with arterial thromboembolectomy, neointimal hyperplasia, or an underlying hypercoagulable state. Generally, patients are seen post the procedure at 3, 6, and 12 months with usual surveillance studies, including clinical examination, ABI, and graft/artery surveillance DUS, as appropriate.[18]

S Endovascular treatment possible?

If an anatomic cause is found for graft thrombosis, it may be amenable to endovascular treatment. Such lesions can include inflow and outflow artery stenoses and mid-vein graft stenosis or missed valve leaflets. Generally, anastomotic strictures should not be treated with balloon angioplasty in the early postoperative period because of the risk of suture disruption and hemorrhage, and the low probability of effectively treating the anastomotic defect.

T Endovascular treatment

Inflow and outflow lesions can be corrected with angioplasty and stents, whereas mid-vein graft stenosis or missed valve leaflets often respond well to balloon angioplasty. Generally, anastomotic strictures should not be treated with balloon angioplasty in the early postoperative period because of the risk of suture disruption and hemorrhage, and the low probability of effectively treating the anastomotic defect. These lesions should be treated with surgical revision. Balloon angioplasty of failed, or failing, infrainguinal bypass grafts results in secondary patency rates of 90% at 2 years. Grafts with multiple stenoses or those requiring revision within 6 months of the index procedure are at higher risk of requiring further interventions.[19]

U Bypass graft revision

If either the proximal or distal anastomosis is stenotic because of technical features, then it should be taken down and revised, often adding a patch to prevent stenosis. If the distal anastomosis is severely compromised or if there is compromised outflow at that level, then a jump graft to a more distal target may be necessary. Short/focal vein graft stenoses can be treated with vein patch angioplasty, whereas longer stenotic lesions should be treated with interposition vein grafting using vein segments from the ipsilateral leg, contralateral leg, or upper extremity. Following bypass revision, intraoperative arteriography of DUS as appropriate should be conducted to exclude any technical problem or other previously undetected defects/stenoses that require treatment during that procedure.

In a contemporary series of patients with failed, or failing, bypass grafts who were treated with surgical salvage interventions including jump grafts, revision of anastomotic stenosis, and thrombectomy, reasonable results were obtained. Primary patency, assisted primary patency, and secondary patency was 57%, 76%, and 82%, respectively, at 12 months and 44%, 70%, and 80%, respectively, at 36 months. Amputation-free survival was 80% at 12 months and 65% at 36 months. Amputation-free survival was similar in salvaged threatened and acutely occluded grafts compared with nonthreatened grafts and better in grafts requiring reintervention later (>6 months from bypass) compared with those requiring early reintervention (<6 months).[20]

REFERENCES

1. Sahin M, El H. External validation and evaluation of reliability of the FARP2 score to predict early graft failure after infrainguinal bypass. *Ann Vasc Surg*. 2018;51:72-77.
2. Davies MG, El-Sayed HF. Objective performance goals after endovascular intervention for critical limb ischemia. *J Vasc Surg*. 2015;62:1555-1563.
3. DeRubertis BG, Pierce M, Ryer EJ, Trocciola S, Kent KC, Faries PL. Reduced primary patency rate in diabetic patients after percutaneous intervention results from more frequent presentation with limb-threatening ischemia. *J Vasc Surg*. 2008;47:101-108.
4. Vierthaler L, Callas PW, Goodney PP, et al. Determinants of survival and major amputation after peripheral endovascular intervention for critical limb ischemia. *J Vasc Surg*. 2015;62:655-664.e8.
5. Siracuse JJ, Menard MT, Eslami MH, et al. Comparison of open and endovascular treatment of patients with critical limb ischemia in the Vascular Quality Initiative. *J Vasc Surg*. 2016;63:958-965.e1.
6. Baer-Bositis HE, Hicks TD, Haidar GM, Sideman MJ, Pounds LL, Davies MG. Outcomes of reintervention for recurrent symptomatic disease after tibial endovascular intervention. *J Vasc Surg*. 2018;68:811-821.e1.
7. Muli Jogi RK, Damodharan K, Leong HL, et al. Catheter-directed thrombolysis versus percutaneous mechanical thrombectomy in the management of acute limb ischemia: a single center review. *CVIR Endovasc*. 2018;1:35.
8. Morrissey NJ. When is embolic protection needed in lower extremity interventions and how should it be done. *J Cardiovasc Surg (Torino)*. 2012;53:173-175.
9. Meecham L, Patel S, Bate GR, Bradbury AW. Editor's choice—A comparison of clinical outcomes between primary bypass and secondary bypass after failed plain balloon angioplasty in the bypass versus angioplasty for severe ischaemia of the limb (BASIL) trial. *Eur J Vasc Endovasc Surg*. 2018;55:666-671.
10. Bradbury AW, Adam DJ, Bell J, et al. Multicentre randomised controlled trial of the clinical and cost-effectiveness of a bypass-surgery-first versus a balloon-angioplasty-first revascularisation strategy for severe limb ischaemia due to infrainguinal disease. The bypass versus angioplasty in severe ischaemia of the leg (BASIL) trial. *Health Technol Assess*. 2010;14:1-210, iii-iv.
11. Roy T, Forbes T, Wright G, Dueck A. Burning bridges: mechanisms and implications of endovascular failure in the treatment of peripheral artery disease. *J Endovasc Ther*. 2015;22:874-880.
12. Bradbury AW, Adam DJ, Bell J; BASIL Trial Participants. Bypass versus angioplasty in severe ischaemia of the leg (BASIL) trial in perspective. *J Vasc Surg*. 2010;51:1S-4S.
13. Soma G, Greenblatt DY, Nelson MT, et al. Early graft failure after infrainguinal arterial bypass. *Surgery*. 2014;155:300-310.
14. Eifell R, Mudawi A. A simple technique to prevent graft kinking during tunneling of a reversed vein femoropopliteal bypass graft. *Surg Today*. 2007;37:356-358.
15. Pejkic S, Savic N, Paripovic M, Sladojevic M, Doric P, Ilic N. Vascular graft thrombosis secondary to activated protein C resistance: a case report and literature review. *Vascular*. 2014;22:71-76.
16. Warkentin TE, Anderson JA. How I treat patients with a history of heparin-induced thrombocytopenia. *Blood*. 2016;128:348-359.
17. Prince M, Wenham T. Heparin-induced thrombocytopaenia. *Postgrad Med J*. 2018;94:453-457.
18. Zierler RE, Jordan WD, Lal BK, et al. The Society for Vascular Surgery practice guidelines on follow-up after vascular surgery arterial procedures. *J Vasc Surg*. 2018;68:256-284.
19. Ali H, Elbadawy A, Saleh M, Hasaballah A. Balloon angioplasty for revision of failing lower extremity bypass grafts. *J Vasc Surg*. 2015;62:93-100.
20. Patel SD, Zymvragoudakis V, Sheehan L, et al. The efficacy of salvage interventions on threatened distal bypass grafts. *J Vasc Surg*. 2016;63:126-132.

Douglas Jones • Jeffrey Kalish

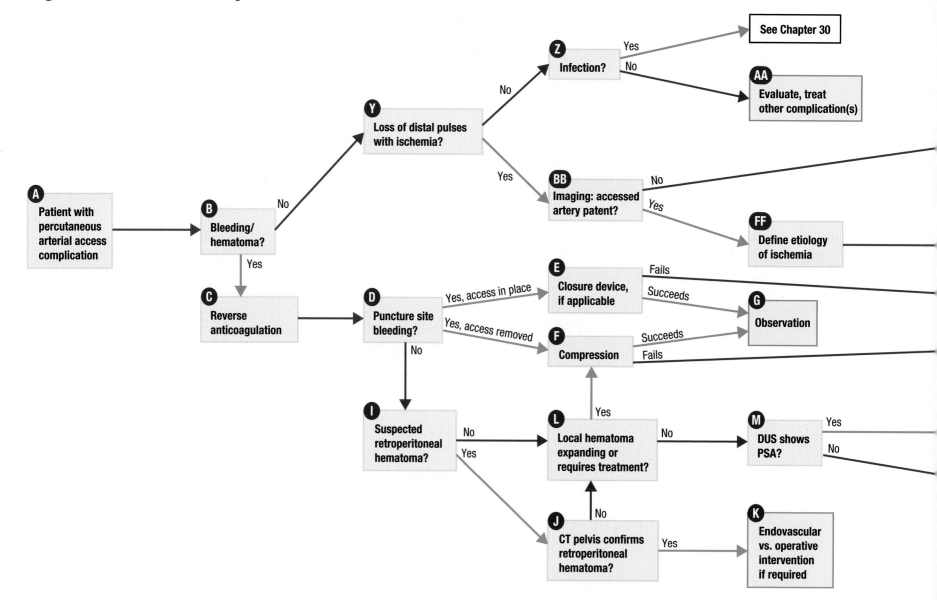

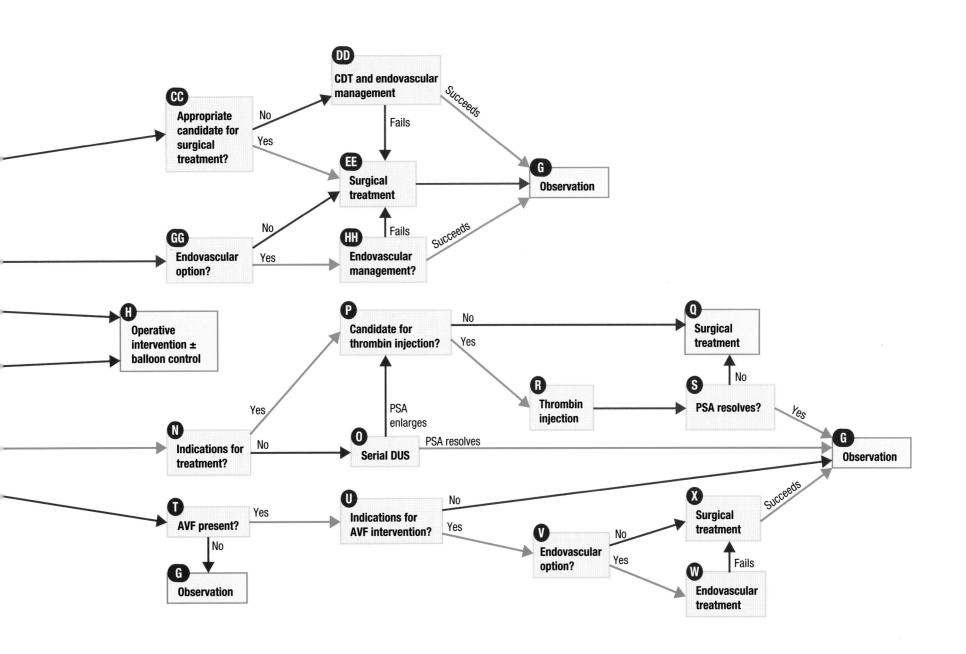

A Patient with percutaneous arterial access complication

With the increasing incidence of percutaneous vascular procedures for the management of vascular pathology, percutaneous complications are inevitable. Ultrasound guidance and use of vascular closure devices (VCDs) have been reported to decrease access site complications.[1,2] Predictors of access site complications include patient factors such as female sex, age >75 years, increased body mass index (BMI), and prior peripheral intervention, and include procedural factors such as sheath size >6F, duration of procedure, urgency of procedure, use of anticoagulants/thrombolytics, antegrade femoral access,[3] and brachial access.[4]

B Bleeding/hematoma?

Bleeding or hematoma following percutaneous arterial access has a reported incidence of 2.0% to 7.9%.[2,5,6] This includes puncture site bleeding, PSA, and retroperitoneal hematoma (after femoral access).

C Reverse anticoagulation

When bleeding occurs following arterial catheterization, it is important to ensure that any periprocedure anticoagulation is fully reversed, unless continued anticoagulation is deemed to be critical by the interventionalist. Protamine should be used to reverse any remaining systemic heparin at a dose of 10 mg of protamine per estimated 1000 units of heparin still in biocirculation (using an approximate half-life of 60 minutes to calculate the amount of heparin remaining in the circulation). Reversal agents are also available for the novel anticoagulants and direct thrombin inhibitors, and these include prothrombin complex concentrate (PCC), idarucizumab, andexanet alfa, and ciraparantag.[7] Before removal of an arterial access sheath, the activated clotting time (ACT) should ideally be <180 seconds.

D Puncture site bleeding?

Decisions regarding the management of puncture site bleeding after arterial access depend on whether the arterial sheath is still in place to allow wire access for a potential closure device or temporary balloon control or stent graft placement, or whether the sheath has already been removed such that new access may be difficult. In some cases of high femoral puncture, retroperitoneal bleeding may occur without apparent bleeding at the puncture site and without visible hematoma in the groin.

E Closure device, if applicable

Multiple studies have examined the role of different VCDs versus manual compression to achieve hemostasis following femoral artery sheath removal after angiography. The largest randomized multicenter trial (ISAR-CLOSURE) demonstrated noninferiority of VCDs for access site complications, shorter time to hemostasis with any VCD compared to manual compression, and lower failure rate with intravascular VCDs compared to extravascular VCDs.[6] There have been reports of increased risk of limb ischemia, arterial stenosis, and need for vascular surgery for arterial complications with the use of VCDs,[8] but standardized protocols for VCD use have the potential to decrease the incidence of access site complications.[9] The Vascular Quality Initiative has identified that use of VCDs decreases the incidence of minor, moderate, and severe access site complications.[2] The choice of which closure device to employ in the setting of bleeding is dependent on operator experience, but suture-mediated closure is preferred over topical agents when the hematoma significantly displaces the anatomy.

F Compression

Bleeding emanating from the puncture site following access sheath removal mandates application of manual compression directly over the puncture site to try and resolve the bleeding. This bleeding may be coming from the artery or a branch artery or from the skin or soft tissue. Usually, bleeding will stop with manual compression unless a hematoma or obesity prevents direct digital compression of the arteriotomy site, or if the puncture site was above the inguinal ligament. For femoral access, compression of the artery over the femoral head (provided the access was appropriately placed in the CFA over the femoral head), can effectively control the artery and associated bleeding. For brachial or pedal access, compression of the soft tissue should be performed without completely occluding the vessel, because this may lead to vessel thrombosis. Rarely, skin bleeding may require additional treatment with a simple suture. If compression is successful, observation is indicated; however, large hematomas that threaten the skin viability or cause neuropathy require operative intervention.

G Observation

After initial treatment of access site bleeding, hematoma, PSA, AVF, or ischemia, patients should be observed in the hospital as needed to ensure complete treatment success. Additional treatment might be required, as discussed in this decision tree.

H Operative intervention ± balloon control

Puncture site bleeding that fails to resolve with manual compression or after failure of a closure device requires operative intervention. If wire or sheath access is still in place, then balloon occlusion control can be accomplished as a temporizing measure before definitive arterial repair. Furthermore, if the access wire and sheath have already been removed, contralateral femoral access can be used in certain cases to obtain rapid balloon occlusion control, especially for a patient who is unstable or has a rapidly expanding or retroperitoneal hematoma. Operative treatment consists of open exposure of the arterial bleeding site and suture closure. If the artery is severely involved with calcific atherosclerosis, then more complex repair, potentially including endarterectomy or, rarely, graft interposition, might be required. Depending on the extent of hematoma and the amount of surrounding tissue that has been affected, wound closure over a closed suction drain or VAC closure may be warranted to prevent postoperative accumulation of serosanguinous fluid in the newly created dead space.

I Suspected retroperitoneal hematoma?

Retroperitoneal hematomas occur in 0.5% to 3.0% of patients undergoing angiography and can occur without an associated groin hematoma.[10] Signs and symptoms of a retroperitoneal hematoma include back/flank pain, abdominal pain, groin pain, or femoral neuropathy, and can be associated with decreasing hematocrit. Hypotension or tachycardia may be present, and patients may have abdominal tenderness. Continued bleeding can lead to ecchymosis in the flanks (Grey Turner sign) or more rarely at the umbilicus (Cullen sign), but these signs usually will not be evident until 48 to 72 hours after the initial bleeding. Retroperitoneal hematoma after high femoral puncture can escape detection for hours and be associated with significant morbidity/mortality if not recognized and treated.

J CT pelvis confirms retroperitoneal hematoma?

Noncontrast CT scan of the pelvis is an expeditious confirmatory test for the presence of a retroperitoneal hematoma. IV contrast is not necessary, but it can provide additional information regarding the bleeding site and the extent of arterial injury. A CT scan should be performed if there is any clinical suspicion of retroperitoneal hematoma because a missed diagnosis can be fatal.

K Endovascular vs. operative intervention if required

Not all patients with retroperitoneal hematoma require intervention, even with a 2- to 4-unit blood loss into the retroperitoneum. Patients with retroperitoneal hematomas should be in an appropriate setting to monitor their vital signs and symptoms, as well as any change in physical examination and serial hematocrit. Initial management includes reversal of any anticoagulation, treating coagulopathy, and transfusion as required. Intervention should be considered for ongoing bleeding refractory to reversal of coagulopathy, hemodynamic instability, acute renal insufficiency in the case of renal displacement from a large hematoma, and femoral nerve dysfunction from compression of the lumbar plexus roots. Evacuation of the hematoma should be considered depending on patient symptoms and signs, with surgical repair via either direct exposure and repair of the bleeding arteriotomy or endovascular management with a covered stent graft. Most patients are treated with open surgery, to avoid placing a stent graft across the CFA, or a small artery used for arm access. However, in very high-risk patients, or a puncture site amenable to stent-graft treatment, this option can be pursued.

L Local hematoma expanding or requires treatment?

Bleeding from an access site can manifest as an expanding hematoma, potentially pulsatile, more diffuse ecchymosis, or external bleeding, depending on how well the arterial bleeding is contained by surrounding tissue. Expanding hematomas are initially managed with local compression but may require operative treatment for control. Stable hematomas after arterial puncture may be associated with PSA, which should be evaluated. Neurologic deficit may result from the hematoma compressing adjacent nerves, including the femoral, median, and deep peroneal or tibial nerves, depending on the access site location. Neuropathy from hematoma compression indicates the need for surgical evacuation to avoid long-term neurologic complications. Similarly, very large hematomas that threaten the viability of overlying skin from compression require surgical evacuation and treatment.

Ⓜ DUS shows PSA?

DUS is the optimal initial modality to evaluate potential access site complications following arterial puncture and has a 95% sensitivity and 95% specificity for detecting femoral arterial PSA[11] and differentiating it from other complications such as an AVF. A PSA exists when active bleeding is contained by surrounding soft tissue and skin only. In such cases, "to-and-fro" blood flow from the artery into the PSA cavity exists and can be detected with DUS, which can also identify the size of the PSA, and the length and diameter of the "neck" (if the PSA sac is separated from the artery, which is often the case). Femoral artery PSAs are reported to have an incidence ranging from <1% up to 3.8% in modern series, with differing and defined risk factors affecting the probability of this complication.[12] PSAs in other puncture locations are possible, but less common.

Ⓝ Indications for treatment?

PSAs may present as a pulsatile mass on physical examination or simply as a hematoma that expands slowly after initial stability. They can be associated with tenderness or compressive symptoms on adjacent nerves. Large PSAs can potentially lead to local skin ischemia and tissue loss. Management strategies have evolved over recent decades and include observation with serial DUS for spontaneous resolution of small PSAs, ultrasound-guided compression, ultrasound-guided thrombin injection, and surgical repair. Current recommendations are to treat PSAs that are >2 cm in diameter with thrombin injection. Although ultrasound-guided compression can be tried, it is usually poorly tolerated because of pain. The incidence of neurologic compression symptoms is higher following brachial artery access than is femoral artery access because of the closer anatomic relation of the artery and nerve at the antecubital fossa compared to the groin.[13]

Ⓞ Serial DUS

PSAs <2 cm in diameter can be observed with follow-up serial duplex examinations unless they cause neuropathy from compression. There are numerous reports of spontaneous thrombosis of small PSAs, with rates ranging from 42%[14] to 89%.[15] Patients on anticoagulants and/or dual antiplatelet agents have higher failure rates for spontaneous thrombosis of femoral PSAs.[14] If a PSA enlarges to a diameter >2 cm, or if any symptoms develop, then treatment is indicated.

Ⓟ Candidate for thrombin injection?

Although an "off-label" use of thrombin, ultrasound-guided thrombin injection has become the treatment of choice to manage PSAs that do not respond to observation or meet the initial criteria for treatment, and do not require urgent operative intervention because of associated bleeding, skin threat, or nerve compression. Thrombin injection is likely more effective for PSAs with narrower and longer necks. Thrombin is contraindicated for patients with suspected/known thrombin allergy, infected PSAs, hemodynamic instability, or ongoing bleeding, overlying skin necrosis or cellulitis, distal limb ischemia, neurologic deficit from compressive effect, and for larger PSAs with wide necks.[16,17] Operative intervention should be considered as first-line treatment in such cases.

Ⓠ Surgical treatment

Surgical treatment of a PSA associated with arterial access involves obtaining proximal and distal control of the artery first, entering the PSA to evacuate the hematoma, and then repairing the arterial defect with a simple suture. With a high inguinal puncture site or a large hematoma, external iliac artery balloon control may be preferable, if this can be obtained from the contralateral or brachial approach. If balloon control is not possible in such cases, surgical control of the EIA must be obtained through a retroperitoneal incision or by transecting the inguinal ligament. In very unstable patients, it may be necessary to directly enter the PSA to obtain digital control of the arterial puncture site, and then obtain additional control if necessary, before repair. However, depending on the site of injury (eg, profunda femoral artery puncture), significant bleeding may occur while attempting digital control such that proximal balloon occlusion is preferred, if possible. Endovascular repair with a stent graft placed across the arterial defect is a second-line method for control of a CFA PSA because it carries a risk of subsequent stent fracture and thrombosis. However, it may be required as a temporizing measure in high-risk patients.

Ⓡ Thrombin injection

Bovine thrombin is reconstituted in normal saline at a concentration of 1000 units/mL. The skin overlying the PSA is prepped with a surgical prep, and then 1% lidocaine is used to anesthetize the puncture site. Under ultrasound guidance, a micropuncture needle is introduced into the PSA sac, and a very small amount of thrombin is injected (as little as 0.1-0.2 mL at first). Care should be taken to avoid injecting thrombin into the neck of the PSA to prevent embolization of the main artery or its distal branches. If there is persistent flow in the PSA by DUS, then additional thrombin can be injected as needed. Distal pulses, or Doppler signals, should be checked before and after the thrombin injection, and patients should remain on bed rest for at least 2 hours following the injection. Reported success of eliminating the PSA with thrombin injection is >97%; complications such as infection or distal ischemia are rare (1%-2%).[18]

Ⓢ PSA resolves?

Recurrence of a PSA after successful thrombin injection is rare (3%).[19] Therefore, the value and timing of repeat DUS to confirm successful PSA thrombosis is variable in the literature and in clinical practice. The time interval for recurrence ranges from 4 to 6 hours[18] to 3 weeks[19] following thrombin injection. Given the low rate of recurrent PSA, most physicians reserve repeat DUS for patients with clinical symptoms or physical examination findings.

Ⓣ AVF present?

AVF is a rare (<1%) complication after arterial puncture, but can result following simultaneous arterial and venous access within the same groin, as well as from through-and-through puncture of the artery into the vein.[1] Risk factors for AVF include HTN, female sex, use of anticoagulants, emergency procedure, and puncture of the left groin.[1,20] AVF can be detected by appreciating a thrill or bruit on physical examination in the area of the arterial puncture. DUS can confirm the arterialization of the venous signal.

Ⓤ Indications for AVF intervention?

AVFs are typically asymptomatic, and reported spontaneous rates of AVF closure range from 38%[20] up to 81%.[15] Intervention is rarely required but is indicated if sequelae develop over time (CHF, limb swelling, or limb ischemia, or if the AVF grows over time and leads to local symptoms). Unless initial treatment is required, AVFs are observed until they resolve or clearly stabilize as asymptomatic.

Ⓥ Endovascular option?

The decision to treat an AVF with operative intervention or endovascular management depends on the location and size of the AVF, the medical comorbidities of the patient that affect operative risk, or in cases where difficulty in surgery is anticipated. This has been described predominantly within the profunda femoral or SFA[21] and care must be taken when close to the distal CFA to avoid coverage of the nearby orifice of the profunda or SFA. There is also a risk of fracture and eventual thrombotic issues if a stent graft is used in the CFA.

Ⓦ Endovascular treatment

Treatment of an AVF involves placement of either a balloon-expandable or self-expanding stent graft within the artery and covering the communication point with the associated vein. Case reports have also described success with embolization of long fistula tracts using different agents, including *N*-butyl-cyanoacrylate (NBCA).[22]

X Surgical treatment

Primary closure of the defects in the artery and vein is the standard of care for operative treatment of AVF. Surgery should also be performed for an AVF in which endovascular management has failed and patients are persistently symptomatic. Accurate preoperative localization of the fistula through imaging is important to guide exposure and control. Depending on the degree of inflammation, dissection around the fistula can be difficult, so obtaining initial proximal arterial control is important. Temporary balloon occlusion can facilitate control if exposure is difficult.

Y Loss of distal pulses with ischemia?

Loss of distal pulses in the extremity ipsilateral to percutaneous access is commonly due to arterial injury at the level of the access site leading to dissection, stenosis, or thrombosis. It is important to document the preprocedure vascular status to recognize a potential change from baseline after access. Patients may complain of distal extremity pain due to ischemia, although an access site injury may be suspected before the development of symptoms on the basis of a change in the postprocedure pulse examination. Access site thrombosis can occur following manual compression or can be caused by VCD. The ISAR-CLOSURE trial and a recent meta-analysis both showed leg ischemia to be very uncommon (<0.5%) after percutaneous femoral access.[6,8] Although some have suggested that the rate of ischemic complications is higher with VCD,[23] this has not been demonstrated in trials or nationwide database reviews.[2] Rates of brachial access site stenosis/occlusion are higher than those seen in femoral access (2.1% vs. 0.4%), which may be mitigated, in some cases, by planned arterial cutdown.[4]

Z Infection?

Percutaneous access site infection is extremely uncommon, occurring in 1 out of >4500 patients in the ISAR-CLOSURE trial.[6] Patients present with local signs of infection: erythema, drainage, or underlying abscess. If infection involves the arterial wall, this can lead to aneurysm formation (see Chapter 30). Once identified, access site infection typically requires antibiotics and source control via drainage, debridement of infected tissue, removal of infected VCD, and possible vascular reconstruction.

AA Evaluate, treat other complication(s)

Patients complaining of access site pain after percutaneous intervention should be evaluated for neurologic changes, bleeding/hematoma, change in distal pulse examination, and signs of local infection. If there is no evidence of these complications, serious underlying pathology is unlikely, and, in most situations, pain will resolve. However, it is important to remember that permanent local nerve injury can be caused by small hematomas, particularly in brachial access cases. As a result, neurologic change may be the only, albeit subtle, sign and should prompt consideration of surgical exploration.

BB Imaging: accessed artery patent?

If distal ischemia is detected during the post-access period, imaging should be immediately obtained to determine the patency of the accessed artery. DUS is widely available and can be used to determine whether there is normal flow across the access site or if the vessel is stenosed or thrombosed from local dissection. If the access site is patent, CTA or DSA through a new access site (such as the contralateral groin) can diagnose potential embolization or dissection not associated directly with the access site. Treatment options for ischemia depend on whether the access site is thrombosed or patent, and if patent what is the underlying cause. For cases where pedal access was utilized, DSA at the time of initial procedure is typically performed following distal sheath removal to determine whether any access site injury has occurred. If a distal access site complication is suspected in a patient with postprocedure limb ischemia, DSA should be performed.

CC Appropriate candidate for surgical treatment?

Once imaging has established access site thrombosis, open surgical treatment is the most expeditious way to reestablish distal perfusion. In cases where a VCD was maldeployed, open repair with VCD removal is mandatory. However, patients undergoing peripheral interventions (particularly cardiac catheterization) can have prohibitive risk for open surgery or have other active, evolving issues such as myocardial ischemia or stroke. Bleeding risk and eligibility for thrombolysis should be determined before pursuing an endovascular approach to thrombosis, because a short period of systemic anticoagulation required for open surgical repair likely incurs lower systemic bleeding risk than catheter-directed thrombolysis.

DD CDT and endovascular management

For high surgical risk patients with access site thrombosis not involving a VCD, a guidewire from an alternative site can usually cross the thrombus, allowing placement of a distal embolic protection device. Underlying atherosclerotic plaque or dissection should be suspected because thrombosis is unlikely to occur in a normal artery with manual compression. Percutaneous mechanical thrombectomy (PMT) can be performed to reveal any underlying lesion. CDT can be considered when significant residual thrombus burden is seen, although this should be undertaken with extreme caution.[24,25] It is important not to oversize any additional PTA or stent to avoid damaging the recently accessed artery. Stent-graft placement or emergency surgical repair may be necessary if any endovascular interventions result in active, uncontrollable contrast extravasation from the access site. Distal embolization can be managed with PMT ± catheter-directed thrombolysis. An endovascular approach to brachial artery access site thrombosis should be discouraged because it will not address any compressive hematoma that may be contributing. Because pedal access is performed in healthy-appearing distal vessels, access site injury is uncommon when performed appropriately. However, DSA may reveal focal thrombosis, which is typically managed with prolonged PTA across the access site. PMT and catheter-directed thrombolysis are not effective in these cases.

EE Surgical treatment

For femoral access site–related ischemia, bleeding from the puncture site is unlikely during surgical arterial exposure. However, care should be taken not to disrupt the VCD, if deployed until vascular control is achieved. A longitudinal arteriotomy should be performed to fully evaluate the intima, allowing for endarterectomy and/or tacking of dissection flaps. For VCD-related thrombosis, bulky posterior wall plaque is often present. As a result, endarterectomy with patch closure is often necessary. When imaging suggests distal embolization, balloon catheter embolectomy is performed via the femoral access site exposure. Brachial artery access site thrombosis is also treated surgically. Pedal access site complications are uncommon and typically managed with endovascular techniques because they are usually detected at the time of the index procedure. However, isolated dissection or thrombosis of a distal access site may require operative intervention if not responsive to endovascular intervention. For these small-caliber arteries, thromboembolectomy should be performed through a longitudinal arteriotomy, which can be closed using a vein patch fashioned from any nearby, suitable vein.

Operative intervention for distal emboli is discussed in Chapter 53.

FF Define etiology of ischemia

If distal ischemia exists but the access site is patent, several possible causes are possible, including a flow-limiting dissection/stenosis at the access site, distal embolization, and more proximal arterial dissection. In such cases, the DSA from a different site (eg, the contralateral CFA) is useful for diagnosis and provides the means for potential endovascular treatment.[24,25]

GG Endovascular option?

Many focal access site dissections can be managed initially via endovascular treatment. If DSA reveals dissection propagation with a long segment of affected artery, open repair may be more efficient and durable. Endovascular techniques should not be attempted for complex dissections or when a wire cannot cross safely into the distal true lumen. In these situations, inadvertent treatment of the false lumen may cause irreparable arterial wall damage. Similarly, local dissection proximal to the access site can usually be treated with endovascular techniques. Distal emboli are usually managed with Fogarty balloon catheter extraction, but in some high-risk patients, thrombolysis may be appropriate (see Chapter 53).

🅗🅗 Endovascular management

Endovascular treatment of access site dissection/stenosis may be safer in the absence of thrombosis, but worsening of access site injury can still occur. After crossing the lesion safely with a wire, prolonged, low-pressure PTA (2-3 minutes) is performed, attempting to "tack down" the dissection flap.[24,25] If there is a residual, flow-limiting lesion seen on DSA, or if a significant residual pressure gradient exists across it, bare-metal stent placement may be necessary to reestablish a normal true lumen. For a femoral artery access site, stent placement in the CFA should only be performed in patients who are not candidates for open surgical repair to avoid potential future stent fracture, distortion, and thrombosis. More proximal dissections causing ischemia can usually be successfully stented. Thrombolysis, if selected for distal emboli, is discussed in Chapter 53.

REFERENCES

1. Kalish J, Eslami M, Gillespie D, et al. Routine use of ultrasound guidance in femoral arterial access for peripheral vascular intervention decreases groin hematoma rates. *J Vasc Surg*. 2015;61:1231-1238.
2. Ortiz D, Jahangir A, Singh M, Allaqaband S, Bajwa TK, Mewissen MW. Access site complications after peripheral vascular interventions: incidence, predictors, and outcomes. *Circ Cardiovasc Interv*. 2014;7(6):821-828.
3. Wheatley BJ, Mansour MA, Grossman PM, et al. Complication rates for percutaneous lower extremity arterial antegrade access. *Arch Surg*. 2011;146:432-435.
4. Kret MR, Dalman RL, Kalish J, Mell M. Arterial cutdown reduces complications after brachial access for peripheral vascular intervention. *J Vasc Surg*. 2016;64(1):149-154.
5. Ohlow MA, Secknus MA, von Korn H, et al. Incidence and outcome of femoral vascular complications among 18,165 patients undergoing cardiac catheterisation. *Int J Cardiol*. 2009;135:66-71.
6. Schulz-Schüpke S, Helde S, Gewalt S, et al. Comparison of vascular closure devices vs manual compression after femoral artery puncture: the ISAR-CLOSURE randomized clinical trial. *JAMA*. 2014;312:1981-1987.
7. Ansell JE. Reversing the effect of oral anticoagulant drugs: established and newer options. *Am J Cardiovasc Drugs*. 2016;16:163-170.
8. Biancari F, D'Andrea V, Di Marco C, Savino G, Tiozzo V, Catania A. Meta-analysis of randomized trials on the efficacy of vascular closure devices after diagnostic angiography and angioplasty. *Am Heart J*. 2010;159:518-531.
9. Goodney PP, Chang RW, Cronenwett JL. A percutaneous arterial closure protocol can decrease complications after endovascular interventions in vascular surgery patients. *J Vasc Surg*. 2008;48:1481-1488.
10. Kent KC, Moscucci M, Mansour KA, et al. Retroperitoneal hematoma after cardiac catheterization: prevalence, risk factors, and optimal management. *J Vasc Surg*. 1994;20:905-910.
11. Helvie MA, Rubin JM, Silver TM, Kresowik TF. The distinction between femoral artery pseudoaneurysms and other causes of groin masses: value of duplex Doppler sonography. *Am J Roentgenol*. 1988;150:1177-1180.
12. Hirano Y, Ikuta S, Uehara H, et al. Diagnosis of vascular complications at the puncture site after cardiac catheterization. *J Cardiol*. 2004;43:259-265.
13. Kennedy AM, Grocott M, Schwartz MS, et al. Median nerve injury: an underrecognised complication of brachial artery cardiac catheterisation? *J Neurol Neurosurg Psychiatry*. 1997;63:542-546.
14. Stone PA, Martinez M, Thompson SN, et al. Ten-year experience of vascular surgeon management of iatrogenic pseudoaneurysms: do anticoagulant and/or antiplatelet medications matter? *Ann Vasc Surg*. 2016;30:45-51.
15. Toursarkissian B, Allen BT, Petrinec D, et al. Spontaneous closure of selected iatrogenic pseudoaneurysms and arteriovenous fistulae. *J Vasc Surg*. 1997;25:803-808.
16. Stone PA, Campbell JE, AbuRahma AF. Femoral pseudoaneurysms after percutaneous access. *J Vasc Surg*. 2014;60:1359-1366.
17. Webber GW, Jang J, Gustavson S, Olin JW. Contemporary management of postcatheterization pseudoaneurysms. *Circulation*. 2007;115:2666-2674.
18. Dzijan-Horn M, Langwieser N, Groha P, et al. Safety and efficacy of a potential treatment algorithm by using manual compression repair and ultrasound-guided thrombin injection for the management of iatrogenic femoral artery pseudoaneurysm in a large patient cohort. *Circ Cardiovasc Interv*. 2014;7:207-215.
19. Stone PA, Aburahma AF, Flaherty SK. Reducing duplex examinations in patients with iatrogenic pseudoaneurysms. *J Vasc Surg*. 2006;43:1211-1215.
20. Kelm M, Perings SM, Jax T, et al. Incidence and clinical outcome of iatrogenic femoral arteriovenous fistulas: implications for risk stratification and treatment. *J Am Coll Cardiol*. 2002;40:291-297.
21. Ruebben A, Tettoni S, Muratore P, et al. Arteriovenous fistulas induced by femoral arterial catheterization: percutaneous treatment. *Radiology*. 1998;209:729-734.
22. Onal B, Ilgit ET, Akpek S, Coskun B. Postcatheterization femoral arteriovenous fistula: endovascular treatment with N-butyl-cyanoacrylate embolization. *Cardiovasc Intervent Radiol*. 2006;29:276-278.
23. Klocker J, Gratl A, Chemelli A, et al. Influence of use of a vascular closure device on incidence and surgical management of access site complications after percutaneous interventions. *Eur J Vasc Endovasc Surg*. 2011;42:230-235.
24. Tsetis D. Endovascular treatment of complications of femoral arterial access. *Cardiovasc Intervent Radiol*. 2010;33:457-468.
25. Samal AK, White CJ. Percutaneous management of access site complications. *Catheter Cardiovasc Interv*. 2002;57:12-13.

Kimberly T. Malka • Jessica P. Simons

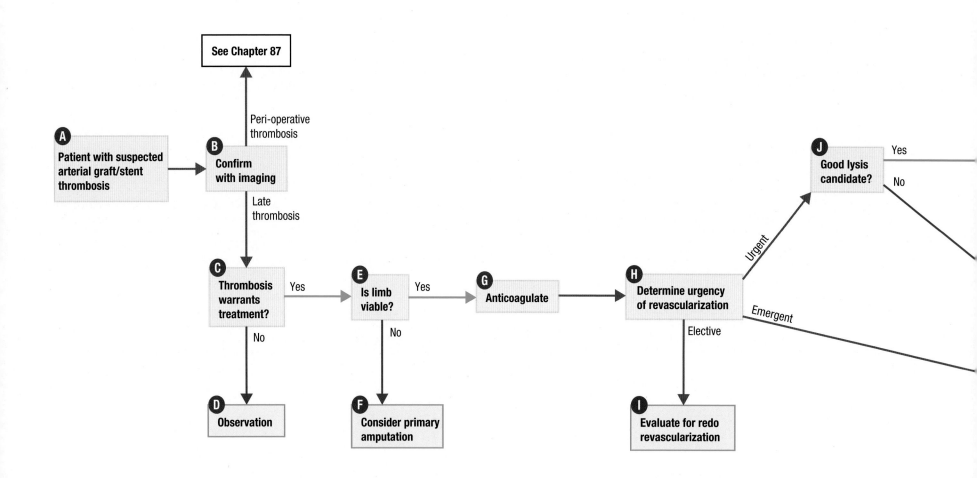

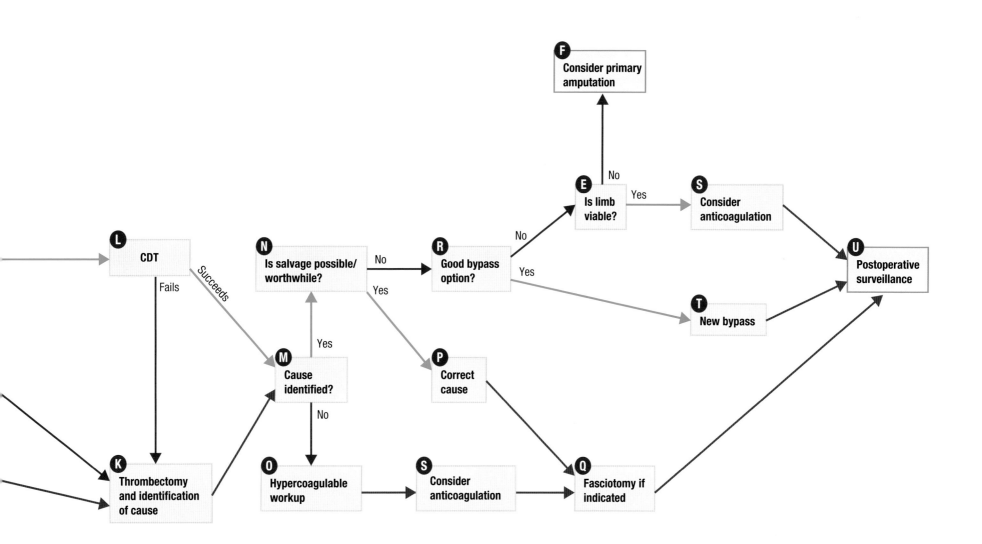

A Patient with suspected arterial graft/stent thrombosis

Patients with late thrombosis of a bypass graft or stent may present with a range of signs and symptoms. Thrombosis may be asymptomatic and incidentally detected, result in profound motor-sensory deficits that require immediate treatment, or have a variety of intermediate presentations between these two extremes. Presentation is largely dependent on chronicity and degree of ischemia. Targeted history should focus on characterizing the time-course of symptoms, functional status, prior surgical history, and indication of previous revascularization. Physical examination, including vascular, neurologic, and skin examination, often confirms thrombosis and dictates timing and necessity for revascularization. ABI is performed to quantify the degree of ischemia.

B Confirm with imaging

Goals of imaging include confirmation of graft/stent thrombosis, and assessment of inflow and outflow. Noninvasive options include DUS, CTA, MRA, or DSA. DUS is noninvasive, with no need for contrast or radiation; however, it is dependent on the availability and skill of the technologist. CTA offers the advantage of being noninvasive, readily available, and with good resolution; the disadvantage is of radiation exposure and the necessity for a nephrotoxic contrast agent. MRA also offers good resolution and can be done without the use of a contrast agent (time-of-flight MRA); however, the time it takes to perform an MRA is often prohibitive in using this as a diagnostic method in patients with a potentially threatened limb. DSA has the greatest utility when endovascular intervention is planned or when other imaging does not provide sufficient anatomic detail, such as for tibial arteries.

Graft or stent thrombosis that occurs shortly after the procedure is discussed in Chapter 87, whereas later thrombosis is considered in this chapter.

C Thrombosis warrants treatment?

Asymptomatic patients with incidentally discovered stent or graft occlusion may be managed conservatively with observation, recognizing that symptoms may progress or manifest later if the patient becomes more active. Those who present with non–lifestyle-limiting claudication are managed conservatively, whereas in patients with lifestyle-limiting symptoms, consideration should be given to simple thrombectomy if it is deemed possible. This approach is favored if it is believed that later intervention is likely to be more extensive. This decision making weighs on prior surveillance imaging. Likelihood of success with simple thrombectomy is lower if low flow, likely caused by poor outflow, has been observed on surveillance imaging.[1] If a better outflow target is known, it may be wise to plan for an alternate bypass. Patients who have had multiple attempts at graft salvage with no identification of reasons for occlusion may not benefit from additional revascularization efforts.

Finally, those who present with a known cause of graft occlusion (operative tourniquet, subtherapeutic anticoagulation levels) should undergo an attempt at graft salvage. In such cases, postoperative imaging is performed to identify an anatomic cause for failure. Patients with CLI (rest pain or tissue loss,) should undergo treatment, with intervention based on acuity, type of symptoms, operative risk, and availability of bypass conduit. Patients who present with acute limb ischemia (ALI) should be considered for urgent revascularization.

D Observation

Observation is considered in cases where the patient is asymptomatic, or when a palliative approach has been decided on. In asymptomatic patients with graft or stent thrombosis, which is incidentally found on surveillance imaging, observation is appropriate. If there is concern about propagation of thrombosis, which is thought to be more common with prosthetic grafts, anticoagulation for several months is recommended, albeit without clear evidence. Asymptomatic patients or patients with claudication should be monitored for development of worsening of symptoms. Patients in whom observation and pain control are part of a palliative approach should be monitored for worsening of tissue loss or development of infection that could require amputation.

E Is limb viable?

Patients who present late with profound paralysis, inaudible Doppler signals, or muscle rigor (Rutherford Class III ALI) are unlikely to benefit from revascularization. Although this does not result until at least 6 hours of severe ischemia has been present, in patients with underlying PAD who have developed good collateral circulation, the time interval before nonviability can be much longer. In patients with a clearly nonviable limb, revascularization may lead to profound and life-threatening rhabdomyolysis and should not be undertaken. Patients presenting with advanced tissue loss or extensive infection may not achieve limb salvage even with revascularization. If viability is uncertain, revascularization is usually the best option unless the patient is at prohibitive risk, recognizing that even in this case, eventual amputation may be required.

F Consider primary amputation

In patients deemed to have a nonsalvageable limb, primary amputation with an eye toward rapid rehabilitation is the best option. Certain protocols have been shown to result in ambulation within 15 days of amputation. These protocols call for placement of a hard plaster cast dressing intraoperatively, and fitting of an immediate postoperative prosthesis.[2] Criteria have been developed to guide patient selection for this approach. When making the decision regarding level of amputation, it is important to ensure adequate perfusion to the affected limb, as well as assess the patient's ambulatory status before their current presentation (see Chapter 48).

G Anticoagulate

For patients who present with graft or stent thrombosis and symptoms of acute ischemia, prompt initiation of anticoagulation is imperative to prevent thrombus propagation. In the acute setting, IV heparin (weight-based dosing, bolus dose of 80 units/kg, followed by infusion at 18 units/kg/h for a goal PTT of 60-80 seconds) is used because it provides rapid onset of anticoagulant activity, is easily titrated, and has a short half-life allowing it to be stopped if necessary during surgery or thrombolysis. Unfractionated heparin is generally the agent of choice because it is easy to regulate and offers a vasodilatory effect in addition to its anticoagulant effect. In patients with a heparin allergy, alternative agents such as direct thrombin inhibitors can be given intravenously. For patients with CKD, argatroban (weight-based dosing, bolus of 350 mcg/kg, followed by infusion at 25 mcg/kg/min) is the agent of choice for anticoagulation in the acute setting because it is metabolized by the liver. Argatroban is, however, contraindicated in patients with hepatic insufficiency. In patients with liver dysfunction and normal renal function, bivalirudin (weight-based dosing, bolus of 0.75 mg/kg, followed by infusion at 0.2 mg/kg/h) may be used because it is degraded by peptidases and partially excreted by the kidneys.

H Determine urgency of revascularization

The time-course of symptom onset (<14 days) and severity of ischemia/neurologic deficit (Rutherford classifications of ALI) dictate much of the management. Generally, treatment priority is assigned on the basis of Rutherford's acute ischemia classification, as elective (Rutherford class I), urgent (Rutherford class IIa), or emergent (Rutherford class IIb or III). Severity at presentation depends on the duration of ischemia and the extent of collateral circulation.

I Evaluate for redo revascularization

Patients with a viable limb, and no evidence of ALI after graft or stent thrombosis, should be evaluated for the need for revascularization, which could consist of thrombectomy and lysis (see J and K) if the graft or stent is salvageable. In many cases, graft or stent thrombosis without acute ischemia is often not detected until late, such that redo bypass is the best option. This should proceed in accordance with standard algorithms for revascularization planning, including evaluation of operative risk, inflow, outflow, and conduit availability.

J Good lysis candidate?

Patients with a viable limb and Rutherford class IIa acute ischemia (minimal sensory loss, no muscle weakness, audible venous Doppler signals) who require revascularization should have it on an urgent basis. Both thrombolysis and surgical revascularization can be considered.[3] Good candidates for lysis include those in whom the symptoms have been present for <14 days (see also Chapter 53).[4] Lysis can be achieved with chemical means using a thrombolytic agent such as tissue plasminogen activator (tPA) or adjunctive mechanical devices. Catheter-directed infusion thrombolysis may avoid the need for open surgery and allow for percutaneous treatment of anastomotic, inflow, or in-graft lesions. Disadvantages of infusion lytic therapy include time required to achieve restoration of flow (24-48 hours); thus, immediately threatened limbs (Rutherford IIB) should not be treated with infusion lysis. Contraindications to lysis include recent major surgery (or minor surgery where bleeding complications would be highly morbid), and known intracranial pathology. When possible, full anticoagulation is reversed before starting lysis treatment, to reduce the likelihood of bleeding complications. Combination of mechanical and chemical lysis may obviate need for the long time required for infusion chemical lysis to work and have been used in patients with immediately threatened limbs, although outcomes with surgical revascularization may be superior.

If symptoms have been present for >14 days, lysis is less likely to be successful, and traditional assessments for revascularization should be undertaken. This 14-day threshold is a guideline that may require adjustment on the basis of patient operative risk versus risk/benefits of lysis. After 14 days, the risks of lysis, in combination with the decreased likelihood of success, did not favor its use in vein grafts, and redo bypass must be considered. However, in the same situation, a prosthetic graft may still be salvaged with open thrombectomy and become durable if the underlying cause of thrombosis can be treated.

Ⓚ Thrombectomy and identification of cause

For those patients who present with immediately threatened Rutherford class IIb (sensory loss with mild to moderate muscle weakness) ischemia, rapid restoration of flow to salvage the limb is needed. Either open surgical revascularization or percutaneous mechanical thrombectomy to prevent limb loss should be performed emergently.[5] Open thrombectomy entails first obtaining proximal and distal control, then passing of an appropriately sized balloon thrombectomy catheter, both proximally and distally. This maneuver should be repeated as many times as needed to achieve two negative passes. Ring strippers have been reported as an adjunct for use in cases of thrombosed prosthetic bypass with very adherent clot. Intraoperative DSA should be performed after thrombectomy to aid in identifying the anatomic cause so that it can be corrected. For patients with stent thrombosis who require emergent revascularization, open thrombectomy and DSA are also appropriate, but open bypass, rather than endovascular intervention, should be considered. For those patients presenting with graft or stent thrombosis and prohibitively high operative risk, an endovascular approach including pharmacomechanical thrombectomy with possible suction embolectomy should be

performed. In either case, the need for fasciotomies must also be determined at the time of revascularization and should be based on the duration of ischemia and likelihood for reperfusion injury.

Ⓛ CDT

Generally, a lysis catheter is placed to infuse tPA at 0.5 to 1 mg/hour. A heparin infusion, at 500 units/hour via the sidearm of the sheath, is used to prevent thrombus development on the sheath. Patients require an ICU, with close monitoring for evidence of a systemic lytic state; this includes serial evaluation of fibrinogen levels, PTT, and complete blood counts. Lysis should be stopped for fibrinogen levels <100 mg/dL, a decrease in fibrinogen levels by >50% within 4 hours, or PTT > 30 (indicating therapeutic levels of heparin). Patients should be monitored for changes in neurologic examination, headache, and nausea because these symptoms can indicate an intracranial hemorrhage. Patients who experience any neurologic symptoms should have lytic therapy stopped immediately and a STAT noncontrast head CT to assess for intracranial bleeding.

Ⓜ Cause identified?

After completion of successful lysis or thrombectomy, it is standard to perform a completion DSA to identify and correct any anatomic cause for the thrombosis. In the absence of a causative anatomic lesion, a hypercoagulable workup should be conducted. The cause for graft or stent occlusion may not always be anatomic in nature. For example, patients undergoing orthopedic procedures may have had a tourniquet placed over a bypass or stent, resulting in graft/stent thrombosis. Patients with recurrent thrombosis may require life-long anticoagulation to preserve stent or graft patency.

Ⓝ Is salvage possible/worthwhile?

Likelihood of durable graft salvage is markedly decreased when the identified cause is poor outflow distal to the distal anastomosis. If a suitable distal target is identified, and conduit is available, there is the potential to salvage the bypass in the context of performing a jump graft to the better target. Likelihood of durable graft salvage is also decreased when the identified cause is a poor conduit, such as a small or diffusely stenotic vein graft. Patients with thrombosed stents, a history of prior stent salvage, or with no identified anatomic cause may not benefit from an additional attempt at stent recanalization.

Ⓞ Hypercoagulable workup

In the absence of an identifiable cause for graft or stent thrombosis, a hypercoagulability workup should be performed as discussed in detail in Chapter 5. If this is positive, or if repeated thrombosis has occurred despite no anatomic cause (suggesting undetected hypercoagulability), anticoagulation should be considered.

Ⓟ Correct cause

Correction of the culprit lesion is imperative to prevent recurrent graft or stent occlusion. Often, inciting lesions can be treated with PTA or stent placement. However, anastomotic stenosis or long lesion graft stenoses may require open surgical revision.

Ⓠ Fasciotomy if indicated

In patients who present with Rutherford level IIa ischemia, the need for fasciotomies must be determined at the time of revascularization and should be based on the duration of ischemia and likelihood for reperfusion injury. Most patients who present with Rutherford level IIb ischemia require fasciotomies. Generally, patients who present with acute ischemia of >6-hour duration or have tense compartments after revascularization should undergo decompressive fasciotomies at the time of surgery. For patients who do not undergo fasciotomies at the time of surgery, postoperative serial examinations to check for compartment syndrome are essential. Loss of sensation in the web space between the first and second toes is the first sign of compartment syndrome, affecting the anterior calf compartment, which is commonly the first to be involved. Other signs include pain with passive dorsiflexion of the great toe, increasing pain coupled with increasing CPK, and any motor or sensory deficits. (Details of fasciotomy are discussed in Chapter 53.)

Ⓡ Good bypass option?

If the initial bypass or stent cannot be salvaged, patients should be evaluated for a reintervention. Inflow and outflow target anatomy can be obtained angiographically at the time of planned graft or stent salvage. Patients should also undergo vein mapping, with mapping including the upper extremities if lower extremity veins are not suitable. In good operative patients with suitable inflow, outflow, and conduit, a new bypass may be the best way to restore limb perfusion.

Ⓢ Consider anticoagulation

The utility of postoperative anticoagulation after surgical treatment for lower extremity thrombotic or embolic events has been well established.[6,7] For first-time thrombosis, 3 to 6 months of anticoagulation is usually sufficient, although this has not been well studied. In patients with recurrent graft/stent thrombosis without an underlying anatomic cause or in whom a hypercoagulable state has been identified, lifelong anticoagulation may be indicated. Although most direct oral anticoagulants are not currently approved for use in cases of arterial thrombosis, they are often prescribed for this condition. Warfarin is the most commonly used anticoagulant for this purpose and does requiring bridging with either heparin or LMWH.

❶ New bypass

Arterial imaging using CTA, MRA, or DSA is the first step in operative planning. For patients with prior endovascular interventions, especially TASC C and D lesions, repeated percutaneous intervention(s) may fail to achieve acceptable patency rates.[8] Surgical bypass should be considered in this patient population. In addition, failure to salvage a stent via endovascular revision may also require conversion to an open procedure. Patients who present with a chronically thrombosed graft may also benefit from a reoperative procedure. Vein mapping, including the upper extremity veins if necessary, is necessary for operative planning.

❶ Postoperative surveillance

Postoperative vein graft surveillance increases bypass graft patency. Many studies have shown that patients with graft or stent thrombosis are at increased risk for requiring a major amputation if no intervention is performed, making graft or stent preservation critical to limb survival.[9] Percutaneous interventions on at-risk grafts can result in patency rates of >80%.[10] DUS can identify both in-stent and in-graft stenoses, as well as anastomotic stenosis, allowing for endovascular interventions aimed at preventing thrombosis. The Society for Vascular Surgery guidelines recommend physical examination, ABIs, and graft surveillance DUS postoperatively (to establish baseline), as well as at 3, 6, and 12 months, and annually thereafter. These guidelines apply to both infrainguinal vein grafts and infrainguinal stents, with optional DUS to be used with infrainguinal prosthetic grafts. Obviously, DUS should be performed expeditiously for any patient presenting with a change in symptoms and prior lower extremity bypass graft or stent(s).[11]

REFERENCES

1. Bandyk DF, Towne JB, Schmitt DD, Seabrook GR, Bergamini TM. Therapeutic options for acute thrombosed in situ saphenous vein arterial bypass grafts. *J Vasc Surg.* 1990;11(5):680-687.
2. Folsom D, King T, Rubin JR. Lower-extremity amputation with immediate postoperative prosthetic placement. *Am J Surg.* 1992;164(4):320-322.
3. Stept LL, Flinn WR, McCarthy WJ III, Bartlett ST, Bergan JJ, Yao JS. Technical defects as a cause of early graft failure after femorodistal bypass. *Arch Surg.* 1987;122(5):599-604.
4. Results of a prospective randomized trial evaluating surgery versus thrombolysis for ischemia of the lower extremity. The stile trial. *Ann Surg.* 1994;220(3):251-266; discussion 266-268.
5. Rutherford RB, Baker JD, Ernst C, et al. Recommended standards for reports dealing with lower extremity ischemia: revised version. *J Vasc Surg.* 1997;26(3):517-538.
6. Tawes RL Jr, Harris EJ, Brown WH, et al. Arterial thromboembolism. A 20-year perspective. *Arch Surg.* 1985;120(5):595-599.
7. Tawes RL Jr, Beare JP, Scribner RG, Sydorak GR, Brown WH, Harris EJ. Value of postoperative heparin therapy in peripheral arterial thromboembolism. *Am J Surg.* 1983;146(2):213-215.
8. Robinson WP III, Nguyen LL, Bafford R, Belkin M. Results of second-time angioplasty and stenting for femoropopliteal occlusive disease and factors affecting outcomes. *J Vasc Surg.* 2011;53(3):651-657.
9. Watson HR, Schroeder TV, Simms MH, et al. Relationship of femorodistal bypass patency to clinical outcome. Iloprost bypass international study group. *Eur J Vasc Endovasc Surg.* 1999;17(1):77-83.
10. Jongsma H, Bekken JA, van Buchem F, Bekkers WJ, Azizi F, Fioole B. Secondary interventions in patients with autologous infrainguinal bypass grafts strongly improve patency rates. *J Vasc Surg.* 2016;63(2):385-390.
11. Zierler RE, Jordan WD, Lal BK, et al. The society for vascular surgery practice guidelines on follow-up after vascular surgery arterial procedures. *J Vasc Surg.* 2018;68(1):256-284.

Katherine Giuliano • James H. Black

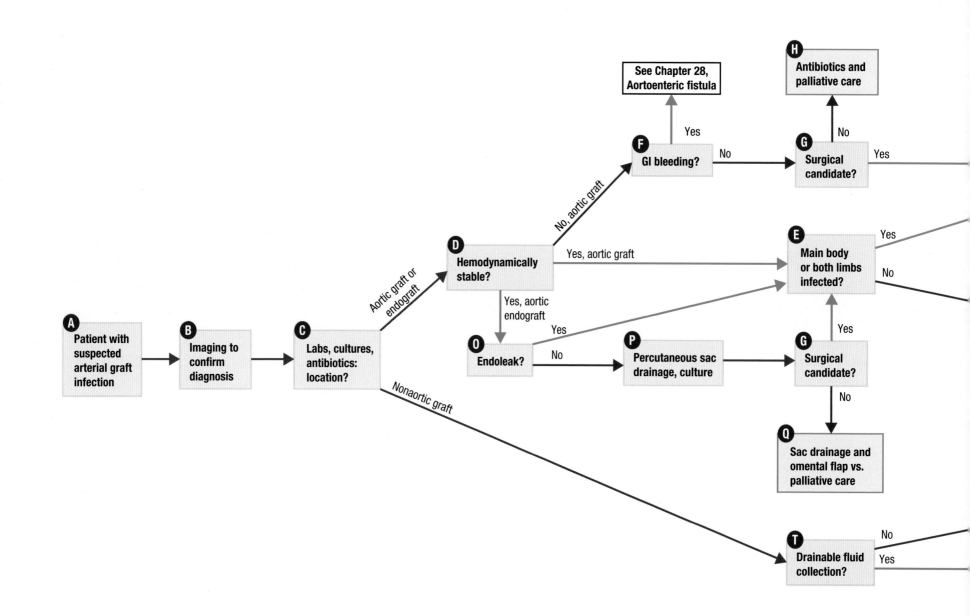

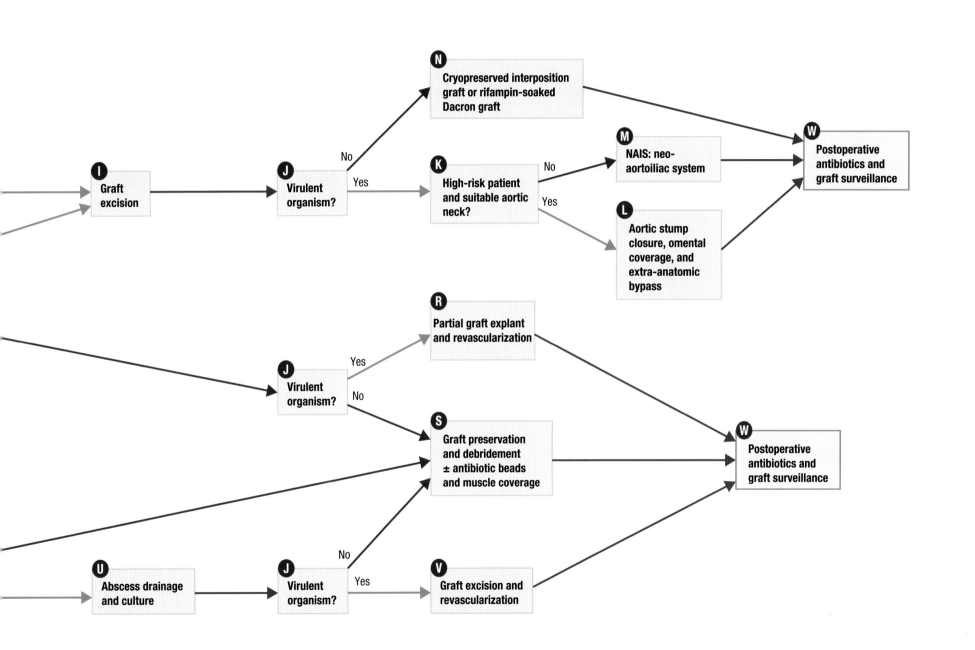

A Patient with suspected arterial graft infection

Prosthetic arterial graft infections occur in approximately 1% to 5% of cases, with the highest rate occurring in the groin.[1-3] Graft infections can present with local signs of infection, systemic illness, or as hemorrhage. Local signs of infection occur primarily at the site of extracavitary prosthetic grafts and include surgical site erythema, swelling, pain, abscess formation, or sinus tract drainage.[4,5] Systemic signs of illness, which is a common presentation of early graft infections (within 4 months of surgery), include fever, chills, and malaise, with leukocytosis, elevated inflammatory markers (ESR and CRP), and, oftentimes, positive blood cultures. Bleeding as a result of a graft infection can be due to anastomotic disruption or PSA.

B Imaging to confirm diagnosis

The imaging modality of choice depends on the location of the suspected graft infection, with intracavitary infections best imaged with CTA. Findings suggestive of graft infection include perigraft air or fluid and surrounding fat stranding.[2,4,6] For extracavitary graft infections, DUS is an inexpensive, minimally invasive, first-line modality of evaluation, with CTA a useful adjunct. DUS findings can include fluid (and, rarely, air) around the graft or anastomotic PSA. If findings are inconclusive, MRI can be helpful in elucidating subtle perigraft inflammatory changes and differentiating infection from hematoma.[4] Uptake on ^{18}F-FDG-PET/CT scan or on tagged WBC studies can also help confirm vascular graft infection in equivocal cases, with PET scan demonstrating added diagnostic accuracy compared with CT alone.[7] Tagged WBC studies have reported sensitivity for detecting graft infection ranging from 60% to 100%, but have a high false-positive rate in the early postoperative period when healing tissue normally contains WBCs.[6] PET scan sensitivity is approximately 90% along with a specificity of 70%.[7]

C Labs, cultures, antibiotics: location?

Workup for presumed arterial graft infection includes a full set of laboratory tests, demonstrating elevated WBC count and inflammatory markers such as ESR and CRP. Peripheral blood cultures should be obtained before initiating broad-spectrum parenteral antibiotics because positive cultures help focus therapy. Although operative intervention should occur promptly for hemodynamically unstable patients, blood cultures should still be obtained if possible. Perigraft and graft tissue should also be cultured intraoperatively, and broad-spectrum antibiotics should be initiated congruent with surgery.[4] Next steps depend on whether the infection involves an aortic graft, an aortic endograft, or a nonaortic graft.

D Hemodynamically stable?

Hemodynamic instability from either sepsis or hemorrhage warrants prompt surgical intervention with proximal and distal control for hemorrhage management and wide debridement for infection control.[4,5]

E Main body or both limbs infected?

When imaging suggests infection of the entire aortic graft or endograft, complete graft excision is necessary, particularly if infection is caused by a virulent organism.[2,3] Graft infection limited to a single limb of an aortobifemoral bypass may be amenable to partial graft preservation.

F GI bleeding?

The presence of GI bleeding in association with aortic graft infection raises the likelihood of a graft-enteric fistula. Rapid diagnosis is needed, because massive bleeding may ensue. Even in the absence of GI bleeding, suspicion should be increased for a graft-enteric fistula in cases of gram-negative bacteremia.[4] For management of an aorto-enteric fistula, see Chapter 28.

G Surgical candidate?

Assessment for a patient's surgical candidacy should include evaluation of their age, medical comorbidities, nutritional status, as well as their preferences and goals of care. Comorbid conditions should be treated as required. When a patient with an aortic graft infection is unstable from bleeding or sepsis, this evaluation must be expeditious, because emergent surgery is required unless the patient is deemed not a surgical candidate.

H Antibiotics and palliative care

If the patients with aortic graft infection have medical comorbidities that preclude operative intervention, they should be managed with intensive antibiotics. Aortic graft infections, however, nearly always lead to death without operative intervention, so involvement of palliative care is advisable.[2,3]

I Graft excision

Surgical treatment of an infected aortic graft involves laparotomy, arterial control, excision of all infected graft components, debridement of adjacent infected tissue, and some type of revascularization, the details of which depend in part on the virulence of the infecting organism.

J Virulent organism?

Most arterial graft infections are caused by gram-positive organisms, most commonly *Staphylococcus aureus*. In gram-negative graft infections, common organisms include *Pseudomonas aeruginosa*, *Escherichia coli*, *Proteus*, and *Klebsiella pneumonia*.[8,9] Virulent organisms include pseudomonas and MRSA, which usually cause more severe infections, present early, and typically require more aggressive management with complete graft excision and revascularization.[4] Less virulent organisms such as *S. epidermidis* are causative in local infections, present late (>4 months postoperatively), and are more amenable to graft preservation.[5]

K High-risk patient and suitable aortic neck?

In a patient with a virulent aortic graft infection, revascularization after graft excision can be performed with either an extra-anatomic bypass or an in situ reconstruction. The decision of which method to pursue is based on a number of factors.[2-5,10] In high surgical risk patients who have a suitable aortic neck for closure, axillofemoral bypass followed by staged graft excision is generally recommended. In patients able to tolerate aortic graft excision and femoral-popliteal vein harvest for aortic reconstruction, this approach reduces the risk of aortic stump blowout and is preferred. Surgical decision making in these cases is complex and must include careful assessment of surgical risk.

L Aortic stump closure, omental coverage, and extra-anatomic bypass

Extra-anatomic bypass, whereby the infected segment of artery/graft is bypassed in a sterile, nonanatomic plane, was the first described method for managing aortic graft infections. In the current era, it is usually reserved for virulent infections in patients at too high risk for an extensive single-stage aortic reconstruction.[11] Typically, in this management strategy, an axillobifemoral bypass is performed first to establish new inflow to the downstream arterial bed, unless the patient required urgent graft excision before the extra-anatomic bypass can be staged. If the aortic graft infection involves the groin, the reconstruction may need to be bilateral axillo-SFA or -popliteal bypass to avoid this infected area. Then, in a second-stage operation, usually the next day, the infected graft is completely excised and tissue debrided. The aortic stump is oversewn and can be buttressed with an omental flap. In this approach, complication rates approach 30%, including risk of aortic stump disruption, reinfection, and lower extremity amputation (see Chapter 48).[3,10-12] Reinfection rates approach 25% and typically occur at the prior infected graft site rather than in the extra-anatomic new bypass graft.[3,13]

M NAIS: neoaortoiliac system

In patients fit for surgery with a virulent aortic graft infection, in situ reconstruction called NAIS (neoaortoiliac system) can be performed with vein harvested from the patient. The femoral-popliteal veins, depending on diameter needed, can be used for arterial reconstruction in the setting of graft infection. Autogenous vein grafting has the benefit of high long-term patency and low risk of reinfection while eliminating the risk of aortic stump blowout that accompanies graft excision. The main disadvantages is the long operative time required to harvest vein, often requiring two surgical teams, and a 15% to 30% incidence of lower extremity severe swelling from venous excision.[14-17] Given its low risk of reinfection (reported as <2%), autologous vein should be considered over cadaveric allografts in the setting of virulent organism graft infection, in patients who can tolerate this procedure.[15,18]

(N) Cryopreserved interposition graft or rifampin-soaked Dacron graft

In patients with aortic graft infection due to a less virulent organism, cryopreserved allografts can be used for aortic reconstruction after graft excision. They provide the benefit of not requiring time to harvest and having a high patency rate, but the downsides include high cost and possibility for late deterioration.[17,19] Synthetic grafts such as Dacron can be soaked in rifampin to provide local antibiotic delivery to sensitive organisms. Such grafts can also be used for infected aortic graft replacement, because data show lower risk of subsequent infection.[14] Polyester grafts are inexpensive and readily available and are often the only reconstructive option immediately available if a NAIS is not feasible.[11]

(O) Endoleak?

If an endoleak is present, the patient with an infected aortic endograft should undergo prompt operative repair to avoid rupture. Treatment options include graft excision versus preservation with the choice based on several factors including the extent of the infection (graft main body vs. graft limbs infected), the virulence of the causative organism, the presence of an anastomotic pseudoaneurysm, and the patient's fitness for surgery.

(P) Percutaneous sac drainage, culture

If the patient with an infected aortic endograft does not have an endoleak and is hemodynamically stable, fluid within the infected AAA sac surrounding the aortic endograft should be percutaneously drained before proceeding with operative intervention if it is accessible to image-guided drainage. If appropriate, the abscess drain can be left in place for continued drainage until definitive treatment is performed. Fluid should be sent for culture to guide antimicrobial therapy.[11,14]

(Q) Sac drainage and omental flap vs. palliative care

If the patient is not a surgical candidate for graft excision, sac drainage provides local control and antibiotics provide systemic therapy. If the patient cannot tolerate the morbidity of a full explant and revascularization operation, but can tolerate a smaller procedure, local debridement of the infected sac with an omental flap can provide coverage of the graft to prevent further sequelae of the infection, assuming good proximal and distal seal zones. Lifelong suppressive antibiotics are recommended in this case. If the patient cannot tolerate any operative procedure, and sac drainage and antibiotics fail to control the infection, palliative care should be undertaken.[11]

(R) Partial graft explant and revascularization

If the entire graft is infected with a virulent organism, complete graft excision is required. If, however, the graft infection is limited to a single limb of an aortobifemoral bypass, this may be amenable to partial graft explantation and revascularization. By preserving the main body and other limb, the morbidity of a more complex operation and an aortic stump are avoided. This procedure is performed in stages to prevent inadvertent contamination of the noninfected graft. Typically, a retroperitoneal incision is used to expose the graft limb proximal to the area of infection. Here, the graft can be divided and oversewn, and this incision closed. The groin is then explored and the infected distal portion of the graft is excised and extra-anatomic, usually axillo-SFA/popliteal revascularization is performed. With a low-virulence organism, in situ replacement of the infected portion of the graft limb can be considered, using autogenous vein, cryopreserved graft, or synthetic graft soaked in rifampin (see O).[2,3]

(S) Graft preservation and debridement ± antibiotic beads and muscle coverage

Graft preservation typically requires debridement of infected and devitalized tissue, often with multiple operations.[4] Medical management with antibiotics is crucial. A technique of placing polymethylmethacrylate antibiotic-impregnated beads in the wound bed has been recommended.[20] With graft infection involving the groin, it may not be possible to obtain good soft-tissue coverage after debriding infected tissue. In this case, coverage of the graft site with a muscle flap increases rate of graft preservation and reduces morbidity, including the rate of amputation.[20-22] Muscle flaps (most commonly sartorius, rectus femoris, rectus abdominis, or gracilis) improve outcomes by filling potential space, increasing vascular supply to promote healing, and protecting the wound and graft from contamination.[4,10,23] In other locations, they may be applicable if soft-tissue coverage of the preserved graft is not possible.

(T) Drainable fluid collection?

If imaging reveals an accessible fluid collection around an infected graft, it should be drained.

(U) Abscess drainage and culture

Extracavitary graft abscesses can be aspirated and the fluid cultured to guide antibiotic treatment.[10,18,20]

(V) Graft excision and revascularization

When nonaortic, peripheral bypass grafts are infected with virulent organisms causing systemic sepsis, are occluded, or are complicated by hemorrhage, they should be treated by excision. Operative intervention should include graft removal, surrounding tissue debridement, and revascularization of the extremity with, preferably, the autogenous vein routed to avoid the area of infection. Alternatively, extra-anatomic bypass in a fresh, uninfected plane using autogenous, cryopreserved, or synthetic material can be performed as a first operation, followed by a second operation for infected graft explantation and debridement.[10,18,20] Graft removal should be complete, especially for prosthetic grafts, because small remnants of graft left at the site of anastomosis can lead to ongoing infection and blowout. This may require patch angioplasty using autogenous or cryopreserved tissue if primary closure of the anastomotic site is not possible without compromising the arterial lumen.

(W) Postoperative antibiotics and graft surveillance

Medical treatment with antibiotics is a key component in the treatment of infected arterial vascular grafts. After obtaining cultures, broad-spectrum parenteral antibiotics with gram-negative and gram-positive coverage should be initiated. Antibiotics can subsequently be focused on the identified organism. The duration of recommended antibiotic therapy is based primarily on the severity of the infection and ranges from 2 weeks to 6 months.[18] Patients' ESR and CRP should be monitored, with rising inflammatory markers a potential harbinger of recurrent infection. Lifelong suppressive antibiotic therapy can also be considered depending on the severity of the infection, the virulence of the causative organism, and other patient-specific risk factors, such as poor candidacy for additional operative interventions.[4,20]

REFERENCES

1. Prendiville EJ, Yeager A, O'Donnell TF Jr, et al. Long-term results with the above-knee popliteal expanded polytetrafluoroethylene graft. *J Vasc Surg*. 1990;11:517-524.
2. Chiesa R, Astore D, Frigerio S, et al. Vascular prosthetic graft infection: epidemiology, bacteriology, pathogenesis and treatment. *Acta Chir Belg*. 2002;102:238-247.
3. O'Connor S, Andrew P, Batt M, Becquemin JP. A systematic review and meta-analysis of treatments for aortic graft infection. *J Vasc Surg*. 2006;44:38-45.
4. Wilson WR, Bower TC, Creager MA, et al. Vascular graft infections, mycotic aneurysms, and endovascular infections: a scientific statement from the American Heart Association. *Circulation*. 2016;134:e412-e460.
5. Kilic A, Arnaoutakis DJ, Reifsnyder T, et al. Management of infected vascular grafts. *Vasc Med*. 2016;21:53-60.
6. Orton DF, LeVeen RF, Saigh JA, et al. Aortic prosthetic graft infections: radiologic manifestations and implications for management. *Radiographics*. 2000;20:977-993.
7. Bruggink JL, Glaudemans AW, Saleem BR, et al. Accuracy of FDG-PET-CT in the diagnostic work-up of vascular prosthetic graft infection. *Eur J Vasc Endovasc Surg*. 2010;40: 348-354.
8. Inui T, Bandyk DF. Vascular surgical site infection: risk factors and preventive measures. *Semin Vasc Surg*. 2015;28:201-207.
9. Pounds LL, Montes-Walters M, Mayhall CG, et al. A changing pattern of infection after major vascular reconstructions. *Vasc Endovasc Surg*. 2005;39:511-517.
10. Zetrenne E, McIntosh BC, McRae MH, Gusberg R, Evans GR, Narayan D. Prosthetic vascular graft infection: a

multi-center review of surgical management. *Yale J Biol Med.* 2007;80:113-121.

11. Fatima, J, Duncan AA, de Grandis E, et al. Treatment strategies and outcomes in patients with infected aortic endografts. *J Vasc Surg.* 2013;58:371-379.

12. Seeger JM, Pretus HA, Welborn MB, Ozaki CK, Flynn TC, Huber TS. Long-term outcome after treatment of aortic graft infection with staged extra-anatomic bypass grafting and aortic graft removal. *J Vasc Surg.* 2000;32:451-459; discussion 460-461.

13. O'Hara PJ, Hertzer NR, Beven EG, Krajewski LP. Surgical management of infected abdominal aortic grafts: review of a 25-year experience. *J Vasc Surg.* 1986;3:725-731.

14. Smeds MR, Duncan AA, Harlander-Locke MP, et al. Treatment and outcomes of aortic endograft infection. *J Vasc Surg.* 2016;63:332-340.

15. Chung J, Clagett GP. Neoaortoiliac System (NAIS) procedure for the treatment of the infected aortic graft. *Semin Vasc Surg.* 2011;24:220-226.

16. Clagett GP, Valentine RJ, Hagino RT. Autogenous aortoiliac/femoral reconstruction from superficial femoral-popliteal veins: feasibility and durability. *J Vasc Surg.* 1997;25:255-266; discussion 267-270.

17. Valentine RJ, Clagett GP. Aortic graft infections: replacement with autogenous vein. *Cardiovasc Surg Lond Engl.* 2001;9:419-425.

18. Samson RH, Veith FJ, Janko GS, Gupta SK, Scher LA. A modified classification and approach to the management of infections involving peripheral arterial prosthetic grafts. *J Vasc Surg.* 1988;8:147-153.

19. Snyder SO, Wheeler JR, Gregory RT, Gayle RG, Zirkle PK. Freshly harvested cadaveric venous homografts as arterial conduits in infected fields. *Surgery.* 1987;101:283-291.

20. Stone PA, Back MR, Armstrong PA, et al. Evolving microbiology and treatment of extracavitary prosthetic graft infections. *Vasc Endovasc Surg.* 2008;42:537-544.

21. Calligaro KD, Veith FJ, Sales CM, Dougherty MJ, Savarese RP, DeLaurentis DA. Comparison of muscle flaps and delayed secondary intention wound healing for infected lower extremity arterial grafts. *Ann Vasc Surg.* 1994;8:31-37.

22. Graham RG, Omotoso PO, Hudson DA. The effectiveness of muscle flaps for the treatment of prosthetic graft sepsis. *Plast Reconstr Surg.* 2002;109:108-113; discussion 114-115.

23. Perler BA, Vander Kolk CA, Dufresne CR, Williams GM. Can infected prosthetic grafts be salvaged with rotational muscle flaps? *Surgery.* 1991;110:30-34.

Timothy K. Liem

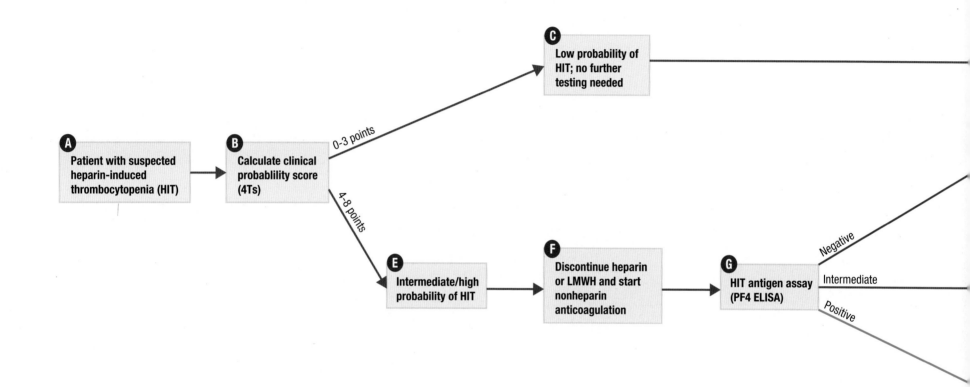

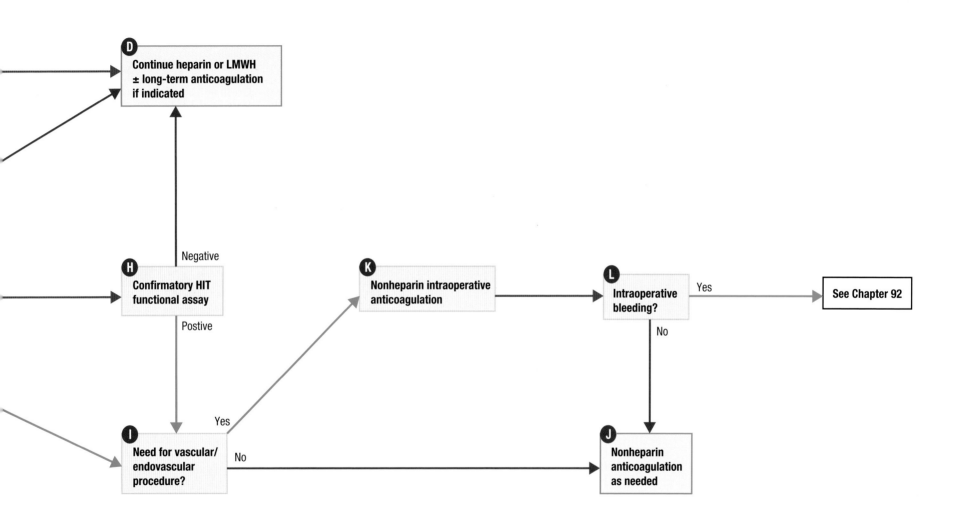

A Patient with suspected heparin-induced thrombocytopenia (HIT)

HIT is caused by the formation of antibodies that recognize a complex of heparin and platelet factor 4 (PF4). Even without antibody formation, heparin/PF4 has the potential to bind B cells and activate direct complement, a process that may be augmented in the presence of inflammation or infection.[1,2] Heparin/PF4, in the presence of HIT antibodies, may cause robust platelet activation (via the FcγRIIA platelet receptor) with subsequent thrombin generation, thrombocytopenia, and thrombosis.

B Calculate clinical probability score (4Ts)

Patients in whom HIT is suspected should be evaluated with the validated "4Ts" clinical scoring system (Table 91-1). Low, intermediate, and high probability scores are 0 to 3, 4 to 5, and 6 to 8, respectively.[3,4] Patients with low clinical probability can continue heparin therapy, whereas those with moderate or high probability require heparin cessation and additional evaluation.

C Low probability of HIT; no further testing needed

The negative predictive value of a low-probability 4Ts score (0-3) is 0.998 (95% CI, 0.970-1.000).[3,4] This allows the clinician to exclude HIT without further diagnostic laboratory testing.

D Continue heparin or LMWH ± long-term anticoagulation if indicated

Patients with a low-probability 4Ts score may safely continue unfractionated heparin or LMWH, if indicated, for the treatment or prevention of arterial or venous thrombosis.

E Intermediate/high probability of HIT

The positive predictive values of intermediate- (4-5 points) and high-probability (6-8 points) 4Ts scores are 0.014 (95% CI, 0.09-0.22), and 0.64 (95% CI, 0.40-0.82), respectively.[4] A 4Ts clinical score cutoff of ≥4 is highly sensitive in detecting HIT [0.99 (95% CI, 0.86-1.00)], but has poor specificity [0.54 (95% CI, 0.43-0.66)].[4] Patients with a 4Ts clinical score of ≥4 require further laboratory testing.

F Discontinue heparin or LMWH and start nonheparin anticoagulation

Patients with intermediate/high-probability 4Ts clinical scores (≥4) should discontinue heparin or LMWH. If the patient is receiving treatment for an acute venous or arterial thrombosis, then the administration of a nonheparin anticoagulant is indicated (see J).

G HIT antigen assay (PF4 ELISA)

Laboratory confirmation of HIT may be performed using either an immunoassay for the HIT antibody or a platelet-activation "functional" assay (see H). Immunoassays (eg, enzyme-linked immunosorbent assays) are more readily available, and technically easier to perform, with high sensitivity (>99%), but only moderate specificity (30%-70%). In patients with a high 4Ts clinical score (≥6) and a positive immunoassay, additional testing is unnecessary, because this confirms HIT. In addition, patients with an intermediate 4Ts clinical score (4-5) and a negative immunoassay also require no additional testing, because this effectively disproves HIT.[1,5]

H Confirmatory HIT functional assay

Functional testing for HIT utilizes heparin, patient plasma, and, typically, donor platelets to detect platelet activation via the release of ^{14}C-serotonin or platelet aggregation assays. These tests are more difficult to perform and, often, are only available in specialized tertiary referral centers. In contrast to immunoassays, these functional assays have a lower sensitivity but a significantly higher specificity and positive predictive value. Functional assays are likely to be most useful in patients who have an intermediate 4Ts clinical score with a positive immunoassay. In these patients, the posttest probability of HIT ranges from 40% to 64%, so there are benefits from functional testing.[1,6] If functional testing is not available, patients with a positive HIT antibody immunoassay and intermediate 4T score should be assumed to have HIT.

I Need for vascular/endovascular procedure?

Some patients with a recent or remote diagnosis of HIT may require a percutaneous or an open vascular procedure. The choice of intraoperative anticoagulation will depend on the platelet recovery and the result of the most recent heparin antibody immunoassay (see K).

J Nonheparin anticoagulation as needed

Regardless of whether a patient requires additional vascular surgery or intervention, the majority of patients with acute HIT will require a course of nonheparin anticoagulation, simply to manage the thrombotic complications of HIT. The American College of Chest Physicians and the British Society for Haematology recommend *4 weeks of anticoagulation for patients with isolated HIT, and 3 months for patients with HIT and thrombosis* (HITT).[7,8]

The choice of anticoagulation remains complex, and consultation with a hematologist is often required. This decision is influenced by multiple factors, including the presence of comorbidities such as CKD or liver dysfunction. Table 91-2 shows the more common nonheparin anticoagulants that have been used in HIT, along with basic pharmacokinetic properties.

Most patients, in whom there is moderate to high clinical suspicion of HIT, can be treated with argatroban, a synthetic direct thrombin inhibitor (DTI) that is administered IV and metabolized by the liver. Argatroban is typically administered via a continuous infusion (2 mcg/kg/min) and monitored with the aPTT (target range 1.5-3× initial baseline value).[9,10] Significant dosage adjustments are required for patients with liver dysfunction.

Bivalirudin is a DTI that is FDA approved for use during percutaneous coronary intervention (PCI) and in patients with HIT who undergo PCI. Although its use outside the PCI setting is considered "off label," bivalirudin is a reasonable option in patients

Table 91-1. 4Ts Clinical Scoring System			
Category	**2 points**	**1 point**	**0 points**
1. Thrombocytopenia	Platelet count fall >50% and nadir ≥20,000/μL	Platelet count fall 30%-50% or nadir 10,000-19,000/μL	Platelet count fall <30% or nadir <10,000/μL
2. Timing of platelet count fall	Clear onset 5-10 d after heparin, or ≤1 d (if prior heparin exposure within 30 d)	Consistent with platelet count fall at 5-10 d (but unclear), or after day 10, or ≤1 d (if prior heparin exposure 30-100 d ago)	Platelet count fall ≤4 d without recent exposure
3. Thrombosis or other sequelae	New thrombosis (confirmed), skin necrosis, acute systemic reaction after intravenous UH bolus	Progressive/recurrent thrombosis, nonnecrotizing skin lesion, or suspected thrombosis	None
4. Other causes of thrombocytopenia	None apparent	Possible	Definite

Low score, 0 to 3; intermediate score, 4 to 5; high score, 6 to 8. Calculate score by adding relevant points (columns) for each of the four categories.
UH, unfractionated heparin.

Table 91-2. Options for Short-Term Anticoagulation in Patients with HIT[7-14]

Anticoagulant	Clearance	Half-Life	Dosage Regimen	Monitoring
Argatroban	Hepatic	40-50 min	IV infusion 2 mcg/kg/min. Decrease infusion rate to 0.5-1.2 mcg/kg/min in liver disease, critical illness, and post cardiac surgery.	Adjust to maintain aPTT 1.5-3× baseline value.
Bivalirudin	Enzymatic/ renal	25 min	Dose not established. 0.15-2.0 mg/kg/h suggested, with dose adjustments with renal and hepatic dysfunction.	Adjust to maintain aPTT 1.5-2.5× baseline value.
Fondaparinux	Renal	17-20 h	Weight-based subcutaneous dosing: 5 mg daily for <50 kg, 7.5 mg daily for 50-100 kg, 10 mg daily for >100 kg	None
Rivaroxaban	Renal/fecal	5-9 h	Dose not established in HIT. Has been used successfully as monotherapy or as a long-term agent after initial parental nonheparin anticoagulation.	None

IV, intravenous; aPTT, activated partial thromboplastin time; HIT, heparin-induced thrombocytopenia.

with acute or subacute HIT who require a percutaneous or open vascular reconstruction. Intraoperative dosing of bivalirudin is discussed in Box K.

Small case series have described the successful use of fondaparinux and direct oral anticoagulants (DOACs) in patients with acute HIT.[9-14] Fondaparinux monotherapy may be used for short- and intermediate-term anticoagulation for HIT, or it may be used as initial anticoagulation before the patient transitions to a vitamin-K antagonist (VKA) or DOAC. Other case series also have described the successful use of DOACs, both as monotherapy, and as a long-term oral agent as patients transition away from parenteral anticoagulation.

VKAs have an established role as a long-term anticoagulant for HIT. However, initiation of VKA therapy should be postponed until the platelet count returns to normal, to avoid the potential for VKA-induced skin necrosis.

🅚 Nonheparin intraoperative anticoagulation

Patients with a confirmed diagnosis of HIT or HITT may require percutaneous or open vascular procedures. In this setting, argatroban and bivalirudin have been used for intraoperative anticoagulation, before arterial clamping.[15-18] The recommended dosing protocols differ from those used outside of the surgical or interventional suite (see Table 91-3). Argatroban and bivalirudin

flush solutions also have been described with dilutions, as shown later.

Patients with a *remote* history of HIT occasionally may receive brief to reexposure unfractionated heparin for vascular or cardiac procedures, but only if the immunoassay test result is negative for HIT and the platelet count has returned to the normal range. Two percent to 5% of patients who do receive reexposure to heparin will develop recurrent HIT.[11,15]

🅛 Intraoperative bleeding?

Despite the lack of any specific reversal agents for argatroban or bivalirudin, significant intraoperative bleeding has not been observed when these direct thrombin inhibitors are utilized during vascular reconstruction, so the risk for major postoperative hemorrhage remains very low.[14-16] Treatment of intraoperative bleeding is discussed in detail in Chapter 92.

Table 91-3. Options for Intraoperative Anticoagulation in Patients with HIT or a History of HIT[15-18]

Anticoagulant	Intraoperative Dosing	Monitoring	Notes
Argatroban	Described dosing regimens: 1. 100 mcg/kg IV bolus, then 2 mcg/kg/min infusion 2. 150 mcg/kg IV bolus, then 5 mcg/kg/min infusion	Adjust to maintain ACT ≥200 s	Argatroban flush solution: 0.5 mg to 10 mg/1000 mL saline
Bivalirudin	Described dosing regimens: 3. 0.75 mg/kg IV bolus, then 1.75 mg/kg/h infusion	Adjust to maintain ACT ≥200 s	Bivalirudin flush solution: 0.1 mg/mL saline
Heparin	Typical UH dosing.	Adjust to maintain ACT ≥200 s	Brief reexposure to UH may be safe if the patient has a remote history of HIT, the platelet count has recovered, and the immunoassay remains negative.

ACT, activated clotting time; IV, intravenous; HIT, heparin-induced thrombocytopenia; UH, unfractionated heparin.

REFERENCES

1. Arepally GM. Heparin–induced thrombocytopenia. *Blood.* 2017;129(21):2864-2872.
2. Khandelwal S, Lee GM, Hester CG, et al. The antigenic complex in HIT binds to B cells via complement and complement receptor 2 (CD21). *Blood.* 2016;128(14):1789-1799.
3. Lo GK, Warkentin TE, Sigouin CS, Eichler P, Greinacher A. Evaluation of pretest clinical score (4T's) for the diagnosis of heparin-induced thrombocytopenia in two clinical settings. *J Thromb Haemost.* 2006;4(4):759-765.
4. Cuker A, Gimotty PA, Crowther MA, Warkentin TE. Predictive value of the 4Ts scoring system for heparin-induced thrombocytopenia: a systematic review and meta-analysis. *Blood.* 2012;120(20):4160-4167.
5. Nagler M, Bachman LM, Ten Cate H, Ten Cate-Hoek A. Diagnostic value of immunoassays for heparin–induced thrombocytopenia: a systematic review and meta–analysis. *Blood.* 2016;127(5):546-557.
6. Nellen V, Sulzer I, Barizzi G, Lammle B, Alberio L. Rapid exclusion or confirmation of heparin-induced thrombocytopenia: a single-center experience with 1,291 patients. *Haematologica.* 2012;97(1):89-97.
7. Linkins LA, Dans AL, Moores LK, et al. Treatment and prevention of heparin–induced thrombocytopenia: antithrombotic therapy and prevention of thrombosis, 9th ed: American College of Chest Physicians evidence–based clinical practice guidelines. *Chest.* 2012;141(2 suppl):e495S-e530S.
8. Watson H, Davidson S, Keeling D. Guidelines on the diagnosis and management of heparin–induce thrombocytopenia: Second edition. *Br J Haematol.* 2012;159(5):528-540.
9. Kelton JG, Arnold DM, Bates SM. Nonheparin anticoagulants for heparin-induced thrombocytopenia. *N Engl J Med.* 2013;368:737-744.

10. Warkentin TE, Pai M, Linkins L. Direct oral anticoagulants for treatment of HIT: update of Hamilton experience and literature review. *Blood*. 2017;130(9):1104-1113.

11. Warkentin TE, Anderson JAM. How I treat patients with a history of heparin-induced thrombocytopenia. *Blood*. 2016;128(3):348-359.

12. Ng JH, Than H, Teo EC. First experience with the use of rivaroxiban in the treatment of heparin–induce thrombocytopenia. *Thromb Res*. 2015;135(1):205-207.

13. Sharifi M, Bay C, Vajo Z, Freeman W, Sharifi M, Schwartz F. New oral anticoagulants in the treatment of heparin–induce thrombocytopenia. *Thromb Res*. 2015;135(4): 607-609.

14. Kunk PR, Brown J, McShane M, Palkimas S, Gail Macik B. Direct oral anticoagulants in hypercoagulable states. *J Thromb Thrombolysis*. 2017;43(1):79-85.

15. Warkentin TE, Pai M, Cook RJ. Intraoperative anticoagulation and limb amputations in patients with immune heparin–induce thrombocytopenia who require vascular surgery. *J Thromb Haemost*. 2012;10:148-150.

16. Ohteki H, Furukawa K, Ohnishi H, Narita Y, Sakai M, Doi K. Clinical experience of argatroban for anticoagulation in cardiovascular surgery. *Jpn J Thorac Cardiovasc Surg*. 2000;48(1):39-46.

17. Hallman SE, Hebbar L, Robison J, Uber WE. The use of argatroban for carotid endarterectomy in heparin-induced thrombocytopenia. *Anesth Analg*. 2005;100:946-948.

18. Kashyap VS, Bishop PD, Bena JF, Rosa K, Sarac TP, Ouriel K. A pilot, prospective evaluation of a direct thrombin inhibitor, bivalirudin (Angiomax), in patients undergoing lower extremity bypass. *J Vasc Surg*. 2010;52:369-374.

Peter J. Lawson • Jeffrey H. Lawson

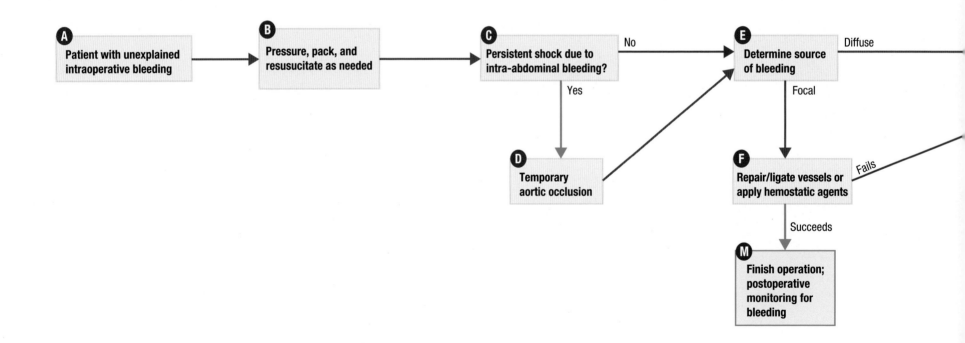

A Patient with unexplained intraoperative bleeding

B Pressure, pack, and resusucitate as needed

C Persistent shock due to intra-abdominal bleeding?

No

E Determine source of bleeding

Diffuse

Yes

D Temporary aortic occlusion

Focal

F Repair/ligate vessels or apply hemostatic agents

Fails

Succeeds

M Finish operation; postoperative monitoring for bleeding

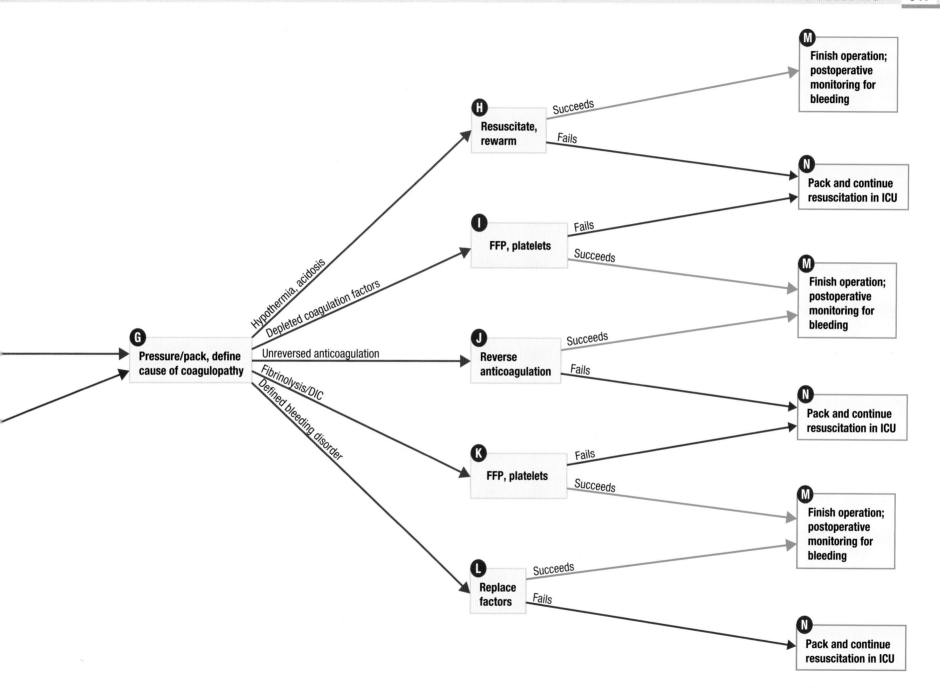

A Patient with unexplained intraoperative bleeding

During surgery, unexplained bleeding can be one of the most difficult operative challenges. The consequences can range from minimal bleeding to life-threatening hemorrhage. Unexplained bleeding may relate to undiagnosed bleeding disorders, nonreversed anticoagulant effects, clotting factor or platelet depletion from operative blood loss, hypothermia, acidosis, or as yet undetected source of bleeding directly related to the operation. An essential first step is to identify that the patient is actively bleeding and that intervention is needed.

B Pressure, pack, and resuscitate as needed

Initial management of intraoperative bleeding requires local pressure or packing to control bleeding to allow resuscitation and transfusion as necessary, depending on the extent of blood loss. Bleeding that requires >4 units of blood/hour or is accompanied by clinical symptoms of hemorrhagic shock warrants activation of the massive transfusion protocol as this has been shown to reduce mortality.[1,2] Although the ratio and cadence of blood product infusion remains debated, PRBCs and thawed fresh frozen plasma (FFP) are essential and the availability of cryoprecipitate and platelet transfusions should be confirmed. Even without shock or massive blood loss, the blood bank should be mobilized to meet the resuscitation needs of the patient until bleeding is controlled. Aggressive resuscitation to reverse shock, and warmed blood products should be used when possible to reduce hypothermia. Resuscitation should be initiated with between a 2:1 and a 1:1 ratio of packed RBC to plasma.[3,4] Further, cryoprecipitate and platelets should also be considered when patients have received greater than six units of transfused RBC.

C Persistent shock due to intra-abdominal bleeding?

If SBP remains <70 mm Hg with ongoing bleeding despite packing and resuscitation, aortic occlusion should be considered if the probable site of bleeding will be impacted by this maneuver.

D Temporary aortic occlusion

During abdominal surgery, proximal aortic control can provide immediate blood pressure support. A hand or blunt instrument can be used to directly compress the aorta while exposure for direct clamping is obtained. Supraceliac exposure can be achieved rapidly by mobilizing the gastrohepatic ligament and exposing the supraceliac aorta between the crus of the diaphragm. In dire situations, a left anterior thoracotomy can be performed with exposure and clamping of the aorta in the chest. In some cases, it may be more expeditious to use REBOA (see Chapter 62).[5] The duration of aortic occlusion should be minimized to prevent distal ischemia while allowing identification and treatment of the bleeding source.

E Determine source of bleeding

After resuscitation and packing/pressure (or aortic occlusion), it is important to characterize the type and source of bleeding. The two major categories are local bleeding from an artery or vein that can be surgically controlled versus diffuse bleeding/oozing from multiple sites suggesting underlying coagulopathy. In some cases, both mechanisms exist, in which case focal bleeding is treated first.

F Repair/ligate vessels or apply hemostatic agents

If a focal artery or vein defect is identified as the source of bleeding, a decision to ligate or repair the vessel is then made. Most small blood vessels can be ligated without consequence, whereas larger ones should be repaired with suture ligation or with a vascular patch, if needed, to prevent stenosis. Small vessels can also be sealed with cautery or harmonic devices. For localized bleeding not involving a discrete vessel, hemostatic dressings such as collagen powder, gelatin sponges, or oxidized cellulose can be applied. These provide a surface for thrombin generation and promote platelet adherence and activation while also promoting upregulation of the contact pathway of coagulation. The use of fibrin sealants or large sheets of oxidized cellulose can be beneficial for larger surface areas and more diffuse bleeding.[6] Shunting of large vessels to maintain perfusion and allow later repair is also an option in patients who are hemodynamically unstable.

Arterial anastomoses that demonstrate persistent bleeding may require revision, if they cannot be corrected with simple or pledgeted sutures. In cases where anastomotic bleeding is diffuse, the area can be wrapped with a thrombin-soaked gelatin sponge, oxidized cellulose, or fibrin (biologic) glue applied. These wraps should be left in place long enough for the assisted hemostasis process to occur, which can often take at least 10 minutes.

G Pressure/pack, define cause of coagulopathy

If bleeding is diffuse, especially widespread oozing from all raw surfaces, underlying coagulopathy is likely. Bleeding should be controlled by pressure and packing while coagulopathy is assessed and treated. There can be multiple causes of coagulopathy leading to diffuse bleeding, including hypothermia, acidosis, depleted clotting factors and platelets, nonreversed anticoagulants, hyperfibrinolysis, and unknown bleeding disorders. Coagulation assessment of the patient should include assays that can measure blood coagulation factors, fibrinogen, platelets, and fibrinolysis. The can be accomplished with a battery of assays including PT-INR, PTT, fibrinogen, complete blood count, or with viscoelastic assessment (TEG or ROTEM). Hemoglobin is also an important factor that can be optimized to improve hemostasis.[7] There are specific viscoelastic assays that can be used to assess for non–heparin-based bleeding using a heparinase to assess for the patients' fibrinogen and platelet function.[8] Specific treatment depends on the etiology

of the coagulopathy defined by results of the assays described earlier.[9]

H Resuscitate, rewarm

After long operations, particularly with associated hypoperfusion, both hypothermia and acidosis are frequent causes of coagulopathy with persistent bleeding. Hypothermia is best prevented by patient and IV fluid warming, but once present, it is difficult to reverse in the operating room. In many cases, packing the surgical site and moving the patient to the ICU for rewarming may be needed before bleeding can be controlled and incisions closed. Acidosis is managed with aggressive resuscitation and cardiac support, as required.

I FFP, platelets

If there has been substantial blood loss during an operation, depletion of plasma coagulation factors and platelets can lead to substantial coagulopathy. FFP and platelet replacement is based on patient weight and extent of PT and platelet abnormality. In addition, after 4 to 6 units of FFP and platelets have been transfused, the use of cryoprecipitate and IV calcium supplementation should be considered.

J Reverse anticoagulation

Heparin is often used during vascular operations and can lead to persistent bleeding if not adequately reversed with protamine. This is best determined by normalization of the activated clotting time. If a patient is on warfarin, weight-based transfusion of FFP is effective. These patients can also benefit from prothrombin complex concentrates (PCCs) if there is a need for rapid reversal such as in the setting of intracranial hemorrhage, and/or if they are unlikely to tolerate the volume of plasma needed for reversal. The most difficult anticoagulants to reverse are the new direct oral anticoagulant medications that bind to and directly inhibit factor Xa or thrombin. Several of these medications have recently developed reversal agents, but these agents are extremely expensive and not immediately available at all hospitals. PCCs have also been proposed to be an alternative strategy to reduce bleeding from these drugs and can be used in the setting where no specific reversal agent is available. In dire situations, dialysis can be considered but is often impossible in the setting of ongoing bleeding and shock. This option should be considered if the patient is able to be packed, rewarmed, and temporarily returned to the ICU.

Antiplatelet agents do not usually increase intraoperative bleeding, but in selected patients on multiple agents, diffuse intraoperative bleeding may result. Platelet transfusion is used when needed in this setting. However, risk and benefit must be assessed in these settings because patients taking these medications for important indications, such as recent drug-eluting coronary stent placement, can have complications such as acute coronary stent thrombosis.

K FFP, platelets

DIC during surgery can be the result of many causes including massive tissue injury, sepsis, ischemia reperfusion syndrome or malignancy. The underlying pathophysiology results in systemic and unregulated activation of the coagulation system, the deletion of blood clotting factors, and a state of hyperfibrinolysis. Intraoperative bleeding due to DIC can be one of the most challenging and difficult situations to manage. Platelet transfusion combined with FFP is initially recommended for bleeding patients with DIC. For continued bleeding despite FFP transfusion, cryoprecipitate and antifibrinolytic agents such as Lysine analogs should be considered. Resuscitation should continue until the underlying cause of DIC is identified and treated.[10]

L Replace factors

On occasion, patients with operative bleeding will have a known specific inherited or acquired bleeding disorder. In this setting, emergent hematology consultation is appropriate for specific transfusion requirements. These bleeding disorders include the classic hemophilias (factor VIII and IX deficiencies), von Willebrand disease, congenital platelet disorders, and autoimmune acquired deficiencies in factors V, VIII, and IX. If the specific coagulation deficiency is known, hematology-directed, factor-specific replacement is recommended. Depending on the nature of the platelet disorder, the use of desmopressin (DDAVP) and platelet transfusions are often required. FFP, cryoprecipitate, and recombinant factor VIIa are beneficial in the treatment of undefined bleeding disorders until the underlying condition can be elucidated.

M Finish operation; postoperative monitoring for bleeding

If hemostasis is achieved and the patient is sufficiently stable, the operation is completed, the incisions closed, and the patient monitored carefully for signs of bleeding, with frequent monitoring of vital signs, hemoglobin, and coagulation factors/platelets.

N Pack and continue resuscitation in ICU

If measures to treat operative bleeding are not completely effective, and especially if hypothermia is present, patients are often best served by packing with temporizing measures to end the operation and move the patient to the ICU for ongoing resuscitation, rewarming, and replacement of blood products. When stabilized, they can then return 12 to 48 hours later for definitive surgery or earlier if they develop uncontrolled bleeding in the ICU despite packing, which would suggest a surgical source of bleeding. Appropriate use of such an approach has been demonstrated to reduce mortality.[11]

Acknowledgments

The authors acknowledge the significant contribution of Dr. Hunter B. Moore (University of Colorado, Denver) in the intellectual and academic development of this chapter. His professional experience and thoughtful input were essential to the completion of this work.

REFERENCES

1. Dente CJ, Shaz BH, Nicholas JM, et al. Improvements in early mortality and coagulopathy are sustained better in patients with blunt trauma after institution of a massive transfusion protocol in a civilian level I trauma center. *J Trauma*. 2009;66(6):1616-1624.
2. Nunez TC, Young PP, Holcomb JB, Cotton BA. Creation, implementation, and maturation of a massive transfusion protocol for the exsanguinating trauma patient. *J Trauma*. 2010;68(6):1498-1505.
3. Nunns GR, Moore EE, Stettler GR, et al. Empiric transfusion strategies during life-threatening hemorrhage. *Surgery*. 2018;164(2):306-311.
4. Borgman MA, Spinella PC, Perkins JG, et al. The ratio of blood products transfused affects mortality in patients receiving massive transfusions at a combat support hospital. *J Trauma*. 2007;63(4):805-813.
5. Stannard A, Eliason JL, Rasmussen TE. Resuscitative endovascular balloon occlusion of the aorta (REBOA) as an adjunct for hemorrhagic shock. *J Trauma*. 2011;71(6):1869-1872.
6. Lawson JH, Tracy ET. Coagulopathy and hemorrhage. In: Sidawy AN, Perler BA, eds. *Rutherford's Vascular Surgery and Endovascular Therapy*. 9th ed. Amsterdam, Netherlands: Elsevier Publishing; 2019:465-483.
7. Holcomb JB, Tilley BC, Baraniuk S, et al. Transfusion of plasma, platelets, and red blood cells in a 1:1:1 vs a 1:1:2 ratio and mortality in patients with severe trauma: the PROPPR randomized clinical trial. *JAMA*. 2015;313(5):471-482.
8. Zmuda K, Neofotistos D, Ts'ao C. Effects of unfractionated heparin, low-molecular-weight heparin, and heparinoid on thromboelastographic assay of blood coagulation. *Am J Clin Pathol*. 2000;113(5):725-731.
9. Gonzalez E, Moore EE, Moore HB, et al. Goal-directed hemostatic resuscitation of trauma-induced coagulopathy: a pragmatic randomized clinical trial comparing a viscoelastic assay to conventional coagulation assays. *Ann Surg*. 2016;263(6):1051-1059.
10. Levi M, Toh CH, Thachil J, Watson HG. Guidelines for the diagnosis and management of disseminated intravascular coagulation. British committee for standards in haematology. *Br J Haematol*. 2009;145(1):24-33.
11. Cotton BA, Reddy N, Hatch QM, et al. Damage control resuscitation is associated with a reduction in resuscitation volumes and improvement in survival in 390 damage control laparotomy patients. *Ann Surg*. 2011;254(4):598-605.

ABBREVIATIONS

AAA	abdominal aortic aneurysm	CTA	computed tomographic angiography	ICU	intensive care unit
ABI	ankle-brachial index	DIC	disseminated intravascular coagulation	IFU	instructions for use
AKA	above-knee amputation	DNR	do not resuscitate	IIA	internal iliac artery
ALI	acute limb ischemia	DRIL	distal revascularization interval ligation	INR	international normalized ratio
ASA	American Society of Anesthesiology	DSA	digital subtraction angiography	IMA	inferior mesenteric artery
ATLS	advanced trauma life support	DSE	dobutamine stress echocardiogram	IV	intravenous
AV	arteriovenous	DUS	duplex ultrasound	IVC	inferior vena cava
AVF	arteriovenous fistula	DVT	deep venous thrombosis	IVUS	intravascular ultrasound
AVG	arteriovenous graft	ECA	external carotid artery	LDH	lactate dehydrogenase
AVM	arteriovenous malformation	ECG	electrocardiogram	LDL	low-density lipoprotein
BEVAR	branched endovascular aortic aneurysm repair	ECHO	echocardiogram	LMWH	low-molecular-weight heparin
BKA	below-knee amputation	ECMO	extracorporeal membrane oxygenation	MAP	mean arterial pressure
BUN	blood urea nitrogen	EF	ejection fraction	MI	myocardial infarction
CABG	coronary artery bypass grafting	EIA	external iliac artery	MRA	magnetic resonance angiography
CAD	coronary artery disease	EMG	eletromyogram	MRI	magnetic resonance imaging
CAS	carotid artery stenting	ePTFE	expanded polytetrafluoroethylene	MRSA	methicillin-resistant *Staphylococcus aureus*
CCA	common carotid artery	ESR	erythrocyte sedimentation rate	PAD	peripheral arterial disease
CDT	catheter-directed thrombolysis	ESRD	end-stage renal disease	PAI	proximalization of arterial inflow
CEA	carotid endarterectomy	EVAR	endovascular aneurysm repair	PE	pulmonary embolism
CFA	common femoral artery	F	French	PET	positron emission tomography
CHF	congestive heart failure	FEV$_1$	forced expiratory volume in 1 second	PFT	pulmonary function test
CI	confidence interval	FEVAR	fenestrated endovascular aortic aneurysm repair	PPG	photoplethysmography
CIA	common iliac artery	FMD	fibromuscular dysplasia	PRBCs	packed red blood cells
CKD	chronic kidney disease	GFR	glomerular filtration rate	PSA	pseudoaneurysm
CLI	critical limb ischemia	GI	gastrointestinal	PSV	peak systolic velocity
COPD	chronic obstructive pulmonary disease	GSV	great saphenous vein	PT	prothrombin time
CPR	cardiopulmonary resuscitation	H&P	history and physical examination	PTA	percutaneous transluminal angioplasty
CRP	c-reactive protein	HDL	high-density lipoprotein	PTT	partial thromboplastin time
CSF	cerebrospinal fluid	HTN	hypertension	PVR	pulse volume recording
CT	computed tomography	ICA	internal carotid artery	RCT	randomized clinical trial

REBOA	resuscitative endovascular balloon occlusion of the aorta
RUDI	revision using distal inflow
SBP	systolic blood pressure
SCA	subclavian artery
SFA	superficial femoral artery
SMA	superior mesenteric artery
SVC	superior vena cava

TAA	thoracic aneurysm
TAAA	thoracoabdominal aneurysm
TASC	TransAtlantic Inter-Society Consensus Document on the Management of PAD
TBI	toe brachial index
TcPO$_2$	transcutaneous oxygen partial pressure
TEVAR	thoracic endovascular aortic repair

TIA	transient ischemic attack
TMA	transmetatarsal amputation
TOS	thoracic outlet syndrome
VAC	vacuum-assisted closure
VCSS	Venous Clinical Severity Score
VTE	venous thromboembolism
WBC	white blood cell

Note: Page number followed by *f* and *t* denote figures and tables.

RRS2006